NEONATOLOGY

DISEASES OF THE FETUS AND INFANT

NEONATOLOGY

DISEASES OF THE FETUS AND INFANT

Edited by

RICHARD E. BEHRMAN, M.D.

Professor and Chairman, Department of Pediatrics, Columbia University College of Physicians and Surgeons; Director, Babies Hospital, The Children's Medical and Surgical Center of New York

Assisted by

JOHN M. DRISCOLL, Jr., M.D.

WITH THE COLLABORATION OF TWENTY-NINE CONTRIBUTORS

with 215 illustrations, including one color plate

The C. V. Mosby Company

Saint Louis 1973

Printed in the United States of America

Distributed in Great Britain by Henry Kimpton, London

Library of Congress Cataloging in Publication Data

Behrman, Richard E 1931-
Neonatology.

1. Fetus—Diseases. 2. Infants (Newborn)—Diseases.
I. Title. [DNLM: 1. Fetal diseases. 2. Infant,
Newborn, Diseases. WS 420 B421n 1973]
RJ254.B45 618.9'201 73-4550
ISBN 0-8016-0578-4

Contributors

PETER A. M. AULD, M.D.

Professor of Pediatrics, New York Hospital–Cornell Medical Center, New York, New York

CONSTANCE U. BATTLE, M.D.

Pediatrician to the Center for Craniofacial Anomalies, Abraham Lincoln School of Medicine, University of Illinois, Chicago, Illinois

RICHARD E. BEHRMAN, M.D.

Professor and Chairman, Department of Pediatrics, Columbia University College of Physicians and Surgeons; Director, Babies Hospital, The Children's Medical and Surgical Center of New York

JAY BERNSTEIN, M.D.

Director of Anatomic Pathology, Beaumont Hospital, Royal Oak, Michigan; Visiting Associate Professor of Pathology, Albert Einstein College of Medicine, Bronx, New York

AUDREY K. BROWN, M.D.

Professor of Pediatrics and Chief, Division of Pediatric Hematology, Medical College of Georgia, Augusta, Georgia

MURRAY DAVIDSON, M.D.

Professor of Pediatrics, Albert Einstein College of Medicine; Director, Department of Pediatrics, The Bronx-Lebanon Hospital Center, Bronx, New York

JOHN M. DRISCOLL, Jr., M.D.

Assistant Professor of Pediatrics, Columbia University College of Physicians and Surgeons; Head, The Neonatal Intensive Care Unit, Division of Perinatology, Babies Hospital, The Children's Medical and Surgical Center of New York

CHESTER M. EDELMAN, Jr., M.D.

Professor of Pediatrics and Director, Division of Pediatric Nephrology, Albert Einstein College of Medicine, Bronx, New York

NANCY B. ESTERLY, M.D.

Director, Division of Pediatric Dermatology, Michael Reese Medical Center; Associate Professor of Pediatrics, Pritzker School of Medicine, University of Chicago, Chicago, Illinois

JOHN M. FREEMAN, M.D.

Associate Professor of Pediatrics and Neurology and Director, Pediatric Neurology Service, Department of Neurology, Johns Hopkins University School of Medicine; Director, Birth Defects Treatment Center, Kennedy Institute, Baltimore, Maryland

MORTON F. GOLDBERG, M.D.

Professor and Head, Department of Ophthalmology, Abraham Lincoln School of Medicine, University of Illinois, Chicago, Illinois

SAMUEL P. GOTOFF, M.D.

Chairman, Department of Pediatrics, Michael Reese Medical Center; Professor of Pediatrics, Pritzker School of Medicine, University of Chicago, Chicago, Illinois

RUTH HARRIS, M.D.

Associate Professor of Clinical Pediatrics, Columbia University College of Physicians and Surgeons; Associate Attending Pediatrician, Babies Hospital, The Children's Medical and Surgical Center of New York

GEORGE R. HONIG, M.D., Ph.D.

Associate Professor of Pediatrics, Abraham Lincoln School of Medicine, University of Illinois; Attending Physician, The University of Illinois Hospital, Chicago, Illinois

L. STANLEY JAMES, M.D.

Professor of Pediatrics, Columbia University College of Physicians and Surgeons; Director, Division of Perinatology, Babies Hospital, The Children's Medical and Surgical Center of New York

JOHN H. KENNELL, M.D.

Associate Professor of Pediatrics, Department of Pediatrics, Case Western Reserve University School of Medicine, Cleveland, Ohio

MARSHALL H. KLAUS, M.D.

Associate Professor of Pediatrics, Case Western Reserve University School of Medicine, Cleveland, Ohio

HARVEY D. KLEVIT, M.D.

Department of Pediatrics, The Permanente Clinic; Clinical Professor of Pediatrics, University of Oregon Medical School, Portland, Oregon

MARTIN H. LEES, M.D.

Professor of Pediatrics, University of Oregon School of Medicine; Head, Division of Pediatric Cardiology, Doernbecher Memorial Hospital for Children, Portland, Oregon

HENRY H. MANGURTEN, M.D.

Director, High-Risk Nursery, Lutheran General Hospital, Park Ridge, Illinois

AKIRA MORISHIMA, M.D., Ph.D.

Associate Professor of Pediatrics and Chief, Division of Pediatric Endocrinology, Columbia University College of Physicians and Surgeons; Associate Attending Pediatrician, Babies Hospital, The Children's Medical and Surgical Center of New York

EDWIN C. MYER, M.B.B.C.H.

Fellow Neurologist, Resident in Neurology, The Johns Hopkins University School of Medicine, Baltimore, Maryland

JOHN F. NICHOLSON, M.D.

Associate Professor of Pediatrics, Columbia University College of Physicians and Surgeons; Director of Pediatric Laboratories and Associate Attending Pediatrician, Babies Hospital, The Children's Medical and Surgical Center of New York

MILES J. NOVY, M.D.

Associate Professor of Obstetrics and Gynecology and Division of Perinatal Medicine, University of Oregon Medical School, Portland, Oregon; Head, Perinatal Physiology, Oregon Regional Primate Research Center, Beaverton, Oregon

HERMINE PASHAYAN, M.D.

Associate Professor, Departments of Pediatrics and Genetics, Center for Craniofacial Anomalies, Abraham Lincoln School of Medicine, University of Illinois, Chicago, Illinois

SAMUEL PRUZANSKY, D.D.S.

Director, Center for Craniofacial Anomalies, Abraham Lincoln School of Medicine, University of Illinois, Chicago, Illinois

JOHN E. READ, M.D.

Resident in Ophthalmology, Abraham Lincoln School of Medicine, University of Illinois, Chicago, Illinois

LAWRENCE M. SOLOMON, M.D.

Associate Professor of Dermatology, Abraham Lincoln School of Medicine, University of Illinois, Chicago, Illinois

WILLIAM T. SPECK, M.D.

Rustin McIntosh Fellow in Pediatrics, Department of Pediatrics, Columbia University College of Physicians and Surgeons and Babies Hospital, The Children's Medical and Surgical Center of New York

ADRIAN SPITZER, M.D.

Associate Professor of Pediatrics, Department of Pediatrics, Albert Einstein College of Medicine, Bronx, New York

TO ANN

for her patience and understanding

Preface

The goal of this textbook of neonatology is to present a comprehensive and detailed description of the diseases that affect infants during the early weeks of life. The emphasis is on the pathophysiology, diagnosis, and treatment of disorders that have their onset in utero or during the neonatal period. Although this aspect of pediatrics continues to change rapidly, a substantial base of clinical knowledge is now established. This rapid acceleration of knowledge about the biology of the fetus and newborn infant and the diversity of problems that must be identified and managed necessitated the collaboration of a number of authors, each with a special area of competence. It is hoped that this book will serve pediatricians, obstetricians, family practitioners, nurses, and special nursery assistants in carrying out their responsibilities for the care of neonatal infants.

Richard E. Behrman

Contents

COLOR PLATE

NEONATOLOGY

DISEASES OF THE FETUS AND INFANT

1 The high-risk infant

The neonatal period is defined as the first 4 weeks of life. It is the period of the greatest mortality in childhood, with the highest risk occurring during the first 24 hours of life. However, the continuing high mortality and morbidity during this period are closely related to the fact that it is part of a continuum of fetal growth and development. Factors acting during gestation and delivery, as well as during the postnatal period, have a major impact on health during the neonatal period. Social, economic, and cultural influences are superimposed on genetic, metabolic, and physiologic intrauterine and extrauterine environmental effects. To encompass these diverse factors the term perinatal is used to designate the period from the twelfth week of gestation through the twenty-eighth day after birth.

The high incidence of disease during the neonatal period and the excessive neonatal and perinatal death rates make it important to identify as early as possible those fetuses and infants who are at greatest risk. Of equal importance is the need to lower the morbidity, especially for handicapping conditions such as mental retardation, resulting from untoward prenatal and natal factors. A reduction in the rate of population growth makes it even more critical to combat diseases that may limit the biologic potential of newborn infants. There is increasing evidence that early recognition of the high-risk pregnancy and high-risk infant and appropriate management in special neonatal intensive care centers will reduce the incidence of handicapping conditions as well as reduce both the perinatal and neonatal death rates. The first part of this chapter discusses the evaluation and treatment of fetal diseases that affect the mortality and morbidity in the neonatal period. The designation of different groups of high-risk infants at birth is then discussed.

RICHARD E. BEHRMAN

EVALUATION AND TREATMENT OF THE FETUS AT RISK

In 1952, Bevis demonstrated that the concentration of bilirubin pigment in the amniotic fluid of Rh-sensitized mothers has prognostic significance for the fetal outcome. Less than 10 years later Liley performed the first successful intrauterine transfusion for erythroblastosis fetalis. These achievements have served as milestones in the development of perinatal medicine, since they showed conclusively that the condition of the fetus is amenable to direct diagnostic and therapeutic intervention. Since then, our knowledge of human growth and development in utero has increased considerably.

Many new methods have been and are continually being developed to determine fetal welfare and to monitor the progress of the fetus during pregnancy and labor. The scope of these activities makes it possible to foresee intensive care for the fetus in the broadest sense of the word. The factors that influence perinatal mortality and morbidity are interdependent; hence any effort that betters the condition of the fetus will be reflected in the condition of the newborn. As a practical matter the high-risk fetus should always be considered a high-risk infant.

The accessibility of amniotic fluid and the slight risk of amniocentesis have led to detection of chromosomal disorders and inborn errors of metabolism before the second half of pregnancy. Biochemical components of amniotic fluid have been directly related to fetal maturity. Other advances include fetal electrocardiography, the sampling of blood from the fetal scalp for determinations of fetal acid-base status, and various measurements of biochemical and endocrine changes in the mother that have been related to fetal or placental function.

In this section the methods and problems involved in evaluating the fetus in utero are discussed whenever possible in the context of fetal growth and development, and the pathophysiology of pregnancy and its complications. Emphasis has been placed on diagnostic and therapeutic procedures that have received recognition and have proved useful or that show exceptional promise in managing the high-risk pregnancy. Most of the criteria and standards for intrauterine diagnosis are based upon the associations of measured parameters and physical characteristics at birth as well as on the prognosis and outcome of the infant in the neonatal period. Before the evaluation of the fetus in utero can be put into proper perspective, the variables seen before and at birth must be appreciated.

Concept of high-risk pregnancy

Most pregnancies represent a state of well-being. Nevertheless, the accompanying cardiovascular and metabolic stresses necessitate physiologic adjustments in virtually every organ system. How the pregnant patients adapts to these stresses will depend on a host of preexisting factors that determine the risk of pregnancy for the mother and fetus.

The high-risk pregnancy can be defined as the pregnancy associated with increased hazards of death or disability for the fetus or neonate because of maternal factors or fetal diseases or abnormalities. In many instances, a substantial risk exists for the mother as well, but a discussion of maternal risks is beyond the scope of this chapter. One of the problems in reducing perinatal wastage is the large number of normal pregnancies, which obscures those requiring special attention. Out of 100 pregnant women beyond the twentieth week of gestation, only 3 will leave the hospital without a living infant. However, a much larger number of infants will survive with mental or physical defects. Clifford has estimated that 3% to 4% of the almost 4 million infants born annually do not achieve an IQ above 70. A promising approach to solving the problem of defective neonates is a system of identifying and separating high-risk from normal pregnancies as early as possible in order to provide special care. Although the prevalence of high-risk pregnancies varies from clinic to clinic, an average estimate indicates that 30% of the patients account for two thirds of the perinatal complications. High-risk factors may not always be apparent at the first visit, yet complications often arise later during pregnancy. This emphasizes the need for thoughtful periodic examination.

A summary of associated findings that have proved useful in identifying the high-risk patient is given in the outline below.*

- I. Demographic factors
  - A. Lower socioeconomic status
  - B. Disadvantaged ethnic groups
  - C. Marital status: unwed mothers
  - D. Maternal age
    - 1. Gravida less than 16 years of age
    - 2. Primigravida 35 years of age or older
    - 3. Gravida 40 years of age or more
  - E. Maternal weight: nonpregnant weight less than 100 pounds or more than 200 pounds
  - F. Stature: height less than 62 in (1.57 m)
  - G. Malnutrition
  - H. Poor physical fitness
- II. Past pregnancy history
  - A. Grand multiparity: 6 previous pregnancies terminating beyond 20 weeks' gestation
  - B. Antepartum bleeding after 12 weeks' gestation
  - C. Premature rupture of membranes, premature onset of labor, premature delivery
  - D. Previous surgical delivery: cesarean section or midforceps delivery
  - E. Prolonged labor
  - F. Infant with cerebral palsy, mental retardation, birth trauma, central nervous system disorder, or congenital anomaly
  - G. Reproductive failure: infertility; repetitive abortion, fetal loss, stillbirth, or neonatal death
  - H. Delivery of preterm (less than 37 weeks) or postterm (more than 42 weeks) infant
- III. Past or present medical history
  - A. Hypertensive or renal disease or both
  - B. Diabetes mellitus (overt and gestational)

*Adapted from Reid, Ryan, and Benirschke: Principles and management of human reproduction, Philadelphia, 1972, W. B. Saunders Co.

C. Cardiovascular disease (rheumatic, congenital, and peripheral vascular)
D. Pulmonary disease producing hypoxemia and hypercapnia
E. Thyroid, parathyroid, and endocrine disorders
F. Idiopathic thrombocytopenic purpura
G. Neoplastic disease
H. Hereditary disorders
I. Collagen diseases
J. Epilepsy

IV. Additional obstetrical and medical conditions
A. Toxemia
B. Asymptomatic bacteriuria
C. Anemia or hemoglobinopathy
D. Rh sensitization
E. Habitual smoking
F. Multiple pregnancy
G. Rubella and viral infections
H. Intercurrent surgery and anesthesia
I. Placental abnormalities and uterine bleeding
J. Abnormal fetal lie or presentation, fetal anomalies, oligohydramnios, polyhydramnios
K. Abnormalities of fetal or uterine growth or both
L. Addiction

Much of our understanding of high-risk factors in pregnancy and the associated perinatal mortality comes from data collected in the 1960's by the British Perinatal Mortality Survey and in the United States by the National Collaborative Study of Factors Related to Cerebral Palsy, Mental Retardation, and other Neurological Disorders. Social and economic factors are clearly implicated in the pathogenesis of the high-risk pregnancy. In the British Perinatal Mortality Survey, the highest mortality was found among the semiskilled and unskilled social classes. In the United States, the perinatal mortality is highest among Indians and Negroes and lowest among those of Japanese and Chinese ancestry.

In many cases, the variation is caused by the educational background, economic status, and the availability and utilization of health services rather than to ethnic differences as such. Although the prematurity rate in Eastern seaboard cities is highest among the black population, in Portland, Oregon, the prematurity rate of whites and nonwhites is about equal. The perinatal mortality in large cities is higher than in rural areas and is correlated with the larger number of births without prenatal care, higher rates of illegitimate pregnancies, and medically indigent patients. The complications of pregnancy are more frequent among the considerable number of unmarried mothers who receive late or no prenatal care. Such patients have a perinatal mortality five times greater than the national average. Maternal age is another factor associated with perinatal mortality, the highest risks being among pregnant teenagers, primigravidas over 30 years of age, and the woman over 40 years of age, who has double the average risk. These patients are more likely to have nutritional problems, toxemia, complication of labor, and a higher incidence of low birth weight infants.

A close relationship exists between the reproductive history of the mother and the outcome of a subsequent pregnancy. A past history of a premature liveborn infant, stillbirth, or neonatal death doubles or triples the risk to a subsequent infant (Fig. 1-1). Some complications of pregnancy recur with significant probability, such as isoimmunization, antepartum or intrapartum bleeding, the incompetent cervical os syndrome, premature onset of labor, dysfunctional or prolonged labor, and complications of delivery related to cephalopelvic

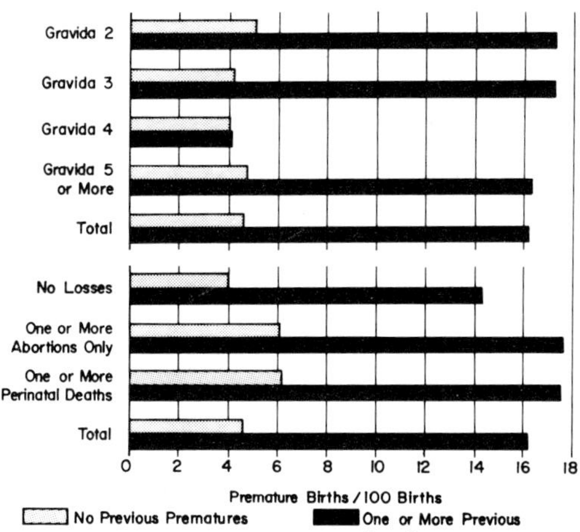

FIG. 1-1. Ontario study covering 18,000 births shows how obstetrical history helps predict probable outcome of subsequent pregnancies. Premature births are much more common in women who have previously delivered a low birth weight infant and are somewhat more common in women with a history of spontaneous abortion or perinatal death. Gravidity as such appears to have little influence (anomalous figures for gravida 4's may be a statistical accident). (From Schneider, J.: Hosp. Pract. 6:133, 1971.)

disproportion and repeated cesarean sections. Obviously, previous coexisting medical diseases or abnormalities predispose the pregnant woman to a higher risk.

Perinatal mortality and morbidity

Although the perinatal mortality in many leading institutions and throughout the country as a whole has substantially decreased over the past 30 years, the rate of decline has leveled in the past decade (Fig. 1-2).* Further reductions in fetal and neonatal wastage will come only with improvements in the identification and management of the high-risk pregnancy, including its socioeconomic implications. The major etiologic factors in the pathogenesis of fetal and neonatal mortality and morbidity are antepartum and intrapartum anoxia, congenital malformations, premature birth, erythroblastosis fetalis, and the respiratory distress syndrome of the newborn. To place the importance of evaluation and treatment of the fetus in utero in proper perspective, we need to review the essential features of perinatal mortality and morbidity.

*In many institutions the perinatal mortality rate is less than 29 to 30 per 1,000 births, a figure that should be within reach of all facilities caring for pregnant women.

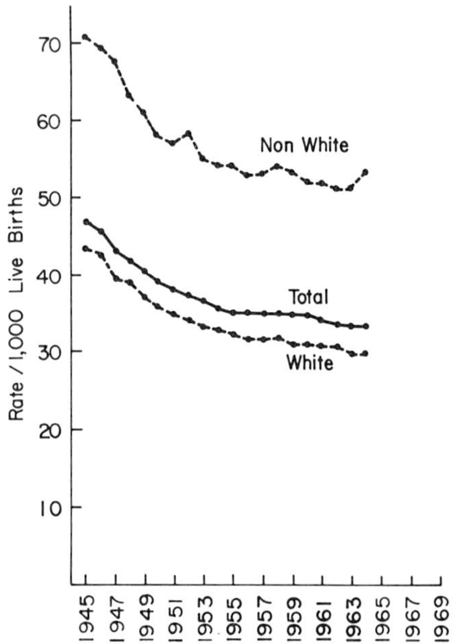

Fig. 1-2. Perinatal mortality (deaths, 20 weeks' or more gestation, plus deaths under 28 days) in the United States. (From Wallace, H. M.: Clin. Obstet. Gynecol. 13:13, 1970.)

Terminology

Fetal death is death that occurs after 20 weeks' gestation and before the product of conception is completely expelled or extracted from its mother and that is indicated by the absence of any signs of life after such separation. Late fetal death is fetal death at 28 or more completed weeks of gestation and is commonly referred to as stillbirth. *Neonatal deaths* occur in the first month of life; early neonatal or postnatal deaths occur in the first week of life. Nearly 75% of infant deaths in the first year of life occur in the early neonatal period.

The *perinatal mortality* is the total number of fetal and early neonatal deaths per 1,000 total births. In some hospitals a weight of 400 to 500 gm is used to distinguish abortions from reportable deaths, a justifiable distinction since the length of gestation is subject to variations in interpretation. International perinatal death rates may not be strictly comparable, since some countries exclude fetuses weighing less than 1,000 gm from their statistics. By this exclusion, however, about 25% of the perinatal mortality is ignored.

Causes of perinatal mortality and morbidity

The experience at the Boston Hospital for Women and the Chicago Lying-in Hospital in the 1950's and 1960's is representative of most major institutions. Total fetal deaths and total neonatal deaths contribute about equally to total perinatal mortality. This similarity and their parallel decline in recent decades emphasize the interdependence of the factors that affect the fetus and neonate. However, when fetal and neonatal deaths in different weight categories are compared, some interesting differences emerge. In the 400- to 1,000-gm and the 1,000- to 2,500-gm categories, neonatal deaths are slightly higher than fetal deaths. However, when the birth weight is over 2,500 gm, fetal deaths constitute a proportionately greater part of the total deaths (Fig. 1-3). In recent years, intrapartum fetal deaths have declined substantially more than antepartum fetal deaths. This may reflect an increasing utilization of fetal monitoring during labor and perhaps also a more liberal use of cesarean section for fetal distress, breech delivery, and other obstetric complications. Likewise, it implies the need for greater sophistication in predicting the maturity and functional reserve of the fetus in utero before the onset of labor.

Neonatal mortality is in general directly proportional to the number of liveborn infants weighing less than 2,500 gm. These low birth weight infants represent about 8% to 9% of all live births, an incidence that has been rising in recent years. During the past few decades, the substantial decrease in neonatal deaths of liveborn infants weighing between 1,000 to 2,500 gm has largely been caused by advances in the intensive care of the newborn. The relatively small decrease in recent years suggests that further substantial reductions in the neonatal death rate will depend on the prevention of low birth weight infants.

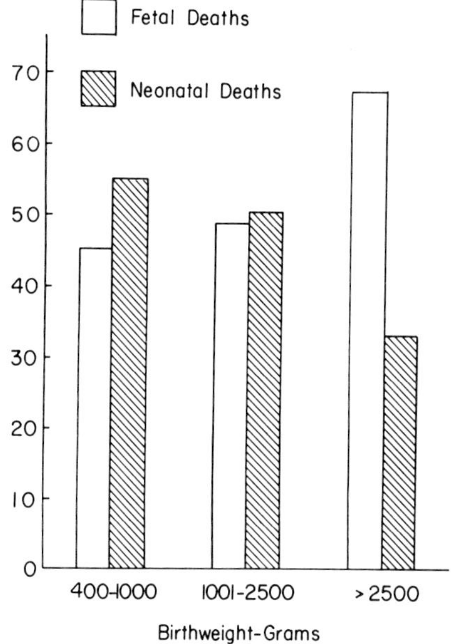

Fig. 1-3. Percent distribution by weight of fetal and neonatal deaths. (From Potter and Davis: Am. J. Obstet. Gynecol. **105**:335, 1969.)

When late fetal and neonatal deaths are taken together, 50% or so occur in infants who weigh more than 2,500 gm; almost one third of the fetal deaths occur in infants weighing more than 2,500 gm. This serves to emphasize that in our attempt to prevent premature labor and delivery of low birth weight infants, we should not overlook the equally significant contribution of the mature fetuses and infants to the total perinatal mortality.

The number of neonatal deaths caused by intracranial hemorrhage and by trauma sustained during labor and delivery has decreased dramatically. Today the majority of neonatal deaths are clinically related to respiratory distress (Table 1-1). Many are associated with pathologic evidence of hyaline membranes or anoxia, but some show no distinct pathologic changes. Intraventricular hemorrhage is a common lesion and contributes significantly to causes of perinatal death. The incidence of intraven-

Table 1-1. Causes of death per 1,000 births among fetuses and infants over 1,000 grams

Causes	1961-1966 Neonatal	Antepartum	Intrapartum	Total
Anoxia	2.8	2.6	1.1	6.1
No abnormality, premature*	2.2	2.8	0	5.0
No abnormality, term*	0.3	2.7	0	2.9
Trauma	0.3	0	0	0.3
Malformations	2.1	0.6	0.4	3.1
Pneumonia	0.6	0.1	0.1	0.8
Erythroblastosis	0.6	0.6	0	1.2
Other	0.1	0.1	0	0.2
Total	8.6	9.5	1.6	19.7

From Potter and Davis, Am. J. Obstet. Gynecol. **105**:335, 1969.

*Among neonatal deaths, this includes infants with various degrees of atelectasis and hyaline membrane disease. Among antepartum and intrapartum deaths, this includes fetuses with no pathologic changes indicative of anoxia or history of known cause.

tricular hemorrhage is five times higher in neonatal deaths than in stillbirths.

Anoxia is the most common cause of perinatal death in cases brought to autopsy; it may be the final common pathway of a variety of abnormal conditions. The diagnosis of anoxia should be based upon findings of petechial hemorrhages in the thymus, pleura, and peritoneum, of visceral congestion and edema of connective tissues, or of aspiration of meconium. In the premature infant, anoxic brain damage occurs predominantly in the deep periventricular tissue, while in the mature newborn infant anoxia leads to patchy areas of infarction in the cerebral cortex. However, frequently the diagnosis is based on the history or on clinical considerations. Lethal congenital malformation (usually of the central nervous system or cardiovascular system) ranks second or third as the cause of fetal and neonatal deaths and accounts for approximately 15% of the total perinatal deaths.

In summary, analysis of the causes of perinatal mortality suggests that the greatest reduction can be brought about by decreasing the number of low birth weight infants and preventing antepartum fetal deaths, a large number of which occur in mature fetuses. Antepartum deaths associated with anoxia or with no known cause and neonatal deaths associated with respiratory difficulties make up more than half the total perinatal mortality.

Prematurity and abnormalities of fetal growth

The weight of the infant at birth can be easily and reliably determined and correlated with perinatal mortality and morbidity. Hence the international definition of prematurity has been based on a birth weight of 2,500 gm or less. In effect, however, this traditional definition obscures some of the differences between fetal age and birth weight. It is now recognized that infants of low birth weight vary greatly in gestational age and maturity and have different postnatal mortality risks. One third of the infants weighing less than 2,500 gm have a gestational age of 37 or more weeks. Thus all infants should be classified according to their gestational age as well as their birth weight.

Gestational age, fetal growth, and fetal maturity are closely related but not synonymous. Maturity is applied to the fetus in a functional sense to indicate the degree to which the newborn organ systems are adapted for the requirements of postnatal life. It is increasingly apparent that the duration of gestation is more closely related than is birth weight to fetal maturity. An infant may be classified as premature if he is born before the thirty-seventh week of gestation, measured from the first day of the last menstrual period. This time interval is commonly expressed in whole weeks. The World Health Organization has recommended that completed weeks (for example, $36\frac{0}{7}$ to $36\frac{6}{7}$ inclusive equals 36 weeks) rather than rounding to the nearest week be used. The Committee on Fetus and Newborn of the American Academy of Pediatrics (1967) has recommended that the duration of gestation be indicated by simple and time-oriented designations such as *preterm* (less than 38 calculated weeks of gestation), *term* (38 to 42 weeks), and *postterm* (more than 42 weeks).

Constructing standards for intrauterine growth and maturation is essential but difficult. Of necessity, these standards must be based on the weights or lengths attained by individual fetuses at the time of their birth and on the premise that the weights of preterm infants reflect normal fetal growth in utero. Ideally, growth charts should accommodate corrections for parity, social class, maternal stature, and various other factors. In addition, there is the problem of applying standards developed in one population group to another. The intrauterine growth curves in most common use today in this country are those reported by Lubchenco. They are based upon measurements of the birth weight, head circumference, and body length of a large number of liveborn infants from Denver, Colorado, born at 24 to 43 weeks' gestation (Fig. 1-4). The mean values for weight and other body measurements in the latter weeks of gestation are lower in the Denver population than in comparable British or Swedish growth curves, which may reflect the lower socioeconomic status of the patients and the altitude in Denver as well as the larger stature of Swedish mothers. The growth curves derived by

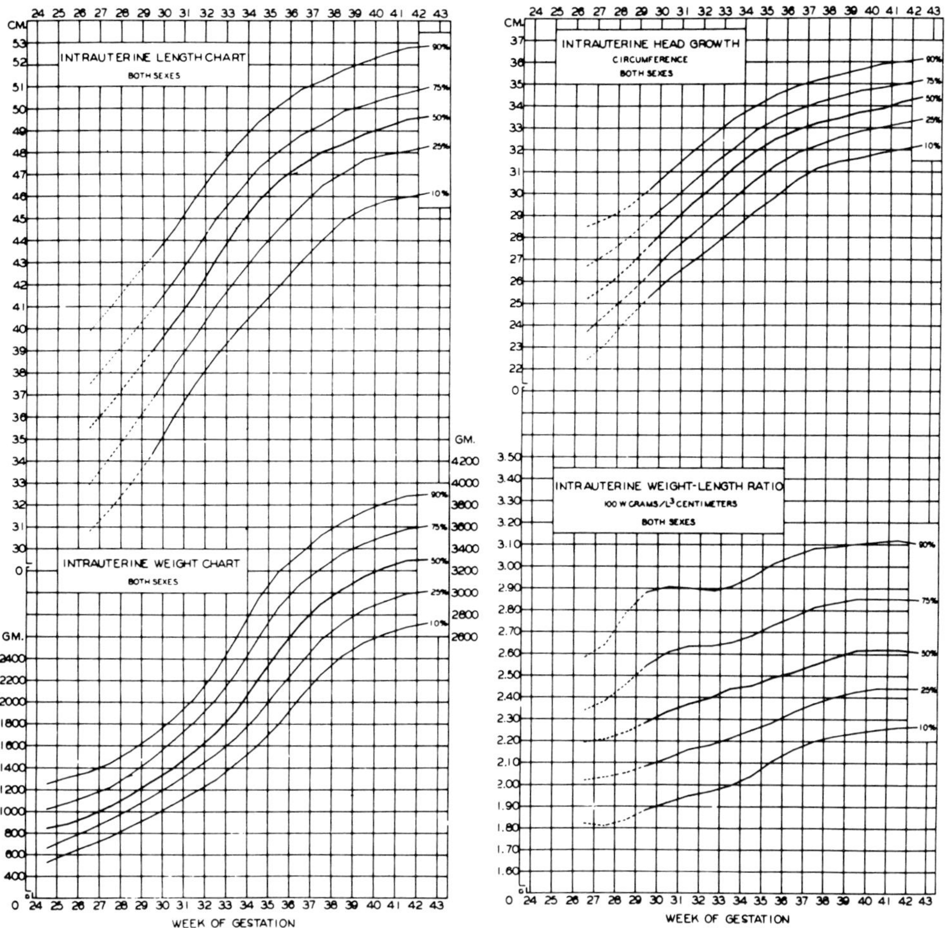

FIG. 1-4. Intrauterine growth curves based upon measurements of birth weight, head circumference, and body length of live-born infants from Denver, Colorado, born at 24 to 43 weeks' gestation. (From Lubchenco, Hansman, and Boyd: Pediatrics **37**:403, 1966.)

Behrman, Babson, and Lessel, from white, middle-class infants born in Portland, Oregon, are more comparable to the British and Swedish figures than are curves from Baltimore or Denver. Birth weights that are low compared with the Denver figures are significantly abnormal when compared with other available data.

Linear measurements such as crown-heel length, crown-rump length, and head circumference are also used to characterize growth at birth. When the relationships of body weight to length are analyzed according to gestational age, it is evident that in normal fetuses the proportion of weight to length increases rapidly in the first 33 weeks of gestation and at a somewhat slower rate up to 38 weeks. A plateau is reached at 39 to 41 weeks; beyond this time in prolonged pregnancy the average fetus again becomes thinner.

When gestational age is plotted as the independent variable, body weight increases rapidly between 28 and 37 weeks' gestation and thereafter is followed by an apparent slowing of the rate of growth. In the newborn infant, the earlier, more rapid rate of growth is resumed, an indication that fetal growth near term is somehow restricted in the intrauterine environment.

Classification of infants at birth by both weight and gestational age provides a more satisfactory method for predicting mortality risks and allows for an optimal plan of management of the neonate (Plate 1). Different clinical problems develop in infants of the same low birth weight but dissimilar gestational ages and in a diabetic mother's infant who is large for his gestational age but functionally immature. The preterm infant who is small for his gestational age will have a lower incidence of the idiopathic respiratory distress syndrome and a lower neonatal mortality than an infant of the same weight born earlier in gestation. However, growth-retarded infants at term have higher neonatal mortality rates than do term babies of normal weight. They also have an increased risk of neonatal hypoglycemia, convulsions, polycythemia, and pulmonary hemorrhage and a higher incidence of major congenital anomalies. The fetal and neonatal death rates in all major categories of postterm infants born more than 3 weeks beyond the expected date of delivery are almost double those of term babies. Postterm infants weighing less than 2,500 gm have a neonatal mortality seven times the rate for prolonged pregnancies. The combined effects of postmaturity and intrauterine growth retardation on intrapartum fetal mortality are shown in Fig. 1-5.

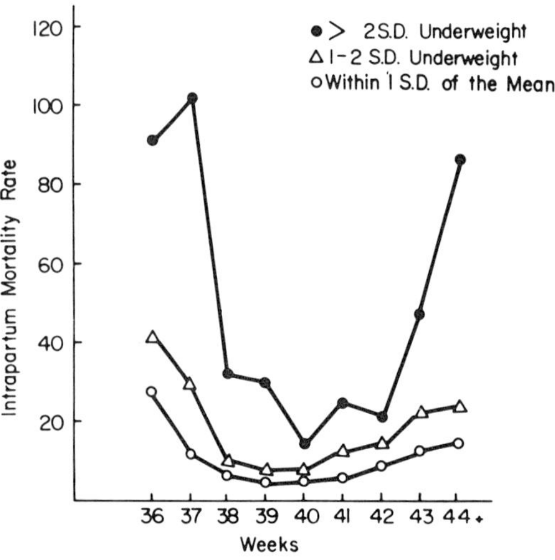

FIG. 1-5. Intrapartum mortality at each week of gestation in babies of average weight and in underweight babies. Intrapartum mortality is expressed as the deaths from asphyxia or trauma or both during labor per 1,000 deliveries. (Adapted fram Dawkins, M.: The "small for dates" baby. In Dawkins, M., and MacGregor, B.: Gestational age, size and maturity. Clinics in developmental medicine, No. 19, Lavenham, England, 1965, Lavenham Press Ltd., p. 34.)

Intrauterine growth retardation

Pathologic growth retardation of the fetus is diagnosed when birth weight is below the tenth percentile for the respective week of gestation, 25% or more underweight for gestation, or below 2 standard deviations (SD) from the mean for gestation (this corresponds roughly to the third percentile). This condition has also been described as dysmaturity, pseudomaturity, placental insufficiency syndrome, fetal malnutrition, and chronic fetal distress. A convenient clinical classification without etiologic implications is simply to refer to these infants as *small for gestational age* (SGA).

Some SGA babies show a proportionate reduction in weight and length and give little overt evidence of malnutrition. They can be distinguished from true premature infants by their alert appearance, well-developed reflexes, and good appetites. These infants reflect long-term deprivation measured roughly in weeks (chronic fetal distress). These terms should not be confused with intrapartum fetal distress (acute fetal distress), which is related to interference with normal fetal oxygenation. (See section on intrapartum fetal monitoring.)

Other SGA infants are long and thin and show wrinkled skin, frequent meconium staining, and evidence of malnutrition. These infants were originally described by Clifford as *dysmature*. Many were associated with prolonged pregnancies and probable placental dysfunction. According to Gruenwald, dysmature infants suffer short-term fetal deprivation before delivery (subacute fetal distress).

Many clinical conditions are associated with the pathogenesis of antenatal growth disturbances; thus it is not surprising that growth-retarded neonates do not constitute a homogeneous group. In addition, the clinical expression of the growth disturbance probably depends on the onset, duration, and severity of the nutritional restriction. The cause of intrauterine growth retardation is complex and incompletely understood, but it is probably related to factors that alter the placental passage of nutrients, including poor placental blood supply to the fetus, multiple gestation, maternal undernutrition, a variety of maternal diseases, and fetal genetic disturbances and intra-

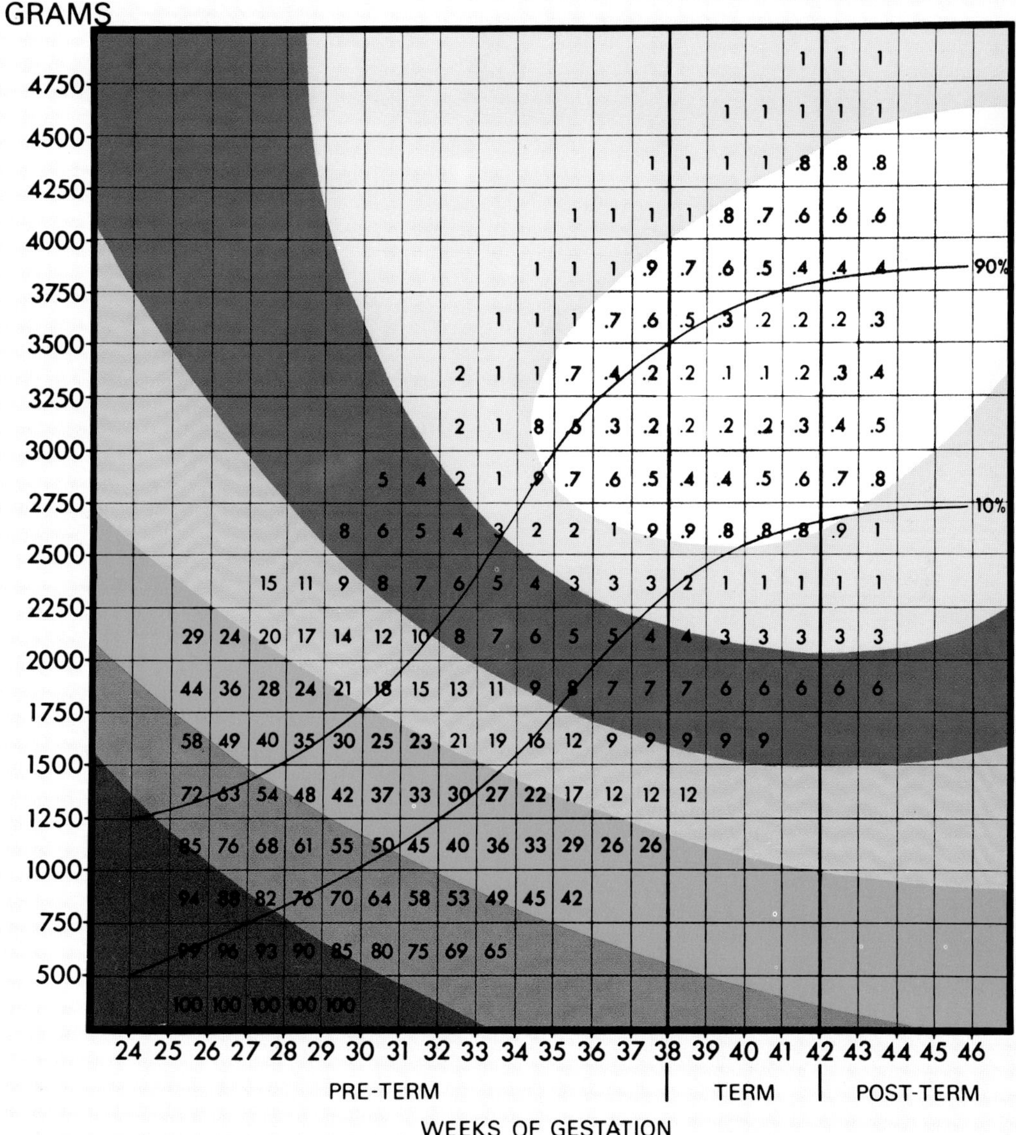

Interpolated data based on mathematical fit from original data
University of Colorado Medical Center newborns, 7/1/58 - 7/1/69

Plate 1. Curvilinear zones of death rates, obtained by connecting blocks having similar death rates. Numbers indicate death rate per 100 newborn infants. Infants below the tenth percentile are *small for gestational age* (SGA), and those above ninetieth percentile are *large for gestational age* (LGA). Those infants with weights for gestational age between the tenth and the ninetieth percentiles are *appropriate for gestational age* (AGA). Different colors indicate zones of risk from least risk (white) to highest risk infants (red). (Lubchenco, L. O., and others: J. Pediatr. **81**:814, 1972; color reproduction in original article made possible through courtesy of Mead Johnson Laboratories, Evansville, Ind.)

uterine infections. These and other factors are listed below.

FACTORS IMPLICATED IN THE CAUSE OF INTRAUTERINE FETAL GROWTH RETARDATION

A. Fetal
  1. Chromosomal disorders (trisomy 21, trisomy 17, 18, trisomy 13-15)
  2. Chronic fetal infection (cytomegalic inclusion disease, toxoplasmosis, congenital rubella, syphilis)
  3. Radiation injury
  4. Multiple gestation
  5. Pituitary failure (?)

B. Placental
  1. Decreased placental weight or cellularity or both
  2. Decrease in surface area
  3. Villous placentitis (bacterial, viral, parasitic)
  4. Infarction
  5. Tumor (chorioangioma, hydatidiform mole)
  6. Placental separation
  7. Twin transfusion (parabiotic syndrome)
  8. Abnormal cord insertions, diffuse fibrosis, and localized transfer lesions

C. Maternal
  1. Toxemia
  2. Hypertensive or renal disease or both
  3. Hypoxemia (high altitude, cyanotic, cardiac, or pulmonary disease)
  4. Malnutrition, chronic illness, or addiction
  5. Sickle cell anemia

D. Experimental
  1. Maternal uterine ischemia—rat
  2. Fetal placental ischemia—sheep and monkey
  3. Maternal protein deprivation—rat, guinea pig, and pig

Except for intrinsic fetal abnormalities, such as genetic defects or chronic fetal infections, which reduce the growth potential of the fetus, the final common pathway is probably a reduced rate or total supply of nutrients to the fetus. There is also the possibility that significant hypoxia plays a role. No pathognomonic lesions have been demonstrated in the placentas of SGA infants. In cases associated with maternal preeclampsia, hypertension, or nephropathy, the characteristic lesions associated with these disorders are recognized in the placenta and include increased fibrin deposition, fibrosis of terminal villi, intravascular sclerosis, and syncytial degeneration.

Despite the heterogeneous features of *placentas* associated with SGA infants, they tend to be lighter in weight than placentas associated with appropriate gestational age (AGA) infants of comparable gestational ages. However, placentas associated with congenital fetal anomalies or infections may be normal in size or even large and edematous. The trophoblastic surface area of the placenta associated with growth-retarded fetuses is diminished. This finding suggests a morphologic and functional index of placental transport capacity. A decreased cell number and DNA content in placentas from growth-retarded fetuses has also been shown by Winick. It is not known whether the observed diminished placental surface area is caused by a primary defect in the placenta or by vascular lesions in the placental bed.

The cellular effects of undernutrition depend on the phase of growth in an organ at the time of stress. During an early phase of growth, which consists primarily of hyperplasia (increase in cell number and total organ DNA content), undernutrition may lead to a permanent reduction in cell number. During a period when hypertrophy predominates (increase in cell cytoplasm and protein/DNA ratio), a slowdown of growth may be caused primarily by a decrease in net protein synthesis. Cheek has shown that when the brain is

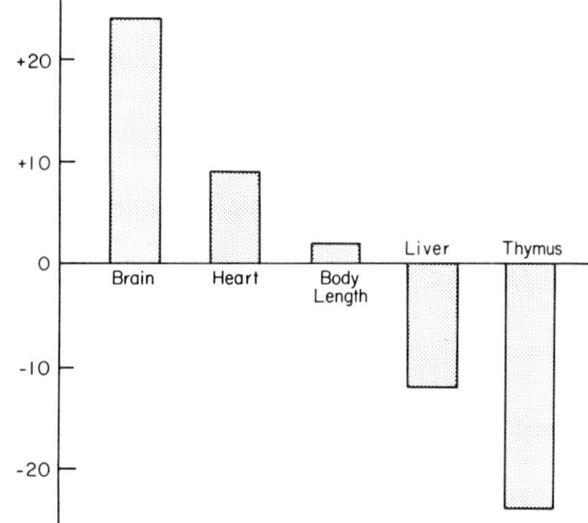

Fig. 1-6. Body length and organ weights of infants who had chronic fetal distress (birth weight below mean minus 2 SD for gestational age) expressed as percent of values for normally grown infants of similar weight. (From Gruenwald, P. In Jonxis, and others, editors: Aspects of praematurity and dysmaturity, Leiden, Holland, 1968, H. E. Stenfert Kroese, N.V.)

affected by intrauterine growth retardation, the cerebellum is most vulnerable, whereas the cerebrum is relatively spared. Growth-retarded infants who come to autopsy show similar changes in organ weights and composition as do experimentally deprived fetuses. The disproportionate effect on the growth of various organs is shown in Fig. 1-6. The liver, thymus, and lungs are on the average smaller than those of truly premature infants of similar weight. The brain is considerably heavier, an indication that the growth of the brain is affected least in the intrauterine growth retardation syndrome.

Maternal protein deprivation affects fetal growth less severely in man than in experimental animals. Even during severe starvation, the mean reduction in birth weight is only a few hundred grams, and no clear association with subsequent *mental subnormality* has been established. Causes of intrauterine growth retardation associated with congenital anomalies or virus infections capable of destroying brain cells are associated with a higher incidence of mental retardation. Other causes of severe intrauterine growth retardation may have a permanent effect on learning ability. Babson studied *monozygotic twins* markedly dissimilar in size at birth and showed that the smaller member had a significantly lower intelligence score at age 8½. A follow-up of postnatal growth also showed that the smaller of the twins at birth retained, in relation to his partner, a small but significant deficit in height, weight, and head circumference at age 4½ to 11. A higher incidence of severe mental retardation has been found in SGA infants weighing less than 1,800 gm (many of whom were also preterm). In these and other cases of severe intrauterine growth retardation, prematurity and extreme undergrowth may have contributed to the results; the observations may not be applicable to the moderately growth-retarded term infant. Other studies have indicated no increase or only equivocally increased long-term morbidity in SGA infants. Recent findings from the Collaborative Study indicate that term infants undersized at birth (below the tenth percentile) and without evidence of fetal infection or malformation have no significant intellectual deficit at age 4 compared with matched controls of normal weight. It is not possible now to definitely answer the question of possible long-term sequelae of intrauterine growth retardation. Prospective studies, ideally extended beyond the period of puberty, will be needed to answer this question, to separate the combined effects of low birth weight, gestational age, and postnatal nutrition, and to determine their associations with maternal factors such as toxemia and antepartum hemorrhage.

Clinical recognition of intrauterine growth retardation

The clinical recognition of intrauterine growth retardation is extremely difficult. Careful measurements of the rate of growth of the uterine fundus in the early months of pregnancy and later estimates of the weight and size of the fetus in relation to the calculated gestational age are essential features of the clinical diagnosis of a SGA fetus. The incidence of birth weights below the tenth percentile is highest in the rapid fetal growth phase, 32 to 40 weeks. At 29 weeks' gestation, both twins have a body weight near that of singletons; after 33 weeks' gestation, twin weights are clearly less than singleton weights. During pregnancy, the average woman gains about double the weight of the products of conception so that a static or falling weight pattern also should alert the clinician to the possibility of a growth-retarded baby. In many patients, a clinical impression based upon palpation or measurements of abdominal girth is not sufficient, and confirmation is best made by other objective estimates of fetal maturity, fetal weight, and tests of placental function.

Indications for assessing fetal maturity

An accurate assessment of fetal maturity is central to many of the clinical problems of fetal medicine and management of the high-risk pregnancy. The obstetrician caring for women with high-risk pregnancies must continually weigh the risks of maintaining the fetus in an adequate or potentially hostile in utero environment against the hazards of delivering the fetus where, despite advances in neonatal supportive care, the risks of prematurity are great. The diagnosis of fetal maturity in utero may not only avoid problems of prematurity and unjustified obstetrical intervention, but it also may permit the appropriate timing of the induction of labor or termination of pregnancy. In addition, the diagnosis of intrauterine growth retardation or other fetal disorders alerts the pediatrician so that coordinated effort and optimum care can be provided to the newborn infant at risk. Induction of labor or delivery of the infant by cesarean section before the onset of labor is frequently the necessary solution to certain complications of pregnancy such as maternal isoimmunization, diabetes, toxemia, infection, premature rupture of the membranes, antepartum bleeding, postmaturity, and fetal growth retardation. Repeat cesarian section and induction of labor for elective reasons is a less urgent but frequent consideration for interrupting pregnancy before the onset of spontaneous labor. On the other hand, in cases of premature rupture of the membranes or premature onset of labor, a decision to stop labor may be made in order to allow a maximal interval of time for further in utero growth and development. The age of the fetus is an important variable in the timing of therapy such as the institution of intrauterine transfusions for erythroblastosis, the attempt to inhibit premature contractions, or the repair of an incompetent cervix in the case of habitual second trimester losses.

Obstetric history and examination

Every effort must be made to accurately define the onset and duration of the patient's last menstrual period. This should be done in the context of the regularity and length of the patient's menstrual cycles, recent use and discontinuation of oral contraceptives, and an attempt to differentiate the last menstrual period from other causes of vaginal bleeding. Sometimes conception takes place during a period of amenorrhea, especially in women who are nursing. In clinical practice, the time of conception is rarely known, and therefore gestational age is customarily calculated on the basis of the first day of the last menstrual period (LMP). The vagaries of establishing LMP by history account for the fact that in about 15% of pregnancies the gestational age cannot be determined by history alone. Reliable estimates by anamnesis indicate that the average duration of human gestation from the first day of the last menstrual period is about 280 days or 40 weeks. However, almost 12% of women do not begin labor until 294 days or more after the start of the LMP. It has been estimated that about 5% deliver on the estimated date of confinement (EDC), or 40 weeks, somewhat more than 50% within 7 days of EDC, and 85% deliver within 14 days of the EDC. Prolongation of pregnancy beyond the expected delivery date is fairly common in patients with menstrual cycles longer than 28 days (about one day for each additional day of the cycle), since the preovulatory phase is likely to be longer in these patients.

It is also important to gain an accurate history of past reproductive performance and of previous birth weights. Sibling birth weights may provide a more reliable index for comparison than absolute growth standards.

An important part of prenatal care in the early weeks and months of pregnancy is to establish a set of obstetrical landmarks that can be used to corroborate the estimated gestational age. Changes in the shape and size of the uterus are most consistent between 12 and 20 weeks' gestation and offer the opportunity for the examining obstetrician to correlate physical findings with the estimated gestational age from the LMP. A closer correlation between uterine size and fetal maturity is generally found before 20 weeks than after. Periodic examinations in the first 20 weeks of pregnancy are most productive in detecting early abnormalities of fetal growth caused by intrinsic fetal defects, multiple pregnancy, hydatidiform mole, or missed abortion. A discrepancy between the gestational age and that based on obstetrical landmarks should be considered a warning of possible intrauterine maldevelopment and not necessarily an error in the reporting of the LMP. The twentieth week is especially important for confirming the duration of gestation. At this time, the uterine fundus is normally at the level of the mother's umbilicus, and fetal movement (quickening) is felt by the mother.

Auscultation of the fetal heart is a reliable procedure in the absence of maternal obesity, and fetal heart tones are usually detected at 18 to 20 weeks' gestation by stethoscopic examination. If fetal heart tones have been present for more than 20 weeks and the uterus is consistent with the patient's EDC, a term pregnancy is virtually assured. Ultrasonic instruments based on the Doppler principle are extremely useful in making the diagnosis of a viable pregnancy at an early age (fetal heart can be heard as early as the third lunar month), but they do not provide a reliable fixed point of reference in time.

At each return visit, it is important to measure and record the fundal height above the symphysis pubis by calipers or tape in a standard manner. Many clinics employ midabdominal girth measurements also. Although there is an inherently large error in the girth measurements, a diminishing or static girth is associated with intrauterine growth retardation. Traditionally the fundus is at the umbilicus at 20 weeks' and the xiphoid by 36 weeks' gestation. However, the height of the fundus palpated in abdomens of different length may be misleading with regard to gestational age. The uterus grows about 1 inch (2.5 cm) every 2 weeks; hence serial observations in the same patient are more valid than absolute measurements. The average height of the uterine fundus above the symphysis pubis with 2 SD at 2-week intervals up to 28 weeks' gestation is shown in Fig. 1-7 and indicates the wide range of measurements. However, the most informative index of fetal maturity is the size of the pregnant uterus assessed by pelvic examination in the first trimester. Of course, serial measurements by the same observer are of even more value.

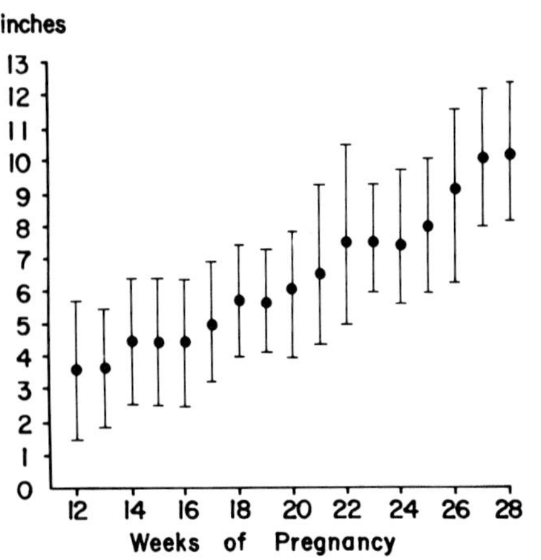

FIG. 1-7. Average height of the uterine fundus above the symphysis pubis, with 2 SD, before 28 weeks' gestation, in patients of abdominal length 12½ to 14½ inches (31.5 to 36.5 cm.). (From Beazley and Underhill, Br. Med. J. 4:404, 1970.)

Radiographic estimates of fetal maturity

Currently, fetal radiographic studies during pregnancy are used most commonly to evaluate fetal position, to identify fetal death or congenital anomaly, and to determine fetal age. The fetus is most sensitive to somatic effects of radiation exposure at 2 to 6 weeks after conception. Fortunately there are few diagnostic problems in obstetrics in which radiologic procedures are of value before the twelfth to sixteenth week, nor can the fetal skeleton be reliably visualized before this time. The possibility of causing mutations or genetic damage in the fetal ovaries is small and varies with the dose administered. Important technical developments such as intensifying screens, high-speed films, and low voltages minimize some of these dangers so that a dose of around 0.1 R to 0.5 R to the maternal ovaries and fetal gonads is standard for most abdominal radiographs used to estimate fetal age. These doses are relatively small compared with those that would eventually cause a doubling of gene mutations. Nevertheless, there is no place in modern obstetrics for *routine* radiologic studies to determine fetal maturity.

Fetal ossification centers. Before 24 weeks' gestation, radiologic estimation of fetal maturity depends upon the size of the fetal head, the length of the fetus, and the rather subjective estimation of the degree of ossification of the skeleton as a whole. Although identifiable epiphyses appear between the twenty-fourth and twenty-eighth weeks of gestation in the calcanium and talus, they may be technically difficult to visualize in utero. The experienced radiologist can estimate the fetal gestational age between 30 and 36 weeks on the basis of skull ossification, size of the vertebral bodies, ankle ossification centers, length of the long bones and lumbar spine, and the development of subcutaneous fat. However, fairly accurate assessments cannot be made until 36 weeks' gestation and thereafter. During or at the end of the thirty-sixth week, the distal femoral epiphyses can be detected as small homogeneous shadows, about 3 mm in diameter and 0.5 cm from the end of the femurs, that grow steadily in size and density until term (Fig. 1-8). Epiphyseal ossification centers begin to appear at the proximal ends of the tibiae at 38 weeks so that normally both distal femoral and proximal tibial epiphyses are present and demonstrable at 40 weeks.

The proportion of infants showing each of the knee epiphyseal centers increases with birth weight (Table 1-2). The distal

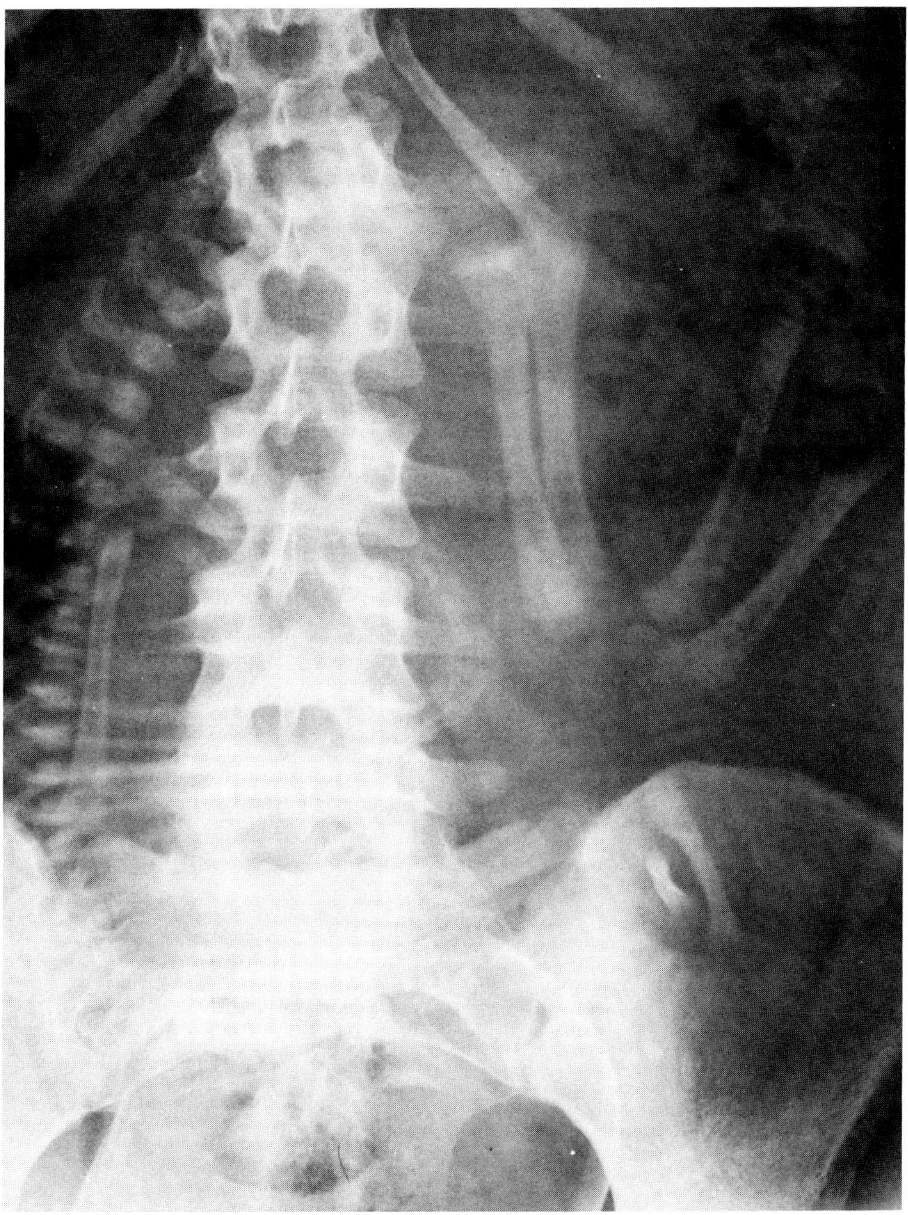

Fig. 1-8. Fetogram for maturity. Both distal femoral and proximal tibial ossification centers are visible, indicating a fetal age of approximately 38 weeks.

Table 1-2. Percentage of roentgenograms of newborn infants in which the presence of an ossification center was clear for various weight groups

Center of ossification, race, and sex	Birth weight in grams					
	Less than 2,000	2,000-2,499	2,500-2,999	3,000-3,499	3,500-3,999	4,000 or more
Distal epiphysis of femur						
White boys	9.1	75.0	85.3	100.0	100.0	100.0
White girls	50.0	91.7	98.0	100.0	100.0	100.0
Negro boys	18.2	88.5	90.7	94.0	100.0	100.0
Negro girls	50.0	93.8	99.0	100.0	100.0	100.0
Proximal epiphysis of tibia						
White boys	0.0	18.8	52.9	78.8	84.1	97.1
White girls	0.0	54.2	75.5	85.7	90.7	90.5
Negro boys	0.0	38.5	62.7	76.0	80.0	92.9
Negro girls	14.3	40.6	76.7	88.1	86.4	100.0

From Christie, A., and others: Am. J. Obstet. Gynecol. **60**:133, 1950.

femoral epiphysis is present in most infants weighing over 2,500 gm. However, it may also be present in 50% of female infants weighing less than 2,000 gm. The proximal tibial epiphysis that develops somewhat later was found in only two infants weighing under 2,000 gm. The appearance of distal femoral epiphyses in a large proportion of low birth weight infants and the correlation of their cross-sectional area with gestational age suggest that development of ossification centers is more closely related to fetal maturity than is the birth weight itself. The appearance of epiphyseal centers is a function of race and sex as well as of gestational age. Negro and female babies show relatively earlier development of the ossification centers. Epiphyses also develop at a faster rate in large babies than in small babies of the same gestational age. This accounts for the general impression that there is a tendency for radiologic estimates of gestational age to underestimate the age of small babies and overestimate the age of large babies.

A marked delay in the appearance of the ossification centers is also seen in babies with evidence of severe intrauterine growth retardation. When present, the epiphyses are much smaller in the malnourished group. Epiphyseal development is of no value in distinguishing the small malnourished term infant from the premature infant.

A few infants (about 2%) with demonstrable distal femoral epiphyses on antenatal films are judged premature by clinical examination. Thus visualization of these ossification centers should not be used as the sole criterion of fetal maturity and should be combined with other diagnostic aids such as amniotic fluid studies. Visualization of both distal femoral and proximal tibial epiphyseal centers on antepartum radiographs provides virtual certainty that the fetus is mature. Postmaturity is suggested when the ossification center of the proximal tibial epiphysis measures at least 7 mm in diameter.

Amniographic techniques. Ethiodan (ethyl[iodophenyl]undecylate), a lipid-soluble contrast medium, has been used to outline the soft tissues of the fetus. When injected into the amniotic cavity, this material is dispersed and adsorbed to the vernix caseosa. Before 38 weeks' gestation, the skin of the fetus is almost completely outlined by the dye. Between 38 and 40 weeks, the outline becomes patchy, and the limbs and abdomen are less clear. At term and thereafter, the outlining virtually disappears from these areas and remains visible only on the back and head. This coincides with the gradual disappearance of the vernix caseosa at term.

Ultrasonic cephalometry

Sound with frequencies above the human audible limit (18 to 1,000 cycles per second) is referred to as ultrasound. Because of their shorter wavelength and high resolution, ultrasonic waves can be focused and propagated in the human body as longitudinal disturbances. The ultrasonic echo images that can be obtained depend upon the physical fact that ultrasound is partially reflected when the beam crosses the interface between tissues of different physical properties. The amount of energy reflected is governed by optical laws and also is determined by the acoustic impedance of the medium (product of the density and velocity of sound in the medium). Sound energy is reflected almost completely at interfaces between gases and solids or liquids. On the other hand, about 30% of the sound energy is reflected at the interface between muscle and bone when the angle of incidence is 90°. Sound waves are produced, and the echoes are returned to a transducer-mounted crystal and are converted by the piezoelectric phenomenon into electrical signals that can be amplified and displayed on an oscilloscope screen. New technical improvements in the equipment make it possible to display sectional images of the human body in rapid succession so that the observer can directly view and film not only stationary positions but also functional changes.

Although the resolution of ultrasonic waves is considerably less than that of x-rays, it is nevertheless possible to visualize with ease the interfaces between soft biologic tissues that can be represented only with considerable difficulty in radiographs. Furthermore, in contrast to radiographs, a sonar image on the B-scan is not a summation image but a true sectional image in which the distances between the various tissue interfaces, including those running parallel to the surface, can be directly measured.

Cephalometry by ultrasound has a distinct advantage over radiologic determinations of fetal age in that it can be repeated at regular intervals to assess the growth rate of the skull in a particular individual. Two display systems are used, the A-scan and the B-scan. In the A-scan, only one dimension can be examined at a time. The echo signals are received in such a way that a vertical deflection is produced on the time base sweep across the oscilloscope screen (Fig. 1-9). The height of the deflection from the baseline corresponds to the strength of the echo, and the position from left to right across the screen corresponds to the depth of its point of origin. The strongest signals are reflected by the proximal and distal tables of the fetal skull and its midline structures. The fetal head in the horizontal plane is an ellipse with only two pairs of parallel surfaces. Therefore, opposing skull margins will yield maximum and equal echoes only when the beam axis passes perpendicular to the occipital-frontal or the biparietal diameter of the fetal skull. In Hellman's study using the A-scan, the absolute mean difference from postnatal measurements of biparietal diameter by calipers was 1.8 mm. Technical errors arise from the difficulty of locating the biparietal diameters because of deep engagement of the fetal head, an exaggerated curvature of the parietal bosses, molding of the head, fetal movement, and calibration of the instrument.

The two-dimensional B-scan makes it possible to locate and outline a section of the fetal skull as an ellipse and to measure the maximum distances that would correspond to the biparietal or occipital-frontal diameters (Fig. 1-10). A midline echo can also be demonstrated. The most satisfactory and accurate measurements of fetal skull diameters are obtained by simultaneous readings of both A- and B-scans. Al-

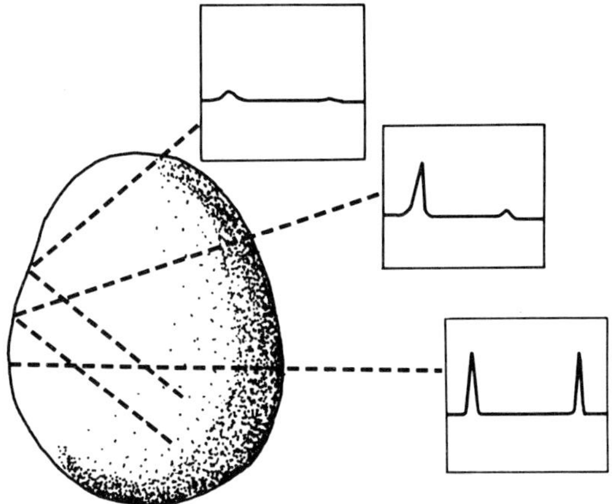

Fig. 1-9. Schematic view of a fetal head in the horizontal plane with ultrasonic A-scan display. Echoes have maximal amplitude when the beam of ultrasound is directed perpendicularly to the parietal bosses and along the biparietal diameter. This serves to identify the biparietal diameter as well as to measure it. (Adapted from Willocks, and others: J. Obstet. Gynaecol. Br. Commonw. **71**:11, 1964.)

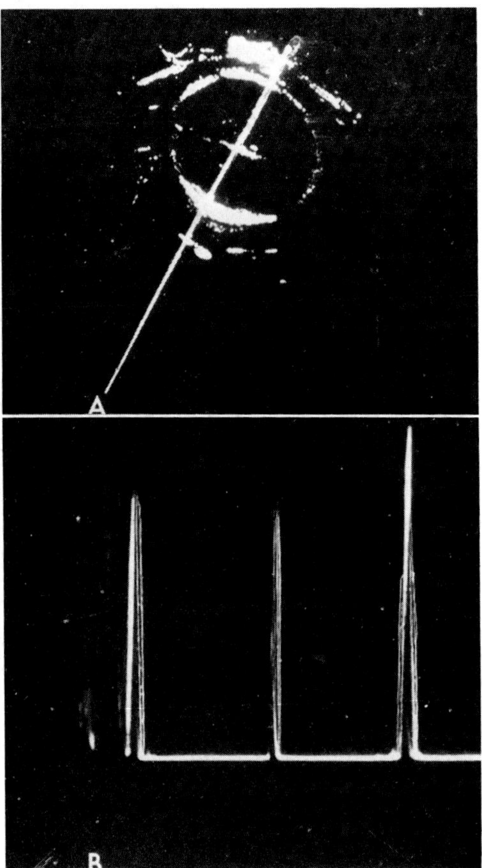

Fig. 1-10. A, A 2-dimensional ultrasonic B-scan of the fetal skull. The fetal biparietal diameter is identified at right angles to the midline echo. **B,** Biparietal diameter measured on A-scan. The midline echo is smaller and equidistant from the echoes from the two parietal eminences. (From Donald, I.: In Wynn, R., editor: Obstetrics and gynecology annual 1972, New York, 1972, Appleton-Century-Crofts, p. 252.)

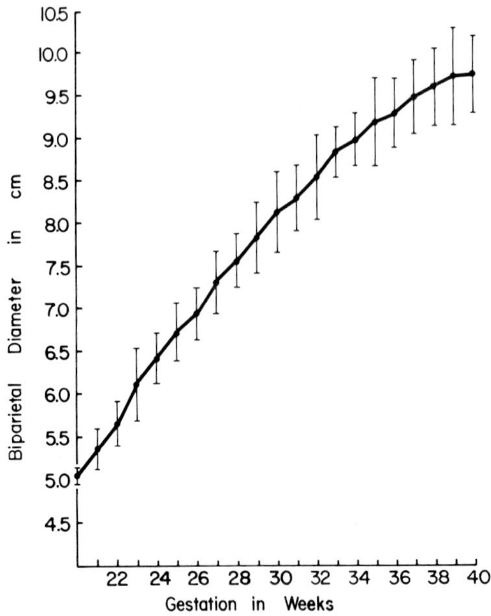

Fig. 1-11. Mean fetal biparietal diameter values equal 2 SD for each week of gestation during the second half of normal pregnancy in 186 patients whose gestation was known (471 individual measurements). (From Campbell: J. Obstet. Gynaecol. Br. Commonw. **76**:603, 1969.)

though birth weight bears a significant linear relationship to the biparietal and occipital-frontal diameters of the fetal head, it is not sufficiently precise to be of great value clinically. However, if the biparietal diameter measures 9 cm or more, 95% of the infants will exceed 2,500 gm.

Ultrasonic cephalometry may be helpful in estimating fetal maturity, in the diagnosis of cephalopelvic disproportion, and in management of the breech labor. Normal growth curves of the biparietal diameter during the second and third trimesters have been obtained from serial studies in patients whose menstrual histories were well defined and who gave birth to infants above the tenth percentile in weight for 40 weeks' gestation. A- and B-scan measurements were obtained simultaneously. The relationship of biparietal diameters to gestational age in weeks is shown in Fig. 1-11. From 20 to 30 weeks' gestation, the growth of the biaprietal diameter is rapid (2.8 mm/wk); in the last 10 weeks it is 1.5 mm/wk. In the later weeks of pregnancy, the values show a wider scatter about the mean. Therefore, for a prediction of fetal gestational age, biparietal diameters appear to be most useful from 20 to 30 weeks' gestation. During this time in 95% of the cases, a given head measurement will predict the true week of gestation ±8.4 days. Although prediction of maturity from biparietal diameter measurements after 30 weeks' gestation is less reliable, clinically useful results can be obtained up to 34 weeks' gestation.

Methods that rely on amniocentesis, chemical indices, or even x-ray studies for estimating fetal gestational age are not specific for a given week but are useful in identifying fetuses who are older than 36 or 37 weeks' gestation. The ultrasonic method of measuring biparietal diameter has the special advantage that it is useful in assessing the gestational age of the fetus earlier in pregnancy. This is important in planning interim or repetitive treatments, such as intrauterine transfusions, in the management of the premature onset of labor, or in planning early delivery of the fetus because of maternal toxemia or diabetes. Most patients attend a prenatal clinic during the second trimester, and most discrepancies between dates and uterine size become apparent at this time; thus ultrasonic measurement of the biparietal diameter in conjunction with estimates of fetal weight may be a useful technique for detecting the syndrome of intrauterine growth retardation. Preliminary evidence suggests that the linear pattern of growth of the biparietal diameter is very similar in normal, diabetic, and hypertensive patients; this measurement may more accurately reflect gestational age and fetal maturity than other techniques.

Safety of diagnostic ultrasound. Direct damage to tissues can be produced by ultrasound of very high energy levels. However, the energy levels used in diagnostic ultrasound are several hundred times lower than those required to produce a minimal rise in tissue temperature. No damaging effects of pulsed ultrasound (as in ultrasonography) or continuous-wave ultrasound (as in fetal heart-rate monitoring) to mothers or their fetuses have been reported. Insonation of fetal and maternal lymphocytes for prolonged periods of time by diagnostic ultrasound does not produce chromosomal damage. However, sonation of fibroblasts in tissue culture has been reported to interfere with their normal growth characteristics.

Amniotic fluid analysis

Amniotic fluid performs various homeostatic functions. It cushions the fetus against trauma and provides a space for normal skeletal growth and fetal development. It also serves as a reservoir for the disposal of fetal secretions and at the same time supplies a medium for fetal swallowing. The possible nutritive significance of swallowed amniotic fluid has been suggested but not documented. There is little doubt that amniotic fluid has multiple origins and that its composition changes during pregnancy. The importance of the different routes of its formation appear to vary with fetal maturity, but the manner in which these processes are integrated and the quantitative aspects of fluid transfer to the amniotic cavity are not well understood.

Regulating the volume of amniotic fluid. Amniotic fluid is elaborated despite the surgical closure of fetal secretory and excretory ducts or even in the absence of the fetus. Presumably, water, electrolytes, and other substances are transferred directly across the membranes or along the umbilical cord. Under normal conditions, transfer across the fetal skin may be important, especially in early pregnancy when the fetus is enveloped by a periderm that has surface microvilli and abundant cytoplasmic organelles. Predictable changes in intrauterine fluid compartments can be produced experimentally by changing tonicity or pressure relationships across the placenta. Under normal circumstances, subtle adjustments of osmotic and hydrostatic pressure gradients between mother and fetus probably control intrauterine water balance and, along with water produced by fetal metabolism, account for a gradual net transfer of water to the fetus as pregnancy advances.

Although there is good evidence that the molecular exchange of water and electrolytes between maternal blood and the amniotic fluid compartment is rapid, volume disturbances created by the withdrawal or addition of fluid may not be corrected for some time. In a patient with hydramnios, amniotic fluid accumulates at a net rate of about 150 ml/24 hr after amniocentesis. Bulk changes in volume are produced in late pregnancy, primarily by an equilibrium between fetal swallowing, replacement by micturition, and the addition of fetal secretions. Respiratory tract secretions may also contribute to the amniotic fluid volume. In the fetal lamb, the net outflow of tracheal fluid is about 5 ml/kg/hr.

The average weekly increment in amniotic fluid volume from 11 to 15 weeks is 25 ml/wk and 50 ml/wk thereafter until the twenty-eighth week of gestation. Although the normal variations in fluid volumes are large, extreme values above 1.5 liters or below 500 ml are abnormal and frequently associated with fetal pathologic conditions. Because of the wide variation during preg-

Table 1-3. Fetal malformations frequently associated with polyhydramnios or oligohydramnios

Polyhydramnios	Oligohydramnios
Anencephaly	Renal agenesis
Meningocele and encephalocele	Ureteral dysplasia
Esophageal or duodenal atresia	Urethral atresia
Pyloric stenosis	Pulmonary hypoplasia
Klippel-Feil syndrome	Amnion nodosum
Multiple anomalies (not central nervous system)	

nancy, measurements of amniotic fluid volume have only a limited value in estimating fetal maturity. A marked decrease in volume postterm is characteristic of fetal postmaturity. Similarly, a decreased volume of amniotic fluid earlier in gestation may provide additional evidence for placental insufficiency.

Severe alterations in amniotic fluid volume are sometimes associated with various congenital anomalies and provide indirect evidence that fetal organs contribute to this pool (Table 1-3). Congenital malformations occur in about one third of the pregnancies associated with polyhydramnios. Defects in the central nervous system of the fetus may interfere with normal fetal swallowing or the production of antidiuretic hormone. Genitourinary tract abnormalities, on the other hand, are associated with oligohydramnios and impaired fetal urine production or micturition.

Composition of amniotic fluid. In view of the diverse origins of amniotic fluid, it is not surprising that it constitutes a heterogeneous system composed of dissolved and suspended constituents. In early pregnancy, amniotic fluid behaves as a dialysate of maternal or fetal blood and as such resembles interstitial fluid. In the latter half of pregnancy, the total osmotic pressure of amniotic fluid is approximately 20 mOsm below fetal and maternal plasma values, largely because of a decrease in sodium and chloride concentrations. No clear changes in calcium, magnesium, or phosphate concentrations have been detected in the amniotic fluid during pregnancy.

The oxygen tension of amniotic fluid is in the range of 10 to 25 mm Hg. The corresponding P_{CO_2} in late pregnancy is 50 to 60 mm Hg, and the range of pH has been recorded as 7.0 to 7.25. The relative acidity of amniotic fluid compared with blood is partly caused by the much lower concentration of protein buffers. Clinically, fetal asphyxia or placental insufficiency cannot be detected by measuring amniotic fluid gases or acid-base status.

The concentration of glucose is less than in maternal or fetal plasma and averages 25 to 40 mg/100 ml. At 28 weeks' gestation, the total protein concentration in amniotic fluid ranges from 400 to 800 mg of protein per 100 ml of amniotic fluid and decreases thereafter to 200 to 300 mg/100 ml at 38 weeks. Albumin accounts for at least 50% of the total protein. After the sixth month of pregnancy, the gamma globulin fraction increases progressively, and the albumin fraction decreases correspondingly. Immunoelectrophoretic studies and transfer studies of labeled materials indicate that many of the proteins in amniotic fluid are of maternal origin. However, fibrinogen appears to be absent from amniotic fluid as are α_2- and β-macroglobulins and α_2-lipoproteins. On the other hand, the globulin, α-fetoprotein, has been found in amniotic fluid and is of fetal origin. Virtually all amino acids are present in amniotic fluid in about the same concentration as in maternal plasma. Although the amniotic fluid protein concentration consistently decreases with advancing gestation, total protein determinations have not been useful indicators of fetal maturity. However, amniotic fluid proteins may be of value in predicting specific fetal diseases. Preliminary findings suggest an increased α-fetoprotein concentration in association with open malformations of the central nervous system, and increases in immunoglobulin G before 34 weeks' gestation have been reported in association with erythroblastosis fetalis and fetal death. Alterations in amino acid metabolism and a number of enzymes have been useful in diagnosing inborn errors of metabolism (p. 22).

Various steroids and protein hormones have been detected in amniotic fluid, including the corticosteroids, estrogens and progestins, and their various metabolites. The concentration of human chorionic gonadotropin in amniotic fluid is similar to that in maternal urine at comparable periods of gestation. The concentration of human placental lactogen in normal amniotic fluid is about one tenth that in maternal serum but significantly more than that present in fetal cord blood. Insulin and thyroxine are detectable by radioimmunoassay, and the erythropoietin concentration in amniotic fluid is correlated with the degree of fetal anemia. Amniotic fluid 17-ketosteroids are elevated in congenital adrenogenital syndrome and decreased in anencephalic pregnancies. In severe erythroblastosis fetalis, amniotic fluid estriol decreases, whereas amniotic fluid placental lactogen increases. Prostaglandins E and F have been detected in amniotic fluid; the latter are known to increase during labor.

Applications and techniques of amniocentesis. The diagnostic and therapeutic uses of amniocentesis during pregnancy are summarized below. Puncture of the amniotic cavity and withdrawal of fluid is a relatively simple and safe procedure in the hands of an experienced operator and can be performed after 14 weeks' gestation on an outpatient basis. The transabdominal route is preferred to the vaginal route in order to minimize the risk of infection and premature rupture of the fetal membranes. The techniques used and precautions taken will vary somewhat with the stage of pregnancy and the indications for the procedure.

APPLICATIONS OF AMNIOCENTESIS DURING PREGNANCY

1. Biochemical and cytogenetic studies in early pregnancy
2. Diagnosis and prognosis of erythroblastosis fetalis
3. Induction of abortion by intraamniotic injection of hypertonic solutions or drugs
4. Treatment of polyhydramnios
5. Injection of radiopaque contrast material for amniography (amniotic fluid volume, hydatidiform mole, multiple gestation, fetal gestational age, fetal deformities, hydrops fetalis, placental localization, fetal function, such as swallowing)
6. Determination of amniotic fluid volume (indicator dilution)
7. Studies of amniotic fluid circulation
8. Determinations of fetal maturity
9. Fetal and placental function study (clearance of injected substances, hormones, and so on)
10. Induction of labor
11. Evaluation of amniotic fluid pressure and uterine contractility in labor
12. Instillation of pharmacologic agents for inhibition of uterine contractions or treatment of the fetus
13. Determination that meconium is present

A suprapubic approach in the midline of the abdomen has much to recommend it in the first two trimesters of pregnancy and for a considerable period thereafter. This technique is easy and safe, provided the bladder is empty and adherent loops of bowel from previous surgery or adhesions can be excluded. The placenta is rarely present in this location, and the danger of fetal trauma is minimized if the fetus can be displaced. Later in pregnancy when the fetus is less mobile, the appropriate puncture site must be selected in reference to the position of the fetus and the placenta. The fetal position should be palpated and the amniotic sac entered in the area posterior to the fetal neck or in the area of the small parts. Placental localization is recommended in order to minimize dangers of hemorrhage and maternal sensitization by fetal blood group antigens. The placenta may be localized by a variety of methods, including thermography, radioisotope techniques, or ultrasonic scanning. Fetal and maternal complications are rare when proper precautions are taken. Complications include fetal or maternal hemorrhage, premature labor, puncture of fetal organs, abruptio placentae, and amnionitis; but serious complications occur in less than 1% of amniocenteses.

Amniotic fluid indices of gestational age. Constituents of amniotic fluid that show useful correlations with gestational age or fetal maturity include creatinine, bilirubin pigment, and phospholipids. From about midpregnancy, osmolality and sodium concentrations of the amniotic fluid fall, and

Table 1-4. Values for osmolality and sodium, urea, and creatinine levels in amniotic fluid with advancing gestation*

Biochemical variable	Gestation in weeks					
	30 or less	31−	33−	35−	37−	39+
Osmolality	275 ± 6.4	269 ± 6.7	268 ± 9.0	264 ± 6.5	261 ± 17.3	259 ± 14.0
Sodium	135 ± 5.2	132 ± 5.6	132 ± 4.7	131 ± 5.1	128 ± 8.4	125 ± 6.0
Urea	20 ± 6.1	21 ± 3.9	21 ± 5.1	24 ± 5.7	29 ± 9.3	32 ± 8.0
Creatinine	0.8 ± 0.18	1.2 ± 0.24	1.3 ± 0.26	1.5 ± 0.28	1.9 ± 0.50	2.0 ± 0.43

Adapted from Lind, T., and Billewicz, W. Z.: Br. J. Hosp. Med. **5**:681, 1971.
*Values are means ± SD.

urea and creatinine levels rise (Table 1-4). These biochemical changes depend largely on the addition of a hypotonic urine to amniotic fluid as gestation advances. Postterm pregnancies continue to decrease in osmolality despite the progressive oligohydramnios that occurs after 40 weeks' gestation.

The amniotic fluid creatinine is well correlated with gestational age but poorly correlated with fetal weight, an indication that the concentration of creatinine reflects maturation of the fetal kidney rather than fetal muscle mass. In 95% of the cases, a creatinine concentration of 2 mg/100 ml in amniotic fluid indicates a fetal gestational age of at least 36 weeks. This relationship is seen despite erythroblastosis, meconium-stained amniotic fluid, or toxemia of diabetes provided that the maternal renal function is normal.

Spectrophotometric analysis of amniotic fluid by the method of Liley (p. 27) is used most commonly as a measure of unconjugated bilirubin in amniotic fluid. The highest values are obtained between 16 and 30 weeks' gestation; thereafter the values decline gradually, and after 36 weeks' gestation most of the samples show no absorption peak at 450 mμ (ΔOD 450). However, positive deviations are found in about 15% of the normal samples of amniotic fluid and in conditions associated with impaired fetal swallowing or vomiting in utero (for example, intestinal atresia). Under conditions of maternal hemolytic disease, sickle cell crises, or hepatocellular dysfunction, an increased maternal serum bilirubin is available for diffusion into the amniotic sac and may lead to a falsely elevated ΔOD 450. Conversely, prolonged exposure of the sample to light will decrease this pigment. Patients with diabetes and toxemia, when an estimate of fetal maturity is especially desirable, have higher ΔOD's 450 than normal for gestational age. However, if the appropriate precautions are taken and the amniotic fluid Δ OD 450 falls to zero, a fetal gestational age of 36 weeks or more is very likely.

Amniotic fluid phospholipids. The concentration of total lipids in the amniotic fluid increases throughout gestation and approaches 60 mg/100 ml at term. The increase in late pregnancy is primarly caused by an increase in phospholipids; the nonpolar lipids that represent 75% of the total lipid content of amniotic fluid do not change appreciably during pregnancy. The placenta is relatively impermeable to maternal lipids, although many free fatty acids cross the placenta rapidly and are then esterified in fetal tissues. The sources of these lipids, besides fetal skin, are amniotic epithelium and tracheal fluid.

At term, lecithin is the most prevalent phospholipid, contributing roughly two thirds of the total phospholipids in amniotic fluid. The functional maturity of fetal lung and its ability to produce surfactant may be reflected in the concentrations of amniotic fluid lecithin. Dipalmitoyl lecithin is the major constituent of alveolar surfactant, and surfactants are synthesized by the fetal lung and secreted into tracheal fluid. Furthermore, amniotic fluid phospholipids are similar to tracheal fluid phospholipids, and the biosynthetic pathways for surfactant production in fetal lung correlate with gestational age and the large increase in lecithin near term. The major pathway for surfactant synthesis matures at 35 weeks and converts cytidine diphosphate choline

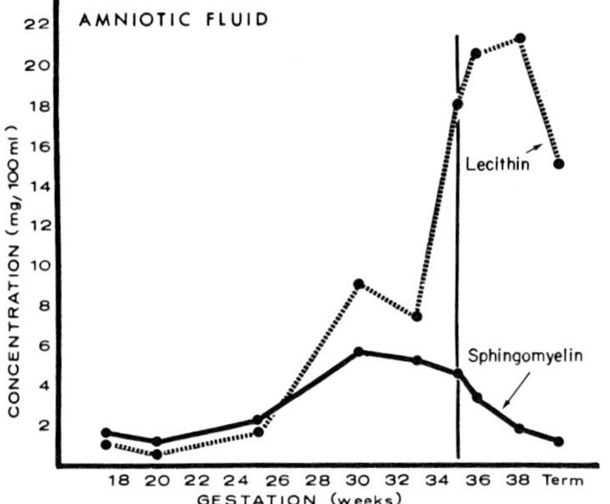

FIG. 1-12. The levels of sphingomyelin and lethicin in the amniotic fluid are plotted against gestational age. There is a significant difference between these two levels at age 35 weeks' gestation. (Gluck, L., and others: Am. J. Obstet. Gynecol. **109**:440, 1971.)

to dipalmitoyl lecithin (phosphocholine transferase). A quantitatively less important pathway involves methylation of phosphatidylethanolamine; it is functional after 20 weeks of gestation but is easily inhibited by perinatal hypoxia or acidosis.

Gluck and his associates noted that the sharp increase in lecithin concentration in amniotic fluid after 35 weeks' gestation is not matched by a parallel increase in sphingomyelin (Fig. 1-12). The lecithin-sphingomyelin ratio (L/S ratio) reflects pulmonary maturity of the fetus; high densitometric ratios of lecithin to sphingomyelin (in excess of 2) are usually associated with the absence of subsequent respiratory distress of the newborn. The interpretation of intermediate and low L/S ratios is uncertain at the present time, since some infants with low ratios do not develop respiratory distress. Sufficient data are not yet available to decide with certainty whether the amniotic fluid L/S ratio is a specific index of fetal lung maturity or the degree to which this ratio may be altered in the presence of obstetrical complications. The possibility of inducing synthesis of lung phosphorylcholine glyceride transferase, which in turn leads to increased synthesis of lecithin in the fetal lung, with corticosteroids and other agents, is being actively investigated.

Cytologic indices of fetal maturity. Identification of fetal squamous cells in the amniotic fluid was originally used for the diagnosis of ruptured membranes during pregnancy. The amniotic fluid cells have a variety of sources, which include fetal skin, amnion, conjunctivas, and genitourinary, alimentary, and respiratory tracts. Cytologic determination of fetal maturity is based upon a change in cellular morphologic characteristics or staining characteristics with advancing gestation. Before 14 weeks the fluid is nearly acellular; between 22 and 32 weeks' gestation, nucleated and anucleated squamous cells are identified in addition to smaller round cells that resemble the parabasal cells seen on vaginal smears. After 30 weeks' gestation the amnion yields large numbers of tall, cylindrical columnar cells with distinct cytoplasmic vacuoles suggestive of secretory activity. Examination of amniotic fluid cytologic factors with the Papanicolaou technique indicates that a consistent increase in cornified cells occurs after 36 weeks' gestation and that anucleated squamous cells predominate in association with keratinization of the epidermis as the fetus approaches term. This method has not found wide application in clinical practice because of the lack of precision in predicting gestational age.

An alternative method makes use of the lipid-staining characteristics of amniotic fluid cells. The percentage of cells in the amniotic fluid sediment that take on an orange appearance or show lipid globules when stained with Nile blue sulfate or oil red O gradually increases after 32 weeks' gestation, with a sharp increase after 36 weeks' gestation. If lipid-stained cells exceed 30% of all cells in the amniotic fluid, 95% of the fetuses will exceed 2,500 gm birth weight or 36 weeks' gestational age. The usefulness of this simple technique is limited somewhat by the virtual absence of lipid-staining cells in a significant number of amniotic fluid samples drawn at term. Amniotic fluid cytologic diagnosis is also limited by our lack of understanding of the precise origins of the cells and their lipid-staining characteristics.

At the present time the usefulness of amniotic fluid analyses in the evaluation of fetal maturity is limited by a lack of clear understanding of the dynamics of the various amniotic constituents and their relation

TABLE 1-5. Hereditary and metabolic disorders detected in tissue culture or by amniotic fluid analysis

Disease	Inheritance	Expression or deficiency	Fibroblasts	Amniotic cells	Diagnosed in utero
Acatalasia	Auto rec	Catalase	+	0	0
Arginosuccinicaciduria	Auto rec	Arginosuccinase	+	++	0
Chediak-Higashi	Auto rec	Cytoplasmic inclusions	+	0	0
Citrullinemia	Auto rec	Arginosuccinic acid synthetase	+	0	0
Congenital erythropoietic porphyria	Auto rec	Uroporphyrinogen III co-synthetase	+	0	0
Cystinosis	Auto rec	Cystine (free)	+	+	0
Cystic fibrosis	Auto rec	Metachromasia	+	+	0
Fabry's disease	Auto rec	Alpha-galactosidase	+	+	+
Fucosidosis	Auto rec	Alpha-fucosidase	+	+	0
Galactosemia	Auto rec	Galactose one-phosphate uridyl transferase	+	++	+
Tay-Sachs disease	Auto rec	Hexosaminidase A	+	++	+
Sandhoff's disease	Auto rec	Hexosaminidase A & B	+	++	+
Generalized gangliosidosis	Auto rec	Beta-galactosidase A, B, & C	+	+	0
Juvenile GM_2 gangliosidosis	Auto rec	Hexosaminidase A	+	+	0
Juvenile GM_1 gangliosidosis	Auto rec	Beta-galactosidase B & C	+	+	0
Gaucher's disease	Auto rec	Glucocerebrosidase	+	+	0
Glucose-6-phosphate dehydrogenase deficiency (Mediterranean form)	Auto rec	Glucose-6-phosphate dehydrogenase	+	++	0
Glycogen storage diseases					
I Von Gierke's disease	Auto rec	Glucose-6-phosphatase	0	0	0
II Pompe's disease	Auto rec	Alpha-one, 4-glucosidase	+	++	+
III Forbes' disease	Auto rec	Amylo-one, 6-glycosidase	+	+	0
IV Anderson's disease	Auto rec	Branching enzyme	+	+	0
V McArdle's syndrome	Auto rec	Myophosphorylase	0	0	0
VI Hers' disease	Auto rec	Hepatophosphorylase	0	0	0
Homocystinuria	Auto rec	Cystathione synthetase	+	+	0
Hyperammonemia	Auto rec	Ornithine transcarbamylase & carbamylphosphate synthetase	0		0
Hyperlysinemia	Auto rec	Lysine ketoglutarate reductase	+	0	0
Hyperornithinemia	Auto rec	Ornithine alpha-ketoacid transaminase	+	+	0
Hypervalinemia	Auto rec	Valine transaminase	+	0	0
I-Cell disease	Auto rec	Inclusions	0	0	0
		Beta-glucuronidase			0

Ketotic hyperglycinemia	Auto rec	Propionyl-CoA carboxylase	+	+	0
Krabbe's disease (globoid leucodystrophy)	Auto rec	Beta-galactocerebrosidase	+	+	0
Lysosomal acid phosphatase deficiency	Auto rec	Lysosomal acid phosphatase	+	+	+
Lesch-Nyhan syndrome	X-rec	Hypoxanthine-guanine phosphoribosyl transferase	+	++	+
Mannosidosis	Auto rec	Alpha-mannosidase	+	+	0
Maple-syrup urine disease (branched chain ketoaciduria)	Auto rec	Branched chain ketoacid decarboxylase	+	+	+
Marfan's syndrome	Auto rec	*Metachromasia*	+	+	0
Metachromatic leucodystrophy	Auto rec	Arylsulfatase A	+	+	0
variant	Auto rec	Arylsulfatase A, B, & C			
Methylmalonic acidemia (B_{12} unresponsive)	Auto rec	Methylmalonyl-CoA mutase	+	+	+
Mucopolysaccharidoses					
I Hurler's syndrome	Auto rec	$^{35}SO_4$ incorporation	+	+	+
		Beta-galactosidase	0	0	0
		*Metachromasia**			
II Hunter's syndrome	X-rec	$^{35}SO_4$ incorporation	+	+	
		*Metachromasia**			
III Sanfilippo syndrome	Auto rec	*Metachromasia*	+	0	0
IV Morquio's syndrome	Auto rec	*Metachromasia*	+	0	0
V Scheie's syndrome	Auto rec	*Metachromasia*	+	0	0
VI Maroteaux-Lamy syndrome	Auto rec	*Metachromasia*	0	0	0
Myotonic dystrophy	Auto dom	*Metachromasia*	+	+	0
Niemann-Pick disease	Auto rec	Sphingomyelinase	+	+	0
Orotic aciduria	Auto rec	Orotidylic pyrophosphorylase	+	0	0
		Orotidylic decarboxylase	+	0	0
Pyruvate decarboxylase deficiency	Auto rec	Pyruvate decarboxylase	+	0	0
Refsum's disease	Auto rec	Phytanic acid alphahydroxylase	+	+	0
Xeroderma pigmentosum	Auto rec	DNA repair enzyme	+	+	0

LEGEND:

Auto dom	Autosomal dominant	X-rec	X-linked recessive
Auto rec	Autosomal recessive	Amniotic cells+	Cultivated amniotic fluid cells
	X-linked dominant	Amniotic cells++	Cultivated and uncultivated amniotic fluid cells

From Maidman, J. E.: Antenatal diagnosis, Obstet. Gynecol. Ann. **1**:65, 1972.

*Metachromasia is listed only where specific studies are unavailable or uncertain or where necessary for completeness in a disease group.

to normal and abnormal fetal development. Nevertheless, it has been repeatedly demonstrated that the accuracy of assessing fetal maturity is greatly improved when two or more diagnostic tests are employed in conjunction with clinical estimates.

Management of specific fetal diseases

Hereditary disorders and congenital abnormalities

With recent advances in tissue culture methods and cytogenetics, hereditary diseases can now be diagnosed early in pregnancy. The obstetrical history should include a thorough review of the details of each birth, fetal or infant death, and chronic illness in siblings or other family members. Prenatal studies of amniotic fluid or of cultured amniotic fluid cells have provided reassurance or guidance to an increasing number of couples who have borne genetically defective infants or who give a family history of inherited disease.

Nearly 50 genetic diseases can now be diagnosed by prenatal testing of amniotic fluid or its cells in tissue culture (Table 1-5). The majority of fetal disorders are diagnosed prenatally by chromosomal abnormalities (for example, Down's syndrome) on karyotype analysis. Some diseases in the fetus manifest themselves by abnormal concentrations of metabolites in the fluid itself (for example, Hurler's disease and adrenogenital syndrome), others by cellular staining characteristics in tissue culture such as metachromatic granules. Many of the amino acid disorders are detected by specific enzymatic deficiencies in amniotic fluid cells before or after culture.

Cultivation of amniotic fluid epithelial cells is most successful before 18 weeks' gestation. Since the interval between amniocentesis and diagnosis from tissue culture is usually 2 to 3 weeks and sometimes longer, early amniocentesis is advisable if interruption of pregnancy is contemplated. Cells are cultured as soon as possible after centrifugation under aseptic conditions for later biochemical and chromosomal studies. An aliquot of cells is separated for immediate sex chromatin determination and for enzyme determinations.

A classification of patients who are at risk for fetal chromosomal aberrations or metabolic disorders and are candidates for amniocentesis has been suggested by Littlefield and is listed below. Genetic counseling in the prenatal period as well as before pregnancy involves a consideration of risk factors based upon the mendelian laws of inheritance and on empirical observations. Autosomal dominant traits (for example, Huntington's chorea) are expressed in 50% of the children because the affected parent is usually heterozygous. Since in most conditions the defect cannot be detected in utero, most couples elect not to undertake pregnancy. In autosomal recessive inheritance, the risk for each sibling is 25%. Most of the inborn errors of metabolism fall into this category. Since the Y chromosome contains no identifiable genes, sex-linked diseases (most are recessive) are carried by the X chromosome, and only males tend to be affected. Females are carriers of the trait (for example, hemophilia and Duchenne's muscular dystrophy) and transmit the disease to one half of their sons. At the present time, in the severe X-linked disorders, all male fetuses would have to be aborted to avoid having an affected child; the only exceptions are Lesch-Nyhan and Hunter's syndromes, in which a specific diagnosis can be made by biochemical analysis. Although errors of sex typing occur in less than 10% of uncultured cells, it is prudent to compare sex chromatin analysis with the karyotype derived later from cultured cells.

IDENTIFICATION OF THE PREGNANCY AT RISK FOR A GENETIC DISORDER*

A. Severe disorder—high genetic risk
   1. Autosomal recessive conditions such as mucopolysaccharidoses and lipidoses (for example, Hurler's and Tay-Sachs diseases), cystinosis, Pompe's disease, usual type of maple syrup urine disease, and certain other metabolic disorders
   2. Familial chromosome translocations
   3. X-linked conditions such as Lowe's, Lesch-Nyhan, and Hunter's syndromes, chronic granulomatous disease, and certain muscular dystrophies

B. Severe disorder—moderate genetic risk
   1. Chromosome disorders in pregnancy of women 40 years of age or older

C. Severe disorder—low genetic risk
   1. Chromosome disorders in pregnancy of women 35 to 39 years of age

*From Littlefield, J. W.: N. Engl. J. Med. **282:** 627, 1970.

2. Recurrence of trisomy 21 after one affected child

D. Treatable disorder—high genetic risk
1. Autosomal recessive conditions such as galactosemia and pyridoxine-responsive homocystinuria
2. X-linked conditions such as hemophilia, nephrogenic diabetes insipidus, and Bruton form of agammaglobulinemia
3. Cystic fibrosis

Chromosomal abnormalities, which occur in about 0.5% of all live births, constitute the largest area where prenatal genetic diagnosis is indicated. The incidence of autosomal trisomies and sex chromosome aneuploidies increases with maternal age. Thus advanced maternal age represents the clearest indication for amniocentesis at the present time. *Down's syndrome* (trisomy 21) is the most common chromosomal abnormality found in live-born infants (1:650 births). Although less than 15% of all pregnancies occur in women over 35, more than 50% of all cases of mongolism result from these pregnancies. The incidence of Down's syndrome births rises to about 1:40 in mothers 45 years of age or older. Most cases of Down's syndrome are caused by nondisjunction of chromosomes during meiosis, which gives rise to some ova with two No. 21 chromosomes. The risks of recurrence are not precisely known, but are probably not more than twice that for other women of the same age. If the mother is young, the risk of recurrence may be less than the risk of amniocentesis. In such cases, a decision for prenatal genetic diagnosis must be made on the merits of each individual case and must take into account emotional and other considerations.

The familial form of mongolism constitutes only a few percent of all cases of Down's syndrome and usually results from the translocation of a portion of chromosome No. 21 to another chromosome in the mother. The mother (a balanced translocation carrier) has only 45 chromosomes and transmits to the ovum the compound 15/21 chromosome as well as a normal chromosome No. 21. The contribution of an additional chromosome No. 21 by the sperm produces in effect the trisomy 21, although the actual chromosome number of the zygote is 46. An assessment of the risks of bearing another child with Down's syndrome requires that the karyotype of both parents be determined. If either parent is a 21/21 translocation carrier, the couple can expect an affected fetus in all cases. The theoretical risk of recurrence for a maternal 15/21 and 21/22 translocation carrier is 1:3. However, in reality the risk is considerably less and has been estimated at 5% to 10%. For a male carrier the risk appears to be even lower. Such patients are appropriate candidates for amniocentesis and prenatal genetic diagnosis. The recent introduction of fluorescent staining of chromosomes by alkylating agents such as quinacrine mustard has provided precise cytogenetic diagnosis, especially of translocations. If fluorescent patterning of the chromosomes succeeds in specifically defining the site of translocation, the recurrence risks for Down's syndromes can be revised with greater accuracy in the future.

The hereditary metabolic disorders often reflect an enzyme deficiency and numerically represent a small fraction of the total pregnant women who are seen for prenatal genetic diagnosis. Usually the family is seen only when a previous child has been affected. The vast majority of these inborn errors of metabolism, as indicated in Table 1-5, are autosomal recessives. Others such a phenylketonuria and histidinemia cannot yet be diagnosed in utero since cultured cells lack the necessary enzymes. Disorders with an ethnic predilection such as Tay-Sachs disease, in which the heterozygote carrier can be detected by serum assay, lend themselves to screening procedures. About one of 40 Ashkenazic Jews are heterozygous for this particular lipid-storage disease. The decision to perform amniocentesis for inborn errors of metabolism will depend upon the severity of the disorder, past reproductive history of the couple, the views of the parents, the availability of therapeutic abortion, and advances in medical treatment. The patient should be informed that significant risks are associated with therapeutic abortion in the second trimester.

Congenital anomalies such as cleft palate, clubbed foot, spina bifida, anencephaly, and many others are the result of interaction of the environment and multiple genetic determinants. The risks of the recurrence of polygenic or multifactoral inheritance of congenital defects is based on empirical observations and differs for each anomaly. However, a number of these anomalies can be diagnosed prenatally. Elevated amniotic fluid bilirubin concentrations have been reported in cases of anencephaly, duodenal atresia, and pyloric stenosis. Ultrasound can be used to diagnose hydrocephalus, microcephaly, or soft-tissue tumors. Amniography has been used for detecting congenital malformations in high-risk pregnancies, particularly in association with polyhydramnios and diabetes mellitus. The in utero detection of congenital anomalies that are secondary to environmental teratogens or infectious agents is being explored. Though possible, examination of the fetus with a fiber optic instrument is still hazardous.

Prenatal genetic diagnosis raises many ethical, medical, and economic issues. The consensus in most centers is that amniocentesis should not be undertaken unless the family is committed to subsequent intervention if appropriate or if treatment can be instituted after diagnosis. Clearly the patient will be best served when there is cooperation between the attending physician, the laboratory, and the geneticist, all of whom should have a special interest and expertise in prenatal genetic diagnosis and counseling.

Erythroblastosis fetalis

Erythroblastosis fetalis (hemolytic disease of the fetus) is caused by maternal immunization against antigens of fetal blood groups (Chapter 9, p. 183). Before modern advances in prevention, erythroblastosis fetalis occurred in about 1% of all pregnancies. Nearly 20% of these fetuses were stillborn, and another 30% died in the neonatal period or suffered permanent brain damage. Today with more effective methods of diagnosis and treatment, including spectrophotometric examination of amniotic fluid, early induction of labor, and exchange transfusion in neonates, the perinatal loss has been reduced to about 10% of affected fetuses. When in select cases these methods are combined with intrauterine transfusion of the fetus, perinatal mortality can be reduced to an estimated 5%. Now that anti-D immunoglobulin can prevent postpartum sensitization in the vast majority of mothers, the incidence of clinically severe erythroblastosis should diminish considerably in the next 10 to 15 years.

Theoretically, any blood group antigen except Lewis and I (which are not present on fetal erythrocytes) can cause erythroblastosis fetalis. The probability of maternal sensitization depends largely on the immunizing dose of blood and the antigenicity of the red blood cell factor involved. AB and Rh_0 (D) are the most potent red blood cell antigens. Less than 2% of all cases of erythroblastosis fetalis are caused by the minor red blood cell antigens. As little as 0.5 to 1.0 ml of Rh-positive blood is sufficient for primary immunization in most individuals. Booster stimuli of 0.1 ml of fetal blood suffice to increase the titer in subsequent pregnancies. Fetal cells enter the maternal circulation sometimes as early as the third month of gestation and can be observed in approximately 20% of pregnancies. However, the primary stimulus occurs at delivery.

Prenatal testing for ABO erythroblastosis is not helpful in predicting which babies will be affected in utero probably because a lower proportion of anti-A and anti-B immunoglobulins cross the placenta. However, a history of previous ABO hemolytic disease in the neonate will allow prompt diagnostic and therapeutic intervention at birth (p. 186). ABO incompatibility accounts for nearly two thirds of hemolytic disease in the fetus and Rh incompatability for about one third, but the hemolytic process associated with A or B incompatability in the fetus is much less severe than that with D incompatability. The blood group antigen Rh_0 (D) is responsible for almost all cases of erythroblastotic stillbirths and almost all early neonatal deaths from erythroblastosis.

Prenatal management of erythroblastosis fetalis. The routine procedures for diagnosing and managing erythroblastosis fetalis during pregnancy are outlined below. During pregnancy all patients should have their ABO and Rh types determined and receive an antibody screening as well. Husbands of all Rh-negative patients should have a full Rh phenotype determination. Testing with the appropriate sera for the five common types determines whether the husband is homozygous or heterozygous for Rh_0 (D). This information is useful in assessing future risks to the family with an infant already affected with erythroblastosis fetalis. If the husband is heterozygous for Rh_0 (D), the chance for each of his future infants to be Rh-negative and free of hemolytic disease is 50%.

PROGRAM OF PRENATAL CARE FOR ERYTHROBLASTOSIS FETALIS

I. All patients on first antenatal visit
   A. History (blood transfusion, previous maternal sensitization, abortion, jaundice, or anemia in a neonate)
   B. ABO and Rh typing
   C. Antibody screening and identification if present
II. Rh-negative patients, unsensitized
   A. ABO and Rh typing and zygosity determination of the husband
   B. Repeat antibody screening at 28 and 35 weeks' gestation and at 6 weeks' postpartum. If negative, deliver at term.
   C. Anti-D gamma globulin postpartum to mother if cord blood is Rh-positive
III. Sensitized patients
   A. History of previously affected neonate or stillbirth
   B. Antibody identification and antiglobulin (Coombs') titer
   C. Repeat indirect Coombs' test and titer at 1-month intervals; repeat at 2-week intervals after 34 weeks' gestation
   D. Amniotic fluid analysis (ΔOD at 450 mμ)
      1. For a "critical" maternal antibody titer (usually 1:32 or greater in the first sensitized pregnancy or 1:16 or greater in a subsequent pregnancy)
      2. For history of previously affected infant or stillbirth
   E. Intrauterine fetal transfusion
      1. Rising amniotic fluid OD (ΔOD 450) in Liley's high zone (III) prior to 34 weeks' gestation
   F. Delivery
      1. Deliver near term for ΔOD 450's consistently in low zone (I)
      2. Induction of labor at 37 to 38 weeks' gestation if maternal titer is low and ΔOD 450 in lower middle zone (II)
      3. Induction of labor or cesarean section at 34 to 36 weeks for rising ΔOD 450 in upper zone II or zone III; or after intrauterine transfusion

Antibody titration in the mother can be achieved by albumin incubation, enzyme treatment of sheep red blood cells, or the antiglobulin (Coombs') test. The greatest serum dilution to cause visible agglutination of test red blood cells is the titer. The critical limit for an antibody titer is that below which intrauterine death rarely or never occurs in the experience of the laboratory or clinic. Because of methodologic differences, this limiting titer varies from one laboratory to another. It follows, therefore, that all antibody titers must be done at the same laboratory. In a first sensitized pregnancy, serial antibody determinations that show a rise in antibody titer indicate that the fetus is Rh-positive and usually reflect the fetal condition. In most centers, no stillbirths or neonatal deaths occur from Rh hemolytic disease within one week of delivery if the titer is 1:16 or less and very rarely with a titer of 1:32. However, in a second sensitized or subsequent pregnancy, the maternal antibody titer cannot be used serially to indicate the severity of fetal disease. Because of these limitations, the antibody titration method is supplemented in clinical practice by analyses for bilirubin pigment in amniotic fluid. The prenatal history is extremely important in determining the fetal prognosis; at the Boston Hospital for Women from 1945 to 1953 nearly three quarters of the patients with a previous history of hydrops or stillbirth had an intrauterine death before 37 weeks of gestation.

Amniotic fluid analysis for bilirubin. (See also p. 187). The yellow discoloration of amniotic fluid obtained from isoimmunized pregnancies produces a characteristic spectral absorption curve with a peak at 450 mμ. This pigment has been identified as unconjugated bilirubin bound to albumin. There is good correlation between the bilirubin content of amniotic fluid and the probability of fetal deterioration or hydrops.

The causes of hydrops fetalis are not precisely known but have been related to hepatorenal dysfunction, cardiac failure, and tissue anoxia associated with severe fetal anemia. Nearly 20% of cases of hydrops fetalis are caused by causes other than blood group incompatibility. Nonimmunologic hydrops fetalis is associated with a variety of diseases or major congenital malformations. (See outline below.) There is a high incidence of polyhydramnios, preeclampsia, and prematurity in cases of idiopathic hydrops fetalis and an association with severe maternal anemia. Fetal anemia or hypoproteinemia is not seen in idiopathic hydrops.

DIFFERENTIAL DIAGNOSIS OF HYDROPS FETALIS

A. Fetal anemia
B. Alpha-thalassemia
C. Maternal anemia (hemoglobin less than 7.5 mg/100 ml)
D. Transfusion syndrome (monochorionic twins, usually affecting the recipient twin)
E. Chorioangioma
F. Adenomatoid hamartoma of the lung
G. E trisomy
H. Parastic fetus
I. Achondroplasia
J. Pulmonary lymphangiectasia
K. Cardiopulmonary hypoplasia
L. Multiple congenital anomalies
M. Infectious diseases
   1. Toxoplasmosis
   2. Cytomegalovirus disease
   3. Syphilis
   4. Leptospirosis
   5. Congenital hepatitis
N. Congenital nephrosis
O. Renal vein thrombosis
P. Idiopathic

The spectral absorption curve of normal amniotic fluid plotted on a semilogarithmic scale describes a nearly straight line; when bilirubin pigment is present, a deviation is seen at 450 mμ (Fig. 1-13). The concentration of bile pigment is derived from the difference between the logarithm of the actual absorbency of the amniotic fluid at 450 mμ and the logarithm of the expected absorbency if no bile pigment were present (Δ OD 450 mμ). The latter value is determined from the point of intersection at 450 mμ of the line drawn tangentially between the logarithm of the absorbencies of the fluid at 365 and 550 mμ.

If amniotic fluid can not be analyzed immediately, it can be frozen and stored after centrifugation. Epithelial cells, vernix, meconium, or hemoglobin will alter its spectrophotometric properties and may invalidate the assay method. Under acid conditions, the bilirubin peak is shifted to shorter wavelengths. Contamination of amniotic fluid with fetal blood and plasma (which usually contains bilirubin at low levels) may invalidate the Δ OD at 450 mμ. If erythrocytes are recovered after centrifugation, blood smears should be prepared and stained for fetal cells by the Kleihauer-Betke technique, which detects HbF; determination of the ABO and Rh type and direct Coombs' test on precipitated fetal erythroctyes may be helpful in anticipating an Rh-positive affected infant in the presence of a normal amniotic fluid curve.

Normally the magnitude of the Δ OD at 450 mμ decreases as gestation advances. In erythroblastosis, the Δ OD 450 may rise, fall, or remain stationary with advancing gestation, depending on the severity of hemolysis. On the basis of his experience with several hundred pregnancies, Liley divided

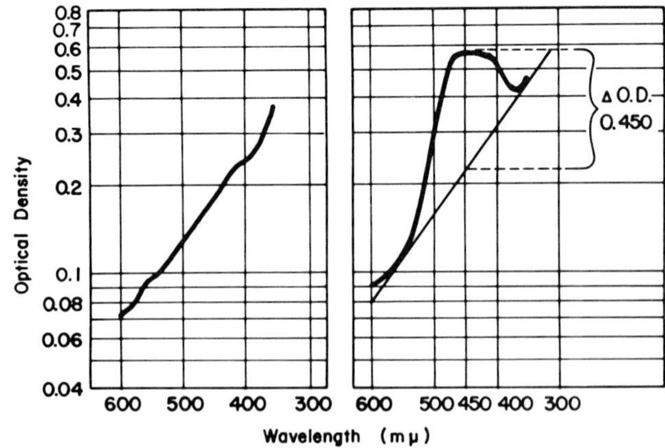

Fig. 1-13. The optical density of amniotic fluid sample is plotted against wavelength. The left side is normal amniotic fluid, the right side is the amniotic fluid of a severely affected erythroblastotic infant. The Δ OD at 0.450 mμ is an index of the degree of severity. (Adapted from Berg, D., Stein, and others: Schwangerschafteratung und Perinatologie, Stuttgart, 1972, Georg Thieme Verlag.)

the values for Δ OD 450 after 27 weeks' gestation into three prognostic zones.

Zone I: Rh-negative fetuses or very mildly Rh-positive fetuses

Zone II: Indeterminate disease. The fetus may be mildly or moderately affected, depending on the magnitude of the Δ OD 450 in the middle zone.

Zone III: Severe fetal disease: impending fetal death within a few days to several weeks. The rapidity of deterioration cannot be predicted.

Fetal prognosis and the institution of therapy should be based on the trend of values obtained from serial analyses of amniotic fluid (Fig. 1-14).

The initial amniocentesis is usually performed at 28 to 29 weeks' gestation. If there has been a previous stillbirth, analysis should be initiated at 22 to 23 weeks' gestation. If the maternal antibody titer is rising rapidly or if there has been a seriously affected child in a previous pregnancy, amniocentesis is begun at 24 to 26 weeks' gestation. An accurate estimate of gestational age is important for the interpretation of amniotic fluid findings.

Amniocentesis is repeated at 1- to 3-week intervals, depending on the results of the previous analysis. Amniotic fluid taps are performed weekly for a Δ OD in the upper portion of zone II; every 2 weeks in the lower portion of zone II; and once every 3 weeks in zone I. A fetus with a consistently low Δ OD in zone I is probably Rh-negative and should be delivered near term to avoid the hazards of prematurity. Falling Δ OD's at the lower portion of zone II indicate that labor should be induced at 37 to 38 weeks' gestation, whereas stationary or rising Δ OD's in the same zone warrant an earlier induction of labor. A Δ OD in zone III before 33 or 34 weeks' gestation is an indication for intrauterine fetal transfusion. Induction of labor or delivery by cesarean section is indicated after 34 weeks' gestation in view of the improved survival rates of premature infants born at this time.

Intrauterine transfusion. In 1963 Liley reported the first successful intrauterine fetal intraperitoneal transfusion for an in-

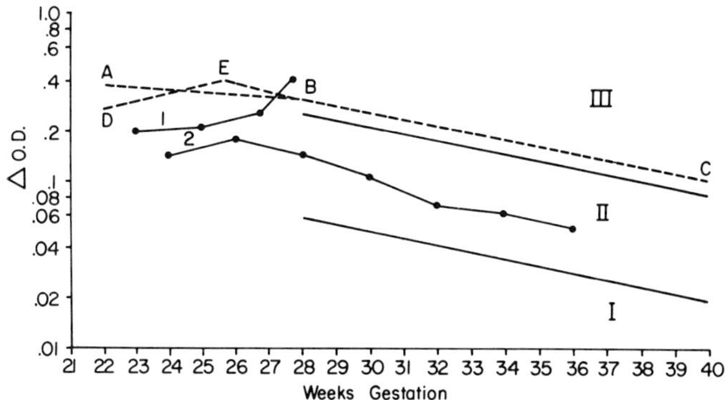

Fig. 1-14. Liley's 3-zone chart for interpretation of amniotic fluid Δ OD at 0.450 mμ. Heavy lines represent Liley's original 3 zones from 28 weeks' to 40 weeks' gestation.

Broken lines A, B, and C represent the upward revision and early extension by Liggins of the line between zones II and III. Broken line DEC represents a similar revision by Umansky. The upward revision of the "danger line" makes criteria for intrauterine transfusion more stringent.

Curves 1 and 2 describe the management of two patients with repeated amniocenteses. Intrauterine fetal transfusion was undertaken in patient 1 at 28 weeks of gestation based on the pattern of change in the Δ OD and the last value for Δ OD in zone III. In patient 2, the results of serial amniocenteses were in zone II, indicating a moderately affected fetus, and labor was induced at 37 weeks of gestation. (From Allen, F. H., Jr., and Umansky, I.: Erythroblastosis fetalis. In Reid, D. E., Ryan, K. J., and Benirschke, K., editors: Principles and management of human reproduction, Philadelphia, 1972, W. B. Saunders Co., pp. 811-832.)

fant with erythroblastosis who, according to the findings on amniotic fluid analysis, was almost certain to die before 34 weeks of gestation. This procedure is now widely accepted for carefully selected patients in whom the risk of premature delivery is greater than the risk of the procedure. Before intrauterine transfusion, an amniogram is performed with a water-soluble contrast medium to determine whether the fetus is grossly hydropic; if it is, intrauterine transfusion is usually considered inadvisable. The amniogram also locates the placental site. After several hours the fetal gastrointestinal tract is visualized by image-intensification fluoroscopy and provides a target for the transuterine puncture of the fetal peritoneal cavity. If the fetal position is favorable, an 18 cm 16-gauge Tuohy needle is inserted while the mother is under local anesthesia through the maternal abdominal wall into the peritoneal cavity of the fetus. A plastic catheter is advanced and its location inside the fetal abdomen is confirmed by radiopaque dye.

Blood for fetal transfusion should be less than 24 hours old, group O, Rh-negative, packed red blood cells, and cross matched against maternal serum. A suitable dosage schedule is 100 ml at 30 weeks' gestation ± 10 ml for each week later or earlier. Intrauterine transfusions are usually performed at intervals of 10 days to 3 weeks. Amniotic fluid analysis is not useful after a fetal transfusion if the fluid becomes contaminated with blood or meconium.

The transfused red blood cells are absorbed into the fetal circulation through diaphragmatic lymphatics, a process that is almost 70% efficient within one week of transfusion and that apparently does not alter the oxygen-binding properties of the transfused blood. Transfused fetuses have had normal growth indices and normal acid-base values at birth even with an adult oxygen dissociation curve. Normal neurologic and developmental performance has been demonstrated in erythroblastotic infants transfused in utero and receiving intensive neonatal care at birth. The usefulness of intrauterine transfusions of adult blood for anemic fetuses can be attributed to the beneficial effect of their large increase in oxygen-carrying capacity.

Results of intrauterine transfusion. The salvage rate of nonhydropic fetuses approaches 50% to 60%; that of hydropic fetuses 10% to 15%. Most of the complications and mortality related to intrauterine transfusion are caused by the mechanics of the procedure or the severity of the underlying disease. The risk of fetal mortality is now estimated as 6% per procedure in most experienced centers, which is less than the hazards of prematurity before 34 weeks' gestation. Fetal injury may occur secondary to needle trauma or misplaced injection of contrast material. The hazard of infection after intrauterine transfusion is low. Graft versus host reaction has rarely, if ever, occurred. Elevated intraperitoneal pressures after transfusion may compromise umbilical vein blood flow and lead to fetal death. In addition, many fetuses are lost after intraperitoneal transfusion because of rupture of the membranes and premature onset of labor. Maternal complications are infrequent; most are caused by bleeding or infection. The success of intrauterine transfusions at 30 to 34 weeks' gestation must be continually compared with the salvage rate of premature delivery and intensive neonatal care, especially as the methods for treating the premature infant or augmenting the synthesis of surfactant develop in the future. Other techniques for intrauterine fetal transfusion that require hysterotomy and direct cannulation of fetal vessels are not recommended.

Prevention of Rh isoimmunization. The postpartum injection of anti-Rh_0 (D) gamma globulin can prevent maternal immunization and subsequent erythroblastosis fetalis. The rationale for this treatment is based upon the observations that maternal immunization usually occurs at delivery and that the passive transfer of anti-Rh_0 (D) gamma globulin (Rh_0GAM) binds Rh-positive antigenic sites on transfused fetal red blood cells.

The risk of maternal Rh immunization rises with the volume of fetal transplacental hemorrhage. The usual amount is less than 0.5 ml of fetal blood. Transplacental hemorrhages of 10 ml or greater are considered large, and hemorrhages of more than 50 ml of fetal blood are massive and occur rarely. The relationship between antibody concentration and circulating red blood cells is not linear, and proportionately more antibody is needed for prevention with a small hemorrhage than for a large hemorrhage. It is generally considered that 25 μg of Rh_0GAM per ml of fetal red blood cells are sufficient to prevent fetal immunization. Thus, in general the standard dose of 300 μg of Rh_0GAM is in excess of the dose necessary for prevention of maternal immunization. A striking neonatal anemia suggests massive transplacental hemorrhage. If the mother is Rh-negative, it is necessary to estimate the amount of fetal blood in the maternal circulation by the Kleihauer-Betke smear in order to estimate the amounts of Rh_0GAM necessary. An alternative to the acid-elution smear is the Du test, which is available in all blood banks; it will detect 20 ml or more of Rh-positive fetal blood in the maternal circulation.

The indications for the clinical use of anti-Rh_0 (D) gamma globulin (Rho_0GAM) are shown below. Du-positive women rarely form anti-D antibodies and thus are not candidates for Rh_0GAM injection. On the other hand, if the baby is Du-positive, the situation is reversed, since the Du antigen may stimulate anti-D formation. It is recommended that an Rh-negative mother who gives birth to a Du child should be given Rh_0 GAM.

INDICATIONS FOR CLINICAL USE OF ANTI-RH_0 (D) GAMMA GLOBULIN (RH_0GAM)

1. Mother Rh_0 (D) negative without Rh antibodies. Baby Rh_0 (D) or Du positive, cord blood Coombs' negative.
2. Administer 1 ml (300 μg) Rh_0GAM intramuscularly to mother within 72 hours of delivery, abortion, or ectopic pregnancy.

A risk of Rh immunization exists for Rh-negative women aborting Rh-positive fetuses. The magnitude of this risk appears to be related to the method of abortion and the gestational age. The incidence of a demonstrable fetomaternal hemorrhage is significantly lower following spontaneous abortion than following an induced abortion and less after abortion by suction currettage than following hypertonic saline infusion or hysterotomy. The average risk of immunization after abortion is approximately one half of the risk incurred by full-term pregnancy and delivery; the latter has been estimated at 11%. Amniocentesis in Rh-negative mothers may increase this risk as will external version of the fetus or abdominal trauma. A single dose of Rh_0 GAM is too small to harm an Rh-positive fetus and may be useful under these circumstances if a fetomaternal bleed is demonstrated. Internal podalic version, cesarean section, and manual extraction of the placenta will increase the likelihood of fetomaternal hemorrhage at delivery. Even though mothers have received Rh_0GAM they should be screened with each subsequent pregnancy since occasional failures are related to inadequate Rh_0GAM administered postpartum or an undetected very low titer in the previous pregnancy.

Tests of fetoplacental function

In addition to transferring oxygen and nutrients and excreting fetal waste products, the placenta shares certain features with the liver and several secretory and endocrine organs. The placenta synthesizes two known protein hormones and together with the fetus produces a wide array of steroid compounds. Since the placenta carries out various physiologic processes, no single test can be expected to provide a total assessment of placental function in health or disease.

Recent evidence indicates that the supply of oxygen and probably of some other nutrients to the fetus is limited more by maternal blood flow than by any other single factor. Reduced blood circulation to the placenta has been implicated in many of the maternal conditions associated with intrauterine growth retardation, and sudden failure of uterine blood flow is a cause of acute fetal distress. Placental lesions such as infarcts, fibrin deposition, or villous abnormalities may reduce the diffusing capacity of the placenta. In preeclampsia and eclampsia, a form of fibrinoid necrosis is found in the spiral arteries supplying the placental cotyledons. In addition, blood flow in the intervillous spaces is reduced in the presence of maternal hypertension. The rate of uteroplacental blood flow also affects the supply of precursors available for hormonal biosynthesis as well as the secretory rate of placental hormones into the maternal circulation. The placenta has a high oxygen consumption owing to its intense metabolic activity; it would not be surprising if its capacity for steroid biosynthesis was reduced in the face of hypoxia secondary to decreased uteroplacental blood flow. The rate of maternal uteroplacental blood flow at cesarean section has been estimated at 500 to 750 ml/min for term singleton pregnancies. However, at the present time, there are no satisfactory noninvasive techniques for quantitative determinations of placental blood flow in clinical practice.

The placental transport capacity or permeability to various substances has been studied in clinical circumstances by the measurement of the transfer of dyes, pharmacologic agents, and metabolic precursors injected into the maternal circulation or into the amniotic cavity. Many of the placental transfer tests have enjoyed a brief period of popularity but have then fallen into disuse. The complexity of the mechanisms involved and the empirical nature of most tests have limited their success in the evaluation of placental function.

There is evidence that the fetus can hear, taste, swallow, detect light, and breathe in the intrauterine environment. Observations in the laboratory of Dawes at the Nuffield Institute in Oxford have shown that the fetal lamb normally engages in shallow irregular and rapid breathing movements during the latter half of gestation. There is little net flow of tracheal fluid during these respiratory efforts because of the high viscosity of fetal lung fluid. Chest movements and diaphragmatic activity are correlated with these respiratory efforts in utero, which occur during rapid-eye-movement sleep. In fetal lambs the presence of prenatal breathing movements is an indicator of health. In human fetuses, breathing movements in utero occur at a frequency of 40 to 70 per minute and can be detected externally by direct observation of the maternal abdomen or by ultrasonic scanning of the fetal chest wall. If the experience in chronic fetal sheep preparations can be shown to apply to man, then observations of breathing movements in utero may provide an additional means of assessing fetal health.

The fetal condition is currently being explored by a number of sophisticated biophysical techniques in addition to the biochemical analyses of amniotic fluid. Congenital disorders of the fetal heart have been detected in utero by electrocardiographic, phonocardiographic, and ultrasonic techniques. The prenatal evaluation of placental oxygen transport relies heavily on continuous electronic fetal heart rate monitoring. The response of the fetal heart rate to a variety of stress tests (maternal exercise, low oxygen inhalation, oxytocin challenge) has been used to evaluate the fetal cardiorespiratory reserve. The interpretation of fetal heart rate changes and their relationship to acid-base balance are discussed at greater length in the section on intrapartum fetal monitoring in the management of labor and delivery. At the present time, hormonal and enzymic indices of fetal and placental function have received the most attention and the widest application in clinical practice.

Estrogen biosynthesis in the fetoplacental unit. The high rate of production of estrogenic hormones is a well-known feature of human pregnancy. However, the specific biologic role of estrogens during pregnancy is still imperfectly understood. Their trophic and vasodilating effect on the female reproductive tract is necessary for maintaining a favorable environment for fetal growth. The correspondingly low concentrations of estradiol and testosterone in fetal tissues suggest that certain mechanisms protect the fetus against exposure to high concentrations of biologically potent estrogens and androgens that might be deleterious to the differentiation of the somatic and central nervous systems. Evidence is also accumulating that estrogens are involved in a complex interplay with progesterone, adrenocortical hormones, and prostaglandins in the mechanism of parturition.

The importance of the fetus for estrogen production during pregnancy is underscored by the sharp drop in maternal urinary estriol when the umbilical circulation is interrupted or the fetus dies. The fetus and the placenta (fetoplacental unit) represent complementary systems for steroid biosynthesis; this has led to the determination of urinary estriol as a clinical test of fetal and placental function.

The placenta can convert dehydroepiandrosterone and other androgenic intermediates to estradiol and estrone. However, the formation of estriol requires an additional hydroxylation at position 16 of the steroid nucleus, and the enzymes necessary for this hydroxylation are lacking in the placenta. Thus the formation of estriol in the placenta requires prior 16-hydroxylation of androgenic precursors in the maternal or fetal compartments. Although the fetal zone of the adrenal gland has a large capacity for dehydroepiandrosterone (DHEA) synthesis, the fetus, like the placenta, cannot convert DHEA to estradiol. A large portion of the DHEA formed in the fetal adrenal gland is available for 16-hydroxylation by the fetal liver. This in turn favors the formation of estriol in the placenta. DHEA of maternal origin contributes less than 10% to the total estriol production. Thus most of the estriol during normal pregnancy is derived from fetal DHEA. Some of the DHEA produced in the fetal adrenal gland escapes 16-hydroxylation and reaches the placenta where it is metabolized to estrone and estradiol. In this way, fetal DHEA is the source of about one half of the maternal estradiol produced during pregnancy and accounts for the low maternal estradiol levels associated with fetal adrenal hypoplasia. The fetus itself produces few, if any, estrogens. Some of the estradiol and estrone produced in the placenta reaches the fetus, but it is conjugated by active sulfokinases in fetal tissue or converted to estriol by the fetal liver. These mechanisms help to explain the low concentrations of the biologically potent estrogens found in fetal fluids and in tissues.

Estriol precursors are present in the fetus in the form of sulfates that must be deconjugated before these steroids can be converted into estrogens. Sulfatase activity is absent in the fetus but abundant in the placenta. Thus the enzymes necessary for estriol production during pregnancy are present reciprocally in the fetus and in the placenta. Normal estrogen production during pregnancy requires that the biosynthetic capabilities of both the fetus and the placenta be integrated.

Application of estrogen assays to assess fetal and placental health. Biologically, estriol is a weak estrogen, but quantitatively it is the most important estrogen in pregnancy. Although it is present in high concentrations in maternal and fetal fluids, its precise biologic role in pregnancy is not known. The daily excretion of estriol rises 1,000-fold as gestation advances and near term reaches values of 10 to 40 mg/24 hr in maternal urine.

In clinical practice, the measurement of maternal urinary estriol is widely used in the management of the high-risk patient. Certain difficulties in interpreting urinary estriol values stem from the wide range of normal values found among pregnant patients (Fig. 1-15) and from the dynamic interchange between fetal, placental, and maternal compartments discussed previously. The day-to-day variability in estriol excretion in the same subject approaches 20%. Thus, isolated determinations of urinary estriols are of limited value; serial estriol determinations are recommended in the management of high-risk pregnancies.

Consistently falling values of urinary estriol are associated with a high risk of fetal death; after 30 weeks' gestation, values of 2 mg/24 hr or less usually indicate fetal

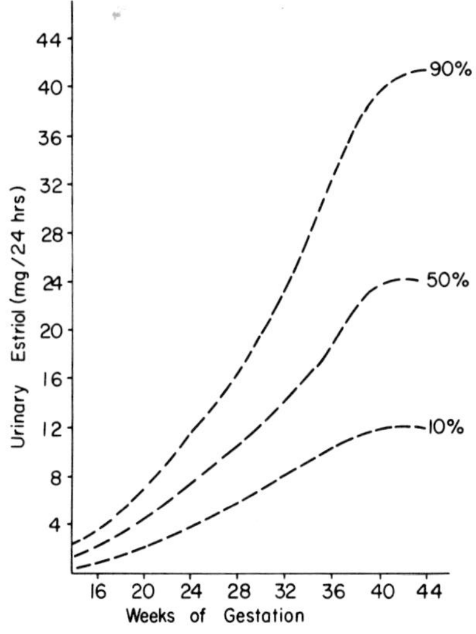

Fig. 1-15. Urinary estriol excretion during pregnancy. The tenth, fiftieth, and ninetieth percentile lines are shown for estriol excreted in 24 hours. Low estriol excretion after 40 weeks' gestation is defined as less than 12 mg/24 hours. (From Beischer, and others: Am. J. Obstet. Gynecol. **103**:483, 1969.)

death. However, several conditions associated with low maternal estriol values do not require active intervention and do not otherwise influence the management of the pregnancy. These conditions must be considered in the differential diagnosis of low maternal urinary estriol values. (See outline below.)

FETAL, PLACENTAL, AND MATERNAL FACTORS ASSOCIATED WITH LOW URINARY ESTRIOL EXCRETION IN LATE PREGNANCY

A. Fetal
   1. Intrauterine growth retardation
   2. Major fetal malformations
   3. Anencephaly
   4. Congenital adrenal hypoplasia or suppression
   5. Hepatitis, cirrhosis
   6. Fetal hypoxia (hypothetical)
   7. Fetal death

B. Placental
   1. Placental sulfatase deficiency
   2. Decreased placental mass or infarction
   3. Decreased intervillous blood flow (hypothetical)
   4. Decreased umbilical blood flow (hypothetical)
   5. Placental hypoxia (hypothetical)

C. Maternal
   1. Hypertension and severe preeclampsia
   2. Severe anemia
   3. Impaired renal or liver function
   4. Drug therapy—mandelamine, meprobamate, anthraquinone, ampicillin, corticosteroids

Inadequate collections of urine or laboratory errors occur commonly. Various maternal medications have also been noted to interfere with the hydrolysis or color development in the assay procedures. Ampicillin sometimes interferes with the actual metabolism of estrogens in the fetoplacental unit. Atrophic fetal adrenals secondary to anencephaly or to suppression by maternal corticosteroid therapy are associated with low urinary estrogens. Corticosteroids administered to the mother cross the placenta, but the quantitative relationship between maternal dose and fetal suppression is variable. With the usual clinical doses of corticosteroids, it is not uncommon to see a depression of the lower limits of normal estriol by 50% or 60%. Placental sulfatase deficiency may result in estriol values ordinarily associated with fetal death, but normal fetuses are found. Low estriol values are sometimes associated with severe anomalies of the central nervous and cardiac systems, occasionally with retarded fetal growth. Major fetal malformations are noted in about 0.1% of pregnancies, and it has been estimated that a fetal anomaly will occur once in 30 pregnancies in which maternal urinary estriol excretion is subnormal. Thus, in some circumstances, a persistently low estriol excretion may indicate radiographic or ultrasonic studies of the fetus.

There is a significant correlation between maternal urinary estriol excretion and fetal weight. High values over 40 mg/24 hr are frequently associated with large fetuses, multiple gestations, or perhaps fetuses with large adrenal glands. Conversely, patients with low urinary estriols have an incidence of growth-retarded fetuses that is many times higher than in the population with normal estriols.

Data from several large retrospective studies indicate that patients with normal urinary estriol excretion have a perinatal mortality of 1% to 4%, whereas patients with estriol values below the tenth percentile have a tenfold higher perinatal mortality rate and a high incidence of intrauterine fetal deaths. Patients with low-normal values that are shown to be declining also seem to be at increased risk. Such observations suggest that urinary estriol determinations be employed routinely as a screening procedure for high-risk patients.

Serial estriol determinations are helpful in the clinical management of severe maternal preeclampsia, intrauterine fetal growth retardation, and the related dysmaturity syndrome in prolonged pregnancy; they aid in making the decision to interrupt or to continue the pregnancy. Urinary estriol values may be misleading when impaired maternal renal function is present; low urinary estriol values may be largely caused by impaired maternal clearance. Calculating the ratio of urinary creatinine to estriol has not provided a solution, probably because creatinine reflects glomerular filtration, whereas estriol is excreted by both tubules and glomeruli. Estriol excretion is often higher after bed rest in the lateral supine position than with standing or lying flat. Such effects probably result from the influence of posture on vena caval compression and on renal and uteroplacental blood flow.

In erythroblastosis fetalis, estriol excretion is not a useful index of fetal condition because urinary estriol values do not always decline before fetal death. Conservative treatment based upon normal estriol measurements is also not recommended with maternal antepartum hemorrhage. Although estriol determinations are widely used, they are of limited value in the management of pregnant diabetic patients. Normal or even rising estriol values are no guarantee of a favorable outcome with maternal diabetes; low estriol levels are helpful in focusing attention on the fetus in jeopardy. The timing of delivery is then decided on the basis of past history, clinical findings such as falling maternal insulin requirements, and amniotic fluid indices of fetal maturity. Optimal management of pregnant diabetics is facilitated by hospital admission 1 or 2 weeks before the planned delivery date.

Many questions remain unanswered with regard to estrogen biosynthesis in abnormal pregnancies. The development of radioimmune assays for measuring different estrogens and their precursors in amniotic fluid and in maternal plasma should widen our understanding of endocrine function in the high-risk patient. Determinations of the metabolic clearance rate of DHEA or other estrogen precursors that indirectly reflect placental blood flow also hold promise of being useful placental function tests. Well-controlled prospective studies are needed to determine if monitoring pregnancy by estriol or related endocrine indices can reduce perinatal mortality and morbidity.

Progesterone and pregnanediol. The corpus luteum is the major source of progesterone in the first 10 weeks of pregnancy. As gestation progresses, it is produced in increasing amounts by the placental trophoblast. Increasing amounts of pregnanediol, the major metabolite of progesterone, are excreted in the urine as pregnancy advances. The excretion of pregnanediol is not significantly reduced in anencephalic fetuses or after fetal death, provided the placenta is intact. Similarly, maternal hypophysectomy or adrenalectomy produces little change in plasma progesterone or in pregnanediol excretion. Progesterone levels in the plasma of the mother are not affected by the sex of the fetus. Despite the inhibitory effect of progesterone on myometrial contractility that has been demonstrated in vitro and in lower animals, the role of progesterone in the physiologic mechanism of human parturition is still controversial. Labor in women is initiated and progresses without any evident relationship to the peripheral progesterone concentration.

The measurement of peripheral plasma levels of progesterone or pregnanediol has been of little value as a sensitive indicator of placental function, and it has not proved to be of value in the management of late pregnancy complications. In early pregnancy, pregnanediol values below the first percentile are generally associated with inevitable abortion. In many such circumstances, it is difficult to determine whether the low pregnanediol value is the cause or the consequence of the pregnancy failure. Well-controlled studies on the use of progestational agents during pregnancy by intramuscular or oral routes have failed to show any beneficial effects on the outcome of threatened or habitual abortion or on premature labor. However, in such extreme conditions as incomplete or missed abortion, hydatidiform mole, or pseudocyesis, pregnanediol assays are helpful in determining the functional state of the corpus luteum or trophoblast. Although pregnanediol output tends to be low in toxemia, pregnanediol excretion is not a sufficiently reliable prognostic index in preeclamptic patients and cannot be correlated with the severity of toxemia or with fetal survival. Neither has pregnanediol excretion been particularly helpful in the management of intrauterine growth retardation, maternal diabetes, or Rh isoimmunization in pregnancy. High-normal or elevated values give no warning of fetal death. The urinary pregnanediol excretion reaches a plateau in the last weeks of pregnancy and declines at term. A persistent fall in pregnanediol excretion in postterm pregnancy may indicate the need for labor induction, but few systematic studies of this assumption have been undertaken.

Placental polypeptide hormones. The human placental syncytial trophoblast produces two polypeptide hormones: human chorionic gonadotropin (HCG) and human chorionic somatomammotropin (HCS). Sensitive and specific immunologic methods have supplanted the previously widely used biologic assays in the measurement of these hormones. However, it is apparent that a dissociation exists between the immunologic and biologic activities of these proteins and that alterations in the subunit structure of these complex hormones may occur in some pathologic states. To date, the most dramatic clinical application of serum and urinary assays of placental protein hormones has been in the diagnosis and treatment of trophoblastic neoplasms.

HCG can be detected in maternal serum and in urine as early as 10 days after conception and provides the basis for the urine pregnancy test in common use. The urinary excretion of HCG reaches a characteristic peak of about 100,000 international units (IU) per day at 8 to 12 weeks of pregnancy and then declines to values that range between 4,000 and 11,000 IU until delivery. The biologic role of HCG is presumed to be the maintenance of the early corpus luteum of pregnancy. Its function in later pregnancy is unknown, although tropic effects on the placenta and on fetal endocrine tissues have been proposed.

Quantitative measurements of urinary or plasma HCG in early pregnancy suggest that concentrations are lower than normal in patients with threatened abortion. Abnormally high levels suggest multiple pregnancy or hydatidiform mole or choriocarcinoma. Low values of chorionic somatomammotropin in association with high levels of chorionic gonadotropin are diagnostic of trophoblastic neoplasms. Later in pregnancy, high-normal or elevated concentrations of HCG are likely to be found in patients with preeclampsia, diabetes, and Rh isoimmunization and may be related to proliferation of syncytial trophoblast under these conditions. However, determinations of HCG are of little value in the assessment of placental function or in the clinical management of such patients.

The placental hormone, HCS, has lactogenic and luteotropic properties as well as metabolic properties that resemble those of human growth hormone. Erythropoietic activity has also been demonstrated. Under basal conditions, but especially during fasting, HCS is thought to promote the mobilization of maternal stores to provide glucose, free fatty acids, and glycerol for placental transfer to the fetus.

The value of HCS as a placental function test is not established. The concentration of HCS in maternal blood increases steadily after the first trimester and reaches 5 to 6 μg/ml at term. Its plasma concentration falls to very low levels within a few hours after separation of the placenta. However, the factors that regulate HCS secretion are still not known. The increase in plasma HCS during pregnancy parallels the increase in placental weight, and values above normal are found with multiple gestations. Maternal values usually correlate with placental weight, although discrepancies have been reported.

There is a tendency for mildly diabetic patients (A and B in the classification of White) to have elevated values of serum HCS, while more severe diabetics with probable vascular disease have normal or lowered values. Intrauterine growth retardation is generally associated with smaller placentas and lowered levels of plasma HCS. There has been no significant correlation with placental weight in erythroblastosis fetalis or in prolonged pregnancy. Abnormally low or falling concentrations in the third trimester suggest but do not establish a failing placental function. Spellacy has reported that stillbirths that occurred in hypertensive and toxemic patients after 30 weeks' gestation had prior HCS levels that fell into the "fetal danger zone" defined as more than 2 SD below the normal mean for the gestational age. Stillbirths associated with diabetes mellitus or erythroblastosis fetalis without associated maternal hypertension did not show these abnormally low values. Others have reported that the majority of patients with levels of HCS consistently below 4 μg/ml at term will show clinical evidence of fetal distress in labor.

Enzymic indices of the fetal environment. The concentrations of most major enzymes in maternal blood remain unchanged during pregnancy. Measurements of cholinesterase, carboxypeptidase, leucine amino peptidase, acid phosphatase, creatinine phosphokinase, lactic dehydrogenase, serum glutamic oxaloacetic transaminase, and isocitric dehydrogenase do not serve as an index of fetal maturity or well-being. However, three maternal plasma enzymes are significantly affected by normal pregnancy and may be further altered in complicated cases: diamine oxidase (histaminase), heat-stable alkaline phosphatase, and oxytocinase (cystine aminopeptidase).

Diamine oxidase (DAO), which inactivates histamine, increases in activity in maternal blood during pregnancy. In general the levels are several hundred times higher in maternal plasma and amniotic fluid than in fetal blood or the blood of nonpregnant adults. A marked linear rise in maternal plasma in the first 20 weeks of pregnancy levels off thereafter and shows a wide range of variability. DAO determinations are sometimes used in the differential diagnosis of pregnancy and trophoblastic tumors (where the concentration is low) and can be helpful in the management of bleeding in the first and second trimesters of pregnancy. However, in the third trimester, plasma levels of DAO are of no practical value in assessing the fetus or placenta.

After 20 weeks of gestation, the activity of *serum alkaline phosphatases* increases and normally reaches values as high as 15 King-Armstrong units at term. The placental phosphatase isoenzyme that can be demonstrated histochemically in the syncytial trophoblast accounts for nearly two thirds of the total alkaline phosphatase activity in maternal serum. In the normal patient the serum heat-stable alkaline phosphatase (HSAP) rises linearly as pregnancy progresses towards term and falls progressively within 3 to 6 days after the placenta is delivered. HSAP is absent in the nonpregnant female and in males and is present in only minimal amounts in cord blood and amniotic fluid. However, at the present time, critical levels of the enzyme at each week of gestation cannot be cited as evidence of failing placental function, and variations from the normal trend are not clinically useful in diagnosing fetal distress.

An *oxytocinase* is produced by the placental trophoblast and increases in maternal plasma during pregnancy. It is absent from fetal blood; the function of serum oxytocinase is still not known. Decreased or falling concentrations of serum oxytocinase have been found in preeclampsia, but the usefulness of this enzyme in predicting fetal maturity or placental function has not yet been convincingly demonstrated.

Intrapartum asphyxia

A significant number of high-risk pregnant patients enter labor with only a narrow margin of safety in the maternal-placental-fetal exchange relationship. The fetuses of these patients are more likely to develop acute fetal distress, a syndrome usually associated with intrapartum asphyxia. Fetal asphyxia interferes with the postnatal cardiorespiratory adjustments of the newborn. Meconium aspiration and a high incidence of respiratory distress and pneumonia are noted after intrapartum asphyxia. Pulmonary hypoperfusion, decreased surfactant synthesis, persistence of right-to-left shunting, heart failure, and even disseminated intravascular coagulation may also follow intrapartum asphyxia. Anoxia remains the most important cause of death in mature fetuses (Table 1-1), and there is increasing evidence that patchy areas of infarction in the cerebral cortex and functional neurologic disturbances in surviving infants often follow hypoxic insults in late pregnancy and during labor. However, the question of when fetal asphyxia will lead to neurologic damage has not been answered. A good biochemical or biophysical index of the functional reserve of the fetus is not available. This is not only the result of technical limitations imposed by the intrauterine environment but also of our incomplete understanding of fetal cardiorespiratory physiology.

Regulation of the fetal circulation. Most of our knowledge of fetal circulatory and respiratory physiology has been obtained from animal models. In fetal lambs and rhesus monkeys, the cardiac output is high by adult standards. In the fetus, the right and left sides of the heart function in parallel, and at term their combined output is nearly 500 ml/kg of body weight. The fetal circulation is so arranged that better oxygenated blood from the umbilical vein is shunted to the left ventricle and then to the coronary circulation and brain, whereas poorly oxygenated blood, mainly from the superior vena cava, is directed to the right ventricle and then distributed to the lower body and placenta through the ductus arteriosus. The distribution of

Table 1-6. Fetal organ blood flows (percent of the cardiac output ± SD)

	Brain	Heart	Lungs	Kidneys	Adrenal glands	Placenta
Control	15.7 ± 2.8	2.7 ± 0.9	10.7 ± 6.4	2.7 ± 1.0	0.4 ± 0.1	47.5 ± 4.9
Fetal distress	30.6 ± 11.3	4.9 ± 1.5	3.2 ± 2.4	1.9 ± 1.4	0.8 ± 0.5	29.2 ± 9.4
Statistical significance	$p < 0.01$	$p < 0.02$	$p < 0.05$	NS*	$p < 0.05$	$p < 0.005$

Adapted from Behrman, and others: Am. J. Obstet. Gynecol. **108**:956, 1970.
*NS is not significant. Mean values ± 1 SD are presented.

cardiac output, obtained by Behrman and others in subhuman primates, is shown in Table 1-6. The myocardium and brain receive about 3% and 15%, respectively, of the cardiac output; the placenta nearly 50%. The less than 3% received by the kidneys is in contrast to the larger share received in the newborn or adult and further emphasizes the importance of placental exchange during fetal life. The mean fetal arterial pressure of 40 to 60 mm Hg in late pregnancy, together with the high rate of systemic blood flow, characterizes the low resistance of the fetal circulation.

In the latter part of gestation, the fetal circulation comes under the control of the autonomic nervous system. Peripheral chemoreceptors and baroreceptors are active in late fetal life, but their interaction with central chemoreceptors is unclear. Both sympathetic and vagal effects are noted. Fetal heart rate and cardiac output increase after α-adrenergic blockade, whereas β-adrenergic blockade causes a slight drop in cardiac output and heart rate. Stimulation of the vagus nerve has a negative chronotropic and inotropic effect.

The direct relationship of fetal cardiac output to the intravascular volume and central venous pressure and to the fetal heart rate follows Starling's relationship. The resting heart rate of the fetus is high (120 to 160 beats per minute) and remarkably stable compared with that of adults. The fetus maintains its stroke volume more effectively at high cardiac rates than does the adult because of the more efficient diastolic filling of the ventricles. Inotropic effects are less prominent in fetuses than in adults, possibly because of lower concentrations of norepinephrine in the fetal myocardium or the low oxygen tension in the fetal coronary circulation.

Under normal cricumstances, umbilical blood flow has been estimated at 200 ml/kg/min. The umbilical circulation shows little or no response to reflex nervous stimulation, to changes in fetal blood gases over a wide range, or to circulating catecholamines in physiologic concentrations. The relative unresponsiveness of the umbilical blood vessels suggests that nearly one half of the fetal cardiac output is directed to a largely passive vascular bed. As a result, umbilical blood flow increases or decreases in proportion to arterial pressure and to the fetal cardiac output. On the other hand, constriction of the umbilical cord vessels is a physiologic event at birth and occurs in response to traction on the longitudinal muscle layer of the umbilical artery and possibly to vasoconstrictor effects of locally released bradykinins nad prostaglandins.

Fetal adaptations to hypoxia. The fetal hemodynamic response to intrauterine asphyxia is largely controlled near term by the aortic chemoreceptors whose afferent nerves run in branches of the vagus. Excitation of aortic chemoreceptors by a decrease in fetal arterial P_{O_2} or in pH results in a tachycardia and peripheral vasoconstriction, an increase in pulmonary vascular resistance, and a rise in blood pressure. The primary circulatory response of the fetus to stress is a diversion of blood flow from the extremities, trunk, kidneys, and gut to the placenta, myocardium, and brain. Myocardial blood flow and cerebral blood flow approximately doubles (Table 1-6). This redistribution of systemic blood flow is a more important fetal adjustment to hypoxia than an increase in heart rate or cardiac output, both of which are already high under normal circumstances.

An increase in heart rate and in blood

pressure can also be produced in the fetus by an infusion of norepinephrine. Comline and Silver have shown that the release of catecholamines (primarily norepinephrine) from the adrenal medulla is directly related to the degree of fetal hypoxemia. A rapid or a large increase in fetal arterial pressure, such as might occur with intense peripheral vasoconstriction or sudden occlusion of the umbilical cord, will lead to reflex fetal bradycardia as a result of activation of the aortic and carotid baroreceptors (depressor or carotid sinus reflex). Selective constriction of the umbilical vein usually leads to an initial tachycardia because of diminished venous return and a decrease in arterial pressure. If this sequence of events is prolonged or if the fetus is already compromised, then a bradycardia will ensue, probably on the basis of myocardial hypoxia. Severe hypoxemia is frequently associated with a fall in heart rate and sometimes in fetal blood pressure. Bradycardia with a falling blood pressure is an ominous sign, since it usually means a decreasing cardiac output and myocardial hypoxia in the fetus. Severe bradycardia also disrupts the streaming effect in the right atrium, and this allows poorly oxygenated blood from the superior vena cava to flow through the foramen ovale and to be distributed to the myocardium and brain.

Both fetal tachycardia and fetal bradycardia have been observed when uterine blood flow has been reduced or when the mother has been given low oxygen mixtures to breathe. Vagal effects on the heart are also elicited by compression of the fontanelles. The factors that determine fetal response to stressful stimuli include the degree and duration of fetal asphyxia that is produced, the existing functional reserve of the fetus, and the manner in which different circulatory reflexes and humoral factors are integrated. The presence of certain drugs or anesthetics will also modify the response.

Compared with adults of the same species, fetal and newborn mammals have a remarkable ability to survive asphyxia. Glycolysis is important for survival during asphyxia, since it is the major source of adenosine triphosphate (ATP) under anoxic conditions. Dawes has shown that the concentration of glycogen in the fetal heart is several times higher than in the adult and relates to the fetal capacity to survive anoxia. The depletion of cardiac glycogen reserves jeopardizes the ability of the fetus to survive successive anoxic episodes.

Acidosis (usually mixed respiratory and metabolic) follows hypoxia and is an additional factor that may compromise the fetus. The initial effects of hydrogen ion accumulation are stimulatory because of sympathetic nervous and adrenocortical activity. Acidemia itself, however, decreases the response to a given dose of catecholamines, and throughout the body the prolonged effects of hydrogen ion excess are depressant; for example, acidosis diminishes myocardial contractility. The accumulation of lactic acid in tissues is several times higher than in blood; and as the pH falls, enzymatic activities are gradually inhibited.

Clinical detection of fetal distress. Historically, the concept of fetal distress evolved from observations that the passage of meconium or marked alterations in fetal heart rate (usually bradycardia) were associated with stillbirths or severely depressed infants at birth. Many of the mothers of such infants had associated findings of antepartum hemorrhage, chorioamnionitis, cephalopelvic disproportion, cord complications, abruptio placentae, or uterine hypertonus. Recent data from the National Collaborative Study of Factors Related to Cerebral Palsy indicate that traditional methods of auscultation of fetal heart tones are unreliable in detecting fetal jeopardy except in extreme cases. In retrospect, the majority of infants with intrauterine asphyxia demonstrate meconium staining, but prospectively the presence of meconium in amniotic fluid is not a reliable index of fetal asphyxia. Transient noxious stimuli to the fetus may cause autonomic discharge and passage of meconium, but recovery may occur before delivery. Meconium in amniotic fluid is an incidental finding with maternal ingestion of laxatives and may be a normal finding in breech presentation. Even when meconium staining is associated with fetal tachycardia or bradycardia, asphyxia at birth is noted in less than 30% of the infants.

Two major advances in the last decade have helped to detect early fetal asphyxia:

the continuous measurement of instantaneous heart rate (electronically computed from the beat-to-beat interval) pioneered by Hon and Caldeyro-Barcia and the fetal capillary blood sampling during labor for acid-base determinations, a technique described by Saling. These techniques have greatly improved obstetrical care during labor, although they are still indirect compared with intensive physiologic monitoring of the adult where parameters of blood pressure, systemic and regional blood flow, arterial blood gases, and oxygen consumption are more easily assessed.

Continuous monitoring of fetal heart rate. Continuous monitoring of the fetal heart rate (FHR) is based upon electrocardiographic, phonocardiographic, or ultrasonic detection of the fetal cardiac activity. The interval between two successive R waves on the ECG or between two heart sounds is electronically computed by commercially available cardiotachometers, and the instantaneous heart rate is recorded. It is customary to record the FHR in conjunction with myometrial contractions, which reduce intervillous space blood flow and thus provide a measure of the fetal response to a stressful stimulus. Before the onset of labor or before cervical dilatation, the FHR can be monitored by external detectors. The frequency and duration of contractions is recorded by a tocograph attached to the maternal abdominal wall. After cervical dilatation, scalp electrodes can be attached for electrocardiographic recording of FHR, which provides a better signal-to-noise ratio. An intrauterine saline-filled catheter is inserted by the vaginal route into the amniotic cavity to obtain a quantitative measure of uterine pressure.

The terminology and interpretation of the clinical significance of FHR patterns are based primarily on the original work of Hon and Quilligan in the United States and Caldeyro-Barcia in Uruguay and studies of Hammacher in Germany. The nomenclature describing FHR patterns on continuous recordings is given in the outline below and in Fig. 1-16. Currently, the system of classifying the FHR patterns is largely empirical and cannot strictly be used to identify their causes. Terms that imply the pathogenetic mechanism of FHR changes such as head compression, uteroplacental insufficiency, and cord compression have been proposed for early, late, and variable decelerations respectively but should be used only as working hypotheses at the present time.

CRITERIA USED FOR THE EVALUATION OF INSTANTANEOUS FHR PATTERNS*

I. *Baseline FHR* is the average rate recorded between uterine contractions. Sustained changes of at least 10 min duration are classified as follows.
   - A. Normal, 120 to 160 beats per minute
   - B. Moderate tachycardia, 181 or more beats per minute
   - C. Moderate bradycardia, 100 to 119 beats per minute
   - D. Marked bradycardia, 99 or less beats per minute

II. *Baseline FHR irregularity* refers to beat-to-beat variations or oscillations about the baseline of less than 20 sec duration but persisting for 10 min or longer.
   - A. Minimal irregularitv (silent or flat), oscillations of 0 to 5 beats per minute
   - B. Average irregularity (narrowed undulatory), oscillations of 6 to 16 beats per minute
   - C. Moderate irregularity (undulatory), oscillations of 11 to 25 beats per minute
   - D. Marked irregularity (saltatory), oscillations of 25 or more beats per minute

III. *Periodic FHR changes* are deviations in the baseline FHR that persist for more than 20 sec but less than 10 min and are above or below the normal range of 120 to 160 beats per minute or are more than 30 beats per minute from the normal baseline. Periodic changes in FHR may occur in relation to fetal movements or during or after uterine contractions.
   - A. Acceleration (periodic tachycardia)
     1. Moderate, 161 to 180 beats per minute
     2. Marked, 181 or more beats per minute
   - B. Deceleration periodic (bradycardia or dip)
     1. Moderate, 100 to 119 beats per minute
     2. Marked, 99 or less beats per minute

IV. *Early deceleration* begins with the onset of a uterine contraction and returns to the baseline near the end of the contraction (type 1 dip).

V. *Late deceleration* begins later in the uterine contraction cycle (usually 20 sec or more after the onset; lag time) and persists for a variable time after the contraction has subsided (type 2 dip).

*The definitions and nomenclature used for FHR patterns follow those of Hon and Caldeyro-Barcia (1968), Hammacher (1968), and Huntingford (1969).

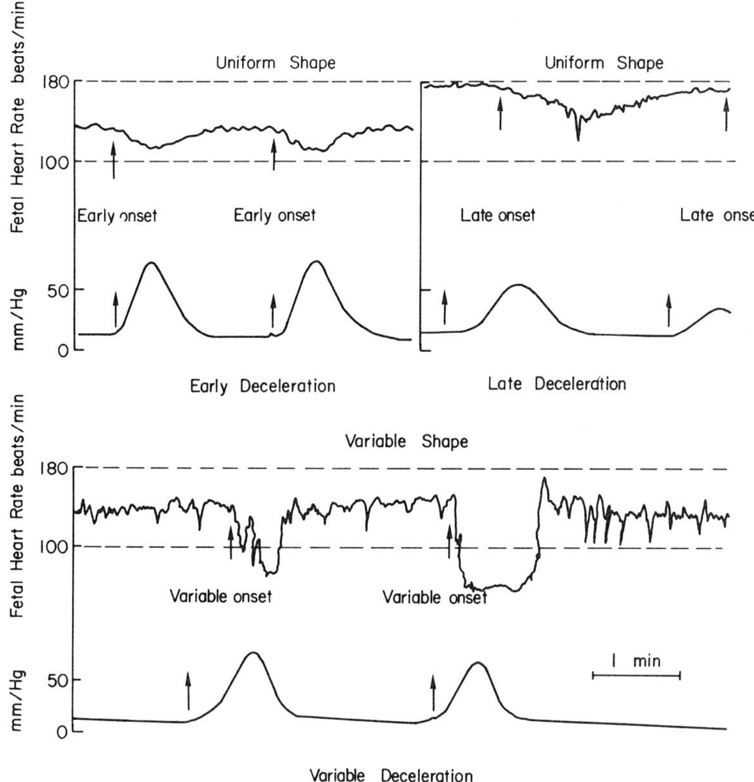

Fig. 1-16. Instantaneous FHR deceleration patterns associated with uterine contractions. *Top left,* Early decelerations are characterized by a uniform shape and an early onset in relation to the rise in amniotic fluid pressure. *Top right,* Late decelerations are similar in form to early decelerations but begin later in relation to the uterine contraction cycle and occur frequently with intrapartum hypoxia. *Bottom,* Variable deceleration patterns are nonuniform and have no consistent temporal relationship to the uterine contraction. This pattern is frequently seen with nuchal encirclement by the umbilical cord and transient compression of the umbilical vessels during labor. (Adapted from Hon and Quilligan: Conn. Med. 31:779, 1967.)

VI. *Variable deceleration* bears no consistent temporal relationship to the onset or duration of the uterine contraction (type 0 dip).

Table 1-7 shows the incidence of different FHR patterns during the first stage of labor in patients with various prenatal high-risk factors or with clinical signs of fetal distress as studied by Beard and others. Normal FHR tracings were obtained in about 30% of the patients. The FHR patterns, which empirically were most often associated in 1-minute Apgar scores below 6 with fetal asphxyia or depression of the newborn, were late decelerations in relation to uterine contractions (Fig. 1-17), loss of beat-to-beat variation (minimal irregularity of the baseline), and baseline tachycardia associated with variable decelerations (Fig. 1-18). The duration, amplitude, and frequency of late decelerations are additional criteria used to make clinical judgments about the severity of fetal distress.

Fetal blood sampling during labor

The concentrations of oxygen in fetal scalp blood vary with tissue metabolism and local blood flow, and the percentage of error is large in measuring oxygen at low pressures. Because of the steep fetal O_2 dissociation curve at low tensions, Po_2 differences of a few mm Hg represent large changes in arterial O_2 saturation. In practice the measurement of scalp blood Po_2 has been largely supplanted by measurements of pH and base excess (BE).

Table 1-7. Distribution of FHR patterns in 356 high-risk patients during one year of intrapartum monitoring

FHR pattern	Percent
Normal trace	29
Acceleration patterns	6
Early deceleration patterns	9
Baseline tachycardia (uncomplicated)	12
Baseline bradycardia (uncomplicated)	12
Variable deceleration patterns	
With normal baseline	9
With abnormal baseline	8
Loss of beat-to-beat variation	
Uncomplicated	6
Complicated	6
Late deceleration patterns*	
Normal baseline	1
Abnormal baseline	2

Adapted from Beard, R. W., and others: J. Obstet. Gynaecol. Br. Commonw. **78**:865, 1971.
*In all, 5% of patients had late deceleration patterns, but some are included under "loss of beat-to-beat variation—complicated." "Complicated" indicates a mixture of fetal heart rate patterns in the tracing.

It is generally agreed that fetal acidemia follows hypoxia. Interference with placental perfusion leads to a mixed acidosis, since fetal hypercapnia is soon followed by the accumulation of lactate and other organic acid products of glycolysis. With the analytical method of Astrup and the nomogram of Siggaard-Andersen, it is now possible to determine fetal and maternal acid-base changes on minute quantities of blood.

Before the onset of labor the maternal acid-base status is characterized as a compensated respiratory alkalosis with an arterial pH of 7.40 to 7.42 and a Pco_2 of 30 to 32 mm Hg. Blood samples obtained at cesarean section or during early labor indicate that maternal and fetal bloods have virtually the same base deficit (about 4 to 5 mEq/liter). A wide range of gas values is noted in umbilical cord blood, even in uncomplicated deliveries. In the umbilical vein, mean Po_2 varies from 25 to 32 mm Hg; mean Pco_2 from 38 to 42 mm Hg; and mean pH values from 7.30 to 7.35. In the umbilical artery, respective values are 12 to 18 mm Hg for Po_2; 48 to 54 mm Hg for Pco_2; and 7.24 to 7.29 for pH. Kubli found that about 20% of babies were born with an umbilical arterial pH of 7.20 or less; about 10% were born with a pH of 7.15 or less; and in about 5% of the fetuses the arterial pH was below 7.10. There is a high correlation between fetal capillary and umbilical arterial blood pH and base deficit.

During normal labor, maternal Pco_2 falls as a result of hyperventilation, whereas fetal Pco_2 rises, probably as a result of impaired placental gas exchange. The base excess in the mother normally decreases by 2 to 3 mEq/liter toward the end of the first stage of labor. Metabolic acidosis is generally more pronounced in the mother than in the fetus so that a change in the pH difference between maternal and fetal blood is normally slight. Concern has been expressed that excessive maternal hyperventilation during labor or delivery may lead to a paradoxical fetal acidosis and depression of the newborn. Such concern is warranted during passive ventilation in patients under anesthesia, which entails a significant decrease in cardiac output. However, voluntary hyperventilation in the awake adult is self-limited and probably without deleterious effects on the fetus.

The Apgar score cannot be predicted from a single scalp blood pH or base deficit measurement with any certainty because other factors such as maternal medications influence the fetal condition at birth. Furthermore, early in labor the fetus sometimes suffers a temporary disturbance that produces an alteration in fetal heart rate or blood gases from which the fetus later recovers. Serial measurements of fetal pH during labor overcome some of the difficulties of assessing the duration of fetal asphyxia. Infants with high Apgar scores can be expected if pH values in repeated blood samples are above 7.20. However, 20% to 50% of the infants with pH values below 7.20 are also vigorous and healthy. Severe fetal acidosis is rare early in labor; fewer than 5% of fetuses have scalp blood pHs below 7.20. This incidence increases to 16% during the second stage according to Kubli. Although it is not possible to give a critical pH value for fetal depression, most infants are born with low Apgar scores if the scalp blood pH is consistently 7.15 or less. A pH below 7.20 that continues to fall on two or more blood samples indicates the need for prompt delivery of the fetus.

Organic acids equilibrate slowly across the placenta. Thus a significant change in

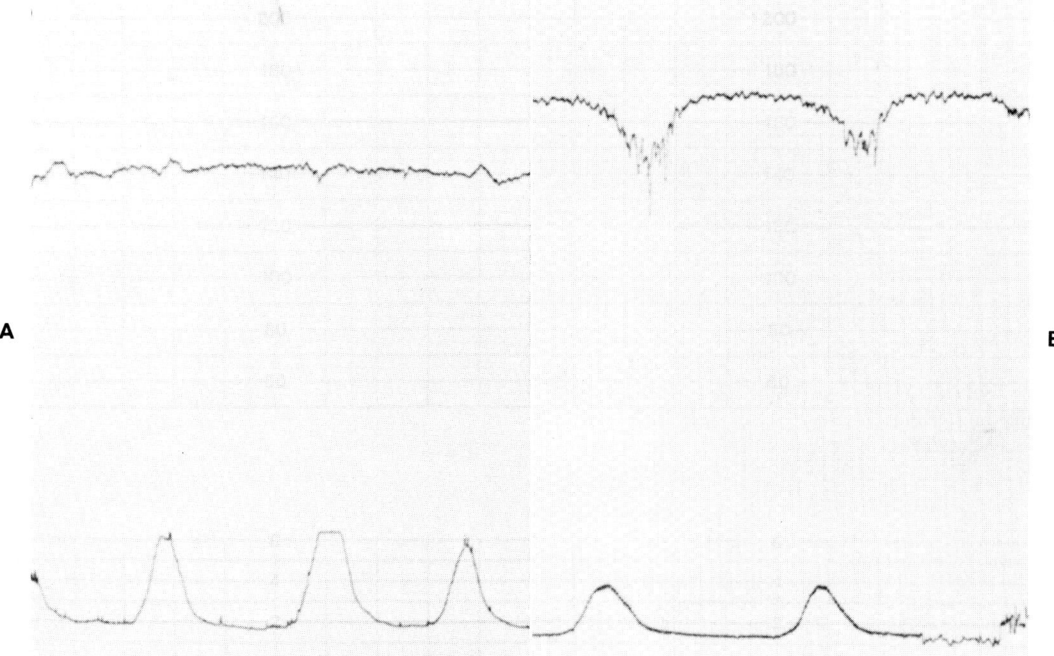

Fig. 1-17. A, Normal baseline FHR with minimal irregularity (loss of beat-to-beat variation) uncomplicated by periodic decelerations or accelerations. **B,** Early decelerations with average baseline irregularity. (From Beard, and others: J. Obstet. Gynaecol. Br. Commonw. **78**:865, 1971.)

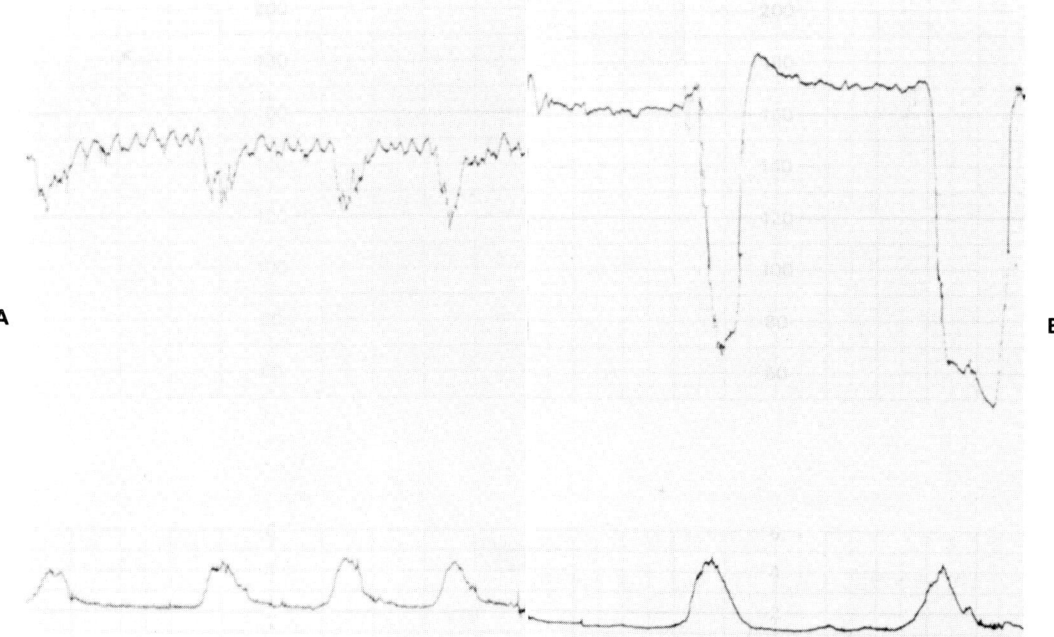

Fig. 1-18. A, Variable deceleration pattern of FHR complicated by baseline tachycardia and loss of beat-to-beat variation. **B,** Late decelerations with a baseline tachycardia. (From Beard, and others: J. Obstet. Gynaecol. Br. Commonw. **78**:865, 1971.)

the metabolic component of the fetal acid-base status probably reflects a change in fetal oxygenation unless there are maternal causes of the fetal acidemia such as excessive muscular activity, starvation, or dehydration. An acidotic fetus whose −BE is greater by 5 mEq/liter or more than the mother's strongly suggests that the fetus has sustained an hypoxic insult. When the fetal BE continues to decrease in the absence of maternal acidosis, continued impairment of fetal oxygenation is apparent.

In current practice, continuous recording of FHR is usually instituted to warn of fetal asphyxia, because it can be applied early in labor and because changes in fetal heart rate usually precede biochemical evidence of acidosis in fetal scalp blood. Major disturbances in the pH of fetal scalp blood are rarely seen in the presence of normal FHR patterns. Presumably, hypoxic brain damage is not likely to occur unless there is biochemical evidence of asphyxia. Fetal electroencephalography (EEG) is being studied in relation to fetal hypoxia with the hope that it will help to prevent brain-damaged infants.

Treatment of fetal distress

The rational management of intrapartum asphyxia depends on the identification of its cause. If such maternal problems as inadequate pulmonary ventilation, hemorrhage, or cardiac failure are present, they must be recognized and treated. Severe anemia or abnormal oxygen-binding properties of blood should be considered in the differential diagnosis. Fetal distress is most often associated wtih obstetrical complications such as abnormal presentations, fetopelvic disproportion, abruptio placentae, umbilical cord compression, and, on rare occasions, massive fetal hemorrhage from the rupture of vasa previa in the fetal membranes.

Immediate cesarean section is indicated in the event of a frank cord prolapse. In many cases, lesser degrees of cord compression can be treated by displacing the fetal presenting part or by changing the maternal position. A change from the dorsal supine to the lateral also relieves pressure on the abdominal vena cava and aorta and improves uteroplacental perfusion. Vasopressors are to be avoided in the treatment of maternal hypotension, but if necessary, agents such as ephedrine, which have less uterine vasoconstrictor activity, should be selected.

Maternal perfusion of the placenta is inversely related to the intensity, frequency, and duration of uterine contractions. It is not surprising, therefore, that prolonged or tumultuous labors and the overenthusiastic use of oxytocin are common causes of fetal asphyxia.

The pharmacologic treatment of fetal distress consists of the administration of oxygen, glucose, and base to the mother and fetus. In most instances, oxygen breathing produces small elevations in fetal blood Po_2 unless maternal hypoxemia is present. Although blood glucose levels in the fetus are rapidly elevated by the infusion of hypertonic glucose solutions to the mother (25 to 50 gm administered intravenously), there is no conclusive evidence at present to indicate that such treatment will replenish fetal glycogen stores or improve fetal acid-base balance. Rapid infusion of concentrated dextrose solutions to the mother can be justified in documented maternal or fetal hypoglycemia (blood glucose less than 40 mg/100 ml), but their general use in the treatment of fetal distress has no firm clinical basis and may even be contraindicated in the diabetic patient.

Unlike glucose, bicarbonate equilibrates slowly across the placenta. Thus the administration of base to the mother is helpful in correcting a maternal acidosis but is not likely to correct a fetal metabolic acidosis in the time desired and may have an untoward effect on the fetus.

If the signs of fetal distress are progressive or persistent and do not respond to corrective measures, prompt intervention is required. The manner and the timing of delivery and the anesthetic management should be decided according to the station of the presenting part, the dilatation of the cervix, severity of fetal asphyxia, and the maturity of the fetus. Since premature and asphyxiated fetuses are more susceptible to sedatives, narcotics, and general anesthetics, this difference in response must be taken into account in maternal premedication and anesthesia for delivery. In order to avoid the aggravation of fetal asphyxia by pharmacologic depression, regional anesthesia is preferred in most cases. However, the depression of the neonate at delivery is related more to the interval from induction of anesthesia to delivery than to the type of anesthesia used, provided it is given by a skillful anesthesiologist.

The ultimate benefits of intrapartum monitoring of FHR and pH to perinatal mortality and morbidity remain to be determined. Reports from large obstetrical services indicate that the intrapartum stillbirth rate is lower in monitored patients than in unmonitored ones despite the fact that the former represent a higher risk group. It is not surprising that the primary cesarean section rate in monitored patients is nearly fivefold higher than in unmonitored patients and in some series approaches 20%. Identifying and singling out the high-risk pregnancy for special care is the basis of the current efforts in obstetrics to reduce the perinatal mortality and morbidity rate. The advances in prenatal care must be made accessible to all patients, and patients and physicians must be educated to effectively utilize them.

MILES J. NOVY

BIRTH WEIGHT, GESTATIONAL AGE, AND NEONATAL RISK

Care can be improved and neonatal mortality and morbidity decreased by identifying those live-born infants who are at high risk during the first few days or weeks of life. A newborn infant should be considered at high risk on the basis of factors associated with pregnancy (outline on pp. 2-3 and discussion on pp. 4-5) or because of his weight or gestational age or both (Fig. 1-5 and Plate 1, p. 8). In regard to the latter, each newborn infant's mortality risk should be predicted as soon after birth as possible by comparison with previous experience of other infants of similar weight and gestational age from a like population. High-risk infants should receive a degree of close observation and intensive care by interested and experienced nurses and physicians commensurate with the estimated degree of hazard of death or injury. The special organization of facilities to care for these infants is discussed in Chapter 5.

The majority of high-risk infants are born either prematurely, are of low birth weight (below 2,500 gm), or are of low weight for their gestational age. In general, the lower the birth weight the higher the neonatal mortality, and for any given weight, the shorter the duration of gestation the higher the neonatal mortality. The highest risk of neonatal mortality is among infants who weigh less than 1,000 gm at birth and whose gestation was less than 30 weeks. Further, some infants presumed to have had a retarded rate of intrauterine growth (pp. 8-9) are born small for their gestational age as calculated from maternal menstrual history, They have a higher mortality than infants of the same gestational age whose weight is appropriate and a lower mortality than infants of the same weight whose gestational age is less but appropriate for this size. The lowest risk of neonatal mortality is among infants with birth weights of 3,000 to 4,000 gm and whose gestational age is 38 to 42 weeks. Neonatal death rates rise sharply for infants whose birth weight is over 4,000 gm and for those whose gestational age is more than 42 weeks. In order to alert the physicians and nurses caring for newborn infants to those infants who are more likely to develop clinical problems, each infant should be classified as appropriate, small, or large for preterm, term, or postterm gestational age (Plate 1). When the gestational age by calculation from the mother's last mentrual period does not agree with that determined by clinical evaluation (p. 97), both should be indicated, and the infant should be considered to be at high risk.

Prematurity and low birth weight infants

Usually the term *premature* is used to designate live-born infants delivered before 37 weeks from the first day of the last menstrual period; these infants with a shortened gestation period are more appropriately called preterm (Plate 1). Infants who weigh 2,500 gm or less at birth are considered to have had either less than the expected rate of intrauterine growth or a shortened gestation period; these infants are called *low birth weight infants*. Prematurity and low birth weight frequently occur together, and both are associated with increased neonatal mortality and morbidity. From 1935 to 1961 a premature infant was defined as a live-born infant weighing 2,500 gm (5 lb, 8 oz) or less at birth and, until recently, much of the available statistical information was based on this definition. In Caucasian populations of the United States the incidence of low birth weight infants is 7.2%; it is approximately 14% among the nonwhite populations. There are about twice as many infants born in the United States weighing less than 1,500 gm than in Sweden. The mortality of this group is approximately 50%. Perinatal and neonatal mortality is lower for black than for white infants in each low weight group. Thus, there is considerable variation in risk from country to country and between different socioeconomic groups.

Until recently, it has not been possible to completely separate factors associated with prematurity from those associated with low birth weight because of failure to record both parameters. About one third of low birth weight infants weigh less than would be expected for gestational age calculated from the mother's last menstrual period; in the remainder the low weight is appropriate for the premature date of delivery. Both prematurity and low birth weight correlate with low socioeconomic status and with high incidences of maternal undernutrition, anemia, and illness; inadequate prenatal care, drug addiction, obstetrical complications, poor reproductive histories, illegitimacy, and multiparity are also associated.

Physical (p. 95) and neurologic signs may be useful in distinguishing those low birth weight premature infants who are of appropriate weight for their gestational age from those who are growth retarded or small for gestational age. Although infants of either group may lack subcutaneous fat, the growth-retarded infant is likely to be shorter than expected for gestational age and to appear to have a more disproportionately large head relative to body size than the premature infant of appropriate weight. Brain growth is generally less affected by factors that adversely influence intrauterine growth than linear or other organ growth, except in the presence of nonbacterial chronic fetal infections and certain chromosome anomalies (pp. 8-9). Thus, the functional development of the fetal nervous system continues to correlate with gestational age and may be used to assess gestational age (p. 97).

Pathology in low birth weight infants

Neonatal deaths among premature and term infants result from the same group of pathologic disturbances (Table 1-1), but the causes of death and morbidity differ in frequency. Problems of major clinical significance associated with prematurity or infants of low birth weight or both include respiratory distress syndromes (hyaline membrane disease, pulmonary hemorrhage, aspiration syndrome, congenital pneumonia, pneumothorax), recurrent apnea, hypoglycemia, hypocalcemia, hyperbilirubinemia, anemia, edema, intracranial hemorrhage, neurologic signs related to cerebral anoxia, circulatory instability and hypothermia, bacterial sepsis and intrauterine infection syndromes with congenital anomalies, persistent viremia with organ localization, and disseminated intravascular coagulopathies. The morbidity of term infants who are small for their gestational age is often caused by fetal distress and central nervous system depression, meconium aspiration, hypoglycemia, chronic intrauterine infections, pulmonary hemorrhage, polycythemia, and congenital anomalies. In contrast, preterm infants whose weight is appropriate for the gestational age have a higher incidence of hyaline membrane disease, nonhemolytic hyperbilirubinemia, neonatal bacterial infections, temperature instability, poor feeding and prolonged weight loss, apnea, cardiac arrythmias, anemia, bleeding (especially intraventricular hemorrhage in infants less than 1,200 gm), and late metabolic acidosis. (See relevant chapters for detailed discussion of these entities.)

Prognosis

The mortality for low birth weight infants who survive to be discharged from the hospital is about three times that of full-term infants during the first 2 years of life. Many deaths are attributable to infection. There is also an increased incidence of the *sudden infant death syndrome* among premature infants. The possible roles of defects in the regulation of the cardiorespiratory system secondary to immaturity and of high environmental risk factors secondary to low socioeconomic status in increasing the mortality has not been delineated.

The incidence of congenital anomalies increases with decreasing birth weight, and they are more common among low birth weight infants who are small for their gestational age than among those of appropriate weight for gestational age. The incidence of congenital anomalies is slightly increased in infants with birth weights above the ninetieth percentile.

In general, the greater the immaturity and the lower the birth weight the greater the likehood of intellectual and other neurologic deficit. There is a high incidence of such handicaps among small premature infants. As indicated, there is also a greater frequency of intrauterine anoxia, intracranial hemorrhage, and adverse socioeconomic factors, such as maternal addiction and poor infant nutrition, than occurs in infants born at term. Mothers of low socioecomonic status tend to have low birth weight babies, and such infants when reared in this environment tend to develop less well than those reared in better environments.

The chances of survival without morbidity, including injury to the central nervous system, is greater in those low birth weight infants with complications who are monitored and cared for in special neonatal intensive care units. In the absence of congenital anomalies, central nervous system injury, or a marked reduction in birth weight for gestational age (severe intrauterine growth retardation), the physical growth of low birth weight infants usually overtakes that of term infants during the second year; this occurs earlier in premature infants of larger size at birth. (See p. 125 for discussion of behavior and personality problems related to prematurity and premature care.)

Postterm infants

Postterm infants are defined as those born after 42 weeks' or more gestation, calculated from the mother's last menstrual period, irrespective of weight. This designation is often used synonymously with the term postmaturity for infants whose gestation exceeds the normal by 7 days or more (approximately 25% of all pregnancies). The cause for the delay in birth is unknown. When the postterm infants are large, their weights correlate poorly with late delivery, but correlate well with the large size of either parent, multigravidity, diabetes mellitus, or the prediabetic or diabetic state of the mother.

Clinical presentation. Postterm infants may be clinically indistinguishable from term infants, or they may appear and behave like infants of 1 to 3 weeks postnatal life. The latter group of postterm infants is sometimes designated as postmature and is characterized by absence of lanugo, decreased or absence of vernix caseosa, long nails, abundance of scalp hair, and white skin, which may be desquamating and parchmentlike. Occasionally, some of these clinical manifestations of postmaturity are observed in term and preterm infants.

Prognosis. There is a significant increase in fetal and neonatal mortality. This has been lowered with improved obstetrical management and intensive neonatal observation and care. Death rates increase with primiparity and increasing maternal age after 25 years.

Treatment. Cesarian section may be indicated in elderly primigravidas who go more than 1 to 2 weeks beyond term.

Placental dysfunction syndrome

The incidence of clinically recognizable placental dysfunction (abnormal fetal heart rate pattern, retarded intrauterine growth, low levels of estriol, amniotic fluid contaminated by meconium) may be as high as 12% of all births. The incidence of clearly recognized manifestations in an infant, yellow staining of the vernix and skin, is about 1.2% of all births. Although this syndrome is frequently confused with postmaturity, only about 20% of infants with placental dysfunction syndrome are postterm; it may occur in term and preterm infants and is frequently associated with preterm low birth weigh infants. The placentas are often small or poorly attached.

Clinical presentation. Clifford has described three clinical patterns of increasing severity in postterm infants with presumed placental dysfunction. *Stage I* infants have signs of postmaturity such as desquamation, long nails, abundant hair, white skin, alert facies, and loose skin giving the appearance of recent weight loss. *Stage II* infants have signs present in Stage I infants plus meconium-stained amniotic fluid, skin, vernix, umbilical cord, and placental membranes. *Stage III* infants have signs of the preceding stages, and their nails and skin are stained bright yellow. The umbilical cord is stained yellow-green.

Prognosis. Stage I infants have an increased mortality that correlates with prolonged gestation. They may also have an increased incidence of respiratory distress or central nervous system irritation or both. Stage II infants are born at the height of intrauterine anoxia or after a moderate to severe hypoxic episode. Approximately two thirds of them have severe respiratory symptoms, possibly from aspiration of meconium-containing amniotic fluid. A smaller number have signs of anoxic cerebral damage. The overall mortality before neonatal intensive care was about 35%. Many stage III infants probably die in utero; the liveborn have presumably survived the acute anoxic phase of stage II. However, they still have a significant mortality as well as morbidity.

Treatment. Therapy depends on the prevention and early diagnosis of fetal hypoxia (p. 40).

High birth weight infants

Perinatal and neonatal death rates decrease with increasing birth weight until approximately 4,000 gm when these rates again increase with higher infant weights. These oversized infants are usually born at term. However, preterm infants whose weights are excessively high for their gestational age also have a significantly higher mortality than infants of the same size born at term. Infants who are very large, regardless of their gestational age, have a higher incidence of birth injuries such as cervical and brachial plexus injuries, phrenic nerve damage with paralysis of the diaphragm, fractured clavicles, cephalohematomas, and ecchymosis of the head and face. The incidence of congenital anomalies is also higher in this group than in term infants of normal weight. Statistically significant evidence for intellectual and developmental retardation has been observed in very high birth weight term and preterm groups of infants on subsequent evaluation at school age in comparison to smaller appropriate weight babies of similar gestational ages. (See p. 441 for discussion of infants of diabetic mothers.)

RICHARD E. BEHRMAN

BIBLIOGRAPHY

Babson, S. G., Kangas, J., Young, N., and Bramhall, J.: Growth and development of twins of dissimilar size at birth, Pediatrics **33**:327, 1964.

Behrman, R. E., Babson, G., and Lessel, M. P. H.: Fetal and neonatal mortality in white middle class infants (mortality risks by gestational age and weight), Am. J. Dis. Child. **121**:486, 1971.

Behrman, R. E., Fisher, D., Paton, J., and Keller, J.: In utero disease and the newborn infant, Adv. Pediatr. **17**:13, 1970.

Bowe, E. T.: Treatment and prophylaxis of Rh disease, Gynec. Invest. (Suppl. 1):13, 1970.

Butler, N. R., and Bonham, D. G.: Perinatal mortality; the first report of the 1958 British Perinatal Mortality Survey, Edinburgh, 1963, E. & S. Livingstone.

Caldeyro-Barcia, R., Casacuberta, C., Bustos, R., Guissi, G., Gulin, L., Escarcena, L., and Mendez-Bauer, C.: Correlation of intrapartum changes in fetal heart rate with fetal blood oxygen and acid-base state. In Adamsons, K., editor: Diagnosis and treatment of fetal disorders, New York, 1968, Springer-Verlag New York Inc., pp. 205-225.

Clifford, S. H.: Postmaturity—with placental dysfunction; clinical syndrome and pathologic findings, J. Pediatr. **44**:1, 1954.

Comline, R. S., Silver, I. A., and Silver, M.: Factors responsible for the stimulation of the adrenal medulla during asphyxia in the foetal lamb, J. Physiol. (Lond.) **178**:211, 1965.

Dawes, G. S.: Foetal and neonatal physiology, Chicago, 1968, Year Book Medical Publishers, Inc.

Dawes, G. S., Fox, H. E., Leduc, B. M., Liggins, G. C., and Richards, R. T.: Respiratory movements and rapid eye movement sleep in the foetal lamb, J. Physiol. (Lond.) **220**:119, 1972.

Dawes, G. S., Mott, J. C., and Shelley, H. J.: The importance of cardiac glycogen for the maintenance of life in foetal lambs and newborn animals during anoxia, J. Physiol. (Lond.) **146**: 516, 1959.

Gluck, L.: Pulmonary surfactant and neonatal respiratory distress, Hosp. Pract. **6**(11):45, 1971.

Hammacher, K., and Werners, P. H.: Über die Auswertung und Dokumentation von CTG-Ergebnissen, Gynaecologia **166**:410, 1968.

Hellman, L. M., Kobayashi, M., Fillisti, L., and Lavenhar, M.: Sources of error in sonographic fetal mensuration and estimation of growth, Am. J. Obstet. Gynecol. **99**:662, 1967.

Hill, D. E., Myers, R. E., Holt, A. B., Scott, R. E., and Cheek, D. B.: Fetal growth retardation produced by experimental placental insufficiency in the rhesus monkey. II. Chemical composition of the brain, liver, muscle and carcass, Biol. Neonate. **19**:68, 1971.

Hon, E. H. G.: Direct monitoring of the fetal heart, Hosp. Pract. **5**:91, 1970.

Jacobson, H. N., and Reid, D. E.: High-risk pregnancy. II. A pattern of comprehensive maternal and child care, N. Engl. J. Med. **271**:302, 1964.

Klopper A.: The assessment of placental function in clinical practice. In Klopper, A., and Diczfalusy, E., editors: Foetus and placenta, Oxford, 1969, Blackwell Scientific Publications Ltd., pp. 471-555.

Kubli, F. W., Hon, E. H., Khazin, A. F., and Takemura, H.: Observations on heart rate and pH in the human fetus during labor, Am. J. Obstet. Gynecol. **104**:1190, 1969.

Liley, A. W.: Liquor amnii analysis in management of pregnancy complicated by rhesus sensitization, Am. J. Obstet. Gynecol. **82**:1359, 1961.

Liley, A. W.: The use of amniocentesis and fetal transfusion in erythroblastosis fetalis, Pediatrics **35**:836, 1965.

Lubchenco, L. O., Delivoria-Papadopoulos, M., Butterfield, L. J., French J. H., Metcalf, D., Hix, I. E., Jr., Danick, J., Dodds, J., Downs, M., and Freeland, E.: Long-term follow-up studies of prematurely born infants. I. Relationship of handicaps to nursery routines, J. Pediatr. **80**: 501, 1972.

Lubchenco, L. O., Searls, D. T., and Brazie, J. V.: Neonatal mortality rates; relationship to birth weight and gestational age, J. Pediatr. **81**:814, 1972.

Nadler, H. L.: *In utero* detection of familial metabolic disorders, Pediatrics **49**:329, 1972.

Novy, M. J., and Edwards, M. J.: Respiratory problems in pregnancy, Am. J. Obstet. Gynecol. **99**:1024, 1967.

Saling, E.: Amnioscopy and foetal blood sampling; observations on foetal acidosis, Arch. Dis. Child. **41**:472, 1966.

Seeds, A. E., and Behrman, R. E.: Acid-base monitoring of the fetus during labor with blood obtained from the scalp, J. Pediatr. **74**:804, 1969.

Tyson, J. E.: Human chorionic somatomammotropin, Obstet. Gynecol. Ann. **1**:421, 1972.

Winick, M.: Cellular growth of human placenta. III. Intra-uterine growth failure, J. Pediatr. **71**: 390, 1967.

Zipursky, A.: The universal prevention of Rh immunization, Clin. Obstet. Gynecol. **14**:869, 1971.

2 Emergencies in the delivery room

Emergencies in the delivery room encompass two main areas: resuscitation of the asphyxiated or depressed newborn infant and the diagnosis of certain congenital anomalies that may require early treatment.

ONSET OF BREATHING AND PHYSIOLOGIC CHANGES AT BIRTH

In order to understand the principles of resuscitation, one must have a knowledge of the normal cardiopulmonary events that take place with the onset of respiration.

Under normal circumstances, the healthy newborn infant will make respiratory efforts within a few seconds of being born; and after the first few breaths, the lungs are almost completely expanded. As the chest emerges from the birth canal, there is an elastic recoil that can draw in between 7 and 42 ml of air to replace fluid squeezed out during the final stages of delivery. This explains the cough that occasionally precedes the first inspiratory effort. Glossopharyngeal muscular movement (frog breathing) may force down an additional 5 to 10 ml. The first inspiration is usually followed by a cry as the infant expires against a partially closed glottis, creating a positive intrathoracic pressure of up to 40 cm H_2O. Within a few minutes, functional residual capacity reaches about three fourths of final aeration.

Although the intrathoracic pressures recorded during the first breaths are high, it is surprising how often initial lung expansion appears to require little effort. The work for initial lung expansion is undeniably greater than that for quiet breathing, but it is not greater than that performed many times a day during vigorous crying.

The first breath appears to be caused by the integrated activity of several stimuli. Of these stimuli, the most important are from hypoxia and acidosis (asphyxia), cord occlusion, and thermal changes. During the final stages of labor and delivery there is a reduction in exchange of oxygen and carbon dioxide between fetus and mother leading to a moderate degree of asphyxia at birth. The average value for oxygen saturation in the arterial blood at birth is 22%, and in nearly one fourth of all neonates it is less than 10%. The relatively low oxygen levels are accompanied by varying degrees of hypercapnia and acidosis, the average carbon dioxide pressure being 58 mm Hg and the average pH 7.28; lower pH and higher carbon dioxide pressure are associated with lower oxygen levels. The respiratory drive during asphyxia depends upon the presence of carotid and aortic chemoreceptors, which are known to be functional in the newborn. Cord occlusion is associated with a prompt rise in blood pressure and stimulation of both the aortic baroreceptors and the sympathetic nervous system. Finally, thermal stimuli immediately after birth are intense. Calculations based on the rate of fall of skin temperature in the first minutes of extrauterine life indicate that at room temperature the newborn human infant loses about 600 calories per minute. It is difficult to avoid this initial heat loss even if the infant is immediately placed under a radiant heater. If this initial stimulus is completely prevented, apnea may follow.

With the onset of respiration and lung expansion, pulmonary vascular resistance falls. This appears to be caused largely by the direct effect of oxygen and carbon dioxide on the blood vessels, resistance decreasing as oxygen tension rises and carbon dioxide tension falls. Lung expansion alone contributes to lowering of the pulmonary vascular resistance. There then follows a gradual transition from the fetal to the adult type of circulation, the foramen ovale and ductus arteriosus remaining open for varying lengths of time.

Pressure in the left atrium falls in the first few hours of life to levels below those in the normal adult; by 24 hours it may be less than 1 mm Hg above that in the right atrium. This small pressure difference probably accounts for the persistence of a right-to-left shunt through the foramen ovale for 24 hours or longer. Pulmonary arterial pressure remains relatively high for several hours. As the pulmonary vascular resistance falls, the direction of blood flow through the ductus arteriosus reverses. In the first hours of extrauterine life, the flow is bidirectional, but the shunt eventually becomes entirely left-to-right and by 15 hours of age is functionally insignificant.

The ductus arteriosus constricts in response to an increase in arterial oxygen tension. Sympathomimetic amines also cause it to constrict. Hypoxemia can cause a constricted ductus to reopen and at the same time may reestablish the fetal pattern of circulation by increasing the pulmonary vascular resistance. This response of the ductus arteriosus to oxygen or hypoxia is thus opposite to that of the pulmonary arterioles, enabling the right ventricle to contribute a variable fraction of its output to placental perfusion during fetal life. The different reactivity of these vessels during hypoxia, although an asset to the fetus, becomes a liability for the newborn infant. Hypoxic episodes in early neonatal life can lead to a rise in pulmonary vascular resistance and opening of the ductus arteriosus, increasing any residual right-to-left shunt.

Failure to breathe at birth

Depression of the fetal central nervous system is the basic cause for failure to breathe at birth. This may be caused by asphyxia, by analgesic or anesthetic agents administered to the mother, or by trauma. Usually there is a combination of these causes.

Fetal asphyxia may be caused by maternal factors. These include compression of the inferior vena cava and aorta by the heavy gravid uterus, particularly if the mother is supine; strong uterine contractions that occlude arterioles leading to the intervillous space impeding blood flow; hypotension caused by regional anesthesia, hyperventilation, or pharmacologic agents administered to the mother for hypertension; and systemic vascular disease including toxemia of pregnancy. Anemia or methemoglobinemia in the mother may also lead to fetal asphyxia.

Fetal factors that may lead to asphyxia include mechanical occlusion of the umbilical cord or fetal hypotension as a result of depressant drugs that have crossed the placenta. Abnormalities of the placenta itself may impair its diffusion capacity; for example, its small size, underdevelopment, aging, edema, infarcts, partial or complete separation, or inflammatory changes.

Neonatal factors may also lead to asphyxia. Most common is depression of the respiratory center from hypnotic, analgesic, or anesthetic agents administered to the mother. Probably the second most common neonatal cause is immaturity of the lung; this may relate to abnormalities in enzyme systems responsible for the release of surfactant to alveolar lining cells, to the vasculature, or to the lung parenchyma itself. The end result is difficulties in lung expansion and establishment of a normal pulmonary circulation. A third category is mechanical airway obstruction from aspiration of meconium and intrauterine pneumonia. Finally, various congenital anomalies may prevent or impede lung expansion; these include choanal atresia, a laryngeal web, hypoplastic lungs (usually associated with diaphragmatic hernias or large abdominal masses), hydrothorax or ascites, certain cardiac anomalies, and congenital myasthenia gravis.

The effect of trauma is more difficult to evaluate and to separate from the effect of asphyxia. It undoubtedly plays a role, particularly in precipitous labors or in difficult forceps deliveries.

Fetal respiratory responses—normal and abnormal

The normal mammalian fetus makes respiratory movements in utero from time to time. These are relatively rapid (80 to 120 per minute) and are noted during the latter half of gestation. It is unlikely that the rapid breathing movements result in a tidal flow of amniotic fluid.

There is a considerable quantity of fluid in the fetal lung prior to delivery. This fluid appears to be an ultrafiltrate of plasma; it is more acidic and has a higher chloride content than plasma or amniotic fluid. With the onset of respiration, reabsorption of this fluid is quite rapid. Its low protein concentration, together with the fall in pulmonary artery pressure occurring when the lung expands, facilitates this process. The difference in composition of tracheal fluid compared with amniotic fluid is strong evidence against aspiration of amniotic fluid occurring as a normal phenomenon.

Cardiovascular, respiratory, and biochemical changes occurring during asphyxia under controlled conditions are predictable. Information on this subject has been obtained experimentally in a variety of newborn mammals. During the initial phase of asphyxia of the unanesthetized newborn primate, respiratory efforts increase in depth and frequency for up to 3 minutes. This period, which is called primary hyperpnea, is followed by primary apnea lasting for approximately 1 minute. Rhythmic gasping then begins and is maintained at a fairly constant rate of about 6 gasps per minute for several minutes. The gasps finally become weaker and slower. Their cessation marks the beginning of secondary apnea.

There is some variation in the period of gasping (time to the last gasp) during the course of complete asphyxiation in different species, depending on the initial acid-base state, drugs given to the mother, environmental temperature, and degree of maturity of the species at birth. At a given environmental temperature the principal determinant of duration of gasping in the nonanesthetized animal is the initial arterial pH. Narcotics and systemic anesthetic agents administered to the mother can abolish the period of primary hyperpnea and prolong primary apnea; large doses can suppress all respiratory efforts. Gasping is always prolonged at lower body temperatures.

During primary apnea a variety of stimuli such as pain, cold, and analeptics can initiate gasping. Once the stage of secondary apnea has been reached these stimuli are without effect. Gasping can, however, be reinitiated by artificial ventilation or correction of acidosis by administration of base. There is a linear relation between the duration of asphyxia and recovery of respiratory function after resuscitation. In newborn monkeys, for each minute after the last gasp that artificial ventilation is delayed, there is a further delay of 2 minutes before rhythmic breathing is established (Fig. 2-1). This indicates that the longer artificial ventilation is delayed during secondary apnea, the longer it will take to resuscitate the infant.

One of the most potent stimuli to gasping in utero is occlusion of the umbilical cord. This has been observed experimentally in both the fetal lamb and monkey. After 2 to 3 minutes of cord occlusion, when the fetus has become partially asphyxiated, deep gasping efforts commence.

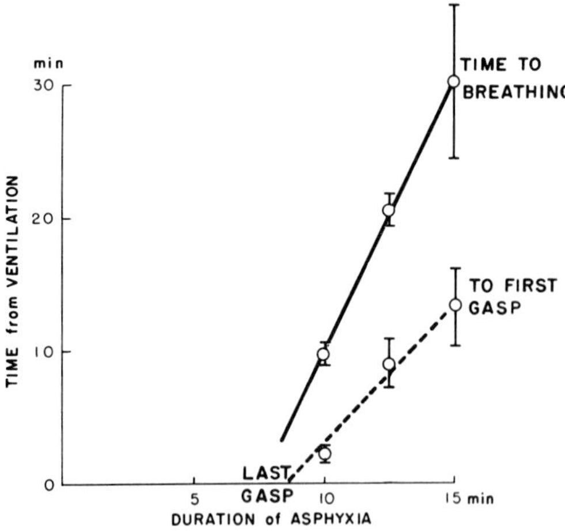

FIG. 2-1. Time from ventilation to first gasp and to rhythmic breathing in newborn monkeys asphyxiated for 10, 12.5, and 15 minutes at 30 C. Mean time from onset of asphyxia until last gasp was 8.42 ±0.24 (SE) minutes. (From Adamsons, K., Jr., Behrman, R., Dawes, G. S., James, L. S., and Koford, C.: J. Pediatr. **65**:807, 1964.)

These respiratory efforts continue for 10 to 20 minutes following release of the cord occlusion. The presence of meconium and squamous cells in the lung periphery of mature infants dying after chronic intrauterine asphyxia indicates that aspiration may occur in the older fetus.

Preparation for resuscitation

The delivery room must be prepared for adequate and prompt treatment of severe asphyxia at birth, whether it is expected or not. All members of the delivery room team should be trained in methods of resuscitation, for both mother and baby may be in difficulty at the same time.

Every piece of apparatus necessary for emergency resuscitation should be carefully checked as present and functioning before each delivery. There should be suction apparatus, a plastic oropharyngeal airway, a laryngoscope equipped with a pencil handle and a blade, and a plastic endotracheal tube with a stylet. Oxygen should be available. In addition, the container for receiving the infant should be warm, and some form of radiant heat should be available to help in maintaining body temperature.

Although thermal stimuli might be important in the initiation and establishment of breathing by increasing the state of activity of the reticular system, prolonged exposure of the naked infant to room temperature has been shown to lead to progressive metabolic acidosis, particularly in the depressed infant or in the infant with impaired pulmonary function. If the depression of the newborn is caused by excessive maternal medication, it is important to recognize that a fall in body temperature will prolong the effect of most analgesic and anesthetic drugs. The mean blood glucose level is also decreased at lower body temperatures.

The fetal heart rate should be determined between every contraction during the final stages of labor. A rate below 100 or above 160 per minute between contractions or the passage of meconium in a vertex presentation is an urgent warning sign of fetal distress. If these signs develop, the staff should be alerted for an emergency and the baby delivered as soon as possible. Analysis of capillary samples from the fetal scalp for pH and blood gases may provide a more precise evaluation of fetal condition (see Chapter 1, p. 42).

EVALUATION AT BIRTH—APGAR SCORE

Immediately after delivery, the baby should be restrained with the head slightly dependent while the cord is clamped and cut. The infant should then be placed supine on a table, the head kept low with a slight lateral tilt. A nurse or assistant should listen to the heartbeat immediately, indicating the rate by finger movement. If help is not available the rate often can be detected from pulsation of the umbilical cord. A strong beat with a rate of over 100 per minute indicates that there is no immediate emergency. A slow rate indicates severe depression, calling for resuscitative measures. While the nurse is listening to the heart, the physician should aspirate the mouth, the pharynx, and the nose with a catheter. This suction should be brief. From birth to completion of suctioning should take about 1 minute. Lightly slapping the soles frequently aids in initiating a deep breath and crying.

During the course of these initial procedures the infant should be carefully observed for any evidence of central nervous system depression or inability to breathe. Particular attention should be paid to the first few breaths and the evenness and ease of respiration. A congenital laryngeal web or bilateral choanal atresia can cause complete airway obstruction; both require immediate treatment. A diaphragmatic hernia with abdominal viscera in the chest, abdominal distention from ascites, congenital cystic lung disease, or intrauterine pneumonia may all cause initial respiratory difficulty and may even prevent lung expansion.

The Apgar score was introduced to quantitate the initial evaluation of the infant. It focuses on five vital signs: heart rate, respiratory effort, muscle tone, reflex irritability, and color, all judged 60 seconds after complete delivery of the infant (Table 2-1). This particular time interval was chosen, since it coincided with maximal depression in our clinic. A score of 0 is given for each of the following: no heart beat, no respiratory effort, no muscle tone, no

TABLE 2-1. Apgar score

Sign	0	1	2
Heart rate	Absent	Slow (below 100)	Over 100
Respiratory effort	Absent	Slow, irregular	Good, crying
Muscle tone	Flaccid	Some flexion of extremities	Active motion
Reflex irritability	No response	Grimace	Vigorous cry
Color	Blue, pale	Body pink, extremities blue	Completely pink

reflex response to a glancing slap on the soles of the feet, and a blue or pale color. A score of 1 is given for a slow heart beat (less than 100), slow or irregular respiratory effort, some flexion of the extremities, a grimace to a glancing slap on the soles of the feet, and a pink body with blue extremities. Finally, a score of 2 is given for a heart rate over 100, good respiratory effort accompanied by crying, fully flexed limbs, a vigorous cry in response to a slap on the feet, and a completely pink coloration.

The majority of infants are vigorous, with a score of 7 to 10 and cry or cough within seconds of delivery. No resuscitative procedures are necessary for these babies. Mildly to moderately depressed infants form the largest group requiring some form of resuscitation at birth. These babies score 4 to 6. They are pale or blue at 1 minute after birth, do not have sustained respirations, and may be nearly flaccid. However, their heart rate and reflex irritability are good. The most severely depressed infants score 0 to 3. They are pale or cyanotic, apneic, hypotonic, have a reduced or absent reflex response, and their heart rates are slow or inaudible; artificial ventilation should be commenced immediately.

Order of disappearance of signs

The foregoing 5 signs disappear in a predictable fashion during asphyxiation of the newborn. In vigorous infants who cry lustily as soon as they are born, heart rate, reflex response, and tone are all present to the full extent; the signs to which the observer has to pay attention are color and respiration. Mildly depressed babies are cyanotic (zero for color), but heart rate and reflex response are usually normal; attention has to be focused primarily on tone and respiration. In severely depressed infants who are pale or cyanotic (zero for color), apneic (zero for respiration), and usually flaccid (zero for tone), attention has to be paid primarily to heart rate and reflex response.

All of the signs but reflex response can be seen—respiration from chest movement, tone from flexed or moving extremities, and heart rate from movement of the index finger of the nurse who listens to the heart with a stethoscope. A normal reflex response is present in all vigorous infants. This sign should be tested for in those infants scoring 6 or less and forms part of the resuscitation procedure during the first minute of life. From a practical point of view, the heart rate is usually slow (under 100) or fast (over 160). In the high score group it is fast, probably in response to catecholamine release and an immediate cold stimulus. In those scoring 6 or less who are not breathing, it is slow either as a result of baroreceptive reflex or from myocardial depression.

Initially, the physician may have some difficulty in evaluating the 5 signs at once. If he makes a mental note of the total clinical picture when 1 minute has elapsed, he can then assign a value for each of the clinical signs.

Value of scoring

Clinical picture at a glance

The scoring system serves many useful purposes. It teaches the delivery room personnel to observe more than one sign at a time and ensures that the infant will be closely observed during the first minute of life.

Need for resuscitation

It has served as a useful guide as to the need for resuscitation; having made his rapid evaluation the physician can decide whether or not the infant should be resuscitated rather than waiting hopefully to see whether the infant will respond spontaneously.

Serial score—index of recovery

A physician or nurse can readily evaluate the infant at 1, 2, 5, and 10 minutes. Thus the scoring system serves as a semiquantitative shorthand method describing the recovery rate of an infant whose condition may change rapidly from moment to moment. This is extremely valuable on a busy obstetric service where there may not be time for detailed notation of the changing clinical state.

Defining infants at high risk

A further advantage of the scoring system is that it will define the infants at high risk, both with regard to mortality and morbidity. The mortality in low score infants is nearly 15 times that in the high score group, and respiratory distress syndrome occurs significantly more frequently in low score than high score infants.

Time to assign the score

A simple alarm timer should be firmly fixed on the delivery room wall and set for 60 seconds. When the head and feet of the infant are visible, the timer is started, and when the alarm sounds at 60 seconds, the score is assigned.

Person to score

Experience has demonstrated that the person delivering the infant should not be the one to assign the score. He or she is usually emotionally involved with the outcome of the delivery and with the family, and may not make an objective evaluation. It is ideal to have a specially trained observer regularly present, whether physician or nurse, but this situation is seldom possible. If a pediatrically oriented person is not routinely present for all deliveries, the anesthesiologist should assign the score, and the infant should be placed in a bassinet near the head of the delivery table.

Five-minute score

The 5-minute score is more predictive of survival or neurologic abnormality at 1 year of age than the 1-minute score. This is not surprising, for it is to be expected that the longer asphyxia exists, the more likely death or permanent damage will occur. However, if the first observation is made as late as 5 minutes, a number of asphyxiated infants will remain untreated, with subsequent higher mortality and morbidity.

Limitations

While this score is useful, it has many limitations. It is no substitute for a careful physical examination or serial observations over the first few hours of life. Although it is of value in estimating the probability of survival in groups of infants, it will not predict neonatal death or survival of individual infants or long-term prognosis.

TREATMENT OF MODERATELY DEPRESSED INFANT

If initial resuscitative measures have produced no response by 1½ minutes after delivery, the progressing asphyxia usually leads to diminished muscular tone and a fall in the heart rate. A small plastic oropharyngeal airway should then be inserted into the mouth and oxygen applied under pressure of 16 to 20 cm H_2O for 1 to 2 seconds. Although this pressure is insufficient to expand the alveoli, some oxygen will reach the respiratory bronchioles. The rise in intrabronchial pressure stimulates pulmonary stretch receptors. This stimulus, added to that of the chemoreceptors, initiates a gasp in about 85% of the cases.

If there is no respiratory effort and the heart rate continues to fall, with the infant becoming completely flaccid, the larynx should be visualized with the laryngoscope and the infant intubated. This is not a difficult procedure, but skill should be obtained by practice on stillborn infants.

Intubation is best accomplished with the infant lying supine on a flat surface. A folded towel under the head and slight extension of the neck will place him in a position resembling a sniffing posture. The head should be steadied with the right hand and kept in line with the body. The laryngoscope is held in the left hand, and the blade is introduced at the right corner of the mouth and advanced between tongue and palate for about 2 cm. As it is advanced, the blade is swung to the midline. This moves the tongue to the left of the blade. The operator looks along the blade for the rim of the epiglottis. The laryngoscope is gently advanced into the space betwen the base of the tongue and the epiglottis. Slight elevation of the tip of the blade will expose the glottis as a vertical dark slit bordered posteriorly by pink arytenoid cartilages.

If foreign material such as small blood clots, meconium-stained mucus, or vernix obstructs the larynx, quick brief suction is indicated. When the glottis is seen to be patent, a curved endotracheal tube is introduced at the right corner of the mouth and inserted through the cords until the flange of the tube rests at the glottis. Care must be taken not to intubate the esophagus. The laryngoscope is then withdrawn. Rarely, the glottis is obstructed by a laryngeal web. If the web is partial or thin, it may be perforated with a stylet, or the opening may be enlarged with an endotracheal tube. The presence of a thick membrane requires immediate tracheostomy.

If stimuli from these procedures have not initiated a spontaneous gasp, positive pressure should be applied to the endotracheal tube. Brief puffs of air blown through the tube with enough force to cause the lower chest to rise gently will usually start spontaneous respiration. If the stomach rises, however, the esophagus has been intubated instead of the trachea, and the position of the tube must be corrected. Pressures between 25 to 35 cm H_2O are necessary to expand normal alveoli initially and can be applied safely for 1 to 2 seconds. Experience in applying this pressure should be gained by puffing into a spring manometer. Oxygen-enriched gas may be delivered to the infant by placing a tube carrying oxygen in the operator's mouth.

If the endotracheal tube is fitted with appropriate-sized adapters, it can be connected to a rubber bag of oxygen or oxygen-enriched gas mixture or to one of the mechanical devices for applying positive pressure.

Artificial expansion of the lungs can initiate a spontaneous gasp. With the first or second application of positive pressure, the infant usually makes an effort to breathe. The endotracheal tube may be withdrawn after the infant has established sustained spontaneous ventilation.

TREATMENT OF SEVERELY DEPRESSED INFANT

No time should be lost in establishing ventilation. The glottis should be inspected immediately with the laryngoscope. If meconium or thick meconium-stained mucus has been aspirated into the trachea, it must be suctioned out at once prior to inflation of the lungs. It is usually possible to accomplish this within 1 minute after delivery. These severely depressed infants may require 3 to 8 minutes of artificial ventilation before a spontaneous gasp is taken. The endotracheal tube can be removed as soon as quiet and sustained respiration is established.

PROCEDURE FOR INFANT RESUSCITATION

During resuscitation, efforts should be made to prevent heat loss by placing the infant under a radiant heat lamp. Three people should be available for emergency resuscitation—one for establishing an airway and ventilating the infant, one for cardiac massage and monitoring the heart rate, and one for umbilical catheterization and the administration of alkali. When possible, the procedure should be carried out under sterile conditions, including sterile gowns and gloves. All equipment, including laryngoscope, endotracheal tubes, and stethoscope, should be sterile. The resuscitation area should be covered with a sterile sheet previously warmed from an overhead heat lamp.

Attention must first be directed to establishing pulmonary ventilation in resuscitating the severely asphyxiated newborn. The steps should be as follows: establishment and maintenance of a clear airway, expansion of the lungs, and continuation of ventilation with 80% to 100% oxygen at a rate of 30 to 40 inflations per minute. Ventilation should be interrupted every six or seven breaths and alternated with periods of cardiac massage as needed to maintain a rate of 120 beats per minute. Both ventilation and cardiac massage may be carried out by one person; if two people are involved, it is important that they coordinate their actions so that cardiac massage and artificial ventilation are not given simultaneously. This can result in the production of a pneumomediastinum or a pneumothorax, since ventilation will be done against a compressed and distorted tracheobronchial tree. While these measures are being initiated, another physician should insert a catheter into the umbilical vein.

Aspiration syndrome

The importance of suctioning meconium from the trachea and bronchi deserves special emphasis. Meconium is passed following an asphyxial episode in utero. If the asphyxial episode is accompanied by prolonged gasping, meconium will be drawn deeply into the lungs. The fetus may recover from this episode with regard to his acid-base state and central nervous system responsiveness, but may yet be born with his lungs full of meconium. Such infants may initially be responsive and vigorously attempt to breathe. It is essential that the larynx be observed in all infants who have passed meconium during labor or who have meconium-stained amniotic fluid as soon as they are born, irrespective of their initial responsiveness. If there is thick meconium at the back of the pharynx, it should be suctioned out under direct vision and the larynx intubated with an endotracheal tube that has a terminal hole (size 12 or 14, French). Suction should then be applied directly to this tube, which is gradually withdrawn while suction is applied. In our unit we use mouth-to-tube suction. Not infrequently, a large piece of meconium, too thick to pass up the endotracheal tube, is observed clinging to the tip of the tube. If this occurs, the trachea should be reintubated immediately and the procedure repeated until only watery mucus is obtained. The fluid normally produced by the fetal lung continues to form and washes out meconium from the deeper radicals of the lung.

If one follows this procedure in all cases of meconium aspiration, many subsequent complications can be avoided.

There are four conditions in which lung expansion is impossible in spite of proper intubation: massive aspiration of meconium that cannot be removed by suctioning, intrauterine pneumonia with organization of exudate, large bilateral diaphragmatic hernias with hypoplastic lungs, and congenital adenomatous cysts of the lung. Infants with the first two conditions are usually severely depressed at birth. However, those with hypoplastic lungs may be vigorous initially and score as high as 7 at 1 minute of age, making strenuous but ineffective respiratory efforts. At present there is no available treatment for this condition. Congenital adenomatous cysts of the lung are usually associated with hydrops fetalis, and the condition is usually fatal.

Cardiac massage

Blood pressure and heart rate fall during prolonged asphyxia. If the blood pressure is unduly low at the beginning of resuscitation, positive pressure ventilation is unlikely to be successful unless cardiac massage is employed. Cardiac massage should not be initiated until after the lungs have been well expanded with two or three inflations. If the hearbeat cannot then be heard or if a slow heartbeat has not increased in rate, cardiac massage should be commenced. External manual compression of the heart between the chest wall and vertebral column forces blood into the aorta. Relaxation of pressure allows the heart to fill with venous blood.

The technique consists of intermittent compression of the middle and lower third of the sternum 100 to 200 times per minute with the index and middle fingers. Initially massage is interrupted every 5 seconds to permit two or three inflations of the lung; subsequently, if the heart is responding, 6 or 7 breaths should be alternated with massage. Cardiopulmonary resuscitation is most successful when there has been no clinical evidence of fetal distress and when a normal FHR has been heard between contractions up to the moment of birth.

Administration of alkali

The rationale for rapid correction of an acid pH from asphyxia is based on experiments in newborn monkeys. The maintenance of a normal pH during asphyxia by rapid intravenous infusion of alkali together with glucose prolongs gasping and delays cardiovascular collapse. Resuscitation is also facilitated if alkali and glucose are infused at the same time as artificial ventilation is started; oxygen consumption is greater, and the time for establising spontaneous breathing is shorter. Cardiac massage is less frequently necessary in the treated animals. The infusion of alkali and glucose alone may cause the blood pressure and heart rate to rise and spontaneous gasping to begin. It has been proposed that the beneficial effects of pH correction are derived from a prolongation and acceleration of anaerobic glycolysis, a restitution of the oxygen-carrying capacity of hemoglobin and the responsiveness of cardiovascular muscle to sympathomimetic amines, and a fall in pulmonary vascular resistance.

The beneficial effects of alkali administration both to asphyxiated newborn monkeys and to adults with cardiac arrest suggest that a rapid correction of pH during resuscitation of severely asphyxiated newborn human infants is of value.

The most severely asphyxiated infants—those with an arterial pH below 7.0—will have a base deficit of 26 mEq/liter or greater in addition to a marked elevation in CO_2 tension. By means of artificial ventilation alone, the base deficit can be reduced by approximately 10 mEq/liter in a matter of 5 to 10 minutes, provided that good alveolar ventilation is achieved and the infant does not remain in circulatory collapse. This change occurs as a result of a significant bicarbonate shift at P_{CO_2}'s greater than 70 mm Hg, which should be taken into consideration in calculations for the initial base administration in order to avoid overcorrection. It is advisable initially to attempt to correct one half of the residual metabolic component of the mixed acidosis. Thus a 3-kg infant would receive 8 mEq of base:

$$\frac{\text{Base deficit (26-10)}}{2} \times \frac{\text{Body weight (3 kg)}}{\text{ECV (3)}}$$

This working formula is only a gross approximation and assumes the estimated circulatory volume (ECV) to be one third of the body weight.

Sodium bicarbonate rather than tris (hydroxymethyl) aminomethane (THAM) is recommended because the latter solution, if given in too great a quantity, occasionally causes depression of the respiratory center and arrest of breathing. Sodium bicarbonate, as it is obtained from the commercial ampule, contains nearly 1 mEq/ml (44.7 mEq in 50 ml, 0.9 molar solution). This solution has an osmolality of 1,400 and a pH of 7.8. It should be diluted in equal parts with distilled water or 5% glucose to reduce its osmolality to 700 and infused at a rate not greater than 2 to 3 ml/min. If the heart rate is slow and irregular, the infusion should be accompanied by intermittent cardiac massage.

The alkali may be infused into either the umbilical vein or artery.

Subsequent alkali administration

The infant's response to alkali administration will vary according to the degree of asphyxia, the effectiveness of ventilation, and the responsiveness of the cardiovascular system. It is important, therefore, to have a measurement of his acid-base state as soon as the initial dose of sodium bicarbonate has been given. This can usually be made by 15 minutes of age. The required amount of sodium bicarbonate for subsequent correction to a pH of 7.3 may then be calculated.

Technique for catheterization of umbilical vein

A straight, soft plastic feeding tube, if advanced to a distance of 7 to 10 cm from the skin surface of the umbilical vein, will lie just beyond the ductus venosus in the inferior vena cava in a mature, term weight infant. If the catheter is even slightly curved, it may be deflected into one of the radicals in the portal system. Any tendency for the catheter to bounce back as it is advanced, should suggest that it is not passing through the ductus venosus. Rapid verification of the correct site can be obtained if the catheter has been previously attached to a strain gauge and a recording polygraph. The moment the ductus venosus is passed, the venous pulsations (A, C, and V waves) can be readily seen, unless there is cardiac arrest. This means of verification of catheter position may be more rapid and suitable for delivery room treatment than the use of an image-intensified roentgenogram.

Technique of catheterization of the umbilical artery

Only fine catheters should be used (3½ or 5, French). They should be nonrigid and pliable with a hole in the tip that is softly rounded. They should also be radiopaque for radiologic localization. The lumen of the artery should be carefully identified after cutting the cord close to the abdominal wall with sharp scissors. Fine, curved, nontoothed forceps should be gently placed in the pinpoint clot that usually marks the vessel opening. Pressure on the forceps is then gradually released to allow the natural spring to open the vessel gradually. This procedure is repeated four or five times, the forceps gradually being advanced to a depth of ¼ to ½ inch. The catheter may then be introduced and will usually pass readily down to the region of the iliac artery. Occasionally, some obstruction is met ½ inch from the skin, but this rarely causes any difficulty. If resistance is felt at the entrance into the internal iliac artery, only moderate pressure should be applied. If the catheter will not advance, 0.5 ml of 0.5% Novocaine may be slowly infused. This may be sufficient to release any spasm and permit further advancement of the catheter. If this maneuver is unsuccessful and resistance persists, the second umbilical artery should be catheterized. If damage to the vessels is to be avoided, resistance in the region of the internal iliac artery should not be responded to aggressively; efforts to catheterize should be discontinued if unsuccessful after three attempts.

Once the venous or arterial catheter is in place, a lateral film should be taken to ver-

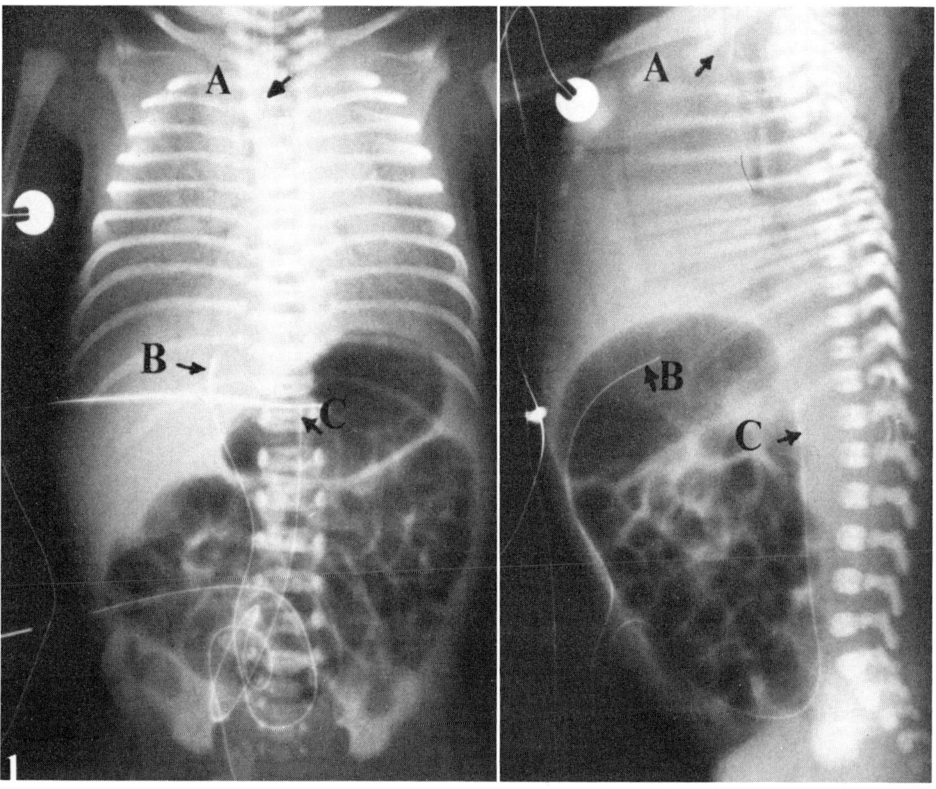

Fig. 2-2. AP x-ray film of infant with thermistors and an umbilical catheter in place; note that maze of wires prevents identification of catheter position in this view. The lateral view clearly identifies that catheter has been inserted into an umbilical vein and is lying in the portal system of the liver. *A,* Endotrachial tube; *B,* umbilical venous catheter at the juncture of the umbilical vein, ductus venosus, and portal vein; *C,* umbilical artery catheter passed up the aorta to T12. (Courtesy Walter E. Berdon, Babies Hospital: Infant with RDS. Note granular lungs, air bronchogram, and air-filled esophagus.)

ify position. In the PA view the catheter cannot be distinguished from the maze of wires attached to the thermistors (Fig. 2-2). A catheter introduced into the umbilical vein may reach a variety of positions. If advanced far enough, it will pass directly through the ductus venosus and foramen ovale into the left atrium. It may also pass into the right or left branches of the portal vein, the superior or inferior mesenteric veins, or even the splenic vein. Lodged in these areas, catheters can occlude blood flow and serve to localize any solutions infused. The ideal position for the umbilical vein catheter is just beyond the ductus venosus in the inferior vena cava.

A catheter introduced into the umbilical artery will usually pass into the aorta from the internal iliac artery. Occasionally it will pass down the femoral artery or into the gluteal artery. The two latter sites are unsuitable for sampling and pressure measurements and also for the infusion of alkali. Either of two positions in the aorta is recommended for the catheter placement—in the lower abdomen below the renal arteries and inferior mesenteric artery or just above the diaphragm. If left in the internal iliac or the region of the aortic bifurcation, the chances of arterial spasm are increased.

The status of the circulation is obviously of great importance when hypertonic or strongly alkaline solutions are administered. For this reason, the relatively rapidly moving bloodstream of the aorta is probably a safer site than the vena cava. From a clinical point of view, blood flow can be fairly reasonably assessed from blood pressure, and, if low, cardiac massage is indicated during injection. If the umbilical vein is used for infusion, the catheter should be just beyond the ductus venosus, and the alkali administered into the inferior vena cava.

Complications from umbilical catheterization

Although catheterization of the umbilical vein and artery are relatively simple maneuvers and allow easy infusion of fluids or blood sampling, the procedures are not without hazard. Complications relate to trauma during insertion, the duration of catheterization, the size of the catheters used, the state of the circulation when solutions are being infused, and the pH or tonicity of the solutions infused. Although the incidence of complications is relatively low, the procedure is not recommended as the usual route for fluid or drug therapy and should only be used in very ill infants or those at high risk when monitoring is essential for diagnosis and therapeutic management.

Acute complications

False lumen and perforation. If the lumen of the constricted artery is not localized accurately, it is possible to create a false lumen in the wall of the vessel. This may be erroneously interpreted as spasm when obstruction is met in the region of the internal iliac artery. If the catheter being inserted is rigid the vessels may be perforated at this point, the catheter passing into the abdominal cavity. If undue force is exerted, even with a soft catheter, it may track extraperitoneally and result in retroperitoneal hemorrhage.

Blanching of the limb or alteration in pulse. This complication occurs in approximately 5% of infants. It is directly related to the relative size of the catheter in the aorta. It has also been seen when a cold solution is rapidly infused into the aorta. The signs will usually disappear upon removal of the catheter. If the limb blanches, the catheter should be removed promptly. We do not advocate warming the contralateral limb as the initial effort to cause vasodilatation of the effected limb because of the higher risk with such delay.

Accidental hemorrhage. This is associated with inexperience. The incidence is negligible when physicians and nursing personnel are accustomed to the use of stopcocks and connections and are experienced in the placement of catheters.

Infection. The incidence of infection is related to the sterility conditions at the time of catheter placement and with maintenance procedures and the experience of the personnel.

Serious complications at necropsy. The incidence of serious complications at necropsy ranges from 1.5% to 7%, and appears as a significant cause of death in less than 2% of cases. The lesions include embolization, thrombosis of hepatic vein, liver necrosis, aortic thrombi, and infarcts. Aortic thrombi are the most common, and their occurrence usually increases the longer the duration of the catheterization. A serious complication observed at Babies Hospital has been thrombosis of the renal arteries and renal shutdown leading to death. In newborn monkeys where the aorta is relatively small, occlusion of the inferior mesenteric arteries by the catheter with infarction of the bowel has been observed; the presenting sign was bloody stool.

Hemorrhagic necrosis of the liver has been observed in asphyxiated newborn infants and newborn monkeys treated with strong alkalis (sodium carbonate or THAM). It was found that if the pH of THAM was lowered from 10.4 to 8.6 by titration with HCl, the hypertonic solution could be administered safely. In relating liver necrosis to catheterization and the infusion of hypertonic solutions, it should be recalled that this complication also occurs following severe asphyxia alone.

DEPRESSION FROM DRUGS VERSUS ASPHYXIA

An infant depressed primarily as a result of maternal analgesics or anesthetics can usually be distinguished by certain clinical signs from one depressed from asphyxia. The infant depressed from medication will not have passed meconium before birth; his skin may be cyanotic rather than pale since he has not received an asphyxial stimulus to cause peripheral vasoconstriction; his heart rate may be slow, but the pulse strong and full, and the cord will be filled with blood since his cardiovascular system has not been depressed by asphyxia; he will usually not be completely hypotonic.

In contrast, the infant depressed primarily as a result of asphyxia may be meconium stained and pale as a result of intense peripheral vasoconstriction; the heart rate will be slow and the sounds soft, distant, and occasionally irregular; the umbilical cord will be limp and contain little blood.

The Apgar score does not distinguish between depression from these two causes. Differentiation is useful since the medicated infant will frequently respond quite promptly to simple resuscitative procedures—stimulation and positive pressure ventilation applied with a mask. Intubation and artificial inflation of the lungs is rarely necessary. On the other hand, the severely asphyxiated infant may require not only intubation, artificial ventilation, and cardiac massage, but also correction of a severe metabolic acidosis by infusion of alkali. Recognition of the infant depressed by medication is also important if drug antagonists are to be administered.

Use of analeptics and drug antagonists

Analeptics and drug antagonists should never be administered before the lungs have been expanded and the infant oxygenated by artificial ventilation. Analeptics, such as nikethamide, are not indicated in resuscitation of the newborn. Although they may shorten primary apnea, they are ineffective in secondary apnea (p. 52) and may cause hypotension and convulsions even if given in the clinically recommended dose. The morphine antagonists nalorphine or naloxone may be of value. The former should not be given unless the infant's respiratory depression is known to be caused by maternal medication with morphine or a related agent, since an overdose can augment the depression of asphyxia. Although crying and restlessness follow administration, this is frequently of brief duration and may be followed by more profound depression. See p. 606 for dosages.

Toxicity from local anesthetics

Rarely, local anesthetics may be injected accidentally into the fetus during an attempted caudal anesthesia or paracervical block. The infant may be profoundly depressed at birth. However, as soon as he is oxygenated during the course of resuscitation and the responsiveness of the central nervous system is partially restored, generalized convulsions may occur. The presenting part of the infant should be carefully examined for a needle puncture if accidental injection is suspected, and the convulsion treated promptly with intravenous phenobarbital, 10 to 15 mg/kg. It may be necessary to repeat the barbiturate and maintain the infant on a ventilator. As soon as possible a 2 to 3 volume exchange transfusion should be performed.

Delayed depression from maternally administered analgesia and anesthesia

Drugs that cross the placenta enter the fetus through the umbilical vein (UV) and the ductus venosus. A variable portion of the UV flow passes to the inferior vena cava through the liver and hepatic veins and not through the ductus venosus. This places the liver in a strategic position for uptake of drugs, particularly those with a high fat solubility. From the liver they can be released slowly over a period of hours. Thus, infants delivered soon after the mother has been given a drug may initially appear vigorous but develop a marked central nervous system depression 2 to 4 hours later. Therefore, when relatively large doses of sedatives or narcotics have been given to the mother and the infant breathes well at birth, he should nevertheless be carefully observed for delayed secondary depression. This may be so severe as to require an exchange transfusion.

Drug-addicted newborn infant

Signs of drug withdrawal are not usually seen for 12 to 24 hours after birth (p. 450). However, if the mother has not taken a dose of narcotic recently, both mother and infant may be in a state of withdrawal at the time of delivery. Early signs include coarse, flapping tremors, jitteriness, irritability, hyperactivity, and exaggerated reflexes. Irritability is reflected in a shrill, high-pitched cry.

Specific therapy should be started only when signs have become manifest. Several drugs have been recommended, including phenobarbital, chlorpromazine, paregoric, and methadone. There is no objective evidence that indicates the superiority of one therapeutic regime over another. Phenobarbital 6 to 8 mg/kg/day in 3 to 4 divided doses is usually effective in controlling central nervous system symptoms.

ACUTE HEMORRHAGE

Acute blood loss may occur under several circumstances: placenta praevia, as a complication of fetal blood sampling, in multiple pregnancy, with cord occlusion, or at cesarean section. If the blood loss has been during the final stages of delivery, the infant will appear pale, but the onset of respiration will not be inhibited. If it has occurred at a longer interval prior to delivery and the fetus has become hypotensive, severe asphyxia will be superimposed, and the infant will be depressed and unresponsive at birth. The mechanism of blood loss in placenta praevia is obvious. Its occurrence as a complication of fetal blood sampling is described below (p. 64). However, in the other three conditions hemorrhage may not be immediately apparent or suspected. In multiple pregnancy, one fetus may bleed into another, or there may be partial placental separation with hemorrhage at the time of delivery of the first infant. Mild cord occlusion sufficient to constrict the vein but not arteries is occasionally seen; under these circumstances, the fetus literally bleeds into the placenta. Such blood loss is usually not severe, being limited by the capacity of the placental vascular bed. Blood loss at cesarean section also occurs into the placenta. When the infant is removed from the uterus, he is usually held up by the feet while the cord is clamped. In a few seconds a considerable volume of blood can flow into the placenta from the arteries, and venous blood can be prevented from returning from the placenta to the infant as a result of the hydrostatic pressure caused by the infant's being held in the air. The venous blood loss by this mechanism is usually not severe. Nevertheless, unless special precautions are taken to prevent this occurrence, such as placing the infant on the mother's abdomen and milking the umbilical cord once or twice toward the infant prior to clamping the cord, the hematocrit of the infant at 3 hours of age will be 6% to 12% lower than that in healthy infants delivered by vagina. This phenomenon does not occur in infants delivered normally, since they are usually held at the level of their mother's perineum, and the uterus, having expelled the infant, is firmly clamped on the placenta.

It is advisable to measure the hemoglobin and hematocrit in all circumstances where blood loss may have occurred if there is any abnormality such as low Apgar score, slow, delayed, or difficult breathing, pallor, or cyanosis. If there is pallor and peripheral vasoconstriction, a hematocrit from the peripheral capillaries will not be reliable and a sample should be taken from the umbilical vein as soon as is practical after delivery. If blood loss has occurred acutely at delivery, it will not be reflected in the hematocrit of central circulating blood during the first minutes of life. Therefore, measurement should be repeated at 3 hours, the time usually necessary for readjustment of blood volume and circulating red blood cells after birth. In normal infants the mean hematocrit usually increases from 48% to 52% during this time. If the hematocrit is below 40% at birth or if there is a significant fall in the first 3 hours of life, accompanied by pallor and respiratory distress, the infant should be given a transfusion of blood.

PNEUMOTHORAX AND PNEUMOMEDIASTINUM

Pneumothorax and pneumomediastinum usually occur spontaneously and in association with aspiration syndromes. Occasionally they may be a result of incorrect or injudicious resuscitative procedures. If mild they will not be recognized clinically and may only be discovered accidentally when a roentgenogram is taken of the infant for another reason.

Pneumomediastinum should be suspected if heart sounds become distant or suddenly cannot be heard in an infant who otherwise appears normal. It should also be suspected if the anteroposterior diameter is increased. No treatment is necessary. The infant should be carefully observed after a chest roentgenogram has been taken, since this complication may progress to pneumothorax.

A tension pneumothorax is a serious complication that requires immediate treatment. It presents as respiratory distress that becomes progressively more severe. The respirations are often rapid rather than labored. The heart will be shifted away from the affected side, which will move little and may appear hyperinflated. The infant usually appears pale rather than cyanotic. Since a diaphragmatic hernia may present similarly, particularly when the stomach and small bowel become filled with air, it is important to first pass a catheter into the stomach and attempt to suck out any air. If symptoms are not relieved by this procedure, a needle should be inserted into the thoracic cavity in the midaxillary line at about the level of the sixth rib and the air pressure released. Following this, a tube should be inserted surgically and connected to underwater drainage. If the pneumothorax is not under tension, it is usually possible to obtain a roentgenogram of the chest to confirm the clinical diagnosis and aid in deciding upon the management, which may require oxygen administration, needle aspiration, placement of a chest tube, or a combination of these therapies (p. 380).

SEVERE ERYTHROBLASTOSIS

In severe cases of erythroblastosis with hydrops, certain emergency procedures in the delivery room may be indicated. These all focus on promptly establishing good cardiopulmonary function and ensuring that the oxygen carrying capacity of the blood is satisfactory. If the infant is born by vagina, a blood sample should be obtained from the cord or from a peripheral venous site for a Coombs test, for determination of hemoglobin or hematocrit, and for crossmatching with compatible blood. It is also possible to obtain a sample of capillary blood from the presenting part prior to delivery. If delivery is by cesarean section, O negative blood compatible with the mother's should be available before delivery. The red blood cells should be partially packed. The blood should be in readiness on the resuscitation table together with umbilical catheters, a laryngoscope, an endotracheal tube, and a 20-gauge needle.

As soon as the infant is delivered he should be intubated, the lungs expanded, and positive pressure ventilation initiated. This is necessary since these infants are prone to develop pulmonary edema because lung capillary permeability is increased and serum proteins are usually low. If there is marked abdominal distension from ascites or a recent intrauterine infusion of blood, a 20-gauge needle should be inserted in the lateral flank to remove fluid and relieve pressure on the diaphragm. We do not recommend removal of fluid from the thoracic cavity as a blind emergency procedure, although it is usually present in such infants. Positive pressure ventilation should be continued until the infant is stabilized in the neonatal intensive care unit and he can be closely observed for the development of pulmonary edema.

During the initial resuscitation, blood should be withdrawn from a clamped segment of the cord for measurement of the central hematocrit and from the umbilical artery for a pH measurement. These results should be available to the physician within 5 to 6 minutes of delivery. If the infant is severely anemic, both umbilical vein and artery should be quickly catheterized and the blood administered through the vein, approximately 20 ml/kg, while an equal quantity is slowly withdrawn from the artery. The speed of infusion and withdrawal should be about 10 ml/min in order to avoid any sudden change in hemodynamics. If a hematocrit has been obtained from fetal capillary blood during labor, catheterization and administration of blood can proceed while the infant is being intubated and ventilated. Freshly drawn heparinized blood is desirable but is rarely available in the delivery room. This will have a pH in the range of 7.3. CPD blood that has a pH of about 7.25 is an adequate substitute for heparinized blood. If only citrated blood is available the pH will be 6.9 or less. This pH should be corrected with sodium bicarbonate or THAM (tris [hydroxymethyl] aminomethane). Citrated blood also has a high potassium content.

During these procedures, every effort should be made to prevent heat loss by having a warm container ready for the infant, with an overhead radiant heat source turned on well in advance of delivery. Prompt oxygenation and restoration of the oxygen-carrying capacity of the blood is essential if these infants are to be given an optimal chance to survive. (For further discussion of erythroblastosis, see p. 183.)

IMMATURE INFANT

Immature infants require the application of all of the principles of resuscitation described above. Because of their relatively large surface area, particular attention should be paid to preventing heat loss by drying the infant promptly and ensuring that the resuscitation area is warmed with a radiant heater and is as draft free as possible. This is sometimes difficult in modern air-conditioned delivery rooms. The small size of the infant and the delicacy of immature tissues demand greater manual dexterity and gentleness if intubation is to be performed rapidly and without trauma. Intubation, if necessary, is facilitated by the physician placing the fifth finger of the left hand, which holds the laryngoscope, over the larynx. Gentle pressure on the larynx as the blade is titled will bring the glottis into view.

COMPLICATIONS OF FETAL BLOOD SAMPLING

Two major types of complications following fetal blood sampling have been observed. The first is abscess formation in the area of the sampling incision, and the second is hemorrhage from the incision itself. These complications have occurred in about 1% of cases.

Abscess formation has been seen where the incision was made in an area that had been previously traumatized, with the subsequent formation of a cephalhematoma, or where the tissue had become traumatized during delivery, either from the application of forceps or a vacuum extractor at the incision site. There also appears to be an increased risk of infection following sampling in the breech presentation since healing of incisions in the sacral region is poor. Although there is no way to be certain that bacteria are introduced at the time of sampling, the fact that abscesses do occur underscores the importance of careful aseptic techniques in the fetal blood sampling procedure.

The second type of complication from fetal blood sampling is hemorrhage from the incision. This may occur if the incision is made over a small artery. It will usually stop when firm pressure is applied, but occasionally the incision may have to be sutured. Hemorrhage from an incision is a potentially lethal complication. It is important that the incision area be observed directly for 2 or 3 contractions after a blood sample has been taken to ensure that hemostasis is present. Clotting studies have been abnormal in a number of infants who have bled from the scalp sampling site. Most of the infants reported to have bled following fetal scalp sampling have suffered from chronic intrauterine asphyxiation, and this is sometimes associated with depletion or deficiency in certain clotting factors, particularly the labile factors V and VII. It is therefore important that neonates who bleed readily from sampling incisions should have at least a screening coagulation study. Postnatal bleeding from a sampling incision may be the first manifestation of a severe neonatal coagulation disorder.

If the scalp appears pale when visualized through the amnioscope and does not blanch when compressed by the instrument, severe peripheral vasoconstriction and hypotension is likely. Under these circumstances it may be difficult to obtain blood when an incision is made. If blood does not flow readily from the first incision, the temptation is to make multiple incisions. However, after delivery and alleviation of asphyxia, the peripheral circulation will improve; the infant then may bleed from several sites and sustain substantial blood loss.

Maternal intrapartum or postpartum infection has been seen more frequently in those infants who develop complications from fetal blood sampling. Therefore, infants whose mothers develop infections should be observed very closely for infection or hemorrhage at the site of a sampling incision.

DIAGNOSIS OF CONGENITAL ANOMALIES

Incidence

The incidence of congenital defects has been estimated to be between 1% and 7% of all live births. This incidence will depend upon the kind of conditions that are included, but it is probably fair to state that 2% to 3% of all live-born infants show one or more significant congenital malformations that may require medical attention soon after birth. Disorders of the skeleton are the commonest of these malformations and comprise approximately one third of all defects. Most of these can be seen or felt and can be verified by roentgenography. However a number of defects are not immediately apparent on visual examination. These may be called the hidden congenital anomalies. Prompt diagnosis of these anomalies in the immediate neonatal period is possible by the use of simple technical maneuvers.

About 20% of deaths in the third trimester of gestation and about 15% in the neonatal period may be attributed to gross congenital malformations. Prompt diagnosis of the anomalies as soon as the patient is born may enable lifesaving medical and surgical treatment to be instituted.

Equipment

A standard clinical stethoscope, a sterile No. 12 soft plastic catheter with two terminal holes and a visible trap, and an infant laryngoscope with a light near the tip of the blade are useful aids in evaluating infants in the delivery room for life-threatening congenital anomalies.

Polyhydramnios

A congenital anomaly should be suspected if the mother has either polyhydramnios or oligohydramnios.

CONGENITAL ANOMALIES ASSOCIATED WITH HYDRAMNIOS

A. Anencephaly
B. Hydrocephaly
C. Microcephaly
D. Spina bifida
E. Mongolism
F. Volvulus
    1. With atretic upper jejunum
    2. With congenital bands of upper jejunum
    3. With common mesentery and herniation of liver
G. Tracheoesophageal fistula with atretic esophagus
H. Imperforate anus
I. Cleft palate
J. Congenital heart disease
K. Pyloric stenosis
L. Genitourinary disease
M. Deformed extremities
N. Agenesis of ears
    1. Oligohydramnios is frequently associated with renal agenesis or other anomalies of the genitourinary tract. (See below.)

Choanal atresia and laryngeal stenosis

During the initial appraisal of the newborn infant, particular attention should be paid to the evenness and ease of respiration. If respiratory difficulty is present and persists after pharyngeal suctioning, choanal atresia or laryngeal stenosis should be suspected. Although rare, these anomalies are emergencies. Choanal atresia is a bony or membranous obstruction between the nose and pharynx. Clinically, although the airway from the mouth to the larynx is patent, this anomaly results in complete respiratory obstruction, since infants are obligatory nose breathers. Respiratory difficulty at birth is usually of such a degree that it requires intubation and artificial ventilation. Once breathing is established, choanal atresia is most simply diagnosed by occluding the mouth and the right or left nostril. It may also be diagnosed by inserting a catheter first into one nostril and then into the other, then ventromedially along the floor of the nose. The catheter should pass with ease for 3 to 4 cm. If this cannot be achieved, atresia is probably present. A temporary airway should be promptly provided. This is best achieved by inserting a small plastic infant airway between the tongue and the palate. Once ventilation is established the infant will then breathe through his mouth while awake. During sleep, however, he will attempt to revert to his obligatory nose breathing. The recommended treatment is prompt surgical removal of the bony obstruction.

If laryngeal stenosis is present, it will be immediately recognized when the glottis is visualized with the laryngoscope. Immediate tracheostomy is imperative. Under these emergency conditions this is most easily done through the cricothyroid membrane.

Diaphragmatic hernia and congenital adenomatous lung cysts

A diaphragmatic hernia with abdominal viscera in the chest or congenital cysts of the lungs may cause immediate respiratory difficulty. The lungs may be hypoplastic if the diaphragmatic hernia is large and bilateral. These two congenital anomalies are likely to be diagnosed during the course of resuscitation. Following intubation for respiratory difficulty, strong resistance is felt when an attempt is made to expand the lungs by positive pressure. Two other conditions must be considered in the differential diagnosis of this type of respiratory obstruction: massive aspiration of meconium that cannot be removed by suctioning and intrauterine pneumonia with organization of exudate. Infants with hypoplastic lungs or congenital adenomatous cysts of the lungs may be vigorous initially and score as high as 7 at 1 minute of age, making strenuous but ineffective respiratory efforts. In contrast, infants with meconium aspiration or intrauterine pneumonia are usually severely depressed at birth. Congenital adenomatous cysts of the lungs may be associated with hydrops.

A small or unilateral diaphragmatic hernia not associated with a hypoplastic lung may not be apparent initially. However, with deep respiratory efforts, additional gut may be drawn into the thorax from the abdomen and prevent lung expansion on one side. This is usually manifest in the first 10 to 15 minutes of life as respiratory difficulty and may be verified by observing asymmetry of chest movement and diminution or absence of air sounds on the affected side.

In some circumstances the diaphragmatic hernia is not apparent for the first 30 to 60 minutes of life or even later. Manifestation of the anomaly in these instances appears to be dependent on the infant's swallowing air and the gradual distention of gut in the thorax by this swallowed air. The diagnosis is then verified by the presence of borborygmus in the chest.

Tracheoesophageal fistula

Atresia of the esophagus with tracheoesophageal fistula should be looked for in every baby. As soon as good ventilation is established, a catheter should be introduced into the mouth on either the left or right side of the tongue and advanced down into the esophagus and stomach. The outline of the tip of the catheter is usually seen in the left half of the abdomen as it is gently advanced. If not, the examiner's hand is placed over the upper quadrant, and a puff of air is blown into the catheter. A bubble is immediately felt. It may also be detected by listening over the stomach with a stethoscope. If the catheter does not enter the stomach, the esophagus probably ends in a blind pouch. The longer this anomaly remains undiagnosed the greater is the risk of aspiration pneumonia. Even if the infant is not fed, this is likely to occur as a result of the acid gastric content passing up the lower segment of the esophagus and through the fistula into the trachea and lungs. An operation should be performed between 12 to 24 hours after birth, the short delay allowing the infant to achieve initial adaptation to extrauterine life. In rare instances a fistula occurs with a patent esophagus. These patients are difficult to diagnose. The anomaly should be suspected if the infant coughs during feeding. It may be verified using a barium swallow and cineradiography.

Anomalies of the upper GI tract

If complete intestinal obstruction is above the midjejunum, the stomach may contain a large volume of fluid. The average volume of fluid found in healthy infants delivered by the vaginal route is 5.7 ml (range 1 to 20 ml); for those delivered by breech, 4.3 ml; and for those delivered by cesarean section, 7.2 ml (range 0 to 50 ml). The smallest amount of fluid that has been associated with a high gastrointestinal obstruction has been 38 ml. A catheter should be passed into the newborn infant's stomach and the contents removed. If more than 15 ml of fluid are present in the stomach, a roentgenogram of the abdomen should be obtained during the first 3 hours of life to detect the presence of gas. The absence of gas below the pylorus may indicate obstruction and necessitate early exploration. Under normal circumstances the upper intestine is filled with air within 3 hours. When obstruction is present the roentgenogram has an even, flat, opaque appearance. A small amount of contrast air is seen only in the stomach. Duodenal jejunal atresia, malrotation of the gut, or an annular pancreas may be the cause.

As noted above, the presence of high gastrointestinal obstructions should be suspected if the mother has polyhydramnios. Normally there is a constant equilibrium of amniotic fluid between the mother and baby. Swallowing of fluid by the fetus and absorption from his intestinal tract into the circulation is one of the principal modes by which fluid returns to the placenta and finally to the mother. Any anomaly of the gastrointestinal tract that interferes with this process may cause amniotic fluid to accumulate and produce polyhydramnios. Central nervous system anomalies that interfere with swallowing may also produce polyhydramnios. In these cases as much as 170 ml of fluid has been aspirated from the baby's stomach.

Perforation of the stomach by the catheter may occur in the newborn period, but this is extremely rare and is usually caused by a deficiency in the muscular wall or a stress ulcer. Provided the catheter used for gastric aspiration is soft and flexible there is little danger of perforation.

Anal atresia

Finally, the catheter should be used to rule out anal atresia. With the infant's thighs flexed, the physician introduces the catheter through the anal opening as far as it can easily be passed. If it passes for 3 cm, obstruction is unlikely. If, however, the cloacal membrane has failed to rupture, there may be no anal outlet. Most rectal atresias occur within the distal 2 cm. They are often accompanied by urologic abnormalities (p. 494). If this anomaly is suspected the urine should be examined for squamous cells or meconium debris that may enter the bladder through an rectovesicular or rectovaginal fistula. Immediate surgery is indicated.

Skeletal anomalies

Following these simple diagnostic procedures with the catheter, the infant should be carefully examined for anomalies of the skeleton. They are usually readily verified visually or by palpation. The association between chromosomal abnormalities and congenital defects particularly relates to the skeletal system; examples are trisomy of chromosomes No. 13 to 15, chromosomes No. 17 to 18, mongolism, Turner's syndrome, Albright's hereditary osteodystrophy, and polydysspondylism. Some patients with triple X chromosomes have been shown to have radioulnar synostosis.

The anterior fontanelle is normally open and should be palpated for size and tension. Bulging is diagnostic of increased intracranial pressure and may indicate hydrocephalus and intracranial hemorrhage. The posterior fontanelle is normally closed and is frequently difficult to outline because of scalp edema. A small or closed anterior fontanelle occurs in craniosynostosis and is not infrequently accompanied by microcephaly or an abnormally shaped head. Soft spots in the skull (craniotabes), usually located in the parietal areas, are present in about one third of all newborn infants. Rarely, a cranial bone may be absent, indicating osteogenesis imperfecta.

The sacral region should be examined for pigmentation and abnormal hair, which is commonly associated with occult spina bifida. If present, a roentgenogram of the spine should be taken.

Cleft palate

The mouth should be carefully examined for the presence of a cleft palate. This may occur even if the upper lip is normal. A small-sized laryngoscope with a premature blade is an ideal instrument with which to visualize both the hard and soft palate. The extent of the defects may vary from a small round hole to a large triangular opening with the base at the site of the uvula. Although treatment for this anomaly is not an emergency, feeding problems and an increased risk of aspiration may be anticipated.

Anomalies of the genitourinary system

Appreciation of the position and shape of the external ear is important because these malformations are associated with renal anomalies. If the ears are low set or the configuration is deformed, the umbilical cord should be examined for the absence of one umbilical artery. The infant should be closely observed for the passage of urine. The abdomen should be carefully palpated, both for the verification of normal position of the liver and spleen and for the presence of abnormal masses. In the first few minutes of life, before the infant has swallowed sufficient gas to distend the gut and while the tone of the abdominal wall is somewhat reduced, the kidneys may be readily felt for verification of their normal position, size, and shape.

Congenital obstruction of the bladder outlet or urethra will usually be associated with a distended bladder readily palpable as a firm, central, dome-shaped structure in the lower abdomen. Finally the umbilical, inguinal, and femoral regions should be examined for hernias. The presence of both testes in the scrotum should be determined and the possibility of hypospadias should be evaluated.

CONCLUSION

The outcome of a difficult and complex resuscitation is not always a happy one. With the introduction of new life-saving techniques that include more effective and efficient artificial ventilation, cardiac massage, and correction of pH, we now have the means of salvaging infants with brain damage who would otherwise have died. The decision not to resuscitate an infant is an extremely difficult one. The answer to this dilemma undoubtedly lies in the development of better means of diagnosing congenital anomalies, assessing the fetal condition prior to the onset of labor, measuring the capacity of the placenta to support the infant during labor, and evaluating the fetus as labor progresses. These measures will provide the obstetrician with more information from which he can make the best judgment in order to deliver the infant in optimal condition. When these advances in preventive medicine are achieved and introduced into obstetric practice, the birth of severely asphyxiated infants requiring a complex resuscitation should become a rare occurrence.

L. STANLEY JAMES

BIBLIOGRAPHY

Adamsons, K., Behrman, R., Dawes, G. S., Dawkins, M. J. R., James, L. S., and Ross, B.: The treatment of acidosis with alkali and glucose during asphyxia in fetal rhesus monkeys, J. Physiol. (Lond.) **169**:679, 1963.

Adamsons, K., Behrman, R., Dawes, G. S., James, L. S., and Koford, C.: Resuscitation by positive pressure ventilation and Tris-hydroxymethylaminomethane of rhesus monkeys asphyxiated at birth, J. Pediatr. **65**:807, 1964.

Adamsons, K., Gandy, G., and James, L. S.: The influence of thermal factors upon oxygen consumption of the newborn infant, J. Pediatr. **66**: 495, 1965.

Apgar, V., Holaday, D. A., James, L. S., Weisbrot, I. M., and Berrien, C.: Evaluation of the newborn infant—second report, J.A.M.A. **168**:1985, 1958.

Apgar, V., and James, L. S.: Further observations on the newborn scoring system, Amer. J. Dis. Child. **104**:419, 1962.

Baker, D. H., Berdon, W. E., and James, L. S.: Proper localization of umbilical arterial and venous catheters by lateral roentgenograms, Pediatrics **43**:34, 1969.

Cockburn, F., Daniel, S. S., Dawes, G. S., James, L. S., Meyers, R. E., Niemann, W., Rodriguez de Curet, H., and Ross, B.: The effect of pentobarbital anesthesia on resuscitation and brain damage in fetal rhesus monkeys asphyxiated on delivery, J. Pediatr. **75**:281, 1969.

Daniel, S. S., Dawes, G. S., James, L. S., and Ross, B.: Analeptics and resuscitation of asphyxiated monkeys, Br. Med. J. **2**:562, 1966.

Gandy, G. M., Adamsons, K., Cunningham, N., Silverman, W. A., and James, L. S.: Thermal environment and acid-base homeostasis in human infants during the first few hours of life, J. Clin. Invest. **43**:751, 1964.

James, L. S.: Acidosis of the newborn and its relation to birth asphyxia, Acta Paediat. (Upps.) **49**(Suppl. 122):17, 1960.

James, L. S.: Physiology of respiration in newborn infants and in the respiratory distress syndrome, Pediatrics **24**:1969, 1959.

James, L. S., and Adamsons, K.: Respiratory physiology of the fetus and newborn infant, New Eng. J. Med. **271**:1403, 1964.

Moya, F., Apgar, V., James, L. S., and Berrien, C.: Hydramnios and congenital anomalies, J.A.M.A. **173**:1552, 1960.

Moya, F., James, L. S., Burnard, E. D., and Hanks, E. C.: Cardiac massage in the newborn infant through the intact chest, Am. J. Obstet Gynecol. **84**:798, 1962.

3 Birth injuries

Birth injuries are those sustained during the birth process (including labor and delivery). They may be avoidable, or they may be unavoidable and occur despite skilled and competent obstetrical care, as in an especially hard or prolonged labor or with an abnormal presentation. Fetal injuries related to amniocentesis, intrauterine transfusions, and fetal scalp vein sampling, and neonatal injuries following resuscitation procedures are not considered birth injuries. Factors predisposing the infant to birth injury include macrosomatia, prematurity, cephalopelvic disproportion, dystocia, prolonged labor, and abnormal presentation.

The incidence of birth injuries is 2 to 7 per 1,000 live births. In a recent autopsy study, Valdes-Dapena and Arey found birth injuries in 2% of all infants studied and in 11% of those weighing over 2,500 gm. Birth injuries rank eighth in importance as a cause of neonatal mortality; in the group weighing over 2,500 gm, they rank fourth. These figures represent a decreased incidence in recent years. This has been attributed to refinements in obstetrical techniques, the increased choice of cesarean section over difficult vaginal deliveries, and elimination (or decreased use) of difficult forceps, vacuum extractors, and version and extraction.

Despite this decrease, birth injuries still represent an important problem to the clinician. They are frequently readily apparent to the parents, provoking anxiety and providing the clinician with the opportunity to provide important counseling and supportive service. Many of the injuries are mild and self-limited; observation is often the best treatment. However, some injuries may be latent and initially subtle, only to develop manifestations suddenly, with rapid progression.

INJURIES TO SOFT TISSUES

Erythema and abrasions

Erythema and abrasions frequently occur when there has been dystocia during labor secondary to cephalopelvic disproportion or when forceps have been used during delivery. Injuries secondary to dystocia occur over the presenting part; forceps injury occurs at the site of application of the instrument. The latter injury frequently has a linear configuration across both sides of the face outlining the position of the forceps. The affected areas should be kept clean to minimize the risk of secondary infection. These lesions usually resolve spontaneously within several days with no specific therapy.

Petechiae

Occasionally, petechiae are present over the head, neck, upper chest, and lower back at birth following a difficult delivery; they are more frequently observed after breech deliveries.

Etiology. Petechiae are probably caused by a sudden increase in intrathoracic and venous pressures during passage of the chest through the birth canal. Infants born with the cord tightly wound around their neck may have petechiae only above the neck.

Differential diagnosis. Petechiae may be a manifestation of an underlying hemorrhagic disorder. The birth history, early appearances of the petechiae, and absence of bleeding from other sites help to differentiate petechiae secondary to increased tissue pressure or trauma from petechiae caused by hemorrhagic disease of the newborn (p. 209). The localized distribution of the petechiae, the absence of subsequent crops of new lesions, and a normal platelet count exclude neonatal thrombocytopenia. The platelet count may also be low secondary to infections or disseminated intravascular coagulation. The former may be clinically distinguished from traumatic petechiae by the presence of other signs and symptoms (p. 131). The latter is usually associated with excessive and persistent bleeding from a variety of sites. Petechiae are usually distributed over the entire body when associated with systemic disease.

Treatment. If the petechiae are caused by trauma, neither steroids nor heparin should be used. No specific treatment is necessary.

Prognosis. Traumatic petechiae usually fade within 2 to 3 days.

Ecchymoses

Ecchymoses may occur after traumatic or breech deliveries. The incidence is increased in premature infants, especially after a rapid labor and poorly controlled delivery. When extensive, ecchymoses may reflect blood loss severe enough to cause anemia and, rarely, shock. The reabsorption of blood from an ecchymotic area may result in significant hyperbilirubinemia (Fig. 3-1).

Treatment. The rise in serum bilirubin that follows severe bruising may be decreased by the use of phototherapy (p. 229). Ecchymoses rarely result in significant anemia.

Prognosis. No local therapy is necessary; the ecchymoses usually resolve spontaneously within 1 week.

Subcutaneous fat necrosis

Subcutaneous fat necrosis is characterized by well-circumscribed indurated lesions of the skin and underlying tissue.

Etiology. Obstetrical trauma is the most likely cause of subcutaneous fat necrosis. Many of the affected infants are large and have been delivered by forceps or after a prolonged, difficult labor involving

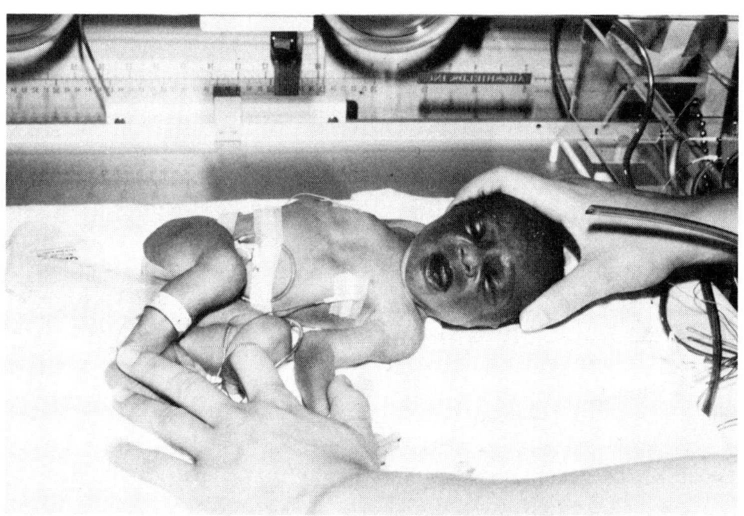

Fig. 3-1. Marked bruising of the entire face in 1,490-gm female born vaginally after face presentation. Less severe ecchymoses were present on the extremities. Despite use of phototherapy from the first day, icterus was noted on the third day, and exchange transfusions were required on the fifth and sixth days.

vigorous fetal manipulation. The distribution of the lesions is usually related to the site of trauma. Other etiologic factors that have been implicated include hypoxia, local ischemia, and excessive cooling.

Pathology. Initially, histopathologic studies reveal endothelial swelling and perivascular inflammation in the subcutaneous tissues. This is followed by necrosis of fat and a dense granulomatous inflammatory infiltrate containing foreign-body-type giant cells with needle-shaped crystals resembling cholesterol.

Clinical manifestations. Necrotic areas usually appear between 6 to 10 days of age but may be noted as early as the second day or as late as the sixth week. They occur on the cheeks, neck, back, shoulders, arms, buttocks, thighs, and feet, with relative sparing of the chest and abdomen. The lesions vary in size from 1 to 10 cm; rarely, they may be more extensive. They are irregularly shaped, hard, plaque-like, and nonpitting (Fig. 3-2). The overlying skin may be colorless, red, or purple. The affected areas may be slightly elevated above the adjacent skin; small lesions may be easily movable in all directions. There is no local tenderness or increase in skin temperature.

Differential diagnosis. The differential diagnosis includes nodular nonsuppurative panniculitis, lipogranulomatosis, and sclerema neonatorum. Panniliculitis is usually associated with fever, hepatosplenomegaly and tender skin nodules. The latter two diagnoses have a grave prognosis.

Treatment. These lesions require only observation. Surgical excision is not indicated.

Prognosis. The lesions slowly soften after 6 to 8 weeks and completely regress within several months. Occasionally, minimal residual atrophy, with or without small calcified areas, is observed.

Lacerations

Accidental lacerations may be inflicted with a scalpel during cesarean section. They usually occur on the scalp, buttocks, and thighs, but may occur on any part of the body. If the wound is superficial, the edges may be held in apposition with butterfly adhesive strips. Deeper, more freely bleeding wounds should be sutured with the finest material available, preferably 7-0 nylon. Rarely, the amount of blood loss and depth of wound require suturing in the delivery room. After repair, the wound should be left uncovered unless it is in an area of potential soiling such as the perineal area; in such locations the wound should be sprayed with protective plastic. Healing is usually rapid, and the sutures may be removed after 5 days.

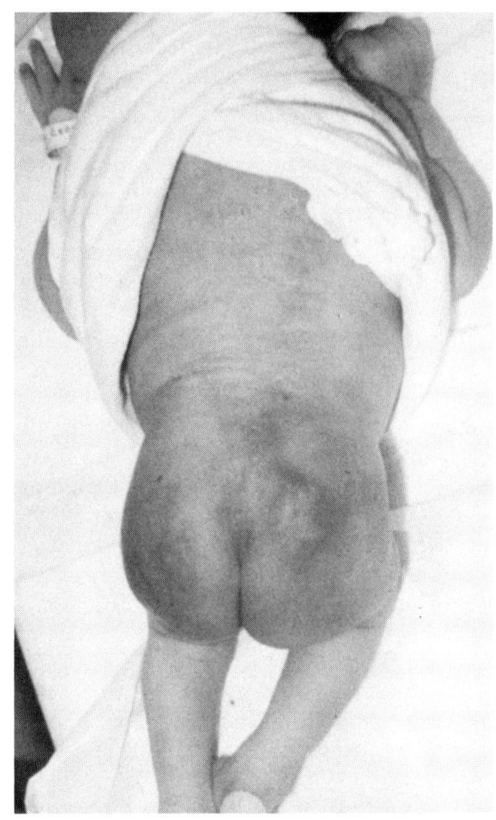

Fig. 3-2. Subcutaneous fat necrosis in 2,900-gm, full-term infant delivered vaginally; pregnancy, labor, and delivery were completely uncomplicated. Note nodular raised lesion over the right buttock that is surrounded by erythema (darkened area). (Courtesy Dr. Rajam Ramamurthy, Cook County Hospital, Chicago.)

INJURIES TO THE HEAD

Skull

Caput succedaneum

Caput succedaneum, a frequent lesion, is characterized by a vaguely demarcated area of edema over that portion of the scalp that was the presenting part during a vertex delivery.

Etiology. Serum or blood or both accumulate above the periosteum in the presenting part during labor. This extravasation results from the higher pressure of the uterus or vaginal wall on those areas of the fetal head that border the caput. Thus, in a left occiput-transverse presentation, the caput succedaneum occurs over the upper and posterior aspect of the right parietal bone; in a right-sided presentation it occurs over the corresponding area of the left parietal bone.

Clinical manifestations. The soft swelling is usually a few millimeters thick and may be associated with overlying petechiae, purpura, or ecchymoses. Because of its location external to the periosteum, a caput succedaneum may extend across the midline of the skull and across suture lines. After especially difficult labors, an extensive caput may obscure various sutures and fontanelles.

Differential diagnosis. Occasionally a caput succedaneum may be difficult to distinguish from a cephalhematoma, particularly when the latter occurs bilaterally. Careful palpation usually indicates whether the bleeding is external to the periosteum (a caput), or beneath the periosteum (a cephalhematoma).

Treatment. Usually no specific treatment is indicated. Rarely a hemorrhagic caput may result in shock and require blood transfusion.

Prognosis. A caput succedaneum usually resolves within several days.

Cephalhematoma

Cephalhematoma is an infrequently seen subperiosteal collection of blood overlying a cranial bone. The incidence is 0.4% to 2.5% of live births; the frequency is higher in male infants and in infants born to primiparous mothers.

Etiology. A cephalhematoma is caused during labor or delivery by a rupture of blood vessels that traverse from skull to periosteum. Repeated buffeting of the fetal skull against the maternal pelvis during a prolonged or difficult labor and mechanical trauma caused by use of forceps in delivery have been implicated.

Clinical manifestations. The bleeding is sharply limited by periosteal attachments to the surface of one cranial bone; there is no extension across suture lines. The bleeding usually occurs over one or both parietal bones. Less commonly it involves the occipital bones and, very rarely, the frontal bones. The overlying scalp is not discolored. Because subperiosteal bleeding is slow, the swelling may not be apparent for several hours or days after birth. The swelling is often larger on the second or third day, when sharply demarcated boundaries are palpable. The cephalhematoma may feel fluctuant and is often bordered by a slightly elevated ridge of organizing tissue that gives the false sensation of a central bony depression. An underlying skull fracture is present in about 25% of cephalhematomas; these fractures are almost always linear and nondepressed.

Roentgenographic manifestations. Roentgenographic manifestations vary with the age of the cephalhematoma. During the first 2 weeks, bloody fluid results in a shadow of water density. At the end of the second week bone begins to form under the elevated pericranium at the margins of the hematoma; the entire lesion is progressively overlaid with a complete shell of bone.

Differential diagnosis. A cephalhematoma may be differentiated from caput succedaneum by: (1) its sharp periosteal limitations to one bone, (2) the absence of overlying discoloration, (3) the later initial appearance of the swelling, and (4) the longer time period before resolution. Cranial meningocele is differentiated from cephalhematoma by pulsations, increase in pressure during crying, and the demonstration of a bony defect on x-ray film. An occipital cephalhematoma may be confused initially with an occipital meningocele and with cranium bifidum because both occupy the midline position.

Treatment. Treatment is not indicated for the uncomplicated cephalhematoma. Rarely, a massive cephalhematoma may result in blood loss severe enough to require transfusion. Significant hyperbilirubinemia may also result, necessitating phototherapy or other treatment of jaundice (p. 225).

The most common associated complications are skull fracture and intracranial hemorrhage. Linear fractures do not require specific therapy, but roentgenograms should be taken at 4 to 6 weeks to ensure closure and to exclude formation of leptomeningeal cysts; depressed fractures require immediate neurosurgical consultation. Specific treatment for blood loss or hyperbilirubinemia or both may be indicated if there has been an intracranial hemorrhage. Incision or aspiration of a cephalhematoma is contraindicated because of the risk of introducing infection. Rarely, bacterial infections of cephalhematomas occur, usually in association with septicemia and meningitis. Focal infection should be suspected when there is a sudden enlargement of a static cephalhematoma during the course of a systemic infection, a relapse of meningitis or sepsis after treatment with antibiotics, or the development of local signs of infection over the cephalhematoma. Diagnostic aspiration may then be indicated. If a local infection is present, surgical drainage and specific antibiotic therapy should be instituted.

Prognosis. Most cephalhematomas are resorbed within 2 weeks to 3 months, depending upon their size; the majority are resorbed by 6 weeks. In a few patients, calcium is deposited (Fig. 3-3), causing a bony swelling that may persist for several months and, rarely, up to 1½ years.

Roentgenographic findings persist after disappearance of clinical signs. The outer table remains thickened as a flat irregular hyperostosis for several months. There may be a persistent (for years) widening of the space between the new shell of bone and the inner table; the space originally occupied by hematoma usually develops into normal diploic bone, but cystlike defects

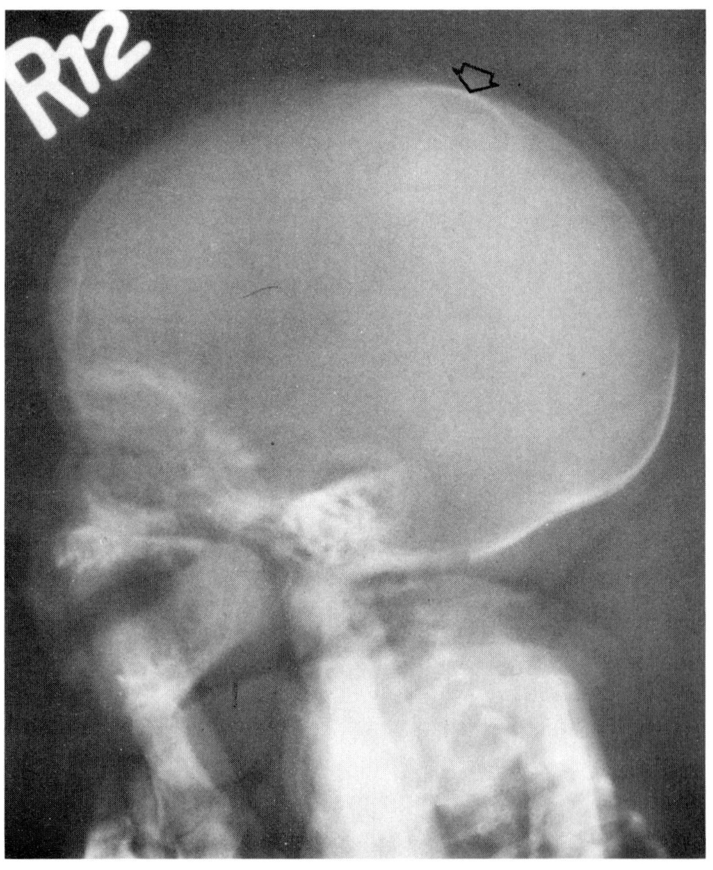

Fig. 3-3. Calcified cephalhematoma in left parietal region of 5-week-old female. Infant weighed 1,410 gm at birth and was delivered rapidly because of prolapsed cord. Hard left parietal swelling was detected at 5 weeks by nurses while feeding the infant.

may persist at the sites of the hematoma for months or years. Rarely, a neonatal cephalhematoma may persist into adult life as a symptomless mass, the cephalhematoma deformans of Schüller.

Skull fractures

Fracture of the neonatal skull is uncommon, since the bones of the skull are less mineralized at birth and thus more compressible. In addition, the separation of the bones by membranous sutures usually permits enough alteration in the contour of the head to allow its passage through the birth canal without injury.

Etiology. Skull fractures usually follow a forceps delivery or a prolonged, difficult labor with repeated forceful contact of the fetal skull against the maternal symphysis pubis, sacral promontory, or ischial spines. Most of the fractures are linear. Depressed fractures almost always result from forceps application. Occipital bone fractures usually occur in breech deliveries as a consequence of traction on the hyperextended spine of the infant when the head is fixed in the maternal pelvis.

Clinical manifestations. Linear fractures over the convexity of the skull are frequently accompanied by soft tissue changes and cephalhematoma. Usually the infant's behavior is normal unless there is an associated concussion or hemorrhge into the subdural or suarachnoid space. Fractures at the base of the skull with separation of the basal and squamous portions of the occipital bone almost always result in severe hemorrhage caused by disruption of the underlying venous sinuses. The infant may develop shock, neurologic abnormalities, and drainage of bloody cerebrospinal fluid from the ears or nose.

Depressed fractures are visible and palpable indentations in the smooth contour of the skull, similar to dents in a Ping-Pong ball. The infant may be entirely asymptomatic unless there is associated intracranial injury.

Roentgenographic manifestations. The diagnosis of a simple linear or fissure fracture is seldom made without roentgenograms, where they appear as lines and strips of decreased density. Depressed fractures appear as lines of increased density. On some views they are manifested by an inward buckling of bone with or without an actual break in continuity. Either type of fracture may be seen on only one view.

Differential diagnosis. Occasionally the fragments of a linear fracture may be widely separated and simulate an open suture. Conversely, parietal foramina, the interparietal fontanelle, mendosal sutures, and innominate synchondroses may be mistaken for fractures. In addition, normal vascular grooves, "ripple lines" that represent soft tissue folds of the scalp, and lacunar skull may be mistaken for fractures.

Treatment. Uncomplicated linear fractures over the convexity of the skull usually do not require treatment. Fractures at the base of the skull often necessitate blood replacement for severe hemorrhage and shock, in addition to other supportive measures. If cerebrospinal fluid rhinorrhea or otorrhea is present, antimicrobial coverage is indicated to prevent secondary infection of the meninges.

Comminuted or large fractures associated with neurologic signs or symptoms usually should be treated by immediate surgical elevation of the indented segment to prevent cortical injury from pressure. Small "Ping-Pong" fractures requiring no treatment may be observed. Several nonsurgical methods exist for elevation of depressed skull fractures in infants:

1. A thumb is placed on opposite margins of the depression and gentle, firm pressure exerted towards the middle. After several minutes of continuous pressure the area of depression gradually disappears.
2. A hand breast pump is applied to the depressed area. Petroleum jelly placed on the pump edges assures a tighter seal, and gentle suction for several minutes results in elevation of the depressed bone.

Since these methods are technically easier and less traumatic, they may be preferable to surgical intervention in an asymptomatic infant with an isolated lesion.

Prognosis. Simple linear fractures usually heal within several months without sequelae. Rarely, a leptomeningeal cyst may develop from an associated dural tear and protrusion of meninges or part of the brain through the fracture. The fracture line may widen rapidly within weeks or a large defect in the skull may be noted many months later. If detected early, the cyst may be excised successfully and brain atrophy prevented. It is, therefore, advisable to repeat skull roentgenograms within 2 to 3 months to detect early widening of the fracture line.

Basal fractures carry a grave prognosis. When separation of the basal and squamous portions of the occipital bone occurs, the outcome is almost always fatal; surviving infants have an extremely high incidence of neurologic sequelae.

The prognosis for a depressed fracture is usually good when treatment is early and adequate. When therapy is delayed, especially with a large depression, death may occur from pressure on vital areas of the brain. Delayed therapy or simple observation of smaller lesions may result in subtle neurologic sequelae that may not become apparent until years later.

Intracranial hemorrhage

See Chapter 17, pp. 527-529.

Face

Facial nerve palsy

Facial nerve palsy in the neonate may follow birth injury or, rarely, may result from agenesis of the facial nerve nucleus. The latter condition is occasionally hereditary but usually sporadic.

Etiology. Traumatic facial nerve palsy most commonly follows compression of the peripheral portion of the nerve, either near the stylomastoid foramen through which it emerges or where the nerve traverses the ramus of the mandible. The nerve may be compressed by forceps, especially when the fetal head has been grasped obliquely. The condition also occurs after spontaneous deliveries following prolonged pressure by the maternal sacral promontory. Less commonly, injury is sustained in utero, often in association with a mandibular deformity, by the persistent position of the fetal foot against the superior ramus of the mandible. An extremely rare cause is the pressure of a uterine tumor on the nerve.

Less frequently than a peripheral nerve injury, a traumatic facial nerve palsy may follow a contralateral injury to the central nervous system such as a temporal bone fracture or hemorrhage or tissue destruction or both to structures within the posterior fossa.

Clinical manifestations. Paralysis is usually apparent on the first or second day, but may be present at birth. It usually does not increase in severity unless there is considerable edema over the area of nerve trauma. The type and distribution of paralysis is different for central facial paralysis compared to peripheral paralysis.

Central paralysis is a spastic paralysis limited to the lower half or two thirds of the contralateral side of the face. The paralyzed side is smooth and full and often appears swollen. The nasolabial fold is obliterated, and the corner of the mouth droops. When the infant cries, the mouth is drawn to the normal side, the wrinkles are deeper on the normal side, and movement of the forehead and eyelid is unaffected. Usually there are other manifestations of intracranial injury, most commonly a sixth nerve palsy.

Peripheral paralysis is flaccid and, when complete, involves the entire side of the face. When the infant is at rest, the only sign may be a persistently open eye on the affected side, caused by paralysis of the orbicular muscle of the eye. With crying the findings are the same as those in a central facial nerve injury, with the addition of a smooth forehead on the involved side. Since the tongue is not involved, feeding is not affected.

A small branch of the nerve may be injured with involvement of only one group of facial muscles. Paralysis is then limited to the forehead, eyelid, or mouth. Peripheral paralysis secondary to nerve injury distal to the geniculate ganglion may be accompanied by a hematotympanum on the same side.

Differential diagnosis. Central and peripheral facial nerve palsies must be distinguished from nuclear agenesis (Möbius' syndrome). The latter frequently results in bilateral facial nerve palsy; the face is expressionless and immobile, suggesting muscle fibrosis. Other cranial nerve palsies and deformities of the ear, palate, tongue, mandible, and other bones may be associated with Möbius' syndrome. Congenital absence or hypoplasia of the depressor muscle of angle of the mouth may also simulate congenital facial palsy and has been associated with an increased incidence of other congenital anomalies.

Treatment. No specific therapy is indicated for most facial palsies. If the paralysis is peripheral and complete, initial treatment should be directed at protecting the cornea with an eye pad and 1% methylcellulose drops instilled every 4 hours. The functional state of the nerve should be followed closely. If there is no evidence of improvement within 7 to 10 days, electrodiagnostic tests should be performed to determine whether there is neuropraxia or degeneration with interruption of the anatomical continuity of the nerve. If the latter condition is present, surgical intervention should be considered. The best surgical results are obtained with decompression or neuroplastry or both. The ideal time for surgery is not known. Occasionally, facial tone may be improved after anastomosis of the facial nerve to the hypoglossal or accessory nerves. Adrenocorticotropic hormone (ACTH) is not indicated.

Prognosis. The majority of facial palsies resolve spontaneously within several days; total recovery may require several weeks or months. Electrodiagnostic testing is of benefit in predicting recovery; repeatedly normal nerve excitability indicates a good prognosis, but decreased or absent excitability early in the course suggests a poor outlook. The subsequent appearance of muscle fibrillation potentials indicates nerve degeneration. The prognosis in surgically treated infants improves with decreasing age at treatment.

Fractures of facial bones

Facial bone fractures may occur during passage through the birth canal, during forceps application and delivery, and during obstetrical manipulation (most commonly the Mauriceau-Smellie-Veit maneuver for delivery of the fetal head in a breech presentation). The latter may result in mandibular fractures and mandibular joint damage but is rarely severe enough to cause separation of the symphysis of the mandible. Fracture of the nose may result in early respiratory distress and feeding difficulties. The most frequent nasal injury is dislocation of the cartilaginous part of the septum from the vomerine groove and columella.

Treatment. Early reduction and immobilization are advised for fracture of the mandible because rapid, firm union may occur as early as 10 to 14 days. Fractures of the maxilla, lacrimal bones, and nose unite even faster, with fixation in 7 to 10 days. Therefore, nasal fractures should be treated even sooner. Since nasal trauma frequently requires extensive surgery, the pediatrician should request immediate consultation with a physician with expertise in nasal surgery. While waiting the pediatrician should provide an oral airway to relieve respiratory distress. Often the surgeon can grasp the traumatized nose and elevate and remold it manually, resulting in relief of respiratory distress. Fractures of the septal cartilage may also be reduced by simple manual remolding, but most are associated with hematomas that should be promptly incised and drained.

Prognosis. If the fracture is reduced and fixated within a few days, rapid healing without complication is the usual course. If treatment is inadequate, missed, or delayed, subsequent developmental deformities are common. Ankylosis of the mandible in the second year of life is thought to result from birth trauma to the temporomandibular joint. Other deformities may not become apparent until adolescence or young adulthood.

Eyes

See also Chapter 12, p. 606.

Mechanical trauma to various regions of the neonatal eye usually occurs during abnormal presentation, in dystocia from cephalopelvic disproportion, or as a result of inappropriate forceps placement in normal deliveries. Most of the injuries are self-limited and mild and require no specific treatment.

Eyelids

Edema, suffusion, and ecchymoses of the eyelids are common, especially after face and brow presentations or forceps deliveries. Severely swollen lids should be forced open by an ophthalmologist for examination of the eyeball; retractors may be necessary. These findings usually resolve within a week without treatment. It is felt by some that these injuries represent a possible cause of congenital ptosis.

Lagophthalmos, the inability to close an eye, is an occasional finding thought to result from facial nerve injury by forceps pressure. It usually is unilateral. The exposed cornea should be protected by an eye pad and methylcellulose drops instilled every 4 hours. The condition usually resolves within a week.

Orbit

Orbital hemorrhage and fracture may follow direct pressure by the apex of one forceps blade, most commonly in high-forceps extractions. In most instances immediate death occurs. Surviving infants demonstrate traumatic eyelid changes, disturbances of extraocular muscle movements, and exophthalmos. The presence of the latter two findings warrants immediate ophthalmologic consultation. Subsequent management may also require neurosurgical and plastic surgery consultations.

Sympathetic nervous system

Horner's syndrome, resulting from cervical sympathetic nerve trauma, frequently accompanies lower brachial plexus injury (p. 81). The syndrome consists of miosis, partial ptosis, slight enophthalmos, and anhidrosis of the homolateral side of the face. Though small, the pupil reacts to light. The presence of neurologic signs indicating brachial plexus injury helps to distinguish this syndrome from intracranial hemorrhage as a cause of anisocoria. Pigmentation of the homolateral iris is frequently delayed to several months of age; occasionally, pigmentation never occurs. Resolution of other signs of the syndrome depends on whether the injury to the nerve is transient or permanent.

Subconjunctival hemorrhage

Subconjunctival hemorrhage, characterized by bright red patches on the bulbar conjunctiva, is a relatively common finding in the neonate. It may be found after a difficult delivery but often is noted after easy, completely uncomplicated deliveries. If the baby is otherwise well, treatment consists of reassuring the parents. The blood is usually absorbed within 1 to 2 weeks. As the blood pigments break down and are absorbed, the color changes from bright red to orange and yellow.

External ocular muscles

Injury involving the external ocular muscles may result from direct trauma to the cranial nerve (in the form of compression or surrounding hemorrhages) or from hemorrhage into the muscle sheath, with subsequent fibrosis. The sixth nerve (abducens) is the most frequently injured cranial nerve because of its long intracranial course; the result is paralysis of the lateral rectus muscle. This injury may follow a tentorial laceration with extravasation of a small amount of blood around the intracranial portion of the nerve. The involvement may be mild and transient; internal strabismus noted at birth may resolve gradually within 1 to 2 months. The seventh nerve may be injured simultaneously with the sixth nerve by compression with forceps. Improvement in lateral gaze of the affected eye may appear within 1 to 2 months. Alternate patching of either eye in the severely affected infant maintains visual acuity until, with time, maximum improvement has occurred. At 6 months the degree of nerve regeneration may be evaluated. Some infants subsequently require surgical repair of their strabismus.

Fourth nerve (trochlear) palsy is uncommon. It may follow small brainstem hemorrhages with nuclear damage. The affected muscle is the superior oblique, which mainly turns the eye inferiorly and medially. This is difficult to identify in the newborn. Surgical correction may be necessary at a later time.

Third nerve (oculomotor) palsy, when complete, causes paralysis of the inferior oblique and medial, superior, and inferior rectus muscles. This results in ptosis, a dilated fixed pupil, and outward and downward deviation of the eye, with inability to adduct or elevate up and in or up and out or to depress down and out. This palsy may also occur in partial form, with or without pupillary involvement. Partial palsies may recover function spontaneously within several months, whereas complete palsies usually require surgical intervention.

Optic nerve

The optic nerve may be directly injured by a fracture in the region of the optic canal or from a shearing force on the nerve, with resultant hemorrhage into the nerve sheath. The latter injury is seldom recognized because of the more apparent and severe changes in the sensorium. Occasionally a fracture through the optic foramen results in formation of callus, which slowly compresses the nerve. A difficult forceps delivery is a frequent preceding event. If optic nerve injury is not diagnosed within several hours with prompt surgical intervention, irreversible damage is likely. The result is optic atrophy and blindness. This is characterized by a blue-white optic disc, in contrast to the grayish disc of the normal newborn. In primary optic atrophy (for example, that caused by birth trauma), the disc margin is well defined, and fine vessels are rarely present in the disc tissue. In secondary atrophy the disc margin is blurred, and, there is a central gray area and evidence of intraocular disease.

Cornea

A diffuse or streaky haziness of the cornea is relatively common. This is usually caused by edema related to the birth process, but may also follow use of a silver nitrate solution more concentrated than 1%. The haziness usually disappears in 7 to 10 days. When it persists, a rupture of Descemet's membrane has probably occurred; usually this results from malpositioning of forceps at delivery. The consequence of a ruptured Descement's membrane is a leukoma or diffuse white opacity of the cornea. This results from interstitial damage of the substantia propia by fluids entering through the tear in the membrane. These leukomas are often permanent and are accompanied by a high incidence of amblyopia and strabismus.

Intraocular hemorrhage

Trauma at birth may result in retinal hemorrhage, hyphema, or vitreous hemorrhage. Retinal hemorrhage is the most common, with a reported incidence of 2.6% to 50% of all births. The extreme variability in incidence is probably related to the infant's age when first examined; the incidence is higher with earlier observations. The cause is most likely compression of the fetal head, resulting in venous congestion. Retinal hemorrhage is more common in primiparous deliveries and after forceps or vacuum extraction; it is rare after cesarean section. It may occur in normal deliveries. The most common lesion is the flame-shaped or streak hemorrhage found mainly near the disc and sparing the macula and extreme periphery; it usually disappears within 1 to 3 days (rarely, 5 days) with no residual effects. Some hemorrhages may take up to 21 days to resolve. Retinal hemorrhages may reduce the resolving power of the macula, either bilaterally to produce nystagmus or unilaterally to produce amblyopia, which may not always respond to prolonged covering of the fixing eye with improvement of the amblyopic eye.

Hyphemas and vitreous hemorrhages result from misplaced forceps and are often associated with ruptures of Descemet's membrane. The hyphema usually is clear of gross blood within 5 days; during this time the infant should be handled gently and fed frequently to minimize crying and agitation. If blood persists or secondary hemorrhage occurs, systemic administration of acetazolamide (Diamox) and surgical removal of blood may be necessary.

Vitreous hemorrhage is manifested by large vitreous floaters, blood pigment seen with the slit lamp, and an absent red reflex. The prognosis is guarded; if resolution does not occur in 6 to 12 months, surgical correction should be considered.

Ears

The proximity of ears to the site of application of forceps makes them susceptible to injury at birth. Most of the injuries are mild and self-limited, but serious injuries may occur because of slipping or misplacement of forceps.

Abrasions and ecchymoses

Abrasions must be cleansed gently to minimize the risk of secondary infection. Ecchymoses, if extensive and involving other areas of the body, may result in hyperbilirubinemia.

Hematomas

Hematomas of the external ear, if not treated promptly, liquefy slowly, followed by early organization and development of cauliflower ear. Wide incision and evacuation of the hematoma may be indicated.

Lacerations

Lacerations of the auricle may be repaired by the pediatrician if they are superficial and involve only skin. After thorough cleansing and draping, the wound edges are sutured with interrupted 6-0 or 7-0 nylon sutures, with exact edge-to-edge approximation. If the laceration involves cartilage, surgical consultation should be obtained because of the tendency for postoperative perichondritis, which is refractory to treatment and leads to subsequent deformities. A sterile field and more meticulous presurgical preparation are essential. A contour pressure dressing is applied postoperatively.

Vocal cord paralysis

Unilateral or bilateral paralysis of the vocal cords is uncommon in the neonate.

Etiology. Unilateral paralysis may be a consequence of excessive traction on the head during a breech delivery or lateral traction with forceps in a cephalic presentation. The recurrent laryngeal branch of the vagus nerve in the neck is injured. The left side is more commonly involved because of this nerve's lower origin and longer course in the neck. Bilateral paralysis may be caused by peripheral trauma involving both recurrent laryngeal nerves, but more commonly it is caused by a central nervous system insult, such as, hypoxia or hemorrhage involving the brainstem.

Clinical manifestations. An infant with a unilateral paralysis may be completely asymptomatic when resting quietly, but crying is usually accompanied by hoarseness and mild inspiratory stridor. Bilateral paralysis results in more severe respiratory symptoms. At birth the infant may have difficulty in establishing and maintaining spontaneous respiration; later dyspnea, retractions, stridor, cyanosis, or aphonia may develop.

Differential diagnosis. Unilateral paralysis of the vocal cords must be distinguished from congenital laryngeal malformations that produce neonatal stridor (p. 374). A history of difficult delivery, especially involving excessive traction on the fetus, may suggest laryngeal paralysis; the diagnosis can only be confirmed by direct laryngoscopic examination. Bilateral paralysis also must be distinguished from a number of causes of respiratory distress in the neonate (p. 355); stridor should suggest the larynx as the site of disturbance. Direct laryngoscopy is necessary to establish the diagnosis.

Treatment. Infants with unilateral paralysis should be closely observed until there is evidence of improvement. Gentle handling and frequent small feedings will aid in keeping the infant quiet and minimizing the risk of aspiration. Bilateral paralysis necessitates immediate tracheal intubation to establish an airway. Tracheostomy is required subsequently in most cases. Laryngoscopic examinations then should be performed at intervals to look for evidence of return of vocal cord function; early extubation may be attempted if there is complete return within a short period of time.

Prognosis. The infant with unilateral paralysis usually improves rapidly without treatment, and complete resolution occurs within 4 to 6 weeks. The prognosis of bilateral paralysis is more variable. If untreated, the infant may develop a funnel deformity in the lower sternal area; this may appear as early as the fifteenth day of life. After tracheostomy a decrease in the severity of the deformity may occur within several weeks. Some of the affected infants subsequently regain normally shaped chests; others may have residual fixed depressions, occasionally severe enough to require surgical correction. The recovery of vocal cord function varies in time and degree. Some infants may show partial recovery within a few months, with several years elapsing before complete movement of the cords is restored. Other infants who have been followed for years show no improvement. Bilateral paralysis of central origin may improve completely if it is caused by cerebral edema or hemorrhage that rapidly resolves.

INJURIES TO THE NECK AND SHOULDER GIRDLE

Fracture of the clavicle

The clavicle is the most commonly fractured bone during labor and delivery. Most clavicular fractures are of the greenstick type, but occasionally the fracture is complete.

Etiology. The major causes of clavicular fractures are difficult delivery of the shoulders in vertex presentations and extended arms in breech deliveries. Usually there has been vigorous, forceful manipulation of the arm and shoulder.

Clinical manifestations. Usually a greenstick fracture is not associated with any signs or symptoms but is first detected after the appearance of an obvious callus at 7 to 10 days of life. Complete fractures and some greenstick fractures may be apparent shortly after birth; there is decreased or absent movement of the arm on the affected side. Deformity and, occasionally, discoloration may be visible over the fracture site with obliteration of the adjacent supraclavicular depression as a result of sternocleidomastoid muscle spasm. Passive movement of the arm elicits cries of pain from the infant. Palpation reveals tenderness, crepitus, and irregularity along the clavicle. The Moro reflex on the involved side is characteristically absent. Roentgenograms confirm the diagnosis of fracture.

Differential diagnosis. A similar clinical picture of impaired movement of an arm with absent Moro reflex may follow fracture of the humerus or brachial palsy. The former is confirmed by roentgenograms; the latter is accompanied by additional clinical findings.

Treatment. Treatment is directed toward minimizing the infant's pain. The affected arm and shoulder should be immobilized with the arm abducted above 60° and the elbow flexed above 90°. A callus forms, and pain usually subsides by 7 to 10 days, when immobilization may be discontinued.

Prognosis. Prognosis is excellent, with growth resulting in restoration of normal bone contour after several months.

Brachial palsy

Brachial palsy is a paralysis involving the muscles of the upper extremity that follows mechanical trauma to the spinal roots of the fifth cervical through the first thoracic nerves, the brachial plexus, during birth. Three main forms occur, depending on the site of injury; (1) Duchenne-Erb, or upper arm, paralysis, which results from injury of the fifth and sixth cervical roots and is, by far, the most common, (2) Klumpke's, or lower arm, paralysis, which results from injury of the eighth cervical and first thoracic roots and is extremely rare, and (3) paralysis of the entire arm, which occurs slightly more often than the Klumpke type.

Etiology. Most cases of brachial palsy follow a prolonged and difficult labor, culminating in a traumatic delivery. The affected infant is frequently large, relaxed, and asphyxiated and, thereby, vulnerable to excessive separation of bony segments, overstretching, and injury to soft tissues. Injury of the fifth and sixth cervical roots may follow a breech presentation with the arms extended over the head; excessive traction on the shoulder in the delivery of the head may result in stretching of the plexus. The same injury may follow lateral traction of the head and neck away from one of the shoulders while attempting to deliver the shoulders in a vertex presentation. More vigorous traction of the same nature will result in paralysis of the entire arm. The mechanism for isolated lower arm paralysis is uncertain; it is thought to result from stretching of lower plexus nerves under and against the coracoid process of the scapula during forceful elevation and abduction of the arm. Excessive traction on the trunk during a breech delivery may result in avulsion of the lower roots from the cervical cord. In most patients the nerve sheath is torn and the nerve fibers are compressed by the resultant hemorrhage and edema. Less commonly, the nerves are completely ruptured and the ends severed, or the roots are avulsed from the spinal cord with injury to the spinal gray matter.

Clinical manifestations. The infant with upper arm paralysis holds his affected arm in a characteristic position, reflecting involvement of the shoulder abductors and external rotators, forearm flexors and supinators, and wrist extensors. The arm is adducted and internally rotated, with extension at the elbow, pronation of the forearm, and flexion of the wrist. When the arm is passively abducted, it falls limply to the side of the body. The Moro, biceps, and radial reflexes are absent on the affected side. There may be some sensory deficit on the radial aspect of the arm, but this is difficult to evaluate in the neonatal infant. The grasp reflex is intact.

Lower arm paralysis involves the intrinsic muscles of the hand and the long flexors of the wrist and fingers. The hand is paralyzed, and voluntary movements of the wrist cannot be made. The grasp reflex is absent; the deep tendon reflexes are intact. Sensory impairment may be demonstrated along the ulnar side of the forearm and hand. Frequently, dependent edema and cyanosis of the hand and trophic changes in the fingernails develop. After some time there may be flattening and atrophy of the intrinsic hand muscles. Usually a homolateral Horner's syndrome (ptosis, miosis, and enophthalmos) is also present because of injury involving the cervical sympathetic fibers of the first thoracic root. Often this is associated with delayed pigmentation of the iris, sometimes of more than 1 year's duration.

When the entire arm is paralyzed, it is usually completely motionless, flaccid, and powerless, hanging limply to the side. All reflexes are absent. The sensory deficit may extend almost up to the shoulder.

Differential diagnosis. The presence of a flail arm in a neonate may be caused by cerebral injury or by a number of injuries about the shoulder. The former is usually associated with other manifestations of central nervous system injury. A careful roentgenographic study of the shoulder (including lower cervical spine, clavicle, and upper humerus) should be made to exclude tearing of the joint capsule, fracture of the clavicle, and fracture, dislocation, or upper epiphyseal detachment of the humerus.

Treatment. The basic principle of treatment is the maintenance of the range of motion about the affected joints. This is accomplished by partial immobilization, appropriate positioning, and an exercise program. Active physical therapy should be avoided initially because of traumatic neuritis, which usually affects the brachial plexus. By 7 to 10 days of age, gentle range of motion exercises may be started.

In upper arm paralysis the arm should be abducted 90° with external rotation at the shoulder, 90° flexion at the elbow, full supination of the forearm, and slight extension at the wrist so that the palm of the hand is turned toward the face. This may be done with a brace or a splint or simply by pinning the sleeve of the infant's garment at the wrist to the undersheet (Fig. 3-4). This position should be maintained for 2 to 3 hours at a time, alternating with periods during which the arm is free. This allows appropriate skin care. After the first few days, gentle massage and passive range of motion exercises are indicated to prevent development of contractures. Immobilization is usually necessary for 6 months intermittently through day and night and, occasionally, for an additional 6 months at night only. The infant must be followed closely, and active and passive corrective exercises continued until normal scapulohumeral rhythm has been reestablished.

In lower arm paralysis, the forearm and wrist should be splinted in a neutral position, and padding should be placed in the fist. Passive range of motion exercises of the wrist, hand, and fingers should be gently performed. When the entire arm is paralyzed, the same treatment principles should be followed: immobilization in a neutral position, padding of the fist, massage, and range of motion exercises.

Routine neurosurgical exploration and repair of the injury are not indicated. Mild injuries are self-limited, and severe injuries usually involve avulsion of the roots from the cord, making suture of the nerves impossible. Dissection of the plexus is so difficult that more damage may be inflicted, resulting in formation of additional scar tissue and symptoms years after the operation. Matson has explored the brachial plexus and performed neurolysis on infants who show no improvement after 3 to 6 months and in whom there was palpable thickening in the supraclavicular fossa or swelling or ecchymosis over the plexus during the acute phase of injury. Although the results have been generally discouraging, several infants have shown a greater degree

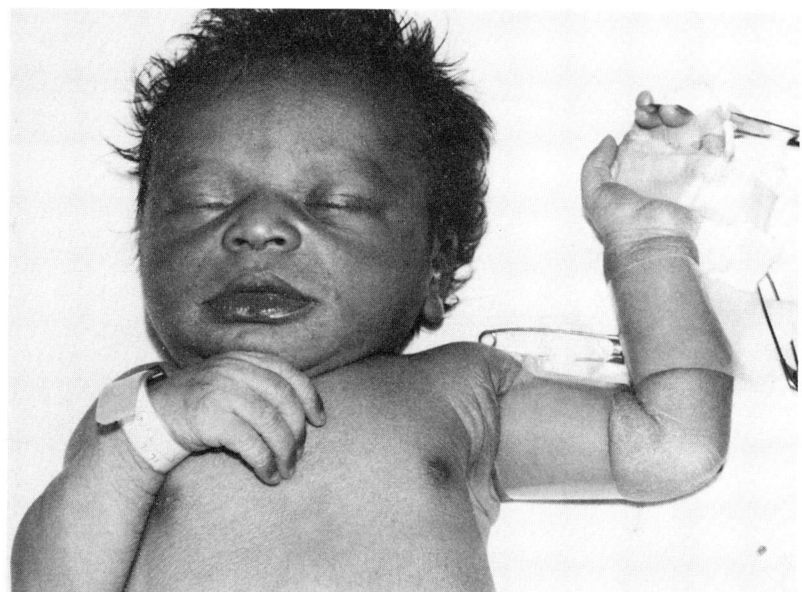

Fig. 3-4. Recommended corrective positioning for treatment of Erb's palsy. Note abduction and external rotation at the shoulder, flexion at the elbow, supination of the forearm, and slight dorsiflexion at the wrist.

of improvements following surgery than would have been expected to have occurred spontaneously.

Prognosis. If the nerve roots are intact, return of function may appear within several days as the local hemorrhage and edema resolve. The rate of recovery varies with the degree of injury. In some infants recovery is complete within a few weeks. The majority of appropriately treated infants will recover completely within 3 to 6 months. An occasional infant with severe injury may show continued improvement over a period of up to 2 years. Even where recovery of function appears complete, close examination will usually reveal peculiar posturing of the arm in abduction at the shoulder, tightness in internal rotation, difficulty in forearm supination, and minimal winging of the scapula.

Lower arm paralysis is associated with a relatively poor prognosis; a claw deformity may develop. Paralysis of the entire arm may show recovery of some function eventually.

Electrodiagnosis is helpful in distinguishing a neuropraxis lesion from a root avulsion. An infant with a severe lesion of the former type may be predicted to have partial, and possibly total, return of function; whereas an infant with an avulsion injury may be predicted to have permanent paralysis. In avulsion injuries and untreated stretch injuries, residual contractures and bony deformities develop. The former may be treated with gentle stretching in the infant and by tenotomies in the older patient. Bony deformities may be treated by osteotomies or tendon transfers. These procedures produce no increase in muscle power but may make motion of the arm less awkward.

Phrenic nerve paralysis

See p. 355.

Phrenic nerve paralysis results in diaphragmatic paralysis and rarely occurs as an isolated injury in the neonatal infant. The majority of injuries are unilateral and are associated with a homolateral upper brachial plexus palsy.

Etiology. The most common cause is a difficult breech delivery. Lateral hyperextension of the neck results in overstretching or avulsion of the third, fourth, and fifth cervical roots, which supply the phrenic nerve.

Clinical manifestations. The first sign may be recurrent episodes of cyanosis, usually accompanied by irregular and labored respirations. The respiratory excursions of the involved side of the diaphragm are largely ineffectual, and the breathing is, therefore, almost completely thoracic so that no bulging of the abdomen occurs with inspiration. The thrust of the diaphragm, which often may be felt just under the costal margin on the normal side, is absent on the affected side. Dullness and diminished breath sounds are found over the affected side. In a severe injury, tachypnea, weak cry, and apneic spells may occur.

Roentgenographic manifestations. Roentgenograms taken during the first few days may show only slight elevation of the affected diaphragm, occasionally so subtle that it may be considered normal. Repeated films will show the more apparent elevation of the diaphragm, with displacement of the heart and mediastinum to the opposite side. Frequently, areas of atelectasis appear bilaterally. Early diagnosis can be confirmed only by fluoroscopy, which reveals an abnormal elevation of the affected hemidiaphragm and seesaw movements of the two hemidiaphragms with respiration (the use of the affected side and descent of the normal side during inspiration); opposite movements occur during expiration. In addition, fluoroscopy reveals the shift of the mediastinum toward the normal side during inspiration.

Differential diagnosis. Careful physical examination should allow differentiation between central nervous system, cardiac, or pulmonary causes of neonatal respiratory distress. Fluoroscopy confirms the diagnosis.

Treatment. Most infants require only nonspecific medical treatment. The infant should be positioned on the involved side, and oxygen should be administered for cyanosis or dyspnea. Intravenous fluids may be necessary the first few days. If the infant begins to show improvement, progressive oral or gavage feedings may be started. Antibiotics are indicated if pneumonia occurs.

Surgical intervention should be considered for the infant with severe or increasing respiratory distress despite medical management, or for the infant who after 3 or 4 months is only mildly symptomatic, but has shown no roentgenographic evidence of recovery of function of the affected hemidiaphragm. The procedure of choice is either plication of or excision of part of the paralyzed diaphragm. This results in a tightening of the diaphragm and brings the dome of the diaphragm down to a normal level, allowing the mediastinum to return toward its normal position.

Prognosis. Most infants recover spontaneously. This may be complete by 6 weeks but usually takes several months. If avulsion of the cervical nerves has occurred, recovery is not possible, and in the absence of surgery the infant is susceptible to pneumonia in the atelectatic lung. Many of these infants die before 3 months of age. Infants treated surgically do well, with no recurrence of pneumonia and no late pulmonary or chest wall complications. The repaired hemidiaphragm remains in a satisfactory position despite permanent paralysis of the phrenic nerve.

Injury of the sternocleidomastoid muscle

Injury of the sternocleidomastoid muscle is also designated muscular torticollis, congenital torticollis, or sternocleidomastoid fibroma. Its cause and pathology have been a matter of controversy for many years.

Etiology. The birth trauma theory suggests that the muscle or fascial sheath is ruptured during a breech or difficult delivery involving hyperextension of the muscle. A hematoma develops and is subsequently invaded by fibrin and fibroblasts with progressive formation of scar tissue and shortening of the muscle. The intrauterine theory postulates abnormal pressure, position, or trauma to the muscle during intrauterine life. Another theory suggests a hereditary defect in the development of the muscle. Still others have noted pathologic findings resembling infectious myositis, suggesting an infection in utero or a muscle injured at delivery.

Clinical manifestations. A mass in the midportion of the sternocleidomastoid muscle may be evident at birth, although usually it is first noted 10 to 14 days after birth. It is 1 to 2 cm in diameter, hard, immobile, fusiform, and well circumscribed; there is no inflammation or overlying discoloration. The mass enlarges during the following 2 to 4 weeks and then gradually regresses and disappears by the age of 5 to 8 months.

A transient torticollis produced by contracture of the involved muscle appears soon after birth. The head tilts toward the involved side, and the chin is somewhat elevated and rotated toward the opposite shoulder. The head cannot be moved passively into normal position. If the deformity persists beyond 3 or 4 years, the skull becomes foreshortened. Flattening of the frontal bone and bulging of the occipital bone occur on the involved side, while the contralateral front bone bulges and the occiput is flattened. The ipsilateral eyebrow is slanted; the clavicle and shoulder become elevated compared to the opposite normal side, and the ipsilateral mastoid process becomes more prominent. If treatment is not instituted, a lower cervical–upper thoracic scoliosis subsequently develops. Rarely, calcification develops in the affected muscles.

Differential diagnosis. Careful roentgenographic examination should be made of the cervical spine and shoulders to rule out Sprengel's or Klippel-Feil deformity, cervical myelodysplasia, and occipitalization of the atlas.

Treatment. Treatment should be instituted as early as possible. The involved muscle should be stretched to an overcorrected position by gentle, even, and persistent motion with the baby supine. The head is flexed forward and away from the affected side, and the chin is rotated toward the affected side. The mother can be instructed to repeat this maneuver several times a day. The infant should also be stimulated to turn the head spontaneously toward the affected side; the crib may be positioned so that he must turn to the desired position of overcorrection in looking for window light or at a mobile or favorite rattle; during sleep the baby should be placed on the side of the torticollis; in this position sandbags should be placed on each side of his body for fixation.

Conservative therapy should be continued for 6 months. If the deformity has not been fully corrected, surgery should be considered to prevent permanent skull and cervical spine deformities. Removal of the tumor is not necessary, and will needlessly deform the outline of the neck. The procedure of choice is lengthening and division of the sternal portion of the muscle from the mastoid process at its origin; the neck outline is preserved. After surgery the head should be immobilized in an overcorrected position for several weeks, followed by an exercise program.

Prognosis. Most infants treated conservatively show complete recovery within 2 to 3 months. If surgery is necessary and if it is performed early, the facial asymmetry will disappear almost entirely.

INJURIES TO THE SPINE AND SPINAL CORD

See p. 528.

Birth injuries to the vertebral spine and spinal cord are now rarely diagnosed. It is not certain whether the low incidence is real, reflecting improved obstetrical techniques, or represents a tendency for postmortem examination to overlook spine and spinal cord lesions.

Etiology. These injuries almost always result from breech deliveries, especially difficult ones utilizing version and extraction. Other predisposing factors include brow and face presentations, dystocia (especially shoulder), prematurity, primiparity, and precipitous delivery.

The injuries are usually caused by stretching of the cord and not by compression. The most common mechanism responsible is probably forceful longitudial traction on the trunk while the head is still firmly engaged in the pelvis. When combined with flexion and torsion of the vertebral axis, this becomes a more significant problem. Occasionally a snap is felt by the obstetrician while exerting traction. Difficulty in delivery of the shoulders in cephalic presentations may result in a similar mechanism of injury. The spinal cord is very delicate and inelastic. Its attachments are the cauda equina below and the roots of the brachial plexus and medulla above. Because the ligaments are elastic and the muscles delicate, the infant's vertebral column may be stretched quite easily. In addition, the dura is more elastic in the infant than in the adult. Consequently, strong longitudial traction may be expected to cause elongation of the spinal column and to stretch the spinal cord and its membranes. The possible result is vertebral fracture or dislocation or both and cord transection. More often, hemorrhage and edema produce a physiologic transection. The lower cervical and upper thoracic regions are most commonly involved, but occasionally the entire length of the spinal canal contains a heavy accumulation of blood.

Clinical manifestations. Affected infants may follow one of three clinical patterns. Those in the first group are in poor condition from birth, with respiratory depression, shock, and hypothermia. They deteriorate rapidly; death occurs within several hours, often before neurologic signs are obvious.

The second group is infants who at birth may appear normal or show signs similar to group one; these infants die after several days. Cardiac function is usually relatively strong. Within hours or days, the central type of respiratory depression, which is initially present, may be complicated by respiratory distress of pulmonary origin, usually pneumonia. The spinal lesion frequently is not recognized for several days, when flaccidity and immobility of the legs are noted. Occasionally urinary retention may be the first symptom. Paralysis of the abdominal wall is manifested by a relaxation of the abdominal wall and bulging at the flanks when the baby is held upright. The intercostal muscles may be affected if the lesion is high enough. Sensation is absent over the lower half of the body. Deep tendon reflexes and spontaneous reflex movements are absent. The infant is constipated. The brachial plexus is involved in about 20% of all cases. The spinal column is usually clinically and roentgenographically normal.

The third group is composed of infants who survive for long periods, some for years. Paraplegia noted at birth may be transient. The lesion in the cord may be mild and reversible, or it may result in permanent neurologic sequelae with no return of function of the lower cord segments. The skin over the involved part of the body is dry and scaly, predisposing the infant to bed sores and ulcers. Muscle atrophy, severe contractures, and bony deformities follow. Bladder distention and constant dribbling perisist, and recurrent urinary tract infections are common. Within several weeks or months this clinical picture is replaced by a stage of reflex activity or paraplegia-in-flexion. This is characterized by return of tone and rigid flexion of the involved extremities, improvement in skin condition with healing of decubiti, and periodic mass reflex responses composed of tonic spasms of the extremities, spontaneous micturition, and profuse sweating over the involved part of the body.

Differential diagnosis. During the first few weeks of life, injuries to the spinal cord may be confused with amyotonia congenita or myelodysplasia associated with spina bifida occulta (p. 532). The former may be differentiated by the generalized distribution of the weakness and hypotonia and by the presence of normal sensation and sphincter control. The latter is usually associated with some cutaneous lesion over the sacral region such as dimples, angiomas, or abnormal tufts of hair; it is always associated with defects in the spinal lamina.

Treatment. Treatment is supportive and usually unsatisfactory. The infant affected at birth requires basic resuscitative and supportive measures. Infants who survive present a therapeutic challenge that can be met only by the combined and interested efforts of the pediatrician, neurologist, neurosurgeon, urologist, physiatrist, orthopedist, nurse, physical therapist, and occupational therapist.

When the infant is reasonably stable, cervical and thoracic spine roentgenograms should be obtained. In the rare occurrence of vertebral fracture or dislocation or both, immediate neurosurgical consultation is necessary for reduction of the deformity and relief of cord compression, followed by appropriate immobilization. Lumbar puncture in the acute period is of little practical value and may aggravate existing cord damage if the infant is excessively manipulated during the procedure. After several days, however, a persistent spinal fluid block may be demonstrated and may be an indication for exploratory laminectomy at the site of trauma. This possibility should be suspected in an infant with partial paraplegia and normal roentgenograms.

Prompt and meticulous attention must be given to skin, bladder, and bowel care. The position of paralyzed parts should be changed every 2 hours. Areas of anesthetic skin should be washed, dried, and gently massaged daily. Lamb's wool covers are helpful in preventing pressure necrosis of skin. Benzoin tincture applications help protect the skin in pressure areas. A decubitus ulcer is treated by scrupulous cleansing and complete freedom from weight bearing and friction. An indwelling urethral catheter should be inserted within several hours after severe cord trauma at any level. In the smaller infant a No. 3 feeding tube may be used. Repeated instrumentation should be avoided. The urine should be cultured at least weekly, and antibiotic therapy employed only in the presence of infection. After several weeks the infant reaches the stage of paraplegia-in-flexion, and urinary retention is usually replaced by regular episodes of spontaneous voiding. If this is accompanied by a decrease in bladder size to normal, the catheter is removed. As urinary tract infection is almost inevitable, frequent cultures should be obtained even after catheter removal. The first infection should be treated with the appropriate antibiotic for 2 weeks. After the neonatal period, this should be followed by suppressive therapy with sulfisoxazole (Gantrisin), 50 to 75 mg/kg/day for 3 to 6 months, assuming that cultures remain negative. Subsequent antibiotic therapy should be governed by the spectrum of sensitivity of cultured organisms. In the infant in whom prompt return of bladder function does not occur, urologic assistance should be sought in catheter management and planning of further procedures (for example, suprapubic cystostomy and wet ureterostomies). Fecal retention is also a common problem, especially after total cord transection. Appropriate dietary balance should aid in keeping the stools soft. Early use of glycerin suppositories at regular intervals will encourage automatic defecation. Digital manipulation may be necessary to relieve fecal impactions. Finally, physical rehabilitation should be instituted early in an attempt to minimize deformity. After several years orthopedic procedures may still be necessary to correct contractures and bony deformities.

Prognosis. The prognosis varies with the severity of the injury. Most severe injuries result in death shortly after birth. Infants with cord compression from vertebral fractures or dislocations or both may recover with reasonable return of function if prompt neurosurgical removal of the compression is performed. Infants with mild injuries or partial transections may recover with minimal sequelae. Infants who exhibit complete physiologic cord transection shortly after birth without vertebral fracture or dislocation have an extremely poor outlook for recovery of function. Many die in infancy of ascending urinary tract infection and sepsis. Long-term survivors have been reported to live into their third decade. These are extremely rare, and although the child may have normal intelligence and learn to walk with special appliances, he faces the late complications of pain, spasms, autonomic dysfunction, bony deformities, and genitourinary, psychiatric, and school problems.

INJURIES TO INTRAABDOMINAL ORGANS

Although birth trauma involving intraabdominal organs is uncommon, it frequently must be considered by the physician who manages neonatal infants because deterioration can be fulminant in an undetected lesion and therapy can be very effective when a lesion is diagnosed early. Intraabdominal trauma should be suspected in any newborn infant with shock and abdominal distention or pallor, anemia, and irritability without evidence of external blood loss.

Rupture of the liver

The liver is the most commonly injured abdominal organ during the brith process. The incidence, obtained from neonatal autopsy studies, has varied from 0.9% to 9.6%.

Etiology. Birth trauma is probably the most significant contributing factor; the condition usually occurs in large infants, infants with hepatomegaly (for example, erythroblastosis fetalis and infants of diabetic mothers), and breech deliveries. Manual pressure on the liver during delivery of the head in a breech presentation is probably a common mechanism of injury. Prematurity and postmaturity have also been felt to predispose the infant to this injury. Other contributing factors include asphyxia and coagulation disorders. Trauma to the liver more commonly results in subcapsular hematoma than actual laceration of the liver.

Clinical manifestations. The infant usually appears normal the first 1 to 3 days and, rarely, for as long as 7 days. Nonspecific signs—that is, poor feeding, listlessness, pallor, jaundice, tachypnea, and tachycardia—may appear early that are related to loss of blood into the hematoma. A mass may be palpable in the right upper quadrant. The hematocrit and hemoglobin level may be stable early in the course, but serial determinations will suggest blood loss. These manifestations are followed by sudden circulatory collapse, usually coincident with rupture of the hematoma through the capsule and extravasation of blood into the peritoneal cavity. The abdomen then may be distended, rigid, and dull to percussion, occasionally with a bluish discoloration in the overlying skin, which may extend over the scrotum. Abdominal roentgenograms may reveal uniform opacity of the abdomen, indicating free intraperitoneal fluid. Paracentesis confirms the presence of free blood in the peritoneal cavity.

Differential diagnosis. This lesion is one of several that can result in hemoperitoneum; others include trauma to the adrenals, kidneys, gastrointestinal tract, and spleen. Presence of a right upper quadrant mass suggests trauma to the liver, but absence of a mass does not rule this out. Abdominal roentgenograms and intravenous pyelography may assist in pinpointing the site of trauma, but ultimately a definite diagnosis can be made only by laparotomy.

Treatment. Immediate management consists of prompt transfusion with whole blood to restore the blood volume and of recognition and correction of any coagulation disorder. Most surgeons agree that this should be followed by laparotomy with evacuation of the hematoma and repair of the laceration with sutures placed over a hemostatic agent. Any fragmented, devitalized liver tissue should be removed to prevent subsequent fatal secondary hemorrhage. Because of the successful treatment of two infants with blood transfusion only and because of hemostatic difficulty in one infant at surgery, it has been suggested that blood transfusion and the tamponade of intraabdominal pressure might be adequate therapy in some infants.

Prognosis. In unrecognized liver trauma with formation of a subcapsular hematoma, shock and death may result if the hematoma ruptures through the capsule, reducing the pressure tamponade and resulting in new bleeding from the liver. Recognition of the possibility of liver rupture in infants with a predisposing birth history, followed by early diagnosis and prompt therapy, should improve the prognosis. Early diagnosis and correction of any existing coagulation disorder will also improve the prognosis.

Rupture of the spleen

Rupture of the spleen in the newborn infant occurs much less often than rupture of the liver. However, recognition of this condition is equally important because of its similar potential for fulminant shock and death if the diagnosis is delayed.

Etiology. The condition is most common in large babies, babies delivered in breech position, and babies with erythroblastosis fetalis or congenital syphilis, in whom the spleen is enlarged and more friable and thereby susceptible to rupture either spontaneously or after minor trauma. An underlying clotting defect has also been implicated. Rupture of the spleen has occurred in normal-sized infants with uneventful deliveries and no underlying disease.

Clinical manifestations. Clinical signs indicating blood loss and hemoperitoneum are similar to those described for hepatic rupture. The hemoglobin and hematocrit decrease and abdominal paracentesis may reveal free blood; several infants have been described in whom the blood was circumscribed within the leaves of the phrenicolineal ligament and, therefore, not clinically detectable. Occasionally a left upper quadrant mass may be palpable, and films of the abdomen may show medial displacement of the gastric air bubble.

Differential diagnosis. Rupture of the

liver must be distinguished. All of the previously mentioned causes of hemoperitoneum should also be considered.

Treatment. Prompt transfusion with whole blood should be followed by immediate exploratory laparotomy and splenectomy. Any coexisting clotting defect should be corrected preoperatively.

Prognosis. With early recognition and emergency surgery, survival should approach 100%.

Adrenal hemorrhage

Neonatal adrenal hemorrhage is more common than previously suspected; some autopsy studies have revealed a high incidence of subclinical hemorrhage. Massive hemorrhage is much less common, and the incidence is difficult to determine, since the diagnosis is often unsuspected and only considered retrospectively years later when calcified adrenals are unexpectedly found on roentgenograms or at autopsy.

Etiology. The most likely cause is birth trauma; the frequency is higher in infants with macrosomia, in infants of diabetic mothers, in breech presentation, in infants with congenital syphilis, and when there is dystocia. Placental hemorrhage, anoxia, hemorrhagic disease of the newborn, prematurity, and, more recently, neuroblastoma have been implicated. Pathologic findings vary from unilateral minute areas of bleeding to massive bilateral hemorrhage. The increased size and vascularity of the adrenal gland at birth may predispose it to hemorrhage.

Clinical manifestations. Signs vary with the degree and extent of hemorrhage. The classic findings are fever, tachypnea out of proportion to the degree of fever, yellowish pallor, cyanosis of the lips and finger tips, a mass in either flank with overlying skin discoloration, and purpura. Findings suggesting adrenal insufficiency include poor feeding, vomiting, diarrhea, obstipation, dehydration, abdominal distention, irritability, hypoglycemia, uremia, skin rash, listlessness, coma, convulsions, and shock.

Roentgenographic manifestations. Initial roentgenographic manifestations may be limited to widening of the retroperitoneal space with forward displacement of stomach and duodenum or downward displacement of intestines or kidneys. In time, calcification may appear. Typically this is rimlike and has been observed as early as the twelfth day of life. After several weeks, the calcification becomes denser and retracted and assumes the configuration of the adrenal gland (Fig. 3-5).

Differential diagnosis. Adrenal hemorrhage must be distinguished from other causes of abdominal hemorrhage. In addition, when a mass is palpable, the differential diagnosis must include the multiple causes of flank masses in the newborn infant, such as genitourinary anomaly, Wilms' tumor, and neuroblastoma. If the infant is large or the delivery is traumatic or breech, an adrenal hemorrhage is most likely. Neuroblastoma may be distinguished by increased excretion of vanillylmandelic acid (VMA) and other urinary catecholamines in 85% to 90% of affected infants. Blood pressure measurements and roentgenograms are also indicated to evaluate this possibility.

Treatment. Significant blood loss should be replaced with whole blood transfusion. Suspicion of adrenal insufficiency may warrant use of intravenous fluids and steroids. The decision for surgical intervention is dictated by the location and degree of hemorrhage. If it appears to be retroperitoneal and limited by the perinephric fascia, some authors recommend blood replacement and careful observation in the hope of spontaneous control by tamponade; often this approach is successful and surgery is not necessary. If paracentesis reveals blood or if blood loss exceeds replacement, exploratory laparotomy is indicated. Surgery may involve evacuation of hematoma, vessel ligation, and adrenalectomy with or without nephrectomy. When the hemorrhagic process extends to the peritoneal cavity, peritoneal exploration and evacuation of clot are indicated.

Prognosis. Small hemorrhages are probably often asymptomatic and have no associated significant morbidity, judging from the unexpected discovery of calcified adrenals on abdominal films taken for other reasons later in infancy and childhood. If hemoperitoneum or adrenal insufficiency or both develops, the outlook depends upon the speed with which diagnosis is made and appropriate therapy in-

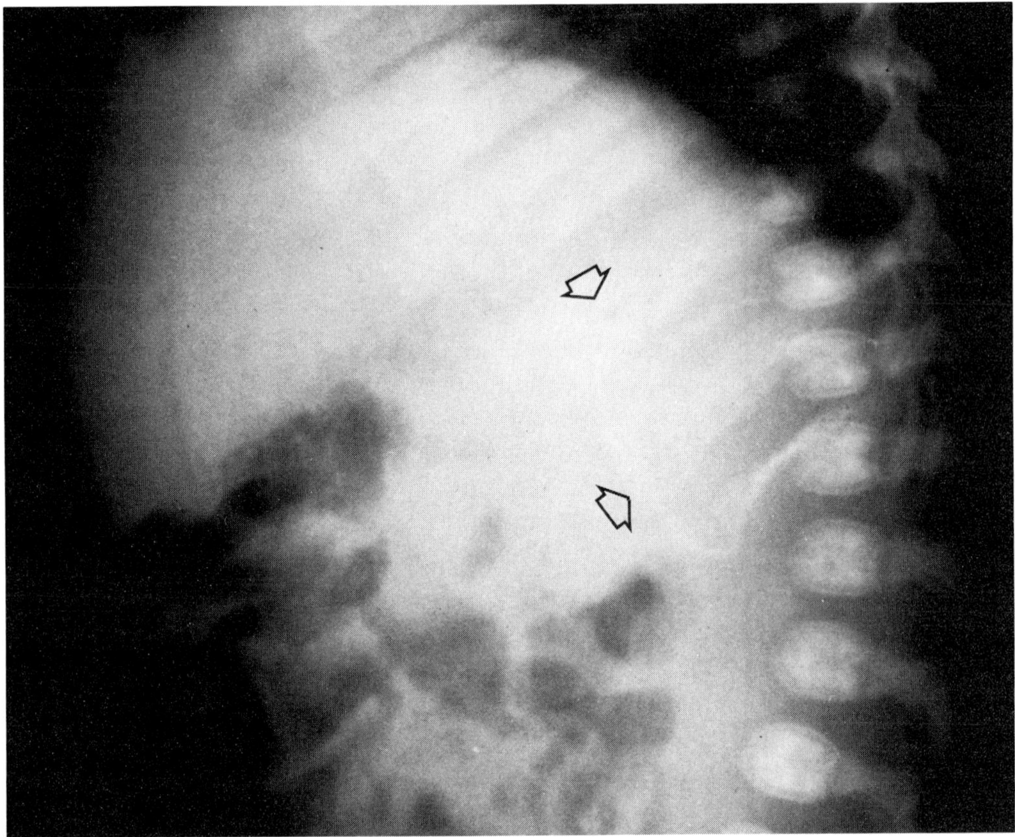

Fig. 3-5. Lateral abdominal roentgenogram of 5,312-gm male delivered vaginally, with difficulty after shoulder dystocia. At 48 hours, fever, icterus, and slow feeding were noted, and a mass was palpable above the left kidney. At 31 days there was dense, retracted calcification, assuming the configuration of the adrenal gland.

stituted. Surviving infants should be followed closely after discharge from the hospital. Adrenal function should be tested with ACTH stimulation at a later date to determine whether a normal response occurs in the urinary excretion of 17-hydroxycorticosterone.

INJURIES TO THE EXTREMITIES

Fracture of humerus

After the clavicle, the humerus is the bone most often fractured during the birth process.

Etiology. The most common mechanisms responsible are difficult delivery of extended arms in breech presentations and of the shoulders in vertex presentations. Besides traction with simultaneous rotation of the arm, direct pressure on the humerus is also a factor. This may account for the occurrence of fracture of the humerus in spontaneous vertex deliveries. The fractures are usually in the diaphysis. They are often greenstick, although complete fracture with overriding of the fragments occasionally occurs.

Clinical manifestations. A greenstick fracture may be overlooked until a callus is noted. A complete fracture with marked displacement of fragments presents an obvious deformity that calls attention to the injury. Often the initial manifestation of the fracture is immobility of the affected arm. Palpation reveals tenderness, crepitation, and hypermobility of the fragments. The homolateral Moro response is absent. Roentgenograms confirm the diagnosis.

Differential diagnosis. Differential diagnosis includes all the previously noted lesions that cause immobility of the arm. An associated brachial plexus injury occasionally occurs.

Treatment. The affected arm should be immobilized in adduction for 2 to 4 weeks. This may be accomplished by maintaining the arm in a hand-on-hip position with a triangular splint and a Velpeau bandage, by strapping the arm to the chest, or by application of a cast.

Prognosis. The prognosis is excellent. Healing is associated with marked callus formation. Moderate overriding and angulation disappear with time because of the excellent remodeling power of infants. Complete union of the fracture fragments usually occurs by 3 weeks. Fair alignment and shortening of less than 1 inch indicate satisfactory closed reduction. Long bone fractures in infants always result in epiphyseal stimulation; the closer the fracture to the epiphyseal cartilage, the greater the degree of subsequent overgrowth.

Fracture of femur

Although a relatively uncommon injury, fracture of the femur is by far the most common fracture of the lower extremity in the newborn.

Etiology. This injury usually follows a breech delivery, when the leg is pulled down after the breech is already partially fixed in the pelvic inlet or when during delivery of the shoulders and arms the infant is improperly held by one thigh.

Clinical manifestations. Usually there is an obvious deformity of the thigh; as a rule the bone breaks transversely in the upper half or third, where it is relatively thin. Less commonly, the injury may not be appreciated until several days postpartum when swelling of the thigh is noted; this may be caused by hemorrhage into adjacent muscle. The infant refuses to move the affected leg or cries in pain during passive movement or palpation over the fracture site. Roentgenograms almost always show overriding of the fracture fragments.

Treatment. Optimal treatment is traction-suspension of both lower extremities, even if the fracture is unilateral. The legs are immobilized in a spica cast; and using Bryant's traction, the infant is suspended by the legs from an overhead frame with the buttocks and lower back just raised off the crib. The legs are extended and the thighs flexed on the abdomen. The weight of the infant's body is enough to overcome the pull of the thigh muscles and, thereby, reduce the deformity. The infant is maintained in this position for 3 to 4 weeks until adequate callus has formed and new bone growth has started. During the treatment period, special attention should be given to careful feeding and protection of bandages and casts from soiling with urine and feces.

Prognosis. The prognosis is excellent; complete union and restoration without shortening are expected. Extensive calcification may develop in the areas of surrounding hemorrhage; this subsequently is resorbed.

Dislocations

Dislocations caused by birth trauma are rare. Often an apparent dislocation is actually a displaced fracture through an epiphyseal plate. Since the epiphyseal plate is radiolucent, a fracture occurring adjacent to an unmineralized epiphysis will give a radiographic picture simulating a dislocation of the neighboring joint. This type of injury has been termed pseudodislocation. Since the humeral and proximal femoral epiphyses are usually not visible on roentgenograms at birth, a pseudodislocation can occur at the shoulder, elbow, or hip.

Of the true dislocations, those involving the hip and knee are probably not caused by the trauma of the birth process. Most likely they are either intrauterine positional deformities or true congenital malformations. A true dislocation resulting from birth trauma is that involving the radial head. This has been described in traumatic breech delivery. Examination reveals adduction and internal rotation of the affected arm, with pronation of the forearm; the Moro response is poor, and palpation reveals lateral and posterior displacement of the radial head. This is confirmed by roentgenograms. With supination and extension the radial head can be readily reduced. This should be done promptly, followed by immobilization of the infant in this position in a circular cast for 2 to

3 weeks. Early recognition and treatment should result in normal growth and function of the elbow.

Epiphyseal separations

Like dislocations, epiphyseal separations are rare. They occur mostly in primiparity, dystocic deliveries, and breech presentations, especially those requiring manual extraction or version and extraction; any delivery associated with vigorous pulling may predispose the infant to this injury. The upper femoral and humeral epiphyses are most commonly involved. Usually on the second day, the soft tissue over the affected epiphysis develops a firm swelling with reddening, crepitus, and tenderness. Active motion is limited, and passive motion is painful. If the injury is in the upper femoral epiphysis, the infant assumes the frog position with external rotation of the leg. Early roentgenograms will show only soft tissue swelling, with an occasional suggestion of dislocation. After 1 to 2 weeks extensive callus appears, confirming the nature of the injury; during the third week subperiosteal calcification appears.

Closed reduction and immobilization are indicated within the first few days before rapidly forming fibrous callus prevents mobilization of the epiphysis. The hip is immobilized in the frog-leg position as in congenital dislocation. Poorly immobilized fragments may require temporary fixation with a Kirschner wire. Union usually occurs within 10 to 15 days. Untreated or poorly treated epiphyseal injuries may result in subsequent growth distortion and permanent deformities such as coxa vara. Mild injuries carry a good prognosis.

Other peripheral nerve injuries

In contrast to the brachial plexus and phrenic and facial nerves, other peripheral nerves are injured less often at birth, and usually in association with trauma to the extremity. Radial palsy has occurred following difficult forceps extractions, both from pressure of incorrectly applied forceps and in association with fracture of the arm. Occasionally the palsy occurs later when the radial nerve is enmeshed within the callus of the healing fracture. Frequently there is associated subcutaneous fat necrosis overlying the course of the radial nerve along the lateral aspects of the upper arm. The presence of isolated wristdrop with weakness of the wrist, finger, and thumb extensors, skin changes overlying the course of the nerve, and absence of weakness above the elbow serve to distinguish this from brachial plexus injury. Palsies of the femoral and sciatic nerves have occurred after breech extractions; the sciatic palsy has followed extraction by the foot. Passive range of motion exercises are usually the only therapy required. Complete recovery usually occurs within several weeks or months.

TRAUMA TO THE GENITALIA

Soft tissue injuries involving the external genitalia are not uncommon, especially after breech deliveries and in large babies.

Scrotum and labia majora

Edema, ecchymoses, and hematomas can occur in the scrotum and labia majora, especially when these are the presenting parts in a breech presentation. Because of laxity of the tissues, the degree of swelling and discoloration occasionally is extreme enough (Fig. 3-6) to evoke considerable concern among the medical and nursing staff, especially regarding deeper involvement (for example, periuretheral hemorrhage and edema), which might hinder normal micturition. However, this has not been a problem, and frequently these babies void shortly after arriving in the nursery. Spontaneous resolution of edema occurs within 24 to 48 hours and of discoloration within 4 to 5 days. Treatment is not necessary. Secondary ulceration, necrosis, or eschar formation is rare unless there is an associated underlying condition such as herpes simplex infection.

Deeper structures

Much less often birth trauma may involve the deeper structures of the genitalia. If the tunica vaginalis is injured and blood fills its cavity, a hematocele is formed. Absence of transillumination distinguishes this form a hydrocele. If the infant appears to be in pain, the scrotum may be elevated and cold packs applied. Spontaneous resolution is the usual course.

The testes may be injured, often in association with injury to the epididymis.

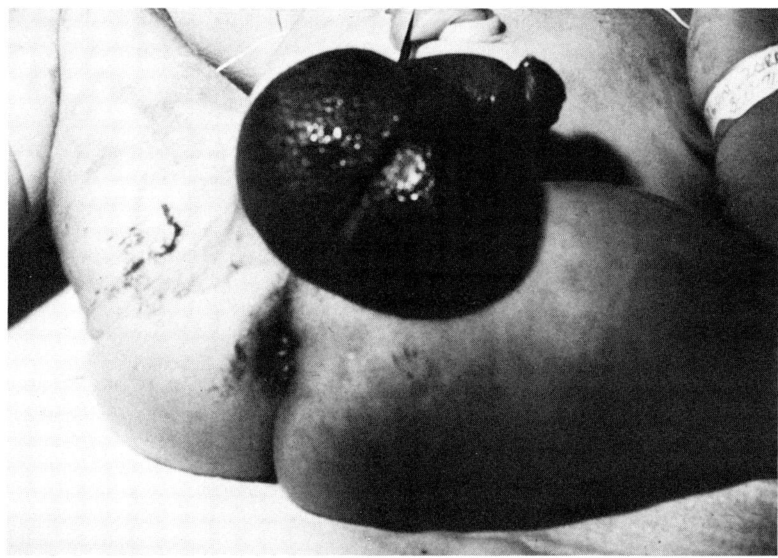

FIG. 3-6. Hematoma of scrotum and penis in 3,895-gm male delivered vaginally after frank breech presentation. The infant voided at 22 hours and regularly thereafter. Swelling diminished appreciably within 5 hours and was gone by the third day. Discoloration was markedly diminished by the second day.

Usually the involvement is bilateral. The testes may be enlarged, smoothly rounded, and insensitive. The infant may be irritable, with vomiting and poor feeding. Urologic consultation is indicated; occasionally exploration and evacuation of blood are necessary, especially with increasing size of the testes. Severe trauma may result in atrophy or failure of the testes to grow. The occasional finding in older children of a circumscribed fibrous area within the testicular tissue is thought to represent old birth trauma to the gland.

RICHARD E. BEHRMAN
HENRY MANGURTEN

BIBLIOGRAPHY

Altemus, L. A., and Ferguson, A. D.: The incidence of birth injuries, J. Natl. Med. Assoc. **58**:333, 1966.

Bingham, J. A. W.: Two cases of unilateral paralysis of the diaphragm in the newborn treated surgically, Thorax **9**:248, 1954.

Birrell, J. F.: The ear, nose, and throat diseases of children, London, 1960, Cassell & Co., Ltd.

Bishop, H. C., and Koop, C. E.: Acquired eventration of the diaphragm in infancy, Pediatrics **22**:1088, 1958.

Breinin, G. M., and Apt, L.: The eyes. In Barnett, H. L., editor: Pediatrics, ed. 14, New York, 1968, Appleton-Century-Crofts.

Cavanagh, F.: Vocal palsies in children, J. Laryng. & Otol. **69**:399, 1955.

Chasler, C. N.: The newborn skull (the diagnosis of fracture), Am. J. Roentgenol. Radium Ther. Nucl. Med. **100**:92, 1967.

Davis, J. A., and Schiff, D.: Bruising as a cause of neonatal jaundice, Lancet **1**:636, 1966.

Drucker, V., and Rodriguez, C. E.: Extensive bilateral calcification within adrenal hemorrhage, Radiology **64**:258, 1955.

Ehrenfest, H.: Birth injuries of the child, ed. 2, New York, 1931, Appleton-Century-Crofts.

Eng, G. D.: Brachial plexus palsy in newborn infants, Pediatrics **48**:18, 1971.

Eraklis, A. J.: Abdominal injury related to trauma of birth, Pediatrics **39**:421, 1967.

Ferguson, C. F.: Congenital abnormalities of the infant larynx, Otol. Clin. N. Am. **3**:185, 1970.

Gross, M., Kottmeier, P. K., and Waterhouse, K.: Diagnosis and treatment of neonatal adrenal hemorrhage, J. Pediatr. Surg. **2**:308, 1967.

Haliburton, R. A., Barber, J. R., and Fraser, R. L.: Pseudodislocation; an unusual birth injury, Can. J. Surg. **10**:455, 1967.

Hepner, W. R., Jr.: Some observations on facial paresis in the newborn infant; etiology and incidence, Pediatrics **8**:494, 1951.

Hodgman, J. E., Freedman, R. I., and Levan, N. E.: Neonatal dermatology, Pediatr. Clin. N. Am. **18**:713, 1971.

Holder, T. M., and Leape, L. L.: The acute surgical abdomen in the neonate, New Eng. J. Med. **278**:605, 1968.

Kendall, N., and Woloshin, H.: Cephalhematoma associated with fracture of the skull, J. Pediatr. **41**:125, 1952.

Labelle, P.: Orthopedic anxieties in the newborn, Appl. Ther. **8**:226, 1966.

Leape, L. L., and Bordy, M. D.: Neonatal rupture of the spleen, Pediatrics **47**:101, 1971.

Lee, Y., and Berg, R. B.: Cephalhematoma infected with bacteroids, Am. J. Dis. Child. **121**: 77, 1971.

McHugh, H. E.: Facial paralysis in birth injury and skull fractures, Arch. Otolaryngol. **78**:443 1963.

Monson, D. O., and Raffensperger, J. G.: Intraperitoneal hemorrhage secondary to liver laceration in a newborn, J. Pediatr. Surg. **2**:464, 1967.

Mortens, J., and Christensen, P.: Traumatic separation of the upper femoral epiphysis as an obstetrical lesion, Acta Orthop. Scand. **34**:239, 1964.

Raynor, R., and Parsa, M.: Nonsurgical elevation of depressed skull fracture in an infant, J. Pediatr. **72**:262, 1968.

Sanerkin, N. G., and Edwards, P.: Birth injury to the sternomastoid muscle, J. Bone Joint Surg. (Br.) **48**:441, 1966.

Schrager, G. O.: Elevation of depressed skull fracture with a breast pump, J. Pediatr. **77**:300, 1970.

Schubert, J. J.: Dislocation of the radial head in the newborn infant, J. Bone Joint Surg. **47**:1019, 1965.

Sezen, F.: Retinal haemorrhages in newborn infants, Br. J. Opthalmol. **55**:248, 1971.

Sieber, W. K., and Girdany, B. R.: Rupture of the spleen in newborn infants, New Eng. J. Med. **259**:1074, 1958.

Towbin, A.: Latent spinal cord and brain stem injury in newborn infants, Dev. Med. Child Neurol. **11**:54, 1969.

.Valdes-Dapena, M. A., and Arey, J. B.: The causes of neonatal mortality: an analysis of 501 autopsies on newborn infants, Pediatrics **77**: 366, 1970.

Vassalos, E., Prevedourakis, C., and Paraschopoulou-Prevedouraki, P.: Brachial plexus paralysis in the newborn, Am. J. Obstet. Gynecol. **101**: 554, 1968.

Walter, C. E., and Tedeschi, L. G.: Spinal injury and neonatal death, Am. J. Obstet. Gynecol. **106**:272, 1970.

Wilson, J. C., Jr.: Fractures and dislocations in childhood, Pediatr. Clin. N. Am. **14**:659, 1967.

4 Physical examination

The initial physical examination of the newborn should be done in the delivery room to detect significant anomalies, birth injuries, and respiratory disorders that may compromise a successful adaptation to extrauterine life. A more detailed examination should then take place in the nursery prior to advising the parents about their infant. The entire examination in the delivery room and nursery should be performed under thermally controlled circumstances to prevent significant heat loss from the infant.

EXAMINATION IN THE DELIVERY ROOM

In the delivery room color is of immediate concern. Generalized cyanosis may indicate significant heart or lung disease or the presence of methemoglobinemia (from a metabolic defect, p. 201, or secondary to misplacement of paracervical anesthesia). Differential cyanosis involving the lower extremities indicates persistence of a right-to-left shunt through the ductus, increased pulmonary vascular resistance, and, on occasion, a preductal coarctation (p. 298). Many normal infants have transient differential cyanosis that clears in the first minutes of life.

The pale infant either has been severely asphyxiated, asphyxia pallida, with the pallor caused by intense peripheral vasoconstriction; or is severely anemic, secondary to acute blood loss from placenta previa, fetomaternal hemorrhage, or to hemolysis from erythroblastosis fetalis (Chapter 9, p. 183). An immediate decision regarding the cause is imperative in the delivery room if shock from acute blood loss is to be reversed by transfusion.

The meconium-stained (green) infant should alert the examiner to the special risks of the acute or chronically asphyxiated infant (p. 52), who is often undergrown (SGA). Jaundice is seldom noted in the delivery room, even in severe erythroblastosis.

After considering the color of an infant, the examiner should evaluate the cardiopulmonary status. Inspection initially determines the respiratory rate. Tachypnea (a respiratory rate greater than 50 breaths per minute) should alert the examiner to possible pulmonary problems; bradypnea (less than 30 breaths per minute) or apnea or both should focus attention on the central nervous system and causes for central nervous system depression. Intercostal retraction, an audible grunt, or nasal flaring are additional signs of respiratory distress commonly present in the delivery room. Inspiratory or expiratory stridor should be noted and when present requires careful direct examination of the upper airway.

Auscultation of the chest reveals the quality of breath sounds bilaterally, the presence or absence of rales, rhonchi or expiratory wheezing, and the ease with which heart tones are heard. (Detailed examination of the cardiovascular system is covered on p. 244.) In the delivery room, each infant's heart rate should be recorded as well as the quality of the heart tones; heart murmurs may be transient, secondary to shunting through the ductus or foramen ovale or both, or may be indicators of significant heart disease. The absence, presence, and quality of peripheral pulses provide additional vital information on each infant.

The abdomen is inspected for protuberance, which may be secondary to abdominal masses or poor muscle tone, or concavity, which may be secondary to displacement of intestinal contents into the chest when there is a diaphragmatic hernia. Palpation and auscultation complete the initial examination of the abdomen. In the delivery room the relaxed muscular tone of the infant often allows the best opportunity for abdominal examination; both kidneys should be palpated to exclude renal anomalies. The umbilical vessels should be counted to exclude the presence of a single umbilical artery, which correlates with an increased incidence of congenital anomalies.

The genitalia are examined to ascertain the sex of the child and to exclude the possibility of ambiguous genitalia before telling parents the sex of their infant (p. 469).

The presence of significant choanal atresia should be excluded by manually occluding the mouth and each nostril and observing the infant for signs of respiratory distress or by passing a suction catheter through each naris into the stomach. The gastric contents should then be aspirated; the presence of greater than 30 cc gastric aspirate should raise the suspicion of upper intestinal obstruction. After the catheter has passed to a level that should be in the stomach, the instillation of 5 to 10 cc of air under direct gastric auscultation may be used to exclude the most common type of tracheoesophageal fistula. After exclusion of choanal atresia and upper intestinal anomalies, the same catheter can be used to establish the patency of the rectum.

The mental state and muscular tone of the infant should then be assessed. The neurologic examination is covered on p. 517.

Prior to releasing the infant from the delivery room, significant anomalies should be looked for; for example, clubfeet, cleft lip or palate, or meningomyelocele.

EXAMINATION IN THE NURSERY

The initial examination should be followed by a more detailed evaluation within the first 12 hours of life. Measurements of head and chest circumference and length, and recording of temperature and of heart and respiratory rate should be included.

Jaundice is the most likely change in skin color to be noted on subsequent examination. In addition, cyanosis and pallor should be reevaluated. The infant should also be carefully examined for the presence of hemangiomas, pigmented or depigmented nevi, and mongolian spots.

The skull should be checked for overlapping sutures, the patency of sutures, caput succedaneum with its poorly defined margins, and cephalhematoma with its clearly demarcated margins. The eyes should be examined (p. 606). Approximately 40% of all infants will have conjunctival or retinal hemorrhages noted in the initial examination. The presence of a red reflex should be established, pupil size and reaction to light recorded, and the lens checked for the presence of cataracts. The size of the globes should be examined for possible microphthalmia.

The face should be examined for any evidence of trisomies or other disorders that may be present with a distinctive facies; for example, cretinism. The symmetry of the face should be evaluated to exclude possible facial nerve injuries following traumatic deliveries or in infants delivered by forceps.

Malformation of the ears may provide evidence of associated renal anomalies, but more often are familial and only of cosmetic concern. The presence or absence of cartilage aids in establishing the infant's gestational age.

With the use of both a finger and a light with good direct visualization, both the soft and hard palates should be checked to exclude a cleft palate. High-arched palates as isolated findings are generally of no significance. Epithelial inclusion cysts are frequently noted along the gum margins and are benign entities requiring only parental reassurance. The tongue should be an appropriate size for its cavity; an inappropriately large tongue should raise the suspicion of a hemangioma or lymphangioma. The large tongue of cretinism is accompanied by other stigmata. The association of macroglossia with Beckwith's syndrome and Pompe's disease (type II glycogen storage disease) is well established. In infants with micrognathia a normal tongue may seem large. The well-known association of micrognathia, glossoptosis, and cleft palate (Pierre Robin syndrome) is often present initially as an upper airway obstruction and later becomes a cosmetic problem (p. 568).

The skin folds of the neck should be checked for webbing or fistulous openings associated with either branchial clefts or thyroglossal duct cysts. While examining the neck, each clavicle should be palpated for possible fracture. An asymmetric Moro reflex will often confirm a suspicious clinical finding noted on palpation.

The chest is examined for its musculature, bony structure, and location of nipples. By feeling for the pectoralis major in the axilla, one excludes absence of this muscle. Pectus excavatum or carinatum are of genuine concern to parents, but only rarely are of clinical or cosmetic significance. The areolar size provides additional evidence on the gestational age of each infant.

The lungs and heart are again examined, but with particular attention to questionable findings previously noted at birth, especially transient heart murmurs or adventitial sounds. Radial, brachial, and femoral pulses should all be palpated and compared. Poor or diminished quality of pulses is an indication of inadequate cardiac output, whatever the cause; absent femoral pulses are associated with coarctation of the aorta. Bounding femoral pulses may be equally grave indicators of congenital heart disease. If pulses are suspect, a blood pressure taken either by flush or by Doppler's technique (p. 245) should be recorded in the upper and lower extremities.

The abdominal examination is also repeated to exclude the presence of a mass. Examination of the genitalia provides additional evidence for establishing gestational age. Males should be checked for hypospadias, to determine the location of the testes, and to exclude either inguinal hernias or hydrocele, the latter being far more common. Most female infants have a mucoid vaginal discharge in the first week of life that occasionally becomes sanguinous secondary to hormonal withdrawal. Either a large penis or clitoris should raise the question of adrenogenital syndrome and there should be appropriate evaluation to exclude the diagnosis and its life-threatening sequelae (p. 472).

The extremities of each infant are ex-

TABLE 4-1. Estimation of gestational age

		Approximate week of gestation when findings present								
	Evaluation	**24**	**28**	**30**	**32**	**34**	**36**	**38**	**40**	
	Head circumference in cm ± 2 SD		**23-28.3**	**25-30.4**	**26.8-32.4**	**28.6-34**	**30.5-35.5**	**32-36.5**	**33-37**	Based on 300 single live births—all Caucasian
CLINICAL	Sole creases	Anterior transverse crease only →					Occasional creases Anterior two-thirds →		Sole covered with creases →	
	Breast nodule diameter	Not palpable—absent →					2 mm →	4 mm →	7 mm →	If small may represent fetal malnutrition
	Scalp hair	Fine and fuzzy → Hard to distinguish individual strands						Coarse and silky → Appear as individual strands		
	Ear lobe	Pliable—no cartilage →					Some cartilage →		Stiffened by thick cartilage →	
	Testes and scrotum	Testes in lower canal Scrotum small—few rugae →					Intermediate	Testes pendulous, scrotum full, extensive rugae →		

From Behrman, R. E., Fisher, D., Paton, J. B., and Keller, J.: In utero disease and the newborn infant. In Schulman, I., editor: Advances in pediatrics, vol. 17, Chicago. Copyright © 1970 by Year Book Medical Publishers. Used by permission. (Adapted from Amiel-Tison, Brett, Koenigsbergh, and Usher.)

amined for the presence of structural anomalies, such as congenital dislocation of hip, clubfeet, and neurologic disorders.

The neurologic examination is covered in Chapter 17.

At the end of the initial examination in the nursery the gestational age of each infant should be estimated. Table 4-1 lists the clinical criteria to establish gestational age. Close examination of sole creases, breast nodule diameter, scalp hair, earlobe, and testes and scrotum provide a rough guide to age that becomes more exact following the neurologic assessment.

Only after this detailed, but to the experienced physician, rapid (~15 minutes) examination, should the parents of the new infant be advised as to his general health. Another examination should be carried out just prior to discharge from the nursery.

JOHN M. DRISCOLL, Jr.

BIBLIOGRAPHY

Behrman, R. E., Fisher, D., Paton, J. B., and Keller, J.: In utero disease and the newborn infant. In Schulman, I., editor: Advances in pediatrics, vol. 17, Chicago, 1970, Year Book Medical Publishers.

Koenigsberger, M. H.: Judgment of fetal age. I. Neurologic evaluation, Pediatr. Clin. N. Am. **13**:823, 1966.

Usher, R., McLean, F., and Scott, K. E.: Judgment of fetal age. II. Clinical significance of gestational age and an objective method for its assessment, Pediatr. Clin. N. Am. **13**:835, 1966.

5 Routine and special care

Care of the newborn infant dramatically changed in the 1960s. Newborn intensive care units (NICU) are now considered as absolute necessities in university or large community hospitals; a need for a transitional care area has been established; and there is increasing evidence of the value of special transportation vehicles that permit care of sick infants in transit.

Each hospital must realistically assess its particular needs and capabilities on the basis of regional population, staff, services, and facilities. Preliminary steps have been taken toward an ultimate goal of regionalization of care for the newborn; but until such time as regional centers are functional, existing services and facilities for the newborn must be continually and critically reassessed in order to deliver the best level of care that is possible with the available resources.

Review of the different facilities established to care for the newborn infant will provide a basic understanding of the role of each unit as it relates to the general care of the infant as well as an appreciation of the specific medical needs of infants requiring a wide range of medical services. Following the definition of each unit, its facilities and staff, aspects of care common to all units are discussed. These suggestions are offered as *minimum standards*. Application of principles of care and definition of the physical location for the delivery of care remains the prerogative and responsibility of each hospital and its medical staff.

NORMAL NEWBORN NURSERY—TYPE I CARE

Characteristics of patients

Infants admitted to this area may include:

1. Well, full-term newborn infants by weight and gestational age who are in the lowest mortality group. They will be 38 through 41 weeks of gestation and 2,500 to 4,000 gm in weight.
2. Well, preterm newborn infants who weigh 2,250 to 2,500 gm and who are at least 37 weeks' gestational age. The capacity to adequately care for these infants depends on the presence of personnel skilled in feeding.
3. Other newborn infants who are at a comparably low mortality and morbidity risk (once this fact has been firmly established), who do not qualify under type II care, and who are well at the time of admission.

Personnel

Registered nurses

One nurse per shift is required; she does not necessarily have to be in constant attendance and may share responsibilities in an adjacent obstetrical area; she *must* be responsible for maintenance of all emergency equipment and know the appropriate physician to call for emergencies.

Paramedical personnel (practical nurses, aides, and others)

One individual must be attending the infants at all times (regardless of census), with a ratio of 1:6 required. These individuals should be trained in routine care, pharyngeal suction, oxygen administration by mask and bag, and routine feeding. They must also understand principles of hemostasis and be able to tie an umbilical cord as an emergency measure. If rooming-in is utilized, at least one person trained in these procedures must be available in an adjacent area at all times.

Physicians

A specific pediatrician should be designated as the physician responsible for general, medical, and administrative policies and routines affecting these infants, and he must regularly review all such matters. Each infant should have a particular physician responsible for his or her medical care.

Facilities and services

1. Infants should be cared for in a unit near the maternity ward or in rooming-in accommodations.
2. Care may be rendered centrally in one large room with a minimum of 18 to 24 inches separation between bassinets and approximately 20 sq ft per infant.
3. The number of bassinets should at least equal the number of postpartum beds plus 10%.
4. Infants should be placed in close proximity to the nursing station for the first twenty-four hr of life to assure more intensive observation during that period.
5. The hospital's laboratory must be able to provide on a 24-hour basis standard bacteriologic studies, urinalysis, hematocrits, white blood cell counts with differentials, blood typing and cross matching, a direct and indirect Coombs test, and microdeterminations of direct and indirect bilirubin, blood glucose, calcium, sodium, potassium, and chloride concentrations. Serology testing for phenylketonuria should also be regularly available during the day shift.
6. Equipment should include foot-controlled sinks and soap dispensers, stethoscopes, sterile umbilical tape, examining equipment, and emergency resuscitation equipment.

Medical policy and administration

1. Hospitals in which 500 or more infants are delivered each year should provide this type of care. Hospitals with less than 500 deliveries should be encouraged to discontinue their obstetrical services and concentrate these services in one regional facility.
2. Special protocols should be established for observation of infants during the first 12 to 24 hr of life.
3. Any infant who becomes ill, in whom a presumptive diagnosis of sepsis is made or whose course requires other than routine care, should be transferred to an area where he can obtain type II care.
4. Unsterile or unregistered deliveries or both not otherwise included under type II care may be admitted to this unit and maintained in an incubator with the special observation protocols used for the first 12 to 24 hr applied throughout their hospitalization.
5. All infants should be examined by a physician within 24 hr of birth and within the 24 hr prior to discharge. In nurseries where babies are discharged within 3 days of birth two examinations should be required within 72 hr.
6. Caps and masks are not required in the nursery. Short-sleeved gowns and hand-to-elbow washing techniques should be used by all visiting personnel. Scrub gowns or freshly laundered uniforms should be worn by nurses.
7. Regular monthly bacteriologic monitoring protocols should be instituted.
8. An area for emergency resuscitation with appropriate equipment, suction equipment, and oxygen must be available in each nursery and available on a portable basis for rooming-in arrangements.

TRANSITIONAL CARE NURSERY—TYPE II CARE

Characteristics of patients

Unless also qualifying for type III care, patients admitted to this unit should include:

A. Infants of high-risk mothers

1. Maternal toxemia, preeclampsia, and eclampsia
2. Maternal diabetes
3. Maternal cardiac or pulmonary disease
4. Maternal hypertension
5. Maternal drug addiction
6. Prepartum mothers with fever or evidence of infection
7. Rh-negative mothers with positive past history and present evidence of sensitization
8. Mothers under 15 and over 40 yr of age
9. Mothers whose infants were delivered by cesarean section
10. Grand multiparas
11. Mothers with evidence of polyhydramnios or oligohydramnios
12. Mothers with any other major medical or surgical complication; for example, thyrotoxicosis, hepatitis, sickle cell disease

B. Infants with birth weights from 1,500 to 2,250 gm
C. Infants with birth weights over 4,000 gm
D. Infants with gestational age by LMP of over 42 weeks
E. Infants with birth weight below the tenth percentile or above the ninetieth percentile for gestational age.

Personnel

Registered nurses

At least one registered nurse must be in attendance on each shift. She should be a part of the pediatric nursing service and should have no nursing responsibilities other than those related to care of these infants. Her overall responsibilities should include the availability and continued maintenance of all emergency equipment.

Paramedical personnel (practical nurses, aides, and others)

These additional personnel must be available to provide a final total personnel-to-patient ratio of 1:3.

Pediatrician

See type I. In addition the pediatrician in charge should make daily rounds with the charge nurse on all patients. Each physician who has admitted a patient should examine and review his patient's course daily.

Facilities and services

1. Infants can be cared for in an area either completely separated or contiguous to the well baby nursery or the newborn intensive care unit. This area may be located in the delivery suite.
2. Care in this area requires 20 to 40 sq ft per infant.
3. There should be accommodations for 3 infants per 100 deliveries.
4. Basic equipment for this area should include all the items required for type I care, in addition to incubators and appropriate monitoring equipment.
5. Infusion pumps should be used to control administration of fluids.
6. There should be 4 to 6 electrical outlets, 2 oxygen outlets, 2 compressed air outlets, and 2 suction outlets per patient care area.
7. The hospital's laboratory should provide the same support as that for type I care. In addition it should provide acid-base, blood urea nitrogen, and P_{AO_2} determinations on a 24-hr basis.
8. A portable roentgen unit with trained technicians must be available to provide radiologic studies in the unit.

Medical policy and administration

1. Hospitals with more than 1,000 deliveries per year should provide this level of care.
2. Administrative policies for type I care are applicable.
3. The duration of stay should be limited to a specific interval (for example, 6 to 8 hr or less if indicated by the infant's condition) with subsequent transfer to type I and type III care as indicated.
4. A transport module that provides oxygen, maintains temperature, and allows easy access to the infant should be available for transfer of infants between areas.
5. A single pediatrician should be responsible for the establishment and enforcement of medical policies and administration of this area.

NEONATAL INTENSIVE CARE NURSERY—TYPE III CARE

Characteristics of patients

Infants admitted to this area should include:

1. Any infant less than 6 weeks of age who requires intensive care. Occasionally, older infants who are small and have special nursing needs (for example, intravenous alimentation of a 3-month-old baby with a short bowel syndrome) may be admitted to this area and cared for in an isolette.
2. All infants with birth weights less than 1,500 gm; if such infants are otherwise normal after 24 to 48 hr, they may require less intensive observation. However, they must be cared for by a staff with skill and experience in feeding and observing low birth weight or premature infants. It may be convenient to group these infants in a subunit of the neonatal intensive care nursery.
3. Any infant less the 6 weeks of age who requires surgery (exclusive of circumcision).
4. Infants with sepsis, meningitis, pneumonia, syphilis, or other infection may remain in this area at the discretion of the director of the nursery with institution of appropriate isolation procedures.

Personnel

Registered nurses

There should be a 2:1 patient-to-nurse ratio with a 1:1 ratio for the sickest infants (for example, an infant requiring mechanical ventilation). Nurses in this area should have no other assignments outside this nursery unless it is on regular rotation to a type II nursery. All nurses in this area should have a closely supervised, well-controlled orientation program with its duration suited to the needs of the particular nurse; nurses without this orientation should not work in this area.

Paramedical personnel (practical nurses and aides)

These personnel should assist in the routine aspects of care, freeing the registered nurses for more technical duties and for more intense care of the sickest infants.

Physician

The director of this unit should be a full-time pediatrician with special training. Twenty-four-hour in-hospital coverage by a pediatric resident staff or a pediatrician is essential, and consultants must be available in all medical and surgical specialties.

Facilities and services

1. Infants must be cared for in an area that is separated from the well-baby nursery, but the area may be contiguous to the transitional care nursery. In designing new units, this area should be adjacent to the delivery suites if possible. Older hospitals may be unable to rearrange existent facilities to provide this access at reasonable costs.
2. A minimum of 60 sq ft per infant is needed to provide this care; 100 sq ft per infant is ideal.
3. Approximately 3 infants per 1,000 deliveries will require artificial ventilation, and 3 to 7 infants per 1,000 deliveries will need intensive care.
4. This area should have all the equipment required for type II care in addition to more extensive monitoring facilities; the question of using open versus closed (isolette) care for sick infants should be resolved by the physician in charge.
5. There should be 8 to 10 electrical outlets, 3 to 4 oxygen and compressed air outlets, and 3 suction sources for each infant.
6. The hospital laboratory must provide all the determinations needed for type I and type II care. In addition to 24-hour service for the aforementioned, determinations of phosphorus, magnesium and total protein levels, platelet counts, and prothrombin times should be available. Where delays in acid-base and particularly, P_{AO_2} are unavoidable because of location of the laboratories or limitation of personnel, a unit to measure pH, P_{O_2} and P_{CO_2} should be available within the nursery.
7. Roentgenographic facilities and trained personnel should be provided on a 24-hour basis in the unit.

Medical policy and administration

1. Hospitals with more than 3,000 deliveries per year should establish intensive care nurseries or have regularized means of transfer to a nearby unit.
2. Administration and medical care of patients in this area should be the responsibility of the director of the unit.
3. Provisions should be made to assure admission for sick infants transferred from smaller services; interhospital transportation of sick infants should be closely supervised by the director of this unit and should be developed to provide regional coverage.

TRANSPORT UNITS

Ideally, infants at risk should be delivered in institutions capable of providing intensive care from the moment of delivery. Nonetheless, it is estimated that 40% of neonatal problems are at present unpredictable. To provide for such emergencies an effective transport system with specially trained nursing personnel is essential. The early transfer of unexpected high-risk infants to a special care unit significantly alters neonatal morbidity and mortality. With present standards, much can be done to protect the infant from the risks involved in such a transfer and to ensure the infant's condition during his transfer. In some areas transport facilities are now available that are capable of initiating therapy in a critically ill infant before effecting transfer to a regional special care unit.

HOSPITAL UNITS

Physical facilities

Lighting

Lighting should allow easy detection of both cyanosis and jaundice and is best provided by fluorescent bulbs emitting 100 to 150 foot candles illuminance at the infant's bedside. This intensity will also alleviate the problems of shadows within the nursery. Spotlights may be provided in selected locations with either portable lamps containing two 150-watt fluorescent bulbs or by ceiling- or wall-mounted spotlights. Such white infrared lamps provide warmth as well as light; ceiling mounts of these lamps permit procedures to be done outside the isolette without the infant losing heat to his environment. The use of ultraviolet lighting in nurseries has been limited because of frequent complaints of nausea and dizziness from personnel working in these units. (See p. 229 for discussion of phototherapy.)

Walls

True skin color is best seen in nurseries having walls that are beige or white; brighter tones of blue and yellow interfere with the ability to evaluate jaundice and cyanosis.

Because of problems with temperature regulation in sick infants and reports of heat loss and overwarming in selected infants, some authorities have suggested elimination of outside windows from neonatal intensive care areas. Air insultation between two glass panes will reduce severe variations in temperature and is a compromise when windows are unavoidable. Outside awnings in parts of the country where radiant heat losses are a problem also reduce these losses.

Storage

Nursing efficiency is increased in a unit where easy accessibility of supplies is guaranteed by design of the unit; modular storage walls can be effectively used to this end.

Temperature control and ventilation

The air temperature in nurseries should be maintained between 28 to 30 F with the relative humidity less than 50%. These temperature and humidity ranges prevent excessive heat loss or gain for the infant and ensure personnel comfort.

The American Academy of Pediatrics suggests a minimum of 12 changes of room air per hour for control of infection. The fresh air input should be located either on or near the ceiling, with the exhaust outlet near the floor; the ventilation unit for the NICU should be separated from the remainder of the hospital system. A slight positive pressure differential between the unit and adjacent hallways should exist within the ventilation system. Most nurseries also incorporate an air-conditioning system within the ventilation system, despite the reluctance of some authorities to use air conditioning. Attention to filtering outside air with adherence to established standards is particularly important in urban nurseries where polluted air is an increasing ecologic problem.

Laminar flow provides direct vertical, sterile air flow more efficiently than presently used ventilation systems. But experience in intensive care units has been limited, and general adoption of this system at this time would be premature. Gluck is presently evaluating a portable laminar flow system to establish water requirements, oxygen consumption rates, and temperature ranges for an infant using such a unit.

Oxygen and compressed air

Oxygen and compressed air are generally supplied to the intensive care unit from a central source. The capability to provide mixtures of air and oxygen producing concentrations from 25% to 100% must be available. These mixtures should be available at both atmospheric pressure and with pressures up to 50 lb per square inch in units where positive pressure ventilators are used. Warning devices to alert personnel to falls in pressure should be part of each system. Compressed air systems require detailed planning and meticulous care once operational. Air should be washed, filtered, and then dehumidified before delivery into the system. All intakes must be closely checked to minimize the introduction of contaminated air. Small compressor units are unreliable and should be avoided; also, compressor units should be operated pneumatically and not electrically, because of an increasing number of power failures in some urban areas.

Acoustics

Design of intensive care units should utilize available methods of sound damping. Monitors, respirators, ventilation systems, and incubators all create noise, and at the present time no safe level of noise has been established. By restricting noise level within the nursery and within the isolette to less than 75 dB, the hearing of both personnel and patients will be protected.

Electricity

The medical profession is generally unaware of electric hazards (cardiac arrests, burns, and so on) related to the use of monitors, and most hospitals have no routine safety testing procedures appropriate for patient safety. In an attempt to minimize electrical hazards, certain recommendations can be made. The use of a single ground of low resistance wire is particularly effective when connected to all outlets in the nursery. Frequent checking of the integrity of this ground and all wiring will prevent the hazard of stray electrical currents. When more than one piece of electrical equipment is used, there must be enough outlets at each isolette to accommodate the equipment, with all units connected to a common ground. Prior to the installation and at regular intervals subsequently, all electrical equipment should be tested and maintained by a qualified engineer to detect defective equipment and current leakage and to specify appropriate safety precautions. Inservice training programs should be initiated to educate all nursery personnel in the proper use of equipment and recognition of potential electrical hazards.

Wash basins

There should be a wash basin adjacent to the door in each area and one basin for each four to six isolettes. All basins should have foot or knee or remote controls for hot and cold water and soap. Scrub brushes and paper towels should be conveniently placed near each basin.

Equipment

Apnea monitors

The availability of an increasing array of monitors has improved the care of the high-risk infant but has placed additional responsibilities on all personnel. The concept of a central nursing area with centralized monitoring, though quite useful in adult coronary units, has not found general application in newborn units.

Most apnea monitors utilize the principle of impedance plethysmography and present problems in proper application and maintenance of leads. The size of the electrodes, the irritation of the electrode paste or tape or both, and the lack of flat areas for application are recurrent problems to the nursery staff. The technique of applying electrodes to the arm of the sick infant offers a promising solution to this problem. The recent introduction of an air-filled mattress with a temperature-sensing device that detects movement of air coincidental with respirations and that sounds an alarm when apneic spells occur is a significant innovation that permits long-term, reliable observation of an infant, without application of electrodes, paste, or tape.

Cardiac monitor

Cardiac monitors either record the heart rate on an established scale or display the electrocardiographic figure on an oscilloscope. Rate changes indicate both ventilation problems and cardiovascular instability. The technical problems of electrode placement and grounding are common to all cardiac monitors. The proper application of the electrode ensures conductivity at the interfaces and minimizes false alarms or alarm failures; but with presently available systems, proper application of leads on the small infant remains a recurrent problem for the nursing staff despite advertisements to the contrary.

Blood pressure recorders

Blood pressure monitoring by direct recording with arterial catheters is often used in neonatal intensive care units. This mode of monitoring demands an awareness of the increased hazard of blood loss, infection, and electrocution and of the need for adequate safeguards. The transcutaneous Doppler method for measuring blood pressure provides a simple, noninvasive method for monitoring blood pressure. The Doppler method detects very weak impulses where the sphygmomanometer would be unable to detect any blood flow; correlations with the direct measurement of blood pressure are not firmly established.

Incubators

Thermal protection, reverse isolation, and complete visual observation of high-risk infants are possible with the use of incubators. The inspired air in such units is filtered, protecting the infant from airborne infections; but the infant, if infected, can still expire his contaminated air into the isolette and nursery, placing infants *outside* isolettes in jeopardy.

Ideally, isolettes should permit easy access to the infant; thus the open-front isolette with a movable patient tray is superior to a unit with a back hinge and front posts in allowing immediate access to the infant. Access holes for intravenous lines, monitor wires, suction tubing, and respirator apparatus are also required.

Monitors and infusion pumps are often placed on the top of an isolette; this damages the isolettes, impairs visual observation of the infant, and causes delays in gaining rapid access to the infant in emergencies. A shelf attached to the isolette itself or mounted on the wall above each unit should be used to avoid accidentally dislodging equipment from the hood of the isolette.

Oxygen or humidity or both may be provided by the isolette itself or via a head box placed within the isolette. The hazard of waterborne organisms and the cost of nursing time to clean water traps should be carefully weighed against the benefits of additional humidity. Each nursery should have a clean, warm isolette on standby at all times for unexpected admissions and emergencies. There also should be a regular check of all isolettes to safeguard against electrical hazards.

Bassinets

Bassinets should allow examination and care of the infant and be easy to clean; each unit should provide a storage area beneath the bassinet for disposable items used in the routine care of infants. A complete, functional unit for each infant provides an additional safeguard against cross-infection within the nursery.

Laboratory support

Intensive care units require responsive and rapid chemistry, bacteriology, and radiology laboratory support; the closer such facilities are to the intensive care area, the more efficient and responsive they are. Continuous communication between the intensive care unit and paramedical laboratory personnel regarding the exact nature of the clinical problems assures a more responsive laboratory and minimizes the problems associated with a heavy demand on the laboratory staff. Regular conferences with laboratory personnel to explain the common problems of the newborn have proved very useful in many nurseries.

Microchemical techniques available 24 hours a day should be an accepted standard for an intensive care facility. The availability of a blood gas analyzer within the intensive care area that can be operated by physicians assigned to the unit not only frees laboratory personnel to complete more complicated tests but also ensures immediate results as a basis for prompt changes in therapy.

The bacteriology laboratory should employ culture and sensitivity techniques that allow rapid identification of pathogens and their antibiotic sensitivities. If the bacteriology laboratory is not near the unit, the provision of a microscope, appropriate stains, and a small incubator will facilitate diagnostic evaluations and improve the efficiency of the staff.

A portable roentgen unit in the intensive care area ensures immediate roentgenologic support while simultaneously avoiding the hazards of hypothermia and hypoxia, which may be involved in the transportation of a sick infant to the radiology department. Newer magnification techniques promise improved quality of roentgenograms and more exact definition of radiologic signs. Proper shielding of patients and personnel is vital.

Control of environment

The establishment of stringent microbiologic environmental control has been the most significant factor in reduction of nosocomial infections in nurseries. Critical evaluation of these controls must be continued, though recent studies permit some modification of previously established standards. Before altering existent procedures and techniques, personnel must realistically compare the type of hospital (for example, university) where the study was conducted to their own institution. Many smaller hospitals have very wisely demanded the continuation of established environmental controls, acknowledging inherent differences between their own facilities and those where innovations have been initiated.

Gowning procedures in nurseries are either strict or modified. The strict version requires physicians and paramedical personnel other than the nursing staff to remove outer coats and jewelry, to scrub hand to elbow, and to gown before entering the unit; nurses change from nursing uniforms to scrub gowns. In modified gowning, personnel may enter the unit without changing their outer garments but, before examination of an infant, must remove their coats and vigorously scrub to the elbow. If an infant is to be removed from his isolette (his own microenvironment), the person must wear a surgical gown that is discarded after completion of the examination. Many authorities still feel that isolettes should be employed if the modified gowning procedure is used, but there is disagreement on this point. However, it is mandatory that nurseries adopting modified gowning procedures supervise and strictly enforce other basic environmental controls.

Thorough hand washing eliminates the most common route of cross-infection within nurseries. It requires accessible antiseptic agents and a sufficient number and proper location of wash basins. A dilute (less than 3%) solution of hexachlorophene is a frequently used solution for personnel even though the iodophors are superior because of their additional effectiveness against gram-negative organisms. Proper technique for washing calls for rolling sleeves above the elbow, initially washing hand to elbow for 2 minutes, and repeating the wash a second time for 15 to 30 seconds. Because of cutaneous sensitizing effects of the iodine-containing compounds, nurseries that use these compounds as the primary agent should always have a second solution readily available.

In addition to gowning and thorough hand washing, random periodic bacteriologic surveillance of intensive care units and personnel offers an additional safeguard against nursery epidemics. However, a survey that is too extensive not only overtaxes the laboratory but provides little useful information for personnel. Spot checks, unannounced to the staff, serve as an effective method for checking efficacy of disinfectant procedures.

The cleaning of equipment requires establishment of specific, detailed guidelines that are well known to all personnel. The aim of cleaning most equipment is disinfection (killing or decreasing the numbers of organisms known to be the potential cause of infection), but sterilization (killing of all organisms) is mandatory for certain items, such as surgical instruments. Gas sterilization has been recommended as the ideal solution to the problems of cleaning and disinfection, but such a gas system is unavailable in most hospitals at the present time. The most commonly used disinfectants are iodophors, chlorine compounds, phenolic compounds, and glutaraldehyde. Before disinfection of equipment, thorough cleaning is necessary in order to remove dust particles and grease that may partially inactivate the disinfectant. To ensure maintenance of certain standards, supervisory personnel should check the disinfectant procedure itself as well as periodically culturing recently disinfected equipment. Specific guidelines for cleaning various equipment used in intensive care units are available in a manual of the American Academy of Pediatrics on hospital care of newborn infants. Meticulous attention to details and supervision of the technique of all personnel are critical for safe, effective microbiologic control.

Temperature control

The effect of appropriate temperature regulation on reducing infant mortality, particularly in premature infants, has been clearly demonstrated. Most isolettes control temperature by using a fan to circulate warm air (forced convection). In these units, the temperature is controlled by a cutaneous, thermistor, usually secured over the liver, which regulates a fan within the isolette. There is generally some warming beyond the set point, and recent reports indicate an increased incidence of apnea during the warming phase of the isolette. For this reason, some investigators have suggested a radiant heat source rather than forced convection, since the former generally provides more sustained and less oscillating heat. The predominance of the forced convection units represents the manufacturers' decisions apparently based on technical and commercial considerations. Contrary to present trends toward more sophisticated equipment, Hey has suggested a more careful evaluation of cots for infants. Whether cots or isolettes are used, it is now possible to calculate the air temperature that provides each infant adequate warmth and simultaneously limits his caloric expenditure. Tables 5-1 and 5-2 are the recent recommendations of American Academy of Pediatrics of useful guidelines for this often neglected aspect of newborn care.

Oxygen therapy

The administration of oxygen to newborn infants requires clinical judgment supported by laboratory determinations. The use of cyanosis alone as a guide to the amount of oxygen that should be administered is potentially hazardous both in terms of underestimating (hypoxic brain injury) and

Table 5-1. Incubator air temperatures—first 24 hours

Birth weight		Temperatures			
		°C		°F	
gm	lb	Median	± Range	Median	± Range
	1	35.5	0.5	96.0	0.9
500		35.5	0.5	96.0	0.9
	2	35.0	0.5	95.0	0.9
1,000		34.9	0.5	94.9	0.9
	3	34.2	0.5	93.6	0.9
1,500		34.0	0.5	93.2	0.9
	4	33.7	0.5	92.7	0.9
2,000		33.5	0.5	92.3	0.9
	5	33.3	0.7	92.0	1.3
2,500		33.2	0.8	91.8	1.4
	6	33.1	0.9	91.6	1.6
3,000		33.0	1.0	91.4	1.8
	7	32.9	1.1	91.2	1.9
3,500		32.8	1.2	91.0	2.1
	8	32.8	1.3	91.0	2.3
4,000		32.6	1.4	90.7	2.5
	9	32.5	1.4	90.5	2.5

From Standards and recommendations for hospital care of new infants, ed. 5, Evanston, Ill., 1971, American Academy of Pediatrics, p. 90.

These tables are recommended for use as a guide when relative humidity is approximately 50%. Temperature should be higher than that in the table for lower humidity and altered in either direction, depending on various factors in the thermal environment and the individual infant's requirements.

Adapted and modified from data published by Scopes and Ahmed and Oliver.

Table 5-2. Temperatures according to age

Birth weight	Under 1,500 gm (3 lb, 5 oz)				1,501 to 2,500 gm (3 lb, 5 oz to 5 lb, 8 oz)				Over 36 weeks' gestation and over 2,500 gm (5 lb, 8 oz)			
Age	°C Median ± range		°F Median ± range		°C Median ± range		°F Median ± range		°C Median ± range		°F Median ± range	
1 da	34.3	0.4	93.8	0.7	33.4	0.6	92.1	1.1	33.0	1.0	91.4	1.8
2 da	33.7	0.5	92.7	0.9	32.7	0.9	90.9	1.6	32.4	1.3	90.4	2.3
3 da	33.5	0.5	92.3	0.9	32.4	0.9	90.4	1.6	31.9	1.3	89.4	2.3
4 da	33.5	0.5	92.3	0.9	32.3	0.9	90.2	1.6	31.5	1.3	88.6	2.3
5 da	33.5	0.5	92.3	0.9	32.2	0.9	90.0	1.6	31.2	1.3	88.1	2.3
6 da	33.5	0.5	92.3	0.9	32.1	0.9	89.8	1.6	30.9	1.3	87.6	2.3
7 da	33.5	0.5	92.3	0.9	32.1	0.9	89.8	1.6	30.8	1.4	87.4	2.5
8 da	33.5	0.5	92.3	0.9	32.1	0.9	89.8	1.6	30.6	1.4	87.0	2.5
9 da	33.5	0.5	92.3	0.9	32.1	0.9	89.8	1.6	30.4	1.4	86.7	2.5
10 da	33.5	0.5	92.3	0.9	32.1	0.9	89.8	1.6	30.2	1.5	86.4	2.7
11 da	33.5	0.5	92.3	0.9	32.1	0.9	89.8	1.6	29.9	1.5	85.8	2.7
12 da	33.5	0.5	92.3	0.9	32.1	0.9	89.8	1.6	29.5	1.6	85.1	2.8
13 da	33.5	0.5	92.3	0.9	32.1	0.9	89.8	1.6	29.2	1.6	84.6	2.8
14 da	33.4	0.6	92.1	1.1	32.1	0.9	89.8	1.6				
15 da	33.3	0.7	92.0	1.3	32.0	0.9	89.6	1.6				
4 wk	32.9	0.8	91.2	1.4	31.7	1.1	89.0	1.9				
5 wk	32.1	0.7	89.8	1.3	31.1	1.1	87.9	1.9				
6 wk	31.8	0.6	89.2	1.1	30.6	1.1	87.1	1.9				
7 wk	31.1	0.6	87.9	1.1	30.1	1.1	86.2	1.9				

From Standards and recommendations for hospital care of newborn infants, ed. 5, Evanston, Ill., 1971, American Academy of Pediatrices, p. 91.
See footnotes on Table 5-1.

exceeding (retrolental fibroplasia) the oxygen demands of a sick infant. The potential complications of oxygen therapy must be weighed against the risks involved in arterial catheterization. In institutions where physicians and nurses are inexperienced with technique, where laboratory support is inadequate, and where transfer to a special care center is impossible, clinical judgment of physical signs alone must be an acceptable compromise. In such cases, by gradually lowering the ambient oxygen concentration to a point where cyanosis is clinically detectable and then increasing the concentration by 10%, the physician has a rough guideline for both preventing hypoxia and avoiding hyperoxia. Regardless of existent institutional limitations, a general knowledge of the physiologic principles governing oxygen therapy is essential for any physician caring for sick infants.

When laboratory service and technical skill with umbilical artery catheterization are available, more exact determination of the oxygenation of a sick infant is possible. The transport and delivery of oxygen to the tissues is a complex process involving many factors: $P_{A_{O_2}}$, hemoglobin concentration, oxygen content, tissue perfusion, and affinity of hemoglobin for oxygen. Periodic measurement of $P_{A_{O_2}}$, hemoglobin, and pH, in addition to close clinical observation, is the most reasonable and accurate approach to minimizing the risk of both hyperoxic and hypoxic insults to a sick infant. When arterial catherization is contraindicated, radial, brachial or temporal artery puncture can be used, but repeated sampling from these sites requires skill and experience. In infants with mild respiratory distress not requiring arterial catheterization and in infants suspected of having significant right-to-left shunts these sites for sampling are particularly useful.

Having determined that an infant requires supplemental oxygen in spite of its potential hazards, the delivery of oxygen should be carefully controlled and monitored. When small increases in ambient oxygen are required, direct delivery into the isolette often suffices. With concentrations exceeding 50%, a head box within the isolette is a simple method for more accurate provision of the correct concentration while simultaneously limiting significant fluctuations in oxygen, especially when the isolette ports are opened. Some isolettes have cut-off mechanisms designed to prevent administration of oxygen exceeding a preset concentration. These controls cannot in general be relied on independently, and the ambient oxygen concentration should be checked at regular intervals by a paramagnetic oxygen analyzer or continuously monitored by means of an oxygen electrode. Orders for oxygen therapy should never be written in terms of flow (that is, liters per minute) but rather in terms of the desired ambient concentration with indicated intervals for routinely checking the concentration.

Oxygen should be humidified and warmed prior to delivery to a sick infant. If dry gas is administered to a patient, it will be humidified by evaporation from the respiratory mucosa. Under normal circumstances, this process presents no problem; but in a sick infant, particularly with respiratory distress, difficulties arise. By drying the respiratory mucosa, the viscosity of pulmonary secretions is increased and effective ciliary action is impaired. With these changes in major airways, airway resistance, already increased in most infants, may be further increased. Such therapy may also aggravate problems of water balance by significantly increasing insensible water losses from the respiratory tract. Oxygen that is not warmed may also be a significant cold stress to the premature infant with respiratory distress syndrome (RDS). Several investigators have demonstrated marked increases in oxygen consumption with the delivery of cold air to the face.

Oxygen may be humidified and warmed through the use of humidifiers and, on occasion, nebulizers. Humidifiers are designed to produce a maximum amount of water vapor, while nebulizers produce water particles of a particular size. Infants requiring nasotracheal intubation need humidifiers in their ventilation, while babies who are breathing spontaneously in head boxes and who have copious secretions are often treated with nebulizers. With nebulizers, exact control of humidity, condensation of water in the tubing, and difficulty of sterilization are common problems. The latter problem and the small droplet size produced by nebulizers have been suggested as possible explanations for the rising incidence of pulmonary infections in patients on respirators. Humidifiers are not difficult to sterilize and therefore are less likely to promote pulmonary infections, but they too are plagued with problems of condensation of water within gas lines and difficulty in controlling the temperature of the gas as it is delivered to the patient. Recent engineering improvements have alleviated the latter problem, but condensation remains a nuisance and demands nursing attention and time for observing and removing partial obstructions caused by condensed water.

Intensive respiratory care

In supporting babies with varying degrees of respiratory distress, certain standards must be established. Continual observation, frequent monitoring of vital signs both clinically and with monitors, and blood gas studies when indicated are essential components of respiratory care. Identification and monitoring of the high-risk infant should be paralleled with a readiness to intubate without delay when there are sudden changes or a gradual deterioration in an infant's course.

Clinical and mechanical monitoring should be supplemented by microblood gas determinations on arterial blood samples. Because of the contrasting risks of hyperoxia and hypoxia, particularly in premature infants, the PA_{O_2} must be measured frequently. The PA_{O_2} should be maintained between 50 to 70 mm Hg, especially if the arterial catheter is beneath the ductus arteriosus; this level of oxygen should eliminate the possibility of a significantly higher PA_{O_2} in blood perfusing the brain and the immature retina. Pulmonary oxygen toxicity is related to both the duration of therapy and ambient oxygen concentration in an unpredictable manner. Therefore each infant should receive only as much oxygen as necessary for as short a period as clinically possible.

Mechanical ventilation

Apnea is an absolute indication for mechanical ventilation, but delay in ventilation to the point of prolonged apnea can result in severe hypoxia that limits the survival from ventilation. The precise laboratory indications for mechanical ventilation are unsettled, and each unit should develop criteria based on a combination of their own experiences and reports from other institutions. Infants with PA_{O_2} less than 50 mm Hg while breathing 100% oxygen are ventilated by most neonatologists, but various combinations of PA_{O_2} and P_{CO_2} are considered as valid indicators for ventilation by others. The use of ventilators by highly skilled personnel has reduced mortality from respiratory distress, but ventilators alone are only partially responsible for this advance. The machines are only as good as the medical and paramedical personnel who operate them and provide total care for the baby.

When an infant is ventilated, the method of delivering a pressure or volume to the airway demands careful consideration. Endotracheal and nasotracheal tubes are used most frequently, but facial and nasal masks are favored by some physicians. Tracheostomy has been abandoned for almost all infants receiving mechanical ventilation because of the problems associated with placement of the tube, particularly in premature infants, and the difficulty in extubating the small infant.

Endotracheal tubes are generally used for resuscitation in the delivery room, but difficulty in fixing the tube for prolonged periods of ventilation limits its usefulness in assisted ventilation in the intensive care unit. Nasotracheal tubes may be easily secured and allow frequent pulmonary toilet during the course of ventilation. The size of the nasotracheal tube is determined by the size of the infant, a 2.5 or 3.0 mm clear portex tube for small (less than 1,500 gm) infants and a 3.5 or 4.0 mm tube for infants with birth weights greater than 2,500 gm.

The usefulness of oral-nasal masks in avoiding intubation is limited by distension of the stomach, large leaks around the mask, and significant facial edema. A mask to fit each infant's nose, using synthetic, rapidly fixing material, has been designed, and this technique may avoid some of these problems. The infant must be able to initiate respiration in order to use oral-nasal masks. No conclusive evidence supporting the superiority of this system to intubation is presently available.

Once ventilation is indicated, there are several types of positive and negative pressure respirators that can be used. The positive pressure ventilators are pressure- or volume-controlled units. The advantage of the volume-controlled units is in their capacity to adjust to changes in compliance of the lung, while the pressure-controlled unit must be manually adjusted as compliance changes. Leaks around the nasotracheal tube may cause problems in estimating the volume to be delivered; a tight-fitting tube limits the leaks and minimizes this problem. The principal problem with pressure-controlled units is development of high intrapulmonary pressures with rupture of blebs and production of pneumothorax and pneumomediastinum. Regardless of the method of ventilation selected, the results must be judged by serial blood gas determinations.

The use of negative pressure respirators is limited to infants greater than 1,500 gm because the effectiveness of ventilation is poor as smaller infants are shifted about within the isolette by the force of the vacuum created by the unit. The standard isolette negative pressure respirator has an additional disadvantage in that oxygen concentrations greater than 50% cannot be achieved in the attached head box. Substitution of a different head box or a transparent bag with additional oxygen sources corrects the problem. Generally speaking, an inspiration-expiration ratio of 1:2 is used with a residual negative pressure of -5 to -10 cm H_2O. The obvious advantage of this method is that artificial ventilation can be achieved without the use of a tube.

The recent introduction of continuous positive and negative airway pressure and positive end expiratory pressure has produced significant reduction in the mortality of infants with RDS (p. 360). The indications for this method of ventilation are the same as previously discussed for mechanical ventilation. The principle is that a continuous positive airway pressure will reexpand atelectatic areas and prevent further progression of atelectasis. This will improve the diffusion of respiratory gases; close monitoring of blood pressure is essential to detect hypotension related to obstruction of venous return to the heart. Because of the poor compliance of the lung, interstitial air, pneumomediastinum, and pneumothorax are a constant threat to the infant. Careful monitoring of each infant and extensive experience with the method have minimized these complications in many centers.

It is important to point out that several workers believe that use of the Ambu bag provides results similar to those from artificial mechanical ventilation while avoiding the problems of intubation. However, a large nursing staff with a 1:1 nurse-patient ratio is required with this method.

The method of delivering the gas and the type of ventilator used are obviously key elements in the successful treatment of sick infants, but without a dedicated, skilled, and experienced team of physicians, nurses, and technicians the former elements will produce mediocre results at best.

FEEDING

The advantage of early feedings in maintaining normal metabolism and growth during the transition from fetal to extrauterine life is clear. As soon as an infant can safely tolerate enteral nutrition, feedings should be initiated. This approach may decrease the incidence of problems such as hypoglycemia, hyperkalemia, hyperbilirubinemia, and azotemia. In the regular nursery, most infants are left without feedings for the first 6 hours of life. At this time, an initial feeding of sterile water is offered, and, if tolerated, the formula of choice is offered subsequently. Animal studies of the pulmonary findings after aspiration have demonstrated equally severe tissue reaction to glucose water and milk formula. When there is any question about tolerance of feeding because of physical or neurologic status of the infant, feeding should be withheld and parenteral fluids substituted.

Most term infants will rapidly progress from 30 cc every 3 to 4 hours to 75 to 90 cc prior to discharge at 4 to 5 days of life. Vigorous premature infants may require smaller (5 to 10 cc) feedings at more frequent intervals (every 2 hours) before progressing to larger, less frequent feedings. Caution and judgment must be continuously exercised in advancing the feedings of a premature infant. Rigid feeding schedules should be avoided and the initial small volume fed gradually and cautiously increased. Table 5-3 is a suggested guideline for initiation and advancement of feedings in premature infants that uses the physiologic capacity of the stomach to approximate the volume of feedings. The rate of increase that is well tolerated varies considerably from infant to infant.

Table 5-3. Average physiologic capacity of the stomach in the first days of life

Day of life	Stomach capacity (ml/kg birth wt)
1	2
2	4
3	10
4	16
5	19
6	19
7	21
8	23
9	25
10	27

From Silverman, W. A.: Dunham's premature infants, ed. 3, New York, 1961, Harper & Row, Publishers, p. 157.

Parenteral fluids

Regardless of birth weight, if the neurologic or physical status of the infant prohibits early feeding, parenteral fluid therapy, rather than starvation, is indicated. The physician must select the intravenous route that minimizes complications and allows the infusate to be delivered with maximum efficiency. In the newborn, the sites routinely used include peripheral veins on the hand or foot, scalp veins, the antecubital veins, and the umbilical vessels. If these sites have been exhausted, a venous cutdown may be inserted, most often utilizing the saphenous vein. The technical expertise and previous experience of the individual physician usually determines the infusion site.

Hypodermoclysis should be abandoned as a route of parenteral therapy. If a saline-glucose solution is infused under the skin, it must enter the functional extracellular fluid to be effective. In dehydration, blood flow is reduced, and thus the rate at which the subcutaneous fluid can enter the circulation is decreased. Furthermore, in some patients not only does the fluid remain in the extravascular tissue, but sodium and water leave the blood volume and enter the clysis fluid, increasing the likelihood of circulatory collapse.

Peripheral veins on the dorsal aspect of the hand or the foot, antecubital veins, and scalp veins are readily available in most newborn infants for routine parenteral therapy. The care utilized in starting the infusion, the subsequent nursing care, and the contents of the infusate are factors in determining the duration of each infusion site. The administration of hypertonic alkaline, or acid solutions through a peripheral vein diminishes the duration of the effective use of that particular site. Because the scalp generally has an abundant supply of superficial veins, these veins have become the most popular route for intravenous delivery of fluids in most nurseries. When entering these vessels, the physician must exercise caution to avoid the fontanelles, bony prominences, and small arteries. Nursery personnel must scrutinize each infusion site frequently to ensure its maximal longevity. If extravasation of acid, alkaline, hypertonic, or calcium-containing solution goes undetected, necrosis and sloughing of the involved area may occur with an increased risk of infection. In critically ill infants requiring long-term parenteral therapy, a venous cutdown is often inserted. In infants receiving intravenous alimentation, Dudrick's method for placing a catheter in the superior vena cava has demonstrated that aseptic technique during insertion of the catheter and meticulous care thereafter will allow constant, long-term infusion of a hypertonic, acidic (pH of 5.5) solution with minimal risk of infection.

Umbilical vessels

The sick neonate receiving supportive oxygen therapy as an intrinsic part of his treatment requires careful, continuous monitoring of the $P_{A_{O_2}}$. Though peripheral arteries (brachial, radial, and temporal) are available, the umbilical artery allows simple insertion of a catheter for continuous monitoring of blood gases. Employing the standards of Dunn (Fig. 5-1), we thread the catheter to a position 1 cm above the diaphragm and carefully secure it with suture or tape. The position is then verified radiologically. The decision to use this route demands constant observation of the umbilicus for bleeding, meticulous care of the catheter to prevent propagation of thrombus or air embolism, continuous

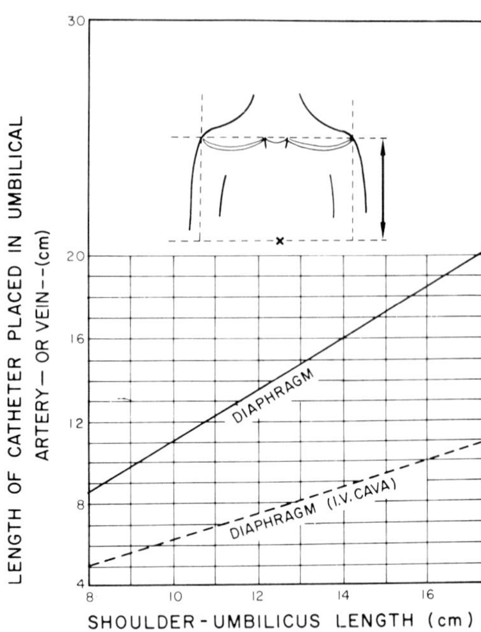

Fig. 5-1. Guide for placement of umbilical catheters.

scrutiny of the lower extremities for evidence of arterial spasm (cyanosis or blanching), and limitation of the duration of catheterization to a period as short as the clinical course allows.

The catheter should be removed cautiously so as to allow proximal arterial spasm for hemostasis. The acute and chronic risks of the umbilical artery catheter should be carefully considered and weighed against the advantages for each individual patient; this route should not be used for routine parenteral therapy.

Realizing the potential complications of the umbilical artery catheter and assuming that there is little risk in utilizing the umbilical vein, many physicians have adopted this route for parenteral therapy. The accessibility, the technical ease of inserting the catheter, and the longevity of the umbilical vein catheter are obvious advantages to this site. However, the umbilical vein catheter may easily pass into the portal vein, and the administration of sodium bicarbonate or THAM through the catheter creates the risk of infusing a hypertonic and strongly alkaline solution directly into the liver. One necropsy series reported a significant incidence (33%) of hemorrhagic liver necrosis in patients receiving THAM via the umbilical vein. Umbilical vein phlebitis, pyemia, and pulmonary embolus were noted by Scott in infants whose therapy was delivered via umbilical vein catheters. There have been recent reports of colonic perforation and peritonitis in infants following exchange transfusion via the umbilical vein. Thus, this route (umbilical vein) of intravascular therapy should be used only when no other is available.

Regardless of the route selected for therapy, certain recommendations are generally applicable. The advantages of the selected route must be weighed against its risks; there must be utilization of the proper technique in starting the infusion to minimize hazards, to safeguard its continuation, and to promote its longevity; proper nursing observation is required during the infusion, including maintenance of intravenous flow records and frequent inspection of the infusion site; and peristaltic pumps should be used to ensure constant flow and to minimize the chance of overhydration of a sick infant.

Gavage feeding

Many debilitated infants who are unable to suck and swallow adequately have evidence of active peristalsis (stools and bowel sounds). Various temporizing measures have been attempted to avoid the complications of parenteral fluid therapy and to take advantage of the infant's functioning intestinal tract. Gavage feeding is the oldest and most established of these techniques but is not entirely free of hazards. In addition to changes in heart rate and blood pressure during passage of the gavage tube, the tube itself may be an obstruction to respiration, particularly in the premature infant. The practice of passing a gavage tube prior to each feeding as opposed to an indwelling tube changed daily depends on the capability and experience of the nursing staff; with an experienced nurse, the indwelling tube is not essential.

A gastrostomy may be helpful in the postoperative period after gastrointestinal surgery. However, a controlled study has demonstrated increased mortality in premature infants fed through a gastrostomy. A *Murphy drip*, an adaptation of the gastrostomy or the gavage feeding, allows slow, controlled introduction of formula into the stomach by partially occluding the feeding tube. This method has enjoyed measurable success, primarily in the postoperative infant. The recent introduction of a *nasojejunal feeding* tube allows slow infusion of formula into the jejunum and circumvents the problems of vomiting, distension, and the dumping syndrome, which may be encountered with the gastrostomy or gavage tube.

Total intravenous alimentation

When enteral nutrition is impossible for prolonged periods of time, intravenous alimentation (IA) allows continuous infusion of sufficient fluid, calories, electrolytes, and vitamins to sustain growth. This technique has been life saving in neonates who have had extensive resection of bowel, but indications for intravenous alimentation in small premature infants are not established.

Under sterile conditions a Silastic catheter is placed proximal to the right atrium after cannulation of either the internal or external jugular vein; when these vessels are not accessible or are already in use, the brachial or subclavian veins may also be cannulated. After the catheter is tightly secured, with particular attention paid to avoiding occulsion of its lumen, the catheter is tunnelled to exit in the posterior occipital region. This maneuver removes the catheter from the wandering hands of the infant and places the exit site beyond the reach of the normal nasal flora of the infant, in an attempt to minimize the hazard of infection. Each area is covered with a pressure dressing and an application of Betadine, an antibiotic and antifungal ointment. The catheter is attached to a 0.22 Millipore filter to eliminate or minimize contamination from any bacteria, fungi, or particulate matter in the infusate. The efficacy of the filter has never been studied in a controlled fashion, but most authorities are reluctant to use the technique without insertion of the filter. The line is then attached to a constant infusion pump that accurately controls the flow of the hypertonic, acid infusate. The dressing is changed aseptically every 2 days as long as the line is used; the filter is changed at the same time. The infusion line is changed daily. In order to decrease the risk of infection, the catheter should be only used for infusion of the alimentation solution; blood should be drawn from other sites.

The infusate should contain a protein equivalent of 2.5 gm/100 ml, and hypertonic glucose in the range of 10 to 25 gm/100 ml, in addition to appropriate quantities of electrolytes and vitamins. There are several sources of protein available, both fibrin and casein hydrolysates and synthetic amino acids (see outline below). The biochemical limitations of each infusate and the needs of the particular patient should be carefully studied before selection of the appropriate protein source. The amino acid composition of the various infusates is not ideal; but until further investigation in this area defines the ideal amino acid solution, the presently available infusates should be used with caution. All solutions should be mixed by a well-trained pharmacist using a laminar flow hood. Mixing of solutions by nursing and house staff should be limited to emergencies to minimize the contamination of the infusate.

The complications of intravenous alimentation are generally confined to problems related to the catheter or to metabolism of the infusate. Sepsis is the most important problem, but several investigators have demonstrated that, with experience, meticulous care of the catheter, and aseptic preparation of the infusate, infection can be controlled. Various mechanical problems, including thrombosis, extravasation of fluid, accidental dislodgment of the catheter, and improper location of the catheter, have been reported. Some are unavoidable; but, once again, with experienced personnel most of these problems can be prevented.

The list of metabolic complications continues to grow as experience with IA increases. Hyperglycemia is most commonly noted in the early stages of IA, particularly in premature infants, when the infant is unable to metabolize the carbohydrates provided; without proper monitoring, the hyperglycemia may lead to significant weight loss caused by an osmotic diuresis. Hyperglycemia occurring later during the course of IA may be an indicator of sepsis and demands a careful examination, particularly in the postoperative infant, for hidden sites of infection. Sudden cessation of the infusion, either by accidental dislodging or thrombosis, may result in hypoglycemia. A peripheral infusion of 10% glycose should prevent this complication.

Hyperammonemia has been associated with IA and has two possible mechanisms With the use of beef fibrin hydrolysates, the hydrolysis of the beef fibrin produces a high level of free ammonia within the solution itself; while with casein hydrolysates, the lack of arginine in the solution may be responsible for the observed hyperammonemia.

Abnormal liver chemistries have been noted in patients receiving beef fibrin hydrolysates, and postmortem examinations in several patients have revealed intrahepatic cholestasis, extramedullary hematopoiesis, and hepatocellular necrosis. Animal studies have also suggested the possibility of the hepatotoxicity of the beef fibrin hydrolysates.

AVAILABLE NITROGEN SOURCES FOR INTRAVENOUS ALIMENTATION

A. Protein hydrolysates
   1. Aminosol (acid-fibrin)
   2. Amigen
   3. CPH
   4. Hyprotigen (enzyme-casein)
B. Synthetic L-amino acid mixtures
   1. Freamine

Despite the fact that most infants do not receive fatty acids, except through transfusion of blood and plasma, fatty acid deficiency is rarely reported.

Metabolic acidosis, a rare complication with protein hydrolysates, was observed in all infants receiving synthetic L-amino acids. Metabolism of cationic amino acids results in an excess of hydrogen ions and an associated hyperchloremic metabolic acidosis. The acidosis can be corrected by decreasing the protein concentration of the infusate or by infusing appropriate amounts of base.

Because of the metabolic complications associated with IA, careful, continuous chemical monitoring of all infants, particularly in the initial stages, is mandatory. This extensive surveillance requires a microchemistry laboratory; without this

Table 5-4. Variables to be monitored during intravenous alimentation, with suggested frequency of monitoring

Variable to be monitored	Suggested frequency	
	First week	Later
Growth variables		
Weight	Daily	Daily
Length	Weekly	Weekly
Head circumference	Weekly	Weekly
Metabolic variables		
Blood measurements		
Plasma electrolytes (Na^+, K^+, Cl^-)	Daily	3× weekly
Blood urea nitrogen	3× weekly	2× weekly
Plasma osmolarity*	Daily	3× weekly
Plasma total calcium and inorganic phosphorus	3× weekly	2× weekly
Blood glucose	Daily	3× weekly
Plasma transaminases	3× weekly	2× weekly
Plasma total protein and fractions	2× weekly	Weekly
Blood acid-base status	Daily	3× weekly
Hemoglobin	Weekly	Weekly
Urine measurements		
Glucose	4 to 6× daily	2× daily
Specific gravity or osmolarity	2 to 4× daily	Daily
General measurements		
Volume of infusate		
Oral intake (if any)	Daily	Daily
Urinary output	Daily	Daily
Prevention and detection of infection		
Clinical observation (activity, temperature, and so on)	Daily	Daily
WBC count and differential	As indicated	As indicated
Cultures	As indicated	As indicated

*Plasma osmolarity need not be determined directly; if the plasma concentration of sodium and glucose are known, osmolarity can be closely approximated by the relationship: plasma osmolarity (mOsm/kg H_2O) = 2× plasma sodium concentration (mEq/l) + plasma glucose concentration (mg/100 ml ÷ 18).

support, IA should not be initiated in infants. Table 5-4 suggests guidelines for chemical monitoring.

Partial intravenous alimentation using peripheral veins should precede IA, especially when a short period of enteral fluid restriction is anticipated. By using 10% glucose and 2.5% protein equivalent, several investigators have minimized weight loss and, in combination with small oral feedings, have achieved weight gain. This technique is far less hazardous and would be particularly useful in the small hospital where the lack of a microchemistry laboratory prohibits IA.

SKIN CARE

Most infants should be bathed with commercial soaps for their initial bath and with either the same preparation or tap water on subsequent days. Until further clarification of the hazards of hexachlorophene by federal authorities, routine use of this agent has been abandoned in infant washing. This change of policy demands close bacteriologic surveillance of nurseries to determine the existent flora and subsequent changes. Judicious use of dilute hexachlorophene (3%) on infants may be indicated for skin infections, and such use has been approved by the FDA.

Nursery personnel may continue to use hexachlorophene in hand washing though other superior iodine-containing preparations are presently available. Skin irritation or allergic reaction may result from the use of these iodine preparations. A rigid requirement of washing from hand to elbow for 2 minutes in the initial wash and for 15 to 30 seconds in the second wash is needed to minimize infection and cross-contamination. Shorter but equally careful washes between handling of each infant should also be mandatory.

CHARTING

Charts should be organized in an orderly fashion so that the clinical problems, therapy, and progress of the patient are obvious to all personnel. In intensive care facilities, nurses' notes, laboratory flow sheets, respirator and oxygen therapy logs, and intravenous therapy sheets should be kept at the infant's bedside. Organization of these records, allowing minimal reduplication and easy recording for the nursing staff, leads to development of concise record keeping and exact documentation of each infant's course. All too often, reconstruction of a significant change in an infant's course is impossible through review of his records. Although continuous electronic recording of vital parameters is increasing, many factors require human observation and demand careful record keeping in order to avoid loss of valuable time when there is an urgent need to document the exact nature of each infant's course. Alternatively, the value of detailed charting must be weighed against the nursing time required to complete flow sheets. The proper balance will increase the efficiency of care and will allow maximal use of time and effort by all personnel involved in delivery of care to sick infants.

PARENTS

The role of parents in any intensive care unit must be a serious concern for the team caring for each infant (p. 121). Maintaining strict environmental control, allaying of parental anxiety, and preventing interference with patient care are no longer acceptable reasons for denying parents access to their critically ill infants. Unlimited visiting privileges for parents should be the goal of every unit, with obvious restrictions of visiting during procedures or medical emergencies; grandparents should be allowed to see infants from the exterior of the unit.

Before a policy of increased parent-child interaction is defined in a particular nursery, there should be a preliminary discussion of each person's role (the attending physician, resident, *and* nurses) in supporting the parents. There should also be a free exchange of ideas among the staff after implementation of such a program. Involvement of parents in the intensive care unit offers a means for personalizing what is often a stark, impersonal setting and for providing greater personal and professional motivation for the entire staff. With these arrangements, the physician partially shares his previously exclusive right of talking to parents with paramedical personnel without compromising his sole responsibility for communication of strictly medical facts to the family. In such a setting, the nursing staff may provide emotional support for a mother that a physician is unable to supply; this support assumes significant proportions in the context of delivery of total care. The death of an infant is made more acceptable for parents when the personnel consider this aspect of care equally important to the salvage of meaningful life.

Premature infants who survive a serious illness but who have prolonged hospitalizations should be in a nursery where parents are actively involved in routine care. Tasks that are often tedious and meaningless to paramedical personnel, (such as diaper changing and washing) are cherished moments for parents who in previous times were separated from their infants. At the time of discharge, the anxiety of parents who have been significantly involved in the care of their child, even at his worst moments, surely must be significantly less than those parents who have been anxious bystanders for 2 months.

JOHN M. DRISCOLL, Jr.
RICHARD E. BEHRMAN

BIBLIOGRAPHY

American Academy of Pediatrics: Hospital care of newborn infants, ed. 5, Evanston, Illinois, 1971, the Academy.

Babson, S. G.: Feeding the low birth weight infant, J. Pediatr. **79**:694, 1971.

Babson, S. G.: Peripheral intravenous alimentation of the small premature infant, J. Pediatr. **79**: 494, 1971.

Chernick, V., and Raber, M. B.: Electrical hazards in the newborn nursery, J. Pediatr. **77**:143, 1970.

Duc, G.: Assessment of hypoxia in the newborn; suggestions for a practical approach, Pediatrics **48**:469, 1971.

Dunn, P. M.: Localization of the umbilical catheter by postmortem measurement, Arch. Dis. Child. **41**:69, 1966.

Gluck, L.: Design of a perinatal center, Pediatr. Clin. N. Am. **17**:777, 1970.

Goldenberg, V. E., Wiegenstein, L., and Hopkins, G. B.: Hepatic injury associated with trometha-mine, J.A.M.A. **205**:71, 1968.

Gregory, G. A.: Continuous positive pressure breathing therapy for neonatal respiratory distress, Hosp. Pract., August 1972, p. 1002.

Gruber, H. S., and Klaus, M. H.: Intermittent bag and mask therapy; an alternative approach to respiratory therapy for infants with severe respiratory distress, J. Pediatr. **76**:194, 1970.

Heese, H. deV., Harrison, V. C., Klein, M., and Malan, A. F.: Intermittent positive pressure ventilation in hyaline membrane disease, J. Pediatr. **76**:183, 1970.

Heird, W. C., Dell, R. B., Driscoll, J. M., Jr., Grebin, B., and Winters, R. W.: Metabolic acidosis after intravenous alimentation with amino acids, New Eng. J. Med. **287**:943, 1972.

Heird, W. C., Driscoll, J. M., Jr., Schullinger, J. N., Grebin, B., and Winters, R. W.: Intravenous alimentation in pediatric patients, J. Pediatr. **80**:351, 1972.

Hey, E.: The care of babies in incubators; recent advances in pediatrics, ed. 4, London, 1971, J. & A. Churchill.

Kitterman, J. A., Phibbs, R. H., and Tooley, W. H.: Catheterization of umbilical vessels in newborn infants, Pediatr. Clin. N. Am. **17**:895, 1970.

Oliver, T. K., Jr.: Temperature regulation and heat production in the newborn, Pediatr. Clin. N. Am. **12**:765, 1965.

Outerbridge, E. W., Roloff, D. W., and Stern, L.: Continuous negative pressure in the management of severe respiratory distress syndrome, J. Pediatr. **81**:384, 1972.

Scott, J. M.: Iatrogenic lesions in babies following umbilical vein catherization, Arch. Dis. Child **40**:426, 1965.

Segal, S.: Transportation of high risk infants, Vancouver, B. C., Canadian Pediatr. Soc. In press.

Segal, S., and Pirie, G. E.: Equipment and personnel for neonatal special care, Pediatr. Clin. N. Am. **17**:793, 1970.

Sinclair, J. C., Driscoll, J. M., Jr., Heird, W. C., and Winters, R. W.: Supportive management of the sick neonate; parenteral calories, water and electrolytes, Pediatr. Clin. N. Am. **17**:863, 1970.

Spaulding, E. H.: Chemical disinfection in the hospital, J. Hosp. Res. **3**:25, 1965.

Stahlman, M. T., Malan, A. F., Shepard, F. M., Blankenship, W. J., Young, W. C., and Gray, J.: Negative pressure assisted ventilation in infants with hyaline membrane disease, J. Pediatr. **76**:174, 1970.

Swyer, P. R.: The regional organization of special care for the neonate, Pediatr. Clin. N. Am. **17**:761, 1970.

Vengusamy, S., Pildes, R. S., Raffensperger, J. F., Levine, H. D., and Cornblath, M.: A controlled study of feeding gastrostomy in low birth weight infants, Pediatrics **43**:815, 1969.

6 Parenteral therapy

Normally water, calories, and electrolytes are provided orally for newborn infants. However, oral intake may be contraindicated by structural anomalies of the gastrointestinal tract, by neurologic or medical problems that impair normal sucking or swallowing, by respiratory distress, by convulsions, or by other acute illness. In these infants, fluid, electrolytes, and calories must be provided parenterally. This discussion focuses on maintenance requirements; that is, the amounts necessary to meet ongoing expenditures but that will not allow growth. Total intravenous alimentation, the provision of calories, fluids, and electrolytes to promote growth, is covered in Chapter 5. General pediatric texts should be consulted for discussions of deficit replacement therapy for dehydration and other exceptional losses.

Parenteral fluid requirements of the newborn are dependent on total body stores and their utilization, which vary with gestational age, postnatal age, and body size. As gestation progresses, intracellular mass increases while extracellular mass decreases; as the fetus grows, extracellular water accounts for a diminishing proportion of total body weight so that the total body water content of a term infant is significantly less than an infant delivered at 28 weeks' gestation. While the total body water decreases as the fetus grows, the protein and fat content increases. At the twenty-eighth week of gestation less than 1% of total body weight is fat, while the fat content of the full-term infant is approximately 15%; the protein stores follow a similar trend. In the last trimester, the glycogen content of the liver, heart, and diaphragm significantly increases so that at birth these organs are twice the adult norms. Carbohydrate is the principal energy source in the early hours of postnatal life. Table 6-1 compares the body composition of three infants.

The metabolic rate of a full-term infant in the first day of life is 30 to 35 calories per kg per day and gradually increases to 43 to 45 calories per kg per day by the third day of life. The premature infant has a lower initial rate (30 calories per kg per day); but by the fourth to sixth week of life, his basal metabolic rate has increased to 60 calories per kg per day. Infants who are small for gestational age have higher metabolic rates than premature infants of similar birth weight; this may be related to the disproportionately large metabolic requirements of the brain. Metabolic rates derived from oxygen consumption studies provide the basis for estimating the basal or resting caloric needs of the infant. Additional calories must be provided for activity, cold stress, specific dynamic action, fecal loss, and growth. Table 6-2 lists the average caloric expenditures for a growing premature infant. Generally, for growth one must double the resting caloric requirements, although there are substantial individual variations in the average caloric requirements necessary to sustain growth (80 to 220 calories per kg per 24 hours). Temperature elevations, hypothermia, increased muscle activity (respiratory distress, convulsions, and so on) increase the caloric requirements.

Fluid and electrolyte requirements are directly related to losses to the environment—evaporation from skin and respira-

TABLE 6-1. Total amounts of water, fat, protein and carbohydrate in the human baby at birth

Constituent	Small premature Amount (gm)	Small premature Percent of body wt.	Large premature Amount (gm)	Large premature Percent of body wt.	Full-term Amount (gm)	Full-term Percent of body wt.
Body weight	1000		2000		3500	
Water	860	86	1620	81	2400	69
Fat	10	1	100	5	560	16
Protein	85	8.5	230	11	390	11
Carbohydrate	4.5	0.5	9	0.5	34	1

Adapted from Widdowson, E. M., by Sinclair, J. C., and others: Pediatr. Clin. North Am. **17**:863, 1970.

TABLE 6-2. Partition of daily caloric expenditure in a typical growing premature infant

Item	Cal/kg/24 hr
Resting caloric expenditure	50
Intermittent activity	15
Occasional cold stress	10
Specific dynamic action	8
Fecal loss of calories	12
Growth allowance	25
Total	120

tory tract (insensible losses)—and to urinary losses. Unless the infant has diarrhea, stool losses are insignificant. Sweat losses are usually negligible. The most significant route for water loss is evaporation. The amount of water lost is dependent on the infant's surface area, air flow over the infant, and vapor pressure differences between the infant's skin and his environment. Water loss from the respiratory tract is dependent on respiratory rate, the minute volume, and the absolute humidity of the ambient air. Evaporative losses from both the skin and respiratory tract can be reduced by increasing the humidity within an isolette; respiratory water losses can be reduced 30% with high humidity. Infants of less than 37 weeks' gestation do not lose significant amounts of water by sweating and evaporation, but term infants can triple their evaporative water losses by sweating.

Water is also lost through urinary excretion. In the first several days of life all infants lose weight. This represents primarily loss of extracellular fluid with corresponding loss of sodium, the main extracellular cation. Though this loss is felt to be physiologic by many authorities and, therefore, does not require replacement, signs of dehydration, both clinical and chemical, will develop if infants do not receive adequate enteral fluids. A reasonable goal is to provide sufficient fluids to prevent the appearance of signs of dehydration. In order to provide this fluid safely, the physician should be aware of certain characteristics of the newborn infant's renal function that may affect his ability to handle the volume and type of fluids provided (Chapter 16, p. 485). First, the tubular capacity to secrete or reabsorb certain substances is limited in comparison to the rate at which the same substances are filtered (for example, glomerulotubular imbalance). In addition, the neonate has a limited diuretic response to water loads. There is also a limitation of renal acidification mechanisms, which in combination with curtailment of ammonium excretion and a reduction in the threshold for bicarbonate reabsorption impairs total renal acidification. All of these factors must be considered in designing parenteral fluids to meet maintenance fluid requirements.

REQUIREMENTS

The aim of maintenance fluid therapy is to match ongoing losses of water, electrolytes, and calories; the former two are easily replaced, but total replacement of caloric losses by parenteral route presents special problems (p. 113). The following list* provides the suggested maintenance

*Adapted from Sinclair, J. C., Driscoll, J. M. J., Heird, W. C., and Winters, R. W.: Pediatr. Clin. N. Am. **17**:863, 1970.

requirements for fluid, electrolytes, and calories.

1. Fluid requirements	Water/kg/24 hours
Insensible water loss	
Lungs	7-10 ml
Skin	14-20 ml
Urine	25-62 ml
Stool	2
Total	48-92 ml
2. Caloric requirements	Calories/kg/24 hours
Resting expenditures	50
Activity	0-15
Cold stress	0-10
Total	50-75 calories
3. Electrolytes	mEq/kg/24 hours
Sodium	0.5-2.0 mEq
Potassium	0.5-2.0 mEq
Chloride	0.5-2.0 mEq
4. Parenteral maintenance solution	
Dextrose 10% and water	100 ml
Sodium	2 mEq
Potassium	2 mEq
Chloride	4 mEq
Rate: 75 ml/kg/24 hours	

The typical fluids should provide 75 ml/kg/day while providing 50 cal/kg/day during the first several days of life. The volume may have to be increased to 100 to 120 ml/kg/day if clinical or chemical signs of dehydration develop. Potassium is usually omitted for the first 24 hours of life because of low glomerular filtration rates and decreased urine output. Therapy should be planned for 12- to 24-hour periods, with close observation of clinical signs and laboratory data determining the adequacy of the initial plan. With loss of weight, development of clinical signs of dehydration, and a diminution in urine output, additional fluids should be provided. Supportive laboratory data (acid-base, electrolyte, and urinary specific gravity determinations) provide additional information to modify initial parenteral therapy. When there are abnormal fluid losses, such as diarrhea and gastric suctioning, an adequate volume with corresponding composition must be replaced.

Practical points in provision of parenteral therapy are covered in Chapter 5.

JOHN M. DRISCOLL, Jr.

BIBLIOGRAPHY

Bruch, R.: Temperature regulation on the newborn infant, Biol. Neonate 3:65, 1961.

Edelman, C. M., and Spitzer, A.: The maturing kidney, J. Pediatr. **75**:509, 1969.

Edelman, C. M. J., and Barnett, H. L.: Role of the kidney in water metabolism in young infants, J. Pediatr. **56**:154, 1960.

Silverman, W. A., and Blanc, W. A.: The effect of humidity on survival of newly born premature infants, Pediatrics **20**:477, 1957.

Sinclair, J. C., Driscoll, J. M. J., Heird, W. C., and Winters, R. W.: Supportive management of the sick neonate; parenteral calories, water, and electrolytes, Pediatr. Clin. N. Am. **17**:863, 1970.

Winters, R. W.: Principles of pediatric fluid therapy. Abbott Laboratories, 1970.

7 Care of the mother

The long period of physical separation common in most nurseries may adversely influence the maternal performance of some women, affecting the formation of affectional bonds and changing mothering behavior months and years after the delivery. This chapter discusses these problems in terms of the history of premature management and the application of new information about prolonged separation to clinical care.

THE HUMAN MOTHER

Pregnancy

Detailed observations of the behavioral changes that take place in a woman during pregnancy have indicated that pregnancy is a process of maturation. A series of adaptive tasks must be completed, each step dependent upon the completion of those preceding (see list below). Two of the most important steps for which an obstetrician should be alert are: (1) acceptance of the pregnancy—a progression from the not uncommon initial rejection of the pregnancy to the woman's acceptance of the fetus as an integral part of herself, and (2) awareness of the fetus as a separate individual. This step usually occurs with the onset of fetal movement, during which time the mother begins to fantasize about the baby, to make preparations for his arrival, and to develop a sense of attachment toward him. At this time, unwanted, unplanned infants may become more acceptable to the mother.

STEPS IN ATTACHMENT

Planning the pregnancy
Confirming the pregnancy
Accepting the pregnancy
Fetal movement
Accepting the fetus as an individual
Birth
Seeing the baby
Touching the baby
Caretaking

A number of stressful factors (for example, the loss of previous children or of other relatives or close friends, a move to an unfamiliar location, or marital infidelity) may leave the mother feeling unsupported or unloved and may retard further bond formation with the infant during pregnancy and cause a delay in further preparation. This in turn may greatly influence a mother's subsequent maternal behavior and, as a consequence, the development of her child.

Delivery

Although surprisingly little data are available for the delivery period, mothers who remain calm and relaxed and have good rapport with their attendants are those who are most apt to be pleased at first sight of their infants. Rejection of the infant is not induced by unconsciousness of the mother during delivery. Affectional ties after birth have been noted before any tactile contact has occurred.

First weeks after delivery

A regular pattern of behavior occurs in the human mother immediately after birth. Filmed observations show that a mother presented with her nude, full-term infant begins fingertip touching on the infant's extremities and then within 8 minutes has proceeded to encompassing, massaging palm contact on the infant's trunk (Fig. 7-

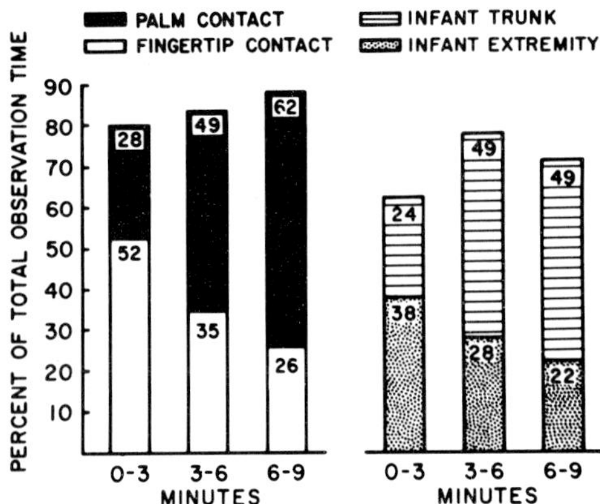

Fig. 7-1. Palm and fingertip contact on the trunk and extremities at the first postnatal contact in 12 mothers of full-term infants. (From Klaus, M., and others: Human maternal behavior at the first contact with her young, Pediatrics **46**:190, 1970.)

1). Mothers of premature infants also follow this sequence, but at a slower rate. Eye-to-eye contact is important to both mothers of full-term and premature infants and appears to be an innate releaser of the maternal caretaking response. The infant's visual pathways are sufficiently developed to attend and follow in the first hours of life.

Minor problems (such as slight hyperbilirubinemia, mild respiratory distress, and poor feeding) resulting in separation during this period may disturb and distort maternal affectional ties. This disturbance of mothering may last for a year or through childhood and beyond, even though the infants' problems were completely resolved prior to discharge.

The introduction of compulsory rooming-in at one hospital resulted in an increase in the incidence of breast feeding and a decrease in frequency of anxious phone calls from mothers after discharge, suggesting that close continual contact after birth may be important in encouraging more relaxed maternal behavior. Mothers who are allowed to visit and touch their infants in the nursery shortly after birth tend to be more skillful in feeding their infants, to hold them differently, and to spend more time cuddling their infants than mothers who are not allowed to touch their infants until 20 days after birth. If early maternal attentiveness does facilitate later exploratory behavior in infants, then the differences in these mothers may strongly affect the later development of their children.

Only mothers who room-in or deliver at home suffer no deprivation of contact with their infants; even mothers of normal full-term infants delivered in a hospital undergo some deprivation. The mother of a premature infant experiences not only severe deprivation of contact with her infant, but faces what has been considered an acute emotional crisis; she progresses through four psychologic stages: (1) anticipatory grief, preparing herself for the infant's death, (2) acceptance of her failure to deliver a full-term infant, (3) resumption of the process of relating to her infant, and (4) learning the special needs of a premature infant.

A mother's ability to endure emotional stress and her ultimate mothering behavior are influenced by a multitude of factors (Fig. 7-2). Some of these may already be unchangeable at delivery (for example, how the mother herself was mothered as an infant, her relationship with the rest of her family, her cultural traditions, and her experiences with previous pregnancies). Other factors may be altered, including the behavior of doctors, nurses, and other hospital personnel, the routine practices of the hospital, and whether the mother and infant are separated after birth. Distortions or disorders of mothering (such as battering, failure to thrive, parents' fears that a normal child will die prematurely, and the behavioral problems of the adopted child) may be related to the above influences on the mother, and a major component of these disorders may be the separation of mother and infant. The disproportionately high percentage of premature infants who return to the hospital with failure to thrive and battering tend to support this contention.

Death of a newborn or stillbirth

Despite advances in neonatal and obstetrical care, a large number of women still suffer early abortion or loss of an infant after birth. Only recently has it been appreciated that a clearly identifiable mourning reaction occurs in both parents after the death of a newborn infant, whether or not the mother has had physical contact with the infant. The same mourning reactions will be observed in parents who have

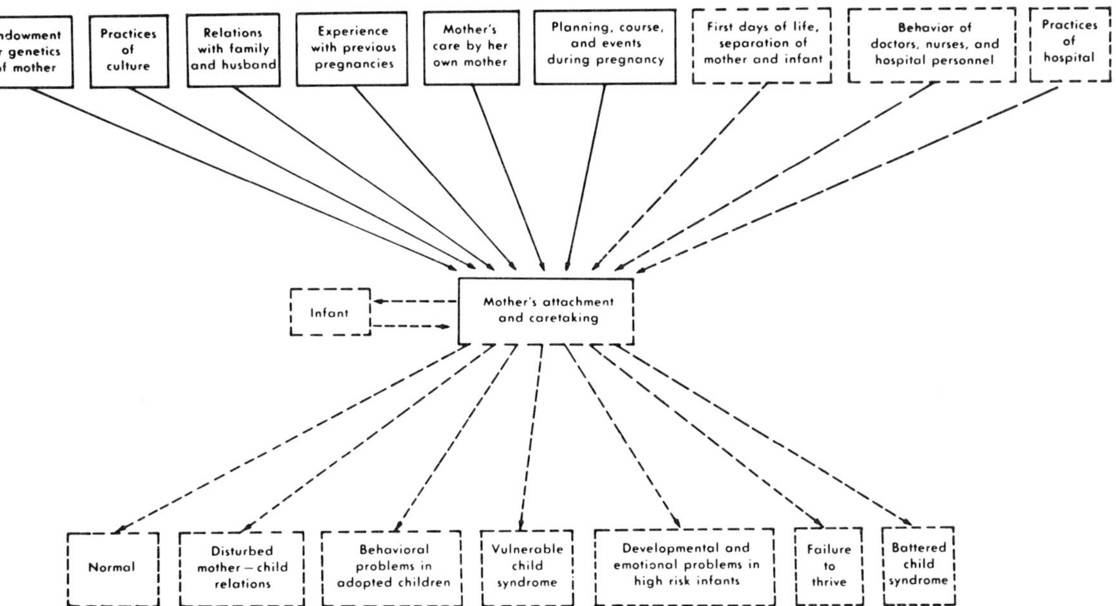

Fig. 7-2. Disorders of mothering; a hypothesis of their cause. Solid lines indicate determinants that are ingrained; dashed lines indicate factors that may be altered or changed. (From Klaus, M., and Kennell, J.: Mothers separated from their newborn infants, Pediatr. Clin. North Am. **17**:1028, 1970.)

lost a newborn as in people grieving the death of a close older relative. The mourning reactions of normal grief comprise a syndrome that includes (1) somatic distress, (2) preoccupation with the image of the deceased, (3) feelings of guilt, (4) feelings of hostility, and (5) breakdown of normal patterns of conduct. These reactions may appear immediately, or they may be delayed or seemingly absent. A painful period of grief is a necessary response; its absence is a signal for alarm.

The frequent observation of a breakdown in communication between husband and wife after the death of a newborn has been a worrisome problem. Parents who, before the loss, communicated well with each other may be unable to express their feelings and therefore never satisfactorily resolve their grief. Since the expression of strong emotion is not encouraged in our society, their reactions to the death may perplex and worry them, causing an even greater barrier to their communication.

Pathologic mourning, believed to be a distortion of normal grief, includes such reactions as (1) overactivity without a sense of loss, (2) acquisition of symptoms belonging to the deceased, (3) psychosomatic reactions such as ulcerative colitis, (4) alterations in relations with others, (5) furious hostility, (6) repression of hostility, (7) lasting loss of patterns of social interaction, (8) activities detrimental to one's own economic and social existence, and (9) agitated depressions.

BASIC CONSIDERATIONS IN ANIMAL BEHAVIOR AND HISTORY PERTINENT TO THE CARE OF THE HUMAN MOTHER

Animals

While certain aspects of behavior vary from species to species, some clearly identifiable common patterns may be observed. Although a literal translation from animals to human beings is not appropriate, it is not unreasonable to consider that extensions may be drawn from trends and patterns in animals to provide additional insight into the behavior of the human mother. In some species, separation shortly after delivery, during what might be termed the maternal sensitive period, may result in the mother's refusal to accept and care for her offspring when the two are reunited. If the separation occurs a few days later for a similar period of time, normal mothering behavior will be resumed when the pair are again brought together. In other species, if separation occurs after delivery, the mother will return to mothering behavior characteristic of her species, but not as skillfully as before. Aberrant mothering that the mother herself received as an infant may also result in distorted maternal behavior, as will intereference with the usual patterns of behavior during and after delivery.

History

The role of the mother in the high-risk and premature nursery has changed greatly since the 1880s, when rooming-in was the accepted mode. The first modern neonatologist, Pierre Budin, recognized the importance of encouraging mothers of premature infants to visit and assist in the care of their infants. However, subsequent nurseries, impelled by the fear of the spread of infection, discouraged visitors and ultimately developed stringent regulations prohibiting visitors and advising limited handling of the infants. The majority of premature centers still do not admit mothers, although recently a few have begun to do so.

RECOMMENDATIONS

Pregnancy

A helpful way to get acquainted with the parents is to obtain a thorough family history. It is particularly important to review the health history, educational background, job, and marital experiences, and fears and concerns of the parents. The following questions are suggested as possible clues to later problems. These should be included in the routine history taking.

1. How long have you lived in this immediate area?
2. Where does most of your family live?
3. How often do you see your mother or other close relatives?
4. Has anything happened to you in the past (or do you have any condition) that causes you to worry about the pregnancy or the baby?
5. What was your husband's reaction to your becoming pregnant?
6. What other responsibilities do you have outside the family?

It is also important to inquire how the mother herself was mothered and by whom. Were her infancy and childhood neglected or deprived, or was her family life warm and intact?

After the second trimester, the obstetrician should look for some outward evidence of preparation for the infant; for example, purchasing clothes or a crib, or selecting a name. If preparations are not being made, this may be evidence of continuing rejection of the pregnancy and should be investigated.

A physician should ask a mother with a condition such as diabetes, hypertension, or heart or thyroid disease what she has heard or read about the course of an infant of a mother with this condition. It cannot be overemphasized how important it is to find out how much such a mother has heard and just where she is in her comprehension of these problems. Even in very high-risk situations, the odds are greatly in favor of the birth of a live baby who will ultimately be normal and healthy; therefore it is reasonable to emphasize the positive and be optimistic. It is a temptation to divulge to the mother all the potential problems, but this will only cause more complications for the mother, the obstetrician, and the pediatrican and may affect the mother's later relationship with her infant, which is in turn extremely important for the child's well-being and development. A prenatal visit with the pediatrician who is to care for the infant provides an opportunity for the mother to get acquainted with the pediatrican and to ask any questions about the baby or his future course that may have been worrying her. The pediatrician should maintain a realistic, optimistic manner, emphasizing that the great majority of infants are normal and healthy. It is valuable to prepare the mother for the events that are likely to occur, but this information should be presented in a positive manner.

Delivery

During delivery and the moments that follow, it is important to let the mother know about the condition of her baby. Communication is helpful, however brief and incomplete.

While baby is in the hospital—first minutes and weeks after delivery

In general, the obstetrician should tell the parents about any problems with the newborn infant since they know and trust him. The obstetrician should introduce the pediatrician and indicate that he is well qualified to care for the infant.

It is hazardous to make a definite statement about the outlook for survival and mental development of a sick newborn infant without observations over a period of several hours. The obstetrician and the pediatrician should avoid comments about an infant's statistical chances of survival. Many predictions made in the first hours after birth prove to be more pessimistic than is warranted by present perinatal mortality statistics and often lead to parental concern that may persist long after the baby has completely recovered. The information available at this time suggests that there has been considerable progress in reducing mortality and improving mental development in the last few years. This and the beneficial effects on maternal attachment if the baby lives suggest the advisability of conveying an optimistic outlook.

The infant with a birth defect

When a baby is born with a congenital defect such as a cleft lip or palate, the obstetrician should tell the mother and father *together* about the problem, preferably with the baby present. He should emphasize the normal, healthy aspects of the baby, then use calm and positive statements about the near perfection of the correction that will be achieved by surgery.

It should be expected that the mother of a sick or malformed newborn infant will undergo a period of mourning for the loss of the perfect infant she has been anticipating. At the same time she must adjust to her new baby and to the realities of his condition. This period of mourning is natural and should not be compressed or suppressed. A strong feeling of guilt is likely and will interfere with the parents' ability to accept the baby fully. The shock of the situation may deafen the parents to the explanations of the physician, so he should be sensitive to their feelings and their questions and should plan to go over his description of the baby's problem, its cause and management, two or three times during the hospital stay and at the baby's first checkups. Frequent visits of the mother with her infant, involving physical contact and caretaking whenever possible, should be arranged to counteract the mother's tendency to withdraw and withhold her full commitment to her infant.

The parents should be encouraged to talk between themselves about the baby's problem and their feelings—disappointment, sadness, anger, guilt, or inadequacy. Their communication with each other should be supported and encouraged. Whenever possible, the physician should talk to both parents together. If this is not possible, he should talk to one on the telephone in the presence of the other. A difference in the shading of reports to one of the parents may block their communication, sometimes with harmful long-term effects.

The physician himself may have feelings of guilt for not having produced a healthy or intact baby for the parents. He may feel that he can be of no help to the mother, while actually it is with this mother that he can be of most assistance.

The premature infant

The mother of a premature infant has been shortchanged of many days of emotional and physical preparation. She may not yet be ready to accept completely the fact that she actually has an infant. She, like the mother of a malformed infant, must go through a period of grieving for the loss of the ideal infant she has been anticipating. In addition, she may feel that the baby is going to die and may start preparing herself for the death before she has established normal affectional bonds with him. If she does not visit the infant and allow the normal process of mother-infant attachment to proceed, she may never be able to relate optimally to her infant and may show distortions of mothering behavior. She may not wish to visit for fear she will "become attached" to the baby only to have it die, but studies have shown that the mother will grieve whether or not she has touched the baby. Therefore, visits to the baby in the premature or high-risk nursery should be encouraged because most babies will live.

Frequently a mother is not able to see her premature infant for the first day or two, while other members of her family may see and even touch and hold the baby. This is often upsetting to the mother, who feels that she is being kept away while others are enjoying the opportunity to become acquainted with her baby. If there is a critical or sensitive period in the human being—and there is increasing evidence to support this—it is within the first few days. A mother's visits to her baby should be encouraged, but she should be allowed to establish a relationship at her own pace.

A mother's room arrangements should be adjusted to her needs. The mothers of premature or critically ill infants should be in private rooms where they are not upset by more fortunate mothers whose infants come to them regularly for feedings. They are often best able to work out their problems when they are alone.

When the mother of a premature or sick newborn asks, "How is my baby doing?" she should be answered in a realistic but optimistic manner. It is common for physicians and nurses to think in a problem-oriented manner and to emphasize the differential diagnosis and the difficulties that may develop, but this can be detrimental to a mother who needs support and encouragement so that mother-infant affectional bonds will develop as optimally as possible. It is often a good idea to ask the mother how *she* thinks the baby is doing, then proceed from there.

The premature nursery, with its attendant tubes, flashing lights, buzzers, hoods, and so on, is bewildering and possibly frightening to a mother. Explanation of the function of these items will be greatly reassuring. A mother should be given advance warning about the equipment, and someone in the nursery should greet her, stand by to give support, and explain the equipment in greater detail at her first visit.

When a mother comes to visit her infant who is under the bilirubin-reduction lights, it is important to remove the infant's eye patches so that she can see his eyes. Patching of the eyes has been extremely upsetting to many mothers.

Arrangements should be made to systematically keep the mother informed about the baby's progress. After the major problems are resolved and the baby is doing well, one conversation a day should be sufficient. The mother should be able to call the nursery at any time for information about the baby.

A consistent picture should be presented to the parents. It is highly desirable that all who are involved with the care of the baby understand the general tenor of the information given to the parents and reply similarly to any questions the parents may ask of them. This of course includes nurses and house officers who can provide additional items without becoming involved in the question of prognosis, which should be tactfully referred to the responsible physician.

The nursery should keep a record of all phone calls and visits by parents. Data have been collected that suggest that when there are fewer than three phone calls or visits during the first 2-week period, there will be a high incidence of subsequent severe mothering disorders. The nurses should feel at ease in reporting any worries or problems they have about a mother's behavior. Frequent meetings of the nursing staff with the physician provide a good opportunity for them to express their problems and concerns.

In determining when an infant can be discharged, more than the infant's weight, physical characteristics, and the presence of a clean bed at home should be considered. The mother's ability to care for the infant in the hospital, her readiness and willingness to take the infant home, and her visiting pattern in the hospital are all indications that aid in making this decision. Preliminary observations have indicated that a good procedure for preparing mothers for caretaking at home is to allow them to room-in with their infants for a few days before discharge. Early discharge may be beneficial if the baby is doing well and the mother is a willing and competent caretaker.

Extended visiting from 1 PM to 7 PM for the mother of a normal full-term infant, when the mother is allowed to handle and completely care for her infant, has been a useful practice, although rooming-in is still preferred.

Death of a newborn or stillbirth

At the time of the baby's death, it is important to tell the parents together about the usual reactions to the loss of a child and the length of time these usually last. A second meeting with both parents prior to the mother's discharge is also desirable.

The shock of the infant's death will usually block the parents' ability to hear and understand what the physician says at the first meeting, so the suggestions should be reiterated at a later time.

Parents appreciate evidence of human concern on the part of the physician. He should not try to repress the sadness he feels and should allow the parents to express their feelings.

The parents should be encouraged to talk together about the loss and not to hold back their feelings. We have found it helpful to prepare parents to expect severe mourning reactions for 2 weeks, with a gradual decrease for 4 to 6 months.

At the postpartum checkup, the obstetrician has an important opportunity to inquire about how the parents are doing and how they are working through their grief. He may also inquire how other children in the family are coping with the situation.

Either the pediatrician or the obstetrician should plan to meet again with the parents 3 to 4 months after the death to discuss the autopsy findings, to check on how the parents are progressing, and to answer any questions the parents may have. At this visit the physician should be alert to abnormal grief reactions, which, if present, may guide him to refer the parents for psychiatric assistance.

The first month at home

It is helpful to consider the events of the perinatal period from the viewpoint of a new mother. She has had a strong and intimate relationship with her obstetrician at visits of progressively increasing frequency up to the time of delivery and during her hospitalization. Suddenly these visits stop. She will usually have only one more appointment 6 weeks after delivery. Cut off from her contacts with the physician who was specifically concerned with her needs, a mother often feels neglected at her visits to the pediatrician, who may tend to focus exclusively on the baby. Actually the pediatrician has three patients—the baby, the mother, and the father. If he can take a little time to inquire about how the mother is doing, praising the efforts she has made to care for the baby and expressing sympathy for the sleep she has missed and the strains she has experienced, he will usually find this more beneficial for the infant than all his admonitions and detailed directions about its care and feeding. Positive reinforcement of a mother's efforts is more effective than corrective and critical statements. The pediatrician's third patient, the father, needs the same attention as the mother. Time spent asking him how he is doing will usually be repaid by the increased support he will provide to his wife.

The affectional bonds a mother establishes with her infant during the first days of life are crucial for his future welfare. When the bonds are solidly established, a mother is motivated to learn about her baby's individual requirements and to adapt to meet his needs and is willing to change diapers thousands of times, to respond to her baby's cries in the night, and to provide perceptual stimulation appropriate in intensity, timing, and quality. Fully developed specific ties keep a mother from striking her baby who has cried for hours night after night—even when she is exhausted and alone. In general, the principles for the care of a mother of a healthy baby are the same as those for the mother of a sick baby.

Whether information is provided by home visits of nurse practitioners or a visiting nurse or by telephone contacts from the physician or his secretary, a physician needs to check on the mother's progress with her baby in the first days at home to provide appropriate support for the mother and infant. For example, a postpartum depression can be particularly damaging to the mental and physical development of a young infant. Intervention may be essential for the welfare of the mother and the baby. At the time of discharge it often helps to tell a mother, with a light touch, that she may be awake throughout the first night, checking on the baby and watching him breathe fast, then slow, loudly, then softly. The physician can add a guarantee that the baby will breathe his way safely through the night.

In the United States, the average woman is poorly prepared for her first baby. Her fantasy about what he will be like at home is often quite different from what she finds. His irregular patterns of sleep, activity, and motor movements, as well as the mysteries of why he cries, may result in worries about what are actually normal aspects of behavior. An inexperienced new mother is usually fortunate if she has her own mother in the home with her or living nearby, as is the case in most of the world. In the United States, however, the pattern of father, mother, and children living as isolated units far away from parents, grandparents, and other relatives intensifies the insecurity and loneliness of a new mother. This is more of a problem if the baby has been ill or has a continuing medical disorder. Whenever appropriate, a physician should assure the parents that the baby's problem is over, that he is healthy, and that he should be handled normally in every respect. It is wise to state this prior to discharge and then repeat it at the first two or three visits. It is natural for parents to look for other evidence to confirm the physician's words and test his convictions. An easy way for the physician to promote this process is to give the same directions to the mother of a high-risk baby as to the mother of a healthy full-term infant; that is, to stress that the baby should be put in a separate room away from the parents' bedroom from the first night on, to emphasize that the mother should plan to leave her baby with someone else, starting in no less than a month, so that she can have free time away from the baby for herself and for activities with her husband; and to remind the parents that the baby will have his first office visit when he is 3 weeks of age. Many physicians choose a 4- to 6-week interval before the first visit, but the intensity of parental concerns, as well as the possibility of detecting an important problem, makes the earlier appointment advisable.

MARSHALL H. KLAUS
JOHN H. KENNELL

BIBLIOGRAPHY

Barnett, C., Leiderman, P., Grobstein, R., and Klaus, M.: Neonatal separation; the maternal side of interactional deprivation, Pediatrics **45**: 197, 1970.

Benedek, T.: Studies in psychosomatic medicine; the psychosexual function in women, New York, 1952, The Ronald Press Co.

Bibring, G.: Some considerations of the psychological processes in pregnancy, Psychoanal. Study Child **14**:113, 1959.

Budin, P.: The nursling, London, 1907, Caxton Publishing Co.

Caplan, G.: Emotional implications of pregnancy and influences on family relationships in the healthy child, Cambridge, 1960, Harvard University Press.

Cohen, R.: Some maladaptive syndromes of pregnancy and the puerperium, Obstet. Gynecol. **27**: 562, 1966.

Deutsche, H.: The psychology of women: a psychoanalytic interpretation. vol. 2. Motherhood, New York, 1945, Grune & Stratton, Inc.

Fanaroff, A.: Follow-up of low-birthweight infants —the predictive value of maternal visiting patterms, Pediatrics **49**:287, 1972.

Harlow, H., and Harlow, M.: The effects of rearing conditions on behavior, Bull. Menninger Clin. **26**:213, 1962.

Harlow, H., Harlow, M., and Hansen, E.: The maternal affectional system of rhesus monkeys. In Rheingold, H., editor: Maternal behavior in mammals, New York, 1963, John Wiley & Sons, Inc.

Helfer, R., and Kempe, C., editors: The Battered child, Chicago, 1968, University of Chicago Press.

Kaplan, D., and Mason, E.: Maternal reactions to premautre birth viewed as an acute emotional disorder, Am. J. Orthopsychiatry **30**:539, 1960.

Kennell, J., and Rolnik, A.: Discussing problems in newborn babies with their parents, Pediatrics **26**:832, 1960.

Kennell, J., Slyter, H., and Klaus, M.: The mourning response of parents to the death of a newborn, New Eng. J. Med. **283**:344, 1970.

Klaus, M., and Kennell, J.: Mothers separated from their newborn infants, Pediatr. Clin. N. Am. **17**:1017, 1970.

Klaus, M., Kennell, J., Plumb, N., and Zuehlke, S.: Human maternal behavior at the first contact with her young, Pediatrics **46**:187, 1970.

Leifer, A., Leiderman, P., and Barnett, C.: Mother-infant separation; effects on later maternal behavior, Child Dev. In press.

Newton, N., and Newton, M.: Mothers' reactions to their newborn babies, J.A.M.A. **181**:206, 1962.

Robson, K.: The role of eye-to-eye contact in maternal-infant attachment, J. Child Psychol. Psychiatry **8**:13, 1967.

Rubenstein, J.: Maternal attentiveness and subsequent exploratory behavior in the infant. Child Dev. **38**:1089, 1967.

8 Infections

GENERAL CONSIDERATIONS, SEPSIS AND SEPTICEMIA

A variety of infectious diseases occur in the neonate; infections may occur in waves, in microepidemics, or as individual sporadic cases. The clinical presentation may differ significantly from that seen beyond the neonatal period. Because of the newborn infant's inability at times to respond to infection in classical fashion, infection in the early stages is often difficult to diagnose. Yet, early diagnosis and appropriate therapy account for the success in therapy of bacterial infections in the neonate.

Prior to parturition, prevention of infection in the fetus depends on sterile amniotic fluid, the integrity of the placenta, and the absence of bloodstream infection in the mother. Transplacental infections are relatively uncommon; but when they occur, they may produce serious illness or death. Viral, bacterial, and parasitic agents may cross the placenta from an infected mother and afflict the infant (Table 8-1).

Amniotic infection also predisposes the neonate to infection. Premature rupture of the fetal membranes, prolonged labor, and excessive manipulation during labor increase the risk of contamination of the amniotic fluid. Rarely, amniotic infection occurs in the presence of intact membranes. Histologic evidence of chorioamnionitis may be found in 7% to 15% of unselected placentas. However, the ratio of amnionitis to systemic infection in the neonate is estimated to be between 30:1 and 100:1. The fetal skin, mucous membranes, and gastrointestinal and respiratory tracts are colonized by organisms from contaminated amniotic fluid or from vaginal secretions swallowed or aspirated either before birth or during passage through the birth canal. These bacteria are usually *Escherichia coli*, *Klebsiella-Enterobacter*, enterococci, and group A and B beta hemolytic streptococci. Infection is presumed to result from some alteration in the gastrointestinal mucosal barrier or from exposure to a large inoculum or both.

Further acquisition of infectious agents occurs in the delivery room or in the newborn nursery through airborne and contact routes. Resuscitation with contaminated equipment in the delivery room or nursery has led to pneumonia and septicemia. Respirators and isolettes using water for humidification have been sources of contamination. Umbilical venous and arterial catheterization is associated with a high incidence of colonization and a lower incidence of bacteremias. While some bacteremias are transient, other cases have been more prolonged and may produce septicemia or focal infections. Recent use of prolonged intravenous catheterization to administer special fluids for hyperalimentation has led to systemic candidiasis as well as bacterial septicemia. In addition to the organisms listed above, staphylococci, *Pseudomonas*, and *Proteus* must be considered in the determination of the cause of septicemia when the predisposing epidemiologic factors are present.

Newborn infants with low birth weights have an increased incidence of infection. This may be the result of intrauterine infection causing growth retardation or premature delivery or of impaired host re-

TABLE 8-1. Fetal and neonatal complications of transplacental transmission of infections

Organism or condition	Teratogenicity	Abortion	Stillbirth	Prematurity	Neonatal disease
Arboviruses	0	0	0	0	+
Bacterial sepsis	0	+	+	+	+
Coxsackievirus B	?	0	?	0	+
Cryptococcosis	0	0	+	+	+
Cytomegalovirus	?	?	+	+	+
Echovirus	0	0	0	0	+
Hepatitis	0	0	?	?	+
Herpesvirus hominis	?	0	0	+	+
Influenza	?	?	?	?	0
Listeria	0	?	+	+	+
Malaria	0	+	+	+	+
Mumps	?	0	0	0	?
Polio	0	+	+	+	+
Rubella	+	+	+	+	+
Rubeola	0	+	+	+	+
Syphilis	0	0	+	+	+
Toxoplasmosis	0	?	+	+	+
Tuberculosis	0	+	+	+	+
Urinary tract infection	0	0	0	+	0
Vaccinia	0	+	+	+	+
Varicella	0	+	+	+	+
Variola	0	+	+	+	+

sistance caused by immaturity. Congenital malformations of the central nervous system and obstructive lesions of the respiratory, urinary, and gastrointestinal tracts may also predispose the infant to infection. There is a greater incidence of infection in males.

While a transient bacteremia may not produce symptoms, septicemia refers to a generalized bacterial infection documented by blood culture, which is usually symptomatic. In contrast, sepsis may occur in a variety of tissues without bacteremia. The many foci of infection in the newborn are presented in the outline below; some of these specific infections are discussed in more detail in the following sections. Viremia, fungemia, and parasitemia may also produce symptoms similar to those of septicemia, but bacterial infections are more common. The following outline lists the etiologic agents in neonatal infections.

FOCAL NEONATAL INFECTIONS

A. Abscesses
   1. Adrenal
   2. Cephalohematoma
   3. Cerebral
   4. Liver
   5. Palmar
   6. Parotid
   7. Prostatic
   8. Retroperitoneal

B. Other infections
   1. Arthritis
   2. Conjunctivitis, cellulitis
   3. Endocarditis
   4. Enterocolitis
   5. Gastroenteritis
   6. Mastitis
   7. Mediastinitis
   8. Meningitis
   9. Myocarditis
   10. Omphalitis
   11. Ophthalmitis
   12. Orchitis
   13. Osteomyelitis
   14. Otitis media
   15. Pericarditis
   16. Peritonitis
   17. Pneumonia
   18. Pyoderma
   19. Urinary tract infection

ETIOLOGIC AGENTS IN NEONATAL INFECTIONS

A. Bacteria
   1. *Alcaligenes fecalis*
   2. *Achromobacter*
   3. *Bacteroides*
   4. *Brucella*
   5. *Diplococcus pneumoniae*
   6. *Clostridium tetani*
   7. *Clostridium welchii*
   8. *Corynebacterium diphtheriae*

9. Enterococci
10. *Escherichia coli*
11. Flavobacteria
12. *Haemophilus influenzae*
13. *Klebsiella-Enterobacter*
14. *Listeria monocytogenes*
15. *Mimeae* species
16. *Mycobacterium tuberculosis*
17. *Neisseria gonorrhoeae*
18. *Neisseria meningitidis*
19. *Proteus* species
20. *Pseudomonas aeruginosa*
21. *Salmonella* species
22. *Serratia marcescens*
23. *Shigella* species
24. *Staphylococcus albus*
25. *Staphylococcus aureus*
26. Streptococci, groups A and B
27. *Vibrio cholerae*
28. *Vibrio fetus*

B. Viruses
1. Arbovirus
2. Coxsackievirus
3. Cytomegalovirus
4. Echovirus
5. Hepatitis
6. Herpesvirus hominis
7. Influenza
8. Parainfluenza
9. Polio
10. Respiratory syncitial
11. Rubella
12. Vaccinia
13. Varicella-zoster
14. Variola

C. Fungi
1. *Candida* species
2. *Coccidioides immitis*
3. *Cryptococcus neoformans*
4. *Histoplasma capsulatum*

D. Protozoa
1. *Plasmodium* species
2. *Pneumocystis carinii*
3. *Toxoplasma gondii*

In the absence of localization of infection, the autopsy findings in neonatal septicemia may be limited to petechiae or ecchymoses on serosal surfaces. With time, inflammatory exudates will be present in the lungs, pleurae, meninges, heart, pericardium, or peritoneum. Placentas infected via maternal bacteremia show septic foci within and between the villi. Inflammation of the chorion occurs in the amniotic infection syndrome and may be seen in almost 20% of randomly examined placentas; inflammation of the cord (funistis) occurs in 10%.

Clinical signs and symptoms

The clinical manifestations of infection in the neonate will vary according to the etiologic agent, localization or major organ involvement, duration, and severity. Certain focal infections such as pyoderma, omphalitis, mastitis, and conjunctivitis are easily recognized. In contrast, early indications of systemic infections may be limited to poor feeding, lethargy, vasomotor instability, and a nurse's comment that the infant is not doing as well as before. These minimal signs of illness and the more serious signs of systemic infections may also be related to noninfectious processes. The signs of septicemia may be related to the involvement of a number of different organ systems (see outline below).

EPIDEMIOLOGIC AND CLINICAL DATA THAT SUGGEST OR SUPPORT A DIAGNOSIS OF NEONATAL SEPTICEMIA

A. History
1. Low birth weight
2. Amniotic infection; for example, foul smelling, cloudy, or purulent amniotic fluid
3. Premature rupture of membranes (>24 hr)
4. Resuscitation problem; especially, intubation and umbilical vessel catheterization
5. Meconium staining of skin
6. Congenital abnormality of urinary tract, CNS, lungs, or heart
7. Bloody secretions in upper airway suggesting aspiration of maternal blood or vaginal secretions
8. Lethargy, "not doing well", poor feeding

B. Signs
1. General
   a. Fever or hypothermia
   b. Sclerema
2. Circulatory system
   a. Pallor, cyanosis, or mottling
   b. Abnormal respirations (apnea, tachypnea, irregular)
   c. Cold, clammy skin
   d. Hypotension
3. Central nervous system
   a. Lethargy
   b. Hyporeflexia
   c. Irregular respirations
   d. Tremors, convulsions, or irritability
   e. Full fontanelle
   f. Apnea
4. Respiratory system
   a. Tachypnea
   b. Dyspnea
   c. Cyanosis
   d. Apnea
5. Gastrointestinal system
   a. Abdominal distention
   b. Hepatomegaly
   c. Vomiting
   d. Diarrhea
   e. Decreased stool

6. Hematologic system
   a. Jaundice
   b. Splenomegaly
   c. Pallor
   d. Purpura
   e. Petechiae
   f. Bleeding

Apnea, tremors, and convulsions are compatible with encephalitis, bacterial meningitis and septicemia, intracranial hemorrhage, anoxia, and intracranial malformations. Infections with *Vibrio fetus* may result in fulminating meningoencephalitis. Dyspnea and tachypnea may be caused by pulmonary or systemic infections or by noninfectious processes. Abdominal distention, vomiting, constipation, and diarrhea may be caused by primary gastrointestinal disease or septicemia. Jaundice, anemia, purpura, and circulatory changes may occur in a variety of infectious and noninfectious disorders of the neonate.

Laboratory tests

Laboratory studies should be requested according to the differential diagnosis in each infant. Leukopenia (<4,000 white blood cells per mm^3) or leukocytosis (>25,000 white blood cells per mm^3) supports a diagnosis of infection. Hemolytic anemia and thrombocytopenia may occur during systemic infection. Localization of the infection and examination of the appropriate body fluid will lead to a rapid diagnosis in meningitis, arthritis, urinary tract infection, and pyoderma. When septicemia is suspected, both urine and cerebrospinal fluid should be examined. The gastric fluid will often show polymorphonuclear leukocytes and bacteria if contaminated amniotic fluid has been ingested. White blood cell counts, differential cell counts, and Gram stains and methylene blue stains of exudates (cerebrospinal fluid, urine, joint fluid, and so on) may provide preliminary identification of bacteria. Final identification is by culture and biochemical reactions. Two blood cultures are indicated when septicemia is considered unless the infant is critically ill, when one culture will suffice. Careful preparation of the skin over a peripheral vein will minimize contamination with organisms from the skin or umbilical cord. In vitro sensitivity tests should be carried out on all gram-negative organisms.

Serologic studies of the infant, and sometimes of the mother, will be helpful in the diagnosis of infections such as syphilis, toxoplasmosis, rubella, cytomegalovirus infections, arbovirus infections, enterovirus infections, and fungal infections. The estimation of serum immunoglobulin (IgM) concentration at birth or in the first week of life may be a useful screening test for prior infection. IgM concentrations are elevated (>17 mg/100 ml) in most infants with chronic intrauterine infections and in some infants with acute perinatal infections. If the IgM level is elevated, the possibility of contamination by maternal IgM should be excluded by obtaining a second sample from the infant.

Diagnosis

A presumptive diagnosis of neonatal septicemia should be made when, in the absence of establishing an alternative diagnosis, sufficient epidemiologic and clinical factors are present to suggest systemic disease that could be caused by bacterial infection. The rapid course of neonatal septicemia is a greater threat to the life of the infant than the undesirable effects of antimicrobial therapy, and a decision should be made to begin therapy on the basis of a presumptive diagnosis after obtaining the appropriate cultures but before the final diagnosis of septicemia is established.

Treatment

The choice of antimicrobial agents for therapy of infections in the newborn should be based on consideration of the most likely pathogen, the effectiveness of the antimicrobial agent against the organism, the site of infection, the metabolism of the drug, and the potential adverse side effects. Bactericidal rather than bacteriostatic drugs are preferred. Susceptibility of gram-negative organisms to various antimicrobial agents often changes with time and particularly with the increased use of a drug. Thus, the physician should be aware of the sensitivity pattern of common bacteria isolated in a hospital and community as well as the relative frequencies of infection with various organisms.

Certain chemotherapeutic agents should be avoided in the newborn period: sulfisoxazole and novobiocin, which are associated with an increased incidence of kernicterus; tetracycline, which may be deposited in teeth and bones, causing discoloration and growth arrest; cephalothin, which may induce a positive Coombs test; and chloramphenicol, which may lead to toxicity and death (gray syndrome). However, in proper doses, chloramphenicol may be used to treat systemic *Salmonella* infections in the neonate.

Dosage schedules for commonly used antimicrobial agents are listed in Table 8-2. While penicillin G has been extensively used in newborn infants, ampicillin may be preferred because of its effect on *H. influenzae, E. coli, Salmonella, Shigella,* and *Proteus mirabilis* as well as streptococci. It is not effective against most *Klebsiella-Enterobacter,* other *Proteus* species, *Pseudomonas,* and some *E. coli* strains. Therefore, it should not be used alone in treating unidentified gram-negative infections. One of the aminoglycoside antibiotics, kanamycin or gentamicin, should be added (Table 8-3). Both agents have potential ototoxicity and nephrotoxicity. Kanamycin has been used more extensively, and, if used in the appropriate dose for a limited time, toxicity is not a serious problem. There is less experience with gentamicin in the newborn infant, but it is currently effective against most gram-negative organisms including *Klebsiella-Enterobacter, Pseudomonas,* and *Serratia.* After 72 hours of life, colonization by staphylococci increases, and these organisms should be considered in deciding upon the therapeutic regimen. Since the majority of staphylococci are resistant to penicillin G, one of the penicillinase-resistant semisynthetic penicillins should be used for treatment. Methicillin, oxacillin, and nafcillin have been used in the newborn infant. While there are differences in blood levels and protein-binding properties, clinical effectiveness in the recommended dosages is comparable. Cephalothin is effective against penicillinase-producing staphylococci and some gram-negative bacteria. However, the semisynthetic penicillins are preferred for treating staphylococci, and an aminoglycoside is recommended for unknown gram-negative organisms. Cephalothin is irritating to veins and is not currently a major

Table 8-2. Commonly used antimicrobial agents for the neonate

	First 5 days, premature			Full-term, over 5 days		
Agent	**Dosage**	**Route**	**Schedule**	**Dosage**	**Route**	**Schedule**
Penicillin G	100,000 μ/kg/d	IM, IV	q 12 h	100,000 μ/kg/d	IM, IV	q 6 h
Oxacillin	100 mg/kg/d					
Methicillin	100 mg/kg/d	IM, IV	q 12 h	200 mg/kg/d	IM, IV	q 6 h
Nafcillin	100 mg/kg/d					
Ampicillin	100 mg/kg/d	IM, IV	q 12 h	200 mg/kg/d	IM, IV	q 6 h
Kanamycin	15 mg/kg/d	IM	q 12 h	15 mg/kg/d	IM	q 12 h
Gentamicin	5 mg/kg/d	IM	q 12 h	5 mg/kg/d	IM	q 8 h
Neomycin	100 mg/kg/d	PO	q 6 h	100 mg/kg/d	PO	q 6 h
Polymyxin B	3 mg/kg/d	IM, IV	q 12 h	4 mg/kg/d	IM, IV	q 8 h
Colistimethate	5 mg/kg/d	IM	q 12 h	8 mg/kg/d	IM	q 8 h
Colistin sulfate	8 mg/kg/d	PO	q 6 h	8 mg/kg/d	PO	q 6 h
Chloramphenicol	25 mg/kg/d	IM, IV	q 8 h	50 mg/kg/d	IM, IV	q 6 h

Table 8-3. Antimicrobial agents for sepsis of unidentified cause

Birth to 72 hours	3 days to 3 months
Ampicillin or penicillin G plus kanamycin or gentamicin	Penicillinase-resistant penicillin plus kanamycin or gentamicin

drug for treating neonatal infections. Carbenicillin has had little use in treatment of the neonate. It is active against *Pseudomonas* and may be useful in combination with gentamicin in treatment of *Pseudomonas* septicemia.

Supportive management of infants with neonatal infections depends on the type of infection and its severity. For most infections, adequate isolation can be obtained with an incubator and strict hand-washing technique. More rigorous isolation in separate rooms is indicated for highly contagious diseases such as varicella and bacterial gastroenteritis. If the infant appears ill, oral feedings should be discontinued, and appropriate fluids with glucose and electrolytes should be given intravenously. The environmental temperature may need adjustment to maintain the infant's rectal temperature between 98.6 and 100.4 F (37 and 38 C). Cool sponge baths should be given to the infant with high fever associated with marked irritability, convulsions, tachycardia, or tachypnea. Oxygen should be administered in sufficient quantities to relieve cyanosis, with intermittent monitoring of arterial oxygen tensions.

Specific complications of severe neonatal infections include shock, adrenal insufficiency, consumptive coagulopathy, congestive heart failure, and hyponatremia. Gram-negative septicemia may result in shock in the neonate. As in older children and adults, this complication should be treated with the immediate administration of whole blood (10 to 20 cc/kg) or other plasma expander in addition to intravenous fluids and antibiotics. Sodium bicarbonate (2 to 3 mEq/kg) and glucose (2 ml/kg of 25% glucose) should be given to counteract metabolic acidosis and hypoglycemia. If the infant remains in critical condition, 10 mg/kg of hydrocortisone succinate is indicated. Persistent hypotension should be treated with a continuous infusion of isoproterenol (4 mg/liter of fluids). If shock is complicated by the onset of disseminated intravascular coagulation, heparinization may be indicated (p. 210).

While there is no evidence of insufficient secretion of adrenal steroids during neonatal septicemia, adrenal hemorrhage has been observed at autopsy. The diagnosis should be considered in infants with shock; and serum sodium, potassium, and glucose levels should be measured. Treatment with hydrocortisone (5 mg/kg every 6 hr) should be given intravenously for presumptive adrenal failure.

INFECTIONS OF ORGAN SYSTEMS

Infections of the skin and mucous membranes

A number of bacterial, viral, and fungal agents cause inflammation of the skin of the newborn infant. The disease may be localized or part of a generalized infection. Fungal infections are discussed elsewhere in this section.

Etiology. *Staphylococcus aureus,* beta hemolytic streptococci, *Pseudomonas aeruginosa,* and *Treponema pallidum* are the most important bacterial pathogens. The viruses pathogenic for the skin include rubeola, varicella-zoster, herpes simplex, vaccinia, and variola. *Candida albicans* may cause an oral infection (thrush) or cutaneous lesions usually limited to the diaper area.

Pathology. Pustules, abscesses, or bullous lesions are commonly caused by *Staph. aureus* and less often by streptococci. Ritter's disease, or the scalded skin syndrome, which is characterized by blistering with progression to confluent bullae and extensive shedding of the epidermis, is frequently caused by a specific toxin from staphylococcal phage types 2, 55/71, and 71. Omphalitis and abscesses of the breast are other common forms of staphylococcal infection. *Pseudomonas* causes ecthyma gangrenosum consisting of yellowish-green pustular-vesicular lesions that rapidly progress to hemorrhagic necrotic ulcers surrounded by an area of cellulitis.

Pathogenesis. Colonization of the infants' skin by *Staph. epidermidis, Staph. aureus,* streptococci, diphtheroid bacilli, and coliform organisms occurs at birth. Other infants and nursery personnel may also serve as sources of staphylococcal and beta hemolytic streptococcal infection. The skin in the diaper region and the umbilical cord are the most common regions for colonization. A number of enzymes released by the staphylococcus probably contribute to the local infection.

Candida albicans colonizes the gastrointestinal tract of most infants at birth. A few infants will have sufficient multiplication of organisms in the buccal mucosa to result in clinical disease (thrush); contamination of the diaper area may lead to a dermatitis characterized by confluent vesicular or pustular lesions with an erythematous base.

Clinical. Diagnosis of cutaneous infections is suggested by the character of the lesion and the associated epidemiologic factors. The bullous lesions caused by staphylococci occur after the first few days of life in contrast to the noninfectious congenital bullous conditions, which may be present at birth (p. 590). The cardinal signs of inflammation make omphalitis and subcutaneous abscesses relatively easy to recognize. Ecthyma gangrenosum should not be confused with other conditions.

An etiologic diagnosis is based on smear and culture of the lesion. Organisms are usually present in pustular and vesicular lesions but may be absent in the bullae in Ritter's disease. Blood cultures may be positive in the staphylococcal syndromes and will be positive in infants with ecthyma gangrenosum. *Candida* dermatitis and thrush are confirmed by demonstration of spores and hyphae on a potassium hydroxide preparation and culture of the organism on Sabouraud's agar.

Treatment. Bacterial infections of the skin in the newborn infant are generally treated with systemic antibiotics. Penicillinase-resistant penicillins are used for staphylococcal infections; penicillin G for streptococcal infections; and gentamicin for ecthyma gangrenosum. A few staphylococcal pustules in a vigorous infant may be treated locally. Saline compresses and intravenous fluid therapy may be necessary in bullous staphylococcal diseases. Some clinicians use steroid therapy in severe Ritter's disease. Warm soaks followed by incision and drainage may be necessary in the management of staphylococcal abscesses. Thrush should respond to the oral administration of nystatin (Mycostatin), and *Candida* dermatitis will improve with saline soaks, 1:5,000 benzalkonium chloride washes, and nystatin cream.

Ophthalmitis

With the routine use of prophylactic silver nitrate at birth, some degree of conjunctivitis is not uncommon in newborn infants. Conjunctivitis caused by infectious agents must be differentiated from chemical conjunctivitis (p. 623).

Etiology. *Neisseria gonorrhoeae* is the most important cause of bacterial conjunctivitis in the newborn infant. Staphylococci, streptococci, pneumococci, the Koch-Weeks bacillus, and *Pseudomonas* organisms may also produce purulent conjunctivitis. Inclusion conjunctivitis or blennorrhea is caused by infection with the trachoma–inclusion conjunctivitis (TRIC) agent, which also causes trachoma.

Pathogenesis. The newborn infant may acquire any of the infectious agents capable of producing conjunctivitis during passage through the birth canal. After birth, infection may result from contact or spread of airborne particles. Chemical conjunctivitis results from the failure to completely irrigate the conjunctivas after instillation of silver nitrate.

Clinical. Chemical conjunctivitis usually occurs within 24 hours after birth. Bacterial conjunctivitis generally appears between 2 and 5 days, and inclusion blennorrhea after 5 days. However, the latter infection may be seen as early as 3 days of age, and the incubation period of bacterial conjunctivitis varies from 1 to 3 days. Physical signs include a thick, whitish-yellow ocular discharge, edema of the lids, and injection of the palpebral conjunctivas. In bacterial infections, unilateral involvement is more common. Inclusion blennorrhea usually affects both eyes and varies from mild to severe. Without therapy, gonococcal conjunctivitis may rapidly progress to keratitis, corneal ulceration, and perforation. *Pseudomonas* infections may also involve other structures of the eye. While inclusion conjunctivitis is usually a self-limited disease lasting 1 to 2 weeks without sequelae, on occasion the infection may persist for months, and permanent scarring may ensue.

Diagnosis. A presumptive diagnosis of the bacterial causes of conjunctivitis may be made by Gram stain of the exudates. Gram-negative diplococci in leukocytes are usually found in gonococcal ophthalmitis, but it may be difficult to differentiate skin contamination by staphylococci or *Pseudomonas.* The lack of response to treatment with neomycin-polymyxin ointment suggests a diagnosis of inclusion conjunctivitis. The specific diagnosis is made when intracytoplasmic inclusions are demonstrated with Giemsa stain in epithelial cells scraped from the tarsal conjunctiva. Inclusions may be single or multiple and are often adjacent to the nucleus.

Treatment. Treatment of gonococcal ophthalmia consists of aqueous penicillin G, 50,000 units/kg, injected intramuscularly daily for 5 days. The conjunctival sac should be irrigated frequently with isotonic saline. Some ophthalmologists recommend topical antibiotics in addition. The other forms of bacterial conjunctivitis may be treated with topical bacitracin-neomycin-polymyxin ophthalmic ointments or solutions for 7 to 10 days. These antibiotics are not effective in treating TRIC infections. Inclusion conjunctivitis should be treated with 1% tetracycline ointment or sulfonamide ointments applied every 3 to 4 hours. Improvement is noted in 24 to 48 hours. Both recurrences and reinfection have occurred. A 2-week course of therapy is recommended, and this should be repeated if signs of infection are noted on follow-up examination.

Prevention. Prophylaxis of gonococcal ophthalmia has been shown to be effective. However, prevention is not complete, probably because of the technical difficulty in topical application of the agent. A 1% silver nitrate solution instilled into the conjunctival sac immediately after birth is most commonly used, although penicillin ointments and solutions and other topical antibiotics may be used instead of silver nitrate if permitted by law. Intramuscular injection of 50,000 to 100,000 units of penicillin is effective, but this may interfere with the bacteriologic diagnosis of sepsis and carries a risk of sensitization.

Otitis media

Although the tympanic membrane of a newborn infant is sometimes difficult to visualize, a diagnosis of otitis media may be made by routine examination with a pneumatic otoscope. It is more common in premature infants and is seen in the majority of infants with cleft palate. Congenital otitis media has also been recorded. Aspirated amniotic fluid has been found in the middle ear without inflammation, but infected amniotic fluid is the most common cause of otitis media in newborn infants. Some cases of otitis media are associated with prolonged rupture of membranes. The infant may aspirate infected fluid during passage through the birth canal. The same organisms that cause sepsis in the newborn infant have been cultured from the middle ear, but not all of the aspirated fluids yield bacteria.

Symptoms of otitis media are often nonspecific. Rhinorrhea and low-grade fever are common. The clinical signs include persistent erythema or dullness of the tympanic membrane, bulging, and reduction of mobility. Perforation of the drum is not infrequent. Examination of the exudate after perforation or myringotomy may reveal polymorphonuclear leukocytes and bacteria. The exudate should be cultured, and the appropriate antimicrobial agents should be selected for parenteral administration on the basis of the initial Gram-stained smear. In the absence of a smear or culture, ampicillin and kanamycin should be given.

Middle ear disease in the neonatal period is associated with a high incidence of chronic otitis media and occasionally mastoiditis and meningitis. Careful follow-up is indicated, and the insertion of plastic tubes may be necessary to ensure adequate drainage and to equalize pressures.

Pneumonia

Pneumonia is always considered in newborns with respiratory distress (p. 355) and is the most common fatal perinatal infection. Pneumonia may be the sole cause of death, but is more often found complicating another disease. The disease may be acquired in utero, resulting in a stillborn fetus or a liveborn infant who is ill from the time of delivery. Naeye and associates classify all pneumonias in stillborn infants, pneumonia death in the first 12 hours of life, and pneumonia in an infant 12 to 72 hours of age associated with chorioamnionitis as congenital pneumonias. Intrauterine pneumonia is found in 5% to 25% of all autopsies in the perinatal period. Pneumonia may be acquired during parturition or at any time thereafter.

Etiology. The organisms causing pneumonia in newborn infants are similar to those causing septicemia. They include *E. coli, Klebsiella-Enterobacter, Pseudomonas, Proteus*, staphylococci, and streptococci.

Viral pneumonias may occur in this period. Fungal and protozoan pneumonias are rare. In Naeye's study, 37% of infants with congenital pneumonia had negative bacterial cultures. Therefore, viral or mycoplasma cause should be considered.

Pathogenesis and pathology. The various pathways leading to neonatal pneumonia are aspirative, hematogenous, and aerogenous. Aspiration may occur in utero as a result of asphyxia. If the amniotic fluid becomes contaminated, aspiration would lead to intrauterine pneumonia. Less commonly, maternal bacteremia or viremia leads to transplacental infection and involvement of the fetal lung. The pneumococcus is the most likely agent in this form of infection. In both cases, the process is diffuse, with almost total involvement of alveoli with polymorphonuclear leukocytes and organisms identifiable with Gram strain. Frequently, bronchitis and bronchiolitis are present. Amniotic debris is usually found, and its absence suggests hematogenous spread. Aspiration of vaginal contents may occur during parturition. In the nursery, the infant may aspirate milk or gastric contents that may predispose him to pneumonia. Aspiration during or following delivery usually leads to a bronchopneumonia. In addition, pleuritis or hemorrhage may be present. Staphylococcal pneumonias are commonly associated with abscesses, empyema, pyopneumothorax, and formation of pneumatoceles. *Pseudomonas* pneumonias may result from septicemia or from inhalation. This infection often complicates the course of patients with other disorders, particularly of a surgical nature. The inflammation is perivascular and characterized by necrosis in the vessel wall and alveoli.

Aerogenic acquisition of viruses, bacteria, fungi, or protozoa may occur at anytime after delivery. In addition to the transmission of infectious agents by droplet infection, the neonate may be at risk from contamination of the resuscitation equipment, respirators, or the humidity-producing apparatus. Epidemics of pneumonia and septicemia have been traced to these sources. The use of antimicrobial agents will alter the infant's flora and make infection with *Klebsiella-Enterobacter, Pseudomonas,* or *Candida albicans* more likely.

Clinical. Any infant may acquire pneumonia in utero but premature infants are more likely to acquire pneumonia during or after parturition. In utero pneumonias are usually associated with obstetrical complications such as maternal infection, prolonged rupture of the membranes, and a difficult labor leading to fetal asphyxia. The infant with pneumonia acquired in utero is usually asphyxiated at birth and will require resuscitation. The umbilical cord and amniotic fluid may be meconium stained. There will be signs of respiratory distress consisting of tachypnea, grunting, and mild to moderate retractions. Premature infants with pneumonia may have fewer signs. The color is poor, respirations are usually irregular, and periods of apnea with cyanosis may ensue. The infant does not cough. Fever may be present, but the premature infant is more likely to be hypothermic. During the physical examination, dullness, decreased breath sounds, and rales may be elicited, but the signs of pneumonia are often absent. Occasionally the course may be complicated by congestive heart failure with cardiac enlargement, hepatomegaly, poor heart sounds, and a gallop rhythm. Neurologic signs are not uncommon in these hypoxic children. Flaccidity, hyperactivity, tremors, and convulsions may be present.

Diagnosis. The diagnosis of pneumonia should be considered in an infant who is not doing well or who exhibits signs of respiratory distress. An initial roentgenogram of the chest is required to distinguish other causes of respiratory distress as well as to diagnose pneumonia. The diagnosis may be established on the basis of physical findings before there is roentgenographic evidence of pneumonia. As in older children, there may be a time lag of 24 to 72 hours in which roentgenographic signs develop. These signs vary from the bilateral homogeneous consolidation seen in in utero pneumonias to a patchy bronchopneumonia, which occurs in postnatal infections. Bronchopneumonia can be differentiated from the discrete opacification seen in segmental or lobar atelectasis. Mediastinal shift and changes in the configuration of the involved hemithorax are often seen with atelectasis. It is difficult to separate the roentgenographic picture of meconium aspiration from bronchopneumonia (p. 371).

In meconium aspiration, the findings are most impressive early and clear over a period of days, while the roentgenographic findings in bronchopneumonia may take a few days to reach their maximal development.

Culture of tracheal aspirates is less helpful in etiologic diagnosis of the neonate than in older infants and children. Cultures most often reveal vaginal flora, but identification of *Staph. aureus* or *Pseudomonas* is important since it affects the choice of antibiotics. Blood cultures are occasionally positive. The white blood cell count is generally in the normal range of 4,000 to 15,000/mm^3, although increased or leukopenic counts may be noted.

Treatment. Treatment of neonatal pneumonia involves the same principles as those in the management of neonatal septicemia. The organisms are most often those found in the maternal birth canal, but the clinician must be sensitive to clues such as concomitant skin infections suggesting a staphylococcal or *Pseudomonas* cause. Ampicillin or penicillin combined with kanamycin are the currently recommended antimicrobial agents. When a staphylococcal cause is suspected, methicillin is substituted for the other penicillin. Gentamicin or polymyxin are used for *Pseudomonas* pneumonias.

Prevention. Obstetrical factors must be considered if intrauterine pneumonia is to be prevented. The diagnosis of ammionitis may be an indication for induction or treatment of the mother with broad-spectrum antibiotics, such as ampicillin, that are capable of crossing the placenta. Many postnatally acquired pneumonias may be prevented by strict attention to sterility in the use of equipment.

Gastroenteritis

Gastrointestinal infections in the newborn infant occur sporadically or in epidemic fashion. In some infants with signs of gastroenteritis, the common stool pathogens are not found, and the etiologic agents are presumed to be viral despite the inability to establish the cause by viral cultures or serologic tests.

Etiology. The same bacteria that cause gastroenteritis in older children may produce disease in neonates. Salmonellae and less commonly shigellae may be found in newborn infants with diarrhea. Certain serologic types of *E. coli* have been associated with epidemic and sporadic diarrheal disease in infancy and have been designated enteropathogenic *E. coli* (EEC). The EEC are divided into two groups, with group A composed of serotypes 026:B6, 055:B5, 0111:B4, and 0127:B8 and group B consisting of types 086:B7, 0112:B11, 0119:B14, 0124:B17, 0125:B15, 0126:B16, and 0128:B12. Group A serotypes, particularly 055:B5 and 0111:B4, have been associated with epidemic disease more frequently than the group B serotypes. Since EEC may be present in the gastrointestinal tract of infants who are asymptomatic, it may be difficult to determine the significance of the presence of group B EEC in a solitary infant with diarrhea. Group A EEC, *Salmonella*, and *Shigella* isolated from infants with diarrhea are generally considered to be etiologically significant, although the carrier state may also exist with these organisms.

Recent studies have shown that serotypes of *E. coli* other than the EEC cause diarrhea in children and adults by elaboration of a choleralike enterotoxin. Thus, further study of *E. coli* enteritis in the newborn may reveal enterotoxin-producing strains. On rare occasions, *Pseud. aeruginosa* or *Staph. aureus* phage group III colonizes the gastrointestinal tract and produces enterocolitis. *C. albicans* may cause gastroenteritis in unusual situations. Amebiasis in a newborn infant is rare. With appropriate cultural and serologic techniques, enteroviruses may be isolated during gastroenteritis in the newborn.

Pathology. Salmonellae may produce acute enteritis and lymphadenitis. Superficial ulceration is not uncommon, but deep ulceration, gross hemorrhage, and perforation are rare. Shigellosis is a less extensive process with inflammation of the mucosa and shallow ulceration. Fibrinous exudates are common and may form pseudomembranes. Rarely, there is pneumatosis intestinales or perforation of the intestine. Mesenteric lymph nodes may show inflammation. A similar histologic picture may be seen in fatal cases of EEC enteritis. However, no pathologic changes have been noted in a number of infants who died with

EEC enteritis. While *Salmonella* enteritis may progress to bacteremia and infection in other organs such as bone and the meninges, bacteremia with shigellae or EEC is extremely rare.

Pathogenesis. The newborn infant's gastrointestinal tract is colonized with organisms from the maternal birth canal. Pregnant women who are symptomatic or asymptomatic carriers of salmonellae, shigellae, or EEC at the time of delivery serve as the major initial source of pathogenic organisms in the nursery. The infant who has acquired the pathogenic strain then serves as a source of infection as the pathogen is spread via the hands of medical personnel or less commonly by fomites or the airborne route. In some nursery outbreaks, asymptomatic carriers among personnel have been incriminated as the source of the epidemic, but it may be difficult to determine whether the suspect acquired the organism in the course of the epidemic. In rare instances, nursery epidemics have been traced to milk or water.

Clinical. Gastrointestinal colonization with pathogenic strains may not produce symptoms. In almost every outbreak, there are asymptomatic carriers. Manifestations of infection vary from the infant who is not doing well to the infant with fever and diarrhea. EEC and salmonellae often produce less severe symptoms than shigellae. Abdominal distention and vomiting may be noted. Blood is commonly present in the stools of infants with shigellosis but is rare in the other infections. A characteristic seminiferous odor has been associated with the feces in infants with EEC enteritis. Dehydration, acidosis, and shock may complicate the course of neonatal enteritis.

Diagnosis. Diagnosis of bacterial gastroenteritis is made on the basis of cultural identification of stool organisms using biochemical and serologic techniques. EEC must be identified using antisera to pool A and to pool B serotypes. Agglutinating colonies are then tested with specific antisera making up the pool. At least ten *E. coli* colonies should be picked before EEC enteritis is excluded. The fluorescent antibody technique may be used for presumptive diagnosis and is useful for screening stool samples. Nonbacterial gastroenteritis may be further studied in virology laboratories. Demonstration of enterotoxin-producing *E. coli* is currently limited to research laboratories.

Diarrheal disease in the newborn may be caused by improper feeding, cow's milk intolerance, or Hirschsprung's disease. Transitional stools may be confused with diarrhea.

Treatment. Enteropathogenic *E. coli* enteritis should be treated with oral administration of neomycin in a dosage of 50 to 100 mg/kg/day in four divided doses for about 5 days. Although bacteriologic relapse is not uncommon, the organisms are suppressed during treatment and the infant may not be infectious. In the unusual case of neomycin resistance, oral polymyxin B or colistin sulfate may be substituted. Mild *Salmonella* gastrointestinal infections do not require antimicrobial therapy. In more severe infections where it is difficult to exclude bacteremia and other organ involvement, full parenteral doses of ampicillin or chloramphenicol should be administered. Appropriate intravenous fluid therapy and correction of acidosis is essential in the management of symptomatic infants.

Prevention. Obstetrical histories should include questioning about recent diarrheal disease in the mothers. Appropriate cultures should be taken and isolation of mother and infant required until the results of the culture are known. Avoidance of overcrowding, proper hand-washing technique, and proper preparation of formulas are essential measures. Personnel with gastrointestinal symptoms should be excluded from the nursery. When EEC epidemics occur, the nursery should be closed to new admissions and all infants treated with neomycin until the time of discharge of the last infant exposed. The nursery may be reopened 48 hours after beginning neomycin therapy.

Urinary tract infections

Infection of the urinary tract is recognized as a frequent concomitant of septicemia in the neonate. Isolated urinary tract infections are occasionally seen, but few reliable estimates are available.

Etiology. The same organisms causing neonatal septicemia may be found in urine. *E. coli* predominates, and specific serotypes of *E. coli* (04 and 06) have been associated with epidemics of urinary tract infections and septicemia in nurseries. These serotypes are generally the most prevalent gastrointestinal serotypes. *Proteus, Pseudomonas, Enterobacter,* and staphylococci are other pathogens in urinary tract infections.

Pathogenesis. Since the kidney receives a major component of the systemic blood flow, it is not surprising that bacteremia results in positive urine cultures in about one third of cases. Ascending infection appears to be much less common. Some newborn infants with urinary tract infection will have demonstrable structural abnormalities, especially congenital obstructive uropathies (Chapter 16). Urinary tract infection, like septicemia, is more common in males in contrast to the incidence in older children and adults.

Pathology. The histology of acute pyelonephritis in infancy is similar to that found at any age. Abscesses may be found throughout the cortex and medulla, or the inflammatory response may be limited to a polymorphonuclear infiltration. In chronic pyelonephritis, lymphocytes, plasma cells, and eosinophils predominate, and pericapsular fibrosis and crescents are seen. Death may occur before the development of scarring and contraction, which is seen in the older child.

Clinical. Urinary tract infections in the newborn infant present manifestations similar to those of septicemia (p. 131). Jaundice has been frequently associated with pyelonephritis. Infants with transient bacteremia resulting in urinary tract infection usually have minimal symptoms such as poor feeding, diarrhea, and fever.

Infants with external features associated with urinary tract malformations, such as single umbilical artery, spina bifida, and low-set ears, should have urine cultures and often roentgenographic studies.

Diagnosis. The urine of a normal newborn contains less than 10 WBC per mm^3 and no bacteria. Leukocytes must be distinguished from tubular epithelial cells. The presence of bacteria in a stained smear of a clean, unspun urine specimen is presumptive evidence for infection. However, the diagnosis is made by culture of the urine. Collection of uncontaminated urine in the newborn infant is difficult; 7% to 30% of clean-voided specimens from normal newborns will contain over 100,000 bacteria per ml. Midstream and catheter specimens decrease contamination, but both are time consuming and the latter involves a risk of secondary infection. While 100,000 bacteria per ml is considered significant, over 1,000 organisms per ml on repeated cultures should be viewed with suspicion. Suprapubic aspiration is the procedure of choice in diagnosing urinary tract infection in the newborn. There is little hazard, and false positives do not occur. The specimen should be prepared within 1 hour or refrigerated to prevent multiplication of bacteria.

Treatment. If the urinary tract infection is part of a generalized infection, the chemotherapeutic agent used to treat septicemia is appropriate. Prior to the culture report, a combination of agents should be given as guided by gram stain of the urine. Ampicillin or kanamycin may be used to treat a sensitive gram-negative organism. Gram-positive cocci in clusters would indicate that an antistaphylococcal agent such as methicillin or oxacillin should be given. Treatment should be continued for 7 to 10 days, and repeated cultures should be obtained after therapy. Relapses are rare in the absence of congenital malformations of the urinary tract.

Arthritis and osteomyelitis

Neonatal osteomyelitis frequently extends into the joint space so both conditions are considered together. These infections are relatively infrequent in the antibiotic era; a busy newborn service may see one or two cases annually.

Etiology. Staphylococci have been the most common organisms in neonatal arthritis and osteomyelitis. Streptococci, pneumococci, *H. influenzae, N. gonorrhoeae* and gram-negative enteric organisms may also cause these infections.

Pathology. Osteomyelitis most commonly affects the metaphyses of long bones. Multiple foci may be found in 10% of cases. The femur and humerus are most susceptible, but the disease may localize in any bone, including the tibia, metacarpals, maxilla, vertebras, and clavicle. Since the cortical bone is very thin, the inflammation generally extends into soft tissue, which saves the cortex from destruction. An extensive involucrum is formed, but sequestration of dead bone is uncommon. Because ossification of the epiphyses has not occurred, the metaphyseal infection frequently penetrates the joint space. In the hip and elbow, the position of the metaphysis on the joint capsule permits direct spread into the joint. There is destruction of cartilage, and pathologic dislocations and fractures may occur. Frequently there is an effect on growth in the involved bone.

Pathogenesis. In the newborn period arthritis and osteomyelitis almost always occur by hematogenous spread. One exception is maxillary osteomyelitis, which has occurred in nursing infants whose mothers have breast abscesses. The initial focus of infection may be an omphalitis or pyoderma, but in many cases there is no obvious source for the bacteremia. Arthritis or osteomyelitis may also occur in infants who are being treated for septicemia or meningitis.

Clinical. High fever with a septic presentation is uncommon. Usually the disease begins with malaise or failure to gain weight. The first signs are localized swelling, limitation of motion of the involved extremity or pain. Fever may not be present. There is usually no redness or heat early in osteomyelitis, but these signs may be present if the process has ruptured into the subcutaneous tissue or the joint space. Roentgenographic changes develop with time; soft tissue swelling appears first, but bone changes are not visible for 7 to 10 days. Periosteal thickening, cortical destruction, irregularities of the epiphysis, cystlike defects, and extracortical new bone formation may be seen.

Diagnosis. The clinical impression of arthritis is confirmed by aspiration of joint fluid and the demonstration of leukocytes and bacteria. In most cases of osteomyelitis, aspiration of bone can also be performed. Cellulitis, syphilis, and scurvy, should be considered in the differential diagnosis.

Blood cultures may be positive in a small percentage of cases.

Treatment. Antimicrobial therapy of arthritis and osteomyelitis depends on the etiologic agent identified by smear or culture of the purulent material or the blood. A penicillinase-resistant penicillin should be used for staphylococcal infections unless the organism is shown to be sensitive to penicillin G. Penicillin G should be given for streptococcal infections, and the combination of ampicillin and kanamycin for gram-negative bacillary infections until culture results and sensitivity patterns permit the selection of a single agent. *Pseudomonas* infections should be treated with polymyxin or gentamicin. Both methicillin (oxacillin or nafcillin) and kanamycin should be administered if there is no information as to cause. Dosages are similar to those used in infants with septicemia. Parenteral therapy is necessary for about 3 weeks, and oral therapy should be continued for a total of 4 to 6 weeks. Intraarticular administration is not indicated.

Decompression may be performed by aspiration or by surgical intervention. Incision and drainage are indicated if signs have been present for more than 72 hours or when the hip is involved. Traction or a brace may be indicated, particularly if there is destruction of bone. The residual damage depends on the joint or bone affected and the extent of disease prior to therapy. While chronic osteomyelitis is rare, marked residual effects may be expected in over 25% of neonates with pyogenic infections of the bones or joints.

Bacterial meningitis

Bacterial meningitis occurs in about 0.4 infants per 1,000 live births. It is four times more common in low birth weight infants. As in septicemia, complications during labor and delivery and maternal peripartum infections predispose the infant to development of meningitis.

Etiology. All of the organisms associated with neonatal septicemia cause meningitis.

Pathology. Exudation is most commonly observed over the base of the brain but may be diffusely distributed over the convexity. There is hyperemia and edema, but herniation is uncommon. Hydrocephalus may be present in half of the autopsied cases. Polymorphonuclear leukocytes predominate in the acute stage of the disease. In the second and third weeks histiocytes and macrophages assume predominance. Vasculitis is characteristic and may be associated with thrombosis and infarction. A glial cell reaction is common, and the cortical cells show diffuse karyorrhexis and loss of nerve cells.

Pathogenesis. Maternal peripartum infection and chorioamnionitis contribute to the development of meningitis via the ascending route. Transplacental hematogenous spread is less common. Congenital malformations of the central nervous system such as meningomyelocele are frequently infected. A number of sites of infection serve as foci for the development of meningitis. Pneumonia, otitis media, skin infections, omphalitis, and urinary tract and gastrointestinal tract infections may be associated with bacteremia and subsequent meningitis. While meningitis may follow approximately a third of the cases of neonatal septicemia, the increased susceptibility of the premature infant remains a subject for speculation. Otila showed increased and more rapid diffusion of an intramuscularly administered dye into the spinal fluid of premature infants which indicates increased permeability.

Clinical. The usual signs are vague and nonspecific. Poor feeding, lethargy, vomiting, increased respiratory rate, hyperthermia or hypothermia, and irritability are common. A bulging fontanelle and stiff neck are late signs of meningitis. The other neurologic signs appearing during the course of meningitis are cranial nerve paralysis, convulsions, abnormal Moro reflex, abnormal cry, and coma. Subdural effusions and hydrocephalus may complicate the acute course. The mortality of neonatal meningitis is over 50%, and 30% to 60% of the survivors will have residua including mental retardation, speech or hearing defects or both, seizures, and neuromotor disabilities.

Diagnosis. The diagnosis of meningitis is made by examination of the spinal fluid. The cell count will vary from a slight increase to over 10,000 cells, depending on the duration of disease and the inflammatory response. The spinal fluid glucose level is usually less than two thirds of the blood glucose level, and the protein concentration is generally elevated, often over 100 mg/100 ml. Bacteria are usually demonstrable on Gram-stained smears, and cultures are positive with few exceptions. Absence of pleocytosis and a negative culture may be found in partially treated meningitis. There are cases of meningitis discovered at autopsy in which the infant received antibiotics for another infection and in which the spinal fluid was sterile and without an increase in cell count. Blood cultures reveal the same organism in more than half the patients.

Treatment. Antimicrobial therapy for bacterial meningitis is similar to treatment for septicemia with the addition of intrathecal therapy for *Pseudomonas* and gram-negative enteric bacteria. In these instances gentamicin may be given intrathecally in a dose of 0.5 to 1.0 mg in 1 ml of saline daily for 3 to 5 days. Supportive therapy is similar to that given for septicemia. Convulsions may be treated with phenobarbital, 5 to 8 mg/kg intramuscularly, or diazepam, 0.1 to 1.0 mg administered slowly intravenously until convulsions are controlled.

Aseptic meningitis and encephalitis

Aseptic infections of the meninges and brain occasionally occur in the neonatal period. Infection results from transplacental transmission or acquisition of the infectious agent during or following birth.

Etiology. The viruses associated with these syndromes include rubella, cytomegalovirus, coxsackievirus B, herpes simplex, arboviruses, polio, and varicella. Syphilis, toxoplasmosis, tuberculosis, and fungi also produce aseptic central nervous system infections.

Pathogenesis. Transplacental passage of virus may occur at various times during pregnancy. If this occurs early in pregnancy, teratogenic effects may be noted, as with rubella. Viremia in the mother just prior to delivery may delay the onset of signs of infection in the newborn. Maternal infection may be asymptomatic, and asymptomatic neonatal infections of the central nervous system have been discovered by screening newborns for elevated serum IgM concentrations. Viruses may be ingested during passage through the birth canal or acquired by contact in the nursery or at home. Mosquito-transmitted encephalitides may also occur in the neonatal period.

Clinical. Aseptic central nervous system infections vary in severity from infants who are asymptomatic to those who have marked involvement with a fatal outcome. Common symptoms are poor feeding, vomiting, irritability, lethargy, hyperthermia or hypothermia, and focal or diffuse seizures. Other manifestations are an abnormal respiratory pattern, circulatory disturbances, and abnormal reflexes. Infants surviving the acute infection in the newborn period have a high incidence of mental retardation, seizure disorders, and neuromotor abnormalities.

Diagnosis. Examination of the cerebrospinal fluid usually reveals abnormalities unless the inflammation does not involve the meningeal surface. A pleocytosis, which rarely exceeds 1,000 leukocytes per mm^3, is usually found, with a predominance of lymphocytes, unless the infection is very acute. The protein concentration is often elevated, and the glucose almost always normal. Gram stain and methylene blue stains are negative, and cultures for bacteria show no growth. Since it is difficult to culture viruses from cerebrospinal fluid, the etiologic diagnosis usually depends on viral isolation from other sources such as throat, urine, or stool, with a rise in specific antibody titers. Syphilis, toxoplasmosis, tuberculosis, and fungal meningitides are discussed elsewhere. Differential diagnosis includes bacterial meningitis, tuberculous meningitis, and vascular malformations of the brain.

Treatment. Specific treatment for syphilis and herpes meningoencephalitis is discussed elsewhere. For the remaining causes of aseptic meningitis only symptomatic therapy is available.

SPECIFIC BACTERIAL INFECTIONS

Listeria monocytogenes infections

Listeriosis is an uncommon infection that has its highest incidence in the newborn period. In some series of neonatal meningitis about 10% of the cases have been caused by *Listeria.* The organism is widely distributed in a variety of animal species. Infections occur in normal children and adults but are much more common in patients with serious underlying disease.

Etiology. *L. monocytogenes* is a short, gram-positive, non–spore-forming rod. It resembles corynebacteria morphologically and has been confused with diphtheroids and discarded as a contaminant. The bacteria are easily decolorized during gram-staining and may be reported as gram-negative rods.

Pathology and pathogenesis. The majority of neonatal infections result from a transplacental bacteremia. The mother's infection may be subclinical, or she may have a brief episode of fever and symptoms suggesting influenza or infectious mononucleosis. Infection early in pregnancy may result in abortion. Listeriosis later in pregnancy often leads to stillbirth or premature delivery. The organisms can be recovered from the cervix and vagina so that ascending infection in utero or infection during parturition is also possible.

At autopsy, the disease may be limited to a diffuse leptomeningitis. The infiltrate is predominantly neutrophilic. In some patients there are miliary microabscesses in the liver, spleen, adrenals, brain, skin, conjunctivas, intestine, and pharynx. This form of listeriosis has been termed granulomatosis infantiseptica. In cases of transplacental infection, there are foci of necrosis in the placenta.

Clinical. *Listeria* has been recovered from the meconium of normal infants. In symptomatic infants, signs vary from poor feeding, lethargy, diarrhea, and vomiting to the infant who appears moribund with dyspnea, apnea, or cyanosis. The disease may have its onset immediately after birth, or symptoms may be delayed for weeks. In most cases of neonatal listeriosis, signs appear by 2 weeks of age. The incubation period for listeriosis is estimated between 8 and 14 days. Mortality is close to 100% if symptoms appear during the first 4 days of life. When symptoms appear beyond the second week of life, the mortality is approximately 10%. If signs appear between 4 and 14 days, the mortality is about 50%. Petechiae, fever or hypothermia, jaundice, bulging fontanelle, or convulsions may be the predominant signs. On examination, hepatosplenomegaly, granuloma of the skin or posterior pharynx, or signs of meningitis or myocarditis may be noted.

Laboratory studies often reveal an increase in polymorphonuclear leukocytes. The urine may contain protein and red and white blood cells. In most cases, cerebrospinal fluid will be purulent with an elevated protein level and decreased glucose content. The organisms are usually seen on smear.

Diagnosis. With the exception of the

granulomatous lesions of the skin and mucous membranes, there is nothing to differentiate listeriosis from other causes of septicemia and meningitis in the newborn infant. The amniotic fluid may have a brownish discoloration, and organisms may be seen on smears of meconium. A definitive diagnosis requires isolation of the organism from blood, urine, cerebrospinal fluid, meconium, or foci of necrosis in tissues at autopsy.

Therapy. The mortality is high despite antimicrobial therapy, and the sensitivity of *Listeria* to different antibiotics is not uniform. Ampicillin or penicillin appears to be the drug of choice in the neonatal period. Tetracycline has been recommended by others. The usual approach to septicemia or meningitis of unknown cause, namely the use of ampicillin (or penicillin) plus kanamycin, is indicated for initial therapy. If the infant fails to respond appropriately, in vitro sensitivity patterns should guide the changes in antimicrobial therapy. Survivors may be normal, but neurologic sequelae and mental retardation are not uncommon.

Syphilis

Syphilis in the neonate is an increasingly important problem. The annual incidence in the United States is rising; approximately five or six infants with syphilis are seen annually in a large newborn service in an urban community.

Etiology. Syphilis is caused by *Treponema pallidum,* an anaerobic spirochetal organism between 4 and 20μ in length. The organism is present in lesions such as the end of the umbilical cord, bullous rash, and infected mucous membranes. *T. pallidum* has not yet been cultured in vitro. The spirochetes are destroyed by temperatures over 40 C and require moisture for survival.

Pathology. Stillbirths occur in approximately one fourth of pregnancies in untreated mothers. In the remaining live births, the nature of the disease depends upon the dose of *T. pallidum,* the gestational age, and the effectiveness of chemotherapy. Since infection occurs beyond the fourth month, there is no interference with organogenesis. Major organ involvement is found in liver, lung, spleen, bone, and bone marrow. The inflammatory response is predominantly one of mononuclear cells and leads to diffuse fibrosis. Plasma cells have been noted. Stillborn infants may show pneumonia alba. The bone lesions depend on the age of the infant and severity. An osteochondritis of the distal metaphysis is seen in advanced disease. In older infants, periostitis is more common. Osteomyelitis usually produces rarefaction at the ends of long bones. Widespread fibrosis occurs in adrenal glands, kidneys and other organs. The cornea, teeth, and central nervous system involvement becomes apparent later in infancy.

Pathogenesis. Syphilis in the newborn infant results from transplacental infection. Organisms are rarely demonstrable in fetuses aborted by women with syphilis prior to the fifth month. If proper therapy is administered to a woman with syphilis before the fifth month of pregnancy, the disease is almost always prevented. Treatment of the mother in the second half of pregnancy will usually cure disease in the fetus, but syphilitic changes may be present if there is a delay in treatment. The liveborn infants of untreated mothers may have no clinical manifestations for weeks or months, and some may escape disease entirely.

Clinical. Severely affected syphilitic newborns may appear hydropic with severe anemia and extramedullary hematopoiesis producing hepatic and splenic enlargement. In most cases there are no clinical manifestations for 1 to 3 weeks. Nonspecific symptoms include fever, poor feeding, and irritability. The usual rash is a diffuse copper-colored maculopapular rash on the face, palms, and soles. Rarely, bullous lesions of the palms and soles are present. Variable rashes often recur and have a predilection for perioral and perianal regions. Perianal condylomata may form. The cutaneous and mucosal lesions are excellent sources of *T. pallidum.* A serous nasal discharge termed snuffles often becomes secondarily infected with excoriation of the lip. There may be generalized lymph node enlargement and hepatosplenomegaly. Syphilitic hepatitis may produce jaundice. The nephrotic syndrome has been described. Painful pseudoparalysis of a limb is uncommon, and bone lesions are usually asymptomatic. By 1 to 3 months over 90% of infants with prenatal syphilis show either osteochondritis at the

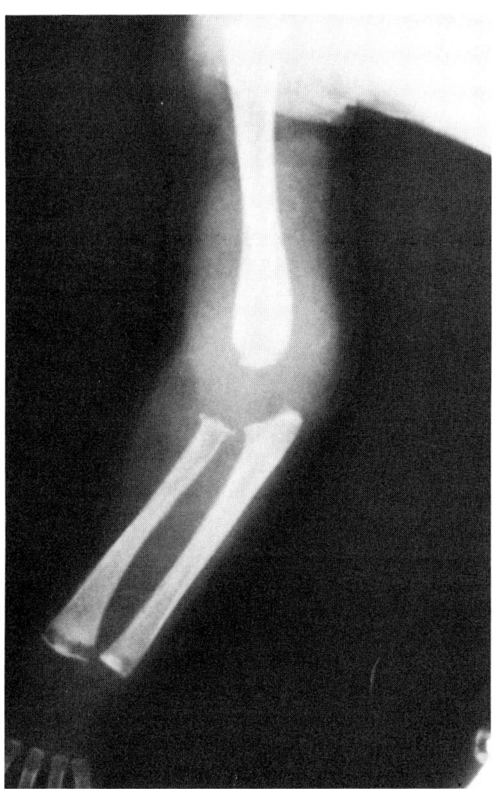

Fig. 8-1. Roentgenogram of the left upper extremity of a newborn with congenital syphilis. Metaphysitis and diaphysitis are present in the radius and ulna. Marked destructive changes of the distal humerus with an extensive periosteal reaction are also noted. (Courtesy E. J. Liebner, University of Illinois.)

metaphysis, periostitis, or osteomyelitis (Fig. 8-1). The humeri are most likely to be involved. Bone lesions may be present despite accepted prenatal treatment and may persist for 3 to 5 months. Central nervous system involvement is rarely symptomatic, but cerebrospinal fluid pleocytosis and increased protein concentration are common.

Diagnosis. Diagnosis may be accomplished by dark-field examination or direct fluorescent antibody staining of a scraping from the umbilical cord, skin, or mucous membrane lesion. Serologic diagnosis is more complicated and requires interpretation. Both specific and nonspecific (reagin) antibodies occur in syphilitic infections. Specific antibody tests include: the *T. pallidum* immobilization (TPI) test, the treponemal antibody (FTA) test, and the fluorescent treponemal antibody-absorption (FTA-ABS) test. The latter is most commonly used to demonstrate specific antibodies to *T. pallidum.* A modification of the FTA-ABS test that detects IgM antibodies to *T. pallidum* has been described.

Serologic tests for nonspecific treponemal antigens utilizing cord blood or maternal serum at the time of delivery are generally adequate for screening in early congenital syphilis. A negative test early in pregnancy does not exclude the diagnosis, and a maternal or cord blood screening test must be repeated at the time of delivery. The nonspecific tests include the VDRL, RPR, Kahn, Hinton, Eagle, Mazzini, Wassermann, and Kolmer tests. A positive VDRL test generally reverts to negative 6 to 12 months after treatment of primary syphilis and 12 to 24 months after treatment of secondary syphilis. The specific tests for treponemal antibody may remain positive for years despite adequate therapy. Both IgG reagin and specific antitreponemal antibody will cross the placenta and appear in cord serum. In the absence of clinical and roentgenographic signs of syphilis, repeated quantitative serial tests are usually performed to determine whether the titer is falling. An elevated cord serum IgM level provides suggestive evidence of infection, and the IgM antitreponemal fluorescent antibody test, in which peripheral blood is used, will give a definite diagnosis. If the later tests are not available, diagnosis usually depends on serial titers that rise or fail to fall over a 2-month period. Some authorities recommend treatment of all newborn infants with a positive serologic test for syphilis. Treatment appears advisable if there is any question of the family's ability to cooperate with follow-up serologic examinations.

The clinical manifestations of prenatal syphilis are varied, and the differential diagnosis should include cutaneous moniliasis, Letterer-Siwe disease, drug rash, epidermolysis bullosa, pyogenic osteomyelitis, toxoplasmosis, cytomegalovirus infection, and the rubella syndrome.

Treatment. Penicillin is the drug of choice administered intramuscularly as aqueous procaine penicillin G, 10,000 units/kg/day for 10 days, or as a single dose of benzathine penicillin G, 50,000 units/kg.

Systemic illness requires daily treatment with aqueous penicillin G. Twenty percent of infants have transient febrile Herxheimer reactions. Successful therapy results in a disappearance of clinical signs, although the roentgenographic signs may persist for months. Blood and spinal fluid serologic tests become negative in a few months. Adequate treatment of the newborn prevents all of the complications of prenatal syphilis.

Complications. Failure to recognize and treat prenatal syphilis may result in late congenital syphilis. Approximately 60% of the infants will have only a positive serologic test for syphilis. The other complications are interstitial keratitis, which usually appears around puberty, Hutchinson's teeth, mulberry molars, eighth nerve deafness, neurosyphilis, sclerotic or gummatous bone involvement, rhagades or fissures about the mouth and nose, and gummas of the skin or other organs.

Tetanus

Neonatal tetanus is essentially limited to certain underdeveloped areas where there is a lack of hygiene. In the United States, 20 to 30 cases occur annually. It is a preventable disease whose eradication awaits only improved delivery of medical care and education.

Etiology. Tetanus is produced by a potent exotoxin released by the anaerobic bacillus, *Clostridium tetani*. The organism is found in soil and the gastrointestinal tracts of man and most animals. The bacilli form highly resistant spores that germinate, proliferate, and release toxin in wounds or necrotic tissues that have lowered oxygen tension.

Pathology. Pathologic changes are found in the brain and spinal cord, particularly in the motor nuclei. Death usually results from asphyxia caused by laryngeal spasm or from prolonged seizures. Cardiac or respiratory arrest may be caused by a direct effect on the medullary centers.

Pathogenesis. Contamination of the umbilical cord stump with soil provides a focus for the proliferation of *Cl. tetani* and the elaboration of toxin. Less commonly, other wounds or skin infections provide a portal of entry. The toxin has an affinity for nervous tissue, affecting the metabolism of acetylcholine. It produces increased irritability of the central nervous tissue and exaggerated motor activity. After toxin is fixed in the nervous tissue, it can no longer be neutralized by antitoxin.

Epidemiology and immunity. *Cl. tetani* has a widespread distribution. The disease itself does not produce immunity, but formalin-treated toxin or toxoid can produce active immunity and complete protection when used properly. Adequate levels of antitoxin are produced after a series of primary immunizations and booster injections every 10 years. The antitoxin crosses the placenta so that infants born to women whose immunization is up to date will have adequate antitoxin levels.

Clinical. The incubation period varies from 3 to 10 days. The initial symptom is difficulty in feeding. Trismus is usually the first sign, followed by diffuse muscle rigidity, jerking spasms, and generalized convulsions. When the interval between trismus and the onset of spasms is over 48 hours, the prognosis improves. Physical examination shows trismus, tonic musculature, and spasms. Opisthotonos may be present. Deep tendon reflexes may be increased or absent during a spasm. Fever, abnormalities in respiratory rate and rhythm, and tachycardia are not uncommon. Mild cases show a stiff upper lip on stimulation of the mouth and clumsy sucking movements.

Diagnosis. The full-blown disease should not be confused with any other diagnosis. Meningitis, brain damage from hemorrhage, congenital defects, anoxia, and kernicterus may produce spasms and convulsions but trismus is absent. In hypocalcemic tetany, there are tremors, seizures, and laryngospasm; however, general rigidity and trismus are absent, and feeding is generally normal in the interim. Phenothiazine derivatives may produce extrapyramidal signs including spasms of the neck and back muscles, trismus, and dysphagia. The symmetrical rapid tonic seizures of tetanus are absent, and the neck spasms usually produce an appearance of torticollis.

Treatment. A clear airway, adequate ventilation, and oxygenation are primary treatments. Barbiturates are indicated for sedation. Meprobamate (50 to 100 mg every 4 hours) is administered for skeletal muscle relaxation. If seizures are not controlled with barbiturates, chlorpromazine

(0.5 mg/kg) is added. Diazepam (0.1 to 1.0 mg) may be used to manage seizures. Overmedication with resulting respiratory depression is not infrequent in patients whose convulsions are difficult to manage.

Tetanus antitoxin is given to neutralize circulating toxin. Human tetanus immune globulin, 1,500 units, is given intramuscularly.

Prevention. Proper care of lesions susceptible to implantation of *Cl. tetani,* such as umbilical cord and circumcision surfaces, require aseptic obstetric and neonatal care. If the mother has been immunized, transplacental antitoxin provides protection to the newborn.

Tuberculosis

Although tuberculosis in the newborn is a rare disease, the management of an infant whose mother has tuberculosis is not uncommon. Prevention of tuberculosis in the young infant is currently a matter of some debate.

The diagnosis of congenital tuberculosis requires demonstration of the organism and either a primary complex in the liver or tuberculous lesions present at or soon after birth. These criteria distinguish congenital tuberculosis from infection acquired in the postpartum period. In 1955, 84 cases of congenital tuberculosis were documented in the literature.

Etiology. *Mycobacterium tuberculosis* var. *hominis* is the cause of congenital tuberculosis. Bovine strains of *M. tuberculosis* are uncommon, and the anonymous or atypical strains of mycobacteria are unlikely to cause systemic disease in normal pregnant women or newborn infants.

Pathology. Hematogenous spread of the acid-fast bacilli via the umbilical vein leads to the formation of a primary complex in the porta hepatis and liver. Miliary tubercles are generally found in the lung, spleen, adrenal, kidney, bone marrow, brain, spinal cord, and serosal surfaces. The placenta is also involved; however, the lesions may be microscopic. When the primary complex is found in the lungs, it is assumed that infection resulted from aspiration of infected amniotic fluid, vaginal secretions, or inhalation of tubercle bacilli in the postpartum period.

Pathogenesis. Three routes of infection may lead to tuberculosis in the newborn. Hematogenous passage of tubercle bacilli may infect the placenta and then the fetus. Most cases of congenital tuberculosis are secondary to hematogenous spread. Generally, miliary tuberculosis is diagnosed in the mother. However, in some instances of congenital tuberculosis the mother's lesion has been reported as mildly active or inoperative. Conversely, normal infants have been born to women with severe miliary tuberculosis. Bacillemia has been demonstrated in cord blood but does not always result in fetal infection. Placental tuberculosis is more common than congenital tuberculosis.

A second route of infection results from aspiration of infected amniotic fluid following rupture of a caseous focus in the placenta or endometrium. In these cases and when infection is acquired during parturition miliary spread is confined to the lungs. Finally, tuberculosis may be contracted after birth from the mother or other household contacts. The onset of symptoms will usually be beyond the neonatal period.

Epidemiology. Tuberculosis is more prevalent in urban populations and lower socioeconomic groups. This influences the management of infants born in nurseries that serve a population where infants are at significant risk from tuberculosis.

Clinical. Symptoms of tuberculosis are usually vague in the newborn period, although a number of sudden deaths in the first 2 weeks of life have been caused by congenital tuberculosis. Anorexia, vomiting, weight loss, or fever is noted after the second week of life. Respiratory symptoms may be absent; in others, cough and respiratory distress are prominent. Some infants have generalized lymphadenopathy. Enlargement of the liver and spleen are common. Obstructive jaundice, osteomyelitis, and meningitis are less common in newborns with congenital tuberculosis. Otitis media and nasopharyngitis are found in newborns who aspirate infected amniotic fluid.

Diagnosis. The diagnosis is suspected if the mother has active tuberculosis during pregnancy. Examination of the placenta may reveal tuberculous granuloma, but the placenta may contain tuberculous foci without spread to the fetus. In some cases of congenital tuberculosis, the placental lesion may be microscopic. The diagnosis can be made by demonstrating acid-fast bacteria in tracheal or gastric aspirates and is confirmed by culture. Histologic examination and culture of material from infected bone marrow, lymph node, or other focus should be carried out when indicated. Roentogenographic examination of the chest provides evidence for pulmonary or miliary tuberculosis. A positive tuberculin test in an infant who did not receive BCG vaccine is diagnostic. While a positive test has been reported at 21 days of life, the tuberculin test may not become positive for months in patients with congenital tuberculosis. Thus, a negative tuberculin test does not exclude the diagnosis. Examination and culture of cerebrospinal fluid or urine will be helpful in infants with meningeal or renal involvement.

Treatment. Untreated congenital tuberculosis is generally a fatal disease, although infants have survived for over a year. Patients have been successfully treated with modern antituberculous chemotherapy. Isoniazid (INH) is the drug of choice (30 mg/kg/day) in conjunction with streptomycin (20 mg/kg/day). Streptomycin may be discontinued after 3 to 4 months, but INH should be administered for 18 months and para-aminosalicylic acid (PAS) substituted for streptomycin. Effort should be made to define the antimicrobial sensitivity of the tubercle bacilli isolated from the infant or the adult source. If INH-resistant organisms are found or the patient fails to respond, the combination of ethambutol and rifampin may be substituted. Kanamycin may be used in place of streptomycin. In seriously ill infants, corticosteroids are indicated in addition to specific antituberculous therapy.

Infants of mothers with active tuberculosis should be separated from their mothers and treated with INH (10 mg/kg/day) in the absence of active infant disease. If a mother with tuberculosis is receiving treatment, either BCG vaccine or INH, prophylaxis should be given. If the mother is known to have sputum containing tubercle bacilli, the infant should be separated from the mother. Pregnant women with tuberculosis should be closely observed during delivery and in the following 6 months for any disease activity since the management of the infant will be affected.

Both BCG vaccination and INH prophylaxis fall short of optimal prevention of tuberculosis. Tuberculosis has occurred in infants immunized with BCG and in infants supposedly receiving INH prophylaxis. Both methods diminish susceptibility in high-risk groups when compared with controls. When the parents are unlikely to obtain or accept long term INH prophylactic therapy, then BCG vaccination is indicated. The objection to BCG is that the development of a positive tuberculin test (which occurs in most cases) eliminates the skin test for diagnosis. However, the skin test after BCG is usually not very large, and other methods may be used for diagnosis.

VIRAL INFECTIONS

Coxsackievirus B encephalomyocarditis

Infection with a number of coxsackieviruses in the newborn period has resulted in myocarditis, encephalitis, or both. While the disease is relatively uncommon, epidemics have been described in newborn nurseries.

Etiology. Coxsackieviruses are enteroviruses now classified in a larger family of viruses called picornaviruses. The viruses are small (15 to 30μ) and have an RNA core. The virus withstands freezing and is inactivated by heating to 60 C for 30 minutes. There are 23 types of coxsackievirus A and six of coxsackievirus B. Coxsackievirus B types 1 to 5 have generally been incriminated in encephalomyocarditis in the newborn.

Pathology. The myocardium typically shows an infiltration of mononuclear cells, degeneration of muscle fibers, and necrosis. Similar inflammatory reactions may be noted in the brain, meninges, liver, lung, and adrenal glands.

Epidemiology. The virus is commonly recovered from feces and occasionally from the oropharynx. In fatal cases the virus has been recovered from myocardium, brain, and other involved organs. Usually, the agent is acquired at birth from the maternal birth canal or from other infants in the nursery. Transplacental transmission has followed an acute febrile illness or pleurodynia in the mother shortly before delivery.

Clinical. The initial manifestations are usually anorexia, fever or hypothermia, vomiting, or diarrhea. These are followed by signs of heart failure, including cyanosis, tachycardia, cardiac enlargement, hepatomegaly, electrocardiographic changes of myocarditis, and shock. Meningeal involvement may be asymptomatic or manifested by signs ranging from lethargy or irritability to convulsions. The cerebrospinal fluid may be xanthochromic, with pleocytosis and elevated protein levels. Pneumonitis is characterized by respiratory distress, cyanosis, rales, and bilateral patchy infiltrates on roentgenographic examination of the chest. Hepatic involvement is manifested by liver enlargement, jaundice, abnormal liver function tests, and occasionally lengthening of the prothrombin time to a degree associated with bleeding in the skin and other organs. Coxsackievirus disease in the newborn is often fatal; however, complete recovery has been reported.

Diagnosis. The association of myocarditis and meningoencephalitis in the newborn strongly suggests coxsackievirus B infection. The diagnosis may be supported by epidemiologic evidence such as pleurodynia in the mother. Isolation of the virus from the blood of the involved organs in fatal cases or from the stool or throat in surviving patients will confirm the diagnosis. Rarely toxoplasmosis will produce myocarditis and meningoencephalitis.

Treatment. No specific therapy is available. Symptomatic treatment for myocarditis, heart failure, and convulsions is covered in the appropriate sections.

Cytomegalovirus infection

Cytomegalovirus infections are common in man and are generally asymptomatic unless host defense mechanisms are compromised. The virus was originally isolated from salivary glands and has been recovered in 10% to 30% of autopsies on adults but in only 1% to 2% of infants. In the newborn, the disease manifestations vary from mild to severe. Approximately four to five cases appear annually in a large newborn service. Disease caused by cytomegalovirus has been referred to as generalized salivary gland virus infection, giant cell inclusion disease, and cytomegalic inclusion disease (CID).

Etiology. The virus has a DNA core and shares characteristics of varicella-zoster and herpes virus. It grows in tissue culture of human cells from a number of sources.

Pathology. Characteristic giant cells with both intranuclear and intracytoplasmic inclusions are found in the salivary glands in 10% to 30% of routine autopsies and in most organs examined in patients with generalized disease. The most frequently involved organs are salivary glands, liver, spleen, lung, brain, kidney, and adrenal. Epithelial cells are typically infected. The cytomegalic inclusion cell measures about 30μ, and the eosinophilic nuclear inclusion measures about 10μ. The tissues show a mononuclear cell infiltration and often diffuse fibrosis. Hemorrhagic areas may be present on the skin and serosal surfaces. Changes in the placenta are nonspecific. In the brain, necrosis of the periventricular region is characteristic with gliosis and secondary calcium deposition.

Pathogenesis. The virus is present in the saliva, blood, and urine of infected individuals. In the newborn, infection is usually the result of transplacental passage; however, postnatal acquisition of virus from relatively intimate contact is not uncommon. The pathologic process will depend on the duration and severity of the infection in the newborn. Longstanding intrauterine infection often may result in the development of microcephaly, cerebral calcification (Fig. 8-2), blindness, or deafness at birth. Other newborn infants may have active inflammatory disease in one or more organs, producing hepatitis, encephalitis, or pneumonia. In these infants, the characteristic chorioretinitis and microcephaly may appear later in infancy. Death may result from respiratory involvement, encephalitis, or hemorrhage. Recovery may be complete or result in mental retardation, convulsive disorder, microcephaly, neuromotor disability, blindness, and deafness.

Epidemiology and immunity. The disease has a worldwide distribution. Approximately half of the women of childbearing age have serologic evidence of prior cytomegalovirus infection. Complement-fixing antibody crosses the placenta and is found in cord blood of infants born to mothers with antibody. If the infant is not infected, the passive antibody disappears during the first year of life. Evidence of acquired infection comes from serologic surveys show-

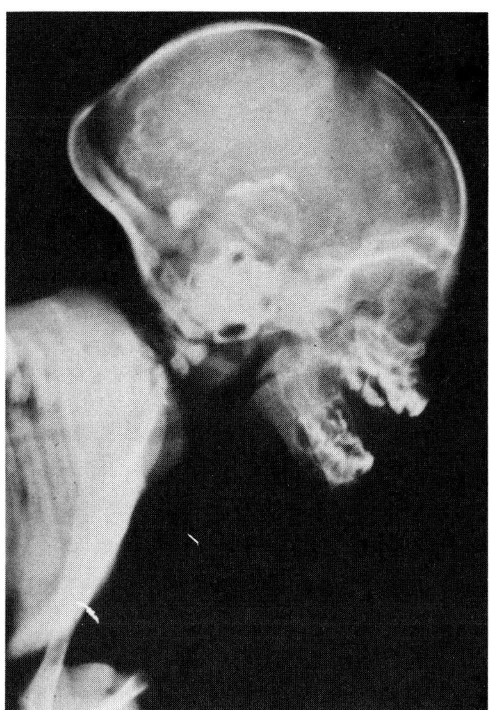

FIG. 8-2. Roentgenogram of the skull of a newborn with cytomegalovirus infection, showing periventricular calcifications.

ing antibody in 15% of infants by the age of 2 years and 30% of children by the age of 10 years. CID virus may be isolated from the urine of 3% to 4% of pregnant women, but the infant born to a woman with viruria is rarely infected. CID in healthy adults is generally asymptomatic. Maternal viruria may persist for months after the delivery of an affected infant. Intrauterine infection occurring in a subsequent pregnancy has been reported but is extremely rare. In infants with CID, virus is commonly excreted for months or years.

In utero infection with cytomegalovirus usually results in fetal synthesis of specific antibody. Since IgM does not cross the placenta, complement-fixing antibody in the IgM fraction of cord serum distinguishes the fetal response from transplacental maternal IgG antibody. Affected infants will continue to produce specific antibody of IgM and IgG classes during infancy.

Clinical. The manifestations of CID in the neonate are extremely varied and range from inapparent infection to severe systemic involvement resulting in death within a few days. CID often results in premature delivery. The severely affected infants often show petechiae and ecchymoses, jaundice, and pallor. Fever may be present. Hepatomegaly and splenomegaly are progressive. Central nervous system involvement is manifested by lethargy, irritability, or convulsions. Chorioretinitis and microcephaly may be present.

Laboratory studies may reveal thrombocytopenia, abnormal liver function, and less commonly hemolytic anemia. Roentgenographic examination may show intracerebral calcifications that are classically periventricular in distribution. Pulmonary infiltrations may be noted and bony sclerosis has been described.

More commonly, infants with CID will have a less severe disease that takes on the appearance of an isolated hepatitis or central nervous system involvement. Thus, CID should be considered in the differential diagnosis of a number of clinical syndromes in the newborn.

Diagnosis. The diagnosis of CID is established by the isolation of the virus from urine, saliva, or tissue, such as liver, obtained at biopsy. Viruria generally persists for months. Inoculation of human tissue culture cells should be carried out with little delay to maximize viral isolation. While isolation of virus from older infants or adults does not incriminate the virus in the disease process, isolation of cytomegalovirus from a sick neonate is generally of etiologic significance.

Typical inclusion-bearing cells may be identified in urine or gastric aspirates. These cells are not always found and may occur in the urine of infants infected with a number of other viruses. CID in the newborn may be documented by a rise in complement-fixing antibody titers or by the presence of antibody in the IgM fraction of cord serum. An indirect fluorescent antibody test for cytomegalovirus IgM antibody is a sensitive diagnostic method.

The differential diagnosis of CID includes bacterial septicemia, toxoplasmosis, rubella, syphilis, generalized herpes simplex infection, and erythroblastosis fetalis.

Treatment. General supportive therapy is the only treatment currently available. Antimicrobial agents, gamma globulin, and corticosteroids have not been effective.

Idoxuridine, cytosine arabinoside, and floxuridine are potential therapeutic agents. Exchange transfusion may be necessary for hyperbilirubinemia. In the future, prevention of CID in the childbearing population may be possible with the development of a vaccine.

Herpesvirus hominis

Neonatal infection with herpesvirus hominis leads to a spectrum of diseases ranging from inapparent infection to fatal encephalopathy. Distribution of these infections is worldwide. The estimated frequency of clinical infections is 1 per 7,500 deliveries.

Etiology. Herpesvirus hominis, or herpes simplex virus, is a DNA virus related to varicella-zoster and cytomegalovirus. On the basis of cytopathic effects two strains have been described. These strains can also be identified serologically. Strain II accounts for over 95% of genitally acquired herpes infections and over 80% of all herpesvirus hominis infections in newborn infants.

Pathology. In the skin, mouth, and esophagus, vesicles result from degeneration of epithelial cells. The fluid contains exfoliated epithelial cells, giant cells, leukocytes, and fibrin. Intranuclear inclusions are found in the floor of the vesicle. With disseminated disease, confluent areas of necrosis surrounded by cells containing inclusion bodies are found in the liver, adrenal cortex, spleen, lymph nodes, brain, stomach, colon, bone marrow, lungs, and heart. There are rare reports of infants with microcephaly and microphthalmia associated with neonatal or maternal herpes lesions, suggesting herpes infection in utero as a possible cause of congenital malformations.

Pathogenesis. If the mother has a primary herpes infection, virus may be transmitted to the fetus transplacentally during the viremic phase. The infection is more commonly acquired from the maternal genital tract through the fetal membranes or at the time of delivery. Following parturition, virus may be spread by direct contact or via the respiratory route. Initial replication occurs at the portal of entry. A primary viremia follows with infection of a few susceptible organs. A secondary viremia leads to widespread organ involvement. In animals, ocular and central nervous system infection may occur without a preceding viremia or evidence of visceral involvement.

Immunity. Humoral antibody develops following primary infection. Type-specific antibodies develop that show some degree of cross-reaction but are not necessarily protective against the cross-reacting type. Herpesvirus antibodies are transmitted transplacentally. While antibody might be expected to neutralize viremia, neonatal herpes has been noted in the presence of transplacental antibody. Maternal antibody may have been produced as a primary response during pregnancy associated with fetal infection. Qualitative or quantitative differences in antibody may not result in protection, or the route of infection may be independent of the bloodstream.

The fetus and newborn with herpes infection usually produces antiherpes antibody in the IgM class.

Clinical. The spectrum of clinical manifestations varies from isolated localized infections of the skin, mouth, eye, or central nervous system to disseminated disease. In one large series, the case fatality rate in those infections diagnosed clinically was 35%.

Signs of disease may be present at birth or delayed for weeks, the median being 6 or 7 days of life. Vesicles may appear on the skin or oral cavity, usually in clusters and sometimes over a dermatome (Fig. 8-3). Conjunctivitis, keratitis, or chorioretinitis may be present. Jaundice or hepatomegaly or both occur in infants with liver involvement. Bleeding from the gastrointestinal tract and elsewhere may be a result of liver damage or may be secondary to disseminated intravascular coagulation. Splenomegaly, pneumonia, and cardiac abnormalities have also been described.

Central nervous system involvement may be asymptomatic but demonstrated by abnormal cerebrospinal fluid or at autopsy. Convulsions are the most common manifestation. Opisthotonus, motor signs, and a bulging fontanelle are less common. The electroencephalogram is abnormal. Cerebrospinal fluid shows an elevation of protein, white blood cells, and often red blood cells.

Diagnosis. The presence of vesicular lesions provides strong evidence for specific diagnosis. In the absence of typical lesions,

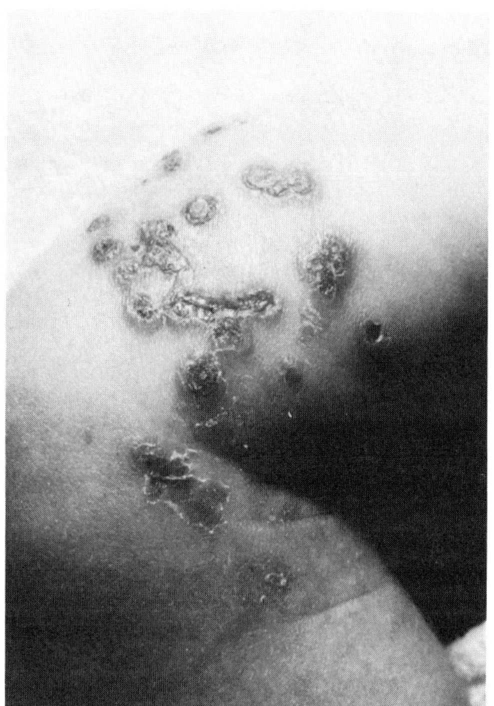

Fig. 8-3. Neonatal herpes simplex infection.

central nervous system infection and disseminated disease may be suspected when there is a history of maternal herpes during pregnancy or genital herpes.

The diagnosis may be made by an examination of cell scrapings from vesicles or from an ulcer for typical intranuclear inclusions and giant cells. Virus may be isolated from vesicles, the oral cavity, conjunctivas and cornea relatively easily and less frequently from blood, CSF, urine, feces, and bone marrow. Finally a rise in type-specific antibody in serial examinations indicates primary infection.

Treatment. The administration of 5-iodo-2-deoxyuridine (idoxuridine) in doses between 50 and 100 mg/kg/day for 5 days is currently undergoing clinical trials in systemic herpes simplex infections. The results are only mildly encouraging, since most infants have either died or been left with neurologic residuals. Prevention is possible in a limited number of cases. If maternal genital herpes is diagnosed, topical idoxuridine may be tried or cesarian section should be carried out. Unfortunately, the genital infection is often inapparent. The administration of gamma globulin has been of no value.

Myxovirus infections

Rubeola and mumps virus may cross the placenta and cause infection in the fetus and newborn infant. Maternal rubeola during gestation contributes significantly to abortion and stillbirths. The relationship of maternal mumps to fetal wastage and congenital malformations is controversial. Some studies have noted an association between delayed hypersensitivity to mumps virus and endocardial fibroelastosis. Influenza virus may produce substantial disease in pregnant women and may lead to increased maternal mortality and fetal wastage. Transplacental passage of influenza virus with a direct effect on the fetus has not been documented.

Etiology. Rubeola, mumps, and influenza viruses are myxoviruses. While the antigenic constitution of rubeola has remained constant, there is significant variation in influenza viruses resulting in multiple epidemic strains. Although mumps virus is classically associated with parotitis, there are other causes, and the specific cause of parotitis should be documented by viral isolation.

Pathology. The pathology of rubeola in the newborn is similar to that observed in the older child. The infiltrate is largely mononuclear, and both intranuclear and intracytoplasmic inclusion bodies are seen in epithelial cells. Interstitial pneumonia and laryngotracheobronchitis are the major life-threatening processes. Congenital parotitis is not a fatal disease, and influenza infection has not been documented in the newborn infant.

Pathogenesis. Transplacental passage of rubeola virus is well substantiated. The measles rash has been recognized in the fetus and newborn infant. The disease is not invariably at the same stage of development as in the mother, suggesting either a prolonged infection in the fetus or the influence of maternal antibody on the disease process.

Transplacental passage of mumps virus is not well documented. While parotitis in the newborn infant has occasionally followed gestational parotitis, virologic evidence of mumps virus infection is lacking. The role of mumps virus as a possible cause of endocardial fibroelastosis is based on delayed hypersensitivity reactions in the offspring of women who have had mumps during pregnancy. A cause and effect relationship has not been substantiated. Influenza virus has not been documented in transplacental or neonatal infections.

Epidemiology and immunity. Most women have had measles during childhood, and the newborn infant receives passive immunity, which lasts for 5 to 9 months. The absence of documented influenza in the newborn period is unexplained. Infections may be subclinical, and transplacental passage of antibody has impaired serologic studies.

Clinical. Rubeola takes its usual clinical form in the newborn infant, although the symptoms may vary from mild to severe. The prodromal symptoms of rhinorrhea, cough, and conjunctivitis with fever and Koplik's spots are followed by the typical morbilliform rash. Congenital measles occurs within 12 days of birth. Most infants have survived without sequelae.

Mumps or parotitis in the newborn period is a mild disease with few systemic signs. Congenital mumps is present at birth or occurs within the first 10 days of life. The pancreatic and central nervous system complications of mumps virus infection have not been described.

Diagnosis. When the mother has had rubeola, neonatal measles can be diagnosed on clinical criteria and by viral recovery or specific IgM neutralizing antibody in less characteristic or subclinical cases. While a presumptive diagnosis of mumps may be based on parotid involvement, the diagnosis rests on recovery of the virus or the demonstration of specific IgM antibody.

Treatment. There is no specific therapy for rubeola or mumps. The latter is a benign infection. Supportive therapy is indicated in infants with rubeola. Secondary bacterial pneumonia should be treated with the appropriate antibiotics. Women exposed to rubeola during pregnancy should receive .25 ml/kg of gamma globulin if they have not had measles in the past.

Poliomyelitis

While poliomyelitis is now a rare disease in the United States and ordinarily occurs in older age groups, it may occur in the newborn period. A review in 1955 reported 58 cases of neonatal poliomyelitis.

Etiology. Polioviruses are members of the enterovirus family in the subgroup of picornaviruses. There are three distinct serotypes, designated I, II, and III. The virus may be grown in a variety of primate cells.

Pathology. Widespread involvement of the gray matter of the spinal cord, medulla, basal ganglia and pons is common with lesser involvement of the precentral gyrus of the cerebral cortex and cerebellum. There is neuronal necrosis, focal and diffuse leukocytic infiltration, perivascular cuffing, and sometimes hemorrhage. Myocarditis has also been observed.

Pathogenesis. The newborn may be infected in utero via the placental circulation during the period of maternal viremia or via contamination with virus-infected feces at delivery or after birth. Since the incubation period is 7 to 10 days, neonatal poliomyelitis manifested after the first week is probably acquired at or following birth. Infection in utero may be associated with fetal death, and the virus has been isolated from fetal blood, tissues, and placenta.

Epidemiology and immunity. Antibody in the maternal serum, as a result of natural infection or immunization, crosses the placenta and provides protection for the first few months of life. Before the introduction of polio vaccine, over 85% of infants had protective antibody at birth. Maintenance of this figure will depend on the level of immunization. Infection may occur in a susceptible pregnant woman and may be asymptomatic or produce only a nonspecific minor illness. Paralytic disease is less common. However, viremia occurs in each infection and may lead to infection in the fetus.

Clinical. Initial symptoms may be irritability, anorexia, vomiting, or diarrhea. Focal or generalized convulsions may indicate the presence of encephalitis. Flaccid paralysis may involve one or more extremities and the muscles of respiration leading to cyanosis. Meningeal involvement is uncommon. The disease is often fatal, but recoveries have been recorded with or without residual paralysis. Subclinical disease has also been documented by culture and neutralizing antibody.

Diagnosis. The virus may be isolated from the throat and feces during life or from internal organs in fatal cases. Serologic tests and viral isolation from the mother and placenta support the diagnosis. The infection is considered congenital if the disease is present at birth or develops within 5 days.

Treatment. There is no specific treatment. The disease is preventable and may be eradicated with widespread immunization programs. Passive immunization and gamma globulin are not recommended. The administration of live, attenuated polio vaccines during pregnancy should be avoided except in epidemic situations.

Rubella

Rubella is a mild infectious disease of children and adults that is rarely recognized as an acquired infection in young infants. The consequences of in utero rubella infection include abortion, stillbirth, teratogenic effects, acute and chronic infection of one or more organs, and asymptomatic infection.

Etiology. Rubella virus has been classified in the paramyxovirus group.

Pathology. Widespread organ involvement occurs in the congenital rubella syndrome. Abnormalities of the cardiovascular system include patent ductus arteriosus, atrial septal defect, pulmonary valvular stenosis, stenosis of pulmonary artery branches, and sclerosis of cardiac valves, aorta, and coronary arteries. Interstitial pneumonia is relatively common. Extramedullary hematopoiesis may produce splenomegaly. The liver usually shows cholestasis, hyalinization and swelling of hepatic cells, some fibrosis, and, in some cases, multinucleated giant cells. Marked alterations in bone growth have been noted, particularly involving the junction of bone and cartilage. Poor mineralization of the metaphysis and diaphysis is apparent radiologically. The brain may show multiple areas of necrosis in the cerebral hemispheres, basal ganglia, and midbrain. Infiltrates are present in the meninges. Subarachnoid hemorrhage, hydrocephalus, and meningomyelocele have been described. The eyes show cataracts, iridocyclitis, or structural abnormalities resulting in glaucoma.

Pathogenesis. Viremia in adults is present 1 week prior to the rash and during the period of the rash. In early pregnancy the chorionic villi may be infected with subsequent fetal viremia. By the fourth month of pregnancy, the fetus appears much less susceptible to rubella infection. Minor abnormalities have been reported following maternal rubella infection in the second trimester. Infection during the second to sixth week after conception, the period of organogenesis, may produce teratogenic effects. Chronic infection causes the diverse signs in the newborn period; namely, hepatitis, thrombocytopenic purpura, and bone lesions. A decrease in the cellular composition of organs has been noted, and rubella infection was found to inhibit mitosis in human embryonic tissue culture cells. These findings would explain the growth retardation in this syndrome.

Epidemiology and immunity. Prior to immunization programs, approximately 20% of women in the childbearing age have no detectable rubella-neutralizing antibody. The risk of rubella-induced malformations is maximal in the first 2 months of gestation, but deafness and mild central nervous system disease may occur when maternal rubella occurs in the fourth month. The incidence of congenital defects as related to gestation is: 0 to 4 weeks, 30% to 50%; 5 to 8 weeks, 25%; and 9 to 12 weeks, 8%.

While abnormalities of immunoglobulin synthesis have been reported in the congenital rubella syndrome, most infected infants form IgM and IgG neutralizing antibody in utero, probably by 20 weeks of gestation. The few studies of cell-mediated immune function that have been performed in these infants indicate an impairment in lymphocyte function. A defect in cell-mediated immunity has been postulated to explain the persistence of virus excretion in the presence of neutralizing antibody. The presence of virus in the throat and urine of infected infants for weeks and months is of considerable hazard to nurses, medical students, and other susceptible health workers.

Clinical. Rubella infection in utero leads to growth retardation so that most infants with the syndrome are small for dates. The classical triad of deafness, cataracts, and congenital heart disease is caused by the teratogenic effects of rubella. Thrombocy-

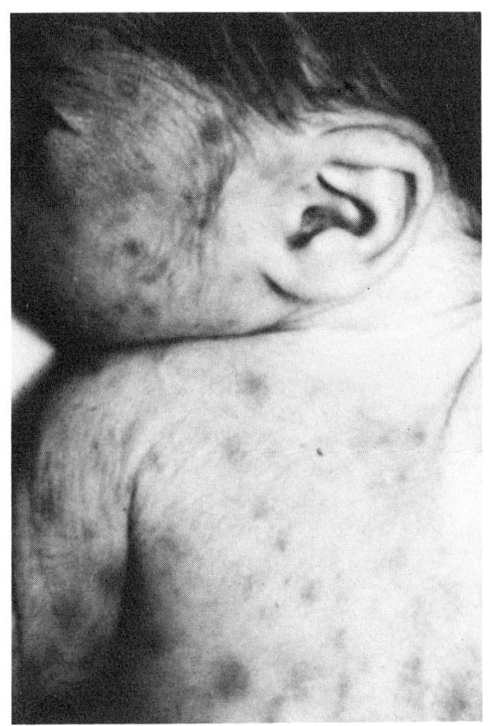

FIG. 8-4. Newborn with the congenital rubella syndrome, showing multiple purpuric lesions over the face, trunk, and upper arm.

topenic purpura (Fig. 8-4), hepatomegaly, splenomegaly, and generalized lymphadenopathy are relatively frequent. Common cardiac lesions include patent ductus arteriosus, atrial septal defect, (ASD), ventricular septal defect (VSD), and peripheral pulmonic stenosis. Cataracts often occur. Glaucoma, self-limited corneal clouding, and retinal pigmentation are also associated with congenital rubella. Bone lesions are characterized by irregular areas of rarefaction in the metaphyseal portion of the long bones. Microcephaly, a bulging anterior fontanelle, and cerebrospinal fluid pleocytosis are early manifestations of central nervous system involvement. Later, varying degrees of mental retardation and gross motor abnormalities may be detected.

Diagnosis. A clinical diagnosis may be made with some certainty in infants with the common teratogenic effects of rubella. A history of rubella in the first trimester provides strong epidemiologic evidence. Those infants with isolated lesions or only a few defects require virologic or serologic diagnosis. Virus has been cultured from the pharynx, urine, cerebrospinal fluid, anterior chamber of the eye, and other organs. Virus excretion decreases with time, but positive cultures may be obtained in over half the infants in the first 4 months of life. A rise in neutralizing antibody titers or the persistence of antibody beyond 6 months in an infant who has not been infected postnatally confirms the diagnosis of congenital rubella.

The differential diagnosis of the congenital rubella syndrome includes idiopathic thrombocytopenic purpura, cytomegalovirus infection, toxoplasmosis, syphilis, and other less common viremic neonatal infections.

Treatment. No specific therapy is available. Treatment of specific organ abnormalities such as glaucoma or congestive heart failure will be indicated. Rehabilitation is often necessary. When hospitalized, these infants should be isolated for a number of months after birth or until their pharyngeal secretions and urine are no longer contagious.

Varicella-zoster

Varicella-zoster infections occur in the neonatal period. In the majority of cases, the disease is mild; but fatalities also occur. The incidence of abortion, prematurity, and congenital malformation associated with varicella in pregnancy is within the expected frequency for normal pregnancies.

Etiology. The viruses causing chicken pox and herpes zoster are identical; this VZ virus is a DNA virus belonging to the same family as herpes simplex and cytomegalovirus.

Pathology. Skin lesions show epithelial cell hyperplasia with intranuclear inclusion bodies that progress to necrotic vesicles and encrustation. Similar lesions may be found in the gastrointestinal tract, forming shallow ulcers in the stomach and intestines. Focal necrosis occurs in lung, liver, pancreas, spleen, adrenals, renal cortex, thymus and bone marrow. Intranuclear inclusions are found in the epithelial elements of these organs.

Pathogenesis. VZ virus may cross the placenta at any time during pregnancy. Intrauterine infection has been documented following clinical varicella in pregnant women during their second and third trimester. However, the placenta provides some protection, since less than half of women with varicella during pregnancy had affected infants. Varicella may also be acquired during passage through the birth canal or postnatally by the airborne route, contact, or fomites.

Epidemiology and immunity. Varicella is predominantly a disease of childhood and is rare in women of childbearing years. Immunity induced by varicella is generally long lasting, but reactivation of the virus may occur in the form of herpes zoster. Immunity to varicella in the newborn appears to be caused by transplacental passage of neutralizing antibody. Protection lasts for 3 to 4 months.

Clinical. The rash may be present at birth or appear later during the neonatal period. Usually 6 to 15 days elapse between the onset of maternal infection and that of the infant. Cases with an onset during the first 10 days are considered congenital varicella, although the incubation period may be as long as 20 days. When the eruption occurs during the first 5 days of life, the course is most likely to be benign. In mild cases only a few vesicular lesions are present, and there are no systemic symptoms. Rarely, the vesicles may have a zosterlike distribution following a radicular topography. In moderately severe cases, symptoms may include fever and poor feeding. Respiratory distress, jaundice, hematuria, and gastrointestinal signs indicate visceral involvement and a more serious prognosis.

Diagnosis. Neonatal VZ infections are usually seen with maternal varicella and the diagnosis is readily apparent. Smallpox has a very limited geographic distribution, and the only disease likely to cause confusion is herpes virus infection. Typical varicella lesions are smaller and less likely to occur in clusters and become confluent. Histologically, viruses of the herpes group produce similar lesions. Final diagnosis rests on the isolation and serologic characterization of the virus.

Treatment. In the majority of cases the course is benign, and no treatment is necessary. There is suggestive evidence that VZ immune globulin given at birth to infants of women with varicella may modify the course of the disease. Severe forms of the disease deserve a trial of 5-iodo-2-deoxyuridine (idoxuridine) or cytosine arabinoside on an experimental basis.

Variola and vaccinia

Variola (smallpox) is presently limited to a few countries in the world. Infection during pregnancy leads to a high rate of abortion, stillbirths, and congenital infections. Vaccinia is an iatrogenic disease that should disappear from the United States now that vaccination is no longer recommended. Vaccinia during pregnancy may result in abortion, stillbirths, and congenital disease.

Etiology. The smallpox virus is a DNA virus in the herpes group. The two types, variola major and minor, vary in the severity of disease produced. Vaccinia virus is a related virus derived from cowpox or variola strains. The vaccine is prepared from vesicles of vaccinated calves.

Pathology. The rash evolves from papules to vesicles and pustules. Microscopically, there is focal necrosis and mononuclear cell infiltration. In variola infections, intracytoplasmic (Guarnieri's bodies) and intranuclear inclusion bodies may be seen. Hematogenous dissemination leads to involvement of lungs, liver, spleen, brain, intestine, kidneys, and adrenals. The placenta shows areas of necrosis and the characteristic inclusion bodies. The lesions are similar in congenital vaccinia; intracytoplasmic inclusion bodies are present, but there are no intranuclear inclusions.

Pathogenesis. Both variola and vaccinia viruses may cross the placenta during any stage of gestation. The infection usually persists in utero, although abortion and premature delivery are common. Transplacental infection may occur in the absence of cutaneous manifestations of disease in the mother. Partial immunity resulting from prior vaccination or natural infection may alter the manifestations of smallpox in the mother; nevertheless viremia and transplacental transmission may occur. Smallpox may also be acquired by contact after birth. The incubation period is about 12 days. While most cases of transplacental vaccinia infection have been secondary to maternal immunization, pregnant women may acquire virus from other vaccinated contacts. In general, fetal infection is unusual, and in many studies vaccination of pregnant women has not resulted in an increased incidence of abortions, stillbirths, or neonatal infections.

Clinical. Infants with congenital smallpox usually have generalized vesicles of varying sizes with a central depression. The infants appear ill and have respiratory distress caused by interstitial pneumonia. The manifestations of disease are similar in congenital vaccinia. There is a very high mortality in both instances.

Diagnosis. The diagnosis of these infections is based on the epidemiologic history and clinical manifestations. Examination of scrapings of the vesicles will reveal the characteristic inclusions. Both intranuclear and intracytoplasmic bodies are found in variola. Recovery of either virus is relatively easy. Specific neutralizing antibody in the IgM fraction can be demonstrated in intrauterine infection.

Treatment. Vaccinia is a preventable disease, and vaccination during pregnancy should be avoided unless there are strong epidemiologic indications. In those countries where smallpox is endemic, congenital variola may be prevented by vaccination during childhood. While N-methylisatin β-thiosemicarbazone and vaccinia immune globulin may alter the course of variola and generalized vaccinia, there is little experience in the use of these agents in neonatal infections.

FUNGAL INFECTIONS

Candidiasis

Candidiasis is usually classified as a deep-seated or superficial infection. Both types of infections have been described in the neonatal period, with oral thrush being relatively common.

Etiology. A number of species of *Candida* (formerly *Monilia*) are pathogenic for man. These include *C. albicans* (the most common), *C. tropicalis, C. stellatoidea, C. pseudotropicalis,* and a few others. *Candida* organisms are yeastlike fungi that produce pseudomycelia in vitro and in tissues. *C. albicans* grows easily on common laboratory media such as Sabouraud's agar.

Pathology. Deep-seated infection refers to abscess formation in the lung, liver, brain, kidney, spleen, myocardium, or endocardium. Bronchopneumonia has been rarely attributed to *Candida.* Superficial infection of the skin or gastrointestinal tract results from invasion of the epithelium by hyphae with penetration of the basement membrane, resulting in congestion and a leukocytic infiltration. In some cases, there is ulceration, pseudomembrane formation, and penetration of veins, leading to thromboses, hematogenous spread, and deep-seated infection. Esophagitis and enteritis may complicate oral disease or occasionally occur in the absence of thrush. *Candida* empyema secondary to esophageal perforation and *Candida* mastoiditis have been described. In congenital systemic candidiasis, the umbilical cord and fetal membranes will be involved. Both superficial and deep-seated lesions are characterized by the presence of budding cells and pseudohyphae (M phase).

Pathogenesis. In normal newborns, the organism is generally acquired from mothers at the time of delivery. *C. albicans* is present in the vaginal flora of approximately 36% of women with or without clinical vaginitis. Secondary transmission occurs from person-to-person spread and rarely from fomites. Recently systemic *Candida* infections have complicated intravenous hyperalimentation in infants with underlying nutritional problems. Congenital candidiasis, both systemic and cutaneous forms, has resulted from *Candida* amnionitis, occasionally in the presence of intact membranes. Surgical wounds, such as gastrostomies, are another common site for *Candida* infection.

Epidemiology. While *C. albicans* is a common commensal in the mucous membranes and the intestinal tract of older individuals, it is generally a pathogen in the newborn. Oral thrush does not appear to be influenced by factors such as prematurity, resuscitation, breast feedings, or antibiotic therapy. Superficial candidiasis is almost always present in infants with combined immunodeficiency disease.

Clinical. The earliest signs of oral thrush are small papules that develop into tiny vesicles. These enlarge and coalesce into the typical white cheesy patches that are found on the tongue, gingiva, and buccal mucosa. There is underlying inflammation; but the infant is generally asymptomatic, and the process usually subsides spontaneously in a few days or weeks. *Candida* esophagitis may appear as difficult feeding, regurgitation during feeding, postprandial vomiting, and hematemesis. There is nothing characteristic about the diarrhea of enteric candidiasis, and the diagnosis depends on the demonstration of mycelian forms in the stool. Deep-seated or systemic candidiasis should be suspected in a newborn infant with systemic disease associated with superficial candidiasis or some predisposing cause such as gastrointestinal tract surgery or the use of hyperalimentation fluids. Disseminated intravascular coagulation may occur as a complication of systemic candidiasis. Cutaneous candidiasis usually begins in the perianal region with spread to the diaper region. Other sites include the neck, axillas, and nails. A more diffuse rash has been described at birth in congenital cutaneous candidiasis. The lesions progress from erythematous macules to papules and vesicles that rupture leaving denuded epithelium with sharply defined, raised, scaling borders. Satellite lesions are common and are highly suggestive of *Candida* dermatitis.

Diagnosis. Oral thrush is a clinical diagnosis, and cutaneous candidiasis may be diagnosed clinically with some degree of confidence. The latter diagnosis should be confirmed by examination of skin scrapings. Cultures of blood, urine, or cerebrospinal fluid are necessary to establish the diagnosis of systemic candidiasis premortem. Mycelian forms should be present in histologic sections. The diagnosis of pulmonary candidiasis is difficult because cultures are easily contaminated with organisms from the oral cavity or esophagus. A pure culture from the trachea or bronchus supports the diagnosis.

Treatment. Deep-seated infection must be treated with a systemic antifungal agent. Amphotericin B is given intravenously in a daily dose of 1 mg/kg over a 2- to 6-hour period for at least 4 weeks. The initial day's dose is 0.25 mg/kg, and this may be increased by a similar increment daily to 1 mg/kg if tolerated. The blood urea nitrogen will generally increase during therapy, and treatment should be temporarily discontinued when the concentration reaches 40 to 50 mg/100 ml. The drug may be resumed, with a lower dosage or alternate day therapy. Intrathecal administration is indicated for *Candida* meningitis that is not responding to intravenous therapy. Candidemia secondary to contaminated intravenous catheters may be transient, and removal of the catheter may be all that is required.

Oral thrush of brief duration and enteric candidiasis will respond to 1 to 2 ml of mycostatin suspension four times a day for 7 to 10 days. Cutaneous candidiasis should be treated with nystatin ointment three times a day for 7 to 10 days. In severe cases, corticosteroid should be added (Mycolog cream or lotion or amphotericin B [Fungizone] lotion).

Prevention. It seems likely that treatment of pregnant women with *C. albicans* in the vagina would affect the incidence of candidiasis in the newborn. While this is appropriate for symptomatic vaginitis, routine cultures of all pregnant women is not an accepted practice. Scrupulous care in the administration of hyperalimentation fluids is an obvious way to prevent *Candida* infection in these newborn infants.

Coccidioidomycosis

Coccidioidomycosis is extremely rare in the newborn period. However, it occurs in the disseminated form and should be considered in the differential diagnosis of systemic infections in endemic areas.

Etiology. *Coccidioides immitis* is a fungus that exists in tissues as a spherule with a doubly refractile capsule containing endospores. In soil and on artificial media the sporangia develop hyphae, and the mycelia become septate; these chlamydospores are highly infectious.

Pathology. Coccidioidomycosis is classically a granulomatous disease, although the lesions resemble abscesses in young infants who expire with disseminated disease. Almost every organ may be involved because of the hematogenous spread. The most frequent sites are lung, meninges, liver, spleen and bone.

Pathogenesis. Infection may result from inhalation of spores carried on clothing or in dust that convert to sporangia and reproduce by endosporulation. Spores may rarely enter through lacerations or abrasions. Since fungemia has been described, the possibility of transplacental passage exists. Placental lesions occur infrequently in pregnant women with disseminated disease. Either transplacental passage or aspiration of infected amniotic fluid may explain intrauterine infections.

Epidemiology. Coccidioidomycosis is endemic in the southwestern United States, northern Mexico, Argentina, Paraguay, and Venezuela; however, one case of neonatal coccidioidomycosis was reported in Chicago. The disease is much more frequent during the dry season. The spherules do not spread from person to person; thus the disease is not contagious.

Clinical. The incubation period ranges from 7 to 21 days. The signs and symptoms depend on the organ involvement. The initial focus of infection is usually in the lungs. Disseminated lesions may appear in the skin, bone, lymph nodes, or meninges. Fever, respiratory distress, and hepatosplenomegaly would be expected. Meningitis and dactylitis have also been reported.

Diagnosis. Examination of a tracheal or gastric aspirate, urine, cerebrospinal fluid, or bone marrow may reveal the spherules. Blood and exudates should be cultured or injected into mice. The white blood cell count is usually elevated with a left shift; spinal fluid findings are similar to those in tuberculous meningitis. Roentgenograms of the chest may show a segmented lesion with hilar involvement or miliary spread. Skin and serologic tests may not be helpful in the immediate newborn period. Complement-fixing antibodies cross the placenta; thus, a rise in the infant's titer is necessary to indicate infection.

Treatment. Disseminated coccidioidomycosis is a fatal disease and should be treated with amphotericin B administered intravenously. Intrathecal or intracisternal therapy is indicated if meningitis fails to respond. Dosage and administration are similar to other systemic fungal infections.

Cryptococcosis

Cryptococcosis rarely occurs in the newborn period. The disease primarily affects the central nervous system, but most organs may be involved. Neonatal infection may occur as a result of transplacental passage.

Etiology. *Cryptococcus neoformans,* or *Torula histolytica,* is the pathogenic fungus in the genus *Cryptococcus,* which includes a number of saprophytic species. In tissue and in culture, it appears as a yeastlike, nonsporulating, nonmycelian budding fungus characterized by a wide capsule. *C. neoformans* is found on the skin and in the oropharynx, gastrointestinal tract and vaginal tract of healthy carriers as well as in food and soil.

Pathology. Hematogenous spread leads to involvement of the central nervous system, liver, spleen, lung, kidney, skin, subcutaneous tissue, joints, and bone marrow. The histologic findings vary from minor inflammatory response to abscess formation. The characteristic lesion is a granuloma. The liver shows hepatitis and cirrhosis. Meningitis often leads to obstruction and hydrocephalus. Granuloma may be found in the brain with calcification.

Pathogenesis. Postnatally, the yeasts enter the host via the respiratory tract. The fetus may be infected transplacentally, or the organisms may be acquired at delivery during passage through the birth canal. Fungemia leads to dissemination of the organisms in many tissues, particularly central nervous system tissue.

Epidemiology. The distribution of *C. neoformans* is worldwide. A number of cases have been associated with pigeon manure. Other than transplacental spread, there is no evidence of human-to-human passage. In most cases, there is a disturbance in the host-parasite relationship, particularly involving defects in cell-mediated immunity.

Clinical. Congenital cryptococcosis has been associated with premature delivery. Newborn infants with the disease feed poorly and generally show signs of central nervous system involvement. Vomiting, irritability, or lethargy may progress to convulsions, opisthotonus, and hydrocephalus. Chorioretinitis or cataracts may be present; one infant had endophthalmitis. An interstitial pneumonia may produce respiratory symptoms. The liver and spleen are usually enlarged, and jaundice may be the initial sign. Ulcerative skin lesions may be noted. Roentgenograms of the skull may show faint, irregular punctate calcific densities along the margins of dilated ventricles and within the brain. The spinal fluid is usually turbid and rarely xanthochromic. The cell count generally ranges between 400 and 1,000 cells but may reach 5,000. Lymphocytes predominate except in the early stage. The protein content is elevated, and the glucose decreased.

Diagnosis. The organism may be identified in spinal fluid examinations using India ink preparations. The fungus appears as a thick-walled, spherical, budding cell 5 to 15 μ in diameter, surrounded by a wide capsule. The fluid should be cultured on blood agar and Sabouraud's media. Organisms may also be isolated from the blood, bone marrow, sputum, or abscess cavities.

Treatment. Current therapy of cryptococcosis consists of the intravenous administration of amphotericin B until there is evidence that the pathogen is eliminated. If meningitis fails to respond to intravenous therapy, the drug should be given intrathecally.

Histoplasmosis

Histoplasmosis in early infancy is a disseminated disease that is generally fatal without treatment.

Etiology. *Histoplasma capsulatum* is a fungus that grows in tissues in a yeast phase with a characteristic capsule.

Pathogenesis. The fungus enters the body through the respiratory tract, gastrointestinal tract, skin, or mucous membranes. The focal lesion then spreads via lymphatics and the bloodstream to involve other organs; including lung, liver, spleen, lymph node, and bone marrow, with formation of granuloma. Transplacental hematogenous spread is possible if dissemination occurs during pregnancy.

Epidemiology. Histoplasmosis is primarily endemic in the Mississippi River basin, but cases have been reported from other areas such as Central and South America. The fungus has been isolated from a numbers of animal species as well as from soil. Except for the possibility of transplacental spread, there is no evidence of transmission from man to man or animal to man.

Clinical. The infant may have signs and symptoms of respiratory distress or gastrointestinal illness. Irritability, failure to gain weight, and fever are common. Enlargement of the liver and spleen is generally noted. Lymph node enlargement may also be found. Meningitis and osteomyelitis are less common complications. The cerebrospinal fluid changes are similar to those in tuberculous meningitis. The peripheral blood shows an anemia, which is occasionally hemolytic. A leukopenia may be present with a predominance of lymphocytes and early myelocytic cells. Thrombocytopenia is a late manifestation.

Diagnosis. Smears and cultures of blood, bone marrow, sputum, or cerebrospinal fluid or biopsies of liver or lymph nodes will usually reveal organisms. Routine Wright's or Giemsa stains may be satisfactory, but the search for organisms will be facilitated by using methenamine silver stain or acridine orange stain and fluorescence microscopy. Complement fixation and precipitin tests are available but may be difficult to interpret if maternal antibody is still present.

Treatment. Untreated disseminated histoplasmosis is a fatal disease, but therapy with amphotericin B has led to recoveries. Administration of the drug is similar to that in systemic candidiasis. Again, intrathecal administration of amphotericin B is indicated for refractory meningitis. Blood transfusion may be necessary when the hemolytic process is severe.

PARASITIC INFECTIONS

Malaria

Epidemic malaria is a major cause of abortion, stillbirth, and neonatal death. Although the disease is largely limited to endemic areas, sporadic cases occur annually in North America. Congenital malaria, which is well documented in malarious regions, has also been reported in the United States.

Etiology. Malaria is caused by protozoan species of the genus *Plasmodium.* Any of the species—*falciparum, malariae, ovale,* or *vivax*—may cause infection in the newborn.

Pathology. Invasion of erythrocytes by malarial parasites leads to adherence to the endothelium of vessels, with subsequent occlusion. The disintegrating red blood cells accumulate in the reticuloendothelial system. Hemolysis produces anemia of varying severity. Parasites may be found in liver, spleen, brain, lung, and intestinal tract. The placenta is involved in the majority of women with malaria during pregnancy.

Pathogenesis. Mosquito-borne disease occurs in the newborn infant as well as in older children and adults. Transplacental transmission of parasites has been documented in endemic regions and in geographic locations where there are no *Anopheles* mosquitos. Women who have been infected may transmit parasites during pregnancy many years after leaving the endemic area. Parasitemia may be subclinical so that in rare instances congenital malaria occurs without a history of an attack during pregnancy.

The placenta serves as an effective protective barrier in many cases of malaria during pregnancy, even in the presence of massive placental infection. In most congenital cases some pathologic damage to the placenta leads to fetal infection; however, there are reports of congenital malaria in which there was no histologic evidence of placental damage. Placental tears during labor or delivery may lead to contamination of the infant's blood with that of the mother.

The major source of malarial parasites in the United States at present is blood donated by servicemen returning from the Far East.

Epidemiology and immunity. Neonatal malaria is a rare disease outside of the tropical zones where the disease is endemic. IgG antibody, which crosses the placenta, provides some protection for several weeks after birth. Antibody augments phagocytosis of merozoites and infected erythrocytes but does not affect the hepatic stage of malaria. Neither the complement fixation titer nor the fluorescent antibody titer is necessarily correlated with protection. Immunity in pregnant women modifies attacks and influences transmission to the fetus, since the frequency of transplacental infections is greater in infants born of nonimmune mothers.

Clinical. The incubation period in postnatally acquired malaria varies from 8 to 30 days according to the plasmodial species, size of the inoculum, and host immunity. In some cases the incubation period is longer; the same variability has been noted in congenital malaria. Signs and symptoms vary from mild illness to the infant born moribund. Fever, gastrointestinal or respiratory tract symptoms, or central nervous system signs may be present. Pallor and jaundice signal the presence of severe anemia. The majority of infected newborns have enlarged livers and spleens. Renal function may be impaired.

Diagnosis. The diagnosis of malaria rests upon the demonstration of parasites in the blood. Thick smears facilitate detection of the parasites; thin smears facilitate species identification.

Treatment. Chloroquine is the drug of choice for treatment of clinical attacks of malaria. It may be given intravenously in a dose of 5 mg/kg diluted in glucose with electrolytes. This dose is repeated once in 12 to 24 hours. By mouth, the dose of chloroquine is 10 mg/kg, followed by 5 mg/kg at 6, 24, and 48 hours. For chloroquine-resistant strains of *P. falciparum,* quinine may be given orally in a dose of 20 to 30 mg/kg/day in 3 doses for 7 to 10 days or intravenously in a dose of 10 mg/kg diluted in electrolyte solution and repeated once after 24 hours. The oral route is preferred because of the drug's toxicity.

Pneumocystis carinii pneumonia

Pneumonia caused by *Pneumocystis carinii* occurs in newborn infants and patients of all ages with impaired host resistance. A few cases have been associated with intrauterine infection.

Etiology. The classification of *P. carinii* as a protozoa is presumptive since the organism has not been cultivated in vitro. However, the morphologic appearance of the cysts in the lungs has been consistent and characteristic, and experimental infection can be induced in animals. The susceptibility of the parasites to pentamidine isethionate further supports this concept.

Pathology. The pathologic changes in *P. carinii* infections are limited to the lungs. The high degree of tissue specificity suggests unique metabolic requirements for the parasite. Infection begins in the pulmonary alveolar spaces. The exudate contains histiocytes, lymphocytes, plasma cells, and polymorphonuclear leukocytes. There is an eosinophilic lacelike appearance that stains with periodic acid–Schiff stain. Cysts are readily found in the alveolar exudates and may be seen in lesser numbers in alveolar septa, bronchioles, and larger airways. They are best demonstrated by silver impregnation techniques. Organisms have not been demonstrated in extrapulmonary tissues.

Pathogenesis. The mode of transmission is unknown, but the epidemics of infections in nurseries suggest contact or airborne spread. While *Pneumocystis* pneumonia has occurred in healthy newborns, impaired host resistance, prior or concomitant infection, and treatment with antimicrobial agents seem to predispose the infant to clinical disease. A few cases of intrauterine infection have been recorded. Disease was limited to the lungs and presumed to be transmitted transplacentally.

Immunity and epidemiology. *Pneumocystis* infections have been reported from all over the world. The occurrence of *P. carinii* pneumonia in newborn and premature infants and its association with immunologic deficiency diseases suggest that disease results from an impaired host-parasite relationship. Latent infections may be activated by suppressing host resistance.

Clinical. The incubation period is about 3 weeks so that few cases will fall within the neonatal period. The onset is usually insidious with progressive tachypnea, dyspnea, cough, and cyanosis. Fever and rales are less common. The roentgenographic findings are bilateral diffuse infiltrates extending laterally from the hila. The white blood cell count is frequently elevated, and eosinophilia is common. Physiologic studies generally are consistent with an alveolar-capillary block.

Diagnosis. The roentgenographic findings are not diagnostic and may be found in interstitial pneumonias of various causes and in pulmonary alveolar proteinosis. The diagnosis rests on the demonstration of *Pneumocystis* cysts. While cysts have been rarely reported in sputum or tracheal aspirates, lung aspiration by needle biopsy is more reliable for diagnosis. Open lung biopsy decreases the risk of pneumothorax. Histiocytes and plasma cells are present except in infants with hypogammaglobulinemia when plasma cells are absent. Gomori methenamine–silver nitrate stain best demonstrates the cysts, which may be seen in some instances with routine stains.

Treatment. Pentamidine isethionate is given in a single dose of 4 mg/kg intramuscularly for 10 to 14 days. The drug is currently available through the Center for Disease Control, Atlanta, Georgia.

Toxoplasmosis

Toxoplasmosis is a systemic disease caused by *Toxoplasma gondii.* Congenital infection follows transplacental spread and often results in the tetrad of chorioretinitis, hydrocephaly or microcephaly, psychomotor retardation, and cerebral calcifications.

Etiology. *T. gondii* is a protozoan that exists as a trophozoite measuring 2 to 4 μ by 4 to 7 μ or as a cyst. There is only one species and only one serotype. It is an obligate intracellular parasite that can inhabit any cell except nonnucleated erythrocytes. The trophozoites are easily stained with Wright's or Giemsa stain.

Pathology. *T. gondii* is widely distributed throughout the body, and cysts may be found in almost every organ. In acute infections, trophozoites may be found as well. Histologic reaction may be minimal, or one may find necrosis in skeletal muscle, heart, lung, liver, and spleen. The microscopic findings are not characteristic, and diagnosis depends on identification of the organism. In congenital toxoplasmosis, the central nervous system, retina, and choroid are frequently involved.

Pathogenesis. Children and adults appear to acquire toxoplasmosis through the ingestion of raw or undercooked meat. Parasitemia follows ingestion, and organisms are widely distributed. The infection may be asymptomatic or mimic infectious mononucleosis. Congenital toxoplasmosis results from hematogenous spread via placental infection and subsequent parasitemia in the fetus. Since toxoplasma can be isolated from the uterus, some workers have suggested that chronic toxoplasmosis is an important cause of abortion, stillbirth, and premature delivery. However, this hypothesis is not proved, and there is agreement that primary infection in a pregnant woman will affect only that offspring. The fetus is most susceptible when maternal infection takes place during the second trimester.

Epidemiology. In the United States, rates of positive toxoplasma dye tests vary from 14% to 35%. Except for maternal-fetal transmission, there is little evidence for any human-to-human transmission.

Clinical. Infants with fetal toxoplasmosis may have signs and symptoms ranging from subclinical infection to widespread systemic illness. Minimal signs of the disease may be chorioretinitis or unilateral cranial nerve paralysis. Newborn infants with active toxoplasmosis develop symptoms at birth or soon after, manifested by fever, maculopapular rash, pneumonia, lymphadenopathy, myocarditis, hepatomegaly, splenomegaly, jaundice, chorioretinitis, convulsions, microcephaly, and hydrocephaly. The acute disease may be fatal or leave residual defects of the central nervous system such as cranial nerve paralysis, chorioretinitis, periventricular calcifications, microcephaly, hydrocephaly, convulsions, or psychomotor retardation.

Diagnosis. In the active stage of toxoplasmosis, organisms may be demonstrated in Wright-stained smears of cerebrospinal fluid. The fluid may also be injected into mice, in which two blind passages should be made at intervals of 1 to 2 weeks before the diagnosis is excluded. Serologic studies on serum from mother and infant should be carried out. A negative test excludes the diagnosis. If the test is positive, a second specimen is obtained from the infant at 2 to 4 months of age to differentiate maternal antibody from that synthesized by the infant.

The dye test has been a specific and sensitive test for measuring antibodies to toxoplasma. Live organisms are mixed with serial dilutions of heat-inactivated test serum. Fresh human serum that does not contain antibody is added as a source of the activator system, which includes properdin and Mg^{++}. After incubation at 37 C for 1 hour, alkaline methylene blue is added, and the numbers of stained and unstained organisms are counted. The titer of the serum is the dilution at which 50% of the toxoplasma are unstained. Active infection produces titers of 1:1,024 or greater. Titers of 1:8 or 1:16 are significant in epidemiologic studies.

More recently an indirect fluorescent antibody test has become available for measuring toxoplasma antibodies. A modification of this test will identify IgM antibodies in the serum of newborn infants, differentiating fetal synthesis from passively transferred IgG antibody. However, false-positive tests may result from leakage of maternal blood across the placenta. If positive, the test should be repeated in 1 or 2 weeks, using peripheral blood from the infant. Complement fixation and hemagglutination tests are used less frequently. Both employ a nonviable antigen, but the tests do not always correlate with the dye test. A skin test antigen is also available; but reactivity is slow to develop, and false-negative reactions are common.

Manifestations of toxoplasmosis may mimic other neonatal infections and erythroblastosis fetalis. No sign is pathognomonic, and serologic studies are needed for diagnosis when direct demonstration of the organism is not possible.

Treatment. Pyrimethamine (Daraprim) and sulfadiazine act synergistically against toxoplasmosis. Pyrimethamine is given in a dosage of 1 mg/kg/day every 12 hours, and a preparation to be administered intravenously is available. Pyrimethamine is a folic acid antagonist that produces reversible bone marrow depression. Triple sulfonamides or sulfadiazine should be given in a dose of 100 to 150 mg/kg/day. While treatment does not appear to affect the chronic form of the disease or central nervous system residual damage, it may affect the acute stage and alter mortality.

IMMUNOLOGIC CONSIDERATIONS

Immunity describes the ability of the host to resist disease produced by foreign cells or their products (see outline below). Host resistance is generally classified into specific and nonspecific mechanisms. Nonspecific mechanisms are those that do not require any specific adaptive change on the part of the host. Nonspecific resistance is provided by the skin and mucous membranes, the reticuloendothelial system, circulating phagocytic cells, and certain humoral factors such as complement, lysozyme, and interferon. Specific immunity is dependent upon the stimulation and responsiveness of a limited cell population that result in some reaction directed against a specific substance or antigen.

Nonspecific immunity

The role of nonspecific immunity in the human newborn infant is not well understood. However, it is obvious that the skin serves as an important barrier, since its disruption leads to increased susceptibility to infection.

The increased frequency of generalized infections with enteric organisms, which are ordinarily not invasive, suggests the possibility that the gastrointestinal mucosa may be a portal of entry. While normally impermeable to bacteria, the intestinal lining may be altered by local or generalized circulatory changes.

The newborn inflammatory response in vivo, which is measured by the cover-slip skin window technique, is comparable to that in the adult, with polymorphonuclear leukocytes predominating in the early cellular response. The shift to mononuclear cells seen after 6 hours in the adult is much slower and less extensive in the newborn infant. In some studies, increased numbers of eosinophils were noted. The significance of these variations is uncertain.

CLASSIFICATION OF PRIMARY IMMUNODEFICIENCY DISORDERS*

A. Thymic hypoplasia with hypoparathyroidism (DiGeorge syndrome)
B. Immunodeficiency with generalized hematopoietic hypoplasia (duVaal)
C. Severe combined immunodeficiency
   1. Autosomal recessive (Swiss agammaglobulinemia)
   2. X-linked (thymic alymphoplasia)
   3. Sporadic
D. Immunodeficiency with short-limbed dwarfism
   1. Severe; with ectodermal inflammation
   2. Cartilage-hair hypoplasia
E. Immunodeficiency with thrombocytopenia and eczema (Wiskott-Aldrich syndrome)
F. Immunodeficiency with exophthalmos-macroglossia-gigantism (EMG) syndrome.

In vitro studies suggest the presence of a quantitative deficiency of chemotactic activity in newborn sera. Moreover, there appears to be a deficient chemotactic response of neonatal leukocytes in the presence of normal chemotactic factor. The role of neonatal phagocytosis in contributing to the newborn infant's increased susceptibility to infection is unknown, and the nitrobluetetrazolium (NBT) dye test appears to be of no practical value.

*Adapted from the World Health Organization classification; limited to diseases that may be diagnosed in the neonatal period.

Nonspecific humoral factors in host resistance include complement, interferon, lysozyme, properdin, and betalysin. Complement activity depends on the interaction of a complex of 11 serum globulins. The bactericidal activity of serum against gram-negative bacteria is caused by the action of complement in the presence of specific antibody. By-products of complement activation play a role in chemotaxis, immune adherence, and other aspects of inflammation. Term and premature infants have approximately 50% of the complement activity present in normal adult serum. Similar deficiencies have been found for the individual complement components, C'_3, C'_4, C'_5. A split product of C'_3, C'_5, and the trimolecular complex of C'_5, C'_6, and C'_7 have chemotactic activity, and the relative deficiencies of these components may contribute to the chemotactic and phagocytic defects in the neonate.

Interferon is a substance that inhibits viral multiplication and is released by cells that are infected with virus or stimulated with substances such as polynucleotides. The interferon-producing capacity of lymphocytes from fetuses, cord blood, and adults is similar. The concentration of properdin, a serum protein that has bactericidal activity against gram-negative bacteria in the presence of complement and Mg^{++} is comparable in cord and adult blood.

Specific immunity

The specific immune response consists of the processing of antigen, the stimulation of lymphoid cells, and an antigen-specific reaction, which can be measured in vitro or in vivo. The reactions are conventionally separated into those mediated by humoral antibody and those that may be transferred by cells and not by serum.

The presence of immunoglobulins in biologic fluids usually signifies that the humoral antibody system is normal. However, in certain disorders of the immunologic apparatus, immunoglobulins, although present, may not be functional. While the quantitative determination of serum immunoglobulins is generally adequate to screen for an immunoglobulin deficiency disease, in some cases the measurement of specific antibody will be necessary.

Lymphocytes are present in the fetus at

8 to 10 weeks. The thymus is the first lymphoid organ to differentiate and is the site of great proliferative activity throughout the fetal and neonatal period. However, most lymphocytes are thought to have their origin in the bone marrow. Some of the bone marrow lymphocytes enter the thymus for a time and then migrate to the mid and deep cortical areas of lymph nodes, Peyer's patches, and the periarteriolar regions of the spleen. These thymic-dependent lymphocytes make up most of the cells in thoracic duct lymph and the majority of the lymphocytes in peripheral blood. The thymic-dependent lymphocytes function in cell-mediated immune responses and cooperate with thymic independent lymphocytes in the antibody response to certain antigens. Cell-mediated immune responses include cutaneous delayed hypersensitivity, allograft rejection, graft-versus-host reactions, and immunity to intracellular infection. Studies of the fetal lamb have shown that cell-mediated immune responses can be demonstrated in the first trimester. The thymic-independent system of cells is also referred to as bone marrow derived or bursal cell system and populates the medullary areas of lymph nodes and spleen, the gastrointestinal lymphoid structures, and germinal follicles. Without antigenic stimulation only minimal amounts of IgM and IgG are synthesized in utero, beginning in the second trimester. If the fetus is stimulated antigenically, significant amounts of immunoglobulins and specific antibody may be produced, and plasma cells can be found in lymphoid tissues.

Both IgG and IgM have been demonstrated in tissue culture studies of fetal spleen. Ordinarily, small amounts of IgM (0 to 17 mg/100 ml) and IgE are present in cord serum at birth. It is difficult to detect the small quantities of IgG produced by the fetus in the presence of maternal IgG in cord serum, yet this has been demonstrated using allotypic markers. IgA and IgD are normally not found in cord serum, but IgA has been detected in cord serum from some infants with intrauterine infections. Antibodies found in external secretions are largely in the IgA class containing a peptide known as secretory piece or transport piece, which is synthesized in epithelial cells. Secretory piece in the absence of IgA is present in the saliva and urine of newborn infants. IgA becomes detectable in secretions in the weeks following birth.

The transfer of IgG across the placenta is an active process that is not related to molecular size since many smaller proteins do not readily cross the placenta. Transfer of IgG occurs largely during the third trimester of pregnancy, and infants born before 34 weeks' gestation may have deficiencies of IgG. Concentrations of IgG in cord serum of full-term infants generally exceed the maternal concentration, and the infant receives whatever specific antibodies are present in the IgG class. Thus, passive protection depends on the quantity of IgG antibody in maternal serum and the sensitivity of the particular infectious agent to antibody. Most newborn infants will receive diphtheria and tetanus antitoxins and antibodies to a variety of bacterial and viral agents. While protection against certain bacterial diseases such as pertussis may last only a month or two, immunity to measles and some other virus infections may persist for 4 to 8 months.

The newborn infant is capable of mounting an antibody response to immunizing agents or naturally occurring infections. In general, the response is less vigorous than that of the older child or adult. Maternal antibody may interfere with active immunization. Secretory antibody in colostrum may inhibit the response to orally administered polio vaccine. Thus, the immunologic responsiveness of the young infant is an important consideration in designing immunization programs, but the role of antibody in recovery from infection remains unclear.

Cell-mediated immune responses are those that may be transferred by lymphoid cells but not by serum. In man, estimation of cell-mediated immune function has been limited to delayed hypersensitivity skin tests until the recent development of in vitro assays. While there is some controversy regarding the interpretation of the in vitro lymphocyte response to mitogens, allogeneic cells, or specific antigens as a pure cell-mediated response, lymphocytes from infants with cell-mediated immunodeficiency diseases have an impaired response to these stimulants as measured by tritiated thymidine incorporation or characteristic morphologic changes.

Lymphocytes from cord blood respond to phytohemagglutinin (PHA), pokeweed mitogen, staphylococcal filtrate, and allogeneic cells in normal fashion. Lymphoid cells from fetuses as early as 14 weeks' gestation may respond to PHA. While other cell-mediated immune functions have not been measured in the human fetus, it is likely that these capacities develop long before parturition.

Delayed hypersensitivity skin tests are more difficult to elicit in the newborn infant.

Immunoglobulin deficiency diseases

Infants with disorders of the immunoglobulin system will not be symptomatic in the first months of life since maternal IgG will provide protection. In families carrying the gene for agammaglobulinemia, the presence of IgM and IgA in the serum of a male infant would tend to exclude the disease. Repeated determinations are necessary, since it is possible for maternal immunoglobulins to cross a defective placenta. The diagnosis can be made in early infancy by histologic examination of a regional lymph node after immunization. Absence of follicles and plasma cells in the antigen-stimulated lymph node is characteristic of agammaglobulinemia.

Thymic hypoplasia (DiGeorge syndrome)

The thymus arises from the third and fourth pharyngeal pouches together with the parathyroid glands during the sixth week of gestation. DiGeorge noted aplasia and hypoplasia of the thymus gland in newborn infants with neonatal hypocalcemic tetany. Since there is no familial occurrence of congenital thymic hypoplasia, the defect appears to be caused by an injury during embryogenesis. Associated congenital malformations include hypertelorism, low set pinnae, a shortened lip philtrum, and nasal clefts. Many of these infants have anomalies of the great vessels. In addition to hypocalcemic tetany, the symptoms that may appear during the neonatal period will be related to bacterial, viral, or fungal infections of the skin or of the respiratory or gastrointestinal tracts. Recurrent candidiasis, diarrhea, and pneumonia are common.

Roentgenograms of the chest reveal an absent thymic shadow. The absolute lymphocyte count may be normal or depressed. Cutaneous delayed hypersensitivity tests are negative. Allograft rejection is delayed or absent. The in vitro peripheral blood lymphocyte response to PHA and other stimuli is markedly abnormal. Immunoglobulin concentrations are usually normal, and the primary and secondary antibody responses are normal in many antigen-antibody systems. The lymphoid tissues contain normal numbers of plasma cells and normal germinal tissue if the infant has had antigenic stimulation. The deep cortical regions of lymph nodes and the periarteriolar sheaths of spleen show a moderate depletion of lymphocytes. The parathyroid glands have either been absent, or hypoplastic remnants have been located ectopically in the neck. In the complete expression of this syndrome, the thymus is absent or markedly hypoplastic. However, many gradations of thymic maturation have been described.

Treatment of congenital thymic aplasia by transplantation of fetal thymic tissue has been successful. The thymic-dependent areas of lymph nodes have been populated, and the tests for cell-mediated immunity become normal.

Combined immunodeficiency disease

Congenital disorders involving both the immunoglobulin and cell-mediated immune systems frequently become symptomatic in the first few months of life. The defect is thought to be one of stem-cell differentiation. The most primitive and most severe form involves the hematopoietic cell as well. This was described as reticular dysgenesis by duVaal. More commonly, combined immunodeficiency disease involves lymphoid cell differentiation. Inherited as an autosomal recessive trait, the first syndrome described was termed the Swiss type of agammaglobulinemia. The sex-linked recessive form was called thymic alymphoplasia. Sporadic cases have also been noted, and some of these infants have short-limbed dwarfism. In some cases, serum immunoglobulins are normal, and certain antibodies are synthesized. Infants with combined immunodeficiency disease are usually symptomatic early in life. Bacterial, viral, fungal, and protozoan infections occur. Pneumonias, gastroenteritis, candidiasis and *Pneumocystis carinii* infections are most common. Vaccination with vaccinia results in vaccinia gangrenosa, and BCG vaccination has led to a generalized reaction.

In the typical infant with combined immunodeficiency disease, immunoglobulins will be of maternal origin, and IgA and IgM will be markedly diminished. Isohemagglutinins will be absent. The absolute lymphocyte count is usually low. Delayed hypersensitivity reactions are negative, although most of the infants have candidiasis. The patients cannot be sensitized with dinitrochlorobenzene and are unable to reject allografts. The in vitro lymphocyte response to phytohemagglutinin is markedly impaired, which is a valuable diagnostic test for this disorder. Some infants with partial deficiencies have shown an in vitro response to allogenic cells. Reconstitution of infants with combined immunodeficiency disease is possible with bone marrow cell transfusions from HL-A identical sibling donors. Mild graft-versus-host reactions (GVHR) may still occur, but the fatal GVHR, which was consistently observed with the use of nonidentical donor cells, can be avoided.

Newborn infants with the Wiskott-Aldrich syndrome may manifest eczema, petechiae, gastrointestinal bleeding, otitis media, and pneumonia. This is inherited as an X-linked disease. Thrombocytopenia may be variable early in infancy. Abnormalities in the immunoglobulin and cell-mediated systems are complex. One patient has received a bone marrow cell transfusion, which resulted in some improvement.

COLLAGEN-VASCULAR DISEASES

Polyarteritis nodosa

Polyarteritis nodosa is an uncommon disorder in infancy that may occur in the newborn period. About 25 cases have been reported to occur during the first year of life. The disease is usually fatal and has rarely been diagnosed premortem. Males are more commonly afflicted. The cause is unknown; both hypersensitivity reactions and viral infection have been postulated.

Pathology. The vascular lesions evolve through a number of stages, and lesions of different stages often coexist. Initially, there is edema of the artery, degeneration of the adventitia, and separation of the muscularis. This is followed by histiocytic and fibroblastic infiltration. The third stage is characterized by necrosis and polymorphonuclear cell exudation, which is often associated with thrombosis and aneurysmal dilatation. Intimal proliferation may occlude the lumen. The reparative phase is one of chronic inflammation, formation of granulation tissue, and scarring.

In infants, the coronary arteries are almost always involved, and this is the most significant lesion. Thrombosis, endarteritis, and aneurysmal dilatation may lead to abnormalities of the conduction system, cardiomegaly, and myocardial infarction. In some cases, the coronary arteries are the only vessels involved. Arterial lesions have been described in multiple organs including kidneys, adrenals, intestines, spleen, pancreas, lung, liver, uterus, testis, epididymis, and prostate. Involvement of skeletal muscle arteries and arteries to the extremities is uncommon. Infarctions in kidneys, spleen, and the extremities have been described.

Clinical. The manifestations of polyarteritis in infancy have been rather consistent. The illness simulates a viral infection, with fever, erythematous rash, and conjunctivitis at the onset. Some infants have cough or difficulty in breathing, abnormal neurologic signs, hypertension, or gangrene of the extremities. Cardiac enlargement and murmurs are occasionally described. Anemia and leukocytosis are common, usually without eosinophilia. The sedimentation rate is elevated, and the serum protein electrophoretic pattern is typical of chronic inflammatory disease. The urine usually shows casts and red blood cells. The spinal fluid may contain an increased protein or mononuclear cell count. The electrocardiogram is almost always abnormal. Left ventricular hypertrophy, S-T segment changes, or arrhythmias have been described. Roentgenographic studies show cardiomegaly and pulmonary infiltrates. The median duration of illness is about 4 weeks, and the disease often terminates in an unexpected cardiac arrest. Diagnosis should be considered in the patient whose viruslike illness persists for more than 5 to 7 days. While muscular arteries are rarely involved, more experience with skin biopsies is needed. The varied clinical manifestations, laboratory alterations, and cardiac findings should lead to the clinical diagnosis. Because the disease has rarely been recognized premortem, there is no experience in the treatment of infantile polyarteritis nodosa. Since this process has been uniformly fatal, a trial of corticosteroids should be instituted early in the course of the disease.

Lupus erythematosus

Lupus erythematosus is a collagen-vascular disease that generally affects older children and adults in systemic form. A variant of the disease limited to patchy erythematous involvement of the skin is termed discoid lupus erythematosus. This form of the disease, associated with certain immunologic phenomena, has been reported in the newborn period. In contrast to systemic lupus erythematosus (SLE), the disease in newborns appears almost entirely benign.

A variety of immunologic reactions have been described in SLE including the LE cell phenomena and antinuclear antibodies (ANA). The antibodies are largely IgG molecules that cross the placenta and enter the fetal circulation. A number of infants born to women with SLE have had circulating LE cell factor and ANA but have been otherwise normal. Seven infants with discoid lupus erythematosus have been born to women with a disease state consistent with SLE during or following pregnancy.

Clinical. Skin lesions are generally present at birth and distributed over the face, scalp, neck, and upper thorax. The borders are irregular but sharply demarcated. The macular, dusky erythematous rash contains areas of atrophy, telangiectasia, and follicular plugging. The infants are otherwise well, without fever or signs of systemic illness. Splenomegaly has been reported in some cases.

Blood counts and erythrocyte sedimentation rate are normal. Urinalysis is negative. ANA tests are positive; the LE cell test is less often positive. Serum alpha-2 globulins may be elevated.

Biopsy shows epidermal atrophy and liquifaction of the basal cell layer. A perivascular infiltration of lymphocytes is present in the dermis.

The course is benign with the lesions gradually receding. Some residual scarring or telangiectasia may remain. The ANA test becomes negative at about 4 months because of the catabolism of maternal IgG antibody. Subsequent attacks of SLE have not been recorded.

At least two exceptions to the usual form of the disease have been reported. An infant of a mother with an exacerbation of SLE at the time of delivery had a severe hemolytic anemia, leukopenia, and thrombocytopenia. He recovered after 3 months. A second infant, whose mother was normal, had thrombocytopenia, Coombs' positive hemolytic anemia, and a positive LE cell preparation. The disease was uncontrollable despite steroid therapy and splenectomy, and the child died.

SAMUEL P. GOTOFF

BIBLIOGRAPHY

GENERAL CONSIDERATIONS, SEPSIS AND SEPTICEMIA

Balagtas, R. C., Bell, C. E., Edwards, L. D., and Levin, S.: Risk of local and systemic infections associated with umbilical vein catheterization; a prospective study in 86 newborn patients, Pediatrics **48**:359, 1971.

Barrett-Conner, E.: Infections and pregnancy. South Med. J. **62**:275, 1969.

Benirschke, K.: Routes and types of infection in the fetus and the newborn, Am. J. Dis. Child. **99**:714, 1960.

Blanc, W. A.: Amniotic infection syndrome; pathogenesis, morphology, and circumnatal mortality, Clin. Obstet. Gynecol. **2**:705, 1959.

Blanc, W. A.: Pathways of fetal and early neonatal infection; viral placentitis, bacterial and fungal chorioamnionitis, J. Pediatr. **59**:473, 1961.

Boeckman, C. R., and Krill, C. E., Jr.: Bacterial and fungal infections complicating parenteral alimentation in infants and children, J. Pediatr. Surg. **5**:117, 1970.

Davis, P. A.: Bacterial infection in the fetus and newborn, Arch. Dis. Child. **46**:1, 1971.

Fierer, J., Taylor, P. M., and Gezon, H. M.: Pseudomonas aeruginosa epidemic traced to delivery-room resuscitations, N. Engl. J. Med. **276**:991, 1967.

Gotoff, S. P., and Behrman, R. E.: Neonatal septicemia, J. Pediatr. **76**:142, 1970.

Klein, J. O., Herschel, M., Therakan, R. M., and Ingall, D.: Gentamicin in serious neonatal infections; absorption, excretion, and clinical results in 25 cases, J. Infect. Dis. **124**:224, 1971.

McCracken, G. H., Chrane, D. F., and Thomas, M. L.: Pharmacologic evaluation of gentamicin in newborn infants, J. Infect. Dis. **124**:214, 1971.

McCracken, G. H., Jr., and Eichenwald, H. F.: Neonatal sepsis, meningitis and pneumonia. In Gellis, S. S., and Kagan, B. M., editors: Current pediatric therapy-5, Philadelphia, 1971, W. B. Saunders Co.

INFECTIONS OF ORGAN SYSTEMS

Alford, C. A., Jr., Foft, J. W., Blankenship, W. J., Cassady, G., and Benton, J. W., Jr.: Subclinical central nervous system disease of neonates; a prospective study of infants born with increased levels of IgM, J. Pediatr. **75**:1167, 1969.

Arthur, A. B., and Wilson, B. D. R.: Urinary infection presenting with jaundice, Br. Med. J.: 539, 1967.

Barson, A. J.: Fatal *Pseudomonas aeruginosa* bronchopneumonia in a children's hospital, Arch. Dis. Child. **46**:55, 1971.

Berman, P. H., and Banker, P. Q.: Neonatal meningitis; a clinical and pathological study of 29 cases, Pediatrics **38**:6, 1966.

Bernstein, J., and Brown, A. K.: Sepsis and jaundice in early infancy, Pediatrics **29**:873, 1962.

Bernstein, J., and Wang, J.: The pathology of neonatal pneumonia, J. Dis. Child., **101**:350, 1961.

Blanche, D. W.: Osteomyelitis in infants, J. Bone Joint Surg. (Am.) **34**:71, 1952.

Bland, R. D.: Otitis media in the first six weeks of life; diagnosis, bacteriology, and management, Pediatrics **49**:187, 1972.

Clarke, A. M.: Neonatal osteomyelitis; a disease different from osteomyelitis of older children, Med. J. Aust. **1**:237, 1958.

Esterly, N. B., and Solomon, L. M.: Neonatal dermatology. II. Blistering and scaling dermatoses, J. Pediatr. **77**:1075, 1970.

Fekety, F. R., Jr.: The epidemiology and prevention of staphylococcal infection, Medicine **43**: 593, 1964.

Goscienski, P. J.: Inclusion conjunctivitis in the newborn infant, J. Pediatr. **77**:19, 1970.

Gower, P. E., Husband, P., Coleman, J. C., and Snodgrass, G. J. I. A.: Urinary infection in two selected neonatal populations, Arch. Dis. Child. **45**:259, 1970.

Groover, R. V., Sutherland, J. M., and Landing, B. H.: Purulent meningitis of newborn infants, N. Engl. J. Med. **264**:1115, 1961.

Haltalin, K. C.: Neonatal shigellosis; report of 16 cases and review of the literature, Am. J. Dis. Child. **114**:603, 1967.

Kenny, J. G., Medearis, D. N., Jr., Klein, S. W., Drachman, R. H., and Gibson, L. E.: An outbreak of urinary tract infections and septicemia due to *Escherichia coli* in male infants, J. Pediatr. **68**:530, 1966.

Melish, M. E., and Glasgow, L. A.: The staphylococcal scalded-skin syndrome; the expanded clinical syndrome, J. Pediatr. **78**:958, 1971.

Naeye, R. L., and Blanc, W. A.: Relation of poverty and race to antenatal infection, N. Engl. J. Med. **283**:555, 1970.

Naeye, R. L., Dellinger, W. S., and Blanc, W. A.: Fetal and maternal features of antenatal bacterial infections, J. Pediatr. **9**:733, 1971.

Nelson, J. D.: Antibiotic concentrations in septic joint effusions, N. Engl. J. Med. **284**:349, 1971.

Nelson, J. D.: Duration of therapy for *E. coli* diarrheal disease, Pediatrics **48**:248, 1971.

Nelson, J. D., and Peters, P. C.: Suprapubic aspiration of urine in premature and term infants, Pediatrics **36**:132, 1965.

Otila, E.: Studies on cerebrospinal fluid in premature infants, Acta. Paediatr. Scand. **35**:3, 1948.

Overall, J. C.: Neonatal bacterial meningitis, J. Pediatr. **76**:499, 1970.

Prophylaxis of gonococcal ophthalmia, The Medical Letter **12**:37, 1970.

Riley, H. D.: Enteropathogenic *E. coli* gastroenteritis, Clinical Pediatr. (Phila.) **3**:93, 1964.

Sack, R. B., Gorbach, S. L., Banwell, J. G., and others: Enterotoxigenic *Escherichia coli* isolated from patients with severe cholera-like disease, J. Infect. Dis. **123**:378, 1971.

Thatcher, R. W., and Pettit, T. H.: Gonorrheal conjunctivities, J.A.M.A. **215**:1494, 1971.

Watson, D. G.: Purulent neonatal meningitis; a study of 45 cases, J. Pediatr. **50**:352, 1957.

SPECIFIC BACTERIAL INFECTIONS

Avery, M. E., and Wolfsdorf, J.: Diagnosis and treatment; approaches to newborn infants of tuberculous mothers, Pediatrics **42**:519, 1968.

Ekelund, H., Laurell, G., Melander, S., Olding, L., and Vahlquist, B.: *Listeria* infection in the foetus and the newborn, Acta. Pediatr. Scand. **51**:698, 1962.

Hughesdon, M. R.: Congenital tuberculosis, Arch. Dis. Child. **21**:121, 1946.

Kendig, E.: Disorders of the respiratory tract in children. Philadelphia, 1967, W. B. Saunders Co., p. 699.

Maguire, B. J., and Riley, H. D., Jr.: Infections due to *Listeria monocytogenes* in infants and children, Am. J. Med. Sci. **254**:421, 1967.

Marshall, F. N.: Tetanus of the newborn; with special reference to experiences in Haiti, Adv. Pediatr. **XV**:65, 1968.

Nichols, W., Jr., and Wooley, P. V., Jr.: *Listeria monocytogenes* meningitis, J. Pediatr. **61**:337, 1962.

Ray, C. G., and Wedgewood, R. J.: Neonatal listeriosis, Pediatrics **34**:378, 1964.

Robinson, R. C. V.: Congenital syphilis, Arch. Derm. **99**:599, 1969.

VIRAL INFECTIONS

Brunell, P. A.: Varicella-zoster infections in pregnancy, J.A.M.A. **199**:315, 1967.

Conchie, A. F., Barton, B. W., and Tobin, J. O'H.: Congenital cytomegalovirus infection treated with idoxuridine, Br. Med. J. **4**:162, 1968.

Debré, R., and Celers, J.: Clinical virology; the evaluation and management of human viral infections, Philadelphia, 1970, W. B. Saunders Co.

Ehrlich, R. M., Turner, J. A. P., and Clarke, M.:

Neonatal varicella; a case report with isolation of the virus, J. Pediatr. **53**:139, 1958.
Monif, G. R. G.: Viral infections of the human fetus, London, 1969, The Macmillan Co.
Naeye, R. L.: Cytomegalic inclusion disease; the fetal disorder, Am. J. Clin. Pathol. **47**:738, 1967.
Nahmias, A. J., Alford, C. A., and Korones, S. B.: Infection of the newborn with Herpesvirus hominis, Adv. Pediatr. **17**:185, 1970.
Newman, C. G. H.: Perinatal varicella, Lancet **2**:1159, 1965.
Oppenheimer, E. R.: Congenital chickenpox with disseminated visceral lesions, Bull. Johns Hopkins Hosp. **74**:240, 1944.
Osborn, J. E., Joo, P. A., Andres, J., and Levy, J. M.: Treatment of cytomegalovirus (CMV) infection with cytosine arabinoside. Presented at Midwest Society of Pediatric Research, November 4-5, 1970.
Overall, J. C., Jr., and Glasgow, L. A.: Virus infections of the fetus and newborn infant, J. Pediatr. **77**:315, 1970.
Pearson, H. E.: Parturition varicella-zoster, Obstet. Gynecol. **23**:21, 1964.
Rawls, W. E.: Congenital rubella; the significance of virus persistence, Progr. Med. Virol. **10**:238, 1968.
Rinvid, R.: Congenital varicella encephalomyelitis in surviving newborn, Am. J. Dis. Child. **117**: 231, 1969.
Sever, J., and White, L. R.: Intrauterine viral infections, Ann. Rev. Med. **19**:471, 1968.
Starr, J. G., Bart, R. D., and Gold, E.: Inapparent congenital cytomegalovirus infection; clinical and epidemiologic characteristics in early infancy, N. Engl. J. Med. **282**:1075, 1970.
Torphy, D. E., Ray, C. G., McAlister, R., and Du, J. N. H.: Herpes simplex virus infection in infants; a spectrum of disease, J. Pediatr. **76**: 405, 1970.
Weller, T. H.: The cytomegaloviruses; ubiquitous agents with protean clinical manifestations, N. Engl. J. Med. **285**:267, 1971.

FUNGAL INFECTIONS

Ajello, L., editor: Symposium on coccidioicomycosis. Tucson, 1967, University of Arizona Press.
Dvorak, A. M., and Gavaller, B.: Congenital systemic candidiasis; report of a case, N. Engl. J. Med. **274**:540, 1966.
Emanuel, B., Ching, E., Lieberman, A. D., and Goldin, M.: Cryptococcus meningitis in a child successfully treated with amphotericin B, with a review of the pediatric literature, J. Pediatr. **59**:577, 1961.
Holland, P., and Holland, N. H.: Histoplasmosis in early infancy, Am. J. Dis. Child. **112**:412, 1966.
Hyatt, H. W.: Coccidioidomycosis in a 3-week-old infant, Am. J. Dis. Child. **105**:93, 1963.
Kozinn, P. J., and Taschdjian, C. L.: Enteric candidiasis; diagnosis and clinical considerations, Pediatrics **30**:71, 1962.
Kozinn, P. J., Taschdjian, C. L., Wrener, H., Dragutsky, D., and Minsky, A.: Neonatal candidiasis, Pediatr. Clin. North Am. **5**:803, 1958.
Neuhauser, E. B. D., and Tucker, A.: The roentgen changes produced by diffuse torulosis in the newborn, Am. J. Roentgenol. **59**:805, 1948.
Rhatigan, R. M.: Congenital cutaneous candidiasis, Am. J. Dis. Child. **116**:545, 1968.

PARASITIC INFECTIONS

Covell, G.: Congenital malaria, Trop. Dis. Bull. **47**:1147, 1950.
Feldman, H. A.: Toxoplasmosis, N. Engl. J. Med. **279**:1370, 1431, 1968.
Harvey, B., Remington, J. S., and Sulzer, A. J.: IgM malaria antibodies in a case of congenital malaria in the United States, Lancet **1**:333, 1969.
Robbins, J. B.: Immunological and clinicopathological aspects of pneumocystis carinii pneumonitis. In Bergsma, D., and Good, R. A., editors: Immunologic deficiency diseases in man, New York, 1968, The National Foundation, pp. 219-244.

IMMUNOLOGIC CONSIDERATIONS

Dossett, J. H., Williams, R. C., Jr., and Quie, P. G.: Studies on interaction of bacteria, serum factors, and polymorphonuclear leukocytes in mothers and newborns, Pediatrics **44**:49, 1969.
McCracken, G. H., and Eichenwald, H. F.: Leukocyte function and the development of opsonic and complement activity in the neonate, Am. J. Dis. Child. **121**:120, 1971.
Miller, M. E.: Chemotactic function in the human neonate; humoral and cellular aspects, Pediatr. Res. **5**:487, 1971.
Rosen, F. S.: The thymus gland and the immune deficiency syndromes. In Samter, M., editor: Immunological diseases, ed. 2, Boston, 1971, Little, Brown and Co.
Stiehm, E. R., Amman, A. J., and Cherry, J. D.: Elevated cord macroglobulins in the diagnosis of intrauterine infections, N. Engl. J. Med. **275**: 971, 1966.
WHO committee report; primary immunodeficiencies, Pediatrics **47**:927, 1971.

COLLAGEN-VASCULAR DISEASES

Benyo, R. B., and Perrin, E. V.: Periarteritis nodosa in infancy, Am. J. Dis. Child. **116**:539, 1968.
Jackson, R.: Discoid lupus in a newborn infant of a mother with lupus erythematosus, Pediatrics **33**:425, 1964.
Nice, C. M., Jr.: Congenital disseminated lupus erythematosus, Am. J. Roentgen. **86**:585, 1962.
Reed, W. B., May, S. B., and Tuffanelli, D. L.: Discoid lupus erythematosus in a newborn, Arch. Dermatol. **96**:64, 1967.
Roberts, F. B., Fetterman, G. H.: Polyarteritis nodosa in infancy, J. Pediatr. **63**:519, 1963.
Seip, M.: Systemic lupus erythematosus in pregnancy with haemolytic anemia, leukopenia and thrombocytopenia in mother and her newborn infant, Arch. Dis. Child. **35**:364, 1960.

9 Disorders of the blood and vascular system

HEMATOPOIESIS IN THE EMBRYO AND FETUS

The hematologic changes that take place during prenatal development form an important basis for consideration of many normal and abnormal blood findings of newborn infants. These events are summarized briefly in this chapter.

Blood cell formation in the human embryo first becomes detectable at about 14 days of gestation. Hematopoietic activity begins within the wall of the yolk sac with the development of blood islands that arise from aggregates of primitive mesenchymal cells. The peripherally situated cells of the blood islands differentiate to form blood vessel endothelium, while those within the interior become the primitive blood cells. A majority of these early blood cells undergo differentiation into erythroblast forms, which morphologically resemble the megaloblasts seen in patients with pernicious anemia. The megaloblastic stage of erythropoiesis gradually becomes replaced by definitive normoblastic erythropoiesis beginning at about the sixth week of gestation.

Hematopoiesis in the blood islands of the yolk sac is succeeded briefly by blood formation in mesenchymal tissue of the body. Subsequently the liver becomes the principal blood-forming organ. The hematopoietic tissue in the liver arises from undifferentiated mesenchyme that proliferates between the parenchymal liver cells. Red blood cell formation by the liver is almost entirely normoblastic and results in the production of mature erythrocytes. Platelets and small number of granulocytes also become evident at this stage. Hematopoiesis in the liver gradually declines, beginning at about the fifth month of gestation, but the liver continues to be a site of blood cell formation throughout the fetal period and into the first week of postnatal life. The spleen, thymus, and lymph nodes function briefly as hematopoietic organs from about the second to fourth months of gestation.

Hematopoiesis in the bone marrow begins in the fifth month, arising from mesenchymal tissue that proliferates with resorption of areas of cartilage within the developing bones. Initially the bone marrow produces predominantly leukocytes, and with the decline of blood formation in the liver, red blood cells and megakaryocytes are produced. Beyond the sixth month of gestation the bone marrow is the principal site of blood cell formation.

THE BLOOD CELLS IN UTERO

By the sixteenth week of gestation the primitive nucleated erythroblasts in the blood are almost entirely replaced by definitive mature red blood cells. The erythrocytes present in the blood at this stage are considerably larger than those present at the time of birth, and the hemoglobin concentration of the blood and the red blood cell count are significantly lower than the normal postnatal levels (Fig. 9-1). A gradual increase in the red blood cell count occurs throughout the fetal period, together with a decreasing size of the red blood cells. Reticulocytosis is prominent in the early fetus, and as much as 80% of the red blood cells may be reticulocytes at 10 weeks of gestation. By 30 weeks the

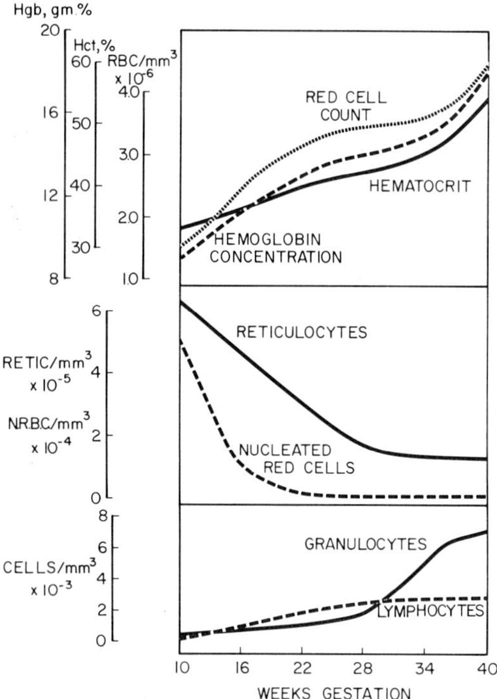

Fig. 9-1. Hematologic changes during prenatal development.

reticulocyte count reaches a minimum of about 4%.

Leukocytes are present only in small numbers during the first half of gestation. Granulocyte counts are less than 50% of adult values prior to the twenty-sixth week and increase prominently in the last 2 to 3 months of fetal life (Fig. 9-1). Lymphocyte counts reach approximately two thirds of the values at term by about 20 weeks of gestation, then increase gradually.

Small numbers of megakaryocytes have been observed as early as the yolk sac stage of hematopoiesis. Platelets are present in the blood by 11 weeks of gestation, and by 30 weeks the platelet count approaches normal adult values.

NORMAL HEMATOLOGIC VALUES

The concentration of hemoglobin in cord blood at birth averages approximately 17 gm/100 ml, with a wide range of values of between 14 and 20 gm/100 ml generally being accepted as normal. Hematocrit values of cord blood average about 55%, with a range of normal of 43% to 63%. The red blood cell count is correspondingly elevated, having a mean of approximately $5.5 \times 10^6/mm^3$. These values may be modified by a number of factors that must be taken into consideration if a meaningful interpretation of hematologic data in the newborn infant is to be made.

An important determinant is the duration of gestation. During the final weeks of intrauterine life the hemoglobin concentration of the blood undergoes a rapid increase (Fig. 9-1), with average increments of from 1 to 3 gm/100 ml occurring between the thirty-eighth and fortieth weeks. This magnitude of change will be reflected in a correspondingly reduced hemoglobin concentration at birth in prematurely born as compared with full-term infants. In a study of a group of premature infants having birth weights of less than 1,200 gm, a mean hemoglobin concentration of 15.6 gm/100 ml was found as compared with a corresponding value of 17.1 gm/100 ml in a group of full-term infants.

The length of time allowed to elapse before the cord is clamped at delivery can have a considerable effect on the blood volume and total circulating red blood cell mass of the newborn infant. It has been estimated that the placental vessels contain approximately 100 ml of blood at term. Transfusion of a major fraction of the blood contained in the placenta can occur under conditions that promote emptying of the placental vessels at delivery. By placing the infant below the level of the placenta and delaying clamping of the cord for several minutes after birth, the blood volume of the infant can be increased by as much as 40% to 60%. In a study by Usher and his associates, newborn infants with delayed clamping of the cord were found to have mean blood volumes of 126 ml/kg as compared with 78 ml/kg in infants whose cords were clamped immediately at birth. In both groups of infants the average hematocrit was the same at birth, but after 48 hours mean hematocrit values of 65% were obtained in the group with delayed clamping of the cord and 48% in the infants in whom placental transfusion was prevented. Increased hemoglobin and hematocrit values can be demonstrated for at least 3 to 4 days in infants with delayed cord clamping.

The effect of transfusion of placental

blood into the infant at birth may result in even greater increases in the blood volume in the case of the premature infant. The quantity of blood in the placenta undergoes little change in the last 2 to 3 months of gestation, during which time the blood volume of the infant increases considerably. The preterm infant can thereby receive a proportionately larger fraction of his blood volume by the addition of the placental blood.

It remains unclear whether the addition of the placental blood to the circulation is advantageous to the infant. It is conceivable that the rapid increase in blood volume that occurs might impose significant stress upon the heart and pulmonary vasculature. Others have claimed a decreased incidence of neonatal respiratory distress in infants in whom clamping of the cord is delayed. What is perhaps of greater importance is that infants having a larger circulating red blood cell mass at birth will gain a valuable storage supply of iron resulting from breakdown of the additional hemoglobin. This supplementary iron can be utilized at a later time for hemoglobin production and will help to prevent iron deficiency if dietary intake is inadequate to supply the iron requirements for rapid growth during later infancy.

In the newborn, hemoglobin values of capillary blood samples obtained by puncture of the infant's heel or finger are usually increased by 2 to 3 gm/100 ml as compared with values of venous blood obtained simultaneously. This difference is attributable to the sluggish peripheral circulation of the newborn infant. Values obtained from venous blood are generally more reliable and reproducible and are preferable for accurate assessment of the hemoglobin concentration during the first fews days of life.

An additional modifying factor that occurs within the first few hours following delivery is a shift in the distribution of fluid to produce a decrease in the circulating plasma volume and a corresponding increase in the red blood cell concentration in the blood. An elevation in the hemoglobin value of approximately 2 gm/100 ml above cord blood values within the first 24 hours is typically observed.

Reticulocyte counts in cord blood of normal infants average 4% to 5% and in most cord blood samples nucleated red blood cell precursors are also present. These findings are accompanied by elevated erythropoietin levels and erythroid hyperplasia in the bone marrow and are interpreted to represent compensatory red blood cell production resulting from conditions of relative hypoxia in utero. The latter is in part a consequence of the decreased oxygen saturation of the fetal blood. An additional contributing factor is the high oxygen affinity of the fetal blood because of the predominance of fetal hemoglobin in the red blood cells; the result of this increase is an impairment of oxygen release to the tissues. In infants with intrauterine growth retardation, hypoxia in utero appears to occur to a more severe extent, and these infants frequently demonstrate higher than normal levels of erythropoietin and a greater degree of erythrocytosis.

The erythrocytes of the newborn infant are considerably larger than those of adults, which is reflected in an increase in the mean cellular diameter and mean corpuscular volume indices (Table 9-1). The red blood cells have an increased hemoglobin content, but the mean corpuscular hemoglobin concentration (MCHC) is within the normal range established for erythrocytes of adults.

A number of physiologic and metabolic characteristics of erythrocytes from newborns also differ from those of red blood cells from older children and adults. Permeability of the fetal red blood cell membrane to sodium and potassium is increased, and glucose utilization and ATP production by the erythrocytes are correspondingly elevated. The latter changes in part appear to represent compensatory activities that serve to maintain normal concentrations of intracellular cations by means of an augmented rate of energy-dependent ion transport.

Red blood cell survival is shortened to a mild or moderate degree in the full-term infant as compared with the normal adult erythrocyte survival time of 100 to 120 days. In the premature infant, shortening of the red blood cell life-span appears to be somewhat greater, although considerable variability has been reported. Available evidence suggests that the reduced

TABLE 9-1. Normal hematologic values in cord blood of the full-term newborn infant

Hemoglobin concentration	14.0-20.0 gm/100 ml
Red blood cell count	4,200,000-5,800,000/mm³
Hematocrit	43% to 63%
Mean cell diameter	8.0-8.3 μ
Mean corpuscular volume (MCV)	100-120 μ³
Mean corpuscular hemoglobin (MCH)	32-40 pg
Mean corpuscular hemoglobin concentration (MCHC)	30% to 34%
Reticulocyte count	3% to 7%
Nucleated red blood cell count	200-600/mm³
White blood cell count	10,000-30,000/mm³
Granulocytes	40% to 80%
Lymphocytes	20% to 40%
Monocytes	3% to 10%
Platelet count	150,000-350,000/mm³
Serum iron concentration	125-225 μg/100 ml
Total iron-binding capacity	150-350 μg/100 ml

life-span of the erythrocytes of the infant may be related to a number of factors that predispose the red blood cells to early destruction. The relatively larger size of the fetal erythrocyte, together with a greater degree of cell rigidity, renders the erythrocytes less compliant and deformable within the small blood vessels and may cause them to be more susceptible to intravascular damage. In addition, the increased permeability of the red blood cell membrane to sodium and potassium predisposes the red blood cells to the development of adverse osmotic changes within the cells, adding further risk of premature cell destruction, particularly within the spleen and other reticuloendothelial organs.

An increase in the activity of a number of glycolytic red blood cell enzymes has also been demonstrated in blood of newborn infants. In many instances, however, these changes may reflect the presence of a larger percentage of young red blood cells rather than a specific characteristic of the red blood cells in infancy. Other enzymes, including carbonic anhydrase and NADPH-dependent methemoglobin reductase, exhibit reduced activity in the red blood cells of the newborn. The decrease in the latter enzyme appears to be a major factor in accounting for the elevated levels of methemoglobin in the blood of newborn infants, particularly in premature infants, as well as the predisposition of young infants to form methemoglobin more readily in the presence of precipitating factors.

From 70% to 90% of the hemoglobin in blood of the fetus and newborn infant consists of fetal hemoglobin. This hemoglobin type continues to predominate through the first weeks of postnatal life, after which it gradually becomes replaced by adult hemoglobin. A functional difference between fetal and adult hemoglobin results from the ability of the latter to interact with low molecular weight phosphorylated compounds in the cell to produce altered oxygen-binding properties of the hemoglobin. When adult hemoglobin combines with these substances, which include 2,3-diphosphoglycerate (2,3-DPG), ATP, and related compounds, a marked decrease in oxygen affinity occurs. Fetal hemoglobin, on the other hand, undergoes virtually no participation in this type of interaction. The result of this difference in the behavior of adult and fetal hemoglobins is a leftward shift of the oxygen dissociation curve of fetal blood as compared with the blood of adults, representing a relatively greater oxygen affinity of the fetal blood. This property may be of considerable benefit to the fetus in utero by facilitating placental oxygen exchange from maternal blood to the fetal erythrocytes. However, because of the high oxygen affinity of the fetal hemoglobin, release of oxygen to the tissues is impeded, which may be disadvantageous to the newborn, particularly if anemia is present.

The leukocyte count at birth averages approximately 20,000/mm³, with a wide range of values occurring in normal infants. Approximately 70% of the white blood cells consist of neutrophils, which often include band forms, and occasionally a small number of metamyelocytes. Phagocytic activity of the neutrophils may be less than normal, but the difference appears to be related to opsonification factors in the serum of the infant rather than to an intrinsic defect of the leukocytes.

Platelet counts of full-term infants range from 150,000 to 350,000/mm^3, which are usually considered to be normal values for adults. Some reports have indicated slightly lower values in some premature infants. In any infant, however, a platelet count of less than 100,000/mm^3 may be considered abnormal.

The bone marrow findings of the newborn infant reflect the extremely active production of blood cells, particularly erythrocytes, which is characteristic of this period of life. The bone marrow at birth is highly cellular and occupies virtually the entire medullary cavity of all of the bones. Consequently, diagnostic bone marrow aspiration in young infants can be performed in long bone areas, such as the tibias, whereas in the older child and adult these bones contain primarily fatty tisue. Erythroid precursors comprise approximately 40% of the cellular elements present in aspirated bone marrow specimens.

HEMATOLOGIC CHANGES BEYOND THE NEONATAL PERIOD

Within hours after birth of a normal infant the low oxygen saturation of the blood increases to reach approximately 95% saturation. The striking changes in erythropoiesis that occur in the first weeks of life are largely attributable to the improved oxygenation of the blood and tissues of the infant. Erythropoietin levels, which are elevated at birth, rapidly fall to undetectable levels. In the bone marrow erythropoietic activity becomes suppressed, with red blood cell precursors comprising less than 10% of the nucleated elements by the end of the first week of postnatal life. The reticulocytosis, which is characteristic at birth, also decreases rapidly to reach less than 1% by 5 to 7 days. Nucleated red blood cell precursors disappear even more rapidly and after 2 to 4 days are usually no longer demonstrable in the blood of normal infants.

The postnatal suppression of erythropoiesis, combined with the expansion of the blood volume of the infant caused by rapid growth, produces a progressive decline in the hemoglobin concentration of the infant, beginning near the end of the first week of life and reaching its low point after 2 to 3 months. This physiologic anemia of infancy may result in a hemoglobin concentration of as low as 9.0 gm/100 ml (11.0 $\pm$ 2.0) in a normal full-term infant. These changes do not represent any abnormality or nutritional deficiency in the infant, and the hematologic events at this stage are not affected by the administration of iron or other hematinic agents. With the resumption of active erythropoiesis following the second to third months, if iron supplies are adequate, the hemoglobin concentration of the infant gradually increases to reach a mean level of 12.5 gm/100 ml, which persists throughout early childhood.

In the premature infant, particularly in infants having birth weights of less than 1,500 gm, the physiologic decrease in hemoglobin concentration develops earlier than in the full-term infant and reaches a lower ultimate level. Minimum values are achieved by 4 to 7 weeks, and hemoglobin concentrations of 7 to 8 gm/100 ml may occur in apparently healthy infants. Resumption of active erythropoiesis in the premature infant is also initiated earlier in postnatal life than in the full-term infant.

The supply of available iron stores in the full-term infant is usually sufficient to sustain normal red blood cell production for approximately the first 6 months of life, even without additional exogenous iron. Thereafter the iron needs related to growth require an intake of approximately 1 mg/kg daily if anemia is to be prevented. In the infant whose iron reserve at birth is diminished, the need for additional iron intake develops earlier. Included in this group are premature infants and infants with blood loss during the fetal or neonatal periods.

Although the iron needs of the normal full-term infant during the first year of life can usually be met by intake of an adequate diet, some of these infants nevertheless develop iron deficiency. It has therefore been recommended that iron supplementation be included in the diet of all infants throughout the first year of life.

Iron-enriched cereals and milk formulas generally provide the most convenient and reliable means for providing this supplementary iron. In the premature infant dietary iron is virtually never adequate to supply the iron needed in the course of rapid growth during infancy, and iron supplementation is mandatory to prevent the development of anemia. In these infants it is desirable to introduce iron-enriched milk formula or other iron-containing preparations into the diet during the early weeks of life. Although exogenous iron is not incorporated into hemoglobin to a significant extent in young infants, orally administered iron is nevertheless absorbed and stored by the infant and can be used for hemoglobin synthesis at a later time when the need for additional iron develops.

ANEMIA IN THE NEWBORN PERIOD

Disorders that result in anemia in the newborn infant often represent abnormalities that are unique to this period of life. Consequences of abnormal fetal-maternal interaction, obstetrical complications, and hematologic changes resulting as manifestations of other neonatal disorders together comprise a major segment of the anemias of the neonatal period. In addition, many of the anemias of the older child and adult may also first make their appearance in the newborn period, and the establishment of a precise diagnosis in an anemic infant may require consideration of a sizable group of disorders and often presents a major diagnostic challenge to the physician. Since it is frequently necessary to institute treatment promptly in an infant with anemia, an accurate diagnosis must be made with a minimum of delay.

An etiologic classification of anemias in the newborn period is indicated in the following outline.

CAUSES OF ANEMIA

A. Hemorrhage
   1. Bleeding in utero
   2. Obstetrical bleeding
   3. Postnatal bleeding
B. Impairment of marrow cell production
   1. Congenital erythroid hypoplasia
   2. Other causes
C. Accelerated red blood cell hemolysis
   1. Erythrocytic enzyme defects
   2. Disorders of the red blood cell membrane
   3. Disorders of the hemoglobin
      a. Hemoglobinopathies
      b. Thalassemias
      c. Methemoglobinemia
   4. Infection
   5. Isoimmune hemolysis
   6. Other hemolytic conditions

Anemia caused by hemorrhage

Fetal-maternal transfusion

Transplacental transfusion of fetal blood into the circulation of the mother has been known for many years to be the basis for maternal antibody formation against fetal erythrocytes in the pathogenesis of isoimmune hemolytic disease. It was first suggested by Weiner that fetal blood loss by this mechanism could occur to an extent sufficient enough to produce anemia at birth. An anemic infant subsequently studied by Chown showed substantial evidence of fetal-maternal hemorrhage; blood from the mother was found to contain an elevated percentage of fetal hemoglobin, and large numbers of erythrocytes were present, having antigenic properties characteristic of the infant's cells but not of those of the mother. The changes in the maternal blood gradually disappeared over a period of several weeks following the delivery. In a survey by Cohen and others of over 600 pregnancies, fetal erythrocytes were detected in maternal blood in approximately 50% of the cases. In about 1% of the pregnancies the transplacental hemorrhage appeared to be of sufficient magnitude to produce anemia in the infant.

Clinical presentation. In most instances of this abnormality the findings in the infant suggest that the fetal hemorrhage occurred a significant interval of time prior to delivery. In a majority of cases the bleeding appears to occur at a slow rate over a prolonged period of time. The degree of anemia in the newborn infant can vary widely, ranging from mild to very severe. Jaundice is characteristically absent, the Coombs antiglobulin test is negative, and the liver and spleen are not enlarged; these findings allow this condition to be readily distinguished from the anemia of isoimmune hemolytic disease. Pallor and tachycardia are present to a degree related to the severity of the anemia. The infant otherwise is usually active and in no ap-

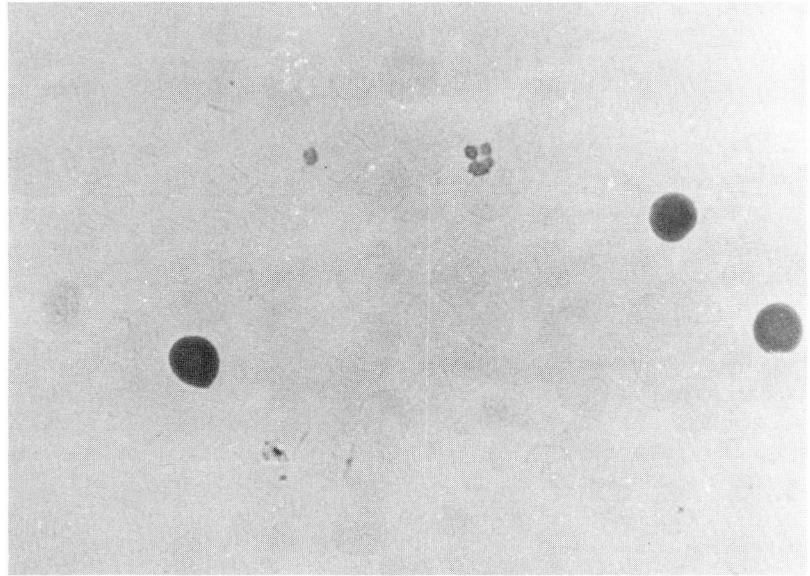

Fig. 9-2. Fetal erythrocytes in maternal blood following a transplacental hemorrhage. The slide was stained following elution of adult hemoglobin by the Kleihauer-Betke procedure. The fetal cells are darkly stained, while those of the mother are barely visible.

parent distress. The anemia is accompanied by polychromatophilia of the erythrocytes, by elevated reticulocyte counts and often by increased numbers of nucleated red blood cells. If the anemia is severe and is the result of chronic long-term hemorrhage, the hematologic findings characteristic of severe iron deficiency anemia will be present, including hypochromia and microcytosis of the erythrocytes, decreased serum iron levels, and an absence of stainable iron in aspirated bone marrow specimens.

If the fetal-maternal transfusion occurs acutely at the time of labor or delivery, the findings in the infant will reflect the rapid reduction in the blood volume (p. 62). Loss of more than 40 ml of blood can be sufficient to produce findings of hypovolemic shock. The infant may appear weak and pale, with tachycardia and labored respirations. Anemia can usually be demonstrated; but if insufficient time has elapsed for compensatory hemodilution to occur, the hemoglobin concentration may not be significantly depressed. Acute blood loss can usually be readily confirmed, however, by the finding of a decreased venous pressure by catheterization of the umbilical vein. The presumptive diagnosis of severe acute blood loss should be considered in any pale neonate in distress when the liver or spleen are not enlarged, and appropriate measures should be undertaken immediately to confirm or disprove this possibility.

Diagnosis. Loss of fetal blood into the maternal circulation can be established as the cause of the anemia by demonstrating the presence of fetal erythrocytes in the mother's blood. A variety of techniques have been employed to detect the fetal cells and have included immunologic methods and procedures to detect increased levels of fetal hemoglobin. The most widely applicable technique is the slide elution procedure of Kleihauer and Betke. In this procedure, which is rapid and easily performed, unstained blood smears are fixed and then incubated in an acidic buffer that causes adult hemoglobin to be eluted from the erythrocytes. Fetal hemoglobin resists elution under these conditions and remains within the intact red blood cells. After staining, the fetal hemoglobin-containing erythrocytes become visible as darkly stained cells, while the erythrocytes of maternal origin, which contain principally adult hemoglobin, appear as clear, ghostlike cells (Fig. 9-2). The presence of even small numbers of fetal cells in maternal blood is readily ascertained by this procedure, and by determination of the percentage of fetal cells present an estimate of the quantity of blood transfused can be made. If major blood group incompatibility exists between the mother and infant, transfused fetal erythrocytes may be rapidly removed from the maternal circulation and may not be detectable in blood smears from the mother. Under these conditions the mother may develop fever or a shaking chill, representing a transfusion reaction to the infusion of incompatible blood. Buffy coat smears of the maternal blood may demonstrate erythrophagocytosis when blood group incompatibility exists and may be helpful in establishing a diagnosis when the slide elution test for fetal cells is negative.

Treatment. Treatment of the infant depends both upon the severity of the anemia and whether the blood loss occurred acutely or over a relatively prolonged period of time. In the infant with a mild degree of anemia, particularly when there is evidence that the blood loss was not acute, no immediate therapy is usually necessary if the infant is vigorous and in no distress. If tachycardia or marked pallor are present, a transfusion of packed red blood cells is indicated. In the severely affected infant with findings of iron deficiency caused by prolonged hemorrhage, incipient heart failure may be present, and transfusion may impose a risk of vascular overload. Under these conditions a partial exchange transfusion using packed red blood cells is preferable. In transfusing these infants it is rarely necessary to increase the hemoglobin concentration to more than 11 to 12 gm/100 ml to achieve complete relief of symptoms of anemia. Iron therapy is essential in subsequent care because of depletion of the iron stores, which is invariably present. Adequate iron supplementation in these infants can be achieved by the regular use of an iron-enriched milk formula or by oral administration of an iron preparation sufficient to provide 2 to 3 mg of elemental iron per kg daily. The iron supplementation should be started in early infancy and continued throughout the first year of life to assure that the iron needs for growth of the infant are fully met.

In the neonate with findings of hypovolemic shock at birth because of acute bleeding into the maternal circulation shortly before delivery, rapid diagnosis and prompt institution of therapy are essential to prevent irreversible changes. Therapy is directed toward rapid restoration of the infant's blood volume and should be started immediately after the condition is recognized. Fresh type O, Rh-negative blood, 10 to 20 ml/kg should be injected rapidly through an umbilical catheter. When blood is not readily available, albumin solutions, plasma, or dextran may be given in the initial infusion, to be followed by whole blood as soon as it becomes available. The response to blood replacement in these infants is usually dramatic. Tachycardia and tachypnea rapidly subside, and tone and activity improve promptly. Subsequent additional transfusions with packed red blood cells are indicated if signs of distress persist or if the hemoglobin concentration falls to less than 8 to 9 gm/100 ml after fluid equilibration in the plasma has taken place. Orally administered iron should be given to these infants and continued throughout the first year.

Blood loss in utero from one twin to another

Newborn monovular twins frequently exhibit large differences in their hemoglobin concentrations at birth, with anemia being present in one twin and polycythemia in the other. In approximately 70% of monovular twin pregnancies the placentas are monochorial and almost invariably contain vascular communications between the fetal circulations. When a significant degree of arterial-venous anastomosis exists between the placental circulation of one twin and the other, the opportunity will exist for the twin on the arterial limb of the communication to infuse blood into the circulation of the other. A study of 130 monochorial twin pregnancies indicated an incidence of at least 15% significant blood loss from one twin to the other. A high mortality of the affected twins occurred, often with death in utero early in the pregnancy. Of 38 of these infants born alive, only 13 survived, suggesting that this complication may be a major factor to account for the higher mortality of monochorial as compared with dichorial twin pregnancies.

In the donor twin, anemia may vary from

mild to severe. Red blood cell hypochromia and microcytosis are often present as a reflection of iron deficiency caused by the prolonged blood loss. Elevated reticulocyte counts and large numbers of nucleated red blood cells represent a compensatory increase of erythrocyte production. The anemia is often accompanied by oligohydramnios and hypotension. If blood loss has been extensive the infant may exhibit pallor, weakness, and tachycardia.

The polycythemic infant presents a ruddy appearance and often is larger than the anemic twin. The infant may show evidence of hypertension, which can be associated with heart failure and pulmonary edema. Hyperviscosity of the blood results from the increased red blood cell mass and can predispose these infants to venous thrombus formation or hemorrhage. Hyperbilirubinemia may accompany breakdown of the increased numbers of red blood cells.

The donor twin may require supportive transfusions if symptomatic anemia is present. With severe anemia a partial exchange transfusion with packed red blood cells minimizes the risk of circulatory overload. If the infant is asymptomatic and the anemia is not severe, orally administered iron will usually be all that is required.

In the polycythemic twin, phlebotomy is indicated if complications arise as a result of hyperviscosity of the blood or from circulatory overload. The hemoglobin concentration can be reduced most effectively by performing a partial exchange transfusion using plasma to replace the blood that is removed. Phototherapy may be useful in minimizing the risk of dangerous hyperbilirubinemia in these infants. Serial determinations of the serum bilirubin level should be performed, and exchange transfusion should be considered if the bilirubin concentration exceeds 20 mg/100 ml.

Obstetrical hemorrhage

It has been estimated that anemia in newborns caused by acute obstetrical hemorrhage occurs at a rate of approximately 1 per 1,000 live births. This complication may result from obstetrical accidents in otherwise normal pregnancies or may be predisposed by abnormalities of the umbilical cord, umbilical vessels, or placenta.

Rupture of the normal umbilical cord has been documented as a cause of neonatal hemorrhage primarily following precipitous, often unattended deliveries. Although this now occurs uncommonly, it should be considered when an anemic infant with a history of an uncontrolled delivery is encountered. When the cord is abnormally short or is entangled with the infant, it may become torn in the course of even a normal delivery. Varices or aneurysms of the umbilical vessels may produce areas of focal weakness that predispose the infant to rupture of the cord. When the placental insertion of the umbilical cord is abnormal, giving rise to anomalous aberrant vessels lying free on the placental surface or to a diffuse velamentous insertion, the unprotected vessels become easily subjected to laceration during the delivery with the risk of considerable blood loss by the infant. A not infrequent anomaly is multilobularity of the placenta, in which one or more accessory lobules exist apart from the main body of the placenta. The lobules are joined by fragile communicating vessels that become easily disrupted during labor and delivery, accompanied by hemorrhage.

In placenta praevia and abruptio placentae, hemorrhage from the placental surface can result in blood loss from the infant as well as from the mother. In these disorders the incidence of stillbirths is high, and surviving infants frequently are severely anemic at birth. Acute blood loss following accidental incision of the placenta at cesarian section is also not uncommon, particularly in placenta praevia. Tearing or separation of the placenta during delivery of the infant through the uterine incision may also lead to significant blood loss.

In anemia developing as a result of obstetrical hemorrhage, the findings in the infant at birth are attributable to acute blood loss, and following severe hemorrhage may include pallor, tachycardia, irregular respirations, decreased tone, and a weak cry. The central venous pressure will often be reduced. The hemoglobin concentration immediately after delivery may not reflect the true magnitude of blood loss; but usually 6 to 12 hours later, after hemodilution has occurred, the anemia will be fully apparent. Treatment for acute hemorrhage is directed toward rapid expansion of the blood volume with transfusions of fresh whole blood whenever possible, as described in the preceding sections. Dietary supplementation with orally administered iron should be started early and in adequate amounts to prevent later development of iron deficiency.

Postnatal hemorrhage

Hemorrhage in the first days of life as a cause of anemia most often results from birth trauma. When a congenital or acquired disorder of hemostasis is present in the infant, postpartum hemorrhage is not uncommon, even in the absence of unusual trauma at delivery. Postnatal bleeding may be apparent or occult, and in either case may result in gradual or rapidly progressive anemia. The sudden onset of shock in a previously well infant may sometimes be the first indication of occult hemorrhage. In any infant who develops anemia beyond the first day of life, without jaundice or other evidence of hyperhemolysis, every attempt should be made to ascertain or exclude the presence of internal bleeding. In premature infants, in cases of multiple births, and following breech or traumatic deliveries the risk of postnatal hemorrhage is increased.

Hemorrhage into the scalp associated with a caput succedaneum occurs commonly (p. 72) but usually subsides within a few days, producing no untoward effect. Occasionally a substantial quantity of blood may be lost into the scalp, resulting in anemia of sufficient severity to require supportive transfusions of packed red blood cells. Subperiosteal hemorrhages (cephalhematomas) frequently arise following fracture of the skull (p. 73). The hemorrhage is often gradual and may continue for 1 to 3 days, after which it usually subsides spontaneously. Massive blood loss requiring transfusion occurs in rare instances. A more frequent complication is the development of hyperbilirubinemia in these infants, following degradation of the extravasated blood. The bilirubin level may become sufficiently elevated to produce kernicterus if the hemorrhage has been extensive.

Intracranial hemorrhage may result as a complication of birth trauma, and is particularly prevalent in premature infants (p. 529). Clinical manifestations primarily reflect neurologic changes and may include hypotonia, poor feeding, vomiting, convulsions, and a high-pitched cry. Subarachnoid or subdural hemorrhage may be of sufficient severity to produce anemia, for which small transfusions of packed red blood cells should be given.

Hemorrhage into the liver, spleen, adrenals, or kidneys, following rupture or laceration of these organs, may also produce anemia in the perinatal period. Predisposing factors includes traumatic or breech delivery, prematurity, disorders of hemostasis, and conditions that produce swelling or distension of the abdominal organs.

The liver is most commonly affected. Hemorrhage may be mild and limited to subcapsular bleeding or may result from rupture of the parenchyma and capsule of the liver, with massive blood loss into the peritoneal cavity. With progressive subcapsular hepatic hemorrhage the infant may appear well until rupture of the capsule ensues, followed by rapid development of hemoperitoneum and hypovolemic shock. (See p. 88 for discussion of clinical presentation and treatment.)

Splenic rupture in the newborn period occurs uncommonly but may follow a traumatic delivery (p. 88). In a majority of the reported examples of this complication, splenic distension associated with splenomegaly caused by isoimmune hemolytic disease was present. Many of the clinical findings are similar to those that accompany rupture of the liver. Transfusions and splenectomy are indicated.

Retroperitoneal hemorrhage involving the adrenals, or less commonly the kidneys, usually follows a traumatic delivery and may produce anemia (p. 89). Findings attributable to blood loss often develop soon after birth and are accompanied by an enlarging flank mass.

In some infants the adrenal hemorrhage may be manifested as unexplained jaundice together with a mass in the flank in an otherwise healthy-appearing infant. The diagnosis can often be established by the finding of a radiolucent suprarenal mass and downward displacement of the kidney on an excretory urogram. These findings may be similar to those of congenital neuroblastoma. Arteriography through the umbilical artery will usually show increased vascularity in neuroblastoma, whereas an avascular lesion is seen in adrenal hemorrhage.

Anemia resulting from decreased production of erythrocytes

Congenital hypoplastic anemia

This unusual form of anemia results from a selective failure of erythrocyte production by the bone marrow. Leukocyte and platelet production are characteristically normal in this disorder, which allows it to be readily distinguished from most other hypoplastic states. The disease has been described under a variety of names, including pure red blood cell anemia, Diamond-Blackfan anemia, chronic congenital aregenerative anemia, and erythrogenesis imperfecta.

Etiology and pathogenesis. A familial incidence has been described in some cases of this disorder, indicating a possible genetic basis for its development. In a small number of affected individuals increased urinary excretion of anthranilic acid and other catabolic products of tryptophan has been observed, which suggests the presence of an associated metabolic abnormality. However, a relationship between these biochemical changes and the anemia in these patients has not been established. Erythropoietin levels are characteristically elevated, demonstrating that the failure of red blood cell production stems from a primary abnormality of the bone marrow rather than from a subnormal degree of erythropoietic stimulation. The occasional presence of other associated abnormalities and the variability in the severity of anemia and in the response to therapy suggest that congenital hypoplastic anemia may represent a group of related disorders rather than a single entity. Acquired erythroid hypoplastic anemia in adults is occasionally accompanied by thymic tumors, but this association does not occur in the congenital hypoplastic anemia of infancy.

Clinical presentation. Evidence of anemia may be present at birth and in most cases is apparent by 3 months of age. Findings in the infant are attributable to anemia and include pallor, irritability, lassitude, loss of appetite, and tachycardia. Jaundice, lymph node enlargement, and bleeding manifestations are absent. The liver and spleen are rarely enlarged early in the course of the disease unless congestive heart failure has supervened. Low birth weight and growth retardation have been noted in a large percentage of affected children. These findings have been attributed to a high rate of prematurity and to corticosteroid-related growth failure in many instances. It appears likely, however, that understature may frequently be an inherent feature of this disorder. A variety of other associated abnormalities have occasionally been described, including malformations of the urinary tract, skeletal defects, and webbing of the neck.

Diagnosis. The anemia is normochromic and normocytic and may be of variable severity. Reticulocytes are greatly reduced or absent, which is a particularly striking finding when observed in the first 48 hours after birth. The leukocyte and platelet counts are normal. The most significant laboratory finding is seen in bone marrow specimens in which there is a marked reduction of nucleated red blood cell precursors in the presence of normal numbers of myeloid elements and megakaryocytes.

Treatment. Most affected infants will require a blood transfusion initially, administered preferably as packed red blood cells. A transfusion sufficient to increase the hemoglobin concentration to 8 to 10 gm/100 ml is usually adequate for relief of symptoms of anemia without causing suppression of erythropoiesis.

Approximately 50% of affected infants will demonstrate a hematopoietic response to treatment with corticosteroids. The probability of obtaining a satisfactory remission appears to be increased if the corticosteroid therapy is started early in the course of the anemia. Optimal results are achieved by initiating therapy immediately after the diagnosis has been established, using prednisone at a dose of 2 to 4 mg/kg of body weight daily. Infants who respond will usually demonstrate reticulocytosis within 1 to 2 weeks, followed by an increase in the hemoglobin concentration to reach a maximum hemoglobin level by 3 to 4 weeks. If little or no response is obtained, the prednisone dosage should be doubled and continued for at least a 4-week period. After a maximum response has occurred, the prednisone dose can be reduced gradually until the smallest dosage is found that is capable of maintaining adequate erythropoiesis. Corticosteroid therapy is usually required for an indefinite period, but very small doses are often adequate to maintain a remission. Undesirable side effects can usually be reduced by administration of the prednisone on an intermittent schedule.

Infants who are unresponsive to corticosteroid therapy usually require periodic transfusions at 3- to 6-week intervals if severe anemia is to be prevented. Progressive accumulation of hemosiderin in the tissues is an inevitable complication of multiple transfusions. The liver and spleen become enlarged, and hypersplenism may result, with the development of leukopenia and thrombocytopenia. Splenectomy has no beneficial effect on the underlying hematologic disorder but may be of value if hypersplenic complications arise.

Prognosis. Occasionally, spontaneous remission of the anemia may occur, particularly at the time of puberty. A remission may develop even if the patient has been unresponsive to corticosteroid therapy. Of 18 unresponsive patients studied by Diamond, 7 eventually achieved remission, in some cases after having received transfusions for a period of many years.

Other causes of bone marrow hypoplasia

Hypoplastic bone marrow changes in newborn infants are uncommon and usually arise as secondary complications of other disease processes. The anemia in these conditions is accompanied by some degree of leukopenia and thrombocytopenia, resulting from a generalized suppression of bone marrow function. Encroachment of normal marrow tissue by metastatic neuroblastoma cells or leukemia can produce pancytopenia in the young infant, and the resulting hematologic changes may provide the first indication of the existance of the underlying disorder. In osteopetrosis (Albers-Schönberg disease), anemia and thrombocytopenia are characteristic findings that may be present at birth. The hematologic abnormalities in this disorder probably result form obliteration of the marrow cavities because of the cortical overgrowth of the bones, but a hemolytic component may also be present. The diagnosis is readily established by radiographic bone studies. Supportive transfusions may be required if anemia is severe.

The syndrome of constitutional aplastic anemia with associated congenital anomalies (Fanconi's anemia) is a familial disorder in which pancytopenia is a characteristic feature. Hypoplastic changes that take place in the bone marrow in this disorder usually have their onset in affected individuals between 4 and 8 years of age, and at birth the infants almost invariably are hematologically normal. Other abnormalities that occur in this syndrome, including skeletal deformities, microcephaly, renal anomalies, and abnormal skin pigmentation, may be readily detected at birth, however, and can be of valuable prognostic importance.

The hemolytic anemias

Anemia caused by an accelerated rate of red blood cell destruction is not uncommon in the newborn period and can accompany a variety of abnormal conditions. Hemolytic disease in the neonate produces a characteristic clinical picture that is unique to this period of life and that stems in large part from hematopoietic and physiologic features that are peculiar to the newborn period.

Hyperbilirubinemia is an almost constant finding in hemolytic disease of the newborn and results from the limited capacity of the neonatal liver for glucuronidation and excretion of the excessive quantities of bilirubin that are produced from the catabolism of hemoglobin. The bilirubin in the serum of these infants is therefore primarily the unconjugated, indirect-reacting type. Bilirubin levels in the neonate can become significantly elevated following the breakdown of an even relatively small quantity of red blood cells; it has been estimated that hemolysis sufficient to reduce the hemoglobin concentration by 1 gm/100 ml will increase the bilirubin level by 35 mg/100 ml if none is excreted. Consequently, jaundice with hyperbilirubinemia frequently will be present before other findings appear to indicate the presence of anemia. In relatively mild hemolytic states that might not require specific measures for management of the anemia, hyperbilirubinemia may nevertheless be sufficiently severe to impose a risk of kernicterus on the infant, and it will frequently be necessary to institute therapy for the management of this secondary complication.

The hematopoietic response to accelerated hemolysis in the neonate is often extremely active, with an extensive outpouring of reticulocytes from the bone marrow. The reticulocytosis is characteristically accompanied by large numbers of nucleated red blood cell precursors. This feature led to the earlier designation of erythroblastosis fetalis for hemolytic disease of the newborn caused by maternal isoimmune antibody. Enlargement of the liver and spleen commonly occurs in hemolytic disorders of newborns and is caused in part by proliferation of hematopoietic tissue within these organs.

Hemolytic anemia in the neonatal period may be caused by congenital hematologic disorders or may be acquired, the latter group accounting for the majority of affected infants. The congenital hemolytic anemias result from intrinsic defects of the erythroctyes and include abnormalities of the structure or function of the red blood cell membrane, deficiencies of essential erythrocytic enzymes, and disorders of the structure or biosynthesis of hemoglobin. In some instances an onset of overt hemolytic anemia may be precipitated by a drug or toxin or by an infection in an infant predisposed to abnormal hemolysis by one of these congenital erythrocyte abnormalities.

Acquired hemolytic disease in the newborn most commonly results from red blood cell damage caused by maternal isoimmune antibody. Hemolytic anemia also frequently accompanies a variety of neonatal infections, including toxoplasmosis, syphilis, cytomegalic inclusion disease, rubella, and bacterial infections, particularly those caused by gram-negative bacilli.

Isoimmune hemolytic disease

This disorder, which is also designated *erythroblastosis fetalis* and *hemolytic disease of the newborn,* results from the transplacental passage of maternal antibody that is active against red blood cell antigens of the infant. The interaction of the antibody with susceptible erythrocytes gives rise to premature destruction of the red blood cells, resulting in anemia and hyperbilirubinemia. This disorder continues to be among the most frequent causes of anemia and of severe icterus in the newborn period.

Pathogenesis. More than 60 different red blood cell antigens have been identified that are capable of eliciting an antibody response in a suitable recipient. With rare exceptions, however, significant isoimmune hemolytic disease is associated only with fetal-maternal incompatibility of the A-B-O factors and the D factor of the Rh group. The latter has been reponsible for most of the severe forms of the disease.

Maternal antibody formation in cases of A-B-O incompatibility can occur when the maternal red blood cells are type O and those of the infant are type A or B, or when the mother is of type A and the infant of type B, or the mother type B and the infant type A. In most instances of A-B-O hemolytic disease the mother is of blood type O, and a disproportionately large percentage of the affected infants have blood type A_1, which appears to be a more highly antigenic factor than either types A_2 or B. However, the antigenicity of all the A-B-O factors is poorly developed in the fetus and newborn, which is probably a major factor in accounting for the relatively unusual occurrence of severe A-B-O hemolytic disease in spite of an estimated 20% incidence of pregnancies in which incompatibilities of these factors exist.

The Rh system was initially thought to involve a single antigen but has subsequently been found to encompass a considerable number of immunogenic entities. The Rh antigenic determinants are genetically transmitted as closely linked traits that are inherited together from each parent as an intact group of factors. The nature of the Rh gene, however, remains controversial. One concept holds that each individual possesses a single pair of genes, each of which determines an Rh type and which in turn directs the production of a number of blood group factors. This theory appears in many respects to be more nearly correct and is more adequate to account for certain findings that otherwise cannot be readily explained.

An alternative theory, however, which

is generally more suitable for clinical applications, maintains that the Rh factors are determined by a group of closely linked genes, each of which determines an individual blood group factor. The Rh factors defined in this system are designated C, c, D, d, E, and e. The two forms of antigen indicated by each of the pairs of letters segregate as alleles, with one form or the other being present normally in each total Rh genome. The d factor is hypothetical and has not been demonstrated, but each of the other factors has been shown to possess a unique antigenic identity and is capable of eliciting a specific antibody response under suitable conditions. A number of variant forms of Rh factors have also been identified, some of which have also been implicated in the pathogenesis of isoimmune hemolytic disease. Included in this group are factors C^W, C^X, and D^u.

Although all of the Rh factors are immunogenic and can therefore produce isoimmune sensitization, the D factor is the only one that is commonly associated with severe hemolytic disease. For practical purposes a satisfactory assessment of the Rh group can be made by determination of the D factor alone. Unless stated otherwise, an individual homozygous or heterozygous for D is considered to be Rh positive, whereas the designation Rh negative is applied only to the presumed genotype d/d. The D antigen is well developed at birth and has been demonstrated to be present as early as the eleventh week of fetal life. This finding undoubtedly is related to the relatively early and severe degree of hemolysis that develops when isoimmunization against this factor occurs. Significant racial differences in the incidence of the D factor have been demonstrated, with approximately 85% of the white population, 93% of the black population, and more than 99% of Chinese people having this factor. This distribution correlates well with the incidence of Rh isoimmune hemolytic disease, which is approximately three times more frequent in white persons than in black persons and is rare among the Chinese.

In addition to the A-B-O and Rh factors, blood group incompatibility involving other red blood cell antigens has occasionally resulted in immune hemolytic disease in newborns. These factors have included Kell, Lewis, M, Duffy, S, Kidd, and rarely others.

Transfusion of fetal erythrocytes into the maternal circulation has been shown to occur in a high percentage of pregnancies, particularly at or near term. In pregnancies in which A-B-O incompatibiltiy could be excluded, Cohen and his associates demonstrated the presence of fetal cells in blood smears of maternal blood in as many as 50% of cases. In most instances, however, the quantity of transfused fetal blood appeared to be less than 0.2 ml, which probably is insufficient in most cases to produce primary immunization. Controlled studies have shown that at least 1.0 ml of blood seems to be required to induce antibody formation in an unsensitized Rh-negative recipient. However, after immunization has initially occurred, considerably smaller doses may be sufficient to stimulate an increase in the antibody titer.

In the case of the A and B factors, individuals who lack either of these blood group antigens normally demonstrate antibody activity against the factors that are absent, even without prior immunization. Thus serum from a type A individual will contain anti-**B**, while serum from a type O individual will contain both anti-**A** and anti-**B**. These "natural" antibodies agglutinate red blood cells in saline suspension, are neutralized by A and B (Witebsky) substances, and are present primarily in the 19 S gamma globulin fraction, which is incapable of crossing the placental barrier. In most type O individuals, however, natural antibody to A factor has been found to be present in both the 19 S and 7 S globulin fractions. The 7 S antibody is a univalent, incomplete antibody that agglutinates type A red blood cells poorly in saline suspension but effectively in a 20% solution of albumin. The albumin-active antibody is not neutralized by A substance, and because of its smaller molecular weight readily traverses the placenta to enter the fetal circulation. This property of the natural antibodies of type O individuals may account for the appreciable incidence of A-O incompatible isoimmune hemolytic disease in firstborn infants, in contrast to the rare occurrence of immune hemolysis in firstborn Rh-positive infants of Rh-negative mothers. Those mothers who have become immunized against the A or B factors from a previous incompatible pregnancy also exhibit antibody activity in the 7 S gamma globulin fraction having the properties described above. These "immune" antibodies are regarded as being the primary mediators of A-B-O isoimmune disease.

Rh-negative individuals, by contrast, do not normally possess serum antibody against the D blood group factor unless immunization has occurred from an incompatible transfusion or from a previous pregnancy. Immunization to the D factor initially gives rise to antibody in the 19 S gamma globulin fraction, which later becomes replaced by 7 S antibody. The latter displays the properties of an immune agglutinin and is the antibody responsible for hemolytic manifestations in the infant. Because transfusion of fetal blood into the maternal circulation occurs to the greatest extent near the time of delivery, Rh-negative mothers pregnant with their first Rh-positive infant rarely become sensitized prior to term, and these infants seldom develop hemolytic complications. In subsequent pregnancies, however, the risk increases considerably and becomes greater thereafter with each Rh-positive infant. Once hemolytic disease has appeared in an infant, succeeding Rh-positive infants are almost invariably affected, often with increasing severity of the disease. The overall incidence of immunization of Rh-negative mothers at risk is nevertheless quite low, with antibody to D factor having been detected in less than 10% of Rh-negative subjects studied, even after five or more pregnancies. In some instances a failure of Rh immunization appeared to reflect an inability to respond to the antigen even when it was introduced in substantial quantities. Thus approximately 10% of Rh-negative subjects who were experimentally injected with Rh-positive cells failed to demonstrate any antibody response. In pregnancies in which Rh incompatibility between the mother and the fetus coexists with incompatibility of an A-B-O factor, the incidence of Rh immunization has been found to be significantly reduced. This protective effect has been ascribed to a rapid lysis of fetal cells that enter the maternal circulation because of the presence of the anti-**A** or anti-**B** antibody, thereby preventing the D factor from exerting an antigenic stimulus sufficient to produce immunization. The presence of certain other Rh antigens with the D antigen has in some cases also been found to diminish the antigenicity of the D factor. The Rh factor e and the combination of C and e have been shown to have this effect.

Clinical manifestations. The severity of the disease in the neonate may vary considerably, ranging from a mild or inapparent hemolytic process to severe anemia accompanied by generalized edema and heart failure and a rapidly fatal course. In hemolytic disease caused by Rh isoimmunization the clinical nature of the disease can often be predicted. If previous infants of the mother were affected, the disease will usually be of equal or greater severity in subsequent Rh-positive infants. A relationship of this kind does not occur in hemolytic disease resulting from A-B-O incompatibility.

Although jaundice is almost invariably a prominent clinical feature of hemolytic disease of the newborn, this finding is usually absent at birth because of the rapid clearance of bilirubin from the fetal circulation across the placental barrier. However, in severely affected infants, icterus may appear within hours after birth and may increase rapidly in intensity. Visible jaundice is usually present within the first 24 hours of life in any case of significant hemolytic disease. Infants who have received one or more intrauterine transfusions often appear jaundiced at birth.

Findings at birth are primarily attributable to the degree of anemia. The most severely affected infants present the picture of *hydrops fetalis,* with marked pallor, edema, and swelling of the chest and abdomen caused by effusion of fluid. The placentas of these infants are often large, pale, and edematous. Manifestations of severe anemia at birth most frequently accompany hemolytic disease resulting from Rh incompatibility. Infants with isoimmune hemolysis caused by A-B-O incompatibility most often develop jaundice during the first 24 hours of life without clinical evidence of anemia.

Enlargement of the spleen and liver is commonly present in infants with isoimmune hemolytic disease. If severe anemia is present, hepatosplenomegaly may in part be caused by congestive changes of heart failure.

In more severe forms of isoimmune hemolytic disease, petechiae and purpura may be present, sometimes accompanied by hemorrhagic complications. These infants often have low platelet counts, and in some instances hypofibrinogenemia and changes in other coagulation factors have been found to suggest the presence of disseminated intravascular coagulation.

Laboratory findings. Findings in the blood reflect a highly active process of red blood cell regeneration. Polychromasia is evident in stained blood smears; the reticulocyte count is elevated, sometimes reaching values as high as 50%; and in most patients considerable numbers of nucleated red blood cells are evident in the peripheral blood. The erythrocytes in Rh hemolytic disease are large and normochromic. In isoimmune disease caused by A-B-O incompatibility, densely staining microspherocytes are often a prominent finding in blood smears and are accompanied by an increased osmotic fragility of the red blood cells. This change may also be observed in some of the forms of isoimmune hemolytic disease caused by uncommon inciting antigens, but spherocytes are characteristically absent in Rh hemolytic disease.

The hemoglobin concentration and hematocrit may be reduced to a moderate or severe degree or may be entirely within the normal range in spite of evidence of an active hemolytic process. The degree of this compensatory change reflects the existing balance between the rate of red blood cell destruction and the capacity of the bone marrow activity to counterbalance the deficit. Although the rate of red blood cell production normally undergoes a rapid decline shortly after birth, in the presence of a hemolytic process it is apparent that the neonate is capable of active, sustained erythropoiesis when it is required. It is known that products of red blood cell lysis are among the most potent of erythropoietic stimulators, and it is likely that this mediating factor is an important one in supporting compensatory red blood cell production in infants with isoimmune hemolytic disease.

The white blood cell count is usually normal but may be elevated, occasionally to a marked degree. Reduction of the platelet count accompanied by other evidence of a hemorrhagic diathesis occurs only in severe hemolytic disease; these changes have been reported, however, to occur in about one third of fatal cases.

Destruction of sensitized red blood cells in the infant takes place primarily in reticuloendothelial organs, and free hemoglobin is not usually detectable in the serum. In cases of severe hemolytic disease, however, intravascular hemolysis may occur to a significant degree, resulting in grossly visible hemoglobinemia and hemoglobinuria.

Bilirubin levels in cord blood seldom exceed 5 mg/100 ml, with virtually all of the bilirubin consisting of the indirect-acting type. Levels of unconjugated bilirubin of greater than 5 mg/100 ml at birth are usually regarded as an indication of unusually severe hemolytic disease. In rare instances a substantial level of direct-acting bilirubin may also be present in the cord blood. Infants having this finding often exhibit prolonged icterus, lasting several weeks or months, together with other changes that suggest the presence of biliary obstruction. Infants who have received an intrauterine transfusion often have elevations of direct- and indirect-reacting bilirubinemia.

Hypoglycemia occasionally occurs in infants with more severe forms of isoimmune hemolytic disease. This finding has been shown to be accompanied by hyperinsulinism and hypertrophy of the pancreatic islets in these infants.

Diagnosis. To establish a definitive diagnosis of isoimmune hemolytic disease, blood group incompatibility between the mother and infant must be demonstrated, together with the presence of antibody bound to the infant's red blood cells. For detection of erythrocyte-bound antibody the direct Coombs antiglobulin test is the single most useful procedure. This test is usually positive in infants with Rh isoimmune disease but may be negative in mild cases. When the red blood cells are heavily coated by anti-**D** antibody the antigenic sites on the cell surfaces may be sufficiently masked so that the erythrocytes will fail to agglutinate with group D typing serum, causing the blood to be falsely typed as Rh negative. With the recognition of this possibility the finding should cause little difficulty in arriving at a correct diagnosis in such infants. The Coombs test on infant cells is usually negative if there have been several intrauterine transfusions. With the availability of improved antiglobulin sera, a positive direct Coombs test can now be demonstrated in a majority of infants with A-B-O isoimmune disease. In a sizeable percentage of these infants, however, the test will give a negative result, and the diagnosis must often remain presumptive. In hemolytic disease caused by incompatibility of the less commonly involved blood group factors a positive antiglobulin test can usually be obtained.

Evidence for the presence of Rh isoimmune hemolytic disease can often be detected prior to delivery by serial determinations for the titer of maternal anti-**D** blood group antibody during the pregnancy. Periodic titers are obtained routinely in each pregnancy of an Rh-negative woman, unless the father is also known to be Rh-negative. A rising antibody titer can be taken as presumptive evidence for the presence of hemolytic disease in the fetus. From the magnitude of the titer as well as from its rate of increase, it is also frequently possible to estimate the severity of the disease. Although the antibody titer is not a highly reliable quantitative indicator, in general the presence of a measurable titer at the beginning of the pregnancy, a rapidly rising titer, or a titer in albumin of 1:64 or greater must be regarded as strongly suggestive evidence of significant hemolytic disease. These findings indicate the need for studies that can yield more specific and reliable information. Antenatal measurement of maternal antibody titers has no predictive value in isoimmune hemolytic disease caused by A-B-O blood group incompatibility.

When the presence of hemolytic disease in utero is suspected on the basis of a high or rising anti-**D** titer or a history of a previously affected infant, a more reliable assessment can be made by analysis of samples of amniotic fluid. Products of hemolysis, primarily bilirubin, accumulate in the amniotic fluid when active red blood cell destruction occurs, and these can be readily detected and quantitated by spectrophotometric procedures. By this type of analysis it has been possible to assess the severity and course of hemolytic disease in the fetus with a high order of reliability, particularly when serial determinations are made. Amniocentesis for this type of study has gained wide acceptance in recent years and has generally been performed without difficulty and with few complications. In rare instances, however, amniocentesis appears to have resulted in fetal hemorrhage with passage of erythrocytes from the fetus into the maternal circulation to give rise to a significant increase in the rate of antibody formation (see p. 26).

Differential diagnosis. A variety of disorders of the neonate may share many of the clinical and laboratory features of isoimmune hemolytic disease. The management and prognosis in these conditions may vary considerably, and an accurate diagnosis must be obtained whenever possible.

Certain congenital infections, including cytomegalic inclusion disease, toxoplasmosis, rubella, and syphilis, often are accompanied by hemolytic anemia with jaundice, thrombocytopenia, and hepatosplenomegaly. Reactions to the direct Coombs antiglobulin test will be negative in all of these conditions, and other findings are usually present in each of them to indicate the identity of the infection. (For a detailed description of these neonatal infections see Chapter 8.)

Homozygous α-thalassemia in the newborn is characteristically accompanied by severe hemolytic anemia and a clinical picture resembling *hydrops fetalis.* This disorder has been reported thus far to occur only in Orientals, in whom Rh isoimmune disease is virtually nonexistant. A negative reaction to the antiglobulin test and hematologic findings characteristic of this disorder (p. 200) serve to establish a correct diagnosis.

Hereditary spherocytosis may initially appear as anemia with hyperbilirubinemia in the newborn period. Although the reaction to the Coombs antiglobulin test will be negative, the presence of spherocytes in peripheral blood smears may suggest a diagnosis of isoimmune hemolytic disease caused by A-B-O or other blood group incompatibility. By a careful family history and examination of blood smears from both of the parents for spherocytes a correct identification of this condition can usually be made.

Erythroblastemia is sometimes a notable finding in infants of diabetic mothers and may be accompanied by hepatomegaly. Findings specific to this disorder and an absence of significant hemolysis usually suffice to prevent diagnostic difficulty.

Bilirubin encephalopathy (kernicterus). Neurologic damage as a result of hyperbilirubinemia is among the most serious complications of hemolytic disease in the newborn infant. The encephalopathy is accompanied by yellow staining of the brain, with the brainstem and basal ganglia usually being most severely involved areas. The pigmentation is caused by the presence of unconjugated bilirubin, which is readily capable of penetrating the brain substance because of its high lipid solubility. Conjugated bilirubin, on the other hand, is poorly soluble in lipid and does not contribute to neurologic damage.

Kernicterus can result from elevated levels of unconjugated bilirubin resulting from any cause; but for reasons that are poorly understood, hemolytic disease appears to impose a greater risk of this complication than nonhemolytic hyperbilirubinemia of a comparable degree. Neurologic damage caused by bilirubin is largely, although not exclusively, confined to the newborn period, primarily because of the infrequency of greatly elevated levels of indirect-acting bilirubin beyond early infancy. Premature infants are particularly at risk for development of bilirubin encephalopathy (p. 227); their increased susceptibility has been attributed in part to a functional immaturity of the blood-brain barrier that facilitates the passage of bilirubin into the central nervous system.

There is substantial evidence to indicate that the risk of development of neurologic damage is directly related to the maximum plasma level of bilirubin that is reached. In general, the hazard for development of kernicterus is regarded as significant whenever the concentration of unconjugated bilirubin in the plasma exceeds 20 mg/100 ml. In the evaluation of an infant with hyperbilirubinemia, however, a number of additional factors must also be considered for a meaningful assessment of risk. A major fraction of the bilirubin present in blood is transported bound to albumin. If the albumin concentration of the plasma becomes reduced, the capacity for binding of bilirubin will become correspondingly lessened and will be exceeded at bilirubin levels of less than 20 mg/100 ml. The excess unbound pigment will be free to diffuse into the tissues, particularly the central nervous system. A number of drugs, most notably salicylates and the sulfonamides, also act to reduce the capacity of the plasma to transport bilirubin by competing for binding sites on the albumin. The effect of any of these drugs is to increase the hazard of neurologic damage, and it is consequently desirable to avoid the use of any of these agents in newborn infants. Other factors that appear to reduce bilirubin binding by the plasma include hypoxia, acidosis, and hypoglycemia. In any of these conditions an increased risk of bilirubin encephalopathy must be anticipated even when the bilirubin level remains substantially less than 20 mg/100 ml. In the premature infant neurologic damage is likely to develop at lower bilirubin levels than in a full-term infant, all other factors being comparable.

Kernicterus is never present at birth and must be regarded as a largely preventable disease. Evidence of encephalopathy in affected infants rarely occurs prior to 36 hours of life; its appearance in newborns with hemolytic disease is most common between 2 and 6 days of age.

Based on the observations of Van Praagh and others, the clinical features that characterize kernicterus can be divided into four phases. Initially, the infant exhibits hypotonia, lethargy, and a poor sucking reflex. The disease in this phase may be fatal, without further progression of the clinical picture. The second phase is characterized by the development of spasticity, often with opisthotonus, and is frequently accompanied by fever. In the third phase, beginning at about 1 week of age, the spasticity diminishes, sometimes with complete disappearance, to leave the misleading impression that kernicterus did not occur. The fourth phase appears beyond the neonatal period and consists of late sequelae, including spasticity, athetosis, partial or complete deafness, and retardation. Any newborn with hemolytic disease, but particularly if the infant is premature, should be observed closely for any evidence of the early changes of kernicterus.

Studies employing animal models have demonstrated conclusively that bilirubin deposited within tissues, including the brain, can be mobilized into the plasma following an exchange transfusion or an intravenous infusion of albumin. Although no clear evidence has been presented that neurologic damage caused by bilirubin can be reversed, prompt institution of measures that reduce the total body pool of bilirubin or that increase the capacity of the plasma to bind bilirubin will offer the greatest chance for reversing or at least minimizing damage to the nervous system. Although the early clinical features of bilirubin encephalopathy are relatively nonspecific and often are seen in sick infants having a variety of diseases, whenever these changes are seen in a newborn infant with hyperbilirubinemia, particularly when hemolytic disease is present, bilirubin encephalopathy must be assumed to have occurred, and appropriate measures should be undertaken without delay.

Although the neurologic sequelae of substantial degrees of hyperbilirubinemia in the newborn period are well known, considerable uncertainty remains concerning the effects of lesser degrees of bilirubin elevation in young infants. A number of studies have suggested that in the neonatal period, levels of bilirubin insufficient to produce overt neurologic damage may nevertheless result in more subtle effects in later childhood, including perceptual impairment, delayed speech development, hyperactivity, and learning difficulties. Although at the present time the criteria used for gauging maximum allowable bilirubin levels are intended to prevent kernicterus, these criteria ultimately may need to be revised to ensure that even more moderate degrees of hyperbilirubinemia are prevented from developing in the neonatal period.

Treatment. The management of an infant with isoimmune hemolytic disease is directed toward two major goals: the prevention of fetal or neonatal disability or death as a result of anemia and the prevention of neurologic sequelae caused by hyperbilirubinemia.

Severe anemia in the fetus, particularly in association with Rh isoimmunization, may give rise to heart failure in utero, often resulting in fetal death. A high incidence of stillbirths has occurred in pregnancies of strongly immunized women, and following an intrauterine death caused by anemia the risk of severe hemolytic disease in subsequent Rh-positive fetuses is considerable. Heart failure as a result of anemia can occur early in fetal life, but nearly one third of stillborns caused by Rh isoimmune disease have been found to have a gestational age of at least 37 weeks. On the basis of this finding early induction of labor, usually at about 37 weeks but in some cases earlier, has been employed as a means for improving the survival rate in this group of infants. The decision to carry out an early delivery, however, must take into account the increased hazards that accompany prematurity in these infants, particularly the added risk of bilirubin encephalopathy. Indications for early delivery of an affected infant include a previous maternal history of a severely affected or stillborn infant, evidence from amniotic fluid analysis of severe involvement of the fetus, or evidence of fetal distress. Early delivery of these infants should be undertaken only if facilities and experienced personnel are available to provide intensive care for a potentially sick premature. Advance preparations must be made for an exchange transfusion to be performed immediately after the delivery and at repeated intervals if necessary.

Prevention of intrauterine death caused by anemia in the previable fetus can also be accomplished by transfusion of the fetus in utero by a technique first introduced by Liley. In this procedure erythrocytes that are compatible with the mother's serum are periodically transfused by means of a catheter introduced into the peritoneal cavity of the fetus under fluoroscopic guidance. Although this form of treatment carries a substantial risk and requires specialized facilities and personnel, a considerable number of pregnancies have been successfully brought to term by the application of these procedures. The need for intrauterine transfusion is becoming increasingly less; and with more extensive application of measures for prevention of Rh immunization, it eventually may cease to be required.

Exchange transfusion. Procedures for exchange or replacement transfusion were

Table 9-2. Indications for exchange transfusion in infants with Coombs-positive hemolytic disease

	Observe	Consider exchange	Do exchange
		At birth	
History of previous offspring	No need for exchange transfusion	Exchange transfusion necessary or kernicterus	Death or near-death from erythroblastosis
Maternal Rh antibody titer	<1 : 64	>1 : 64	—
Clinical situation at birth	Apparently normal	Induced or spontaneous delivery of premature infant	Jaundice Fetal hydrops
Cord hemoglobin	>14 gm/100 ml	12-14 gm/100 ml	<12 gm/100 ml
Cord bilirubin	<4 mg/100 ml	4-5 mg/100 ml	>5 mg/100 ml
		After birth	
Capillary blood hemoglobin	>12 gm/100 ml	<12 gm/100 ml	<12 gm/100 ml and falling in first 24 hours
Serum bilirubin	<18 mg/100 ml	18-20 mg/100 ml	20 mg/100 ml in first 48 hours or 22 mg/100 ml on 2 successive determinations at 6-8 hour intervals after 48 hours
			Clinical signs suggesting kernicterus at any time or any bilirubin level

From McKay, R. J., Jr.: Pediatrics **33**:763, 1964. See Chapter 10 for indications in premature infants.

first employed extensively in the early 1950s and currently comprise the principal therapeutic measure available for the treatment of hemolytic disease of the newborn. As a result of an exchange transfusion, erythrocytes that are subject to premature destruction are replaced by donor cells that are not affected by the antibody present; a major fraction of the antibody itself is removed; and a significant quantity of bilirubin bound to albumin in the plasma is also withdrawn. If anemia is present, the red blood cell concentration can be increased during the course of the exchange transfusion by replacement with packed red blood cells for part of the blood that is removed.

An exchange transfusion is indicated in a newborn infant with hemolytic disease if severe anemia is present, if the bilirubin level is sufficient to impose a risk of neurologic damage, or if the hemolytic process is sufficiently severe so that either of these complications is likely to develop. A practical guide for evaluating the need for an initial exchange transfusion was devised by R. J. McKay and is outlined in Table 9-2. In general, an initial exchange transfusion serves chiefly to remove a major fraction of the antibody-coated erythrocytes and to correct existing anemia. Subsequent exchange procedures are primarily of benefit for the removal of bilirubin.

Blood used for an exchange transfusion optimally should be freshly drawn or in any case not older than 2 days if at all possible. Blood that is stored for longer periods is likely to contain potentially dangerous quantities of free potassium and is more readily subject to hemolysis, which will further contribute to hyperbilirubinemia in the infant. Erythrocytes in stored acid-citrate-dextrose (ACD) anticoagulated blood also become readily depleted of intracellular ATP and 2,3-diphosphoglycerate, which produces adverse changes in the oxygen-binding properties of the intracellular hemoglobin. Suitable donor cells must be compatible with both the infant's and mother's serum, and whenever possible crossmatching against both serums should be performed. In most instances of hemolytic disease caused by Rh isoimmunization, type O, Rh-negative blood from a donor having a low titer of anti-**A** and anti-**B** is most suitable. For exchange transfusion of an infant with A-B-O hemolytic disease, type O blood of the same Rh type as that of the infant is appropriate. It is a wise precaution to be certain that the blood donor does not carry sickle cell trait; an instance of fatal intravascular sickling was reported to have occurred when blood from such a donor was administered to a newborn infant in an exchange transfusion.

In a full-term infant an exchange transfusion with 500 ml of blood will achieve a 2-volume exchange, based on an estimated blood volume of about 250 ml in a 3 kg infant and will result in a replacement of approximately 85% of the erythrocytes by those of the donor blood. In a small premature or a full-term infant in poor condition, the initial exchange transfusion will often need to be limited to a smaller volume. Whole blood is used if the infant is not significantly anemic. If anemia needs to be corrected, packed red blood cells can be substituted for the whole blood during part of the procedure.

The exchange transfusion should be performed under rigidly aseptic conditions. The infant is restrained, ideally in a heated mantle, and leads are attached for continuous monitoring of the heartbeat. Except under unusual circumstances, a catheter inserted in the umbilical vein is used for withdrawing blood from the infant and for infusion of donor blood. In this procedure, aliquots of 10 to 20 ml of blood are removed, followed each time by replacement with an equal volume of the donor blood. Volume adjustments are made periodically as indicated, based on changes in the venous pressure; the latter is determined by measurement of the height of the fluid column in the umbilical catheter. When ACD-anticoagulated blood is used in the exchange transfusion, careful administration of 1 ml of 10% calcium gluconate solution after each 100 ml of blood infused is a useful precaution for prevention of hypocalcemia.

At the conclusion of the procedure, blood samples are taken for determination of the hemoglobin concentration and bilirubin level. Administration of antibiotics following an exchange transfusion is not warranted ordinarily in the absence of a specific indication.

Subsequent exchange transfusions are indicated if bilirubin levels become excessively elevated or whenever there is evidence of kernicterus. Bilirubin determinations should be performed at 4- to 8-hour intervals following each exchange transfusion and continued as long as the level remains significantly elevated. In exchange transfusions the efficiency of bilirubin withdrawal can be substantially increased by an infusion of albumin prior to the exchange procedure. The additional albumin augments the capacity of the plasma to bind bilirubin and can result in a transfer of a considerable quantity of bilirubin from tissues into the blood. Salt-poor albumin, in a dose of 1 gm/kg body weight, is infused 1 to 2 hours prior to the exchange transfusion in order to achieve a maximal effect. Albumin should never be administered to an infant with severe anemia, edema or other evidence of congestive failure, or cardiovascular overload, because of the hazard of producing dangerous hypervolemia.

Phototherapy. This form of treatment has recently come into wide use as an adjunct to exchange transfusions in the management of infants with hemolytic disease. Phototherapy is potentially of value in these infants whenever hyperbilirubinemia is likely to be the major indication for an exchange transfusion. Infants with Rh isoimmune disease of a moderate to severe degree may benefit from phototherapy following an initial exchange transfusion, and mildly affected infants without significant anemia may be spared the necessity of an exchange transfusion entirely. Hemolytic disease caused by A-B-O incompatibility, in which elevated levels of bilirubin often comprise the only important element of risk, may be the most appropriate indication for phototherapy within this group of disorders (p. 232). Studies of the effectiveness of phototherapy in A-B-O hemolytic disease have shown it to be capable of achieving a significant reduction in bilirubin levels, and undoubtedly it has reduced the need for exchange transfusions in some of these infants. (For a description of phototherapy and its applications see p. 229.)

Late complications of isoimmune hemolytic disease

Anemia. Following one or more exchange transfusions, development of a mild to moderate degree of anemia is a frequent occurrence. In most instances the anemia appears to result from a persistence of the hemolytic process, superimposed upon a reduction of the red blood cell mass of the infant caused by the exchange transfusion. The anemia in these infants is usually self-limiting and requires no specific therapy in most cases. If the hemoglobin concentration of the infant falls below 8 to 9 gm/100 ml prior to hospital discharge, a small transfusion of packed erythrocytes is indicated. Any infant receiving an exchange transfusion at birth should also be given adequate dietary iron supplementation in order to compensate for the decrease in iron stores caused by the loss of erythrocytes from the exchange procedure.

In some infants with isoimmune hemolytic disease, particularly those not requiring exchange transfusion, a precipitous fall in the hemoglobin concentration may occur, most commonly between 10 and 20 days of age. The complication is particularly frequent in premature infants. The cause of this late anemia is obscure. In most instances the anemia subsides without therapy, but in some cases it may be sufficiently severe to require supportive transfusions of packed erythrocytes. Because of the risk of anemia of rapid onset in affected infants not requiring exchange transfusion, close observation of these infants for 4 to 6 weeks after their discharge from the hospital is recommended.

Persistent jaundice. A small percentage of infants with isoimmune hemolytic disease exhibit prolonged jaundice for weeks or months beyond the neonatal period. A major fraction of the bilirubin in the plasma of these infants is of the direct-acting type, and the jaundice is accompanied by findings suggestive of biliary obstruction, including acholic stools and the presence of bile in the urine. In many instances an elevation in the concentration of direct-acting bilirubin in these infants can be detected at birth in cord blood samples. This syndrome has been designated the inspissated bile syndrome and formerly was thought to occur by plugging of bile duct canaliculi as a result of excessive bilirubin production. This mechanism is no longer thought to be correct, although the pathogenesis of this syndrome in most instances remains unknown. In some infants with these findings, evidence of hepatocellular disease has been found. No specific therapy is usually required, and the infants almost invariably recover completely by 3 to 6 months of age.

Prevention of Rh isoimmunization. Advances over the past decade have led to the development of highly effective means for the prevention of primary isoimmunization of Rh-negative mothers to the D blood group antigen. The basis of this treatment was derived in part from the earlier observation that Rh isoimmunization was rare in mothers whose infants were also A-B-O incompatible (p. 30).

For prevention, gamma globulin is prepared from plasma of Rh-negative individuals who are immunized to achieve high titers of anti-**D** activity. By administration of the gamma globulin to Rh-negative mothers immediately after delivery of each Rh-positive infant, sensitization can be entirely prevented in a very large percentage of patients. The effectiveness of the gamma globulin treatment is probably caused chiefly by destruction by the antibody of fetal erythrocytes in the maternal circulation, thereby interfering with their antigenic effectiveness. The entry of fetal cells into the maternal blood occurs primarily at the time of delivery, and the perinatal period is therefore the time of greatest risk for immunization. With routine administration of anti-**D** gamma globulin to Rh-negative women following each delivery, it appears likely that it will be possible in coming years virtually to abolish Rh isoimmune hemolytic disease as a cause of infant morbidity and mortality.

Hemolytic anemia caused by congenital deficiencies of red blood cell enzymes

Metabolic properties of erythrocytes of the newborn. The maturation of nucleated red blood cell precursors leading to the formation of mature erythrocytes is normally accompanied by the loss of a considerable number of metabolic processes of the red blood cell. Biosynthesis of nucleic acids, protein, and lipids can no longer proceed in the fully mature erythrocyte; and because of the absence of mitochondria at this stage, heme synthesis, the tricarboxylic acid pathway, and the cytochrome-linked electron transport system are also lacking. As a result of these changes, maintenance of the necessary metabolic functions of the mature red blood cell depends upon a very limited number of energy-yielding and related biochemical pathways. The virtual absence of alternative metabolic pathways for most of the energy-yielding reactions causes the red blood cell to be unusually susceptible to adverse changes whenever any of the existing enzyme-dependent metabolic processes is defective.

Energy for cellular functions of the mature red blood cell is derived almost exclusively from the metabolism of glucose. The Embden-Meyerhof glycolytic pathway accounts for approximately 90% of the glucose consumed by red blood cells under normal conditions. Glucose catabolism by this pathway results in the formation of lactate as a final product with two moles of ATP generated per mole of glucose metabolized. Other important products of the Embden-Meyerhof pathway include 2,3-diphosphoglycerate, which serves as a source for potential ATP formation as well as a regulator of the oxygen affinity of hemoglobin, and NADH, which is the major cofactor required for maintaining the heme iron of hemoglobin in the reduced state.

The hexose monophosphate shunt pathway, although quantitatively less significant in the erythrocyte, is nevertheless essential in the economy of the cell because it provides the only means for generation of NADPH. This cofactor is specifically required for the enzymatic reduction of glutathione, a sulfhydryl-containing tripeptide. This substance serves to prevent oxidative damage to cellular components largely by its function as a cofactor for glutathione peroxidase, an enzyme that catalyzes the reductive decomposition of hydrogen peroxide. There is considerable evidence that peroxide formation in the red blood cell is the principal mediator of adverse oxidative changes that occur in the course of certain infections and from drugs, chemicals, and toxins. The peroxide formation is thought to result from interaction of the oxidative agents with oxyhemoglobin within the erythrocytes.

Red blood cells of the newborn differ from those of the adult by a number of quantitative differences in these metabolic pathways, and as a result of these changes the cells are more susceptible to certain adverse conditions. A majority of the enzymes of the glycolytic pathways have been found to be elevated in erythrocytes of newborn infants. These changes, however, probably reflect a younger average population of circulating red blood cells in the infant rather than a specific finding unique to this period of life. The overall rate of glucose consumption by red blood cells of newborns is increased, and ATP levels in the cells have been found to be normal or elevated. The incorporation of inorganic phosphate into ATP was shown to be reduced in comparison with cells from adults, and the intracellular ATP is subject to a more rapid rate of depletion when the cells are incubated. Although the basis for these findings has not been precisely determined, a major factor may be a reduction of phosphofructokinase activity, which was shown to occur in the neonatal period and which could impose a significant rate-limiting effect on ATP production.

The hexose monophosphate shunt enzymes are also increased in activity in red blood cells of the newborn, and glucose catabolism by this pathway has been shown to be capable of increasing considerably in response to oxidative stimuli. Instability of reduced glutathione has been demonstrated when erythrocytes of newborns were incubated with phenylhydrazine, but this change was prevented when additional glucose was added to the cells. In spite of apparently normal activity of the hexose monophosphate shunt pathway in red blood cells of newborns, normal infants and especially prematures nevertheless exhibit a significant risk of abnormal hemolytic reactions from drugs or chemicals having oxidant properties. When the erythrocytes are exposed to these agents, increased numbers of Heinz bodies form, reflecting precipitation of oxidatively-damaged hemoglobin. In erythrocytes of adults, excessive Heinz-body formation under these conditions occurs only when an intrinsic red blood cell abnormality is present. Red blood cells of the newborn have been found to have a reduced activity of glutathione peroxidase, which may account in part for the abnormal response of these cells to oxidative stress. Catalase, another enzyme that removes peroxide, is also reduced in activity in erythrocytes of newborns.

Glucose-6-phosphate dehydrogenase (G-6-PD) deficiency. More than 50 variant forms of erythrocytic G-6-PD have thus far been identified, and considerably more are likely to be found. The enzymatic activity associated with these mutant forms is variable, ranging from a considerable increase over the activity of the normal enzyme to a reduction of a mild, moderate, or severe degree, in some instances with an almost total absence of enzymatic activity. Enzyme forms having deficient activity occur with particularly high frequency in certain racial groups, including Sephardic Jews, black persons, Southern Europeans, Arabs, Chinese, and Southeast Asians.

The genetic determinant of this enzyme is inherited as an X-linked trait. Significant degrees of enzyme deficiency are therefore encountered primarily in males. In American black persons, however, the incidence of G-6-PD deficiency may be as high as 14%, and homozygous females are also occasionally seen. Even among heterozygous females, a moderate to severe degree of enzyme deficiency may be found, presumably reflecting X-chromosome inactivation chiefly involving chromosomes that bear the normal G-6-PD gene.

The *clinical expression* of G-6-PD deficiency depends largely on the degree of reduction of enzyme activity in the red blood cells. Three principal forms of clinical disease have been recognized in this disorder.

Drug-induced hemolysis is the most characteristic clinical manifestation of relatively mild G-6-PD deficiency and is the form most often seen in black persons. Affected individuals usually demonstrate no hematologic abnormality under normal conditions, but when they are exposed to certain drugs or chemicals (see outline below) or in the course of an infection they may develop an acute episode of hemolytic anemia. The anemia will sometimes be severe in these patients but usually requires no treatment and is self-limiting.

DRUGS AND CHEMICALS KNOWN TO PRODUCE HEMOLYSIS IN PATIENTS WITH G-6-PD DEFICIENCY

A. Analgesics
   1. Acetanilid
   2. Acetylsalicylic acid
   3. Acetophenetidin (Phenacetin)
   4. Antipyrine
   5. Aminopyrine (Pyridon)
B. Sulfonamides and sulfones
   1. Sulfanilamide
   2. Sulfapyridine
   3. N^2 acetylsulfanilamide
   4. Sulfacetamide
   5. Sulfisoxazole (Gantrisin)
   6. Thiazolsulfone
   7. Salicylazosulfapyridine (Azulfidine)
   8. Sulfoxone
   9. Sulfamethoxypyridazine (Kynex)
C. Antimalarials
   1. Primaquine phosphate
   2. Pamaquine naphthoate
   3. Pentaquine phosphate
   4. Quinacrine hydrochloride (Atabrine)
D. Nonsulfonamide antibacterial agents
   1. Furazolidone
   2. Nitrofurantoin (Furadantin)
   3. Chloramphenicol
   4. Paraaminosalicylic acid
E. Miscellaneous
   1. Naphthalene
   2. Vitamin K (water-soluble analogues)
   3. Probenecid
   4. Trinitrotoluene
   5. Methylene blue
   6. Dimercaprol (BAL)
   7. Phenylhydrazine
   8. Quinine
   9. Quinidine

Congenital nonspherocytic hemolytic anemia is a less common form of clinical expression of G-6-PD deficiency and reflects a more severe reduction of enzyme activity in the erythrocytes. Affected individuals exhibit lifelong hemolytic anemia accompanied by splenomegaly and jaundice. The hemolytic process becomes greatly accelerated following exposure to oxidant drugs or chemicals or during infections.

Favism is a poorly understood form of hemolytic anemia that occurs as severe episodes of hemolysis following ingestion of fava beans or exposure to pollen of the fava bean plant. Affected individuals all demonstrate a severe deficiency of G-6-PD in their erythrocytes. Acute hemolytic episodes have been described in young breast-fed infants deficient in G-6-PD following fava bean ingestion by their nursing mothers.

The clinical consequences of G-6-PD deficiency in the newborn depend on the degree of deficiency of the enzyme and on the presence of other precipitating factors. Normal full-term black infants with mild G-6-PD deficiency have not been found to demonstrate an increased incidence of hyperbilirubinemia. On the other hand, in premature infants and in full-term infants having more severe forms of enzyme deficiency, a higher than normal incidence of hyperbilirubinemia in the absence of other precipitating factors has been reported. Hyperhemolysis and jaundice in the newborn period can occur in infants with any of the forms of G-6-PD deficiency following exposure to oxidant drugs or chemicals. Drug-induced hemolysis may follow administration of the offending agent to the infant or may result from medications given to the mother late in the pregnancy or during lactation. In some instances, however, severe neonatal jaundice occurs in infants with G-6-PD deficiency in the absence of any apparent precipitating factor.

The clinical severity of hemolytic reactions may be affected by a number of other factors, including the maturity of the infant, the presence of hypoxia, hypoglycemia, or infection, and the dosage of the offending agent. In most instances hemolytic episodes are relatively mild and result in hyperbilirubinemia without a severe degree of anemia. In some instances, however, anemia may develop rapidly and with life-threatening severity. Hyperbilirubinemia may be of sufficient magnitude to produce kernicterus unless suitable measures are taken to prevent this complication.

Laboratory findings include a variable degree of anemia, hyperbilirubinemia consisting mainly of the unconjugated bilirubin fraction, and reticulocytosis. Severe hemolytic episodes usually are also accompanied by changes in the morphologic characteristics of the red blood cells, including poikilocytosis and cellular fragmentation. Increased numbers of Heinz bodies in the erythrocytes can be demonstrated by supravital staining. Deficiency of G-6-PD activity can be readily detected with the use of any of a number of simple screening tests. A positive reaction should also be confirmed by a specific analysis for quantitation of enzyme activity. Occasionally when the reticulocyte count is substantially elevated, particularly following an acute hemolytic episode, deficiency of the enzyme may be temporarily obscured because of the increased activity of G-6-PD in reticulocytes and young erythrocytes.

The anemia in these infants is usually self-limiting and seldom requires any specific measure. Hyperbilirubinemia is most often the major complication. A screening test for G-6-PD deficiency is indicated in any infant with unexplained hyperbilirubinemia, and those identified as being affected should be observed closely, with frequent determinations of the serum bilirubin concentration. Bilirubin levels of greater than 20 mg/100 ml are generally regarded as an indication for exchange transfusion. Phototherapy may be sufficient to prevent dangerous hyperbilirubinemia in infants with milder degrees of hemolysis and may be particularly useful in prematures. Medications known to precipitate hemolytic reactions in this disorder should be carefully avoided.

Other erythrocytic enzyme abnormalities that predispose the infant to drug-induced hemolysis. A number of other less common enzyme deficiency disorders have been identified that also produce hemolytic episodes following exposure to certain drugs and chemical agents (see the outline on p. 194). This group includes deficiencies of the enzymes glutathione synthetase, glutathione reductase, and glutathione peroxidase. Some of these disorders have been implicated as causes of anemia and hyperbilirubinemia in newborn infants. This group of disorders can be readily identified by the presence of a decreased concentration of glutathione in erythrocytes or by glutathione instability following incubation of the cells with acetylphenylhydrazine. Activity of G-6-PD is normal. Specific enzymatic assays are required to establish a precise diagnosis. Principles of management are the same as for G-6-PD deficiency.

Pyruvate kinase deficiency. This disorder results from any of a number of abnormalities of the erythrocytic enzyme pyruvate kinase and is expressed as a hemolytic anemia with a variable degree of severity. All of the forms of this disorder are inherited as an autosomal recessive characteristic. Heterozygous carriers exhibit reduced activity of the enzyme in their erythrocytes but are hematologically normal. The hemolytic process in homozygous individuals stems from a reduced capacity of the cells to produce ATP.

Anemia and jaundice in the newborn period have been reported in a large percentage of patients with this disorder. Hyperbilirubinemia may be of sufficient magnitude to produce kernicterus if untreated.

The anemia is accompanied by increased numbers of reticulocytes in the blood and often by erythroblastemia. The diagnosis is established by a specific enzymatic assay for pyruvate kinase activity. A simple rapid screening test for detection of a deficiency of this enzyme is also available.

As with other hemolytic disorders that occur in the newborn period, hyperbilirubinemia is potentially among the most serious complications. One or more exchange transfusions may be required to prevent neurologic damage and are indicated whenever the concentration of unconjugated bilirubin in the serum reaches a level of 20 mg/100 ml. If the anemia is severe, supportive transfusions of packed red blood cells may be required initially and later at periodic intervals. In older children splenectomy will sometimes be of value, particularly in reducing the transfusion requirement.

Hemolytic anemia caused by deficiencies of other glycolytic enzymes. Deficiencies in the red blood cells of a number of other glycolytic enzymes have also been implicated as the basis for congenital hemolytic disease. Most of these disorders are inherited as autosomal recessive traits, and all of them are uncommon. Identification of each individual entity requires specific determinations of enzymatic activity. A deficiency of the enzyme 2,3-diphosphoglycerate mutase has been documented as a cause of anemia and jaundice in the newborn period. Deficiencies of other glycolytic enzymes are also likely to produce similar findings. Management of affected infants is as described for pyruvate kinase deficiency.

Hemolytic anemias caused by intrinsic abnormalities of the erythrocyte membrane. A group of congenital hemolytic disorders has been demonstrated to have as a common feature an intrinsic defect of the erythroctyes that apparently involves the cellular membrane. The precise nature of the abnormality has not been ascertained in any of these conditions, but a number of studies have shown that defective membrane function exists, which causes the erythrocytes to be excessively permeable to electrolytes. Because of their increased ion permeability the cells are more susceptible to adverse osmotic changes, which in turn are thought to produce premature hemolysis. In most of these conditions the affected erythrocytes exhibit distinctive morphologic changes that often permit these disorders to be readily identified.

Hereditary spherocytosis. This disorder is characterized by the presence of variable numbers of spherocytic erythroctyes and hemolytic anemia. The abnormal red blood cells in this condition exhibit an increased susceptibility to lysis under hypotonic conditions and have been shown to be abnormally permeable to sodium and potassium. Glucose consumption and ATP production occur at a more rapid rate than in normal erythrocytes, apparently representing compensatory energy-yielding reactions. The additional ATP appears to be required to support an increased rate of active ion transport, which is needed to maintain normal sodium and potassium concentrations within the cells. Although the primary defect in this disorder stems from an intrinsic erythrocyte abnormality, red blood cell destruction occurs almost exclusively in the spleen, and splenectomy will usually terminate the hemolytic process. The disorder is transmitted as a dominant trait, but in as much as 30% of cases spherocytes will not be present in blood smears of either parent. However, in some of these apparently unaffected parents other evidence of abnormal erythrocyte permeability to cations can be demonstrated, suggesting incomplete expression of the abnormal gene.

A significant percentage of affected individuals demonstrate evidence of spherocytosis in early infancy (Fig. 9-3). Pallor can be noted in the neonatal period in some affected infants, although the anemia is rarely severe. Hyperbilirubinemia is a frequent complication, however, and may necessitate one or more exchange transfusions to prevent kernicterus. Splenomegaly is a usual finding in patients with spherocytosis, but may not be apparent in the neonate.

Laboratory findings include hyperbilirubinemia and a variable degree of anemia. Elevation of the reticulocyte count is a typical finding, even in the absence of a significant degree of anemia, and in most cases spherocytes are readily observable in stained smears of peripheral blood. Al-

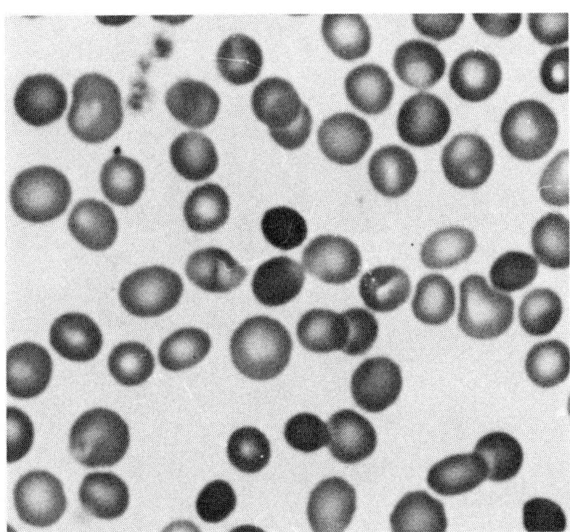

Fig. 9-3. Blood smear of a patient with hereditary spherocytosis. The spherocytes appear as densely stained cells with an absence of central pallor.

though increased osmotic fragility is a prominent characteristic of the erythrocytes in hereditary spherocytosis, the osmotic fragility test may not be reliable for diagnostic purposes in the newborn because of a variable and generally greater resistance of the red blood cells to osmotic lysis in the neonatal period.

In most instances a presumptive diagnosis may be readily confirmed on the basis of a positive family history or by the demonstration of spherocytes in a blood smear of one of the parents. In the event that these avenues are unrewarding it may be difficult or impossible to distinguish this disorder with certainty from mild isoimmune hemolytic disease. A direct Coombs test with red blood cells of the infant and a blood type of both the infant and the mother should always be performed when spheroctyes are detected in a newborn; these tests will usually allow a correct diagnosis to be made. Persistence of spherocytes beyond infancy will confirm a diagnosis of hereditary spherocytosis.

Anemia in the newborn period is rarely severe in this disorder. Occasionally, however, the hemoglobin concentration may fall to less than 7 gm/100 ml, and a transfusion of packed red blood cells will be required. Infants with jaundice must be observed carefully, and bilirubin determinations performed at frequent intervals. Elevation of the indirect-reacting bilirubin fraction to 20 mg/100 ml is an indication for exchange transfusion of these infants. Phototherapy is a valuable measure in less severely affected infants and may obviate the need for exchange transfusion in some instances.

Splenectomy is the definitive therapeutic measure in hereditary spheroctyosis and usually results in elimination of all of the untoward consequences of the disorder. However, splenectomy is contraindicated in infants less than 2 years of age because of a risk of serious infections at this age following removal of the spleen. Infants beyond the neonatal period may require periodic transfusions of packed red blood cells if the anemia is severe.

Hereditary elliptocytosis. This abnormality is characterized by the production of erythrocytes of which variable numbers are elliptical in shape. The defect is transmitted as an autosomal dominant trait. In most forms of this disorder the morphologic change is not associated with a measurable shortening of red blood cell survival. In other forms hemolytic anemia is present, often accompanied by jaundice and splenomegaly. Available evidence suggests that the hemolytic forms of this disorder result from a red blood cell membrane defect with abnormal ion permeability similar to that described in hereditary spherocytosis.

Hemolytic disease caused by elliptocytosis in the neonatal period results in a variable degree of anemia with reticulocytosis and jaundice. Elliptocytes can usually be found without difficulty in blood smears of these infants, although in some cases the erythrocytes may not demonstrate the distinctive morphologic changes characteristic of this disorder for a period of several months. Management of these infants is as described for hereditary spherocytosis.

Congenital stomatocytosis. A diverse group of hemolytic disorders share as a common feature a morphologic abnormality of the erythrocytes characterized by the presence of one or more slitlike areas of central pallor that produce a mouthlike appearance (Fig. 9-4). Variable degrees of anemia have been found in association with these abnormalities, and in some cases a familial incidence has been described. These disorders may appear in the neonatal period with findings resembling those of infants with hereditary spherocytosis. Sim-

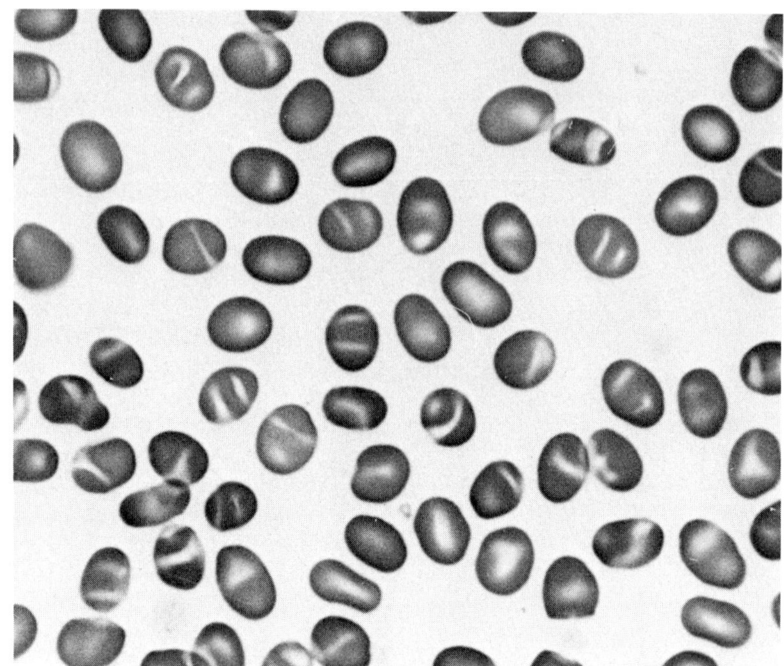

Fig. 9-4. Blood smear of an infant with a form of hereditary stomatocytosis.

ilar principles of management are appropriate.

Hemolytic anemia of vitamin E deficiency in premature infants. A moderately severe degree of hemolytic anemia has been observed in premature infants demonstrated to be deficient in vitamin E. The anemia in these infants was frequently accompanied by the appearance of variable numbers of irregularly contracted erythrocytes in smears of peripheral blood. Increased numbers of reticulocytes were characteristically present, and platelet counts were often increased. Severe edema unassociated with cardiovascular dysfunction or hypoproteinemia has also been observed in a group of these infants. Administration of vitamin E in the form of α-tocopherol produced a rapid reversal of the abnormal findings in these infants.

Disorders of hemoglobin structure, biosynthesis, and function

Human hemoglobin molecules are made up of four subunit components, each of which contains a globin protein chain and an iron-porphyrin moiety. The latter forms the site for the reversible binding of oxygen. Each of the normal human hemoglobins demonstrates unique characteristics that result from differences in the amino acid composition of the globin chain proteins.

Beyond the first year of life hemoglobin A (adult hemoglobin) forms a major hemoglobin component in the erythrocytes of normal individuals. This hemoglobin contains a pair of subunits designated α and a pair of β subunits ($\alpha_2\beta_2$). A minor hemoglobin, hemoglobin A_2, is also present in adult life but normally does not comprise more than 3% of the total. This hemoglobin is composed of a pair of α subunits identical to those of hemoglobin A and a pair of δ-chains unique to this hemoglobin type ($\alpha_2\delta_2$).

Hemoglobin production during the embryonic and fetal periods is characterized by the synthesis of two unique hemoglobin types. In the earliest stages of erythropoiesis a primitive hemoglobin type is elaborated for a very brief period. This form is designated embyronic hemoglobin and is composed of α and ϵ globin chains. Beyond approximately 12 weeks of gestation this hemoglobin is no longer detectable. The predominant hemoglobin produced during intrauterine development is hemoglobin F (fetal hemoglobin), which has a composition $\alpha_2\gamma_2$, the α-chains being identical to those of other hemoglobins. Hemoglobin F is characterized by resistance to denaturation by alkali, a property that forms the basis for a simple method for its detection and quantitation (p. 177). Fetal hemoglobin exhibits very little interaction with 2,3-diphosphoglycerate and other intracellular anions that normally bring about a reduction of the oxygen affinity of most of the other hemoglobin types. As a result of this difference, erythroctyes containing mainly hemoglobin F ordinarily exhibit a higher oxygen affinity than do red blood cells containing hemoglobin A. The increased oxygen affinity of fetal blood may facilitate transplacental oxygen transport to the fetal circulation.

The concentration of fetal hemoglobin in cord blood from full-term infants normally varies from 65% to 95% of the total hemoglobin, the remainder being almost entirely hemoglobin A. In premature infants the percentage of fetal hemoglobin is generally higher than in term infants. Hemoglobin A can be detected in the fetus as early as 10 weeks of gestation. Significant quantities of this hemoglobin are not produced, however, until after 30 weeks, when the fetal hemoglobin gradually begins to be replaced by the adult forms. By 6 months of age hemoglobin F makes up only a small percentage of the hemoglobin of the normal infant, and by 2 years of age it comprises about 1% to 2%, a level that persists for the remainder of adult life. Hemoglobin A_2 production is closely linked to that of hemoglobin A and represents about 2.5% of the hemoglobin A present at any period of development.

Congenital disorders that primarily affect the hemoglobin molecule have been classified broadly into two major categories: the hemoglobinopathies, which represent structural changes in the molecule as a result of amino acid substitutions in the globin chains, and the thalassemias, which denote a reduced synthesis of individual globin chains, the structures of which are normal. These abnormalities may involve globin chains of any of the hemoglobin types.

Because of the variation in the hemoglobin composition of the blood at different stages of development, abnormalities of a particular globin chain will be expressed only in the period during which the involved hemoglobins are produced in significant quantities. Consequently, abnormalities of the γ-chains are expressed almost exclusively during the fetal and neonatal period. β-chain abnormalities, on the other hand, generally produce no adverse effects until the infant is 3 to 6 months old, at which time a predominance of hemoglobin A first develops. Because all of the normal hemoglobins contain α-chains, abnormalities of this globin component are expressed throughout fetal and postnatal life.

Abnormalities of hemoglobin structure (hemoglobinopathies)

γ-Chain abnormalities. A number of hemoglobin variants have been described in which an amino acid substitution was demonstrated in the γ-chains of fetal hemoglobin. Every reported instance of these abnormalities was discovered in the course of electrophoretic surveys of cord blood hemoglobins, and none has been associated with known pathologic consequences. Consistent with evidence that multiple pairs of allelic γ-chains genes are normally present, hemoglobins containing abnormal γ-chains all have been found to comprise only a small fraction (usually 10% to 15%) of the total fetal hemoglobin. Beyond 3 to 6 months of age these abnormalities can no longer be detected.

β-Chain abnormalities. Structural changes affecting the β-chain account for a substantial majority of the known variant hemoglobins. In the United States, however, all except sickle cell disease and hemoglobin C are of rare occurrence. Because of the relatively small percentage of adult hemoglobin in blood of the neonate, none of the β-chain abnormalities are known to have produced clinical manifestations at birth.

By means of electrophoretic methods, most notably a procedure of agar gel electrophoresis carried out at pH 6.2, sickle hemoglobin and other β-chain variants can be identified with a high order of reliability in hemoglobin prepared from cord blood. Moreover, in most instances the presence of hemoglobin S in the newborn can be confirmed by a sickling test using metabisulfite as a reducing agent. On the other hand, hemoglobin solubility tests such as the Sickledex method are generally not suitable for the detection of sickle hemoglobin in cord blood, because a positive result can be readily obscured by the presence of a large quantity of hemoglobin F.

In a number of hospitals it has been established as a routine procedure to perform screening tests for sickle hemoglobin in all black obstetrical patients because of the high incidence (7% to 12%) of sickle hemoglobinopathy in this population. A positive result in the mother may be taken as a suitable indication for electrophoretic studies of cord blood hemoglobin from the infant. Although these studies are more easily performed after the infant is several months old, a diagnosis at birth affords an opportunity for improved management of infants with sickle cell disease as well as for providing genetic counseling for the parents.

Thalassemias. *β-Thalassemia* (Cooley's anemia; Mediterranean anemia) is now known to consist of a group of related disorders in which the synthesis of β-chains of hemoglobin A is selectively impaired. The severity of the defect can vary widely among the various forms of β-thalassemia, and any of these disorders may exist in either a heterozygous or homozygous state. The most severe homozygous forms produce a degree of anemia for which periodic transfusions are required to sustain life.

Because only hemoglobin A is affected in this disorder, the synthesis of fetal hemoglobin is not impaired in affected individuals. Hemoglobin production in the fetus and newborn is therefore only minimally suppressed. In most instances findings related to anemia first become apparent when the infant is beyond the age of 2 to 6 months. A diagnosis can be established in most cases by demonstrating an elevated percentage of hemoglobin A_2 in red blood cell hemolysates or a persistence of elevated levels of hemoglobin F beyond the first months of life. With the application of specialized procedures for assessment of rates of globin chain synthesis it has been possible to establish a diagnosis of β-thalassemia at birth.

α-Thalassemias result from a selective deficiency of α-chain synthesis and comprise a diverse group of disorders. Because α-chain synthesis is required for production of fetal as well as of adult hemoglobins, these disorders are manifested during the fetal and neonatal periods as well as in adult life.

The highest incidence of α-thalassemia has been found in blacks and in Oriental populations. Available evidence has suggested that the varieties that occur most commonly in black persons represent a relatively mild biosynthetic defect. The genetics of α-chain inheritance remain to be clarified, and the genetic nature of α-thalassemia is therefore also not well defined. It appears likely that at least in some individuals four independent α-chain genetic loci exist. Based on this model four possible forms of expression of an α-thalassemia gene have been postulated. These include (1) a "silent carrier" state without any apparent hematologic disorder, (2) a mild abnormality accompanied by hypochromic anemia, (3) hemoglobin H disease, an anemic disorder characterized by the presence of variable amounts of hemoglobin H (β_4) and hemoglobin Barts (γ_4), and (4) a severe condition apparently incompatible with extrauterine survival, in which α-chain synthesis is virtually or completely absent.

Clinical presentation. Mild to moderately severe forms of α-thalassemia in the newborn period commonly appear as a relatively mild hemolytic state accompanied by hypochromia of the erythrocytes and reticulocytosis. The diagnosis is established by hemoglobin electrophoresis, with the demonstration of hemoglobin Barts (γ_4), a fast-moving electrophoretic fraction. Small quantities of hemoglobin H (β_4) may also be detected in cord blood samples. With the normal transition from γ-chain production to the production of β-chains, hemoglobin Barts may undergo gradual replacement by hemoglobin H. In the milder forms of α-thalassemia most commonly present in blacks, hemoglobin Barts gradually disappears over the first few weeks with the disorder persisting as a mild hypochromic anemia without any abnormality demonstrable by hemoglobin electrophoresis.

The most severe clinical forms of α-thalassemia have been known to occur only in

Orientals; recent findings have shown that α-thalassemia in Oriental populations is accompanied by a particularly profound degree of suppression of α-chain synthesis. The clinical picture presented by these infants at birth resembles that of severe hydrops fetalis caused by isoimmune hemolytic disease. The infants are pale and edematous and exhibit marked hepatosplenomegaly. In every reported case the infant was stillborn or died shortly after birth.

Laboratory findings. The hemoglobin concentration in blood samples from these infants is reduced, often to a severe degree. The erythroctyes are hypochromic and, with supravital staining, demonstrate intracellular inclusion bodies representing precipitated hemoglobin. Reticulocytosis and an extreme degree of erythroblastemia are typical findings in stained smears of peripheral blood. Reaction to the direct Coombs test is negative, which allows this disorder to be readily distinguished from isoimmune hemolytic disease. Hemoglobin electrophoresis demonstrates the presence almost exclusively of hemoglobin Barts (γ_4), with trace amounts of hemoglobin H and normal adult hemoglobin. Sickling of the erythrocytes, a consequence of the γ_4 hemoglobin, can also be demonstrated in blood samples that are allowed to stand at room temperature for several hours.

The adverse consequences of this disorder appear to stem principally from two pathogenic mechanisms: instability of the abnormal hemoglobin forms results in hemoglobin precipitation intracellularly, which in turn leads to an accelerated rate of red cell destruction; the presence of hemoglobin Barts (γ_4), which has also been shown to produce a greatly increased oxygen affinity of the blood, results in a severe impairment of oxygen delivery to the tissues. The nature of the adaptation, which allows survival with this disorded during fetal life but not beyond the neonatal period, is not understood.

Methemoglobinemia. Methemoglobin is an oxidized form of hemoglobin in which the heme iron is in the ferric state rather than in the normal ferrous form. Methemoglobin is totally nonfunctional as an oxygen carrier and normally makes up no more than 2% of hemoglobin in blood. When greater than 10% of the hemoglobin is in this form, the skin color becomes dusky, and the blood develops a brown discoloration that persists following oxygenation.

Pathophysiology. Methemoglobin formation apparently occurs at a slow rate under normal conditions, but the oxidized hemoglobin undergoes reduction to the normal form by enzymatic action in the erythrocytes. Quantitatively the most important of the reductive enzymes is an NADH-dependent diaphorase designated NADH-methemoglobin reductase. Activity of this enzyme is known to be substantially reduced in erythrocytes of newborns, particularly in premature infants. The deficiency is reflected by a higher concentration of methemoglobin in blood during infancy and an increased suspectibility to formation of this hemoglobin form in young infants. A variety of drugs and chemicals have been found to precipitate acute episodes of methemoglobinemia in newborns. These have included nitrites, which may be a contaminant of well water, aniline and its derivatives, phenacetin, certain sulfonamides, and a variety of other benzene derivatives.

Diagnosis. Acute methemoglobinemia may develop a variable period of time following exposure of the infant to the offending agent. Although a marked degree of cyanosis may accompany this condition (p. 262), symptoms are usually mild. Occasionally methemoglobin levels may exceed 30% to 50%, and the infant may develop respiratory distress and tachycardia. When this diagnosis is suspected it can be rapidly confirmed in most cases by a simple screening test. A drop of blood from the patient and from a normal control are collected on filter paper that are agitated in the air for about 30 seconds to aerate the samples. A persistent brown color in the blood sample from the affected infant is usually an indication of a methemoglobin concentration of at least 10%. Quantitation of the abnormal hemoglobin form can be readily achieved by a spectrophotometric procedure.

In addition to acute drug- or chemical-induced methemoglobinemia, a number of congenital forms have also been identified, all of which produce lifelong cyanosis. Congenital deficiency of NADH-dependent methemoglobin reductase activity has been found to be associated with a variety of abnormalities that affect this enzyme. These disorders are inherited as an autosomal recessive trait, and examples of their occurrence in more than one member of a family have been described. In blood of affected individuals 20% to 50% of the hemoglobin exists as methemoglobin resulting in cyanosis, which is often apparent at birth. The diagnosis of this disorder is established by the demonstration of reduced activity of the enzyme in the erythrocytes. Studies of kinetic properties and electrophoretic mobility of the abnormal enzymes form the basis for more definitive identification of the abnormality.

Congenital methemoglobinemia may also result from structural abnormalities of the hemoglobin molecule. In these variant forms of hemoglobin, amino acid substitutions are present in regions of the globin chains at which the heme groups are attached. Because of the altered protein-heme interactions that result, the affected heme groups remain in the oxidized state and are unable to bind oxygen. A number of these abnormal hemoglobin forms have been identified, which are classified collectively as hemoglobin M disease. Affected individuals, all of whom have been heterozygous for the abnormality, exhibit lifelong cyanosis but have an asymptomatic course. Forms of hemoglobin M disease that result from amino acid substitutions in the α-chains may produce cyanosis at birth; β-chain abnormalities become apparent only after 2 to 6 months of age. The abnormal hemoglobin forms are identified by electrophoresis and spectrophotometric analysis.

Treatment. Acute methemoglobinemia resulting from the effect of drugs or chemicals will often subside spontaneously after exposure to the agent is discontinued. If the infant is symptomatic, the abnormality can usually be corrected rapidly by intravenous administration of a 1% solution of methylene blue in a dose of 2 mg/kg. However, excessive doses of methylene blue must be avoided because this material itself may cause methemoglobin formation as well as hemolytic anemia when given in large amounts. Ascorbic acid, 100 to 200 mg, is also effective in the reduction of methemoglobin, although its action is less rapid. Ascorbic acid is specifically indicated in the presence of G-6-PD deficiency, because in this condition methylene blue is ineffective. Administration of either of these agents on a continuing basis will effectively reduce the methemoglobin concentration in patients with congenital deficiency of NADH-dependent methemoglobin reductase. In hemoglobin M disease, on the other hand, the methemoglobinemia is refractory to these reducing agents.

Heinz-body anemias. Heinz body formation can result from any of a variety of conditions that produce intracellular hemoglobin precipitation. Although this process apparently occurs to a small extent in normal erythroctyes, Heinz bodies are not ordinarily demonstrable in blood because of selective removal of the precipitated protein by reticuloendothelial elements of the spleen. Following splenectomy, however, or in individuals with splenic agenesis, these cellular inclusions are commonly present. The Heinz bodies are not visible in blood smears prepared with Wright's stain but can be readily detected by supravital staining of erythrocytes with methyl violet or brilliant cresyl blue (Fig. 9-5).

Acute hemolytic anemia accompanied by the presence of large numbers of Heinz body–containing erythrocytes has been described in the older literature to occur in newborns, particularly in premature in-

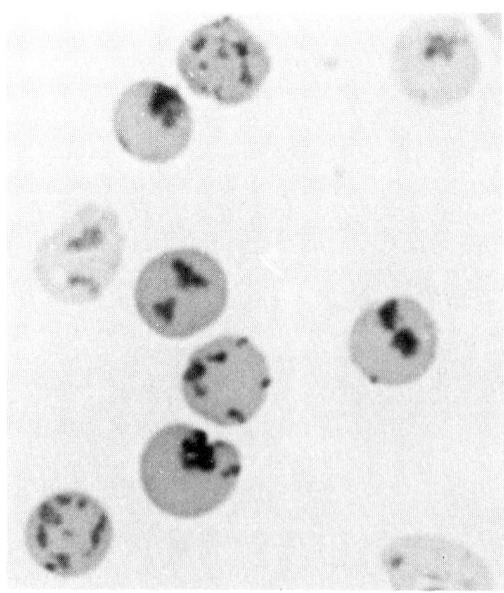

Fig. 9-5. Heinz bodies in erythrocytes of a patient having congenital Heinz-body anemia caused by an unstable hemoglobin (hemoglobin Abraham Lincoln).

fants. These reported cases appear largely to have represented examples of the hemolytic action of oxidant drugs and chemicals in the newborn (p. 194) and may well have also included infants having G-6-PD deficiency.

Congenital forms of Heinz-body anemia were also identified that are now known to represent a form of hemoglobinopathy characterized by instability of the hemoglobin molecule, leading to its intracellular precipitation. Hemolytic anemia of a variable degree occurs in many of these conditions. In one of these disorders, hemoglobin Zürich disease, protein instability and intraerythrocytic precipitation are greatly accentuated by oxidant drugs and chemicals to produce acute hemolytic episodes resembling those seen in patients having G-6-PD deficiency. Unstable hemoglobin forms can be identified by electrophoresis or by evidence of abnormal protein precipitation in a hemoglobin heat stability test.

Disorders of the leukocytes

Abnormalities that primarily affect the leukocytes are an uncommon cause of significant disease in the newborn. Correct identification of these disorders and their differentiation from other neonatal abnormalities having similar clinical findings depends upon a cognizance of the normal leukocyte values of the newborn as well as changes that occur under conditions of stress. Interpretation of leukocyte values of newborn infants must be made with the recognition that white blood cell counts are extremely variable at birth, that the differential count differs substantially from that of older infants and children (p. 172), and that the white blood cell and differential counts normally undergo considerable change during the first weeks of life.

Changes in the leukocyte and differential counts caused by infections or other inflammatory or stressful conditions follow a less predictable course in the neonate than in older children or adults, either leukocytosis or leukopenia being known to occur under these conditions. Rapid mobilization of leukocytes in the newborn as a result of infection or other inflammatory disease may produce a greatly exaggerated "leftward shift" in the white blood cell differential count, with the appearance of significant numbers of immature granulocytes, including metamyelocytes, myelocytes, and occasionally earlier forms.

Leukemia. Leukemia appearing in the neonatal period is rare. Infants with mongolism have accounted for a disproportionate number of these cases, and in some of the others a familial predisposition may have been present. Leukemia in a mother during a pregnancy has never been known to result in congenital leukemia appearing in a newborn infant.

Clinical presentation. Infants with leukemia may exhibit evidence of the disease at birth or may appear normal in the neonatal period, with clinical and hematologic signs becoming apparent later in infancy. Clinical findings are variable and may include pallor, hemorrhagic manifestations, enlargement of the liver and spleen, and the appearance of nodular infiltrations in the skin. The cutaneous nodules are a frequent and characteristic feature of congenital leukemia and typically present as firm, discrete, easily movable tumors ranging in size from 0.2 to 3.0 cm in diameter. The skin manifestations may develop prior to the appearance of other recognizable features of the disease.

Diagnosis. Leukemia of the newborn is mainly of the acute myelogenous form, although examples of the lymphocytic variety in the neonatal period have also been described. Leukocytosis is almost invariably present, with leukocyte counts frequently being greater than 100,000/mm^3. Immature white blood cell forms, including myeloblasts and promyelocytes, usually are present in large numbers. The platelet count is almost invariably reduced. Anemia may be found at the outset or may develop subsequently, with rapid progression. The bone marrow is hypercellular and predominantly contains early white blood cell forms with reduced numbers of red blood cell precursors and megakaryocytes.

Difficulty may arise in establishing a diagnosis of leukemia in a newborn infant because of the similarities of the clinical and laboratory findings occurring in this disease to those in a number of neonatal infections. A variety of other conditions affecting the newborn also may be accompanied by the presence of immature leukocyte forms in the perpiheral blood and may suggest a diagnosis of leukemia. Neonatal disorders that must be considered in the differential diagnosis of leukemia include isoimmune hemolytic disease, toxoplasmosis, congenital syphilis, viral infections, and bacterial sepsis.

Treatment. The response of neonatal leukemia to treatment with chemotherapeutic agents has generally been poor. In most cases the infants have survived no more than a few weeks or months following diagnosis, with hemorrhage or infection being the most common cause of death. Experience with newer agents that are effective for treatment of acute myelogenous leukemia in older children and adults (daunomycin, arabinosylcytosine) has not yet been reported in leukemia of the neonate, and it is possible that these drugs may produce beneficial results in affected infants.

Infants with mongolism are known to have a considerably increased risk of developing leukemia. In most instances the leukemia is of the undifferentiated stem cell type and has its onset beyond the neonatal period, but a disproportionate number of neonatal cases of leukemia have also occurred in association with mongolism. The latter have usually been of the myelogenous form, similar to that occurring in other patients with neonatal leukemia. Infants with mongolism and congenital leukemia have shown the usual clinical and laboratory features of leukemia, but in contrast to the almost invariably fatal outcome of neonatal leukemia a number of these infants have developed spontaneous remissions, in some instances without recurrence of the disease. It has not been determined if these cases represent a spontaneously curable form of leukemia or a nonmalignant disorder indistinguishable from leukemia in its clinical manifestations.

Granulocytopenic disorders. Serious infections in newborn infants may be accompanied by a reduction of the white blood cell count, occasionally with a severe degree of neutropenia. In most instances these changes are thought to represent a toxic suppression of bone marrow activity, occurring as a consequence of the infectious process. In newborns a variety of conditions also have been identified in which neutropenia occurs as a primary abnormality, which in turn predisposes the infant to the development of infection. This group of disorders accounts for only a small percentage of severe neonatal infections but should receive careful consideration in the evaluation of any infant with infection exhibiting granulocytopenia.

Transplacental transfer of maternally formed antileukocytic antibody has been shown to be one of the mechanisms for the development of neonatal granulocytopenia. This disorder may arise as a consequence of any of a number of conditions in the mother that result in the formation of leukocyte-agglutinating antibody. These may include systemic lupus erythematosus, lymphomas, infectious mononucleosis, and drug-induced antibody formation in which the drug acts as a hapten to stimulate the production of antibody capable of agglutinating leukocytes. Granulocytopenia in the mother is present in any of this group of conditions because of the nonspecific character of the leukocyte antibody, and it provides a ready means of identification of the cause of leukopenia in the newborn infant.

Formation of maternal antibody active against leukocytes of the infant may also occur by a mechanism analogous to that of isoimmune hemolytic disease. Antibody formation in the mother is initiated by the passage of fetal leukocytes into the maternal circulation and may be further stimulated during subsequent pregnancies. Because the antibody is specifically directed toward leukocyte antigens of the infant, the white blood cell count of the mother is not affected. Agglutinating antibody against leukocytes of the infant has been detected in serums of approximately 20% of nontransfused mothers who were studied, but instances of significant neonatal neutropenia attributable to this mechanism appear to be rare. Granulocytopenia of the neonate arising as a result of maternally-formed leukocyte antibody is a transient condition, which usually subsides spontaneously within 2 to 4 weeks, in parallel with the disappearance of antibody activity. Protection of the infant from sources of infection and careful observation and prompt use of appropriate antibiotics if infection develops will usually assure a favorable outcome.

A number of congenital forms of granulocytopenia may also appear in the newborn period. A marked reduction or absence of circulating granulocytes has been identified as the primary basis for a severe congenital disorder characterized by serious and frequent bacterial infections often beginning in early infancy. A familial occurrence has been reported in some patients with this disorder, which has been designated *infantile genetic agranulocytosis*. Eosinophilia and monocytosis are frequently present in these infants, and the red blood cell count and platelet count are usually normal. A characteristic finding in the bone marrow in this disorder is a marked diminution or absence of granulocytic precursors more mature than the promyelocyte or early myelocyte stage. Many of the reported patients with this disease died in infancy as a result of infection, and few have survived beyond early childhood.

A less severe form of congenital neutropenia, *chronic benign granulocytopenia,* may also become apparent in infancy. Although a marked degree of neutropenia is characteristic of this disorder, increased numbers of granulocytes may appear in the blood following the onset of an infection. Affected infants exhibit a greater than normal degree of susceptibility to bacterial infections, but infections are usually relatively mild and respond well to antibiotic therapy. Some patients may require continuous antibiotic administration to remain free of infection, but in most cases the prognosis is good. Spontaneous remission with complete recovery has been reported in some affected children.

Other forms of congenital granulocytopenia that may appear in the newborn period include *cyclic neutropenia*, neutropenia in association with thymic alymphoplasia, and neutropenia as part of a syndrome characterized by bone marrow hypoplasia and pancreatic insufficiency.

Hemostasis and hemorrhagic disorders

Normal hemostatic mechanisms. The series of events that normally occurs to prevent excessive blood loss following injury to blood vessels involves the participation of vascular reactions, platelets, and blood clotting factors derived from the tissues and from the blood plasma. The diagram in Fig. 9-6 demonstrates the most important reactions of the overall process of hemostasis

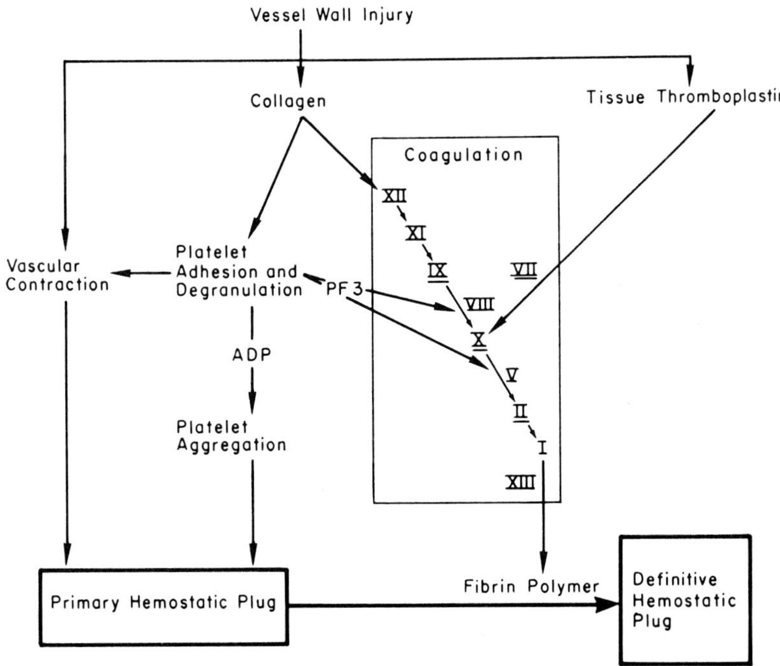

Fig. 9-6. Components of the hemostatic mechanism. (From Bleyer, W. A., Hakami, N., and Shepard, T. H.: J. Pediatr. **79**:838, 1971.)

and some of the major interrelationships between the components of the hemostatic system.

Hemostasis. The hemostatic mechanisms of the normal newborn infant show a number of quantitive changes in comparison with those of the older child and adult. Many of these changes are particularly accentuated in prematures, and in these infants may be sufficient to impose a significantly higher risk of hemorrhagic complications. Table 9-3 summarizes the most important of the hemostatic changes seen in the premature and full-term newborn infant.

It is generally accepted that platelet count values of the normal full-term infant are within the normal range as established for older children and adults. In the premature infant a somewhat lower range of values may be considered normal, but in infants of any age a platelet count of less than 100,000/mm^3 must be regarded as an abnormal finding.

Recent studies have also demonstrated that a number of aspects of platelet function are poorly developed at birth and may be particularly deficient in the premature infant. These include platelet aggregation in response to collagen or epinephrine and platelet factor 3 availability, a measure of the clot-promoting activity of the platelets. It has also been demonstrated that platelet aggregation in the newborn can be significantly affected by a diverse group of pharmacologic agents at levels considerably less than those that affect platelets in adults. The implications of these findings are thus far unclear; but it has been suggested that because of these platelet functional characteristics, the newborn, and particularly the premature infant, may have an increased susceptibility to intracranial bleeding and other hemorrhagic manifestations.

Changes in the plasma levels of a number of the coagulation factors are also observed in the normal newborn infant. Factors V, XI, and XII may be reduced to a variable extent in the normal newborn, but rarely if ever are the levels of these factors

TABLE 9-3. Hemostatic function

Hemostatic factor or component	Premature infant	Full-term infant	Age adult level is attained
Vascular and platelet function			
Vasoconstriction	Present	Present	At birth
Capillary fragility	Increased	Normal	At birth
Bleeding time	Normal	Normal	At birth
Platelet count	Normal	Normal	At birth
Platelet function	↓ ↓ Aggregability	↓ Aggregability ↓ Clot retraction ↓ Platelet factor 3 availability	Not established
Coagulation			
Whole blood clotting time	↑	↓ Or normal	At birth
Partial thromboplastin time (PTT) (adult normal 35-45 sec)	70-145 sec	45-70 sec	2-9 months
Prothrombin time (PT) (adult normal 12-14 sec)	12-21 sec	13-20 sec	3-4 days
Thrombin time (TT) (adult normal 8-10 sec)	11-17 sec	10-16 sec	Few days
Thrombotest (II, VII, IX, X)	30-50%	40-68%	2-12 months
XII (Hageman factor)	Not established	25-70%	9-14 days
XI (PTA)	5-20%	15-70%	1-2 months
IX (PTC)	10-25%	20-60%	3-9 months
VIII (AHF)	20-80%	70-150%	At birth
VII (Proconvertin)	20-45%	20-70%	2-12 months
X (Stuart-Prower factor)	10-45%	20-55%	2-12 months
V (Proaccelerin)	50-85%	80-200%	At birth
II (Prothrombin)	20-80%	25-65%	2-12 months
I (Fibrinogen)	60-90%	60-90%	2-4 days
XIII (Fibrin-stabilizing factor)	100%	100%	At birth

From Bleyer, W. A., Hakami, N., and Shepard, T. H.: J. Pediatr. **79**:838, 1971.

sufficiently decreased to impair hemostasis. The levels of the vitamin K–dependent factors (II, VII, IX, X) may be profoundly decreased in the newborn so that serious hemorrhagic complications result. (These changes are discussed on p. 208.)

Laboratory evaluation of hemostasis. With application of appropriate laboratory procedures, an accurate analysis of each of the known components of the hemostatic system can be performed. This may include determination of platelet numbers and function, assay of the individual coagulation factors, and assessment of fibrinolytic and anticoagulant activity of the plasma. These studies, however, are often time consuming and costly and may require special facilities. For most purposes a clinical assessment of the hemostatic system can be accomplished with readily available screening tests, with the more specific procedures being reserved for diagnostic problems requiring more exact definition.

Most of the screening tests in common use assess the collective activity of a number of individual components of the hemostatic system, and few of these tests are therefore specific. However, when an appropriate group of these tests are performed together, it is often possible to obtain highly specific information that may allow a precise diagnosis to be made directly or may indicate a limited number of specific determinations that will then allow a diagnosis to be made. The most useful of the hemostatic screening tests are summarized below.

The *platelet count* provides a specific indication of platelet numbers in the blood, and in thrombocytopenic hemorrhagic states is sufficient to establish the cause of the bleeding. The *bleeding time* provides an assessment of the vascular component of hemostasis as well as the contribution of the platelets. A prolonged bleeding time will occur in qualitative platelet disorders as well as in thrombocytopenic states. In the presence of a significant reduction in the platelet count a bleeding time test usually is not indicated. The *partial thromboplastin time* (PTT) screening test is the most widely available means of assessment of the plasma coagulation factors. The results of this test is prolonged with a deficiency of any of the coagulation factors except for the rarely occurring deficiencies of factor VII, or factor XIII. The *prothrombin time* (PT) becomes prolonged with deficiencies of the extrinsic coagulation pathway, comprising factors VII, V, X, II (prothrombin), and fibrinogen. This screening test is particularly useful in detecting decreased levels of vitamin K–deficient factors. Rapid screening tests are also available to detect abnormal levels of fibrinogen, factor XIII, and increased fibinolytic activity.

Congenital deficiency of coagulation factors. From available evidence it appears unlikely that coagulation factors are transferred to any significant extent from the maternal circulation to that of the fetus during gestation. Factor IX, however, may be a possible exception. As a consequence, a predisposition to hemorrhage in this group of disorders can be expected to be present in the infant from the time of birth. Severe forms of *factor VIII deficiency and factor IX deficiency* account for a majority of hemorrhagic problems of the newborn caused by congenital coagulation abnormalities. Both of these disorders are inherited as X-linked characteristics and therefore affect males almost exclusively. Congenital deficiencies of other coagulation factors occur rarely, with most of them having an autosomal recessive mode of transmission, males and females being equally affected.

Significant clinical bleeding has been reported to occur within the first week of life in nearly 50% of infants having a severe *deficiency of factors VIII or IX.* Bleeding following circumcision has accounted for a majority of these episodes. Hemorrhage associated with birth trauma may also occur in these infants, producing intracranial bleeding, visceral hemorrhage, or bleeding into joints or soft tissues. Congenital deficiencies of other coagulation factors often produce a similar clinical picture in the newborn period.

Laboratory findings in these deficiency states may include a variable degree of anemia if hemorrhage has been extensive, often with accompanying reticulocytosis. Hemorrhage into soft tissues may also produce a significant degree of jaundice, with hyperbilirubinemia caused by heme pigment degradation. The platelet count is characteristically within the normal range, and the bleeding time is also normal. The latter should be deferred, however, if a severe coagulation defect is suspected, because of the risk of protracted secondary hemorrhage. The coagulation abnormality in these disorders is most readily detected by the findings of prolongation of the PTT together with a normal PT value. It is important to note, however, that a meaningful assessment of the results of these laboratory screening tests in the newborn cannot be made unless vitamin K deficiency in the infant can be excluded with certainty. In other congenital deficiency states of coagulation factors, prolongation of both the PTT and PT screening may be present.

Congenital deficiency of factor XIII (fibrin-stabilizing factor) is an unusual disorder, which may appear in the newborn period, frequently appearing as umbilical cord hemorrhage. Both the PTT and PT screening tests are characteristically normal in this condition; and if this abnormality is suspected, a specific screening test based on clot solubility in urea or acetic acid provides a simple and reliable means of detection. Whenever the presence of a congenital deficiency of a coagulation factor is suggested by abnormal screening test results, specific laboratory studies to determine the precise coagulation abnormality are essential. An exact diagnosis will be required in order to assess the degree of the deficiency and therefore the risk of hemorrhagic complications, to provide a sound basis for correct therapy when it is needed, and to furnish accurate genetic information for the parents of the child.

The management of bleeding episodes in infants and children with coagulation factor deficiencies has been greatly facilitated in recent years with the availability of concentrated forms of coagulation factors. With the use of these preparations it is possible to replace the deficient factor and temporarily restore the hemostatic function of the patient to normal. The relatively low protein content of most of these materials allows them to be given in large doses if needed, without the risk of hypervolemia, a complication that imposes a strict limitation when whole plasma is administered as a source of coagulation factors. Factor VIII deficiency can be treated with a variety of commercial preparations of this factor or by administration of plasma cryoprecipitate. The latter is often less expensive but has the disadvantage of having unknown and variable potency. Intravenous administration of 30 to 50 units of factor VIII per kg of body weight once daily will usually provide a hemostatic level of the factor and will be effective for management of hemorrhage in factor VIII–deficient patients. Larger dosages are required in more serious hemorrhage or for surgery. Concentrated commercial preparations of the vitamin K–dependent factors (II, VII, IX, X) are also available (Konyne, Proplex). Bleeding episodes in factor IX–deficient patients can usually be managed by a daily infusion of 50 to 100 units per kg of this material. Congenital hypofibrinogenemia similarly can be temporarily corrected by administration of fibrinogen infused in a dose of 50 to 100 mg/kg once daily. Hemorrhage caused by deficiency of other coagulation factors can usually be treated effectively by infusion of fresh or fresh-frozen plasma in a dose of 10 ml/kg, 2 to 4 times daily.

Neonatal vitamin K–deficiency. At birth, plasma levels of the vitamin K–dependent coagulation factors (II, VII, IX and X) are significantly reduced from normal adult values. Over the first 2 to 3 days of life these coagulation factors may become further reduced if vitamin K is not available, and a small percentage of deficient infants will develop a severe bleeding diathesis designated hemorrhagic disease of the newborn. Available evidence indicates that vitamin K stores are virtually absent in the newborn infant. In addition, because of the absence of intestinal microflora that produce vitamin K and the limited intake of vitamin K–containing foods in the first days of life, newborn infants may be frequently at risk of developing this complication. Breast milk has been shown to be a particularly poor source of vitamin K, and hemorrhagic complications have most commonly appeared in breast-fed infants. Infants receiving cow's milk on the first day of life, on the other hand, seldom have become vitamin K deficient.

Because the vitamin K–dependent group of coagulation factors is produced by the liver, severe liver disease in the neonate as well as in older children may be associated with a deficiency of these factors, even when adequate amounts of the vitamin are given. Small premature infants may also respond poorly to vitamin K, presumably because of immature biosynthetic activity of the livers of these infants. It also has become evident in recent years that a particularly severe deficiency of the vitamin K–dependent coagulation factors may occur in infants born to mothers who received anticonvulsant medications during the pregnancy. Drugs that have been associated with this complication include phenobarbitol and diphenylhydantoin. The bleeding manifestations have been severe in many of these infants, and the onset of hemorrhage frequently occurred within the first 24 hours of life. Vitamin K was found to be effective for correction of the coagulation abnormality in most cases, but in some of the infants the response was poor and sometimes was delayed.

The platelet count and fibrinogen levels are characteristically normal in uncomplicated deficiency of the vitamin K–dependent factors and serve readily to distinguish this condition from most of the other acquired hemorrhagic disorders of the newborn. Both the PTT and the PT screening tests will be prolonged in the presence of significant vitamin K deficiency. Specific assays of levels of the individual coagulation factors are rarely indicated, but if carried out will usually demonstrate a marked degree of reduction of all the vitamin K–dependent group.

A newborn with hemorrhagic disease resulting from vitamin K deficiency will usually respond dramatically to administration of the vitamin. Bleeding will usually cease within 2 to 4 hours, and by 24 hours the vitamin K–dependent factors will be nearly normal in most infants. Water-soluble forms of vitamin K are among the group of agents known to precipitate hemolysis in newborn infants, particularly when G-6-PD deficiency is present (p. 194). For treatment of newborn infants, natural forms of vitamin K (Aqua-mephyton, Mephyton, Konakion) should be used exclusively, in a dose not to exceed 2 mg. Intramuscular administration of vitamin K in this manner within the first 24 hours of life is now carried out as a routine procedure in many hospital nurseries in order to assure an adequate supply of the vitamin in the neonatal period.

For infants whose mothers received anticonvulsant medications during pregnancy, special precautions may need to be taken if hemorrhagic complications are to be prevented. It is recommended that cord blood be obtained at delivery from the infants for a PT determination, followed by intravenous administration of 1 to 2 mg of vitamin K. If the PT is greatly prolonged and fails to improve after administration of the vitamin K, an infusion of fresh plasma in a dose of 10 ml/kg body weight may be given to supply the deficient coagulation factors. Plasma infusions may also be required for premature infants and infants with liver disease who are unresponsive to vitamin K. Concentrated forms of the vitamin K–dependent coagulation factors should be avoided in this group of infants because these products may carry a considerable risk of transmitting the virus of serum hepatitis.

Intravascular coagulation disorders. A diverse group of entities has been identified that may be accompanied by inappropriate activation of the coagulation mechanism. As a result of this process soluble fibrinogen becomes converted to fibrin to form thrombi within blood vessels. In addition, blood coagulation factors that are normally consumed in the coagulation process become depleted in the circulating plasma. The latter includes particularly factors II, V, VIII, X, and XIII, as well as fibrinogen and platelets. The reduction of the platelet count and depletion of coagulation factors may result in serious hemorrhagic complications.

Pathogenesis. The pathogenesis of intravascular coagulation may vary, depending on the underlying condition. In intravascular coagulation in the neonate caused by abruptio placentae, amniotic fluid embolism, or a dead twin fetus, infusion of thromboplastic material into the fetal circulation appears to be the major factor responsible for initiation of the coagulation process. Severe infection with endotoxin-producing organisms is probably the most common clinical condition of young infants associated with the intravascular coagulation syndrome. It appears likely that the pathogenic mechanism in these infants may be similar to that of the Shwartzman reaction, which is induced by injections of endotoxin into experimental animals. Antigen-antibody complexes may also act as triggering agents for intravascular coagulation agents and may be a major factor responsible for the examples of this complication in infants with severe isoimmune hemolytic disease and in a group of infections including disseminated herpes simplex, rubella, and cytomegalic inclusion disease.

Clinical presentation. Clinical findings in an infant with the intravascular coagulation syndrome may be variable, depending on the underlying disease process. Hemorrhagic manifestations are often evident, with prolonged oozing at venipuncture sites probably being the most common initial finding. Serious hemorrhagic complications may occur if thrombocytopenia or coagulation changes are severe.

Laboratory findings. The most important laboratory abnormalities that accompany intravascular coagulation can be detected by readily available screening tests. The platelet count is usually significantly reduced, and the PTT and PT are prolonged. Young infants with the intravascular coagulation syndrome, and particularly those with gram-negative infections, typically demonstrate a marked reduction of the plasma fibrinogen level, a change that can be readily detected by simple screening tests. Reported studies of newborn infants with septicemia have shown an incidence of over 50% having evidence of intravascular coagulation, and it is a worthwhile precaution in any neonate with a severe bacterial infection to perform a platelet count, PTT, and PT to look for evidence of this complication. It is important to note, however, that significant thrombocytopenia may often accompany bacterial septicemia without intravascular coagulation being present.

The presence of fibrin thrombi in small blood vessels as a result of intravascular coagulation often results in fragmentation and distortion of red blood cells that pass through the affected vessels. This microangiopathic process can produce a significant degree of hemolytic anemia accompanied by hyperbilirubinemia and reticulocytosis. The morphologic characteristics of red blood cells may be strikingly abnormal even in the absence of the significant anemia, with fragmented cells being present in large numbers. Fibrin deposition in the blood vessels as a result of intravascular coagulation also results in stimulation of the fibrinolytic mechanism. The euglobulin lysis time or other tests for measurement of fibrinolysis are shortened, and degradation products of fibrin may be detected in blood and urine of the infants.

Diagnosis. In most instances it will be possible to establish accurately a diagnosis of intravascular coagulation without the aid of specific coagulation factor assays. The presence of thrombocytopenia together with a prolongation of the PTT and PT screening tests and evidence of the red blood cell fragmentation in an infant having bacterial septicemia or other known predisposing orders can usually be considered presumptive evidence of intravascular coagulation. Occasionally the findings in some infants, particularly those having infections together with liver disease or with vitamin K deficiency, can produce considerable diagnostic difficulty. In these infants, specific assays to detect reduced levels of factor V and fibrinogen will usually be the most helpful subsequent studies.

Treatment. Management of the infant with intravascular coagulation is directed toward the following objectives: (1) control of the underlying disorder, (2) termination of the intravascular coagulation process, and (3) control of bleeding. If the underlying disorder can be brought under control, particularly in such conditions as infection, shock, or isoimmune hemolytic disease, the abnormal coagulation changes will often subside spontaneously. In an infant showing any evidence of intravascular coagulation syndrome a careful effort should always be made to identify the underlying cause, with particular emphasis placed on the possibility of infection and shock. If a treatable condition can be shown to exist, prompt, aggressive therapy of the disorder is indicated.

Regardless of the cause of coagulation abnormality, specific measures to control the intravascular coagulation process itself are indicated when there is evidence of a severe degree of consumption of coagulation factors, when clinical bleeding is present, or when the infant is severely ill. For this purpose, anticoagulant therapy is instituted, usually by administration of heparin, to interrupt the intravascular coagulation process and thereby prevent the consumption of platelets and clotting factors. Paradoxically, when the anticoagulant therapy is effective, hemorrhage rapidly subsides. Heparin is administered intravenously in an initial dose of 100 units per kg and is repeated at 4-hour intervals. Indications for discontinuing heparin therapy are: (1) a sustained increase in the platelet count and a significant reduction toward normal of the PTT and PT screening tests, and (2) evidence of control or clear improvement in the underlying disease process that is presumed to have initiated the intravascular coagulation. When severe depletion of coagulation factors has occurred as a result of intravascular coagulation or whenever hemorrhage is present, heparin therapy should be supplemented by a source of coagulation factors. For this purpose fresh whole plasma is most generally useful and may be administered in a dose of 10 ml/kg body weight. This dose may be repeated at 6- to 8-hour intervals if required. For the initial dose we have found it convenient to infuse the fresh plasma containing heparin, 10 units/ml, as the anticoagulant. Alternatively, an exchange transfusion with heparinized blood may be indicated.

Platelet disorders

Abnormalities of platelet function. A variety of hemorrhagic disorders have been described in recent years in which the underlying defect consists of one or more abnormalities of platelet function. The platelet count is characteristically normal in this group of disorders, and usually no coagulation defect is demonstrable. Prolongation of the bleeding time is a finding common to all of these conditions.

Thrombasthenia, the most severe of this group of disorders, is a rare familial abnormality transmitted as an autosomal recessive trait. Severe hemorrhagic complications may occur in the neonatal period in the affected infant, with ecchymoses and mucous membrane bleeding being the most common manifestations. The bleeding time is greatly prolonged, and clot retraction is poor or absent. The diagnosis is established by demonstration of an absence of platelet aggregation in response to collagen or adenosine disphosphate. Platelet factor 3 availability is also characteristically reduced.

A heterogeneous and generally less severe group of hemorrhagic disorders are the *thrombopathies*. These disorders may be of sporadic occurrence or inherited as an autosomal dominant trait. The bleeding tendency is variable but may be severe. A normal platelet count with prolongation of the bleeding time is characteristic of the more severe forms. Platelet aggregation in response to adenosine disphosphate is unaffected, but collagen-induced aggregation and platelet factor 3 availability are usually abnormal.

Acquired platelet function abnormalities have also been reported in newborn infants whose mothers received aspirin or promethazine late in their pregnancy or during labor. No evidence of abnormal hemorrhage was observed in these infants, but studies of their platelets showed severe impairment of platelet aggregation in response to collagen and epinephrine.

In *von Willebrand's disease* hemorrhagic manifestations and prolongation of the bleeding time appear to be attributable to abnormal platelet function. The primary abnormality of this disorder, however, is not within the platelets themselves, but appears to represent a deficiency of a plasma protein factor that is required for normal platelet function. This disorder is transmitted as an autosomal dominant trait and may equally affect males and females. Platelet aggregation studies are usually normal in this condition, but platelet adhesion as measured by platelet retention by a glass bead column is abnormal. An additional feature of the disorder in most affected individuals is a reduction in the level of factor VIII, a finding that may present diagnostic difficulty in the differentiation of this condition from hemophilia. The bleeding time, platelet adhesion value, and factor VIII level are characteristically variable in von Willebrand's disease and may need to be determined repeatedly in some patients in order to establish a diagnosis.

Neonatal thrombocytopenia. A reduction of the platelet count in the newborn period sufficient to produce hemorrhagic manifestations may result from a variety of causes. These may include congenital abnormalities affecting platelet production, a variety of neonatal conditions that secondarily affect platelet production or result in platelet destruction, and acquired abnormalities resulting from adverse maternal factors. The most important of these conditions are summarized in the outline below.

CAUSES OF THROMBOCYTOPENIA

A. Congenital defects of platelet production
   1. Congenital megakaryocytic hypoplasia
   2. Wiskott-Aldrich syndrome
   3. Deficiency of megakaryocyte maturation factor
B. Accelerated platelet destruction caused by maternal antibody
   1. Maternal lupus erythematosus or thrombocytopenic purpura
   2. Isoimmune thrombocytopenia
   3. Maternal drug ingestion
C. Thrombocytopenia secondary to other conditions
   1. Neonatal infections
   2. Leukemia
   3. Intravascular coagulation

Congenital megakaryocytic hypoplasias. A group of congenital thrombocytopenic disorders has been identified in which affected infants demonstrate greatly reduced numbers of megakaryocytes in their bone marrow. In most reported examples of this condition the hematologic abnormality was accompanied by one or more associated congenital anomalies. Most common in this group has been the absence of both radii, but other anomalies have also included microcephaly, cardiovascular malformations, and a variety of orthopedic abnormalities. The disorder is rare and usually occurs sporadically, although familial examples have been reported. Thrombocytopenia is usually severe and frequently results in hemorrhagic manifestations in the neonatal period. Anemia is present only as a result of hemorrhage. White blood cell counts are often normal in the newborn period, but many of these infants have subsequently developed a striking elevation of their leukocyte count within the first weeks of life. The prognosis is generally poor in this condition, the majority of affected infants having died within the first months of life as a result of hemorrhage.

Wiskott-Aldrich syndrome. This disorder is inherited as an X-linked recessive trait and is characterized by the triad of thrombocytopenia, eczema, and recurrent infections. Hemorrhage, often presenting as bloody diarrhea, is the most frequent finding and may occur in the newborn period. Eczema usually appears later in infancy and in most cases will not be present at birth. Purulent infections occur periodically and often are life threatening. The platelet count is reduced to a variable degree. Reported bone marrow findings in this disorder have been inconsistent. Reduced numbers of megakaryocytes having an irregular, fragmented appearance have been described in some patients; in others, usual numbers of normal-appearing megakaryocytes have been reported. The predisposition to infection appears to be the result of abnormalities of both the humoral and cellular immune mechanisms. Absence of isoagglutinins has been observed in many affected children, and some have also been found to have reduced levels of IgA or IgM. It has become increasingly apparent that defective cellular immunity is of particular significance in the cause of infection in these infants. A deficiency of thymus-dependent lymphocytes has been demonstrated in this disease, and the immunologic response to polysaccharide antigens has been shown to be decreased or absent. Administration of an extract ("transfer factor") from lymphocytes of immunologically normal donors has been reported to improve the immunologic reactivity of some of these children, with a resulting reduction in the frequency of their infections. An additional feature of the Wiskott-Aldrich syndrome is an increased risk of the development of lymphoreticular malignancy, a possible consequence of the immunologic impairment in this disorder.

Congenital deficiency of megakaryocyte maturation factor ("thrombopoietin"). This rare disorder described by Schulman and others is characterized by severe congenital thrombocytopenia, apparently caused by a failure of megakaryocytic maturation in the bone marrow. Bone marrow smears demonstrate large numbers of early megakaryocyte forms. Following transfusion of normal plasma, which evidently supplies a deficient factor, megakaryocyte maturation proceeds with the production of large numbers of platelets within 2 to 4 days. The diagnosis of this condition is established by the characteristic response to plasma transfusions, followed by recurrence of the thrombocytopenia 3 to 4 weeks later if the transfusion is not repeated.

Neonatal immune thrombocytopenia. In a variety of neonatal thrombocytopenic states a reduced platelet count in the infant is attributable to the transplacental passage of antiplatelet antibody produced by the mother. In one group of these disorders, the antibody production reflects an immunologic abnormality in the mother. Maternal disease states that may produce this effect include systemic lupus erythematosus, the idiopathic thrombocytopenic purpura syndrome, and drug purpura caused by quinidine or other drugs that are known to act as haptens to stimulate the formation of antibody active against platelets. In all of these conditions thrombocytopenia will be present in the mother, which provides a ready means for ascertaining the cause of the disorder in the infant. A possible exception may be a splenectomized mother with the idiopathic thrombocytopenic purpura (ITP) syndrome in whom the platelet count may not be significantly reduced in spite of continued antibody production.

In other cases of neonatal thrombocytopenia, an isoimmune mechanism appears to be the basis of antiplatelet antibody production. Transfusion of fetal platelets into the maternal circulation during pregnancy is known to occur in a manner similar to the passage of erythrocytes in the development of isoimmune hemolytic disease. A variety of immunogenic antigens have been identified in platelets, and it appears likely that the platelets include the entire complement of histocompatibility antigens of the individual. In spite of the high frequency of fetal-maternal incompatibility that can be anticipated, significant thrombocytopenia of the newborn caused by an isoimmune mechanism nevertheless appears to be an uncommon occurrence. The platelet count of the mother is characteristically normal in this form of neonatal thrombocytopenia because of the specificity of the antibody toward platelets of the infant. Multiple offspring of a mother may develop this form of thrombocytopenia, but for unexplained reasons a substantial majority of identified cases have been in firstborn infants. The diagnosis is established by the demonstration of antibody against platelets of the infant in serum from the mother, usually by means of a complement fixation test.

Thrombocytopenia caused by other neonatal disorders. Thrombocytopenia may accompany a variety of neonatal conditions that may produce hemorrhagic sequelae as the first clinical sign of disease in the infant. Conditions in which thrombocytopenia is often of major significance include neonatal leukemia (p. 203) and the group of disorders including neuroblastoma and osteopetrosis (p. 204), in which a generalized suppression of bone marrow function may develop. These conditions can usually be differentiated from other neonatal thrombocytopenic states on the basis of additional distinguishing characteristics.

Thrombocytopenia is also a frequent finding in a wide variety of neonatal infections. Included in this group are congenital rubella, cytomegalic inclusion disease, congenital syphilis, toxoplasmosis, disseminated herpes simplex, and all forms of severe bacterial infection. The thrombocytopenia may arise by a variety of mechanisms in the various forms of infections. In some forms a suppression of platelet production seems to be the major cause, while in others accelerated destruction of platelets appears to be the principal mechanism. A variety of infectious processes may also produce thrombocytopenia in the newborn by acting as a triggering mechanism for the onset of intravascular coaguation. It is axiomatic that thrombocytopenia in a newborn with infection should prompt a search for evidence of the intravascular coagulation syndrome (p. 209). Thrombocytopenia of a substantial degree usually accompanies intravascular coagulation in the newborn resulting from any cause, and this entity must be considered in the differential diagnosis of neonatal thrombocytopenia of unknown cause.

Significant degrees of thrombocytopenia have also been observed in a number of infants born to mothers who received chlorothiazide or related drugs in the latter weeks of pregnancy. The cause of this complication is unknown, but it appears not to be mediated by an immune mechanism. The platelet count of the mother remained within the normal range in the reported examples of this complication.

Management of neonatal hemorrhage caused by platelet disorders. Severe degrees of thrombocytopenia or impairment of platelet function may impose a risk of life-threatening hemorrhage in the neonate. In most instances, however, findings are limited to minor hemorrhagic sequelae, including the development of petechiae and bruising and prolonged bleeding at injection sites. More severe complications may include gastrointestinal hemorrhage, hematuria, and intracranial hemorrhage. The last accounts for most of the fatalities resulting from neonatal platelet disorders and probably stems primarily from trauma to the head during delivery. Careful observation for signs of intracranial hemorrhage is indicated in any newborn infant with significant thrombocytopenia or platelet function abnormality. These signs may include apneic spells, rigidity, irritability, convulsions, a high-pitched cry, and bulging of the fontanelle.

Whenever a platelet abnormality or thrombocytopenia is found in a newborn infant a careful effort to establish a precise etiologic diagnosis is indicated. Thrombocytopenia secondary to many forms of infections, certain intravascular coagulation disorders, and other treatable conditions will often respond well to proper management of the underlying condition.

In most instances the neonate with a platelet function defect or thrombocytopenia will not require any form of specific therapy. As in the management of the older child with thrombocytopenia, a low platelet count is not an indication for treatment in the absence of significant hemorrhage. Many forms of neonatal thrombocytopenia, particularly those arising as a result of maternal antibody, are of a transient nature; if the infant is protected from trauma they will usually resolve permanently after several weeks, without need for any specific treatment.

When hemorrhage occurs in these conditions several forms of therapy may be employed. *Corticosteroids* are of most general value. The corticosteroids appear to exert an effect on capillary vessels, increasing their resistance to injury, and in addition may interfere with antibody-mediated mechanisms of platelet destruction. Corticosteroid therapy in the newborn is usually administered in the form of prednisone, 1 to 2 mg/kg body weight in daily divided doses. Thrombocytopenic bleeding resulting from maternally formed antiplatelet antibody may also be benefited by removal of antibody from the infant's circulation by means of *exchange transfusion.* The considerations for this procedure parallel those for the infant with isoimmune hemolytic disease (p. 189).

Transfusion of platelets may also provide substantial benefit in many forms of neonatal thrombocytopenia. In the immune types of thrombocytopenic purpura, transfused platelets may be rapidly destroyed, but nevertheless they may be of value when hemorrhage occurs. Platelet transfusions are specifically indicated for thrombocytopenic bleeding arising as a result of bone marrow failure or in platelet function abnormalities such as thrombasthenia. Daily administration of platelets derived from 1 to 2 units of fresh blood will usually be adequate for the control of hemorrhage in neonatal thrombocytopenia, although more frequent transfusions may be required in immune forms. For most purposes, particularly in transient forms of neonatal thrombocytopenia, platelets from red blood cell–compatible donors are usually satisfactory. In conditions that carry a lifelong risk of hemorrhage with a potential need for repeated platelet transfusions, as in thrombasthenia, special measures are indicated to prevent the formation of platelet antibodies. In these conditions careful tissue typing and the use of compatible, close relatives as platelet donors will produce an optimal long-term clinical response.

GEORGE R. HONIG

BIBLIOGRAPHY

HEMATOPOIESIS IN THE EMBRYO AND FETUS

Schulman, I.: Characteristics of the blood in foetal life; oxygen supply to the human foetus, Oxford, 1959, Blackwell Scientific Publications, Ltd., p. 43.

Thomas, D. B., and Yaffey, J. M.: Human foetal haemopoiesis. I. The cellular composition of the foetal blood, Br. J. Haematol. 8:290, 1962.

Walker, J., and Turnbull, E. P. N.: Haemoglobin and red cells in the human foetus and their relation to the oxygen content of the blood in the vessels of the umbilical cord, Lancet **2**:312, 1953.

NORMAL HEMATOLOGIC VALUES

Gairdner, D., Marks, J., and Roscoe, J. D.: Blood formation in infancy; the normal bone marrow, Arch. Dis. Child. **27**:128, 1952.

Gairdner, D., Marks, J., and Roscoe, J. D.: Blood formation in infancy; normal erythropoiesis, Arch. Dis. Child. **27**:214, 1952.

Humbert, J. R., Abelson, H., Hathway, W. E., and Battaglia, F. C.: Polycythemia in small for gestational age infants, J. Pediatr. **75**:812, 1969.

Iron nutrition in infancy, 1970, Sixty-second Ross Conference on Pediatric Research, Chicago, Ill.

Maurer, H. S., Behrman, R. E., and Honig, G. R.: Dependence of the oxygen affinity of blood on the presence of foetal or adult haemoglobin, Nature **227**:388, 1970.

O'Brien, R. T., and Pearson, H. A.: Physiologic anemia of the newborn infant, J. Pediatr. **79**: 132, 1971.

Oski, F., and Naiman, J. L.: Hematologic problems in the newborn, Philadelphia, 1966, W. B. Saunders Co.

Oski, F. A., and Smith, C.: Red cell metabolism in the premature infant. III. Apparent inappropriate glucose consumption for cell age, Pediatrics **41**:473, 1968.

Schulman, I.: The anemia of prematurity, J. Pediatr. **54**:663, 1959.

Usher, R., Shephard, M., and Lind, J.: The blood volume of the newborn infant and placental transfusion, Acta Paediatr. Scand. **52**:497, 1963.

Xanthou, M.: Leucocyte blood picture in healthy full term and premature babies during neonatal life, Arch. Dis. Child. **45**:242, 1970.

ANEMIA CAUSED BY HEMORRHAGE

Chown, B.: Anaemia from bleeding of the fetus into the maternal circulation, Lancet **1**:1213, 1954.

Cohen, F., Zuelzer, W. W., Gustafson, D. C., and Evans, M. M.: Mechanisms of isoimmunization. I. The passage of fetal erythroctyes in homospecific pregnancies, Blood **23**:621, 1964.

Eraklis, A. J.: Abdominal injury related to the trauma of birth, Pediatrics **39**:421, 1967.

Goodall, H. B., Graham, F. S., Miller, M. C., and Cameron, D.: Transplacental bleeding from the fetus, J. Clin. Pathol. **11**:251, 1958.

Kirkman, H. N., and Riley, H. D., Jr.: Posthemorrhagic anemia and shock in the newborn, Pediatrics **24**:92, 97, 1959.

Leonard, S., and Anthony, B.: Giant cephalohematoma of newborn, Am. J. Dis. Child. **101**:170, 1961.

Miles, R. M., Maurer, H. M., and Valdes, O. S.: Iron-deficiency anemia at birth; two examples secondary to chronic fetal-maternal hemorrhage, Clin. Pediatr. (Phila.) **10**:223, 1917.

Neligan, G. A., and Russell, J. K.: Blood loss from the foetal circulation, a hazard of lower segment caesarean section in cases of placenta praevia, J. Obstet. Gynaecol. Br. Commonw. **61**:2, 1954.

Neligan, G. A., and Smith, M. C.: Prevention of haemorrhage from the umbilical cord, Arch. Dis. Child. **38**:471, 1963.

Pachman, D. J.: Massive hemorrhage in the scalp of the newborn infant; hemorrhagic caput succedaneum, Pediatrics **29**:907, 1962.

Rausen, A. R., and Diamond, L. K.: Enclosed hemorrhage and neonatal jaundice, Am. J. Dis. Child. **101**:164, 1961.

Rausen, A. R., Seki, M., and Strauss, L.: Twin transfusion syndrome; a review of 19 cases studied at one institution, J. Pediatr. **66**:613, 1965.

Rose, J., Berdon, W. E., Sullivan, T., and Baker, D. H.: Prolonged jaundice as presenting sign of massive adrenal hemorrhage in newborn; radiographic diagnosis by intravenous urography with total-body opacification, Radiology **98**: 263, 1971.

Siddall, R. S., and West, R. H.: Incision of the placenta at cesarian section; cause of fetal anemia, Am. J. Obstet. Gynecol. **63**:425, 1952.

Weiner, A. S.: Diagnosis and treatment of anemia of the newborn caused by occult placental hemorrhage, Am. J. Obstet. Gynecol. **56**:717, 1948.

CONGENITAL HYPOPLASTIC ANEMIA

Allen, D. M., and Diamond, L. K.: Congenital (erythroid) hypoplastic anemia; cortisone treated, Am. J. Dis. Child. **102**:416, 1961.

Diamond, L. K., Allen, D. M., and Magill, F. B.: Congenital (erythroid) hypoplastic anemia; a 25 year study, Am. J. Dis. Child. **102**:403, 1961.

Minagi, H., and Steinback, H. L.: Roentgen appearance of anomalies associated with hypoplastic anemias of childhood; Fanconi's anemia and congenital anemia (erythrogenesis imperfecta), Am. J. Roentgenol. **47**:100, 1966.

Nilsson, L. R.: Chronic pancytopenia with multiple congenital abnormalities (Franconi's anaemia), Acta Paediatr. **49**:518, 1960.

Sjölin, S.: Studies on osteopetrosis. II. Investigations concerning the nature of the anaemia, Acta Paediatr. **48**:529, 1959.

ISOIMMUNE HEMOLYTIC DISEASE

Bowman, J. M., and Pollock, J. M.: Amniotic fluid spectrophotemtry and early delivery in the management of erythroblastosis fetalis, Pediatrics **35**:815, 1965.

Chessells, J. M., and Wiggelsworth, J. S.: Haemostatic failure in babies with rhesus isoimmunization, Arch. Dis. Child. **46**:38, 1971.

Cohen, F., Zuelzer, W. W., Gustafson, D. C., and Evans, M. M.: Mechanisms of isoimmunization. I. The transplacental passage of fetal erythrocytes in homospecific pregnancies, Blood **23**: 621, 1964.

Dunn, P. M.: Obstructive jaundice and haemolytic disease of the newborn, Arch. Dis. Child. **38**: 54, 1963.

Farquhar, J. W., and Smith, H.: Clinical and biochemical changes during exchange transfusion, Arch. Dis. Child. **33**:142, 1958.

Freda, V. J., Gorman, J. G., and Pollack, W.: Suppression of the primary Rh immune response with passive Rh IgC immunoglobulin, N. Engl. J. Med. **277**:1002, 1967.

Grundbacher, F. J.: ABO hemolytic disease of the newborn; a family study with emphasis on the strength of the A antigen, Pediatrics **35**:916, 1965.

Hsia, D. Y., Allen, F. H., Jr., Gellis, S. S., and Diamond, L. K.: Erythroblastosis fetalis. VIII. Studies of serum bilirubin in relation to kernicterus. N. Engl. J. Med. **247**:668, 1952.

Hsia, D. Y., and Gellis, S. S.: Studies on erythroblastosis due to ABO incompatibility, Pediatrics **13**:503, 1954.
Liley, A. W.: Diagnosis and treatment of erythroblastosis in the fetus, Adv. Pediatr. **15**:29, 1968.
Lucey, J. F.: Current indications and results of fetal transfusions, Pediatrics **41**:139, 1968.
McKay, R. J., Jr.: Current status of use of exchange transfusion in newborn infants, Pediatrics **33**:763, 1964.
Odell, G., Cohen, S. N., and Gordes, E. H.: Administration of albumin in the management of hyperbilirubinemia by exchange transfusion, Pediatrics **30**:613, 1962.
Pochedly, C.: Etiology of late anemia of hemolytic disease of the newborn, Clin. Med. **78**:30, 1971.
Raivio, K. O., and Osterlund, K.: Hypoglycemia and hyperinsulinemia associated with erythroblastosis fetalis, Pediatrics **43**:217, 1969.
Robinson, G. C., Phillips, R. M., and Prystowsky, M.: Spheroctyosis and increased fragility occurring in erythroblastosis fetalis associated with ABO incompatibility, Pediatrics **7**:164, 1951.
Sisson, T. R. C., Kendall, N., Glauser, S. C., Knutson, S., and Bunyaviroch, E.: Phototherapy of jaundice in newborn infants. I. ABO blood group incompatibility, J. Pediatr. **79**:904, 1971.
Van Praagh, R.: Diagnosis of kernicterus in the neonatal period, Pediatrics **28**:870, 1961.
Walker, W., and Ellis, M. I.: Intrauterine transfusion, Br. Med. J. **2**:223, 1970.
Waters, W. J., Richert, D. A., and Rawson, H. H.: Bilirubin encephalopathy, Pediartics **13**:319, 1954.

GLUCOSE-6-PHOSPHATE DEHYDROGENASE DEFICIENCY

Beutler, E.: Glucose-6-phosphate dehydrogenase and nonspherocytic congenital hemolytic anemia, Semin. Hematol. **2**:91, 1965.
Brown, A. K., and Cevik, N.: Hemolysis and jaundice in the newborn following maternal treatment with sulfamethoxpyridazine (Kynex), Pediatrics **36**:742, 1965.
Eshaghpour, E., Oski, F. A., and Williams, M.: The relationship of erythrocyte glucose-6-phosphate dehydrogenase deficiency to hyperbilirubinemia in Negro premature infants, J. Pediatr. **70**:595, 1967.
Ifekwunigwe, A. E., and Luzzatto, L.: Kernicterus in G-6-PD deficiency, Lancet **1**:667, 1966.
Lopez, R., and Cooperman, J. M.: Glucose-6-phosphate dehydrogenase deficiency and hyperbilirubinemia in the newborn, Am. J. Dis. Child. **122**:66, 1971.

OTHER ERYTHROCYTE ENZYME ABNORMALITIES THAT PREDISPOSE THE INFANT TO DRUG-INDUCED HEMOLYSIS

Jaffé, E. R.: Hereditary hemolytic disorders and enzymatic deficiencies of human erythrocytes, Blood **35**:116, 1970.
Necheles, T. F., Boles, T. A., and Allen, D. M.: Erythrocyte glutathione-peroxidase deficiency and hemolytic disease of the newborn infant, J. Pedaitr. **72**:319, 1968.

HEMOLYTIC ANEMIAS CAUSED BY INTRINSIC ABNORMALITIES OF THE ERYTHROCYTE MEMBRANE

Cutting, H. O., McHugh, W. J., Conrad, F. G., and Marlow, A. A.: Autosomal dominant hemolytic anemia characterized by ovalocytosis; a family study of seven involved members, Am. J. Med. **39**:21, 1965.
Wolman, I. J., and Ozge, A.: Studies on elliptocytosis. I. Hereditary elliptocytosis in the pediatric age period; a review of recent literature, Am. J. Med. Sci. **234**:702, 1957.
Zarkowsky, H. S., Oski, F. A., Sha'afi, R., Shohet, S. B., and Nathan, D. G.: Congenital hemolytic anemia with high sodium, low potassium red cells, N. Engl. J. Med. **278**:593, 1968.

HEREDITARY SPHEROCYTOSIS

Jacob, H. S.: Hereditary spherocytosis; a disease of the red cell membrane, Semin. Hematol. **2**:139, 1965.
Truccoo, J. I., and Brown, A. K.: Neonatal manifestations of hereditary spherocytosis, Am. J. Dis. Child. **113**:263, 1967.

HEMOLYTIC ANEMIA OF VITAMIN E DEFICIENCY IN PREMATURE INFANTS

Ritchie, J. H., Fish, M. B., McMasters, V., and Grossman, M.: Edema and hemolytic anemia in premature infants; a vitamin E deficiency syndrome, N. Engl. J. Med. **279**:1185, 1969.

DISORDERS OF HEMOGLOBIN STRUCTURE, BIOSYNTHESIS, AND FUNCTION

Huntsman, R. G., Metters, J. S., and Yawson, G. I.: The diagnosis of sickle cell disease in the newborn infant, J. Pediatr. **80**:279, 1972.
Jaffé, E. R., and Heller, P.: Methemoglobinemia in man, Progr. Hematol. **4**:48, 1964.
Minnich, V., Cordonnier, J. K., Williams, W. J., and Moore, C. V.: Alpha, beta, and gamma polypeptide chains during the neonatal period with description of a fetal form of hemoglobin Da-St. Louis, Blood **19**:137, 1962.
Necheles, T. F., and Allen, D. M.: Heinz-body anemias, N. Engl. J. Med. **280**:203, 1969.
Ranney, H. M.: Clinically important variants of human hemoglobin, N. Engl. J. Med. **282**:144, 1970.
Weatherall, D. J.: The thalassemia syndromes, Oxford, 1965, Blackwell Scientific Publications, Ltd.

LEUKEMIA

Engel, R. R., Hammond, D., Eitzman, D. V., Pearson, H., and Krivit, W.: Transient congenital leukemia in 7 infants with mongolism, J. Pediatr. **65**:303, 1964.
Pierce, M. I.: Leukemia in the newborn infant, J. Pediatr. **54**:691, 1959.
Reimann, D. L., Clemmens, R. L., and Pillsbury, W. A.: Congenital acute leukemia; skin nodules, a first sign, J. Pediatr. **46**:415, 1955.

GRANULOCYTOPENIC DISORDERS

Kostmann, R.: Infantile genetic agranulocytosis; a new recessive lethal disease in man, Acta Paediatr. (supp. 105) **45**:1, 1956.

Lalezari, P., Nussbaum, M., Gelman, S., and Spaet, T. H.: Neonatal neutropenia due to maternal isoimmunization, Blood **15**:236, 1960.

Miller, D. R., Freed, B. A., and Lapey, J. D.: Congenital neutropenia; report of a fatal case in a Negro infant with leukocyte function studies, Am. J. Dis. Child. **115**:337, 1968.

Stahlie, T. O. V.: Chronic benign neutropenia in infancy and early childhood, J. Pediatr. **48**:710, 1956.

HEMOSTASIS AND HEMORRHAGIC DISORDERS

Aballi, A. J., Puapondh, Y., and Desposito, F.: Platelet counts in thriving premature infants, Pediatrics **42**:685, 1968.

Bleyer, W. A., Hakami, N., and Shepard, T. H.: The development of hemostasis in the human fetus and newborn infant, J. Pediatr. **79**:838, 1971.

Corby, D. G., and Schulman, I.: The effects of antenatal drug administration on aggregation of platelets of newborn infants, J. Pediatr. **79**:307, 1971.

Hathaway, W. E.: Coagulation problems in the newborn infant, Pediatr. Clin. North Am. **17**: 929, 1970.

CONGENITAL DEFICIENCY OF COAGULATION FACTORS

Baehner, R. L., and Strauss, H. S.: Hemophilia in in the first year of life, N. Engl. J. Med. **275**: 524, 1966.

Cade, J. F., Hirsh, J., and Martin, M.: Placental barrier to coagulation factors; its relevance to the coagulation defect at birth and to hemorrhage in the newborn, Br. Med. J. **2**:281, 1969.

NEONATAL VITAMIN K DEFICIENCY

Dam, H., Larsen, H., and Plum, P.: The relation of vitamin K deficiency to hemorrhagic disease of the newborn, Adv. Pediatr. **5**:129, 1952.

Keenan, W. J., Jewett, T., and Glueck, H. I.: Role of feeding and vitamin K in hypoprothrombinemia of the newborn, Am. J. Dis. Child. **121**: 271, 1971.

Mountain, K. R., Hirsh, J., and Gallus, A. S.: Neonatal coagulation defect due to anticonvulsant drug treatment in pregnancy, Lancet **1**:265, 1970.

INTRAVASCULAR COAGULATION DISORDERS

Abildgaard, C. F.: Recognition and treatment of intravascular coagulation, J. Pediatr. **74**:163, 1969.

Hathaway, W. E., Mull, M. M., and Pechet, G. S.: Disseminated intravascular coagulation in the newborn, Pediatrics **43**:233, 1969.

ABNORMALITIES OF PLATELET FUNCTION

Corby, D. G., Zirbie,, C. L., Lindley, A., and Schulman, I.: Thrombasthenia, Am. J. Dis. Child. **121**:140, 1971.

Hirsch, J., and Doery, J. C. G.: Platelet function in health and disease, Progr. Hematol. **7**:185, 1971.

NEONATAL THROMBOCYTOPENIA

Anthony, B., and Krivit, W.: Neonatal thrombocytopenic purpura, Pediatrics **30**:776, 1962.

Eisenstein, E. M.: Congenital amegakaryocytic thrombocytopenic purpura, Clin. Pediatr. (Phila.) **5**:143, 1966.

Hall, J. G., Levin, J., Kuhn, J. P., Ottenheimer, E. J., van Berkum, K. A. P., and McKusick, V. A.: Thrombocytopenia with absent radius, Medicine **48**:411, 1969.

Pearson, H. A., Shulman, N. R., Marder, V. J., and Cone, T. E., Jr.: Isoimmune neonatal thrombocytopenic purpura; clinical and therapeutic considerations, Blood **23**:154, 1964.

Schulman, I., Pierce, M., Lukens, A., and Currimbhoy, Z.: Studies on thrombopoiesis. I. A factor in normal human plasma required for platelet production; chronic thrombocytopenia due to its deficiency, Blood **16**:943, 1960.

10 Jaundice

NEONATAL HYPERBILIRUBINEMIA

Jaundice, probably the commonest symptom in the newborn, results from accumulation of unconjugated bilirubin in the serum and tissues. About 50% of all full-term infants and about 80% of all preterm infants become jaundiced in the first few days of life unless measures are taken to prevent its appearance. Even in the infant without visible jaundice, bilirubin levels are higher than those observed under normal circumstances at any later period of life. Cord bilirubin values range from 1.8 to 2.8 mg/100 ml, and the level of bilirubin usually rises for the first 48 to 72 hours in full-term infants and for as long as 7 days after birth in premature infants.

It has become obvious in recent years that many factors influence what has been accepted as normal patterns of "physiologic" bilirubinemia in both full-term and preterm infants. Nursery practices such as the time of the first feeding, the amount of exposure to light, and the administration of certain drugs modify these patterns of jaundice, so that the distinction between what may be considered physiologic and what is considered pathologic jaundice will depend in part upon the nursery circumstances and practices. Despite this, one of the most important tasks within the nursery is to distinguish the degree and type of jaundice that is acceptable as physiologic from that which is pathologic in its extent and which may herald a specific disorder in the newborn.

Concept of physiologic jaundice

Since some degree of jaundice or bilirubin accumulation is to be expected in the newborn, it has become customary to consider its occurrence physiologic and to relate this phenomenon to a transient limitation in the infant's capacity to metabolize and excrete bilirubin in the immediate neonatal period. The type of pigment that accounts for physiologic jaundice is unconjugated bilirubin, a nonpolar, lipid-soluble pigment that requires conjugation, usually as a glucuronide, to render it ready for excretion from the hepatic cell into the biliary system. As understanding of the pathways of bilirubin formation, metabolism, and excretion has gradually increased, differences have become apparent between the nature and extent of bilirubin metabolism in the fetus and newborn and that in the adult.

The limitations in bilirubin metabolism that have been identified in the newborn infant appear to result from an extension into extrauterine life of fetal bilirubin metabolism. At the time of birth the transition from fetal to adult metabolism usually is incomplete. A brief discussion of this transition is necessary for the understanding of physiologic jaundice.

Adult versus fetal type of bilirubin metabolism

In the adult, bilirubin is produced from the daily degradation of hemoglobin. About 1% of the hemoglobin mass is converted to bilirubin each day; each gram of degraded hemoglobin produces 35 mg of bilirubin. The enzymatic sequence by which hemoglobin is ultimately converted to bilirubin first involves the conversion of hemoglobin to biliverdin through the action of hemeoxygenase. This enzyme is most plentiful in the liver and spleen. Biliverdin is then reduced to bilirubin through the action of biliverdin reductase. The nonpolar bilirubin is then transported, bound to albumin, to the hepatic parenchymal cell.

A second protein is needed for the intracellular transport of bilirubin to the hepatic microsomes. Here, lipid-soluble bilirubin is converted to water-soluble bilirubin diglucuronide through the action of the hepatic microsomal enzyme glucuronyl transferase. In this reaction the specific glucuronide donor is uridine diphosphoglucose through the action of uridine diphosphoglucose dehydrogenase (UDPG dehydrogenase). This metabolic step requires the normal antecedent carbohydrate, as well as uridine, metabolism.

In conjugated soluble form, bilirubin diglucuronide is excreted from the hepatic cell into the biliary system and into the gastrointestinal tract. The intestine, in a sense, completes the excretory function of the liver, since substances rendered water soluble and polar by the hepatic conjugating systems are not usually reabsorbed across the intestinal mucosa but pass out of the body in stool. If there is delay in passage of bilirubin through the intestine, some deconjugation of bilirubin may take place, rendering the pigment again nonpolar. In this lipid-soluble state the pigment can be reabsorbed across the mucosa. It is recycled via the enterohepatic shunt and ultimately metabolized and excreted again by the liver.

During maturation of the fetus the system for elimination of the degradation products of hemoglobin varies; throughout gestation the sequence differs from that in later adult life. Limitation of bilirubin excretion via the adult route is, of course, more exaggerated in the immature, preterm infants than in those born at term.

The major characteristics of fetal bilirubin metabolism are depicted in Fig. 10-1. Early in fetal life (16 to 20 weeks), biliverdin can be found in the amniotic fluid. This pigment may be the major end product of bilirubin in the fetus until conjugated bilirubin is formed. How or why bilirubin enters amniotic fluid from about 20 weeks' until 36 weeks' gestation is not yet known; the concentration of the pigment decreases with advancing gestation, unless there is either hemolytic disease or some disorder that interferes with the normal circulation of the amniotic fluid. Such disorders include high intestinal obstruction and anencephaly; the latter probably affects fetal swallowing of amniotic fluid.

The major difference between the fetal and adult system for bilirubin clearance appears to hinge upon the fact that, in the fetus, the major pathway for elimination is via the placenta; elimination of waste products via the fetal intestine is not a well-developed or even a desirable route. Utilization of the fetal pathway requires that bilirubin remain in a nonpolar form in order to cross the placenta.

In general, the limited functions of the fetus with regard to the metabolism of bilirubin are those that would result in the formation of a pigment that would not cross the placental membranes. In the fetus the bilirubin is not readily conjugated to a glucuronide; the capacity to excrete it from the hepatic cell is not fully developed; and relatively little bilirubin enters the intestine for excretion. In addition, the fetus also has a high concentration of β-glucuronidase in the intestine. This enzyme further ensures placental excretion, since it can deconjugate bilirubin glucuronide that has been formed and excreted into the intestine; deconjugation renders the bilirubin lipid soluble, once more permitting intestinal reabsorption. The limited mobility of the fetal gut promotes reabsorption of deconjugated (nonpolar) bilirubin across the intestinal mucosa and offers another opportunity for placental clearance of the circulating pigment. Two other features of fetal metabolism also contribute to the varying degree of physiologic jaundice in the neonate: increased red blood cell degradation and decreased hepatic perfusion.

Red blood cell degradation

The major source of bilirubin even in fetal life is the degradation of red blood cell hemoglobin. Most studies indicate that

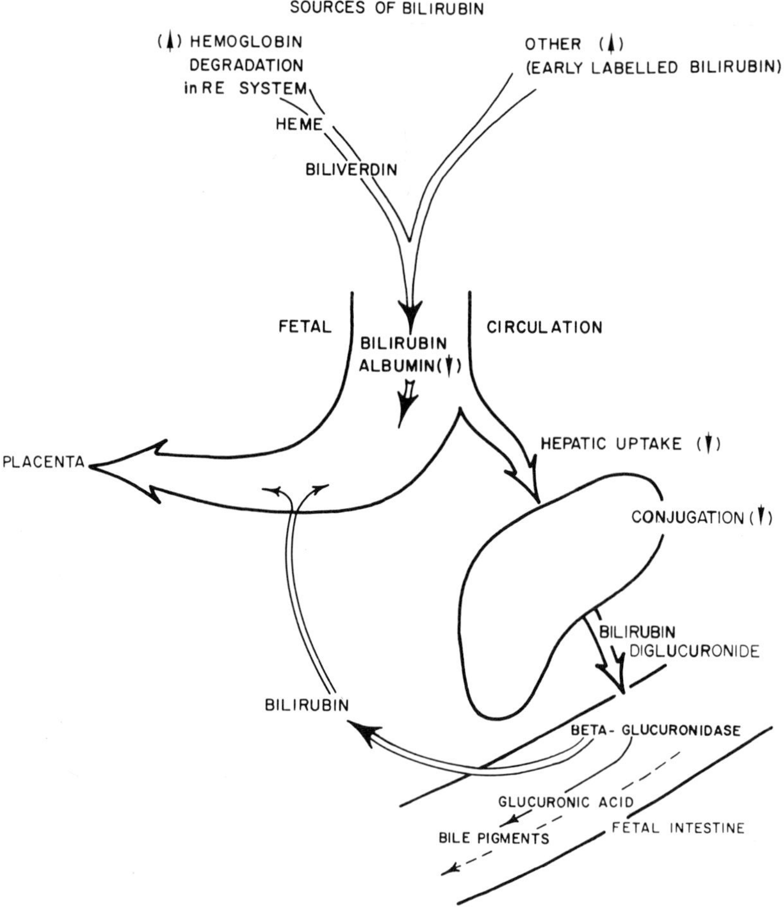

Fig. 10-1. Fetal metabolism of bilirubin. Arrows (above or below) indicate relative increase or decrease in function.

the survival time of the erythrocytes of preterm infants is shorter than that of adults; red blood cell survival in the full-term infant is only slightly decreased. The more immature the infant, the greater is the likelihood of an increased contribution of hemoglobin degradation to the load of bilirubin imposed on the marginally functioning hepatic conjugating system. From recent studies in which the endogenous production of carbon monoxide from heme has been measured, it has been calculated that the normal newborn produces bilirubin from hemoglobin at a rate of 6 to 8 mg/kg/24 hr. This rate is more than twice the rate of production in the adult. Such an increase in hemolysis in the adult would not produce hyperbilirubinemia, since adults have reserve capacity for hepatic metabolism of bilirubin. In the infant, however, the marginal capacity for bilirubin metabolism is easily exceeded, and even minimal increases in the pigment load often lead to hyperbilirubinemia.

Hepatic perfusion

In many abnormal clinical situations such as hypoxia or hyaline membrane disease, the perfusion of the liver may be reduced. This may be related to patency of the ductus venosus through which portal blood may bypass hepatic sinusoidal circulation.

Summary

With advancing gestation, there is a gradual increase in the capacity of the fetus to metabolize bilirubin according to the adult pathway. However, since the major portion of bilirubin continues to be excreted via the placenta, a route of clearance that requires that bilirubin remain non-polar, it is not surprising to find that the capacity to conjugate and excrete the polar form of bilirubin remains limited until late in gestation when the fetus readies himself for extrauterine existence. The infant is born in this transitional phase and must quickly convert from the fetal to the extra-uterine pattern of bilirubin metabolism. Thus gestational age at birth and the degree to which he has developed the adult patterns of the functions of heme catabolism, bilirubin transport, conjugation, and excretion as well as the degree to which the enterohepatic shunt contributes to the bilirubin load on the liver will in large measure determine the degree to which the neonate will manifest physiologic jaundice.

Limits of physiologic jaundice

The limits of physiologic jaundice have been set largely by experience. The parameters by which these limits are determined include consideration of the time of appearance and disappearance of jaundice as well as the nature, rate, and degree of accumulation of serum bilirubin. Since the time of disappearance of jaundice, as well as the extent of bilirubin accumulation, varies with the degree of maturity of the infant, different limits are usually set for the preterm infant. The accumulation of conjugated (direct-reacting) bilirubin is never considered physiologic jaundice.

Full-term infants

Cord indirect reacting bilirubin levels range from 1.8 mg/100 ml to 2.8 mg/100 ml in the normal infant. Higher values of serum bilirubin from umbilical cord samples are almost always indicative of intrauterine hemolytic disease (p. 190). In full-term infants, there is a gradual rise in bilirubin from birth until 48 to 72 hours of life; the rate of increase is less than 5 mg/100 ml/24 hr. In the normal infant no jaundice will be visible until after 24 hours of age, since jaundice is not apparent in the neonate until more than 5 mg/100 ml has accumulated in the serum. Jaundice in the first 24 hours of age can never be caused by physiologic processes alone, either in full-term or preterm infants.

In full-term infants a peak bilirubin level of about 5 mg/100 ml is found at about 72 hours, and then there is a gradual decrease. By the end of the first week of life full-term infants should not have levels of bilirubin in excess of 1 to 2 mg/100 ml. Jaundice does not persist into the second week. Normal values for the expected degree of bilirubin in the neonate vary considerably, since many nursery practices with regard to feeding, lighting, and so on may influence bilirubin metabolism. The mean values for serum bilirubin levels in appropriately grown (AGA) full-term infants compared with undergrown (SGA) infants as well as with preterm infants is seen in Fig. 10-2. In the Collaborative Study, in which data was gathered over many years in 12 institutions, the extent to which hyperbilirubinemia occurred in large populations of white and black infants was documented. Less than 3% of full-term infants developed bilirubin levels greater than 15 mg/100 ml (Table 10-1). It is likely that even within this limited number with excessive jaundice, factors other than physiologic jaundice accounted for the bilirubinemia.

Preterm infants

Cord bilirubin levels for preterm infants are similar to those found in full-term infants under normal circumstances. The rate of bilirubin accumulation is also identical to that found in full-term infants during the first 24 to 48 hours of life. The preterm infants, however, continue to accumulate bilirubin longer than the full-term infant,

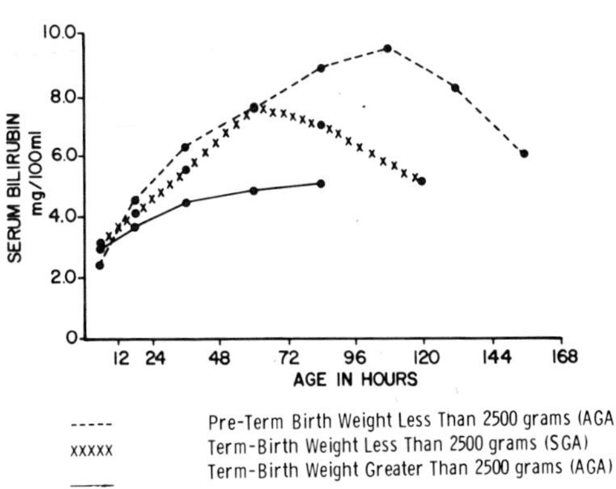

FIG. 10-2. Mean serum bilirubin levels in relation to age in three groups of infants.

TABLE 10-1. Highest total serum bilirubin of newborn by birthweight (white)

Bilirubin mg/100 ml	Under 2,500 gm (1,142) percent of infants	Over 2,500 gm (17,292) percent of infants	Overall percent
0-7	42.73	73.73	71.69
8-12	29.42	20.08	20.70
13-15	11.21	3.29	3.81
16-19	9.98	1.95	2.48
20+	6.65	0.95	1.32

Adapted from Niswander, K. R., and Jordan, M., editors: The Collaborative Perinatal Study of NINDS, Philadelphia, 1972, W. B. Saunders Co.

even though the rate of accumulation remains about the same (less than 5 mg/100 ml/day). The peak of the bilirubin concentration, as well as the time it takes for jaundice to become maximal and then recede, varies from infant to infant, depending on the time it takes for that infant to fully assume the extrauterine functions needed for the clearance of bilirubin.

In our nursery, the mean peak bilirubin level among preterm infants is about 8 mg/100 ml, which occurs on the fourth day of life (Fig. 10-2). In the Collaborative Study 16.6% of low birth weight (presumably preterm) white infants were found to have bilirubin levels greater than 15/ mg/100 ml; only 7.9% of black infants of similar weight had such extreme degrees of hyperbilirubinemia (Table 10-2). Occasionally in very immature infants, some degree of physiologic bilirubinemia may persist into the second week of life. Jaundice is extremely rare after the tenth day of life.

Only unconjugated bilirubin in the blood can be accounted for by the concept of physiologic jaundice. Accumulation of any direct-reacting, or conjugated, bilirubin in the blood is a reflection of impaired excretion of conjugated bilirubin from the hepatic cell or biliary tree and should always be looked upon as an index of pathologic jaundice.

A summary of the clinical criteria for the limits of physiologic jaundice is outlined in the list below. These same limits, when exceeded, form the basis of selecting those infants whose jaundice requires investigation. The pattern of expression of jaundice (too early, too high, too late, and so on) is helpful in arriving at a diagnosis.

LIMITS OF PHYSIOLOGIC JAUNDICE: CRITERIA FOR INVESTIGATION OF JAUNDICE

1. Jaundice in the first 24 hours of life
2. Serum bilirubin rising at a rate *greater* than 5 mg/100 ml/day
3. Serum bilirubin greater than 12 mg/100 ml in full-term infants
4. Serum bilirubin greater than 15 mg/100 ml/day in preterm infants
5. Persistence of jaundice after the first week of life
6. Presence of direct-reacting bilirubin (> 1 mg/100 ml) at any time

Pathologic jaundice

Jaundice is pathologic if the nature of the pigment and its degree or time of appearance or disappearance are incompatible with the above criteria for physiologic jaundice or if the degree of jaundice, even if accumulated within the patterns described for physiologic processes, is sufficient to produce a significant risk of damage to the infant. For example, a preterm infant with a bilirubin level of 12 mg/100 mg may have accumulated this bilirubin by a physiologic process, but might develop kernicterus with this degree of bilirubinemia.

The differential diagnosis of hyperbilirubinemia in the early neonatal period is extensive because many factors can upset the tenuous balance between bilirubin formation and the infant's capacity for bilirubin clearance. However, the vast array of causes of jaundice can usually be consolidated into major categories. These include those factors that augment the production of bilirubin, such as hemolysis, hematomas, polycythemia; those factors that impair or inhibit hepatic microsomal conjugating capacity; and those factors that interfere with or obstruct hepatic excretion

TABLE 10-2. Highest total serum bilirubin of newborn by birthweight (black)

Bilirubin mg/100 ml	Under 2,500 gm (2,261) percent of infants	Over 2,500 gm (18,015) percent of infants	Overall percent
0-7	50.29	74.48	71.45
8-12	31.80	21.00	22.36
13-15	9.95	2.62	3.54
16-19	5.0	1.28	1.75
20+	2.96	0.62	0.91

Adapted from Niswander, K. R., and Jordan, M., editors: The Collaborative Perinatal Study of NINDS, Philadelphia, 1972, W. B. Saunders Co.

of bilirubin. Table 10-3 outlines the major causes of hyperbilirubinemia in relation to their clinical patterns of expression. The time of appearance of jaundice and rate of accumulation of bilirubin are useful indices of the nature of the underlying cause of jaundice.

Increased production of bilirubin

Jaundice appearing in the first 24 hours of life is almost always an index of hemolysis or of other disorders, such as enclosed hemorrhage, hematoma, and polycythemia, that increase the load of bilirubin presented to the liver.

Rh hemolytic disease (p. 183) is characterized by a positive reaction to a direct Coombs test. The anemia and the reticulocytosis are variable, ranging from extreme anemia, with associated hepatosplenomegaly and even hydrops, to little or no anemia and a reticulocyte count that may be within the normal range for the gestational age. Rh hemolytic disease can occur in any situation in which the infant possesses an Rh antigen (CDE; cde) that the mother does not have.

A-B-O hemolytic disease (p. 184) is usually associated with a positive reaction to a direct Coombs test in the first week of life, but when this reaction is negative the infant's serum can be shown to give a positive reaction to an indirect Coombs test against adult cells of his own type (A or B). Spherocytes are usually obvious on the peripheral smear. Anemia is modest, and only on rare occasions does the hemoglobin fall below 12 gm/100 ml. Reticulocytosis of a mild degree may exist (6% to 10%). The associated jaundice is disproportionate to the degree of anemia. Kernicterus may occur.

Congenital spherocytosis (p. 196), which is more common among white than black infants, can produce a clinical picture identical to that of erythroblastosis associated with isoimmune disease. Reaction to the Coombs test is negative, and spherocytes are identifiable on smear. The spleen may be palpable. Anemia and jaundice may be modest or extreme. Kernicterus has been reported in neonates with this disorder. (Other congenital defects in red blood cell metabolism that may be present with jaundice in the neonatal period are discussed in Chapter 9.)

Glucose-6-phosphate dehydrogenase (G-6-PD) deficiency (p. 194) occurs in 10% to 14% of the black male population. Hyperbilirubinemia and kernicterus have been reported among G-6-PD–deficient newborns from many parts of the world, including China and Greece. Surveys of black full-term infants who are G-6-PD deficient have not revealed an increased incidence of hyperbilirubinemia. However, among black premature infants with G-6-PD deficiency, an increased incidence of hyperbilirubinemia has been documented. The increased incidence of jaundice in such G-6-PD–deficient infants may be the result of hemolysis, but in many instances no offending drug or other factor has been identified as the triggering agent. In some of these infants mild sepsis is diagnosed in association with a degree of hyperbilirubinemia disproportionate to the degree of apparent illness. Reticulocytosis, even in the absence of anemias is a very common finding, probably reflecting erythropoietic compensation for subtle hemolysis. When there is hemolysis, fragmented red blood cells as well as spherocytes and pyknocytes are common. Early in the

TABLE 10-3. Diagnostic features of the various types of neonatal jaundice

Diagnosis	Nature of van den Bergh reaction	Jaundice		Peak bilirubin conc.		Bilirubin rate of accumulation	Remarks
		Appears	Disappears	Mg %	Age in days	Mg %/day	
1. "Physiologic jaundice":							1. Usually relates to degree of maturity
Full-term	Indirect	2-3 days	4-5 days	10-12	2-3	<5	
Premature	Indirect	3-4 days	7-9 days	15	6-8	<5	
2. Hyperbilirubinemia due to metabolic factors, etc.:							2. Metabolic factors: hypoxia, respiratory distress, lack of carbohydrate Hormonal influences: cretinism, maternal hormones Genetic factors: Crigler-Najjar syndrome, transient familial hyperbilirubinemia Drugs: vitamin K, novobiocin
Full-term	Indirect	2-3 days	Variable	>12	1st wk.	<5	
Premature	Indirect	3-4 days	Variable	>15	1st. wk.	<5	
3. Hemolytic states and hematoma	Indirect	May appear in 1st 24 hours	Variable	Unlimited	Variable	Usually >5	3. Erythroblastosis: Rh, ABO. Congenital hemolytic states: spherocytic, nonspherocytic. Infantile pyknocytosis Drugs: vitamin K, enclosed hemorrhage—hematoma
4. Mixed hemolytic and hepatotoxic factors	Indirect and direct	May appear in 1st 24 hours	Variable	Unlimited	Variable	Usually >5	4. Infection: bacterial sepsis, pyelonephritis, hepatitis, toxoplasmosis, cytomegalic inclusion disease Drugs: vitamin K
5. Hepatocellular damage	Indirect and direct	Usually 2-3 days	Variable	Unlimited	Variable	Variable: can be >5	5. Biliary atresia; galactosemia; hepatitis and infection as in (4)

From Brown, A. K.: Pediatr. Clin. North Am. **9**(3):589, Aug. 1962.

course of hemolysis, supravital stains reveal Heinz bodies within the red blood cells. Normal newborn infants have increased levels of red blood cell G-6-PD, so that the finding of markedly reduced levels of this red blood cell enzyme is evidence of the inherited deficiency. The mothers of these infants can be identified as carriers of this sex-linked inherited defect.

Other factors increasing the production of bilirubin. Other disorders that produce early jaundice or a rapidly rising bilirubin level include polycythemia, enclosed hemorrhages, and extensive bruises or petechiae. In polycythemia, while the rate of hemoglobin degradation may not be increased, degradation at the normal rate (1% or 2%) of the increased hemoglobin mass each day leads to hyperbilirubinemia. It is important to recognize that even minimal apparent hemolysis can be associated with extreme jaundice. The major indices of hemolysis are exaggerated reticulocytosis (75%) and early jaundice rather than a percipitous fall in hemoglobin.

Because of the wide range of normal values for both hemoglobin and reticulocytes in the newborn it is important for the physician, when trying to evaluate the presence of hemolysis, to record whether the sample was venous or capillary and to compare the patient's hematologic findings with normal values for both the gestational and the postnatal age (p. 172).

Hyperbilirubinemia without hemolysis

Persistent jaundice beyond the time when it usually is expected to disappear may be related to hormonal or pharmacologic agents that depress or delay the infant's capacity to metabolize bilirubin. Such agents include drugs such as novobiocin or hormones such as altered pregnanediol in the breast milk of a small percentage of women. In the perinatal period such agents may be administered directly, or they may pass from mother to infant prenatally or in breast milk.

The commonest cause of pathologic jaundice is probably accentuated physiologic jaundice caused by immaturity. Delayed initial feeding of infants also may be associated with accentuated jaundice. The practice of delayed feeding of premature infants of diabetic mothers has been shown to influence the degree of hyperbilirubinemia encountered in these infants. Late feeding may also contribute to hyperbilirubinemia by delaying normal intestinal activity and thus promoting recycling of bilirubin through the enterohepatic shunt. Comparison of bilirubin levels in early- and late-fed groups of infants is seen in Fig. 10-3.

Direct-reacting bilirubin—obstructive jaundice

Another major index of the pathologic nature of jaundice in the newborn is the presence of direct-reacting bilirubin. If more than 1 mg/100 ml of bilirubin is detected by a 1-minute direct diazo reaction, an abnormal process such as hepatitis or biliary obstruction, sepsis, or pyelonephritis should be suspected. The urine is positive for bile; even minor amounts of direct-reacting, water-soluble bilirubin in the serum are associated with urinary excretion of this pigment. The presence of direct-reacting bilirubin even with a total bilirubin level within acceptable limits is an index of a pathologic condition.

Several clinical circumstances in the neonate appear as obstructive jaundice with an elevated (> 1 mg/100 ml) direct reacting bilirubin level, indicating that bilirubin glucuronide is being "regurgitated" into plasma rather than being cleared from the hepatic cell. Some of these circumstances are rare, such as trisomy 18 and Dubin-Johnson syndrome (p. 236). Others, such as sepsis (p. 129), hepatitis (p. 233), and pyelonephritis (p. 139), are relatively common. The presence of direct-reacting bilirubin may herald the presence of a systemic disorder, including congenital bacterial, spirochetal, protozoal, or viral infections that impair the hepatic cellular capacity to excrete conjugated bilirubin. There is no clinical circumstance in which direct-reacting bilirubinemia is a good sign. Its presence is not evidence of increased conjugating capacity, rather it is a signal that the hepatic excretory capacity is impaired or has been damaged.

It is common to find conjugated (direct-reacting) bilirubin in severely anemic *infants with erythroblastosis fetalis;* and in

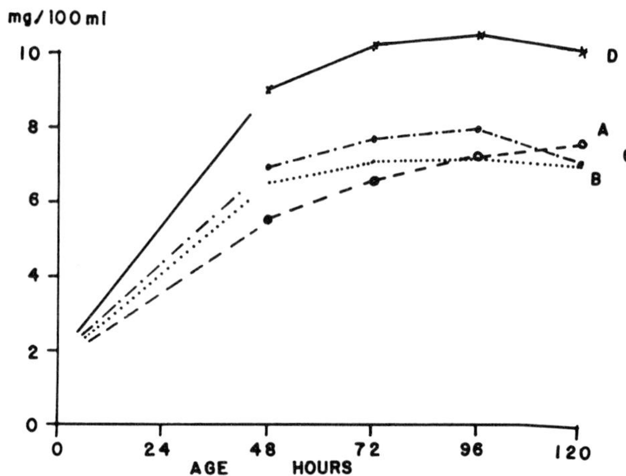

Fig. 10-3. Comparison of average plasma bilirubin concentrations of infants in the various study groups during the first 5 days of life. Groups *A*, *B*, and *C* were fed early; group *D* received no feedings until 48 hr of life. Thereafter, infants in all groups were fed the same standard evaporated milk formula.

recent years, infants severely affected with hemolytic disease who have survived intrauterine transfusion have frequently exhibited elevations of direct-reacting bilirubin. This finding probably reflects some degree of hepatic injury during severe anemia and hypoxia, but also may represent intrahepatic mechanical obstruction to bile flow. Modest elevations of direct-reacting bilirubin are commonly associated with pyelonephritis (often with septicemia) caused by *E. coli.* Attention to this phenomenon has led to rapid, early diagnosis of such infections, often before the actual total bilirubin level was elevated beyond otherwise acceptable limits of physiologic bilirubinemia.

Neonatal hepatitis (p. 233), whether viral, bacterial, protozoal, or spirochetal, is associated with an elevated direct-reacting bilirubin level. Testing for the presence of bile in the urine usually produces an abnormal finding, even when associated with only modest elevations (1 mg/100 ml) of this pigment in the infant's serum. Elevation of direct-reacting bilirubin in the serum may be the initial sign of the presence of congenital viral infections. Biliary atresia (p. 237) would be diagnosed much earlier if the clinical significance of direct-reaction bilirubin were more widely appreciated and acted upon.

One of the most difficult diagnoses for the pediatrician to make is to differentiate mechanical obstruction of *extrahepatic biliary atresia* (p. 234) from that of obstructive jaundice occurring as part of the manifestations of neonatal hepatitis. One of the main reasons for this difficulty is the physician's failure to investigate the early signs of obstructive jaundice. It is far easier to differentiate between neonatal hepatitis and atresia in the first week of life than at 6 weeks of life. In the first or second week one has the benefit of observing clinical signs of hepatitis prior to a fully obstructive phase. These signs include (1) whether any of the early stools contain bile pigments, (2) whether the SGOT and SGPT are markedly elevated (> 500 units), (3) whether there is early splenomegaly (common early in hepatitis), and (4) whether there is early evidence of hemolysis and of reticulocytosis or fragmented cells or both (common in hepatitis). As the infant becomes older, there is increasing hepatic damage in the child with extrahepatic atresia, and the clinical picture blends with primary disorders affecting the hepatic parenchyma.

Choledocal cysts may appear early, with an elevation of direct-reacting bilirubin. There are usually acholic stools, and a right upper quadrant mass can be both palpated and transilluminated.

Cystic fibrosis of the pancreas may produce obstructive jaundice within the first month of life, and even at this age the elevated sweat chloride level is discernible in this disorder.

Kernicterus

Although an elevated level of unconjugated bilirubin is the sine qua non for the development of kernicterus, there is no precise level above which each infant will develop brain damage. Many factors potentiate the movement of bilirubin into susceptible tissues, while other factors protect against this threat. As these factors have been recognized, it has become possible to develop approximate predictive indices of the degree of threat to individual infants. Many studies have demonstrated an increasing risk of brain damage as the level of bilirubin rises. More than one third of the infants with untreated hemolytic disease and bilirubin levels in excess of 20 mg/100 ml will develop toxicity. In all infants the occurrence of motor disturbances increases as bilirubin levels rise above 15 mg/100 ml in the neonatal period.

Overt signs of kernicterus are rarely observed in the first day of life, probably because bilirubin levels are rarely greater than 15 mg/100 ml. When hemolysis is present, signs of kernicterus may become apparent from the second to the fifth day of life, corresponding to the time of occurrence of the early high levels of bilirubin in hemolytic disorders. Among premature infants without additional pathologic conditions, kernicterus was first recognized as "seventh day disease," corresponding to the time when bilirubin levels would gradually rise to pathologic levels even by physiologic mechanisms. Excessive bilirubinemia anytime during the first few weeks of life poses the threat of kernicterus, although there is some protection associated with maturation.

Factors that increase the likelihood of kernicterus at a given level of bilirubin are listed in Table 10-4. The majority of the factors that have been identified augment the movement of bilirubin into tissues, including brain, by decreasing the available binding sites on albumin necessary to keep bilirubin in the vascular space.

Prematurity

While prematurity is listed as a major responsible factor, specific host cell susceptibility has not yet been demonstrated. It is common to find that the albumin levels of preterm infants are low; the total capacity for binding bilirubin to its transport protein may thus be diminished. Further, many of the diseases that occur in preterm infants involve, in part, common pathophysiologic conditions such as hypoxia that may lead to acidosis and thereby decrease the binding of bilirubin to the limited amount of albumin available.

Drugs such as sulfisoxazole can potentiate the effect of bilirubin, since they compete for the binding sites on albumin. Hemolysis may also exert an effect by contributing nonbilirubin pigments that compete for binding sites. Hypoglycemia, starvation,

TABLE 10-4. Factors influencing the risk of kernicterus

	Reduced albumin binding capacity	Competition for binding sites	Increased cell susceptibility to bilirubin toxicity
Prematurity	+	−	?
Hemolysis	−	+	?
Asphyxia	+	−	+
Acidosis	+	−	?
↑ NEFA	−	+	−
Cold stress	−	+	−
Starvation	−	+	−
Hypoalbuminemia	+	−	+
Hypoglycemia	−	+	?
Infection	+	−	?
Drugs	−	+	−
Male sex	−	−	?

From Bergsma, Hsia, and Jackson, editors: Birth defects. Original article series: Bilirubin metabolism in the newborn, The National Foundation—March of Dimes **6**(2), 1970.

and chilling lead to increased production of nonesterified fatty acids (NEFA); these substances also compete for bilirubin-albumin binding sites. Male infants are more susceptible than female infants to the toxic effects of bilirubin.

Factors that tend to protect infants from the threat of kernicterus at a given level of bilirubin are in general those that increase the availability of albumin binding sites for bilirubin.

Many of these factors have influenced the management of hyperbilirubinemia. Some treatments are directed toward removing the pigment; others are directed toward reducing the serum bilirubin level. Newer approaches are directed toward altering the nature of bilirubin so that it is no longer toxic. Other efforts have been directed toward elimination of those factors that potentiate damage. The potential danger of the combined effects of several high risk factors on the presence of hyperbilirubinemia has prompted earlier action in these situations. In addition, intravenous infusions of albumin have been used both to reduce the immediate threat of brain damage by reversing the tendency of bilirubin to move into neural tissues and to increase the amount of bilirubin removed during exchange transfusion.

Principles of prevention and management of hyperbilirubinemia

The principles upon which management of neonatal hyperbilirubinemia is based include the demonstration that:

1. Unconjugated hyperbilirubinemia can lead to cellular damage, particularly to brain damage.
2. Toxicity is largely proportional to the concentration of serum bilirubin attained, and even at serum bilirubin levels of 15 mg/100 ml (and occasionally lower) residual central nervous system damage may occur.
3. Bilirubin exists in plasma bound to albumin; only a small amount appears to be free and diffusible.
4. The toxicity of bilirubin is largely determined by the size of the diffusible fraction.
5. Many factors including pH, hypoxia, and the presence of organic anions that complete with bilirubin for albumin binding sites can influence the dissociation of the bilirubin-albumin complex and increase the potential diffusion of bilirubin.
6. Premature (particularly male) infants, as well as infants with hemolytic disease (of any type), are most susceptible to bilirubin encephalopathy. Hypoxia, acidosis, and cold stress aggravate this risk.
7. The proportion of the population at risk of developing significant hyperbilirubinemia (> 15 mg/100 ml) is approximately 3% of full-term infants, 9% of preterm black infants, and 17% of preterm white infants (in the United States).
8. The methods of treatment, whether involving removal of bilirubin (exchange transfusion), alteration of bilirubin (photodecomposition), or enhancement of hepatic metabolism and excretion of bilirubin by enzyme induction (phenobarbital, alcohol, morphine, and so on), all carry identified and potential risks that must be weighed against the risk of kernicterus. Each of these modes of therapy has been employed either to prevent hyperbilirubinemia or to treat it. In addition, attempts have been made to directly prevent brain damage, even when the bilirubin level was high, by administration of albumin to augment the bilirubin binding capacity of the plasma. The experience with some of these newer approaches to prevention and treatment of hyperbilirubinemia and kernicterus deserve special mention. (See p. 189 for discussion of exchange transfusion.)

Prevention of hyperbilirubinemia

Early feeding. The simplest method of reducing the extent of physiologic jaundice is the introduction of early feeding, as opposed to a 48-hour delay (Fig. 10-3). The reasons for the associated limited degree of physiologic jaundice under these circumstances are not clear. It is possible that early feeding stimulates the motility of the intestine and induces more rapid elimination of meconium, thus diminishing the potential absorption of bilirubin across the intestinal mucosa and thereby decreasing enterohepatic circulation of bilirubin (which reimposes this bilirubin load on the liver). Many substances other than food that enter through the gastrointestinal tract early may have a similar effect on total serum bilirubin levels. This effect has been demonstrated when charcoal or agar has been fed to infants in the first day of life; these agents probably also exert a nonspecific effect on the potential reabsorbtion of bilirubin from the intestine.

Another mechanism by which early feeding may affect bilirubin metabolism is the introduction into the intestine of bacteria that can reduce bilirubin to urobilinogen.

Other possible deleterious effects of fasting on bilirubin metabolism include: (1) the possibility of increased production of bilirubin, since microsomal hemoxygenase, which promotes the conversion of heme to bilirubin in the liver, is increased during starvation, and (2) some evidence that fasting decreases the hepatic capacity for extraction of bilirubin from plasma. Fasting may also lead to jaundice because of decreased availability of glucose and diminution of the availability of uridine diphosphoglucuronic acid, the glucuronide donor for bilirubin.

Phototherapy. The exposure of newborn infants to a high intensity of light is associated with a diminution in the incidence of neonatal jaundice, a decrease in levels of serum bilirubin, and a decreased frequency of exchange transfusions. A decline of 1 to 4 mg of serum bilirubin can be expected in jaundiced nonhemolytic infants, following 8 to 12 hours of exposure. Infants in widely different geographical settings have been found to have a similar response to light, and this mode of therapy has been increasingly used in the United States for both the prevention and treatment of hyperbilirubinemia. However, there is limited information concerning the mode of action of light in jaundice of the neonate, and the potential hazards associated with its use are poorly defined.

There is, of course, great interest in how and where such a reaction takes place in the human neonate and in whether the decomposition products are safer than unconjugated bilirubin itself. There is also a need to examine the effects of light on other substances, since bilirubin may not be the only target of the intensified light. This section contains a summary of present concepts concerning the mode of action of light on bilirubin as well as the potential hazards of such radiation. Guidelines for the limited use of this type of therapy and other treatments in the prevention and management of hyperbilirubinemia are then presented.

The photochemical reaction of light. The instability and decomposition of bilirubin in the presence of light are well documented, but neither the mechanism nor the products of these reactions in the human being are fully known.

McDonagh has presented evidence that bilirubin photooxidation is a self-sensitized reaction involving an excited state of molecular oxygen (singlet oxygen) that proceeds as follows:

$$\text{Bilirubin} \longrightarrow (\text{Bilirubin})$$
$$(\text{Bilirubin}) + {}^3O_2 \longrightarrow \text{Bilirubin} + {}^1O_2$$
$${}^1O_2 + \text{bilirubin} \longrightarrow \text{Bilirubin products}$$

During the in vitro exposure of bilirubin (in chloroform) to visible light (high-pressure mercury lamp) there is a progressive decrease in absorbance over the range of maximum absorbance (440 to 460 mm) of bilirubin. The evidence that this destruction of unbound bilirubin involves singlet oxygen in the reaction includes the observation that the reaction is accelerated in the presence of methylene blue as well as other compounds known to photosensitize the production of singlet oxygen. In these in vitro experiments photodestruction of protein-bound bilirubin is also accelerated by addition of methylene blue, but under these conditions the rate of increase is smaller than with unbound bilirubin, presumably because of competition by the protein for singlet oxygen. Further supportive evidence that this is the way bilirubin and light interact is derived from the observation that quenchers of singlet oxygen, such as trans-β-carotena, effectively inhibit the photodecompositon of bilirubin. In addition, trapping of singlet oxygen (with 2, 3-dimethyl-2-butene) leads to competitive inhibition.

The main products of decomposition occurring through such a mechanism would be colorless dipyrrylmethane. This is in agreement with previous studies in which products were qualitatively examined in vitro and in vivo, but not fully identified.

Mechanisms of in vivo action of phototherapy. It is presently postulated that in vivo photodegradation of bilirubin takes place principally in the peripheral tissues and probably involves singlet oxygen as demonstrated by the in vitro experiments. However, photooxidation may not be the only, or even the major, mechanism that accounts for the observed in vivo decrease in serum bilirubin in infants exposed to light. Recent studies of the effect of light on bilirubin clearance in a child with Crigler-Najjar syndrome, as well as studies in Gunn rats, imply that phototherapy may also promote the hepatic excretion of (presumably) unconjugated bilirubin. No quantitative assessment like this has been performed in infants with neonatal hyperbilirubinemia. It is not known whether the bilirubin excretion from the intestine increases during phototherapy or whether the decrease in serum bilirubin is accounted for only by the photodestruction of bilirubin.

Phenobarbital. Phenobarbital, an inducer of microsomal enzymes, has been shown to increase hepatic bilirubin conjugation and excretion in newborn and adult animals. It also decreases serum bilirubin levels in patients with type II Crigler-Najjar syndrome. Controlled studies of the use of phenobarbital to prevent physiologic jaundice in infants have demonstrated that phenobarbital, either given to a mother prior to delivery, to an infant, or to both of these, is effective in limiting the development of physiologic jaundice in the newborn and in decreasing the number of exchanges done for hyperbilirubinemia of the premature. Phenobarbital has been administered to already jaundiced infants, but significant lowering of bilirubin requires 4 or 5 days of treatment. Premature infants respond less well than do full-term infants, and some infants do not respond at all when they are already jaundiced.

There is serious question as to whether phenobarbital should be used at all in newborn infants. Phenobarbital leads to proliferation of the endoplasmic reticulum and enchances enzymatic activity of the enzymes located in the smooth endoplasmic reticulum of the liver cell. It has been postulated that its use might lead to greater susceptibility of the hepatic cell to hepatotoxic drugs and that it may accelerate metabolism of many compounds and perhaps decrease the effectiveness of drugs administered to the infant. It may alter steroid metabolism. One of its major drawbacks is also the fact that the excretion of barbiturates is extremely variable in neonates. Infants of epileptic women who were taking barbiturates have been found to have severe depression of vitamin K factors, and this has led to neonatal bleeding.

In general, there is very little indication to use phenobarbital in the neonatal period to prevent jaundice and no indication to use it to treat jaundice. Phenobarbital requires a much longer time, 3 or 4 days, for similar decrement in overall serum bilirubin level than that obtained with phototherapy. In areas other than the United States (for example, Hong Kong and Greece) where a specific problem exists because of a very high percentage of infants who develop hyperbilirubinemia and kernicterus, it has been suggested that programs of prophylactic therapy using this agent might prove beneficial. In the United States, however, there is little indication at the present time to utilize this largely experimental method of dealing with the problem of hyperbilirubinemia.

Other drugs that influence jaundice. Other agents that appear to stimulate the mechanism of conjugation also decrease anticipated bilirubin levels in newborn infants. For example, the intravenous administration of 100 to 115 gm of ethanol to women 3 to 96 hours prior to delivery has led to a significant reduction in hyperbilirubinemia on the third to fifth day of life in their offspring. It has also been found that infants of heroin addicts have lower than expected levels of bilirubin. Chlorophenothane (Dicophane), nikethamide (Diethylnicotinamide), and uridine diphosphoglucose also lower bilirubin levels in newborn infants. The toxicity and side effects of these agents contraindicate their use in preventing or managing neonatal jaundice.

Guidelines for the management of hyperbilirubinemia

Fig. 10-4 outlines suggestions for the management of hyperbilirubinemia, taking into account the age of the infant and the bilirubin concentration, as well as some of the factors that augment the toxic effect of any given level of bilirubin. The purpose of these guidelines is to offer an approach to the management of hyperbili-

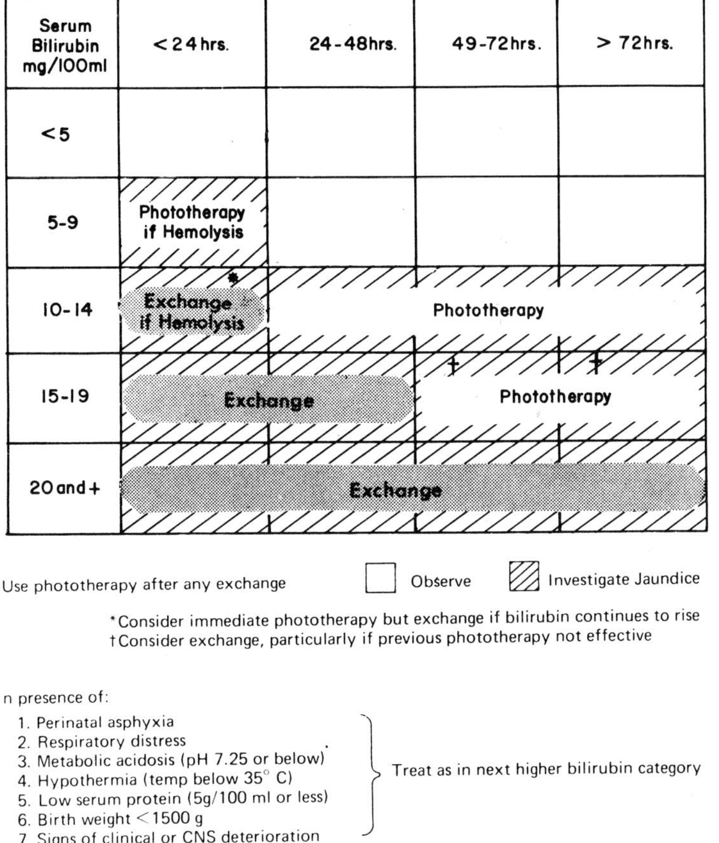

Fig. 10-4. Guidelines for the management of hyperbilirubinemia.

rubinemia in the first few days of life, combining the best of what we now know of the use of exchange transfusion and of phototherapy so that appropriate indications for these two most common methods of therapy can be applied.

Investigation of jaundice. No therapy, including phototherapy, should be used without a knowledge of the cause of the infant's jaundice. Appropriate diagnostic efforts must be made in any infant with a pattern of jaundice beyond that acceptable for physiologic jaundice. Such investigation implies the use of ordinary clinical or laboratory means to rule out the most common treatable or potentially life-threatening cause of pathologic jaundice, sepsis or hemolysis or both. This requires a detailed history and physical examination and the pursuit of information concerning the presence of anemia (hematocrit, reticulocyte count, and blood smear) and infection (urinalysis, blood cultures, urine cultures, and a clinical or laboratory search or both for evidence of viral disorder). Appropriate measures also should be undertaken to determine the underlying cause (p. 223 and Table 10-3).

The indications for investigation of jaundice are based on exceeding the limits of physiologic jaundice (see list on p. 222). The indications include jaundice in the first 24 hours, increases in serum bilirubin levels exceeding 5 mg/100 ml/day, a bilirubin level of 12 mg/100 ml at any time in a full-term infant, 15 mg/100 ml in a preterm infant, the presence of direct bilirubinemia, or the persistence of jaundice beyond the first week. These are all diagnosed as hyperbilirubinemia and not physiologic jaundice; a specific cause is then sought.

The vast majority of infants who have an abnormal pattern of jaundice are found to have a cause or a complex of causes for their hyperbilirubinemia if investigations are made to explain this abnormality. The explanation should be available prior to starting phototherapy or any other therapy in order to ensure that the basic cause of the jaundice is treated rather than merely masking its presence.

Phototherapy: hemolytic versus nonhemolytic jaundice. It is also essential to distinguish those infants who have hyperbilirubinemia in association with hemolysis from a variety of causes from those who have no element of hemolysis; the response of these two groups to phototherapy is very different. While some infants with A-B-O hemolytic disease can respond to phototherapy even after jaundice has appeared, in general the response of infants with hemolysis to phototherapy is highly variable and unreliable. While in some instances, even in the presence of hemolysis, an initial trial of phototherapy may be useful, the rate of photodecomposition or elimination of bilirubin is usually not sufficient to compensate for the increment in bilirubin production in the presence of increased hemolysis.

The guidelines in Fig. 10-4 take these considerations into account. Phototherapy is not recommended initially in the hemolyzing infant if the bilirubin is already above 10 mg/100 ml during the first 24 hours, or above 14 mg/100 ml between 24 and 48 hours, or above 20 mg/100 ml at any time. In addition, it is also important to realize that the hemolysis still goes on in infants whose jaundice may respond to light; anemia in such infants must be carefully monitored during the first 6 weeks of life. In contrast the effect of exchange transfusion on hemolysis is twofold: the hemolytic process is decreased (Chapter 9), and there is a removal and limitation of further rise in bilirubin. The adjunct of phototherapy has been extremely useful in reducing the need for reexchange of infants with hemolytic disease and in precluding the necessity of exchange of infants whose hemolysis is mild.

Untoward effects of phototherapy include eye injury, loose stools, skin rashes, overheating, chilling, delayed diagnoses (that is, anemia, sepsis), and the bronze baby syndrome. The latter skin discoloration is associated with bilirubinoid pigments in the serum and may last 2 to 4 months with no sequelae if there is no associated liver disease. (See p. 234.)

AUDREY K. BROWN

BIBLIOGRAPHY

Bernstein, J., and Brown, A. K.: Sepsis and jaundice in early infancy, Pediatrics **29**:873, 1962.

Bergsma, Hsia, and Jackson, editors: Birth defects. Original article series: Bilirubin metabolism in the newborn, The National Foundation—March of Dimes **6** (2), 1970.

Brown, A. K.: Bilirubin metabolism in the developing liver. In Assali, A., editor: Biology of gestation, vol. 2, New York, 1968, Academic Press, Inc.

Brown, A. K.: Bilirubin metabolism with special reference to neonatal jaundice, Adv. Pediatr. **12**:121, 1962.

Brown, A. K.: Neonatal jaundice, Pediatr. Clin. North Am. **9**:575, 1962.

Brown, A. K., and Zuelzer, W. W.: Studies on the neonatal development of the glucuronide conjugating system, J. Clin. Invest. **37**:332, 1958.

Maisels, M. J.: Bilirubin—on understanding and influencing its metabolism in the newborn infant, Pediatr. Clin. North Am. **19**:447, 1972.

McDonagh, A. F.: The role of singlet oxygen in bilirubin photo-oxidation, Biochem. Biophys. Res. Commun. **44**:1306, 1971.

Thaler, M. M.: Perinatal bilirubin metabolism, Adv. Pediatr. **19**:215, 1972.

Wennberg, R. P., Schwarts, R., and Sweet, A. Y.: Early versus delayed feeding of low birth weight infants; effects on physiologic jaundice, J. Pediatr. **68**:860, 1966.

LIVER DISEASE

The liver is the primary site of a number of abnormalities that affect the metabolism and excretion of bilirubin. Jaundice may be the initial sign of these disorders.

Crigler-Najjar disease

Crigler-Najjar disease is characterized by a deficiency of glucuronyl transferase in the liver.

Diagnosis. The diagnosis is established clinically by evidence of a strong family history and extreme elevation of unconjugated, indirect-reacting serum bilirubin in the neonatal period without evidence of hemolysis or any direct-reacting bilirubin fraction. No hepatosplenomegaly occurs. Bilirubin is absent from the bile, and the liver is unable to form bilirubin glucuronide. Bilirubin is partially degraded by other mechanisms. In these patients there is also a reduced excretion of glucuronic acid conjugates of the metabolites of ^{14}C cortisone after infusion of the steriod as well as reduced excretion of glucuronides of menthol, chloral hydrate, trichloroethanol, and salicylate.

Pathology. The pathology consists mainly of bile staining of all organs. The liver appears grossly normal with bile plugs in the canaliculi and occasional large ductules. The Kupffer cells are prominent and distended with bile. Bromsulphthalein clearance is normal, and intravenous cholangiography shows gallbladder visualization.

Treatment. These patients have been separated into two groups. The patients in group I have higher serum bilirubin levels (20 to 30 mg/100 ml) and essentially colorless bile and more readily develop kernicterus. The defect is transmitted as a recessive characteristic, and the bilirubinemia is not decreased by the administration of phenobarbital. Group II patients have lower levels of bilirubin, develop kernicterus less readily, and have small amounts of bilirubin glucuronide in the bile. These patients are benefited by phenobarbital administration in amounts varying from 30 to 120 mg daily. This trait appears to be transmitted as an autosomal dominant character, and it has been suggested that drug treatment may induce glucuronyl transferase activity. Treatment of both groups may require exchange transfusion in the neonatal period, followed by controlled phototherapy to maintain bilirubin levels in a nontoxic range.

Glucuronyl transferase inhibition

Transient unconjugated hyperbilirubinemia that cannot be explained by factors creating increased bilirubin production, dehydration, fasting, heart failure, or hepatic cell uptake may be caused by inhibition of glucuronyl transferase activity. Arias observed several families whose offspring developed severe neonatal unconjugated bilirubinemia and a high incidence of kernicterus. Examination of the blood of these mothers during the last trimester of pregnancy showed a factor, probably a steroid, that inhibited glucuronyl transferase in vitro. This factor disappeared about 2 weeks after delivery. Exchange transfusion should be used to prevent kernicterus.

Gilbert's syndrome

Chronic nonhemolytic acholuric jaundice may result from defective glucuronide formation. It is a benign disorder that is seen after the neonatal period with unconjugated bilirubin levels between 6 and 20 mg/100 ml and mild gastrointestinal symptoms.

Breast milk jaundice

A small proportion of breast-fed full-term babies have persistent unconjugated bilirubinemia beyond the physiologic limits. Jaundice occurs about the seventh to tenth day of life and may disappear in as short a time as 5 days after cessation of breast feeding. There are no other clinical abnormalities. Although rare, unconjugated bilirubin levels may reach as high as 24 mg/100 ml; kernicterus has not been reported. In these patients maternal milk is capable of inhibiting glucuronyl transferase activity in vitro; the urine, during lactation, has the same inhibiting capacity. There is normal excretion of bilirubin into the stools. Two thirds of the breast-fed siblings in an involved family showed prolonged jaundice, while formula-fed infants were unaffected. Arias and his associates isolated pregnane-3(α), 20(β)-diol from breast milk of mothers of these infants and showed that feeding the steroid to two full-term infants produced a reversible unconjugated hyperbilirubinemia unrelated to hemolysis or evidence of general liver dysfunction. However, Ramos, Silverberg, and Stern studied a number of neonates with addition of the same steroid and failed to show any hyperbilirubinemia. Others have found a variable relationship between breast milk jaundice and pregnanediol.

Treatment consists of substituting a formula for the breast milk. The decrease in serum bilirubin levels is then closely monitored. Persistent low bilirubin concentrations may not be an indication to discontinue breast feeding. Phototherapy or enzyme stimulation by drugs is contraindicated.

Intrauterine and neonatal hepatitis

Etiology. There may be a history of maternal illness or contact with infectious hepatitis virus, rubella, varicella, or herpes simplex. Cytomegalovirus, coxsackievirus

B, toxoplasmosis, and syphilis may also be etiologic agents. Bacterial sepsis may on rare occasion result in hepatitis. Appropriate viral and bacterial cultures and antibody titers should be obtained (Chapter 8, p. 148). Positive reactions to tests for Australian antigen have not been associated with neonatal hepatitis. Their usefulness in predicting chronic liver disease in these infants is unknown.

Clinical presentation. Only fulminant intrauterine infections of the liver are usually recognized as such within the first few days of life. Microcephalus, petechiae, and large liver or spleen or both may be associated clinical signs. Infants with trisomy 21 (Down's syndrome) and trisomy 17, 18 may have a higher incidence of neonatal hepatitis.

Usually jaundice is the problem appearing in the neonate with hepatitis. The serum indirect and direct fractions of bilirubin are elevated, and the urine appears dark. Phototherapy for neonatal hyperbilirubinemia may result in "bronzing" of the skin of an infant with neonatal hepatitis and should alert the physician to the possibility of hepatic cellular damage. Liver dysfunction may only be suspected because of prolongation of physiologic jaundice with the later development of an obstructive component to the inflammation in the liver. However, after the first week of life the initial jaundice may disappear; jaundice may then recur or be recognized for the first time during the obstructive phase of liver involvement at 4 to 6 weeks of age. A pattern of jaundice persisting from the first week of life helps to distinguish hepatitis from biliary atresia (p. 237). Dark yellow staining of the diapers with urine and light- or buff-colored stools may also indicate progression of the disease process to an obstructive stage. There is no single test available to clearly differentiate hepatic cellular damage caused by hepatitis from abnormalities caused by an obstruction to bile flow because of biliary atresia. Initially other causes of hyperbilirubinemia must be evaluated (p. 222).

Laboratory findings. Prothrombin time is a sensitive test of hepatic protein synthesis and early cell injury. Serum transaminases are usually only mildly abnormal (100 to 300 IU) in cholestatic processes while values associated with parenchymal damage may range between 300 to 1,000 IU in young infants. Transaminase levels between 100 and 200 IU within the first week of life may reflect hemolysis during blood sampling. High levels of γ-glutamyl transpeptidase and 5′-nucleotidase are commonly associated with biliary obstruction. Serum cholesterol levels over 200 mg/100 ml often occur in infants under 2 months of age who have cholestasis. Serum alkaline phosphatase values in the neonatal period may be elevated because of rapid infant growth and are not a reliable index of biliary obstruction.

Appropriate studies should be carried out to diagnose galactosemia (p. 423), tyrosinosis (p. 412), fructosemia (p. 424), and cystic fibrosis (sweat test), which may present as icterus. Low α-1, antitrypsin levels have been found in individuals with cirrhosis and a history of neonatal hepatitis. How early this can be detected is not known.

In neonatal infections blood and urine amino acid patterns may show the severity of liver damage by mildly elevated methionine and tyrosine levels; high levels should suggest specific metabolic disturbances of amino acid metabolism. A high immunoglobulin M level (over 20 mg/100 ml) suggests intrauterine infection.

The bile content of meconium in the normal infant during the first 24 hours after birth is quite low (40 to 100 mg) and increases twofold to threefold over the next 2 days. Stool bile consists almost entirely of bilirubin during the first 6 weeks, with gradual conversion to urobilinogen in the fecal content from 6 weeks to the fourth month of life, depending on the bacterial flora and the speed of transport of the fecal material through the bowel. Consequently, urinary studies in young jaundiced infants will show only bilirubin, not urobilinogen, in either parenchymal disorders or obstructive problems.

Radioactive iodine–tagged rose bengal liver scans, particularly when used with the Anger camera, may effectively demonstrate homogeneity of liver biliary function. If excretion from the liver is obvious by 6 hours or 24 hours, the degree of cholestasis can be readily quantitated; sometimes focal accumulations of bile can be recognized either in the gallbladder or in a common duct cyst. The longer 3-day collection of stool and urine for direct measurement of rose bengal output is difficult and less reliable in neonates because of loss of specimens and cross contamination; it also gives no information about a surgically correctable cystic lesion that may partially or intermittently obstruct bile flow (p. 238).

Pathology. Viral infections produce a generalized distortion of the parenchymal liver pattern, with swollen hepatocytes and binucleate and giant cell transformation; there is also some cell necrosis, with cholestasis and portal duct proliferation. Depending on the degree of red blood cell turnover, the magnitude of the infectious process, and maturity of the neonate, extracellular hematopoiesis will be present. Certain infections have definite patterns. In syphilis there are giant cell cords bound in a loose stroma of mononuclear cells, and with coxsackievirus there may be only a few discrete areas of focal necrosis. The lesions may be so small that a percutaneous biopsy only shows normal parenchyma. In some infections the degree of intracytoplasmic cholestasis and plugging of canaliculi and intralobular bile ducts may be very difficult to differentiate from an extrahepatic obstruction.

Percutaneous liver biopsy in young infants with normal reactions to coagulation studies has a morbidity of less than 1% and no mortality. It provides a means of following histologic changes over a long interval of time and may provide a means of direct identification of bacterial or viral agents. There is significant morbidity associated with surgical biopsy, but it provides fuller evaluation of the liver and the extrahepatic duct system.

Treatment. Good nutrition should be maintained. In the presence of severe liver dysfunction with a low blood glucose level and increased plasma methionine and tyrosine, the neonate should be maintained on glucose. The protein content of the diet should be reduced to a daily intake of 1.5 gm/kg and maintained at this level until improvement has occurred. Blood and albumin administration may be required for general support and to maintain serum protein levels. In the presence of severe liver damage with poor excretion of bile and bile salts, absorption of fat soluble vitamins is poor. Double or triple the usual requirement must be given to maintain adequate absorption of vitamins A and D, and possibly E. A prolonged prothrombin time should be restored by parenteral administration of vitamin K_1; continued correction should be supplied until the liver has recovered sufficiently so that absorption of vitamin K is normal. Specific etiologic therapy for hepatitis is not satisfactory except for syphilis and bacterial infections. Since rubella virus may be transmitted from the affected newborn, specific isolation and other preventive measures should be taken (p. 154).

Cholestasis

A slowed excretion of conjugated bilirubin (cholestasis) may occur in the hepatocyte, in the canaliculi, or in the portal ducts. Impaired transport of bile salts may be associated with the condition. The rapidity of appearance of symptoms of obstructive jaundice depends on the degree of prehepatic overload, the maturity of function at the site of stasis, and possibly the pattern of liver perfusion, which may be related to the circulatory changes after birth.

In hemolytic disease the prehepatic bilirubinemia may be recognized by high levels of unconjugated circulating bilirubin associated with anemia. With hepatic cell enzyme disorders, high levels of unconjugated bilirubin occur early and are not accompanied by anemia. Abnormalities of excretion from the liver cell are less obvious clinically and, depend upon the capacity of the liver cell to swell, retain the pigment, and still function. Because of the large capacity of the liver, disorders of cell excretion may require weeks or months before they become evident; histologic examination may be a more important approach at an early phase of these disorders. Canalicular stasis alone is rarely seen but has been demonstrated in animals. In most metabolic problems intracellular and intracanalicular pigment deposition occurs. In extrahepatic obstruction, bile usually accumulates in or near portal areas first; then as the process becomes more chronic, cellular pigment becomes obvious.

The inspissated bile syndrome

Inspissated bile syndrome can occur in two situations. First, an infant who had moderately severe hemolytic disease requiring several exchange transfusions may have persistent low-grade jaundice for 1 or 2 months. An elevation of direct-reacting bilirubin is often noted early in life. There may be persistent hepatosplenomegaly. Stools may vary in color from pale to dark yellow. Cholesterol levels are over 250 mg, and transaminases between 200 to 300 IU. It may not be possible to distinguish cholestasis from infectious hepatitis following blood transfusions without liver biopsy, unless the Australia antigen is present in the blood. Second, a rare infant with unrecognized hemolytic disease of the newborn may have a chronic overload of bilirubin and develop clinical signs of cholestasis at 2 to 3 months of age. The persistence of a positive reaction to the indirect Coombs test, anemia, and maternal-infant red blood cell incompatibility should establish the diagnosis. Unfortunately, this disorder may lead to irreversible biliary cirrhosis. Treatment should consist of adequate fluid intake, double or triple the usual intake of fat-soluble vitamins, and if necessary to maintain growth, a formula containing medium chain triglycerides. Phenobarbital, 5 to 10 mg/kg daily, has been used in an attempt to improve bile flow; if effective, a decrease in serum bilirubin levels should occur within 1 or 2 weeks.

Cholestatic liver disease associated with heart disease

Infants dying in the first week of life from left-sided cardiac anomalies, such as coarctation of the aorta or hypoplastic left heart, may have centrolobular hepatic necrosis and some midzone necrosis. Many of these infants also have periportal hemorrhages. The histologic picture is different from that seen in congestive heart failure with dilated sinusoids. Similarly, some patients with intrahepatic biliary atresia have associated cardiovascular lesions, such as abnormal mitral valve, aortic stenosis, medial calcification of the hepatic artery, and tetralogy of Fallot. Jaundice may be present within the first 2 to 3 weeks of life before a heart murmur has been detected. The hepatic lesions associated with left-sided cardiac problems may be hypoxic in origin.

Cholestasis in the Amish

Cholestasis may present in the neonatal period in descendants of the Amish family of Jacob Byler, who settled in western Pennsylvania and eastern Ohio. These infants have defects in the ability to transport bromsulphalein, conjugated bilirubin, and bile salts across the bile canalicular membrane. They have mild jaundice in the neonatal period but become irritable, with loose bowel movements and recurrent jaundice, by the third to sixth month of life. The symptoms of diarrhea are related to the bile salt abnormality. The neonatal jaundice may be recognized as an important part of the disease only when the family history is known.

There is moderately severe deposition of bile pigment in parenchymal cells and in canaliculi. Electron microscopy shows dilation of rough endoplasmic reticulum and large vacuoles in hepatocytes. Microvilli lining canalicular surfaces may be decreased or appear as swollen blebs projecting into the lumen.

Depending on the progression of the disease, treatment of this disorder may include cholestyramine, medium chain triglycerides, and phenobarbital (8 mg/kg/day) to decrease bilirubin levels.

Dubin-Johnson disease and Rotor's syndrome

Dubin-Johnson disease and Rotor's syndrome, two relatively benign familial syndromes, may present in the neonatal period only with conjugated hyperbilirubinemia. Total bilirubin concentrations may range from 2 to 24 mg/100 ml. It is important to distinguish these entities from other chronic liver diseases with jaundice that may progress to cirrhosis and from causes of neonatal unconjugated hyperbilirubinemia. In Rotor's syndrome the liver is histologically normal. In Dubin-Johnson disease the liver is usually, but not invariably, macroscopically black with dark brown pigmented granules in parachymal cells. Patients with this disorder may have dark urine and develop hepatomegaly. The excretion of cholecystographic agents may be abnormal, but tests of hepatocellular function are usually normal. Abdominal pain, weakness, nausea, vomiting, anorexia, and diarrhea may develop later in childhood.

Familial biliary cirrhosis

Familial biliary cirrhosis, a disorder of varying and unknown cause, usually does not become manifest before 3 to 6 months of age. Pruritus is often the initial symptom, followed by signs of clinical obstructive type jaundice at a later period ranging up to 3 years of age. Abnormalities of bile acid metabolism occur early in the course of the illness.

Intrahepatic atresia

Intrahepatic atresia, a relatively rare problem, may appear as unexplained obstructive jaundice within the first few weeks of life. Clinical signs include claylike stools, deep orange urine, and an elevation of direct-acting and total bilirubin. It is usually associated with extrahepatic biliary atresia.

Clinical presentation. The liver is mildly enlarged, firm, and smooth. The spleen becomes large later in life in relation to the degree of portal hypertension. These infants usually survive for relatively long periods, up to 12 years of age. During the first 3 years of life xanthomatosis of hands, feet, back, ears, eyes, and nose may become disfiguring. The development of xanthomatosis parallels the high serum cholesterol and phospholipid levels in these children; this hyperlipemia begins to decrease from ages 4 to 6, and the xanthomatosis may decrease at this time.

Diagnosis. The diagnosis is made histologically by the paucity or absence of bile ducts within the portal triads and the relative lack of fibrous tissue in the portal areas. While some fibrosis exists, it is not the proliferative scarring that is seen in the cirrhosis associated with extrahepatic biliary atresia. Extrahepatic ducts may also be deficient.

Because of the presence of a few bile ducts at the portal triads, and if the extrahepatic ducts are intact, ^{131}I rose bengal excretion from the liver may occur. Without a liver biopsy such a finding in the neonate might support a diagnosis of neonatal hepatitis.

Treatment. Treatment consists of a low-fat diet, and administration of cholestyramine and extra fat-soluble vitamins as needed. Phenobarbital may lower serum bilirubin levels in some patients.

Prognosis. Early death is often related to intercurrent infections. With longer survival, problems of severe osteoporosis develop. Portal hypertension occurs, despite the fact that the degree of hepatic fibrosis is much less than that in extrahepatic atresia. If hypersplenism accompanies this, removal of the spleen may be followed by a sharp drop in serum bilirubin. A central splenorenal shunt may effectively decompress the portal system; the risk of overwhelming infection increases if the spleen is removed. Superior mesenteric vein to inferior vena cava shunt is often preferred in children.

Extrahepatic biliary atresia

Extrahepatic biliary atresia causes 30% to 50% of all obstructive jaundice in the neonate. The obstruction of the extrahepatic bile ducts may be complete, partial, or may consist of skipped areas with dilatation of sacculated obstructed segments that appear cystic. In most instances these abnormalities appear without a history of maternal illness or unusual medications taken during pregnancy. Other siblings are not usually affected. Biliary atresia has also been seen with abnormalities of chromosome Nos. 17-18, No. 13, and with partial deletion of one chromosome. The cause of extrahepatic atresia is not established, but an association with a defective blood supply has been postulated, similar to experimental segmental intestinal atresia (p. 393).

Clinical presentation. Characteristically, the baby with extrahepatic biliary atresia appears normal at birth and does not develop hyperbilirubinemia during the first week of life. Rarely, there are reports of abnormal clay or light-colored stools within the first week. The jaundice is seldom recognized before the end of the first month. The abnormality in stool color is usually observed about the same time. A combination of low-grade icterus (bilirubin levels between 6 to 12 mg/100 ml with 50% to 70% conjugated bilirubin), elevated cholesterol and/or γ-glutamyl transpeptidase and/or 5′-nucleotidase, and mildly elevated transaminases and serum proteins support this clinical diagnosis. Prothrombin time is within normal limits.

Diagnosis. ^{131}I rose bengal liver scan should indicate no excretion from the liver for over 24 hours or excretion into discrete areas near the liver, compatible with collection into a cystic structure. This latter localization should be confirmed by ultrasonogram. If a cystic structure is partially patent there may be intermittent presence of bile in the stool; an upper gastrointestinal series should help exclude the possibility of cysts. Percutaneous liver biopsy may suggest a block in excretion at the level of the larger bile ducts and show minimal giant cell changes. There is no extramedullary hematopoiesis. Definitive diagnosis requires surgical exploration, which is usually advised betwen 2 and 4 months, depending on the course. If surgery is contemplated, a 24-hour preoperative regimen of orally administered neomycin is suggested to diminish intestinal flora. At exploration, following inspection of the liver, a wedge biopsy should be taken before further manipulation. The hilar region should be carefully explored to identify the normal structures and exclude aberrant cystic structures. If observations are made by direct cholangiography without dissection, the dangers of injury to normal structures by inadvertent interference with local blood supply can be avoided. It is also important to needle into liver substance in search if dilated cystic structures that could be used subsequently for anastomosis.

Treatment. Two types of anastomoses are used, either anastomosis directly to the duodenum or by the Roux-en-Y technique to the jejunum. Ascending cholangitis is the most common and serious complication and may occur more often with the duodenal anastomosis. Jejunal anastomosis has been the more successful procedure. Alternatively, Japanese surgeons have advocated anastomosing a loop of jejunum around microscopically proved fine hepatic ducts in the hilum when no external duct structures can be found. Bile fistulas and pseudocyst formation are serious surgical complications. The development of ascites following exploration should always be viewed as a possible result of bile seepage; the bilirubin levels of this fluid are higher than blood values.

Adequate hydration and use of orally administered magnesium sulfate and bile salts to stimulate bile flow are important therapeutic adjuncts. Ascites from portal hypertension may occur temporarily and can be adequately controlled by use of spironolactone, chlorothiazide, and intravenously administered albumin (at dosage of 1 gm/kg body weight per day) with mild salt restriction. If cholangitis occurs, it may be difficult to identify the offending organisms. Blood culture and percutaneous liver biopsy for culture (if clotting parameters are normal) are the most likely means for establishing such identity as a basis for antibiotic therapy.

Prognosis. Long-term survival depends on the degree of liver damage before the problem is recognized, the degree of cirrhosis, and the relative success of the repair. If intrahepatic ducts are also deficient and fibrosis is minimal, the unsuccessfully treated patient with extrahepatic obstruction may survive from 2 to 10 years.

Common duct cysts

Common duct cysts are abnormal areas of dilatation of the biliary system. They may be outpouchings from an obstructed common bile duct, which may be sausage shaped or saccular in appearance. Such cysts may represent a developmental anomaly or erosion of the wall of the biliary tree with loss of endothelial lining, following distention from distal obstruction of the bile duct. Common duct cysts are often seen in girls, with a 4:1 preponderance. Symptoms may appear in the neonatal period or at any time during childhood and young adult life. Obstructive jaundice, episodes of vomiting, abdominal pain, fever, jaundice, itching, and acholic stools are characteristic. The physician should carefully search for cysts during surgical exploration in infants with signs of extrahepatic obstruction. Surgical correction is by anastomosis of the cyst to the jejunum. Cysts may develop in the liver and protrude from the surface in infants with atresia of the bile ducts. This usually happens in the latter half of the first year when there has not been corrective surgery. Such bile lakes provide unsatisfactory sites for anastomosis because of the stasis and limited hepatic drainage of bile.

Perforation of the common bile duct

Rare instances of perforation of the common duct occur in the first or second month of life.

Clinical presentation. Perforation of the common bile duct may be observed as an acute episode with fever, irritability, abdominal rigidity, or signs of shock. There may be roentgenographic evidence of air under the diaphragm. Commonly, there is increasing abdominal distention from fluid accumulation in the peritoneal cavity, minimal clinical jaundice, and intermittent to complete absence of bile in the stools. Surprisingly, in the young infant leakage of bile into the peritoneal cavity is often not as life threatening as it would be in an adult.

Alternatively, the neonate may simulate an extrahepatic atresia with mild obstructive-type jaundice, light-colored stools, and dark urine. The presence of ascites and a normal-sized liver should alert the physician to an unusual situation. The bilirubin content of ascitic fluid is elevated. Occasionally, perforation occurs into the lesser sac or may be localized elsewhere by pseudocystic production in inflamed tissue.

Pathology. A perforation of the bile ducts may arise from distal stenosis of the common duct or abnormal regurgitation of pancreatic juice into the bile ducts with subsequent erosion. Stasis at the ampulla of Vater or aberrant pancreatic ducts also have been suggested as possible causes.

Treatment. Surgical closure of the perforation over a T-tube is the preferred treatment, but an anastomosis to a loop of jejunum to divert the flow of bile may be required when the hole is too large. Secondary bacterial peritonitis should be treated with antibiotics, and bile drainage during the recovery phase should be re-fed to stimulate bile flow. Deficits of fluid and electrolytes should be replaced intravenously.

Prognosis. If surgical repair is accomplished, chances for complete recovery are excellent. Late intestinal obstruction from adhesions is a serious complication.

Bile plug syndrome

Thick, impacted accumulations of bile secretions and bilirubin may obstruct the outflow of the common bile duct near the ampulla of Vater. These patients have relatively higher levels of unconjugated serum bilirubin than those with biliary atresia. They may also be anemic and have symptoms suggesting pain. Liver biopsy shows histologic changes compatible with extrahepatic obstruction. Diagnosis is confirmed by operative cholangiographic demonstration of obstruction with distortion of the column of opaque material, suggesting a mass. Evacuation of the bile plug relieves the signs and symptoms. Normal spasm of the cystic duct may cause difficulty in injecting saline or radiopaque dye into the gallbladder. Sudden relief of such spasm should not be confused with the supposed ejection of a bile plug through the duct system. Care should be taken to rule out cystic fibrosis in such patients.

Intestinal obstruction and jaundice

The association of jaundice with various types of intestinal obstruction in the neonate has been recognized for a long time and has been assumed to result from a combination of stasis and dehydration. The association of hyperbilirubinemia with hypertrophic pyloric stenosis has been observed by several investigators; liver biopsy showed normal tissue, but Arias found decreased glucuronyl transferase activity in the liver. Liver uridine diphosphate glucuronyl transferase activity is depressed in jaundiced neonates with gastrointestinal obstruction but not in anicteric obstructed infants.

Infants with *cystic fibrosis,* both with and without meconium ileus, may have hepatic cellular and intracanalicular bile stasis. Confusion with neonatal hepatitis should be clarified by a sweat test. The bile stasis is usually temporary.

RUTH HARRIS

BIBLIOGRAPHY

Arias, I. M., and Gartner, L. M.: Production of unconjugated hyperbilirubinaemia in full-term new-born infants following administration of pregnane-3 (alpha), 20 (beta)-diol, Nature (Lond.) **203**:1292, 1964.

Arias, I., Schorr, J. B., and Fraad, L. M.: Clinical conference—congenital hypertrophic pyloric stenosis with jaundice, Pediatrics **24**:338, 1959.

Arias, I. M., Wolfson, S., Lucey, J. F., McKay, R. J.: Transient familial neonatal hyperbilirubinemia, J. Clin. Invest. **44**:1442, 1956.

Bakken, A. F. Bilirubin excretion in newborn human infants, Acta Paediatr. Scand. **59**:148, 1970.

Bernstein, J., Braylan, R., and Brough, A.: Bile plug syndrome, Pediatrics **43**:273, 1969.

Clayton, R., Iber, F. L., Ruebner, B. H., and McKusick, V.: Byler disease; fatal familial interhepatic cholestasis in an Amish kindred, Am. J. Dis. Child. **117**:112, 1969.

Crigler, J. F., and Najjar, V. A.: Congenital

familial nonhemolytic jaundice with kernicterus, Pediatrics **10**:169, 1952.

Fleischner, G., and Arias, I. M.: Recent advances in bilirubin formation, transport, metabolism and excretion, Am. J. Med. **49**:576, November 1970.

Huang, P. W., Rozdalsky, B., Garrard, J. W., Goluboff, N., and Golman, G. H.: Crigler-Najjar syndrome in 4 of 5 siblings with post mortem findings in one, Arch. Pathol. **90**:536, 1970.

Kantrowitz, P. A., Jones, W. A., Greenberger, N. J., and Isselbacher, K. J.: Severe post-operation hyperbilirubinemia resembling obstructive jaundice, N. Engl. J. Med. **276**:591, 1967.

Kasai, M., Kimura, S., Asakura, Y., Suzuki, H., Taira, Y., and Ohashi, E.: Surgical treatment of biliary atresia, J. Pediatr. Surg. **3**:665, 1968.

Lou, M., Schmutzer, K. J., and Regan, J. F.: Congenital extrahepatic biliary atresia, Arch. Surg. **105**:771, November 1972.

Newman, A. J., and Gross, S.: Hyperbilirubinemia in breast fed infants, Pediatrics **32**:995, 1963.

Niswander, K. R., and Jordan, M., editors: The Collaborative Perinatal Study of NINDS, Philadelphia, 1972, W. B. Saunders Co.

Poland, R. L., and Odell, G. B.: Physiologic jaundice; the enterohepatic circulation of bilirubin, N. Engl. J. Med. **284**:1, 1971.

Ramos, A., Silverberg, M., and Stern, L.: Pregnanediols and neonatal hyperbilirubinemia, Am. J. Dis. Child. **111**:353, 1966.

Severi, F., Rondini, G., Zaverin, S., and Bruschelli, M.: Prolonged neonatal hyperbilirubinemia and pregnane-3(alpha), 20(beta)-diol in maternal milk, Acta Paediatr. Scand. **59**:451, July 1970.

Shiraki, K.: Hepatic cell necrosis in the newborn, Am. J. Dis. Child. **119**:395, 1970.

Stiehl, A., Thaler, M. M., and Admirand, W. H.: The effects of phenobarbital on bile salts and bilirubin in patients with intrahepatic and extrahepatic cholestasis, N. Engl. J. Med. **286**:858, 1972.

Weinberg, A. A., and Boland, R. P.: The liver in congenital heart disease—effects of infantile coarctation of aorta and hypoplastic left heart syndrome in infancy, Am. J. Dis. Child. **119**:390, 1970.

Williams, C. N., Kaye, R., Baker, L., Hurwitz, R., and Senior, J. R.: Progressive familial cholestatic cirrhosis and bile acid metabolism, J. Pediatr. **81**:493, 1972.

11 Diseases of the cardiovascular system

Congenital cardiovascular disease constitutes a major health problem in the newborn. The newborn with a severe cardiac malformation will usually have difficulties in the neonatal period or at least in the first 6 months of life. If he survives this critical period without problems, it is likely that he will remain asymptomatic for many years (as in patients with mild pulmonic or aortic stenosis) or decades (as in patients with an atrial septal defect).

The practice of pediatric cardiology thus tends to be partitioned, on the one hand, into care of the older child with easily identifiable, electively correctable heart disease (such as atrial and ventricular septal defects, patent ductus arteriosus, aortic and pulmonic stenosis, postductal coarctation of the aorta, and most cases of tetralogy of Fallot) and, on the other hand, into care of the newborn with such life-threatening malformations as transposition of the great arteries, hypoplastic left heart syndrome, preductal coarctation of the aorta, and a host of complex malformations. As a generalization, one may say that the outlook for the older child with one of the seven commonest malformations noted above is now excellent, while the prognosis for the sick neonate with cardiac disease may vary from excellent (as in infants with transposition of the great arteries with low pulmonary arterial pressure or severe isolated pulmonic stenosis) to bad (as in infants with a hypoplastic left ventricle with diminutive aortic arch).

This chapter is entirely concerned with those severe lesions that present problems in the first month of life. It should be remembered, however, that the majority of infants born with heart disease manifest no problem in the neonatal period and that recent advances in diagnosis and corrective surgery allow survival with normal life expectancy in the majority of children with congenital heart disease.

INCIDENCE OF STRUCTURAL CONGENITAL HEART DISEASE

Precise figures of the incidence of structural congenital heart disease will probably never be attainable. Some cardiac defects (such as ventricular septal defects [VSD] and patent ductus arteriosus [PDA]) close spontaneously, while others (such as atrial septal defects [ASD]) may not become manifest until late in childhood. In other disorders (such as endocardial fibroelastosis and muscular hypertrophic subaortic stenosis) a congenital origin is in doubt. A recent study of 56,109 births followed an average of 3 years disclosed an incidence of 8.14 infants with congenital heart disease per 1,000 births. Approximately one third of all infants born alive with a congenital heart defect die within the first month of life. However, many of these infants have multiple cardiac defects together with congenital defects of other organ systems.

ETIOLOGY OF CONGENITAL HEART DISEASE

Although several causes of congenital heart disease have been firmly identified, in the great majority no antecedent factor can be determined. Some cardiac malformations (such as PDA) are more common in girls, while others (such as aortic stenosis) are more common in boys; the overall sex ratio is approximately 1:1. Prematurity, calculated by both gestational age and weight, has been found to be approximately 2½ times more frequent in infants born with heart disease. However, it has been suggested that infants with transposition of the great arteries tend to be heavier than average; but this finding has been questioned.

Factors known to be associated with congenital heart disease include maternal ingestion of thalidomide and probably of many other drugs, maternal infection with rubella virus and possibly with other viruses, season of the year, high altitude (PDA only), major chromosomal disorders such as Down's syndrome and Turner's syndrome, disorders of connective tissue such as Marfan's syndrome and Ehlers-Danlos syndrome, and maternal diabetes. The influence of ionizing radiation is unknown.

Common major chromosomal disorders

The incidence of structural congenital heart disease is high in infants with major chromosomal disorders. For trisomy D_1 the incidence is approximately 80%; for trisomy 18 it is 10% to 50%. Since only 10% to 20% of infants with the major trisomies survive to 1 year of life, hemodynamic studies and surgery of heart disease are rarely warranted.

Heart disease is also common in Down's syndrome (40%) and in Turner's syndrome (approximately 44%). In Down's syndrome the heart defect is frequently severe (for example, common atrioventricular canal). Since the mental and life-span prognosis is unpredictable in neonates with this syndrome, we have evolved a policy of investigation and treatment identical to that of the chromosomally normal infant. The presence of Down's syndrome or Turner's syndrome in the neonate should not influence one's diagnostic or therapeutic approach—such infants withstand cardiac catheterization and cardiac surgery well. Occasionally a Turnerlike syndrome (Noonan's syndrome) is encountered. In this instance the child has the phenotypic features of Turner's syndrome, but no demonstrable chromosomal abnormality; heart disease, especially pulmonic stenosis, is common.

Heart disease caused by maternal rubella

The frequency of fetal infection from mothers having rubella during the first trimester is about 50%. The heart may be affected in a variety of ways: PDA, peripheral pulmonary artery stenoses, systemic arterial stenoses, and myocarditis are common. Recognition that cardiovascular disease is part of a general disorder is paramount to the multidisciplinary approach necessary for the adequate management of associated mental retardation, deafness, cataract, and glaucoma, although, in general, the presence of other system malformations does not alter the treatment of the cardiovascular problem.

Infantile hypercalcemia and vascular disease

A broad maxilla, full prominent upper lip, and a small anteverted nose characterize the face of the infant with idiopathic infantile hypercalcemia. The hypercalcemia, when detected, is generally present only in infancy, and the association with vascular disease is based on the observation that a number of children with supravalvular aortic stenosis (stenosis of the ascending aorta) or peripheral pulmonary artery stenoses or with both have a very similar facial appearance. The disease can occur in siblings, but it remains to be established whether treatment of idiopathic hypercalcemia in infancy will prevent the occurrence of arterial stenoses or the often associated mental retardation.

Hereditary disorders of connective tissue

The cardiac defects associated with Marfan's syndrome (aortic regurgitation, aortic aneurysm) do not usually lead to problems in infancy. Similarly, neonatal problems are unusual with Ehlers-Danlos syndrome. Spontaneous rupture of a renal artery has been described in a 6-day-old infant with osteogenesis imperfecta.

Glycogen storage disease

Pompe's disease (α-glucosidase deficiency) is the only type of glycogen storage disease causing cardiac symptoms in the newborn period. The disease is suggested by a positive family history, large tongue, hepatosplenomagaly, and muscular hypotonia. The left ventricle is grossly enlarged. Definitive diagnosis can be made by biochemical and enzymatic examination of skeletal muscle.

Other syndromes associated with cardiovascular disease

In addition to the syndromes already referred to, a number of cardiac anomalies are associated with recognizable patterns of human malformation.

Genetics and congenital heart disease

The question frequently asked of the pediatrician is: what is the risk of a malformed heart when a first-degree relative (mother, father, sibling, or child of index case) has congenital heart disease? The question becomes even more timely now that many patients who would previously have died before reproductive age undergo successful surgery. Nora and associates studied the children of 308 adults with ASD or VSD, most of which had been surgically corrected. Parents with ASD had 2.6% of their children affected with ASD, which is 37 times greater than the estimated population frequency. For VSD, 3.7% of the children of parents with this heart defect were similarly affected. The data were found to approximate closely the predictions of the multifactorial inheritance hypothesis. This hypothesis states that the incidence in first-degree relatives of an individual with a malformation transmitted by multifactorial inheritance approaches the square root of the population frequency of that lesion (for example, if the population frequency is .001 [1 per 1,000], the increase is to $\sqrt{.001}$ [.032, or 32 per 1,000]). For ASD the number of offspring affected is very close to the multifactorial prediction; for VSD the 3.7% of children with cardiac malformations approximates the 4.2% prediction. In the future, more marriages will occur between adults who both have corrected or uncorrected congenital heart disease. The risk will presumably be further increased, as has been shown to occur in the case of cleft lip and palate.

TABLE 11-1. Less common syndromes sometimes associated with cardiovascular abnormality

Syndrome	Congenital heart defect
Cerebrohepatorenal	PDA with or without septal defect
Holt-Oram	ASD and other types of congenital heart disease
Hurler's	Cardiomyopathy
Friedreich's ataxia	Cardiomyopathy
XXXXX	PDA
Carpenter's	PDA, VSD; transposition
Cornelia de Lange	Variable
Cri-du-chat	Variable
Ellis–van Creveld	Septal defects
Radial aplasia and thrombocytopenia	Variable
XXXXY	PDA
Laurence-Moon-Biedl-Bardet	Tetralogy of Fallot

Despite the multiple factors known to cause or to be associated with congenital heart disease, in approximately 75% of infants afflicted no cause is evident: the family history is negative, pregnancy has been uncomplicated, and no other disease exists in the baby. In the majority, therefore, the disease is unexpected and is not repeated in siblings. Environmental factors such as ionizing radiation or undiagnosed fleeting infections during embryogenesis also influence the incidence of congenital heart disease. The question frequently asked by the mother who has just given birth to a heart-diseased infant is, naturally, what is the risk for future infants? At the present state of our knowledge a general answer should be that the risk is approximately 1:25, unless there are additional first- or second-degree relatives with congenital heart disease, in which case an assessment cannot be given. There are occasional families in which congenital heart disease occurs at a rate greatly exceeding the multifactorial inheritance hypothesis prediction.

SIGNS OF SERIOUS CARDIOVASCULAR DISEASE IN THE NEONATE

The presence of cyanosis or the signs of heart failure are overwhelmingly the most frequent reasons for suspecting serious heart disease in the newborn. Less commonly, heart disease appears as a shock-like picture, with pallor, flaccidity, and hypoactive arterial pulses; and occasionally the presenting abnormality is an arrhythmia, especially paroxysmal atrial tachycardia or complete heart block.

Table 11-2. Reasons for study of 100 neonates proved by cardiac catheterization and angiocardiography to have cardiovascular disease*

Condition	Number
Cyanosis	66
Heart failure	7
Cyanosis and heart failure	23
Cardiogenic shock	2
Arrhythmia (complete heart block)	1
CNS abnormality (A-V fistula)	1

*The overwhelming indication was cyanosis with or without heart failure. Analysis of the reasons for cardiac catheterization of infants in the 2- to 4-month age range reveals a much higher incidence of heart failure (mostly from left-to-right shunts) and of failure to thrive.

Uncommon signs of serious neonatal heart disease include isolated tachypnea, isolated liver enlargement, a loud cardiac murmur in a temporarily asymptomatic infant, "failure-to-thrive," prenatal stethoscopic detection of a loud heart murmur or arrhythmia, hyperdynamic cardiac impulse, abnormal arterial pulses, unsuspected electrocardiogram or x-ray film abnormality, and central nervous system (CNS) symptoms secondary to a cerebral arteriovenous fistula or cerebral hypoxia. Bacterial endocarditis is almost nonexistent in the newborn.

An analysis of the symptoms of 100 consecutive neonates with heart disease undergoing cardiac catheterization in our institution is indicated in Table 11-2.

PHYSICAL EXAMINATION OF THE INFANT SUSPECTED OF HAVING CARDIOVASCULAR DISEASE

History

The family history should be reviewed for evidence of congenital heart disease, connective tissue disorder, glycogen storage disease, hypercalcemia, or unusual hereditable disease. Questions relating to the present pregnancy should include inquiries about rubella, coxsackievirus infection, unusual radiation exposure, or threatened abortion.

General appearance

The pedigree, history, and general appearance of the infant may reveal evidence of a major chromosomal defect, hypercalcemia, rubella, connective tissue disorder, glycogen storage disease, or rare syndrome. Early recognition that heart disease is but one manifestation of a complex disorder is essential to proper management.

Behavior of the infant

A general appraisal of the infant's spontaneous activity and response to stimuli often provides insight into the seriousness of his disease. A baby with reduced oxygen delivery to the tissues—whether from cyanotic heart disease or from heart failure—may show little spontaneous movement, presumably in an attempt to conserve available oxygen for basal metabolic requirements. In the extreme case, a newborn with severe heart failure from myocarditis or the hypoplastic left heart syndrome may be flaccid and apathetic and show almost no response to external stimuli.

Breathing patterns

Tachypnea, altered depth of respiration, intercostal retractions, flaring of the alae nasi, grunting, stridor, and apneic spells may all be observed in infants with cardiovascular disease. *Tachypnea* is the least specific sign. A sustained respiratory rate of over 45 per minute is compatible with many types of heart disease, lung disease, or mechanical interference with lung function. A sleeping respiratory rate of over 45 per minute in the full-term infant or over 60 per minute in the low birth weight infant, however, indicates at least that something is wrong.

Increased depth of respiration is most characteristic of infants with cyanotic heart disease and *decreased* pulmonary blood flow. Much of the ventilation is wasted because the alveoli are grossly underperfused. Increased depth of respiration is also seen in neonates with primary pulmonary hypertension, multiple pulmonary artery thromboses, alveolar proteinosis, and pulmonary oxygen toxicity and in some infants with Wilson-Mikity syndrome. *Decreased depth of respiration* is characteristic of neonates with severe heart failure, cardiogenic shock, intracerebral hemorrhage, subdural hemorrhage, gross intracranial malformation, meningitis, encephalitis, and septicemia. Underventilation is usually caused either by stiff, noncompliant lungs or by interference with the normal servomechanisms whereby blood gas abnormalities and cerebrospinal fluid pH regulate respiration.

Intercostal retractions are characteristic of primary lung disease and mechanical interference with lung function. Retractions are also seen in severe heart failure when there is bronchiolar obstruction caused by alveolar transudate (pulmonary rales and rhonchi). Intercostal or subcostal retraction implies airway obstruction or noncompliant lungs. In the newborn the sign is most typical of hyaline membrane disease (HMD) and pneumonia, but it is seen in a wide variety of diseases.

Flaring of the alae nasi is seen most typically in infants with HMD, pneumonia, and heart disease with pulmonary overcirculation and with uncomplicated pneumonia. Flaring during inspiration probably represents an attempt by the infant to reduce total airway resistance, much of which is accounted for by the small nasal passages.

Expiratory grunting is typical of primary lung disease (especially HMD and pneumonia). It appears likely that it represents an attempt at maintaining an increased positive pressure in the alveoli until the last possible moment before inspiration (p. 356).

Stridor suggests mechanical interference with lung function and is characteristic of vascular rings compressing the trachea. It is also observed in tracheomalacia, epiglottitis, Pierre Robin syndrome, cystic hygroma, mucous plugs in the airway, diaphragmatic hernia, pneumothorax, abnormal thoracic cage, bronchogenic cyst, and mediastinal masses. The common denominator is obstruction of the airway during inspiration.

Apneic spells in full-term infants suggest a pathologic condition in the CNS but also occur in the exhaustion phase of lung and heart disease. Apneic spells are also characteristic of hypoglycemia; a number of infants with the hypoplastic left heart syndrome have severe hypoglycemia, and within this group apneic spells are common.

Arterial pulses and measurement of blood pressure

The radial, posterior tibial, and dorsalis pedis pulses are readily palpable in the normal newborn. Feeling one strong foot pulse that is synchronous with the radial is sufficient to rule out significant adult-type postductal coarctation. In contrast, it *is* necessary to feel both radial pulses, since supravalvar aortic stenosis, aortic isthmus stenosis, and juxtaductal coarctation may all lead to an increased pressure in the right arm as compared with pressure in the left. A reasonable approach therefore is for the physician to feel both radial (or brachial) pulses simultaneously and then to palpate a radial and foot pulse simultaneously, feeling for evidence of pulse delay in the leg (characteristic of mild or moderate coarctation). It should be stressed that the more common form of coarctation found in sick neonates is the juxtaductal or preductal form, in which the lower half of the body is perfused with blood originating from the right ventricle. In this situation, the femoral and foot pulses are often normal, and one should be able to observe cyanosis of the feet as compared with the appearance of the hands. In practice this sign is often missed until after the angiocardiogram has disclosed the true anatomy. If hyperactive pulses are suspected, one may move peripherally and feel the palmar pulses or even the digital pulses (not normally palpable).

If the pulses are adjudged equal in arm and leg it is necessary to measure only brachial blood pressure. Arm blood pressure can usually be measured with a 1- to 2-inch cuff and with a stethoscope over the brachial artery; however, the recent availability of the Doppler technique is a significant advance in the accurate measurement of systolic blood pressure in sick neonates, premature babies, and in infants in neonatal intensive care units. A major advantage of this technique is that one can easily detect systolic blood pressures with accuracy in the 20- to 40-mm Hg range. The systolic measurements obtained have been shown to correspond accurately with simultaneously obtained intravascular measurements (r = 0.905). The diastolic measurements showed a slightly less close correlation with intravascular pressure (r =

0.871). There seems little doubt that this will become the standard noninvasive method for the measurement of blood pressure in newborns. The flush technique for measurement of blood pressure remains useful for the detection or confirmation of postductal coarctation. The normal blood pressure (descending aorta) was found by Moss and associates (1963) to average 72/47 mm Hg for the resting full-term infant and 64/39 mm Hg for the premature. Crying caused an elevation of approximately 20 mm Hg in both systolic and diastolic measurements. Clearly, therefore, a baby in whom coarctation is being considered should be quiet while upper and lower limb pressures are measured.

Venous pressure

In contrast to the examination of arterial pulses in the newborn, assessment of venous pressure is of very limited diagnostic aid. Burnell compared a group of infants not in heart failure with a group in clinical right heart failure (hepatomegaly) undergoing cardiac catheterization. The group in heart failure had a central venous pressure of approximately 6 mm Hg, whereas the group not in heart failure had a mean pressure of 3 mm Hg. The explanation of the difference between the behavior of the venous pressure of the adult in heart failure as compared with venous pressure of the infant seems to be in the compliance of the liver. The newborn liver appears to act as a readily distensible sponge, giving rise to gross hepatomegaly rather than allowing much rise in central venous pressure. Occasionally, one may observe distended neck veins in the upright infant and, rarely, a prominent A wave, suggesting obstruction to right atrial emptying (for example, tricuspid atresia or Ebstein's anomaly of the tricuspid valve).

Liver size

Ordinarily the liver may be palpable 2 and sometimes 3 cm below the right costal margin, measured in the nipple-umbilicus line. Fortunately, the size of the liver is a highly reliable index of the severity of right heart failure; in this condition it is frequently 5 or 6 cm below the costal margin. Liver enlargement occurs in a number of other neonatal conditions, including congenital rubella, toxoplasmosis, cytomegalic inclusion disease, metastases of neuroblastoma, and hemolytic anemias. However, the observation of an enlarged liver should lead to a strong consideration of heart failure even in the absence of cyanosis or heart murmur. A centrally placed or left-sided liver, if associated with levocardia, frequently is associated with complex congenital heart disease.

Spleen

Splenic enlargement is not a sign of heart failure; however, congenital absence of the spleen, when associated with an abnormally placed liver and evidence of heart disease, frequently portends a complex inoperable abnormality. Congenital absence or hypoplasia of the spleen is suggested by excessive numbers of Heinz bodies within the red cells. Heinz bodies, however, are seen in a variety of situations in the newborn, and their presence especially in the premature infant should be interpreted with caution.

Peripheral edema

Occasionally, the backs of the hands and dorsum of the feet may show pitting edema as a consequence of heart failure. Rarely, there is more widespread edema, with sacral pitting and puffy eyelids. In general, however, the lack of a major rise in central venous pressure in infants in congestive heart failure appears also to preclude the development of marked edema presumably because the high systemic capillary pressures occurring in adult congestive heart failure are not found in infancy. Severe, widespread peripheral edema is, accordingly, a more ominous sign in infants than in adults. The lymphedema characteristic of Turner's syndrome, especially if associated with organic heart disease, may give the erroneous impression of heart failure.

Ascites, pleural and pericardial effusion

If ascites is observed in the newborn, heart failure is an unlikely cause, presumably because of the rarity of high systemic capillary pressures. Before ascribing ascites to heart failure, one should give careful consideration to primary liver disease, primary kidney disease, chylous ascites, and peritonitis. Similarly, pleural effusion should prompt consideration of chylothorax and lung disease rather than heart failure. Pericardial effusion or pericarditis in the newborn period is rare and is usually caused by bacterial sepsis.

Precordial impulse and thrills

Considerable information can be gained by laying a warm hand over the infant's left chest. The cardiac impulse of a normal full-term baby is barely palpable, so that if the impulse is readily felt, ventricular volume overloading as from a left-to-right shunt or valvular regurgitation is likely. Right ventricular enlargement and overactivity are suggested by an impulse that is felt in the subcostal angle and left parasternal area, while left ventricular overactivity is indicated by a hyperdynamic

Table 11-3. Peripheral arterial pulse abnormalities (excluding arrhythmias)

Condition	Characteristics
Full-term infants resting	72/47 mm Hg (aortic); brachial, femoral, radial, and dorsalis pedis pulses easily felt when baby is warm and still
Premature infants resting	64/39 mm Hg (aortic); Brachial and femoral pulses easily felt; radial and dorsalis pedis pulses felt with difficulty when baby is warm and still
Patent ductus arteriosus Aortopulmonary window Peripheral arteriovenous fistula Truncus arteriosus Hyperthyroidism Aortic regurgitation	Widened pulse pressure; typical value 90/30 mm Hg; radial and foot pulses bounding; palmar and digital pulses often palpable
Severe aortic stenosis Hypoplastic left heart syndrome Cardiogenic shock (especially myocarditis) Hemorrhagic or endotoxin shock Advanced heart failure	Narrowed pulse pressure; typical value 55/45 mm Hg; foot and wrist pulses impalpable; Brachial and femoral pulses barely palpable; Doppler technique may be only accurate noninvasive method for obtaining blood pressure
Postductal coarctation (adult type)	Arm pulses normal or increased; typical value 90/50 mm. Hg; leg pulses absent, diminished, or delayed; flush or Doppler technique usually necessary for lower limb (foot); typical value 60/50 mm Hg; adequacy of collaterals, as well as severity of coarctation, determines gradient
Preductal coarctation Juxtaductal coarctation	Arm and leg pulses may be normal if ductus is open; right ventricular blood perfuses descending aorta; differential cyanosis present but hard to recognize; when ductus is closed, pressure is as with postductal coarctation; absolute values depend on length of coarcted segment, degree of heart failure, and presence of associated lesions (frequent)
Supravalvar aortic stenosis Aortic isthmus stenosis	Right arm pressure may be higher than left arm pressure; typically 80/50 (right) versus 65/50 (left)
Pericardial tamponade Constrictive pericarditis	Pulsus paradoxus; arterial pressure falls by more than 10 mm Hg during inspiration (Doppler technique needed); very rare in infancy, tamponade more likely to be suggested by rapidly increasing venous pressure and liver size
Left ventricular failure	Pulsus alternans; strong pulses alternating with weaker ones; reflects rapidly failing left ventricle; occasionally observed in infants with myocarditis and terminal congenital heart disease

quality at the cardiac apex. A hypodynamic or impalpable heart suggests tetralogy of Fallot if the infant is not in heart failure. If heart failure exists, the observation of a hypodynamic impulse may simply reflect low cardiac output.

A number of thrills are diagnostically very useful in the newborn and constitute "hard" physical signs. Fig. 11-1 indicates the site, location, significance, and timing of the four commonest systolic thrills.

Although these thrills are diagnostically useful, in many cases they simply indicate part of the diagnosis; for example, a pulmonic stenosis thrill with tetralogy of Fallot or a VSD thrill with tricuspid atresia. Isolated diastolic thrills are uncommon in the newborn period but may occasionally be felt with congenital valvular regurgitation, especially of the pulmonary valve. A continuous or near-continuous thrill suggests a PDA; the thrill and its accompanying murmur may be maximal in the second, third, or fourth left intercostal space. When the pulmonary artery pressure is sufficiently low to cause a continuous "run-off" of blood from the aorta through a PDA, the continuous murmur or thrill is nearly always accompanied by bounding arterial pulses.

Heart rate and regularity in normal infants

The heart rate in quiet full-term infants averages 130 beats per minute, but the range may vary from 70 to 180 beats per minute during the first week of life. A mild sinus arrhythmia occurs in most newborns and is more pronounced in premature infants. The use of long-term ECG recordings in full-term newborns has revealed the existence of clinically unsuspected and presumably benign arrhythmias. A study of 56 full-term infants revealed isolated sinus arrest in one baby, a few premature supraventricular beats in 3, and ventricular premature beats in 2, one of whom had a premature ventricular beat every fourth beat but who had a normal ECG by age 14 days. A similar study of 20 premature infants revealed sinus bradycardia in 8 and very marked sinus bradycardia (rate below 50 beats per minute) with nodal escapes in an additional 5. All infants with birth weights below 1,500 gm had one or more periods of marked sinus bradycardia with or without nodal escape; none of the 50 full-term infants studied by the same group had sinus bradycardia (below 70 beats per minute) or had a nodal rhythm.

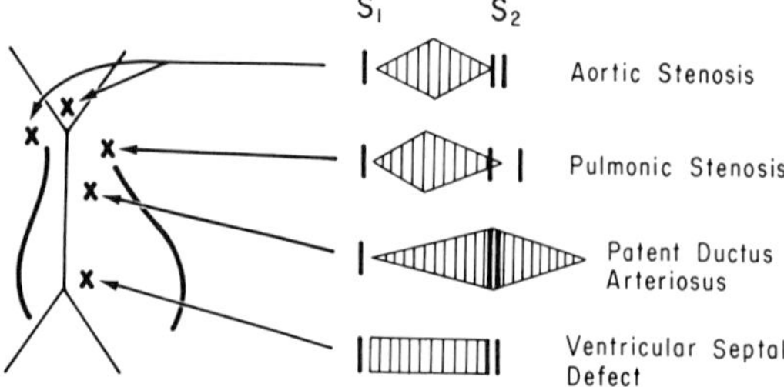

Fig. 11-1. Site, location, significance, and timing of the four commonest systolic thrills felt in the newborn.

The finding, therefore, of an occasional premature beat or of a short period of sinus bradycardia or sinus tachycardia is not of itself ominous. However, in the presence of severe heart disease such arrhythmias may portend serious trouble. The introduction of long-term ECG tape recording and the use of continuous ECG monitors equipped with a memory loop, whereby the minute preceding and including an arrhythmia can be printed out, have greatly facilitated the unravelling of intermittent arrhythmias in newborns.

Heart sounds

The diaphragm side of the stethoscope is usually preferable for auscultation of both heart sounds and murmurs since it is not necessary for the whole diaphragm (in contrast to the bell) to make contact with the chest wall. There is no advantage to use of the pediatric size, but it is of help always to use the same type of stethoscope, preferably one of longer length to manipulate through incubator portholes.

Infant heart sounds have a "tic-tac" quality because of the more equal duration of systole and diastole (with faster heart rates), the presence of slight pulmonary hypertension (for the first few days), and the proximity of semilunar valves to the chest wall. Compared with that in older children, the infant's apical first sound is particularly well heard, and the small size of the chest allows simultaneous assessment of first and second sounds with the stethoscope at the lower left sternal border. In the normal infant, splitting of the first sound is not obvious. Apparent splitting of the first sound should lead one to suspect that one is hearing either a fourth sound (atrial sound) plus a first sound or a first sound plus an ejection click (as in aortic or pulmonic stenosis). Narrow splitting of the second sound is apparent in most babies; widening and narrowing of the second sound with respiration is usually apparent when the respiration rate is normal. An unusually obvious persistent wide splitting of the second sound may indicate an ASD or total anomalous pulmonary venous return.

Ejection clicks, though uncommon, are useful physical signs, since when loud and obvious they are characteristic of aortic and pulmonic valvular stenosis. Soft ejection clicks are sometimes heard in normal babies. The ejection click is heard at the onset of an ejection murmur and resembles in timing, though not in character, a widely split first heart sound. The two may be distinguished, if necessary, by the recording of a simultaneous ECG and phonocardiogram; the ejection click is characteristically at least 0.09 seconds after the Q wave of the ECG, while the first heart sound (mitral and tricuspid valve closure) finishes earlier.

Cardiac murmurs

Certain murmurs are of major diagnostic help in the newborn period; however, the frequent presence of "innocent" murmurs and of transient ductus arteriosus murmurs renders their interpretation more difficult and more subject to error than in the older child. The situation is complicated by the fact that there are no absolute criteria for loudness, and the fast heart rate of babies sometimes makes it difficult to differentiate ejection from pansystolic murmurs. Characteristic heart murmurs of common heart defects appearing as problems in the neonatal period are discussed later in this chapter when specific lesions are considered. Serious heart disease may exist without any murmur, and conversely a grade 5 or 6 murmur may indicate a benign closing ventricular septal defect.

An organic systolic murmur present at the initial physical examination is more likely to be caused by an obstructive lesion such as aortic stenosis, pulmonic stenosis, or coarctation, while a murmur that is first heard at 2 or 3 months of age suggests a septal defect or ductus arteriosus, since the left-to-right shunt "opens-up" as pulmonary vascular resistance falls in the first days and weeks of life.

Chest x-ray film

Every newborn suspected of having serious heart disease requires a well-centered anteroposterior chest x-ray film and preferably a lateral film in addition. The lateral film may disclose left atrial enlargement or an unsuspected pathologic condition in the lung that is not evident on the anteroposterior film. The chest x-ray film serves two broad purposes: (1) to evaluate the type and severity of heart disease and (2) to detect some of the many simulators of heart disease, including a wide variety of primary lung diseases and mechanical interference with lung function (Chapter 12). In the evaluation of heart disease the following features should be considered.

1. *Expansion of the lungs.* Atelectasis or hypoventilation may give the spurious impression of cardiomegaly; correspondingly, overaerated lungs (as in lobar emphysema) may disguise cardiac enlargement.

2. *Heart size.* Unfortunately, no firm criteria exist with which to assess cardiomegaly, and except in gross situations (such as a cardiothoracic ratio greater than 0.75) pronouncements are mostly intuitive. A normal-sized heart is compatible with serious heart disease (such as transposition of the great arteries in the first day of life or anomalously draining pulmonary veins, with obstruction of the common pulmonary vein collecting trunk). A very large heart may be present without heart disease, as is the case in hypoglycemia or high hematocrit syndrome, or the heart may appear spuriously large because of the thymus gland.

3. *Shape of the heart.* The shape is often of considerable help, as in the "egg-on-side" heart of transposition (Fig. 11-15), the boot-shaped heart of tetralogy of Fallot (Fig. 11-23), the globular heart of Ebstein's anomaly (Fig. 11-28), or the "snowman" heart of total anomalous pulmonary venous return into the left superior vena cava (Fig. 11-31). Much of the time, however, the heart is simply large; such useful signs as prominence of the ascending aorta (aor-

tic stenosis) (Fig. 11-18), prominence of the main and left pulmonary artery (pulmonic stenosis), square-shaped heart of tricuspid atresia (Fig. 11-26), and the high origin of the pulmonary arteries (truncus arteriosus) (Fig. 11-29) have often not had time to develop or are obscured by the thymus gland.

4. *Pulmonary vascularity.* Three basic abnormalities can be recognized: oligemic lungs, hyperemic lungs, and lungs in which there is obstruction to pulmonary venous return. The pulmonary venous distension of this last category may lead to a "ground-glass," "snowstorm," or reticulated pattern. It is quite different from the pulmonary hyperemic appearance where prominent large vessels appear to emanate from a single source, the hilum, and reflect a different spectrum of pathologic conditions (mitral valve disease, total anomalous pulmonary venous return with obstruction, cor triatriatum).

5. *Specific appearances.* In the scimitar syndrome one lung, usually the right, is supplied by systemic arteries, and a single large pulmonary vein (the "scimitar" on the x-ray film) joins the inferior vena cava just below the diaphragm (Fig. 11-2). Usually the affected lung is hypoplastic, and the heart is shifted to the right (dextroposition).

A

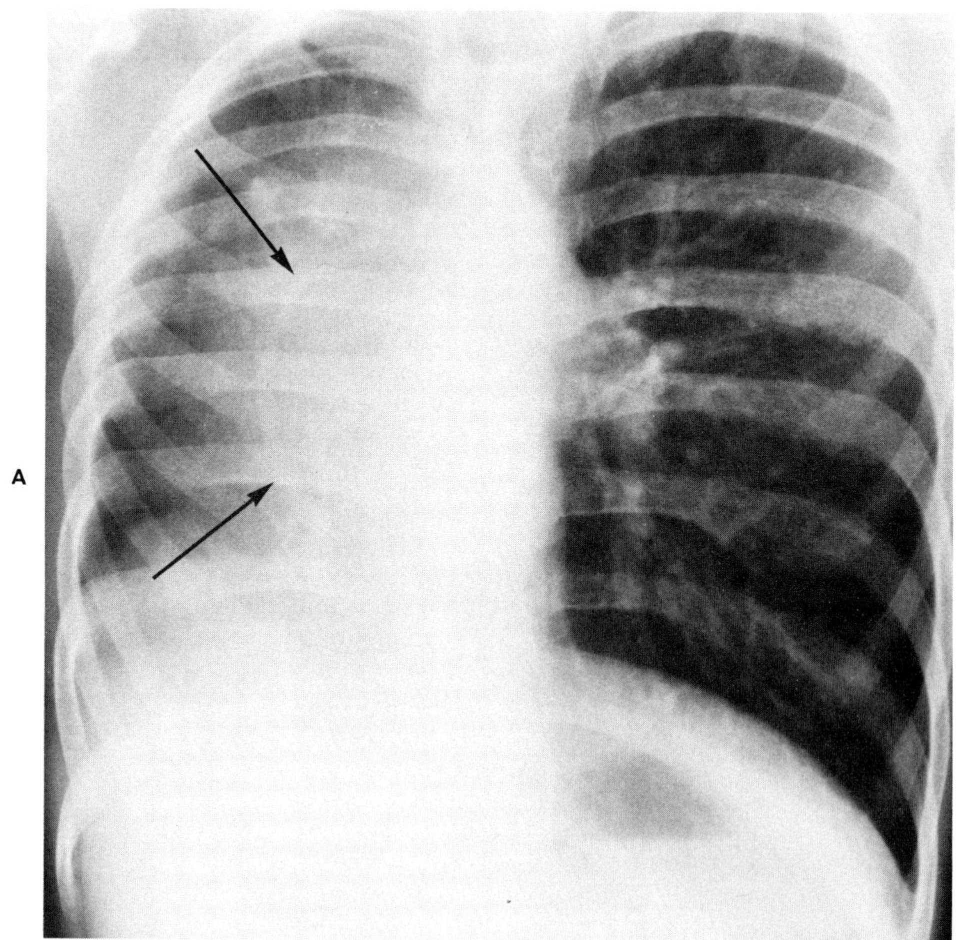

Fig. 11-2. "Scimitar" sign. **A,** With hypoplastic right lung. **B,** In an older child with normal right lung. In both cases the "scimitar" (arrow) represents the conjoined right pulmonary veins curving downward to enter the inferior vena cava below the diaphragm.

The electrocardiogram

The neonatal ECG and especially the ECG taken during the first 24 hours of life show great variability within the range of normal. The changes probably are secondary to the rapidly changing circulation (closing foramen ovale and ductus arteriosus, removal of the low-resistance placenta from the systemic circulation, and the falling pulmonary artery pressure). Other influences are the infant's gestational age, pH status and the levels of sodium, potassium, and calcium. Despite the wide variability of the normal newborn electrocardiogram, it is still an extremely useful diagnostic tool; and since it is such a simple noninvasive procedure, it is mandatory in the assessment of any neonate suspected of having cardiovascular disease. The electrocardiogram in the normal newborn infant has been well described by Hastreiter and Abella.

The QRS complex. The newborn's ECG exhibits prominent and prolonged anterior forces resulting in a tall and broad R wave in the right chest leads and often a deep

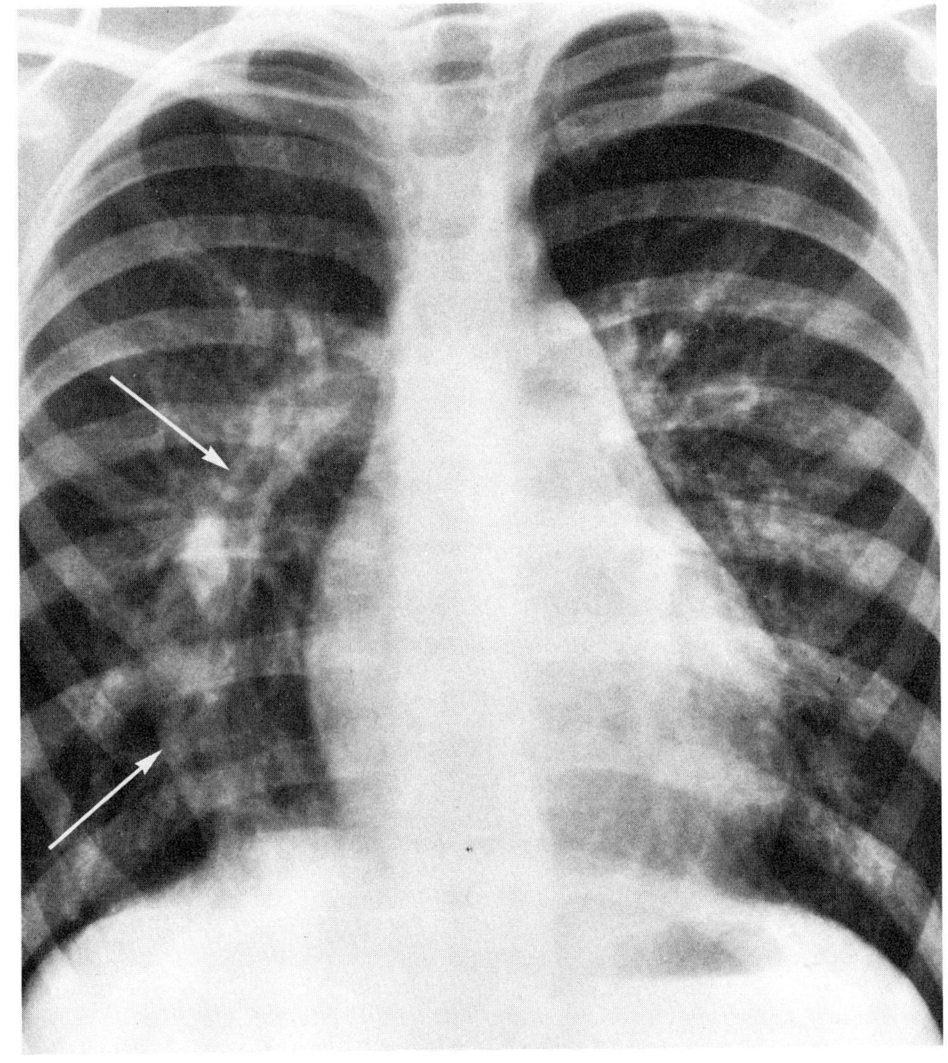

Fig. 11-2, cont'd. For legend see opposite page.

S wave in the left chest leads. The leftward vector in the newborn infant is small; consequently, the R wave in the left precordium has low amplitude initially, but increases rapidly in the first few months. The posterior vector, although variable, is frequently small in the newborn period and appears late. Thus, the S wave in leads V_1 and V_2 is small.

The initial, or septal, vector may be to the left in the newborn period (less so in the premature infant). Rarely, this may result in a qR complex in lead V_4R or even in V_1 and absent or small Q waves in the left chest leads. With aging, the initial vector extends further to the right, and the Q wave increases in the left precordium. The terminal rightward force is prominent in the newborn infant and gradually decreases over months to years. This explains the deep S wave in the left chest leads, which decreases with age. The newborn's ECG almost invariably demonstrates clockwise rotation in the frontal plane and usually (but less often) also in the horizontal plane.

The QRS patterns in the chest leads are classified into:

1. Adult R/S progression—S wave has higher amplitude than R wave in right chest leads and smaller than R wave in left chest leads
2. Partial reversal of R/S progression—R wave amplitude is higher than that of S wave in both right and left chest leads
3. Complete reversal of R/S progression—R wave is larger than S wave in the right and smaller than S wave in the left chest leads (Fig. 11-3)

The newborn has either complete (50%) or partial reversal (50%) of R/S progression in the precordial leads, but no adult progression (with rare exceptions) of the R/S ratio is seen. By 1 month of age complete reversal disappears, and adult R/S progression is common. A pure R wave in lead V_1 is rare, and a qR is only exceptionally seen in newborns.

T vector. Major changes occur in the T vector following birth. Within the first 5 minutes following birth this vector is oriented to the left anteriorly and minimally inferiorly; by 1 to 6 hours it has shifted much more inferiorly and to the right.

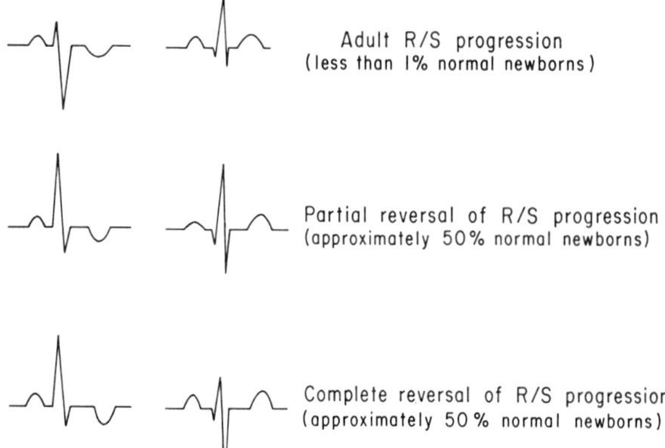

Fig. 11-3. QRS patterns in V_1 and V_6 of normal newborn infants. Note that adult R/S progression is sufficiently unusual to prompt consideration of left ventricular hypertrophy (or underdevelopment of the right ventricle).

Over the next several days the vector rotates markedly to the left and eventually becomes oriented to the left and posteriorly. In the series of Hasteriter and Abella, during the first 24 hours the T vector was still oriented to the left anteriorly and inferiorly; at 2 to 7 days it was oriented to the left posteriorly and inferiorly. These changes explain the upright T in lead V_1 and the negative or flat T in lead V_6 that are characteristic of the very early neonatal period.

Electrocardiographic time intervals. Fast paper speeds (100 or 200 mm/sec) increase the accuracy of the measurement of the short time intervals found in the newborn. For practical purposes, however, the standard 25 mm/sec is quite adequate. At birth the average heart rate is 140 beats per minute, but the rate drops to approximately 120 in the quiet infant during the first several hours. Premature infants have slightly higher heart rates. Although variations in heart rate from 70 to 200 beats per minute are compatible with a normal cardiovascular system, extremes should prompt ECG confirmation that the rhythm is sinus tachycardia or bradycardia. In general, one should be concerned if the *resting* rate is below 90 beats per minute or above 170. The P-R interval should be recorded as the longest observable in a standard or unipolar limb lead (usually the longest is lead

II). The normal range is between 0.07 and 0.12 seconds, influenced slightly by heart rate and the time of cord clamping. The QRS duration averages 0.065 seconds at birth, falls to about 0.055 seconds at the end of the first week, and gradually increases to 0.068 seconds at 12 months. The Q-T interval is greatly influenced by heart rate and is, therefore, expressed as Q-T observed or Q-Tc (Q-T corrected to a heart rate of 60). At birth the average observed Q-T interval is relatively long (0.30 seconds), decreasing to 0.24 seconds at 3 weeks and to 0.27 at 1 year. The Q-Tc is much more constant, averaging 0.40 seconds.

Electrical axes of the newborn heart. A consideration of the frontal plane QRS axis (assessed from the standard and unipolar limb leads) can be of considerable diagnostic help. The normal newborn has a QRS axis of approximately +35° to +180°. The normal P wave axis should lie between 0° and +90° (that is, upright in leads I and AVF). The T wave axis in the frontal plane is much more labile after birth than is the P or QRS axis. The T axis averages +7° at 1 to 5 minutes after birth, then shifts to +115° at 2 to 4 hours after birth; this is followed by a gradual return to approximately the previous level (+10°) during the following 2 to 7 days. From the first week to the beginning of the third month of life the frontal T wave axis gradually increases to reach a maximum of +60°. The T wave, therefore, should always be upright in lead I except for a brief period in the first 24 hours of life, when it may be biphasic or, on rare occasion, inverted. The T waves are frequently of low amplitude during the first week of life. In the horizontal plane (that is, the precordial leads V_4R through V_6) the mean QRS axis has an average value of +130° during the first day of life and decreases gradually to about +110° at the end of the first week; it remains stationary throughout the first month. Thus, in all but an occasional infant the QRS axis is registered as a predominantly positive deflection in the right precordial leads. The T wave is usually negative in V_1 immediately after birth but becomes positive in this lead at 2 to 6 hours, after which it usually becomes negative successively in V_1, V_2, V_3, and V_4. On occasion, the T wave may be partially negative (biphasic) in V_5 and V_6. This characteristic has been correlated with a left-to-right shunt through the ductus arteriosus in the first 10 hours of life. After the first month of life, the T wave should always be upright in V_6. A clearly negative T wave in V_5 or V_6 should suggest an abnormality such as myocarditis, left ventricular hypertrophy, conduction abnormality, or electrolyte disturbance. Whatever the cause of a negative T wave in V_6, follow-up ECGs are indicated.

The ECG of the premature and postmature infant. A number of comprehensive studies have failed to resolve the question of whether or not the premature infant's ECG has characteristic features different from those of a mature newborn. In part this is because the premature newborn's ECG shows even more variability than that of the full-term infant. Generally, however, there is less right ventricular dominance (also lower right ventricle–to–left ventricle weight ratio) in the ECG of the premature and more right ventricular dominance in the postmature infant.

The ECG in diagnosis during the newborn period. Despite wide variability of the ECG in newborns, it is a valuable adjunct to diagnosis in the neonatal period. The ECG is most useful in the unravelling of an arrhythmia, the detection of gross atrial and ventricular hypertrophy, and the occasional almost pathognomonic finding, such as myocardial infarction indicating an anomalous left coronary artery (Fig. 11-38), or left axis deviation and left ventricular hypertrophy typical of tricuspid valve atresia (Fig. 11-27). The ECG plays a supportive role in the detection and assessment of severity of electrolyte disorders and myocardial disorders (Figs. 11-4, 11-34, 11-35, 11-36, 11-38, and 11-39).

The major area of uncertainty is in the diagnosis of right ventricular hypertrophy. This is related to the rapidly changing hemodynamics and individual right:left ventricle weight ratios. Later in infancy and in childhood (when the left ventricle far outweighs the right) the opposite is found: the ECG is a sensitive indicator of right ventricular hypertrophy, but the voltage criteria for left ventricular hypertrophy are unreliable.

Diagnosis of atrial hypertrophy. Since the terms atrial and ventricular hypertrophy are deeply entrenched, they are used here; alternative terms are overwork and enlargement. The diagnosis of atrial hypertrophy is relatively straightforward. A P wave that is peaked and more than 3 mm (0.3 millivolts) in any standard or unipolar lead indicates probably right atrial hypertrophy (p pulmonale); if the P wave is 4 mm, right atrial hypertrophy is certain. Left atrial hypertrophy is characterized by broadening and notching of the P wave, so that the duration (in a limb lead) is 0.10 seconds or greater, and the Macruz index (the ratio of P wave duration to the remainder of the P-R interval) is increased (greater than 1.6:1).

Diagnosis of ventricular hypertrophy. The following outline shows the criteria for the diagnosis of ventricular hypertrophy. No single measurement is diagnostic; all values are possible in normal newborns but are statistically unlikely.

CRITERIA FOR RIGHT AND LEFT VENTRICULAR HYPERTROPHY IN THE NEWBORN

A. Right ventricular hypertrophy
   1. An R in lead AVR of greater than 7 mm
   2. A qR pattern in V_1
   3. An RV_1 greater than 28 mm
   4. SV_6 greater than 13 mm
   5. A pure R wave (no q or S) in V_1 of 10 mm or greater
   6. Positive T in V_1 after day 5

B. Left ventricular hypertrophy
   1. R in AVL greater than 9 mm
   2. R in V_6 greater than 17 mm in first week
   3. R in V_6 greater than 25 mm in first month
   4. Inverted TV_6 or T_1 with voltage changes
   5. Adult R/S progression; that is $SV_1 > RV_1$ and $RV_6 > SV_6$ (before day 3)

Electrolytes and the electrocardiogram in the neonatal period. Although abnormal serum calcium and serum potassium levels are sometimes associated with characteristic ECG abnormalities, undue reliance should not be placed on the ECG to *detect* electrolyte disturbances, since intracellular as well as extracellular electrolyte levels are responsible for the disordered wave form. Magnesium and sodium ion levels and pH disturbances are not generally considered primary determinants of the ECG wave form but are thought to act predominantly by their effects on the intracellular and extracellular levels of potassium.

Hyperkalemia produces a succession of changes in the ECG, with tall, narrow, "tented" T waves progressing to S-T segment depression, QRS widening, and a lengthened P-R interval (Fig. 11-4). Finally, with severe hyperkalemia the QRS blends with the T wave to produce the "sine-wave" effect. This type of ECG is often observed in the dying neonate, especially following external cardiac massage. *Hypokalemia* leads to S-T depression, low-voltage T waves, and development of a prominent U wave (Fig. 11-4). The P-R interval may be prolonged with prominent P waves. The changes are much less apparent than those of hyperkalemia.

Serum calcium changes. It is now realized that the levels of intracellular and extracellular calcium ions are basic determinants of the speed of myocardial depolarization and repolarization. Hypocalcemia lengthens the Q-T interval, while hypercalcemia shortens it.

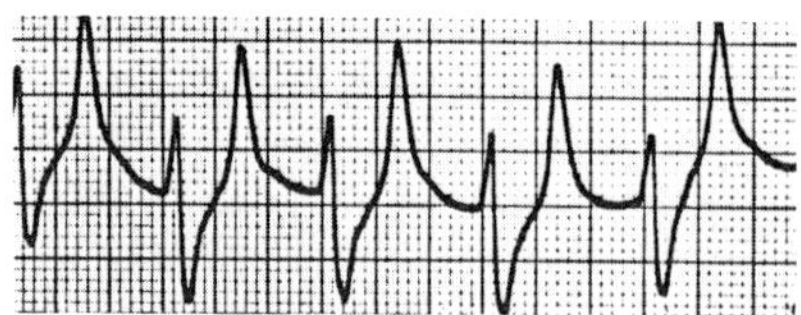

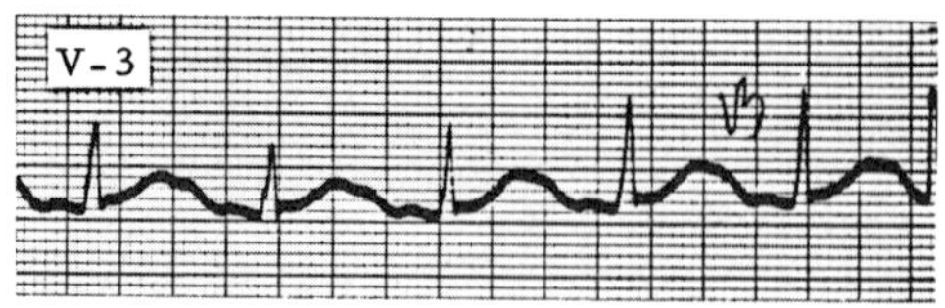

Fig. 11-4. ECG changes of advanced hyperkalemia (lead II). Note tall "tented" T waves, S-T depression, and barely visible P waves on downslope of T wave. In the example of hypokalemia (lead V_3) there is a prominent U wave—the second component of what appears to be a double-peaked T wave. In other examples there would be P-wave prolongation or prominence, S-T depression, or low-voltage T waves. The changes of hypokalemia are much less distinctive than those of hyperkalemia.

Significance of common electrocardiographic abnormalities in the neonate

Sinus arrhythmia may be obvious in the full-term neonate and very marked in the premature. Clinically extreme sinus arrhythmia requires electrocardiographic confirmation.

Tachycardia (rate over 170 beats per minute) may reflect fever, hyperthyroidism, or excessive activity or may on occasion be physiologic. Sinus tachycardia rates up to 200 beats per minute in the full-term infant and 210 beats per minute in the premature infant have been described. However, these fast rates (over 170 beats per minute) necessitate an ECG to distinguish between sinus tachycardia, paroxysmal supraventricular tachycardia, atrial flutter with 2:1 A-V conduction, and paroxysmal ventricular tachycardia. The major problem that arises is the distinction between paroxysmal atrial tachycardia (PAT) and sinus tachycardia (see section on PAT).

Bradycardia (rate under 90 beats per minute)—rates down to 90 beats per minute in the full-term infant and 70 beats per minute in the premature have been found in the absence of disease. Even lower rates occur during defecation and breath holding with crying. The ECG will distinguish pathologic sinus bradycardia (from apneic spells, pathologic conditions of the CNS, gross hypoxia, and so on) from specific bradycardias (such as complete heart blocks, second-degree A-V block, and atrial flutter or PAT with a high degree of A-V block).

Prolongation of the P-R interval indicates first-degree A-V block. If the P-R interval is constant, no treatment is required; but one should be alerted to the possibility that first-degree A-V block may progress to second-degree A-V block especially if digitalis is being administered. One should also consider hyperkalemia, hypokalemia, and acidosis as possibilities. In most instances no abnormality exists, and the condition is a benign variant.

Shortening of the P-R interval indicates an ectopic atrial pacemaker (close to the A-V node) or the Wolff-Parkinson-White syndrome (short P-R, broad QRS) (Fig. 11-12).

Variation of the P-R interval with equal atrial (P) and ventricular (QRS) rates may indicate premature atrial beats or, if the P-R interval has three or more different durations with P waves of varying forms, the benign "wandering pacemaker."

Absence of the P wave usually indicates an A-V nodal pacemaker.

Variation of the P-R interval, atrial rate faster than ventricular rate—a P wave rate in excess of the QRS rate, when there is no relationship between the two, indicates complete heart block (third-degree A-V block), incomplete A-V dissociation with ventricular captures, or second-degree heart block.

Variation of the P-R interval, atrial rate slower than ventricular rate—this rare situation (sometimes called A-V dissociation by interference) implies that a lower pacemaker (usually A-V nodal) beats somewhat faster than the sinoatrial (S-A) pacemaker. Hence the ventricular rate is rarely as slow as in complete heart block. The most common causes are digitalis intoxication and myocarditis.

A wide QRS indicates right or left bundle branch block, complete A-V block, or the Wolff-Parkinson-White syndrome. Random wide QRS complexes indicate ventricular ectopic beats or supraventricular beats with aberrant ventricular conduction. Hyperkalemia, hyponatremia, acidosis, and drugs such as quinidine and diphenylhydantoin (Dilantin) sodium may broaden the QRS.

A shortened Q-Tc interval is characteristic of hypercalcemia and of digitalis effect. Hyponatremia may also cause slight Q-Tc shortening.

A lengthened Q-Tc interval is characteristic of hypocalcemia, hypokalemia, drug intoxication (especially from quinidine and phenothiazine derivatives), and of patients with cerebrovascular disease. Q-T prolongation is also seen in children with congenital deafness, and a heritable form of Q-T prolongation is associated with syncopal spells and sudden death.

Right axis deviation (+90° to +180°) is a normal finding in the first month of life.

Normal axis (0° to +90°)—an axis between +35° to +90° is normal in the newborn period. Axes between 0° and +35° are occasionally seen in a newborn and suggest left ventricular hypertrophy, aortic stenosis, endocardial cushion defects, or tricuspid atresia.

Left axis deviation (0° to −90°) is excessively rare in a normal infant and is highly suggestive of endocardial cushion defects (ostium primum ASD, common atrioventricular canal) and tricuspid atresia.

A north-west axis (−90° to −180°) if close to −90° usually represents extreme left axis deviation, if closer to −180°, usually extreme right axis deviation. Clockwise inscription of the vector loop in the frontal plane implies the latter, counterclockwise inscription the former.

Right atrial hypertrophy is common with tricuspid atresia and Ebstein's anomaly. It is less common with transposition, tetralogy of Fallot, pulmonary hypertension, and any situation where the right ventricle is operating at systemic pressure. Right atrial hypertrophy is also seen where pulmonary hypertension is secondary to lung disease or when heart failure is present, as in PAT.

Left atrial hypertrophy is common with mitral insufficiency and may occur with left ventricular failure (especially secondary to isolated aortic stenosis).

Right ventricular hypertrophy is, unfortunately, shown in the ECG in a wide variety of conditions in which the right ventricle operates at systemic pressure. It is also seen in many neonates with pulmonary disease. Extreme right ventricular hypertrophy suggests isolated pulmonic stenosis.

Left ventricular hypertrophy strongly supports a diagnosis of tricuspid atresia (especially if there is associated left axis deviation). Other possibilities include isolated severe aortic stenosis. Secondary T wave changes (inverted TV_6 or T_1 or both) may be present with either diagnosis.

The Wolff-Parkinson-White syndrome may be a chance finding and in most cases indicates no underlying heart disease. There is, however, a strong association with PAT and with a pathologic condition of the CNS. A wide variety of organic heart disease may be associated, but especially common are Ebstein's anomaly and corrected transposition.

A myocardial infarction pattern (abnormal Q waves) is almost diagnostic of anomalous origin of the left coronary artery from the pulmonary artery (Fig. 11-38). Endocardial fibroelastosis may on rare occasions produce the ECG pattern of infarction, secondary to widespread myocardial fibrosis.

Arterial blood gases and pH

Estimation of arterial P_{CO_2}, P_{O_2}, and pH will aid in the quantitative assessment of the seriousness of the condition of infants suspected of having heart disease. If the infant's heel is warm and blood is free flowing, a heel prick provides a worthwhile estimate of arterial P_{CO_2} and pH. Measurement of P_{O_2} from capillary blood is less accurate, since the oxygen tension of blood rapidly increases on exposure to room air. However, if the sample can be collected from the center of drops of blood, one may obtain a rough indication of oxygen tension. In the evaluation of the effect of 100% O_2 breathing on O_2 tension it is necessary to sample arterial blood. In the postnatal period this usually can be obtained from the umbilical artery, but in older infants the right brachial artery is preferable. Arterial blood collected from anywhere distal to the ductus arteriosis may be "contaminated" by right-to-left ductal shunting and consequently does not accurately reflect pulmonary function. In order to obtain truly "arterial" blood it is necessary to sample a pulmonary vein, since in many cyanotic babies the right-to-left shunt is at the atrial level.

Certain deductions may be made from a consideration of the arterial P_{CO_2} and P_{O_2} while the infant is breathing room air and from the P_{O_2} while the infant is breathing 100% O_2 (Table 11-4). A more complete analysis of the cause of a lowered arterial O_2 tension requires measurement of alveolar gas tensions for Pa_{O_2}, Pa_{CO_2}, Pa_{N_2}, and arterial Pa_{N_2} (p. 348). Diffusion problems have been ignored, since they have not been shown to exist in infants with heart disease. A "perfect" lung would provide a Pa_{O_2} of approximately 650-670 mm Hg during 100% O_2 breathing; however, one is not administering 100% O_2 when the conventional "hutch" face mask is used.

It is commonly stated that if an infant becomes pink in oxygen, the hypoxemia is pulmonary in origin, while if he remains blue it is cardiac (that is, the problem is a right-to-left shunt). Unfortunately, this

TABLE 11-4. Blood gases in the three common mechanisms for arterial unsaturation*

Mechanism	Pa_{O_2} room air (mm Hg)	Pa_{CO_2} room air (mm Hg)	Pa_{O_2} 100% O_2 (mm Hg)
Alveolar hypoventilation	Decreased (<60)	Increased (>50)	Normal (>300)
Right-to-left shunt	Decreased (<60)	Normal† (35 to 45)	Decreased (<100)
Ventilation/perfusion unevenness	Decreased (<60)	Normal† (35 to 45)	Normal (>300)

*Pa_{O_2} (room air) provides an estimate of the severity of the problem. A diminished Pa_{CO_2} (room air) implies alveolar hypoventilation, and failure of the Pa_{O_2} to increase significantly on 100% O_2 implies right-to-left shunting as the problem.
†Rises slowly with prolonged right-to-left shunting or ventilation/perfusion unevenness.

is an oversimplification. For example, first, there are large intrapulmonary and foramen ovale right-to-left shunts in many neonates with lung disease, who therefore fail to achieve high arterial Po_2 in 100% O_2 (especially true in HMD). Second, an infant with isolated PDA may be cyanotic from heart failure, alveolar transudate, and obstructed small air passages. He will become pink in 100% O_2 because the mechanism of his hypoxemia is alveolar hypoventilation; yet heart disease (PDA) is his problem. Finally, if an infant with transposition is very cyanotic in room air but becomes considerably pink in 100% O_2, the explanation is not that the cause of his cyanosis is pulmonary but that 100% inspired O_2 has lowered his pulmonary vascular resistance, allowing better mixing through an existing foramen ovale or patent ductus or both. He may clinically appear to become pink, but his arterial Po_2 will never approach 300 mm Hg. Blood gases and the response to 100% O_2 breathing are, therefore, only to be considered as indicative of the disordered pathophysiologic mechanism and the seriousness of the problem rather than as an identification of the problem as pulmonary or cardiac.

Measurement of the arterial or capillary pH is also of value because it supplies an estimate of the severity of the problem. When the plasma bicarbonate level and arterial Pco_2 tension are known, rational treatment to return the pH toward normal values can be instituted. A slight degree of respiratory acidosis (perhaps to pH 7.25) need not be corrected. Correction of severe acidosis may be partially achieved by the use of sodium bicarbonate or tris (hydroxymethyl) aminomethane (THAM) buffer. It should be remembered, however, that the use of sodium bicarbonate adds to the total body stores of sodium and of carbon dioxide, and the use of THAM buffer is occasionally associated with respiratory depression or even apneic spells. Temporary and partial correction of acidosis is often, however, indicated as a prelude to cardiac catheterization and surgery; if sodium bicarbonate is used, 2 to 6 mEq/kg should be administered over a 1- to 2-minute period into as large a venous pool as possible. Frequently, we have used this method of pH adjustment at the beginning of a cardiac catheterization; the usual indication is a sinus bradycardia in a dying infant, and pH is usually 7.1 or lower.

Other laboratory tests

Hypoglycemia

The initial evaluation should include a screening test for hypoglycemia (Dextrostix); and when the blood glucose level is low, a clinical determination of true blood glucose should be made. Hypoglycemia may simulate structural congenital heart disease very closely, with cardiomegaly and cyanosis. Hypoglycemia frequently also complicates serious neonatal heart disease, especially the hypoplastic left heart syndrome. The hypoglycemia should be treated with intravenous glucose while investigation and treatment of the underlying heart disease are proceeding.

Serum electrolytes

Serum sodium, potassium, and chloride, levels should be measured both because electrolyte abnormalities can occur in the infant with serious neonatal cardiovascular disease and because adrenal insufficiency may closely mimic heart disease. Sommerville and colleagues reported three neonates and one 6-week-old baby (all male) in whom cyanosis and cardiac arrhythmias simulated heart disease. In two of the infants the finding of serum potassium levels of 10 and 11 mEq/liter together with the electrocardiographic features of hyperkalemia led to the correct diagnosis of congenital adrenal hyperplasia (p. 472).

Methemoglobinemia

Congenital or acquired methemoglobinemia may closely simulate cyanotic congenital heart disease. The infant appears a peculiar lavender or slate blue, and blood from a heel prick appears chocolate colored. Blood from an infant with methemoglobinemia fails to become pink when placed on a glass slide and exposed to room air. The diagnosis can be confirmed by spectroscopy (a characteristic absorption peak at 634 mμ) and by the rapid response to intravenous methylene blue (1 to 2 mg/kg). For long-term medication ascorbic acid (300 to 500 mg/day) administered orally may be preferable but is sometimes less completely effective.

Vectorcardiography

The study of vector cardiography has contributed enormously to our understanding of the scalar ECG (normal 12- or 13-lead ECG). The scalar ECG depicts in two dimensions what is actually a three-dimensional event—the P loop, followed by the QRS and T loops. The ECG can be constructed from the VCG and vice versa, with certain imperfections because of the differences in lead systems. The VCG is an excellent teaching tool and for the student of pediatric cardiology adds to informed scalar ECG reading; however, the small amount of additional information gained from the VCG does not warrant its routine use in the diagnosis of the neonate suspected of having serious heart disease.

Phonocardiography

In the newborn period good phonocardiograms are hard to record because of the rapid respiratory rate of the newborn and because the frequency content of diastolic sounds is similar to that of background electronic noise. We have found the phonocardiogram most useful in the unravelling of multiple additional sounds in the cardiac cycle and on occasion in the demonstration that a second sound has a constant fixed split or that a murmur is "pansystolic" or "ejection" in timing. In children and adults it is usual to decide clinically whether a sound or murmur is systolic or diastolic and to decide what it represents; in the neonate with faster heart rate and lack of easily observable reference pulses (carotid or jugular pulse), a phonocardiogram with simultaneous recording of the ECG, carotid pulse, or respiration may be necessary to resolve a problem.

CYANOSIS OF THE NEWBORN INFANT*

A blue or dusky hue in the newborn infant is frequently brought to the physician's attention by an experienced nurse. Since the causes may vary from trivial to life threatening, rapid evaluation is essential; those newborn infants who have persistent central cyanosis usually deteriorate rapidly.

Recognition of cyanosis

Clinical cyanosis is chiefly dependent on the *absolute* concentration of reduced hemoglobin in the blood, rather than on the ratio of reduced hemoglobin to oxygenated hemoglobin. Central cyanosis implies significant arterial unsaturation, while "peripheral" cyanosis implies normal arterial saturation. In the latter, cyanosis is visible only in the skin of the extremities where a wide arteriovenous oxygen difference leads to a "capillary" reduced hemoglobin content of greater than 4 to 6 gm/100 ml of blood. It is sometimes stated that it is necessary to have 5 gm of reduced hemoglobin in *arterial* blood before central cyanosis is detectable visibly; clinical experience indicates that this provides a very coarse basis for detection of arterial unsaturation. Were this the case, an infant with a total hemoglobin content of 15 gm/100 ml of blood would be visibly cyanotic only at an arterial saturation of 67% or less, whereas

*Adapted from Lees, M. H.: Cyanosis of the newborn infant, J. Pediatr. **77**:484-498, 1970.

central cyanosis is detectable by inspection of the tongue and mucous membranes at arterial saturations of 75% to 88% in the presence of about 3 gm of reduced hemoglobin in arterial blood (Fig. 11-5).

Central versus peripheral cyanosis. Infants suspected of being cyanotic are best inspected when they are quiet or sleeping in a thermoneutral environment under a white light, preferably daylight. Central cyanosis is defined as cyanosis of the tongue, mucous membranes, and peripheral skin in the presence of 3 gm or more of reduced hemoglobin in arterial blood. It may be physiologic or pathologic.

Peripheral cyanosis is defined as blue discoloration or duskiness confined to the skin of the extremities; it too may be physiologic or pathologic, but the arterial blood will be normally saturated (that is, greater than 94%). Clearly, there are intermediate conditions in which arterial saturation may be in the range of 90% (for example, 2 gm of reduced hemoglobin out of a total of 20 gm of hemoglobin), and the tongue may appear pink and the extremities cyanotic. Such a baby clinically has peripheral cyanosis as a result of a central disturbance. The clinical distinction of central from peripheral is therefore not always absolute, and elucidation frequently requires the measurement of arterial oxygen saturation or oxygen tension (Pa_{O_2}).

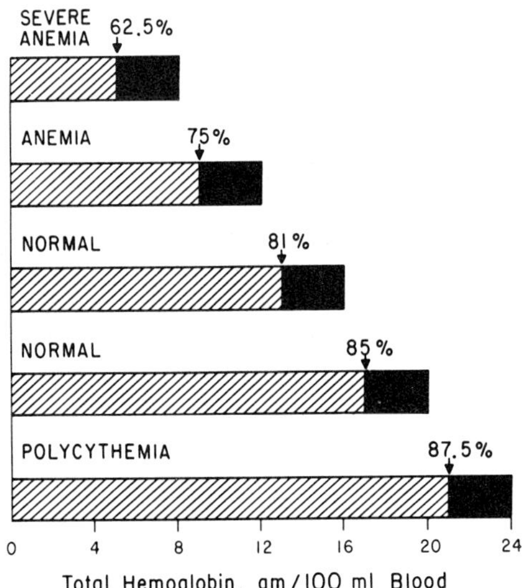

Fig. 11-5. The percentage arterial saturation of blood (diagonally lined portion of each column) when cyanosis will be detected at different total hemoglobin concentrations in the presence of 3 gm/100 ml of reduced hemoglobin. It is evident that central cyanosis is detectable at higher arterial saturations when the total hemoglobin concentration is high. With severe anemia, as for example 8 gm/100 ml of hemoglobin, central cyanosis may not be apparent until arterial saturation falls to nearly 62%. (Adapted from Lees, M. H.: J. Pediatr. 77:484, 1970.)

Clinical confirmation that cyanosis of extremities is peripheral in origin may often be obtained by immersing the baby's foot in a pan of 100° F water for 5 minutes; vasodilatation will occur, and the foot will become pink. Reflex vasodilatation may also occur in the other foot. The color of the rapidly flowing capillary blood ("arterialized") obtained by puncture of a warmed heel often makes it immediately apparent whether there is arterial saturation or unsaturation. If doubt still remains, it is then necessary to obtain an arterial blood specimen. Arterial blood may be from various sites; single samples may be obtained from the temporal or radial arteries, or a No. 3½ or 5 Fr feeding tube may be placed in the umbilical artery and left for sequential sampling. The relative safety of the latter has been questioned. If the infant's condition requires that arterial blood be obtained to determine the Pa_{O_2} value, the pH, Pa_{CO_2}, and oxygen saturation values should also be obtained. Significant arterial unsaturation (central cyanosis) should be considered to be present if the Pa_{O_2} is below 75 mm Hg at 24 hours of age or if the arterial oxygen saturation is below 94%. This does not infer that a Pa_{O_2} of 75 mm Hg or less necessarily represents a pathologic state, but it does mean that the infant either has alveolar hypoventilation or has an alveolar-arterial oxygen difference of about 25 mm Hg (see section on physiologic central cyanosis).

Peripheral cyanosis. Peripheral cyanosis is common in the neonate and may persist for hours, days, or even weeks. It is usually ascribed to "vasomotor instability" and may come and go in an unpredictable fashion. In some instances, peripheral cyanosis is clearly caused by cold environment, by a high total hemoglobin content, or by local venous obstruction (for example, cord around the neck). In other instances, the cause is obscure. The most bizarre expression is that of the "harlequin" infant, in whom one quadrant or one side of the body may be cyanotic while the other half is pink; the hands and feet feel warm despite their appearance. Peripheral cyanosis with cold extremities in a relatively warm environment suggests the possibility of peripheral vasoconstriction caused by shock or heart failure. "Differential" cyanosis—that is, pink upper half and blue lower half of the body, or vice versa—is always indicative of serious heart disease.

Physiologic central cyanosis. An arterial saturation of less than 94% is usually regarded as abnormal in the awake healthy adult or older child breathing atmospheric air at sea level. However, the critical level of saturation for a newborn depends upon his postnatal age, the proportion of adult to fetal hemoglobin, and whether he is crying when the blood sample is taken. With regard to age, Oliver and associates found that normal newborns have an arterial P_{O_2} of 19.5 ± 12.3 mm Hg at 2 to 5 minutes, 48.7 ± 15.9 mm Hg at 6 to 10 minutes, 56.3 ± 12.1 mm Hg at 11 to 20 minutes, 56.7 ± 7.7 mm Hg at 21 to 40 minutes, and 61.7 ± 13.8 mm Hg at 41 to 64 minutes. The calculated mean percentage oxygen saturations at these times were 27%, 83%, 90%, 92%, and 95%, respectively. The great majority of infants, therefore, would not be expected to manifest physiologic central cyanosis later than 20 minutes after birth, and many would have a pink tongue and mucous membranes before 10 minutes. An occasional normal (by other criteria) full-term infant may require a longer time to achieve a Pa_{O_2} of 60 mm Hg.

The ratio of fetal to adult hemoglobin varies from infant to infant, and the proportions of each hemoglobin greatly affect the oxygen saturation resulting at any given Pa_{O_2}. Thus, if a baby with a pH of 7.4 and a temperature of 37 C, has mostly adult hemoglobin, central cyanosis (arterial saturation 75% to 85%) will be observed at a Pa_{O_2}, of 42 to 53 mm Hg, whereas if the baby has mostly fetal hemoglobin, central cyanosis will be observed at a Pa_{O_2} of 32 to 42 mm Hg. *Thus the newborn with a high proportion of fetal hemoglobin may have a serious reduction in oxygen tension before central cyanosis is clinically apparent.* Therefore, measurement of oxygen tension is considerably more discriminatory than measurement of oxygen saturation.

The effect of crying on the arterial saturation of the newborn infant must be considered. Infants aged 1½ hours to 3 days have variable responses; 66% have a decrease in oxygen saturation, 27% an increase, and 6.8% no change. Older infants, between 4 to 9 days of age, respond differently: 21% have a decrease in saturation, 59% an increase, and 22.4% no change. Right-to-left shunting through the ductus arteriosus or foramen ovale is thought to be the most likely explanation.

Pathologic mechanisms of central cyanosis. When a resting or sleeping newborn has central cyanosis that persists longer than 20 minutes after birth, an explanation is required. Categories of disease that should be considered are: (1) congenital heart disease with right-to-left shunting and diminished pulmonary blood flow, (2) congenital heart disease with right-to-left shunting and increased pulmonary blood flow, (3) congenital heart disease with alveolar hypoventilation secondary to heart failure, (4) primary lung disease, (5) mechanical interference with lung function, (6) primary pulmonary hypertension, (7) central nervous system disease, (8) methemoglobinemia, (9) hypoglycemia, (10) a high hemoglobin level, (11) shock and sepsis, and (12) miscellaneous conditions.

Physiologists recognize five mechanisms whereby arterial unsaturation may occur in an adult or child who is breathing atmospheric air and is not at high altitude: (1) alveolar hypoventilation, (2) diffusion impairment, (3) right-to-left shunting, (4) ventilation/perfusion unevenness, and (5) inadequate transport of oxygen by hemoglobin.

A diagnostic approach to central cyanosis

Once it is decided that an infant has central cyanosis (by examination of the tongue, warmed heel-prick blood, ear oximeter, or direct measurement of arterial P_{O_2} or O_2 saturation), it is necessary to determine the cause, since the responsible disease process is rarely self-limiting.

The examination of the cyanotic neonate should proceed along the lines discussed earlier in this chapter, with particular emphasis on the respiratory pattern; spontaneous movement; response to 100% O_2 breathing; arterial pH, Po_2, and Pco_2; chest roentgenogram; and electrocardiogram.

Use of heel prick blood to screen for hypoglycemia (Dextrostix) and methemoglobinemia (failure of blood to become pink in air) takes but a moment and rules out two immediately correctible causes of central cyanosis. Measurement of serum electrolytes may reveal hyperkalemia, raising the possibility of adrenal insufficiency or unsuspected sodium or chloride abnormality.

Certain clinical patterns may suggest one of the twelve groups of conditions detailed below. However, the clinical signs are capricious, and infants sometimes do not manifest typical findings. The following associations of clinical signs may be helpful (see also Table 11-5); however, cardiac catheterization and angiocardiography are almost always required for the precise anatomic diagnosis of congenital heart disease. An aggressive diagnostic approach is always justified, since in the majority of instances treatment is available.

Congenital heart disease with right-to-left shunt and diminished pulmonary blood flow without heart failure. This pattern is characterized by only a slight increase in respiratory rate (to 40 to 50 per minute), an increase in depth of respiration (tidal volume), no response to 100% O_2 breathing, a normal capillary pH or acidosis in the presence of extreme hypoxia, normal or low capillary Pco_2, diminished vascularity on roentgenogram of the chest, and an abnormal ECG. Common cardiac lesions include tetralogy of Fallot, pulmonary atresia, tricuspid atresia, extreme pulmonic stenosis, and Ebstein's anomaly of the tricuspid valve.

Congenital heart disease with right-to-left shunt and increased pulmonary blood flow without heart failure. This pattern is characterized by a moderately increased respiratory rate (to 60 to 100 per minute), a slightly reduced tidal volume, a minimal response to 100% O_2 breathing, a normal or acidotic capillary pH, a normal capillary Pco_2, and increased pulmonary vasculature on chest roentgenogram, usually with cardiomegaly. The ECG is usually abnormal. Common lesions include transposition of the great arteries, the hypoplastic left heart syndrome, preductal coarctation of the aorta, total anomalous pulmonary venous return, truncus arteriosus, very large VSD or common ventricle, and atrioventricular canal.

Congenital heart disease with heart failure. Heart failure frequently occurs when one of the cardiovascular anomalies listed in the preceding category are present. In addition, a newborn with a large PDA, a VSD, a severe aortic stenosis, a postductal coarctation, or PAT may rapidly develop heart failure. Cyanosis occurs secondary to alveolar hypoventilation, and it is easy to be misled into thinking that the baby has one of the forms of heart disease with right-to-left shunting. Perhaps the most common example of this is the large PDA; heart failure with hypoventilation may closely simulate transposition of the great arteries. Infants are often flaccid and unresponsive. Cyanosis is mild to moderate. Tachypnea is extreme, with rates up to 120 per minute. There is marked hepatomegaly and inappropriate sweating. The chest film shows cardiomegaly, except when there is obstruction to pulmonary venous return. Pneumonia is frequently present clinically and radiographically. The electrocardiogram is almost always abnormal. In these circumstances the tidal volume is greatly decreased. Alveolar ventilation is reduced because of increased dead space/tidal volume ratio, with a consequent elevation of alveolar and arterial carbon dioxide tensions. Signs of respiratory distress (grunting, retractions, and audible wheeze) are frequent and are caused by bronchiolar transudate or pneumonia or both. The response to oxygen breathing is unpredictable, but usually there is a noticeable improvement in color since alveolar hypoventilation is the major cause of hypoxemia.

Primary lung disease. (See also p. 359). When cyanosis is the result of primary lung disease, there is usually moderate-to-marked tachypnea; if there is obstruction of the airway, intercostal retractions are prominent. An expiratory grunt and flaring of the alae nasi are typical of pneumonia. The administration of 100% O_2 appreciably increases the arterial oxygen saturation; the cyanosis is usually secondary to alveolar hypoventilation or ventilation/perfusion ($\dot{V}/\dot{Q}$) unevenness rather than right-to-left shunting. In contrast, intrapulmonary right-to-left shunting becomes a major factor in the production of cyanosis and unsaturation in severe hyaline membrane disease. This cyanosis is not abolished by 100% O_2.

Cyanosis caused by pulmonary disease is usually associated with an elevated $P_{A_{CO_2}}$ secondary to either alveolar hypoventilation or to $\dot{V}/\dot{Q}$ unevenness, especially when there are areas of well-ventilated but poorly perfused lung. The pH of capillary blood is frequently depressed, usually caused by a combination of respiratory and metabolic acidosis. The initial roentgenogram of the chest is often diagnostic and helps to exclude conditions causing mechanical interference with lung function.

Mechanical interference with lung function. When the airway is partially obstructed, stridor and intercostal retractions are prominent. When lung tissue is compressed, the signs may closely mimic primary lung disease. Usually there is a positive response to the breathing of 100% O_2 because alveolar hypoventilation is the major cause of cyanosis; the Pa_{CO_2} provides a useful measure of the degree of alveolar hypoventilation. Frequently a chest film is diagnostic. In the immediate newborn period, mucous plugs, aspiration, and gross congenital malformations are common. If the infant's nasal airway appears blocked, choanal atresia should be excluded by passage of a rubber tube, which may then be passed on into the stomach to rule out the more common varieties of tracheoesophageal fistula. A nasal tube should not be passed routinely, since it may sometimes lead to bradycardia and apnea. Radiographic examination is useful to determine whether the mediastinum is shifted (as in lung agenesis, lobar emphysema, atelectasis, cystic adenomatoid malformation, diaphragmatic hernia, hydrothorax, pneumothorax, and tumor) or whether it is midline (as in aspiration syndrome, pulmonary hemorrhage, HMD, pneumonia, pulmonary dysplasia, transient tachypnea of the newborn, abnormal thoracic cage, and airway obstruction caused by vascular rings).

Primary pulmonary hypertension. The designation primary pulmonary hypertension is used for those infants with severe elevation in pulmonary artery pressure, no structural heart disease, and nonspecific histologic changes in their lungs when no alternative diagnosis can be established. The infants have increased total and alveolar ventilation, with rapid respiratory rates and increased tidal volumes. Much of the ventilation is wasted; there is a large arterial-alveolar CO_2 difference, suggesting the presence of many overventilated, under perfused alveoli. The cyanosis frequently responds to 100% O_2 breathing initially, with a large increase in pulmonary vein oxygen saturation and a decrease in pulmonary artery pressure. Subsequently, there is a progressively diminishing response to oxygen breathing in most patients. The report by Gersony and associates provisionally entitled the persistence of the fetal circulation (PFC) syndrome and of Roberton and associates describing respiratory distress and gross hypoxemia in term babies have certain similarities to this entity.

Central nervous system disease. When cyanosis is a manifestation of central nervous system disease, it is indicative of gross alveolar hypoventilation. Hypoventilation may be intermittent in association with sporadic periods of apnea, or it may be persistent and characterized by either a decreased respiratory rate or a reduced tidal volume. The administration of 100% oxygen will increase arterial saturation. Often in these patients there are signs of gross intracranial disturbance such as hydrocephalus, tense fontanelle, or seizures.

Methemoglobinemia. Typically, these infants have an alarming lavendar hue but are not in distress; the respiratory pattern is normal. If the percentage of methemoglobin is greater than about 50%, however, tachypnea becomes apparent. Administration of 100% O_2 does not signicantly affect the baby's arterial saturation, and blood withdrawn from a heel prick will not become pink on exposure to air or oxygen. The diagnosis is confirmed by absorption spectroscopy or by intravenous administration of methylene blue (1 to 2 mg/kg).

Hypoglycemia. Cyanosis and cardiomegaly are sometimes observed in association with neonatal hypoglycemia, especially when the infant is born to a diabetic mother or is small for gestational age. We have observed three hypoglycemic infants with cardiomegaly and cyanosis in whom intravenous infusion of glucose produced rapid resolution of cyanosis and gradual resolution of cardiomegally. The cyanosis was not affected by breathing 100% O_2 therefore, it was probably caused by right-to-left shunting. The capillary pH and Pa_{CO_2} were within normal limits. The Dextrostix is a useful screening procedure, but chemical determination of the blood glucose value is indicated when this test is abnormal or equivocal. Hypoglycemia frequently coexists with congestive heart failure secondary to structural congenital heart disease in the newborn period, especially with the hypoplastic left heart syndrome. The infusion of glucose may improve cardiac function as well as abolish the hypoglycemia.

High hemoglobin concentration. The infant who is cyanotic as a result of a high hemoglobin concentration usually appears plethoric; the color is somewhat more purplish than the usual cyanosis. In some patients there may be roentgenographic evidence of cardiac enlargement, slightly increased respiratory rate, and borderline right atrial and right ventricular hypertrophy by ECG. The tongue and lips of such babies become pinker after breathing 100% O_2 and blood from a warmed heel has a normal pH, Pa_{CO_2}, and Pa_{O_2}, and an increased hematocrit. Usually no treatment is indicated, but phlebotomy has been suggested if seizures or other neurologic symptoms occur.

Shock and sepsis. Hypovolemic, septic, cardiogenic and adrenal insufficiency shock all may be responsible for central cynosis and are almost invariably associated with peripheral cyanosis. Peripheral vasoconstriction often leads to cold extremities resulting in a peculiar blotchy cyanosis or an exaggeration of the normal "marbling" response to cold. There is usually little spontaneous movement; babies are limp and apathetic, and warming the infant's heel fails to change its color appreciably. Variable degrees of acidosis and hypercapnia occur, depending on the underlying causes. The roentgenogram frequently shows cardiomegaly and the ECG a low-voltage or "myocarditis" pattern. The central cyanosis in shock is caused by alveolar hypoventilation, by ventilation/perfusion unevenness (resulting from low pulmonary artery pressure and pulmonary artery blood flow), or by right-to-left shunting. The response to oxygen breathing is variable.

Miscellaneous conditions producing generalized cyanosis or differential cyanosis. Cyanosis may occasionally be caused by alveolar hypoventilation secondary to respiratory depression from drugs given to the mother during labor or to the newborn. Transient tachypnea of the newborn may occasionally cause mild cyanosis in addition to extreme tachypnea (see p. 370). The process is self-limiting, and the cause is unknown. Neuromuscular disorders, such as Werdnig-Hoffmann disease or incoordination of swallowing with aspiration, may appear as cyanosis of unexplained cause (see p. 532). Anomalous systemic venous return to the left atrium produces cyanosis; classically there are no other symptoms. A pulmonary arteriovenous fistula may be responsible for quite marked arterial unsaturation; such fistulas are frequently multiple and are usually visible on the chest roentgenogram. A bruit is often, but not always, present.

Differential cyanosis implies that the upper half of the body is pink and the lower half blue, or vice versa. Preductal coarctation of the aorta with the right ventricle supplying the descending aorta with venous blood via a PDA is the commonest cause of cyanosis restricted to the lower half of the body. The less frequent opposite pattern—that is, cyanosis restricted to the upper half of the body—usually occurs in association with transposed great arteries, a PDA, or pulmonary hypertension.

Clinical spectrum of generalized cyanosis

The spectrum of disease producing cyanosis, obvious and severe enough to lead to a provisional diagnosis of cyanotic congenital heart disease, is presented in Table 11-6. Clearly, experience will differ greatly in different hospitals. The 56 infants here analyzed represent consecutive newborns of 2,500 gm or over for whom a cardiology consultation was obtained because a physician considered cyanotic congenital heart disease to be present. Obvious cases of HMD, pneumonia, diaphragmatic hernia, and identifiable noncardiac lesions are

TABLE 11-5. Elucidation for cause of cyanosis from clinical signs and simple laboratory tests*

Category and pathophysiology	Common underlying disorder	Activity and respiratory pattern	100% oxygen breathing
1. Congenital heart disease Right-to-left shunt; decreased pulmonary blood flow	Tetralogy of Fallot; pulmonary atresia; tricuspid atresia; extreme pulmonary stenosis; Ebstein's anomaly	Respirations 20-50/min; increased tidal volume; total ventilation and alveolar ventilation both increased	No response because pulmonary capillary blood is almost completely saturated
2. Congenital heart disease Right-to-left shunt; increased pulmonary blood flow	Transposition; hypoplastic left heart; preductal coarctation; TAPVR; truncus arteriosus; very large VSD; atrioventricular canal	Respirations 30-60/min; tidal volume normal; total ventilation and alveolar ventilation normal or moderately increased	No response because pulmonary capillary blood is almost completely saturated
3. Congenital heart disease Severe heart failure; shunt or no shunt; alveolar hypoventilation	All in category 2; isolated PDA; isolated VSD; severe aortic stenosis; postductal coarctation; paroxysmal atrial tachycardia	Flaccid with severe heart failure; cyanosis moderate; respirations 40-120/min with rales and rhonchi; decreased tidal volume; total ventilation usually normal with greatly reduced alveolar ventilation, that is, increased dead space/tidal volume	Usually good response because increasing alveolar oxygen tension to 650 mm Hg overcomes pulmonary capillary unsaturation secondary to alveolar hypoventilation
4. Primary lung disease Alveolar hypoventilation; intrapulmonary right-to-left shunt; $\dot{V}/\dot{Q}$ unevenness; diffusion barrier (HMD)	Atelectasis; atypical HMD; aspiration syndrome; pulmonary hemorrhage; pneumonia; Wilson-Mikity syndrome; lymphangiectasia; pulmonary agenesis; adenomatoid malformation; bronchopulmonary dysplasia	Respirations 30-120/min; typically there is distress, with flaring of alae nasi, grunting, intercostal and sternal retraction; with severe pathology, tidal volume and alveolar ventilation are greatly decreased; decreased compliance increases work of breathing	Response unpredictable; lack of response indicates intrapulmonary or intracardiac right-to-left shunting as a major factor
5. Mechanical interference with lung function Alveolar hypoventilation	Mucous plugs; lobar emphysema; diaphragmatic hernia; pneumothorax; chylothorax; abnormal thoracic cage; vascular ring; tracheoesophageal fistula; bronchogenic cyst; choanal atresia; Pierre Robin syndrome; mediastinal masses	May closely mimic primary lung disease if lung tissue is compressed; when the airway is partially obstructed, stridor and intercostal retractions are prominent; unreliability of signs underscores need for x-ray film in every infant with cyanosis	Usually good response because alveolar hypoventilation is often the major mechanism of cyanosis
6. Primary pulmonary hypertension Gross $\dot{V}/\dot{Q}$ unevenness; intrapulmonary right-to-left shunt	Cause often undetermined even after autopsy; consider *Pneumocystis carinnii*; multiple pulmonary thromboses or emboli; alveolar proteinosis; oxygen toxicity; "persistence of the fetal circulation"	Hyperventilation with increased tidal volume and rate is usual; much of the ventilation is wasted, since it is to underperfused or unperfused alveoli	Variable response depending on the degree of $\dot{V}/\dot{Q}$ unevenness (good response) and intrapulmonary right-to-left shunt (no response); less oxygen responsiveness with passage of time

TAPVR = total anomalous pulmonary venous return; VSD = ventricular septal defect; PDA = patent ductus arteriosus; RVH = right ventricular hypertrophy; HMD = hyaline membrane disease.
*Categories 1, 2, 3, and 6 usually require catheterization and angiography for definitive anatomic diagnosis.
†Heart may be normal in size in certain varieties of TAPVR.

Heel-prick blood exposed to air	Dextrostix, hematocrit	Arterial pH, arterial P_{CO_2}	Chest x-ray film	ECG
ark; becomes pink in air	No abnormality	pH normal unless hypoxemia is extreme; Pa_{CO_2} normal or low	Decreased pulmonary vascular markings; heart may be large or normal	Abnormal
ark; becomes pink in air	Hypoglycemia may be present especially with hypoplastic left heart syndrome	pH normal unless hypoxemia is extreme; Pa_{CO_2} normal	Increased pulmonary vascular markings; heart may be of normal size at first but after a few days is almost always enlarged†	Abnormal
ark; becomes pink in air	Hypoglycemia is frequent, especially with hypoplastic left heart syndrome	Acidosis and elevated Pa_{CO_2} reflect increasing airway obstruction and alveolar hypoventilation	Enlarged heart; increased vascular markings; often pneumonia	Abnormal
ark; becomes pink in air	May be hypoglycemia if glycogen reserves are becoming depleted	Acidosis and elevated Pa_{CO_2} characterize most of these conditions and indicate severity	Each condition has a rather characteristic x-ray appearance, but exceptions occur	Normal or RVH
ark; becomes pink in air	Normal	Elevated Pa_{CO_2} that may or may not be compensated; in severe instances acidosis is present	Characteristic x-ray film in most instances; contrast visualization studies may be needed	Normal or RVH
ark; becomes pink in air	Normal	Elevated Pa_{CO_2} usually because of a large arterial-alveolar CO_2 difference caused by the presence of overventilated but underperfused areas; pH depressed	Generally have "snowstorm" or "ground-glass" appearance; heart usually normal in size	Normal or RVH

Continued.

TABLE 11-5. Elucidation for cause of cyanosis from clinical signs and simple laboratory tests-

Category and pathophysiology	Common underlying disorder	Activity and respiratory pattern	100% oxygen breathing
7. Central nervous system disease Alveolar hypoventilation	Intracerebral hemorrhage; subdural hemorrhage; gross intracranial malformation; meningitis or encephalitis; primary seizure disorder	Apneic spells alternating with periods of normal breathing or there may be continuous hypoventilation with small tidal volume or bradypnea or both; infant is often apathetic and unresponsive; seizures common	Good response, providin tidal volume is appreciably greater than anatomic dead space and frequency of breathing is not too slow
8. Methemoglobinemia Reduced oxygen-carrying capacity of blood because of abnormal hemoglobin	Sepcific enzyme deficiency; abnormal hemolgobin	Infants though lavender blue show little distress until over 50% of hemoglobin is methemoglobin; in severe cases, tachypnea and hyperventilation closely mimic heart disease	No response
9. Hypoglycemia Probably right-to-left shunting through foramen ovale; hypoventilation	Infant of diabetic mother; small for date baby; idiopathic; heart failure, especially from hypoplastic left heart syndrome	May be apathetic and limp; jitteriness or seizures common; infant may have moderate tachypnea or repetitive apneic spells	Good response to hypoventilation component of cyanosis; no response to right-to-left shunt, that is, variable
10. High hemoglobin content Increased absolute amount of reduced hemoglobin; arterial blood normally saturated but increased viscosity and stagnant capillary flow may produce apparent central cyanosis	Maternofetal transfusion; twin-to-twin transfusion; high hematocrit value plus unusually large "placental transfusion"	Usually normal behavior and respirations, but myoclonic jerking, moderate tachypnea, or apneic spells have been reported	Good response because o almost total saturatior of hemoglobin when alveolar PO_2 is raised to 650 mm Hg
11. Shock and sepsis Alveolar hypoventilation; $\dot{V}/\dot{Q}$ unevenness	Blood loss; septic shock; septicemia; myocarditis; adrenal insufficiency	Apathetic, hypotonic, and underresponsive to stimuli; respirations rapid and shallow or frequent apneic spells (hypoventilation); low pulmonary artery pressure and blood flow ($\dot{V}/\dot{Q}$ unevenness)	Good response unless hypoventilation or $\dot{V}/\dot{Q}$ disturbance or both are extreme

therefore for the most part excluded, and the experience is heavily weighed in favor of congenital heart disease. Nevertheless, only 36 (64%) of the infants proved to have cyanotic congenital heart disease with right-to-left shunt (that is, the referral diagnosis). Six had left-to-right shunts (PDA or VSD), with heart failure and alveolar hypoventilation causing cyanosis, and 14 had no structural abnormality of the heart. The relative incidence of the various categories listed in Table 11-6 will vary greatly according to whether small infants are included and whether the consultant is a neurologist, cardiologist, neonatologist, or specialist in pulmonary disease.

HEART FAILURE IN THE NEONATAL PERIOD*

The recognition of heart failure during the first days of life is not always straight-

*Adapted from Lees, M. H.: Heart failure in the newborn infant, J. Pediatr. **75**:139-152, 1969.

ont'd

Heel-prick blood exposed to air	Dextrostix hematocrit	Arterial pH, arterial P_{CO_2}	Chest x-ray film	ECG
ark; becomes pink in air	Normal	Elevated Pa_{CO_2}; combined respiratory and metabolic acidosis is usual	Normal or may show pneumonia	Normal
nocolate-colored blood; does not become pink in air or oxygen	Normal	Normal pH; Pa_{CO_2} may be slightly decreased if infant hyperventilates	Normal	Normal
ark; becomes pink in air	Dextrostix indicates extreme hypoglycemia; confirm by another method	Pa_{CO_2} frequently elevated secondary to hypoventilation; pH variable	Mild to massive cardiomegaly	Normal
ark; becomes pink in air	High hematocrit value (75-85%)	Normal	Normal or mild cardiomegaly	Normal or mild RVH
ark; becomes pink in air	Normal hematocrit value; hypoglycemia is frequent; hyperglycemia may also occur	Elevated Pa_{CO_2} and acidosis common	Cardiomegaly frequent	Normal or myocarditis pattern

forward. Heart failure may simulate disease of other organs or systems, and conversely other disease entities may appear with some of the clinical signs of heart failure. Though heart failure is usually the result of structural congenital heart disease or of myocardial disease, it may on occasion be secondary to arrhythmia, respiratory disease, CNS disease, anemia, high hematocrit, systemic or pulmonary hypertension or septicemia. Thus when heart failure is diagnosed, it is necessary to determine whether primary structural heart disease is responsible or whether the heart failure is secondary to some other disease.

Recognition of heart failure

Heart failure may be defined as a state in which the heart does not maintain a circulation adequate for the needs of the body despite a satisfactory venous filling pressure. In the newborn, heart failure gives rise to a distinctive clinical syndrome. Common symptoms and signs are feeding

TABLE 11-6. Final diagnoses of 56 newborns of over 2,500 gm suspected of having structural cyanotic congenital heart disease with right-to-left shunt

Diagnosis	No.
Heart disease	
Transposition of great arteries	13
Hypoplastic left heart syndrome	7
Left-to-right shunt with left heart failure (PDA or VSD)	6
Tetralogy of Fallot	4
Isolated pulmonary stenosis or pulmonary atresia	3
Double outlet right ventricle	3
Tricuspid atresia	3
Preductal coarctation	2
Truncus arteriosus	1
Total	42
No structural heart disease	
"Primary pulmonary hypertension"	3
Wilson-Mikity syndrome	3
Atypical "hyaline membrane" syndrome	2
Hypoglycemia	3
High hematocrit	1
Myocarditis and cardiogenic shock	1
Septicemia	1
Total	14

difficulties, tachypnea, tachycardia, pulmonary rales and rhonchi, liver enlargement, and cardiomegaly. Less common manifestations include measurable increase in systemic venous pressure, peripheral edema, ascites, pulsus alternans, gallop rhythm, and inappropriate sweating. Pleural and pericardial effusions resulting from heart failure are exceedingly rare. The distinction between left heart failure (characterized by tachypnea, tachycardia, pulmonary rales, and cardiomegaly) and right heart failure (characterized by liver enlargement, tachycardia, and cardiomegaly) is less obvious in the newborn than it is in the older child or adult. This difference is caused in part by the fact that many of the lesions producing failure give rise first to left ventricular failure, the results of which are elevated left atrial pressure and secondary pulmonary arterial hypertension, which in turn causes right ventricular failure. On occasion, one observes "pure" right-sided failure; for example, the newborn with severe isolated pulmonic stenosis, or "pure" left-sided failure, as in the early stages of heart failure associated with aortic stenosis. The signs and symptoms of heart failure in the newborn are considered here in the approximate order of their frequency of occurrence and reliability.

Physical signs of heart failure

Tachypnea. The earliest sign of left heart failure is an increase in respiratory rate to above 50 per minute. It is important that respirations be counted while the baby is sleeping, since the slightest movement or agitation will temporarily elevate the respiratory rate. There is no increase in the depth of respiration (tidal volume), and the baby is not distressed; that is, there is no grunting, flaring of the alae nasi, or intercostal retraction. When a respiratory infection coexists or when cardiac failure has resulted in the accumulation of pulmonary transudate, the signs of respiratory distress often appear.

Tachycardia. An increase in the resting heart rate to 140 to 180 beats per minute is characteristic of heart failure. The rate tends to be constant, and the R-R interval on the electrocardiogram varies little. A rate of over 180 beats per minute suggests the possibility of PAT.

Liver enlargement. Liver enlargement is best assessed if one measures the distance between the liver edge and the right costal margin in a line joining the right nipple and umbilicus. When measured in this way, the normal liver may extend as much as 2 cm below the costal margin, but in heart failure it is frequently 3 to 5 cm or more below the costal margin.

Cardiomegaly. The silhouette of the heart as seen on the chest roentgenogram must be carefully interpreted. In the normal newborn the cardiac diameter may seem to be as much as 75% of the thoracic diameter. A large thymus gland interferes with an evaluation of heart size. In addition, cardiomegaly is not present in all neonates with heart failure; for example, the heart is frequently small when the failure is caused by total anomalous pulmonary venous drainage with obstruction to pulmonary venous return.

Pulmonary rales and rhonchi. In the early stages of the formation of a pulmonary transudate, fine crepitant rales are present at the lung bases. As left heart failure progresses and the transudate reaches the bronchioles, the clinical signs often change to those of obstructive airway disease with rhonchi and sometimes with audible wheezing. If the baby is first seen at this stage, the clinical pattern may simulate that of bronchiolitis.

Feeding difficulties. At birth the infant with severe heart disease usually appears well nourished, since the fetal circulation often minimizes the effect of structural heart disease as long as the infant is in utero. After birth, however, the increasing tachypnea and exhaustion of heart failure make it difficult for the infant to suck, and calorie and fluid intakes are below the daily requirements. Mothers frequently say that the infant tires or goes to sleep after the first 1 to 2 ounces, and experienced nurses quickly recognize the poor feeding performance and exhaustion of the newborn with heart disease.

Peripheral edema. Systemic edema may appear as puffiness on the backs of the hands, on the dorsa of the feet, or around the eyes. Sometimes pitting edema may also occur over the tibia or sacrum, but it is unusual for edema to become widespread.

Elevated systemic venous pressure. Because of the short squat conformation of the infant's neck, elevation of venous pressure is not easily detected by inspection of the jugular veins. When venous pressure is extremely high, the scalp veins may occasionally appear distended when the infant is in the sitting position.

Measurements of venous pressure made during cardiac catheterization indicate that it is rarely more than 7 or 8 mm Hg even in the presence of gross liver enlargement from congestive heart failure. This paradox is probably caused by the marked compliance or distensibility of the neonatal liver when compared with that of the older child or adult.

Inappropriate sweating. Inappropriate sweating at normal room temperature is a frequent sign of heart failure in the older infant (3 to 4 months) and is occasionally observed in the newborn. It is probably caused by the excessive production of catecholamines associated with heart failure.

Gallop rhythm. A protodiastolic gallop rhythm (accentuated third heart sound) is suggestive of primary myocardial disease, especially myocarditis, but it is also observed late in the course of left ventricular failure from a variety of other causes.

Pulsus alternans. Alternate strong and weak peripheral pulses are usually evidence of severe left ventricular failure and are particularly common in primary myocardial disease.

Ascites. Ascites due to heart failure in the newborn is uncommon; and when it does occur, the amount of fluid in the peritoneal cavity is usually small.

Electrocardiogram. The electrocardiogram may be helpful in supplying supportive evidence of heart failure, but no single electrocardiographic sign is pathognomonic. Tall-peaked P waves (greater than 0.3 mm in the standard limb leads) are common in right heart failure but also are found in situations such as tricuspid atresia, where the right atrium is hypertrophied but heart failure is not present. Wide-notched P waves (in the standard limb leads) are often associated with left heart failure but are also seen, for instance, with mitral regurgitation (as in the endocardial cushion defect complex) when heart failure, as judged by other criteria, is not present.

Despite the difficulties thus far mentioned, the diagnosis of heart failure in the neonate is not difficult in the majority of instances. Usually there is obvious evidence of severe structural congenital heart disease; for example, unequivocal central cyanosis, loud heart murmur, abnormal peripheral pulses, abnormal chest roentgenogram, or abnormal electrocardiogram. Difficulties arise, however, under three circumstances: (1) when the heart failure has progressed to a near-terminal stage at the time of the first examination, (2) when heart failure is secondary to a cause other than structural heart disease, and (3) when noncardiac disease simulates one or more of the features of heart failure.

Advanced, near-terminal heart failure. Heart failure may progress very rapidly in the first hours and days of life. The delay of long-distance transportation, suboptimal environmental temperature, aspiration pneumonia, and other complications may lead to the hospital admission of a near-moribund infant in heart failure. Frequently, there is no heart murmur, and the clinical picture is more one of advanced cardiogenic shock, with pallor, apathy, minimal spontaneous movement, greatly diminished peripheral pulses, bradycardia, and diminished heart sounds. The respiratory rate may be very rapid with widespread rales, or the infant may have become exhausted with slow respirations or apneic periods. The liver is usually very large, and the spleen may also be enlarged. Sometimes there is peripheral edema.

The clinical picture may closely simulate that of septicemia, meningitis, bronchiolitis, or pneumonia. However, the presence of a very large liver and gross cardiomegaly usually indicate that heart failure is the major problem.

Heart failure without structural congenital heart disease

The following are situations in which heart failure occurs without structural congenital heart disease.

Myocarditis. Myocarditis in the neonatal period is usually the result of coxsackievirus infection (see p. 324).

Endocardial fibroelastosis. See p. 324.

Glycogen storage disease. See p. 326.

Congenital heart block. See p. 282.

Paroxysmal atrial tachycardia. See p. 279.

Other arrythmias. Other important arrhythmias that occasionally occur in the neonatal period include atrial fibrillation (p. 281), atrial flutter (p. 281), and second-degree atrioventricular block (p. 283).

Respiratory disease. Heart failure may occur late in the course of the respiratory distress syndrome. One sequence is for hypoxia and acidosis, secondary to the respiratory disease, to produce pulmonary vasoconstriction. The greatly increased pulmonary vascular resistance may cause right heart failure or right-to-left shunting, or both, through the foramen ovale or ductus arteriosus. Another sequence is for heart failure to develop in association with left-to-right ductal shunting. In some instances, however, the situation may mimic certain forms of structural heart disease, such as cor triatriatum, and the diagnosis can only be established by catheterization and angiocardiography. When doubt exists as to whether the condition is primarily respiratory or primarily cardiac and the baby's condition is deteriorating, the hemodynamic studies are often justified, since the risk to the baby is small and the diagnosis can be clarified so far as ruling out the existence of an operable surgical lesion, such as PDA.

CNS disease. Heart failure may be a consequence of pulmonary hypertension secondary to alveolar hypoventilation or apneic periods or both that are caused by cerebral hemorrhage or other major CNS disease. An intracranial arteriovenous fistula may cause heart failure with or without clinical evidence of CNS disease. (See p. 323.)

Anemia. Severe anemia (hemoglobin less than 3.5 gm/100 ml) occasionally causes heart failure because of the sustained attempt to maintain an increased cardiac output. The commonest example is hydrops fetalis caused by Rh incompatibility.

High hematocrit value. Infants with very high hematocrit values may manifest some of the signs of heart failure, with cardiomegaly, slight liver enlargement, and tachypnea; on occasion venesection with volume replacement is justified.

Systemic hypertension. See p. 336.

Pulmonary hypertension. Pulmonary hypertension may result from many disease entities. The clinical picture and hemodynamic findings may be secondary to multiple small pulmonary emboli originating from peripheral venous thrombosis, to thrombi building up on a Spitz-Holter valve (used in the treatment of hydrocephalus), or to emboli that are septic in origin. Pulmonary hypertension may also be secondary to the acidosis and hypoxia associated with obstructive airway disease (for example, choanal atresia and tracheomalacia), to multiple peripheral pulmonary artery stenosis (common in the rubella syndrome), or to obstructive disease of the left heart (for example, cor triatriatum, mitral stenosis, and so on). In occasional instances the cause of pulmonary hypertension cannot be determined even at autopsy and depending on the pathologist's interpretations, death may be attributed to oxygen toxicity, pulmonary alveolar proteinosis, Hamman-Rich syndrome, pulmonary lymphangiectasia, or other assumed causes. In severe cases of pulmonary hypertension not only is the baby in heart failure, but he is also usually deeply cyanotic as the result of right-to-left shunting through the ductus arteriosus or foramen ovale.

Septicemia. (See also p. 129.) Septicemia may be responsible for heart failure in the neonatal period by infection of the myocardium or by the effects of bacterial toxins on the myocardium. The liver and spleen are usually grossly enlarged; the baby is pale and apathetic and may have apneic spells. If the baby is first seen in the near-moribund state, the distinction between heart failure caused by structural heart disease and heart failure caused by septicemia may be especially difficult. Blood culture, white blood cell count, and chest roentgenography may resolve the issue, but often it is necessary to institute aggressive medical treatment for both septicemia and heart failure. When the baby's condition continues to deteriorate and death seems inevitable, a rapid hemodynamic and angiocardiographic study is warranted if there is a clinical suggestion of existing structural congenital heart disease that might be treated by surgical correction.

Noncardiac diseases simulating heart failure

It is not uncommon for noncardiac disease to appear with one or more of the physical signs of heart failure. In some cases, particularly respiratory disease, the resemblance may be so close that definitive diagnosis requires cardiac catheterization and angiocardiography. This is particularly likely to happen if the baby is first observed when he is a few days or a few weeks old and the early postnatal history is not available.

Hypoglycemia. Infants born to diabetic mothers and low birth weight infants sometimes become hypoglycemic shortly after birth. Hypoglycemia in these and other seemingly normal infants is usually manifested by jitteriness, pallor, apneic spells, and convulsions. Sometimes there is marked cyanosis, cardiomegaly, and hepatic enlargement.

Respiratory disease. The signs of the respiratory distress syndrome may be erroneously interpreted as indicative of left heart failure. However, hepatic enlargement usually occurs only in the terminal phase of the respiratory distress syndrome as evidence of right heart failure.

Left heart failure may be simulated by such diverse respiratory conditions as obstruction of the airway by a vascular ring, an anomalous left pulmonary artery, choanal atresia, tracheo-esophageal fistula, or tracheomalacia. Pulmonary conditions such as congenital lobar emphysema, Wilson-Mikity syndrome, and pulmonary lymphangiectasia may also create diagnostic difficulties. Diaphragmatic hernia, with the partial displacement of abdominal contents into half of the thoracic cavity, may also on occasion be difficult to differentiate from heart failure.

Renal disease. Renal agenesis rapidly gives rise to metabolic acidosis with secondary extreme tachypnea and alveolar hyperventilation. The liver is not enlarged, and the kidneys cannot be palpated. Characteristically, arterial pH is depressed to below 7.0, and Pa_{CO_2} is lowered to 15 to 20 mm Hg. The condition can be definitively diagnosed by abdominal aortography. Later in the neonatal period, cystic disease of the kidney, pyelonephritis, hydronephrosis, and other renal malformations may give rise to metabolic acidosis and mimic the tachypnea of left heart failure. The presence of primary renal disease and its effect can usually be established by urinalysis, blood urea nitrogen, and palpation of the kidneys. Pyelography or renal arteriography or both are often required for definitive anatomic diagnosis.

Rubella syndrome. (See also p. 154.) Intrauterine infection of the fetus with the rubella virus may cause cataracts, microcephaly, deafness, growth retardation, and congenital heart defects. Common rubella-induced cardiac defects are PDA and peripheral pulmonary artery stenosis. Heart failure may occur from these lesions in the neonatal period.

The baby may also be born with active rubella. In this case, a rather distinctive syndrome of hepatomegaly, splenomegaly, failure to thrive, and purpura may be manifested, and the hepatomegaly may be mistaken for a sign of heart failure. The situation may be further complicated by the presence of rubella myocarditis or valvulitis, in which case true heart failure may exist.

Liver enlargement. Hepatomegaly associated with galactosemia, toxoplasmosis, cytomegalic inclusion disease, metastases of neuroblastoma, and a number of other conditions may at times simulate right heart failure. Neuroblastoma, in particular, may invade the right hemithorax, causing tachypnea and dyspnea, as well as hepatic enlargement.

Factitious cardiomegaly. Apparent cardiomegaly may be caused by a normal thymus gland, mediastinal disease, or a narrow chest. The thoracic component of the cardiothoracic ratio may be altered by atelectasis, pectus excavatum, asphyxiating thoracic dystrophy, or some other gross chest deformity.

The heart may be enlarged even though there is no evident cardiac dysfunction. This occurs with left-to-right shunts, valvular regurgitation, and any form of structural congenital heart disease that leads to volume overload of one or both ventricles. By fluoroscopy one may observe that the overloaded (but nonfailing) ventricle is hyperdynamic, whereas with heart failure there is little difference in apparent size during systole or diastole. However, it is often difficult to determine the exact point at which decompensation occurs; perhaps the most useful guideline in this situation is liver enlargement.

Peripheral edema and ascites. Peripheral edema is never observed as the sole manifestation of heart failure. The lymphedema characteristic of Turner's syndrome, especially if associated with organic heart disease, may on rare occasions give the erroneous impression of heart failure.

If ascites is observed in the newborn, heart failure is one of the least likely causes. Before ascribing ascites to heart failure, the physician should give careful consideration to primary liver disease, primary kidney disease, chylous ascites, and peritonitis.

Management

General considerations: indications for cardiac catheterization

When clinical evidence indicates that structural heart disease is the cause of heart failure in a newborn infant, medical treatment should be initiated immediately, and preparations should be made for diagnostic cardiac catheterization and angiocardiography. Rarely is medical treatment alone sufficient to produce permanent improvement or is it possible to be so certain of the diagnosis from clinical signs that surgical treatment can be confidently planned without special studies. The timing of diagnostic studies is therefore critically important. The objective is to perform such studies when the infant is in the best possible condition. Fortunately, optimal timing is usually age related. If heart failure occurs during the first 2 or 3 days of life, the course is usually relentlessly downhill, and if the responsible lesion is to be surgically corrected, diagnostic studies should be performed within a few hours. The infant who has traveled a long distance to the hospital has probably become cold and hungry and has not been breathing an oxygen-enriched atmosphere; he therefore may be an exception to this rule. In these circumstances a "watch and wait" approach may be justified.

The infant with structural congenital heart disease who develops heart failure for the first time at 3 or 4 weeks of age has already demonstrated his viability. Commonly at this time heart failure appears to be precipitated by an episode of pneumonia, dehydration, or some other untoward event. Correct management of the older neonate includes a rapid assessment of whether the baby's condition is improving, deteriorating, or stable. The accurate charting of physical signs is most helpful in this respect. Continuing deterioration during the first 12 to 24 hours of medical management is usually an indication for immediate cardiac catheterization; a classic example is the 3- or 4-week-old infant with a large PDA, pneumonia, and heart failure. In this situation thoracotomy and ductus ligation represent lesser risks than continued intensive medical treatment.

An occasional infant in severe heart failure has such classic clinical signs (for example, transposition of the great arteries, coarctation of the aorta, large PDA) and is so sick that immediate surgery without diagnostic studies is indicated. Usually, however, foreknowledge of the precise anatomy is essential for informed effective surgery.

When heart failure is clearly identified

as being the result of some nonstructural cause, such as PAT or myocarditis, appropriate medical treatment is indicated rather than hemodynamic studies.

Routine measures

Chart. A chart for recording the baby's major physical signs, and drug dosages at 4 hourly intervals is of great assistance in evaluating the response to medical treatment. The chart may be conveniently taped to the top of the incubator. Respiratory rate (basal or sleeping), heart rate, liver size (centimeters), weight, rales (+ to +++), dose of digoxin (oral or parenteral), doses of other drugs, and other pertinent physical signs such as gallop rhythm, puffy hands or feet, and intercostal retractions should be recorded. The development of apneic periods or apathy and lethargy in a baby with heart failure usually indicate that he is becoming exhausted, probably from the additional work of respiration and lack of sufficient oxygen transfer across the lungs to maintain necessary oxidative metabolism. It is also possible that the glycogen reserve in the diaphragm becomes exhausted, as has been described in the respiratory distress syndrome.

Digitalis. Every infant with heart failure should receive digitalis, unless the heart rate is below 100 per minute. Many preparations are available; we prefer digoxin (Lanoxin). This drug is available in a pediatric elixir and in a parenteral solution. The 24-hr digitalizing dose depends on the age and maturity of the infant (Table 11-7). The newborn and especially the premature are more liable to digitalis toxicity than is the older infant. Any suspicion of digitalis intoxication (arrhythmia, tachycardia, or bradycardia) is an indication for an electrocardiogram and possibly for temporarily withholding the drug and then reducing the dose of it.

Incubator. An up-to-date incubator aids in the management of a neonate in heart failure in several ways. The baby can be clothed only in a diaper so that his chest movements can be observed from across the room. He can be easily positioned to lie on a 10° to 30° head-up incline. The oxygen-enriched atmosphere necessary to minimize cyanosis can be provided, and at the same time heat loss and oxygen consumption can be minimized by controlling the environmental temperature. The incubator also allows maintenance of optimal humidity, protects the infant from nursery infections, and facilitates the use of intravenous infusions and of cardiac and respiratory monitoring equipment.

Monitoring. Infants who have bradycardia or arrhythmia or who have had a cardiac arrest require continuous electrocardiographic monitoring, and those subject to apneic periods require respiratory monitoring.

Feeding. Infants who tire easily often benefit by being fed smaller volumes every 3 or even every 2 hours. Moderately sick infants find even short periods of feeding difficult because of dyspnea, and they may aspirate milk. Gavage feeding is often useful to lessen this danger. A low-salt milk such as Lonalac (Mead Johnson Labs), 100 to 120 ml/kg/day, may be used for a few days, but there is a danger of salt depletion from continued use of such formulas. A good compromise between high- and low-salt formulas is a milk moderately low in mineral content, such as Similac PM 60/40 (Ross Labs). Increasing the concentration to 25 calories per ounce (30 ml)

Table 11-7. Twenty-four–hour digitalizing dose (oral digoxin)

Age	Digitalizing dose (oral digoxin) first 24 hours (mg/kg)
Premature infants 0-2 weeks	0.03
Premature infants 2-4 weeks	0.04
Term newborn infants 0-1 week	0.05
Term newborn infants 1-4 weeks	0.07

The parenteral dose should be two thirds of the oral dose. The 24-hr maintenance dose is approximately one fourth of the digitalizing dose. For urgent digitalization give one half of the digitalizing dose initially, followed by 2 doses of one quarter each after 8 hours and 16 hours, respectively. The schedule will be safe in at least 95% of infants, but frequent clinical and electrocardiographic examinations are mandatory to detect such signs of toxicity as second degree atrioventricular block, sinus bradycardia of less than 100 beats per minute, and multiple ectopic beats. Digitalis toxicity is potentiated by hypokalemia. Because of individual variations in the amount of digitalis that is required to be effective, increases in the projected digitalizing dose will be needed in many instances.

may be desirable in order to increase caloric intake. Frequently even gavage feeding provokes vomiting and aspiration. Under these circumstances it is important for the baby to receive his fluid requirements intravenously even though his caloric intake will fall short of normal daily requirements; at best the goal is to approach daily basal requirements. Severely ill infants should be given intravenous infusion initially.

Thermal environment. The newborn infant in heart failure is best observed clothed only in a diaper. He should be maintained in a neutral thermal environment. For the average-sized infant the neutral environmental temperature varies from 84 to 92 F depending on body weight, thickness of subcutaneous fat, metabolic rate, presence or absence of fever, and other incompletely understood considerations. Environmental temperature within the incubator should be manually controlled to maintain a deep rectal temperature of approximately 98.6 F and skin temperature of approximately 97 F (abdominal skin). A more convenient method is to use an incubator equipped with a "skin thermistor servocontrol" (Air-Shields, Inc.). With this device the environmental temperature is automatically adjusted to maintain a skin temperature of 97 F.

Posture. Young infants in heart failure should lie on a 10° to 30° incline inside the incubator. This allows venous blood to pool in the legs and probably decreases the work of breathing by lessening the compression of the diaphragm by the abdominal contents. If the slope is steeper, it may be necessary to put tape from the axillae to the mattress in order to avoid sliding.

Humidity. A 3-kg newborn infant, when placed in a standard-sized incubator with normal air flow and a flow of oxygen of 3 or 4 liters/min, generates (by insensible fluid loss) a relative humidity of 40% to 50%. If the relative humidity falls below 40% (because of unusually dry nursery air), it may be necessary to augment water vapor tension by a humidifying device; but excessive humidity (60% to 70%) should be avoided. Excessive humidity makes thermal control more difficult, and water condensation encourages bacterial growth.

Oxygen. The infant with heart failure may benefit considerably from breathing an oxygen-enriched atmosphere, generally 30% to 35%. Even if pulmonary venous and arterial blood are fully saturated, additional dissolved oxygen can be carried in physical solution in plasma, thus decreasing the circulatory needs by a small factor. In the premature infant this additional advantage must be weighed against the risk of retrolental fibroplasia. Arterial blood Po_2 should be monitored.

Treatment of anemia. The oxygen-carrying capacity of blood will be increased by correcting anemia. The optimal hematocrit value for the acyanotic baby with heart failure is probably between 40% and 50%. A transfusion is usually indicated if the hematocrit reading is below 30% when the the infant's state of hydration is normal. Transfusions should be given very slowly as packed cells in increments of 5 ml/kg, while continuously and carefully observing the response (respirations, liver size, and so on). Heart failure can be aggravated by hypervolemia from transfusion.

Diuretics. (Table 11-8.) Meralluride (Mercuhydrin), 0.1 ml/10 lb of body weight, is usually an effective diuretic in the management of heart failure in infants. Maximal diuresis, however, is often delayed for 4 to 8 hours, a delay that is unacceptable in the treatment of acute pulmonary edema. Further, with the use of mercurials there is a real danger of potassium depletion, which may potentiate the action of digitalis and lead to digitalis toxicity. Thus it is important to check the serum potassium and, if necessary, supply oral potassium chloride.

Ethacrynic acid may also be used in infants and children with congestive heart failure. The suggested dose is 1 mg/kg of ethacrynic acid diluted as 2 mg/ml in 5% dextrose in water and administered intravenously over a 5- to 10-minute period. The drug can be given orally; however, the circumstances that require its use usually also require the rapid diuresis that occurs with intravenous administration. Thus where a rapid response is mandatory, intravenous ethacrynic acid is the diuretic of choice, but when a slower (4 to 8 hour) response is acceptable, an alternative to ethacrynic acid is furosemide, 3 to 5

Table 11-8. Drugs useful in the treatment of heart failure in the neonatal period (for digitalis see Table 11-7)

Drug	Administration	Dosage	Frequency	Indications, response, complications
Meralluride (Mercuhydrin)	IM injection	0.1 ml/5 kg	May be repeated daily but usually only given 1-2/wk	For diuresis; 4-8–hr response with risk of hypokalemia
Ethacrynic acid (Edecrin)	IV over 5-10 min	1 mg/kg diluted as 2 mg/ml in 5% dextrose and water	A second dose is rarely indicated	For diuresis; ¼-3–hr response; risk of deafness if renal failure is present
Furosemide	IV over 2 min	3-5 mg/kg	Can be repeated after electrolyte check	For diuresis; 1- to 1½-hr response; risk of deafness if renal failure present
Hydrochlorothiazide (Hydrodiuril)	Oral (in 2 divided doses)	0.5 to 0.75 mg/kg/day	Suitable for long-term therapy	For diuresis; slow response; risk of hypokalemia
Sodium bicarbonate	IV over 12-hr period	Desired bicarbonate concentration (usually 23 mEq/liter) minus existing bicarbonate concentration × 0.6 × body weight (kg) = mEq bicarbonate dosage	Usually given once before planned therapy	For partial correction of metabolic acidosis; risk of hypernatremia, water retention, and alkalosis
Sodium bicarbonate	Large vein (umbilical) or intracardiac; over ½-1 min	2-5 mEq/kg	Administer one time	Last resort as a resuscitative procedure in cardiac arrest or extreme bradycardia
THAM buffer	IV into large vein, over 5-10 min	2-5 ml/kg as a 0.3M solutation in 5-10 glucose at pH 8.4	Administer one time usually before planned surgery	For partial correction of metabolic acidosis; an alternative to sodium bicarbonate when hypernatremia is present; risks of hypoglycemia, respiratory depression, and severe local irritation at site of administration
Morphine sulfate	Subcutaneously	0.5 to 1 mg/5 kg	Rarely administered more than once	Useful where signs of left heart failure predominate and the baby is very restless and agitated; risk of respiratory depression
Epinephrine	IV or intracardiac	1 ml of 1:10,000 solution	One time	Last resort for cardiac arrest or extreme bradycardia
Isoproterenol	IV infusion by pump	0.1-0.4 μg/kg/min	Continuous administration during cardiogenic shock	Cardiogenic shock or severe failure especially when associated with bradycardia; requires slow weaning
Calcium chloride or calcium gluconate	Intracardiac	1-2 ml of 10% solution	One time	Last resort for cardiac arrest or extreme bradycardia

mg/kg as an intravenous dose. Meralluride is a reliable drug and is safe, providing its hypokalemic effects are appreciated. Long-term diuretic administration is rarely indicated in the management of the newborn infant; however, hydrochlorothiazide (Hydrodiuril) may be useful occasionally. Infants under 6 months of age require 0.5 to 0.75 mg/kg/day in 2 doses. Care should be taken to avoid the development of hypokalemia. Patients on long-term thiazide therapy should also have determination of hematocrit, white blood cell, and platelet counts repeated at monthly intervals. The principal occasion for the use of hydrochlorothiazide is in the infant with chronic congestive heart failure for whom nothing surgical can be done, or for whom surgery would at best be temporarily palliative.

Fluid and electrolytes. Despite the presence of heart failure, the newborn has continued need for fluid to replace insensible and urinary water losses and for electrolytes to maintain normal body fluid tonicity. Serum sodium, potassium, and chloride levels should be measured as soon as possible; the amount and type of fluid administered intravenously will depend on serum electrolyte concentrations and the estimated degree of fluid retention. In general, fluid restriction should not be as aggressive as in the older child or adult with heart failure. The problem of prolonged intravenous fluid therapy does not often arise, because the newborn with heart failure who is sick enough to require intravenous fluids generally requires rapid hemodynamic assessment and often surgery. Approximately 80 to 100 ml/kg/24 hr of fluid will be required. The requirement for sodium will vary from 1 to 4 mEq/kg/24-hr and that for potassium from 0 to 3 mEq/kg/24 hr, depending upon the serum electrolyte levels. The neonate in heart failure cannot tolerate sudden increases in circulating blood volume. If these daily requirements are distributed evenly throughout the 24 hours and a careful check is kept on the presence of pulmonary rales, the liver size, systemic edema, and weight, their administration will not worsen the baby's heart failure by producing hypervolemia and hyponatremia and will prevent him from developing hypernatremia from too severe water restriction. If the baby is first seen when heart failure is in an advanced state with evidence of peripheral edema and widespread pulmonary rales, then intravenous administration of fluid should be reduced to 40 to 80 ml/kg/24 hr pending the baby's improvement from medical measures or following surgery.

Acid-base status. (Table 11-5.) Heart failure may produce acidosis, carbon dioxide retention (high Pa_{CO_2}), and hypoxia (low Pa_{O_2}). When severe heart failure is present, alveolar and bronchiolar transudates give rise to a situation analogous to obstructive airway disease. There are rhonchi, rales, and signs of respiratory distress. Alveolar ventilation is reduced, and the work of breathing is increased. As a result of alveolar hypoventilation, there is failure of gas exchange in the lungs, with resultant retention of carbon dioxide and hypoxia. Respiratory acidosis may then be complicated by metabolic acidosis if hypoxia is extreme. Under these circumstances the infant resorts to anaerobic metabolism, with consequent increased production of lactic acid and derivatives, hence metabolic acidosis.

In the baby with mild heart failure there is commonly no disturbance of pH or Pa_{CO_2} but there may be some lowering of Pa_{O_2} owing to intrapulmonary right-to-left shunting or to uneven perfusion of the lung. When one is faced with a baby in severe heart failure and acidosis, the use of sodium bicarbonate or THAM buffer intravenously is sometimes justified. The amount of bicarbonate may be determined by the following formula: desired bicarbonate concentration (usually 23 mEq/liter) minus existing bicarbonate concentration × 0.6 × body weight (kg) equals milliequivalents of bicarbonate that would be expected to totally correct the metabolic acidosis. Often an adequate clinical response is obtained when the patient has received only part of the required milliequivalents estimated for total correction. The sodium bicarbonate should be given over a 12-hour period. Normally this kind of therapy will be used as a prelude to surgery, since its benefits are only temporary. The use of THAM buffer to correct acidosis is more controversial because of its tendency to produce hypoventilation or apneic spells, but THAM may be the buffer of choice when hypernatremia is already present. If THAM is given it should be infused intravenously into a large vein as a 0.3M solution at pH 8.4; the dose is in the range of 2 to 5 ml/kg.

Antibiotics. Some neonates with heart failure have increased pulmonary perfusion, which makes them more susceptible to respiratory infections. Even after auscultation, roentgenography, and white blood cell count, it is often difficult to be sure whether or not pulmonary infection is present. Flaring of the alae nasi, grunting, or intercostal retractions suggest the presence of pneumonia and the need for antibiotic therapy.

Emergency measures

If the condition of the infant is deteriorating rapidly, more aggressive measures may be indicated, particularly if the baby has an operable heart lesion.

Rotating tourniquets. Medical venesection by tourniquets placed around the upper arms and thighs can be a life-saving measure. The major indication is pulmonary edema. A tourniquet is applied tightly to three of the extremities to obstruct venous but not arterial circulation, and one of these tourniquets is moved every 10 minutes so that the circulation of each limb is unobstructed for 10 out of every 40 minutes.

Rapid infusion of sodium bicarbonate by syringe. This is occasionally indicated. The bradycardic, bradypneic, flaccid infant with severe heart failure is severely acidotic. A sudden elevation of pH can be achieved by injection of 2 to 5 mEq/kg sodium bicarbonate into a large central vein (usually the umbilical vein) or, in an extreme situation, directly into the heart by chest-wall puncture. The effects can be dramatic, presumably because the myocardium suddenly receives coronary artery blood of more nearly normal pH and because pulmonary vasoconstriction is relaxed by perfusion of blood with a higher pH value. The effects are usually transient (10 to 30 minutes); therefore, the major objective of rapid correction of acidosis is to keep the baby alive while preparing for surgery or to permit a more effective response to other and longer range medical therapy.

Infusion of β-adrenergic drugs. Infants with severe heart failure from left-to-right shunts may improve temporarily following infusion of catecholamines. These agents act by direct inotropic effect.

A suitable β-adrenergic stimulator is isoproterenol. This may be particularly useful when bradycardia is present in advanced cardiogenic shock. The initial dose is approximately 0.1 μgm/kg/min increasing to 0.4 μgm/kg/min until a heart rate of approximately 140 to 160 beats per minute is achieved. Isoproterenol should be continued throughout anesthesia until the underlying cause of heart failure has been corrected. It should then be discontinued slowly during monitoring of the blood pressure and recording of the ECG.

Peritoneal dialysis. This procedure should be reserved for the rare infant with severe refractory heart failure for whom other therapies have been unsuccessful.

Resuscitative measures. These measures are indicated as last resort procedures when extreme bradycardia or cardiac arrest occur in an infant who has an operable heart lesion. Usually they will take place on the operating table while the surgeon is preparing for the operation. They are external cardiac massage, pulmonary venilation via an endotracheal tube, intracardiac injection of epinephrine (1 ml of 1:10,000 solution), and intracardiac injection of calcium chloride or calcium gluconate (1 to 2 ml of 10% solution).

Morphine sulfate. (Table 11-8.) Morphine sulfate is indicated in very rare instances where a baby in heart failure is extremely restless and agitated. Such occasions are more likely to occur in a 3- to 4-week-old infant in whom signs of left heart failure predominate. The dosage is 0.5 to 1 mg/5 kg body weight, subcutaneously. The risk of respiratory depression must be considered when one is using this drug.

Summary

Heart failure in the newborn is characterized by tachypnea, tachycardia, feeding difficulties, pulmonary rales and rhonchi, hepatic enlargement, and cardiomegaly. Less common signs include visibly elevated systemic venous pressure, peripheral edema, ascites, pulsus alternans, gallop rhythm, and inappropriate sweating.

When heart failure occurs in the first days and weeks of life it is usually caused by structural congenital heart disease or by primary myocardial disease. It may on occasion, however, be secondary to arrhythmia, respiratory disease, CNS disease, anemia, systemic or pulmonary hypertension, or septicemia.

The distinction between left heart failure and right heart failure is less obvious in the newborn than in the older child or adult. The newborn with advanced near-terminal heart failure is often pallid and apathetic. He has minimal spontaneous movements, diminished peripheral pulses, bradycardia, apneic periods, splenic enlargement, widespread peripheral edema, and gross cardiomegaly. Near-terminal heart failure may closely simulate septicemia, meningitis, bronchiolitis, or severe pneumonia.

Certain noncardiac conditions may also simulate heart failure. Such conditions include hypoglycemia, many forms of respiratory disease, renal disease, the rubella syndrome, liver enlargement caused by a variety of diseases, factitious cardiomegaly, cardiomegaly not caused by heart failure, peripheral edema caused by hypoalbuminemic states or lymphedema, and ascites caused by escape of chyle or liver disease.

The management of heart failure in the newborn requires a rapid assessment of the effect of the medical measures described. Deterioration or failure of the infant to improve within 12 hours is usually an indication for cardiac catheterization and angiocardiography. In general, the younger the infant the more urgent are diagnostic studies and surgery, if indicated. The use of an incubator is essential for optimal care.

A number of emergency measures are available for the critically sick newborn with heart failure. The usual objective of these more drastic measures is to produce a temporary improvement so that other measures that may provide longer-range benefit may be utilized.

ARRHYTHMIAS IN THE NEONATAL PERIOD

Benign arrhythmias

Benign arrhythmias are frequent in the neonatal period, especially in premature infants. Many of the arrhythmias go unrecognized unless there is continuous recording of the ECG. These benign phenomena include transient periods of sinus bradycardia, especially with straining, micturition, or crying (Valsalva physiology), and of sinus tachycardia, especially with activity and crying. Rates below 90 or above 180 beats per minute for more than 15 seconds should be regarded as pathologic and require electrocardiographic confirmation of normal P waves and a normal PQRS relationship.

As a general statement one can say that bradycardia is a more serious finding than tachycardia. Although it is clear that an infant with complete heart block (with, for example, a rate of 60 beats per minute) can remain asymptomatic, an infant with a sinus bradycardia of 60 beats per minute associated with structural heart disease or CNS disease frequently develops low-output heart failure and requires treatment. Tachycardia up to 200 beats per minute is tolerated much better than bradycardia, (sinus tachycardia or PAT). If structural heart disease or other reason for circulatory compromise is present, however, heart failure may rapidly develop, at rates of 200 to 220 beats per minute.

Aside from sinus tachycardia and sinus bradycardia, other abnormalities often encountered are premature supraventricular and ventricular beats, brief periods of sinus arrest, ectopic atrial rhythm, and the so-called wandering pacemaker, in which the P-wave shape and the P-R interval will be seen to change from beat to beat in the same lead.

Before embarking on the treatment of a tachycardia, bradycardia, or irregular heartbeat, one must decide (1) if the abnormality is benign and is likely to resolve spontaneously or (2) if the arrhythmia is symptomatic and there is underlying noncardiac serious disease, such as CNS disease, sepsis, hypoglycemia, drug intoxication (especially digitalis toxicity), severe tissue hypoxia, or adrenal insufficiency (especially congenital adrenal hyperplasia). Fever, excessive activity, or hyperthyroidism cause tachycardia. If the arrhythmia is secondary, treatment of the underlying disorder is of major importance, although treatment of a secondary bradycardia may also be lifesaving. One must also decide if the treatment is likely to be more dangerous than the arrhythmia; for example, one occasionally encounters a baby with very frequent or even short runs of ventricular ectopic beats in whom the use of quinidine or lidocaine is more dangerous than allowing the arrhythmia to continue. In deciding to treat or not to treat, one should consider whether the ventricular rate and rhythm are compatible with a normal cardiac output.

Pathologic arrhythmias

Paroxysmal supraventricular tachycardia and complete (third-degree A-V) heart block numerically dominate the spectrum of pathologic arrhythmias and consequently are discussed here in detail. Both arrhythmias are potentially lethal—especially when structural heart disease is present—and both are treatable.

One reasonable classification of arrhythmias of the newborn is into tachyarrhythmias (over 180 beats per minute), bradyarrhythmias (below 90 beats per minute), and irregular arrhythmias. These categories correspond to nurses' observations of disordered heartbeat as they are likely to be reported to the physician. The classification is certainly not esthetically or etiologically satisfying to the electrophysiologist.

Tachyarrhythmias (rate over 180 beats per minute)

The major causes of tachyarrhythmias (after simple sinus tachycardia) are paroxysmal supraventricular tachycardia (PST), atrial flutter with frequent ventricular response, atrial fibrillation with frequent ventricular response, and ventricular tachycardia. PST is the most common.

Paroxysmal supraventricular tachycardia. In most instances the rapidly discharging ectopic focus is in the right atrium (hence, PAT); in a small minority the focus is in the A-V node (no P waves visible) or rarely in the left atrium.

Clinical presentation. PAT is common and is often discovered before birth by detection of an unusually rapid fetal heart rate. The newborns who are discovered to have PAT are either those in whom the arrhythmia is discovered during the first few days after birth when they are relatively asymptomatic or those infants who are brought into the hospital in heart failure, having had the arrhythmia for probably 3 to 4 days. Many neonates who are asymptomatic develop short periods of PAT.

The history usually reveals that the infant has become anxious, restless, tachypneic, or "not well" 1 to 2 days before there is serious concern. Neonates then usually become "wheezy," and at this stage it is easy for both parent and physician to diagnose a lower respiratory tract infection; as the PAT persists, the infant becomes pale, apathetic, and obviously very sick, with signs of congestive heart failure (pulmonary rales, hepatomegaly) and poor skin perfusion. Even at this stage it is possible for one to overlook, because of noisy respiration, the fact that the heart is beating at 300 per minute.

The time taken for an infant to develop heart failure depends mainly on the ventricular rate (180 to 300 beats per minute) and the presence or absence of structural heart disease. An infant with serious cyanotic heart disease who develops PST during the course of cardiac catheterization may seriously worsen in a few minutes, while an infant with a normal heart may tolerate a rate of 220 beats indefinitely.

Diagnosis. Recognition of PST is based upon (1) a persistent ventricular rate of over 180 beats per minute, (2) a fixed or almost fixed R-R interval on the ECG, (3) abnormal P-wave shape, P-wave axis, or P-R interval or total absence of P waves (usually implying A-V nodal ectopic pacemaker), and (4) little change in heart rate, with activity, crying, breath holding, or gentle eyeball compression. There is rarely any difficulty in diagnosis when the rate is over 210 per minute, but frequently the question arises to whether a tachycardia is sinus or paroxysmal supraventricular when the rate is 180 to 210 per minute. Often the question can be resolved by gentle eyeball pressure. With sinus tachycardia the rate slows somewhat, and P waves become more obvious; with PST there is usually no effect, or occasionally there is reversion to sinus rhythm, maintained after eyeball pressure is discontinue. In cases of doubt, and where a persistent *sleeping* rate of over 180 beats per minute exists, a therapeutic trial of digitalis is indicated.

Treatment. PST in the neonate with

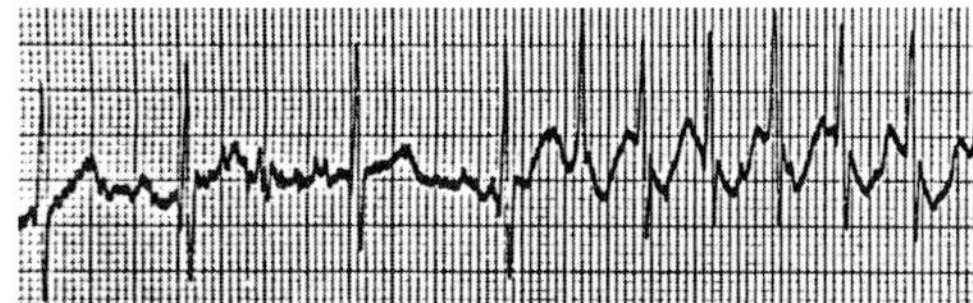

Fig. 11-6. Onset of PAT. Tracing obtained by telemetry. The rate increases from 75 to 200 beats per minute. Note the unchanging R-R interval in the last 6 complexes and that the P waves are masked by the preceding T waves. (Courtesy Dr. Herbert Semler.)

heart failure can usually be satisfactorily treated. The availability of DC countershock makes conversion to sinus rhythm possible in virtually all cases. The following therapies are available.

1. *Vagal stimulation.* There is doubt concerning the advisability of eyeball pressure, because of both the possibility of injury to the eye and the ineffectiveness of the procedure in the newborn. However, initial gentle eyeball compression is indicated to distinguish sinus tachycardia from PST and in the hope of an occasional conversion. Carotid sinus compression and persistent eyeball compression are not indicated.

2. *Digitalis.* One half of the 24-hour digitalizing dose of digoxin (Table 11-7) should be administered parenterally, intramuscularly if heart failure is only moderate, and intravenously if the baby is in severe heart failure or cardiogenic shock. If the intravenous route is used, the ECG should be watched continuously and the injection given over a 30-second period. Conversion commonly occurs 15 to 20 minutes after the intravenous injection and 2 to 3 hours after the intramuscular injection. Digitalization can be completed if one gives one fourth of the digitalizing dose after 8 hours and then the final one fourth 16 hours later.

3. *Propranolol hydrochloride.* This drug is a β-adrenergic blocker and may be tried in the control of PST unresponsive to digitalis if the neonate's condition is not critical. It may be given intravenously; but intravenous administration requires ECG monitoring, since it may cause the heart rate to drop to unexpectedly low levels and may cause a significant fall in blood pressure. The recommended dose is 0.05 to 0.15 mg/kg body weight. Half of the calculated dose may be given intravenously at a rate not to exceed 1 mg/min. If after 2 minutes there is no response, the other half may be given at the same slow rate of less than 1 mg/min. Atropine sulfate and isoproterenol (Isuprel) hydrochloride should be immediately available to treat complicating bradycardia. If necessary, atropine sulfate should be given intravenously at a dose of 0.01 mg/kg. The dosage of intravenous isoproterenal required to produce a 50% increase in heart rate varies widely but is usually between 0.1 and 0.4 *micrograms* per minute per kilogram of body weight.

4. *DC countershock.* In the event that digitalis or propranolol does not cause conversion within the first few hours, one may proceed to the use of countershock, if the infant's condition is deteriorating, or wait for the effect of digitalis if his condition is stable. Whenever possible, DC countershock should be used in the catherization laboratory setting. A transvenous pacemaker catheter should be at hand (in case of cardiac standstill), along with instruments for a rapid cutdown, for catheterization of the femoral vein, and for airway intubation, and with cardiac resuscitation drugs (epinephrine, isoproterenol, sodium bicarbonate, lidocaine). If the infant appears moribund in the emergency room, then the physician should use DC countershock as a life-saving measure without waiting to move the baby or assemble the equipment mentioned above. With external DC countershock, 20 watt-seconds is almost always sufficient, although it may be necessary to repeat 3 or 4 times.

5. *"Overdrive" pacing.* In the extremely unlikely circumstance that a PST is refractory to cardiac drugs and to DC countershock, overdrive pacing may be indicated in an attempt to slow the heart rate of a moribund infant. We are unaware of any reports of its use in neonates with refractory supraventricular tachycardia, though its use has been reported in adults. In overdrive pacing a curved-tip electrode catheter is lodged in the right atrial appendage or in the apex of the right ventricle.

6. *Other drugs.* With the advent of DC countershock in the treatment of PST, quinidine, phenylephrine (Neo-Synephrine) hydrochloride and other previously used agents are no longer indicated.

7. *Maintenance treatment.* A newborn

who has had one attack of PAT has an approximately 20% recurrence risk, and continued maintenance of digoxin for 6 months is indicated. Recurrences are more likely in those with underlying Wolff-Parkinson-White syndrome, and in these patients continued maintenance of digoxin, sometimes supplemented by quinidine, may be indicated. Prophylactic propranolol in oral dose of 0.2 to 0.5 mg/kg may be tried in recurrence-prone infants; however, there is extreme variability of response, and the correct individual dose should be established while the baby is hospitalized.

Prognosis. Nadas and associates have divided infants into prognostically useful clinical groups. The first group consists primarily of male infants under 4 months of age without structural heart disease; the second group is composed of older infants of both sexes with or without heart disease. Recurrences after the age of 1 year are unlikely with the first group; but recurrences are frequent with the second group, particularly if the Wolff-Parkinson-White syndrome is present.

Atrial flutter with frequent ventricular response. This arrhythmia is rare in the neonate; but in contrast to PAT it is very likely to be associated with organic heart disease, especially mitral valve disease and endocardial fibroelastosis. Atrial flutter is recognized from these features: (1) the atrial rate, which is 220 to 400 per minute, (2) the regularity of the atrial mechanism, and (3) the characteristic sawtooth pattern of the flutter waves in leads II and III. When the atrial rate is 200 to 250 per minute and there is A-V block, the distinction between atrial flutter and PAT depends upon the configuration of the atrial activity (sawtooth in atrial flutter). Recognition is sometimes difficult when the ventricles respond to every second atrial beat, since the extra P wave is hidden in the T wave. This issue can be resolved if one records an intracavitary right atrial electrogram or observes flutter fluoroscopically.

Treatment is generally successful; but because there is usually underlying heart disease with a large left atrium, the arrhythmia tends to recur. Digoxin and, if necessary, propranolol should be tried first, as indicated for PST. If unsuccessful or if the arrhythmia appears to be contributing to

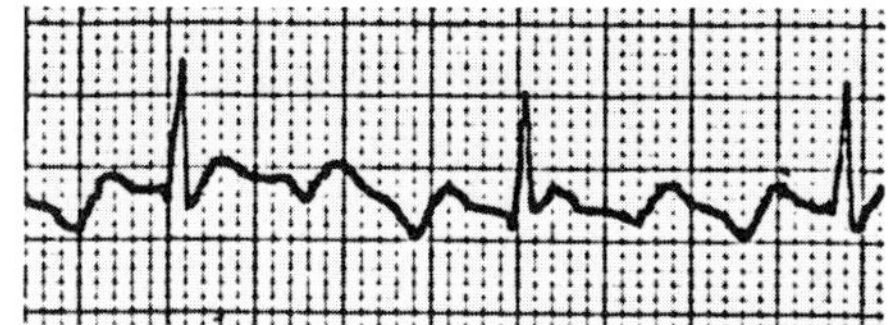

Fig. 11-7. Atrial flutter with 3:1 ventricular response. Ventricular rate is 80, atrial rate 240. The flutter waves have a "sawtooth" appearance.

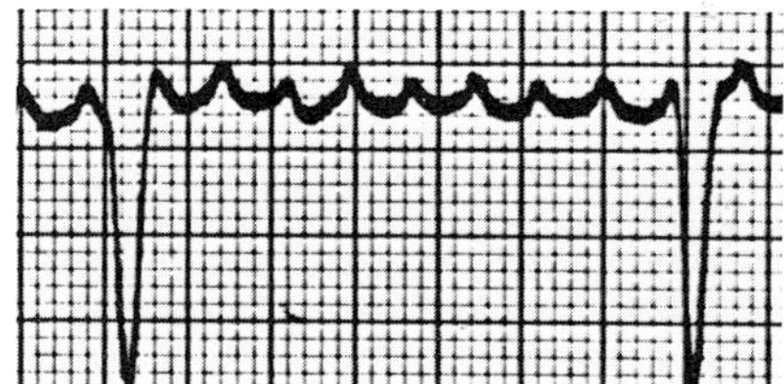

Fig. 11-8. Atrial fibrillation (12-year-old child). Ventricular rate 50 per minute, atrial rate ("f" waves) 400 per minute. On a long tracing it would be seen that the ventricular response is totally irregular.

the infant's deterioration, DC countershock (20 watt-seconds) should be used, with the precautions previously outlined. Occasionally, overdrive atrial pacing may be necessary to convert atrial flutter either to atrial fibrillation or to sinus rhythm. The prevention of recurrence is difficult in the presence of organic heart disease; it may be indicated first to digitalize an infant (Table 11-7) and then give him quinidine orally at a dosage sufficient to keep the infant's blood level at 4 to 8 mg/liter (20 to 30 mg/kg/day in four divided doses).

Atrial fibrillation. Atrial fibrillation is extremely unusual in the neonate. As in the case of atrial flutter, it is likely to be associated with serious organic heart disease, especially with those conditions associated with left atrial enlargement. The arrhythmia may appear clinically as a tachycardia, but it is more likely to be recognized as a chaotic rhythm. The ECG shows characteristic fibrillation "f" waves and irregular QRS response. If the ventricular rate is greater than 160 per minute, the infant should be digitalized to slow conduction through the A-V node and to slow the ventricular rate to 110 to 140 per minute. Conversion may be attempted by the use of DC countershock, preferably on the already digitalized patient. Conversion is usual; but, unfortunately, atrial fibrillation tends to recur.

Ventricular tachycardia. Ventricular tachycardia may presage ventricular fibrillation or by itself produce an ineffective cardiac pumping action. Ventricular tachycardia most commonly occurs in the presence of organic heart disease. The atrial aid to ventricular filling is lost, and the sequence of ventricular depolarization is abnormal. In infancy, ventricular tachycardia is most likely to be encountered with myocarditis and endocardial fibroelastosis. Ventricular tachycardia is suggested when the ECG shows a series of broadened aberrant QRS complexes, with a rate of 150 to 250 beats per minute, and atrial activity is not discernible.

With the type of tracing shown in Fig. 11-9 there are four possibilities: (1) ventricular tachycardia, (2) supraventricular tachycardia with bundle branch block (unlikely in the neonatal period), (3) aberrant intraventricular conduction complicating supraventricular tachycardia, and (4) Wolff-Parkinson-White syndrome with supraventricular tachycardia. When this type of tracing is observed, hyperkalemia should also be considered.

If doubt exists (as it frequently does), it is probably best to proceed directly to DC countershock (unless digitalis toxicity is thought to be present). If a confident diagnosis of ventricular tachycardia can be made, lidocaine (Xylocaine) may be tried at a dosage of 1 to 2 mg/kg as a single rapid intravenous injection. If conversion is successful, recurrences may be prevented by the intravenous infusion of lidocaine, 20 to 30 μgm/min., with continuous cardiac monitoring to warn of premature ventricular contractions or a recurrence of ventricular tachycardia. A number of other medical measures, including diphenylhydantoin (Dilantin), propranolol, bretylium tosylate, and quinidine, have been used in adults.

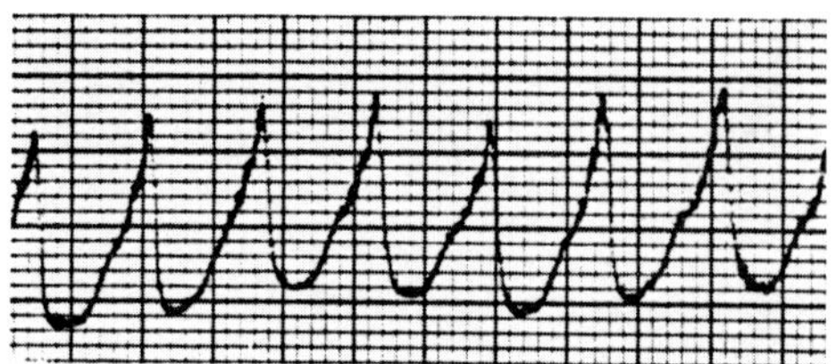

Fig. 11-9. Ventricular tachycardia. Rate is 200 per minute, and there is grossly abnormal ventricular conduction with wide, bizarre QRS complexes. (For differential diagnosis, see text.)

Bradyarrhythmias

The heart rate of the full-term, and especially the premature, neonate may fall to 90 or 70 beats per minute, respectively. Nevertheless, the finding of a bradycardia of less than 90 per minute in a sleeping neonate certainly merits an ECG to rule in or out complete A-V block. As previously noted, surprising degrees of transient sinus bradycardia frequently occur with defecation, micturition, and crying. Bradycardia secondary to digitalis intoxication is discussed on p. 337.

Congenital complete A-V block. This arrhythmia is commonly referred to as complete heart block. With the advent of long-term electronic pacing it has assumed major importance as a totally controllable (when necessary) heart lesion. Complete heart block may on rare occasions be "acquired," secondary to myocarditis or other myocardiopathy.

Congenital complete heart block in children is often considered to be rather benign, in contrast to the acquired form common in adults (usually associated with coronary atherosclerosis). It is now clear that the low-risk infants represent a selected group who have already demonstrated their viability. A cooperative study from 12 pediatric cardiac centers disclosed the natural history of 192 children from infancy to young adult life. Associated cardiac anomalies, diagnosed in 64, contributed to death in 22. Sudden unexpected death occurred in 10, 7 of whom had no evidence of heart disease. The natural history was favorably influenced in 15 by cardiac surgery and in 9 by pacemaker implants for heart failure or Stokes-Adams attacks. The risk of premature death is highest in the first 6 months, especially in those infants with serious associated heart disease.

Diagnosis. The ventricular rate is below 50 per minute in half of the babies, and the block is recognized in utero in nearly one third. The block remains unrecognized until after the age of 1 year in approximately

50%. In cases where bradycardia does not lead to the recording of the diagnostic ECG, complete heart block may be discovered by the investigation of exercise intolerance, cardiomegaly, Stokes-Adams attack, or heart murmur. Heart murmurs are frequently secondary to bradycardia and increased stroke volume. Increased systolic and diastolic blood flow through the semilunar and A-V valves may closely simulate organic valvular heart disease.

The ECG is diagnostic (Fig. 11-10); the P wave rate exceeds the QRS rate, and there is no relationship between the two. The QRS is usually (two thirds of cases) less than 0.08 seconds in duration, indicating that the pacemaker is probably in the bundle of His. There is often moderate cardiac enlargement.

Treatment. The occurrence of Stokes-Adams attacks indicates the need for long-term treatment by pacing. If the losses of consciousness are frequent and the situation is urgent, a temporary transvenous pacemaker catheter may be inserted via the saphenous, superficial femoral, or the external jugular vein for temporary control while preparations are being made for thoracotomy and permanent transvenous pacemaker implantation. The other group of neonates who may require pacemaker implantation are those with a persistent bradycardia (less than 40 beats per minute). These infants frequently have serious organic heart disease and heart failure. Increasing their heart rate from 40 to 120 may resolve the heart failure and can allow heart surgery under more optimal conditions.

Isoproterenol infusion is sometimes successful in increasing the heart rate of neonates with complete heart block and severe bradycardia; it may be given by intravenous infusion (constant-speed infusion pump) at a dose of 0.1 to 0.3 μgm/kg/min, with cautious increases in dose until a heart rate of 60 to 70 beats per minute is achieved. Our experience with isoproterenol or other chronotropic agents in this age group, however, has not been encouraging; usually only a very minor increase in rate is achieved, and ventricular pacing is necessary to control heart failure. Isoproterenol is of no benefit in preventing Stokes-Adams attacks.

Prognosis. The average life-span of a permanently implanted pacemaker is about 3 years. It is likely that the next few years will see major advances in the use of pacemakers.

S-A block and A-V dissociation. A situation in which the ventricular rate exceeds the atrial rate is extremely uncommon in neonatal pediatrics. The phenomenon may result when the impulse fails to leave the S-A node or to be propagated normally through the atrial tissues (S-A block) or when the automaticity of ventricular tissue exceeds that of atrial tissue. Digitalis intoxication should be considered as a possible cause. In the unlikely event that the superior ventricular automaticity is insufficient to prevent heart failure, acceleration of the heartbeat might be achieved by vagal suppression (atropine) or β-adrenergic stimulation (isoproterenol). A trial of atrial pacing will determine whether or not A-V nodal function is normal.

Second-degree A-V block. A bradyarrhythmia may occur with second-degree A-V block of the Mobitz type, in which there is intermittent A-V block with or without P-R prolongation in the conducted beats (Fig. 11-11); its presence suggests

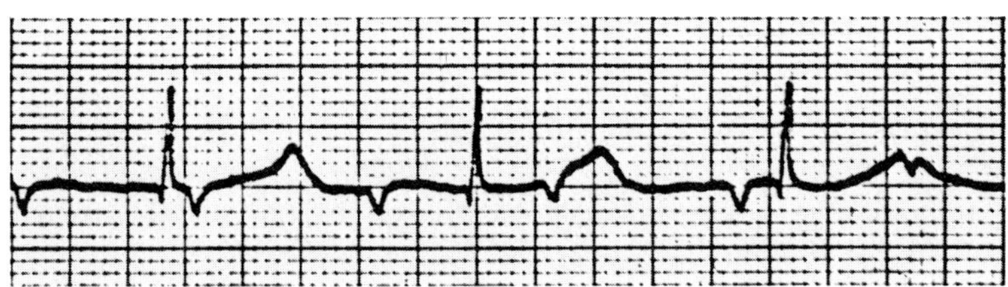

Fig. 11-10. Complete (third-degree) A-V block. Note that the P wave rate exceeds the QRS rate and that there is no constant P-R interval.

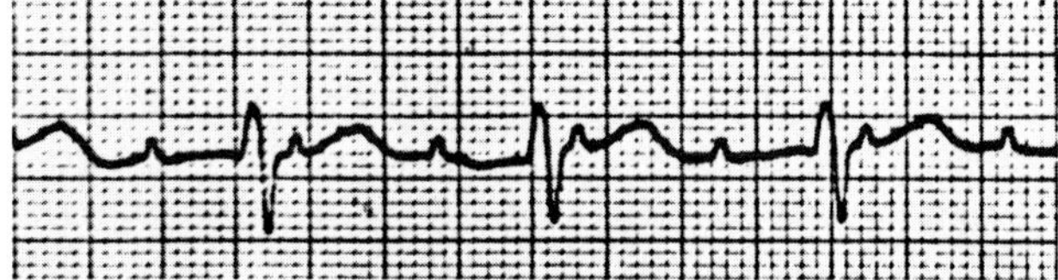

Fig. 11-11. Second-degree A-V block (Mobitz type II). Every second P wave gives rise to a QRS complex after a long P-R interval.

digitalis intoxication. Pacing may be required if Stokes-Adams attacks occur or if it progresses to complete heart block.

Bradycardia in the dying neonate. One is not infrequently faced with the problem of a progressive sinus bradycardia secondary to hypoxemia, acidosis, electrolyte imbalance, or sepsis complicating a wide variety of neonatal conditions. Occasionally, the infusion of isoproterenol or electronic pacing is indicated if the situation appears reversible; such situations may include adrenal insufficiency, myocarditis, meningitis, encephalitis, and septicemia. Since fluoroscopy will usually be required, careful clinical judgment will be needed to balance the risk of moving the baby (usually receiving assisted ventilation) against the possible advantages of a faster heart rate.

Irregular arrhythmias

Benign conditions include marked degrees of sinus arrhythmias, occasional sinus arrest, premature atrial and ventricular contractions, and sinus bradycardia with nodal escape. All are common in premature infants.

Pathologic irregular arrhythmias are usually caused by atrial flutter or fibrillation with varying A-V conduction. Less frequent causes are runs of atrial or ventricular ectopic beats. Atrial flutter and fibrillation have been discussed on p. 281. Multiple ectopic beats usually pose no threat to life unless they occur within the framework of organic heart disease (usually myocardial disease). Thus the infant with tight valvular pulmonic stenosis may remain out of heart failure until multiple ectopic beats start to develop; the relative inefficiency of the ectopic beat leads to lowered cardiac output. By contrast, normal infants may have alarming runs of ectopic beats, yet be asymptomatic.

In general, ventricular ectopic beats should be regarded more seriously than atrial ectopic beats, since strings of ventricular ectopic beats may portend the development of ventricular tachycardia or fibrillation. Unfortunately, suppression of ventricular ectopic beats with lidocaine, quinidine, diphenylhydantoin, or propranolol is rarely successful. They have a negative inotropic action, and their use should be considered only if it appears that cardiac output will be increased more by a stable rhythm than it will be decreased by a negative inotropic drug. Bretylium is not yet released by the FDA, but is said to have a positive inotropic action on the heart.

Documented ventricular tachycardia is a rarity in the neonate (except in the dying infant and the infant with myocardial disease). Therefore, unless the infant *is* symptomatic, treatment of frequent ventricular ectopic beats is not indicated. When followed over a period of time, the arrhythmia usually ceases spontaneously, or it can be demonstrated that sinus rhythm occurs with exercise.

The Wolff-Parkinson-White syndrome

The Wolff-Parkinson-White syndrome (short P-R, deformed and widened QRS) is caused by preexcitation of the ventricles either by an anomalous conducting bundle or an area of accelerated conduction through the A-V node. Recognition of the syndrome is important because of (1) the high incidence of PAT, (2) the frequent misinterpretation of the ECG as ventricular infarction or hypertrophy, and (3) the high incidence of associated CNS disease.

PAT is usually manifest in infancy. At this time the signs of the Wolff-Parkinson-White syndrome are often subtle and are frequently only diagnosed in retrospect with gradual widening of the QRS and emergence of the characteristic delta wave.

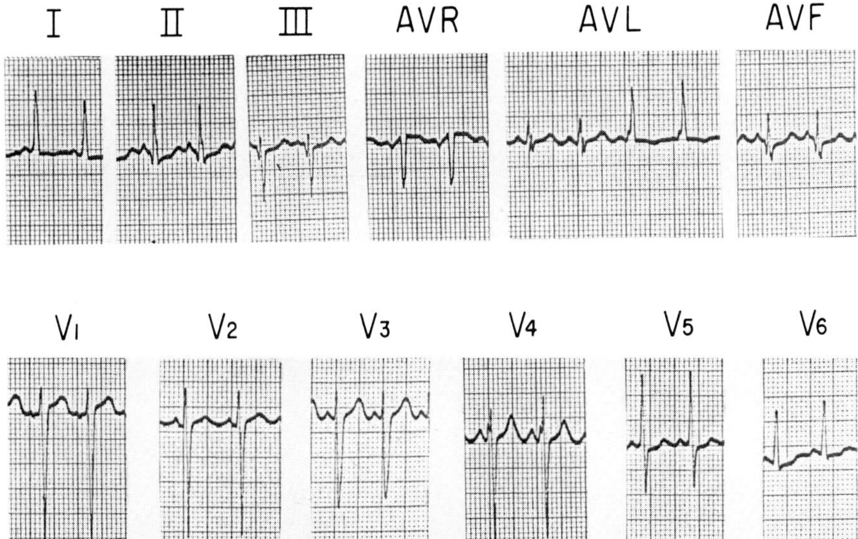

Fig. 11-12. Wolff-Parkinson-White syndrome in the neonate. P-R interval is shortened (evident in most leads). QRS is slightly prolonged to 0.08 seconds (leads II, III, and AVF), and there is a slurred upstroke in the R wave (lead I). The first two complexes in AVL show normal ventricular excitation, while the next two show Wolff-Parkinson-White (ventricular preexcitation) syndrome.

The PAT associated with this syndrome is harder to control than PAT with normal ventricular excitation. The combination of digoxin and quinidine is most effective. Organic heart disease occurs in approximately 40% of children diagnosed as having the Wolff-Parkinson-White syndrome (doubtless many more are undiagnosed). Ebstein's anomaly, corrected transposition, and primary myocardial disease predominate.

CARDIOGENIC SHOCK

The term cardiogenic shock implies acute primary failure of the heart as a pump. The distinction between cardiogenic shock and severe heart failure is somewhat arbitrary; yet the two do appear as different clinical pictures. In the adult, myocardial infarction is overwhelmingly the commonest cause of cardiogenic shock. In the neonate the clinical picture of cardiogenic shock is encountered infrequently, but it is perhaps most common with myocarditis and overwhelming septicemia (especially meningococcemia). The infant with congenital heart disease who has been in heart failure for a number of days may appear with signs identical to those in an infant who has been transferred over a long distance and has become cold, hypoglycemic, and hypoxemic.

Pathogenesis. Clues to indicate that primary failure of the heart as a pump is the cause of shock are (1) the elevation of systemic venous pressure to 10 to 15 cm of water, as compared with the low venous pressure associated with endotoxin and hemorrhagic shock, (2) the presence of a triple or quadruple rhythm, (3) enlarged liver or pulmonary rales, (4) gross cardiomegaly evident on the chest roentgenogram, (5) low-voltage QRS complexes indicating rapid dilatation of the heart, (6) primary T wave abnormalities on the ECG, and (7) severe acidosis.

Diagnosis. Arterial pulses are almost impalpable; the infant is bradycardic and tachypneic, and blood flow through the blanched skin is extremely slow. Often the whole skin has a mottled blue-white appearance. The liver may be enlarged, and there may be rales in the lungs, but these signs of heart failure may be absent if the heart has failed very rapidly and peripheral circulatory failure with deficient tissue blood flow is extreme. The picture, then, is dominated by evidence of greatly reduced tissue perfusion rather than traditional heart failure. The resemblance to endotoxic shock and to hemorrhagic shock is close.

The need for urgent treatment of the bradycardic, mottled, dying baby precludes a complete diagnostic evaluation. Cardiogenic shock is often caused by viral myocarditis, but the differential diagnosis should also include the following possibilities: (1) bacterial sepsis with myocarditis and pericarditis, (2) end-stage left ventricular failure from congenital heart disease, (3) anomalous left coronary artery arising from the pulmonary artery, causing myocardial infarction, (4) adrenal insufficiency, especially that caused by congenital adrenal hypoplasia, (5) extreme hypoglycemia with and without heart disease, (6) bacterial or viral myocarditis, (7) primary thoracic conditions such as bilateral pneumothorax or congenital lobar emphysema, (8) hemorrhagic shock with concealed bleeding, as in ruptured spleen, and (9) complete heart block with very slow rate.

Treatment. The following plan is suggested for the emergency room management of the moribund infant with the clinical diagnosis of cardiogenic shock.

Record the ECG to rule out complete heart block and to monitor heart rate. Insert a central venous catheter (umbilical vein or femoral vein to right atrium). Measure the central venous pressure (express in centimeters of water). Withdraw blood for immediate blood glucose (Dextrostix) and serum electrolyte determination. (Increased potassium and decreased sodium suggests adrenal insufficiency.) Blood culture (bacterial and viral), hematocrit reading, complete blood count, blood urea nitrogen level, pH and P_{CO_2}, blood type, and crossmatch should also be obtained. If the venous pressure is low (less than 4 cm of water), give blood or blood substitute. In endotoxic or hemorrhagic shock very large volumes (up to 40 ml/kg) may be needed to raise the central venous pressure and increase cardiac output. If the venous pressure is high (over 12 cm in a neonate), cardiogenic shock is probably present, in which case digitalize the baby, and start an isoproterenol infusion. (Dose is highly variable. Mix 1 mg in 100 ml 5% dextrose to give 10 mg/ml. This solution can then be infused by pump at 1/10 ml/min. or 1 μgm/min. Isoproterenol is a powerful β-adrenergic stimulator with chronotropic and inotropic actions. A satisfactory response is indicated by a falling venous pressure and a rise in heart rate to 100 to 140 beats per minute. If the blood glucose level is low, infuse 10% dextrose in addition to maintenance fluid. A high serum potassium or low sodium level is highly suggestive of adrenal insufficiency. These findings may require treatment by rehydration, salt replacement, and the administration of adrenocorticoids (p. 479). Take a chest and abdominal film as soon as possible to exclude diagnoses such as pneumothorax, peritonitis with free air in the peritoneal cavity, and so on. A lumbar puncture may be indicated, depending on whether there is a strong possibility of meningitis. Correction of acidosis may require assisted ventilation rather than alkali therapy. Myocarditis, if present, is usually of viral origin. However, once the cultures are taken, if myocarditis is presumptively diagnosed, antibiotics such as penicillin and kanamycin are indicated because of the remote possibility of a bacterial cause. The death rate from viral myocarditis appearing as a shock-like state in the neonate is approximately 75%. If one is faced with an obviously dying infant, corticosteroids such as hydrocortisone hemisuccinate 50 mg/kg may be tried; and if the heart rate is slow (below 80 per minute), transvenous pacing should be considered. If anomalous origin of the left coronary artery is a possible diagnosis, consider an emergency aortogram. Ligation of the anomalous vessel at its site of origin in the pulmonary artery can be a life-saving maneuver.

CARDIAC ARREST AND EXTREME BRADYCARDIA

Apparent cardiac arrest—that is, lack of audible heartbeat, cardiac impulse, or peripheral pulse—is usually caused by ventricular asystole or extreme bradycardia rather than by ventricular fibrillation (Fig. 11-13). Either of these two events may be the result of primary respiratory failure. Ventricular asystole and ventricular fibrillation can be distinguished by an ECG. However, it is essential that treatment be started immediately without losing valuable minutes locating an ECG machine and attaching leads. In many neonates there

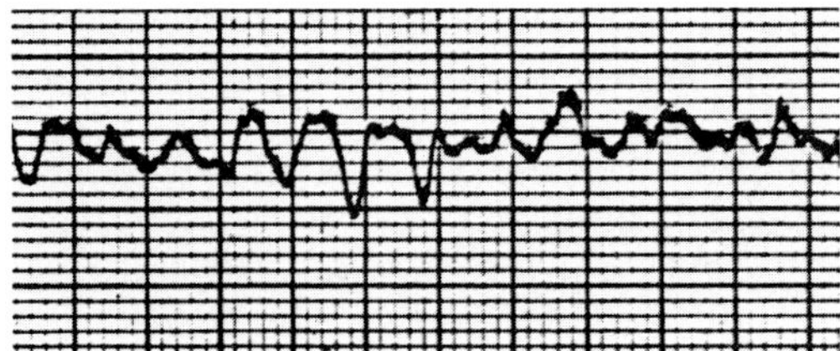

FIG. 11-13. Ventricular fibrillation. Chaotic electrical ventricular activity associated with complete ineffectiveness of ventricular contraction.

is no doubt as to whether cardiac arrest has occurred. The majority of sick neonates are already on heart rate monitors, and the alarm is set to sound at a rate of 80 per minute. By the time someone reaches the baby, the rate may have fallen to 60 and be continuing to decrease. Treatment should be initiated without waiting for the infant to deteriorate further.

It needs first to be determined whether bradycardia or cardiac arrest is primary or is secondary to respiratory failure. In many immature and sick infants, bradycardia is secondary to respiratory arrest, and prompt respiratory resuscitation takes first priority and often restores the heart rate to normal. When respirations cease, heart rate and cardiac output fall. In other instances the neonate has become too hypoxemic and acidotic for respiratory resuscitation alone to restore the heartbeat. In this situation cardiac resuscitation is required. Pupillary dilatation begins within 45 seconds after circulation stops and is complete by about 1 minute and 45 seconds.

Respiratory resuscitation of the neonate

In respiratory resuscitation of the neonate, the following procedures should be initiated.

A thump with the fist on the wall of the isolette may cause the neonate to gasp and reinitiate respiration. A few seconds of proprioceptor stimulation, massaging the infant's legs and moving his knee and hip joints, is frequently successful, especially in the case of immature neonates. Determine that the airway is clear, and then apply positive pressure ventilation (to 30 cm water) by face mask and oxygen. A suitable device should be in each isolette. If adequate pulmonary ventilation cannot be achieved by mask-to-face breathing, rapid endotracheal intubation is essential, followed by mouth-to-tube ventilation, bag-to-tube ventilation, or positive pressure ventilator. All of these measures should occupy less than 1 minute.

Cardiac resuscitation of the neonate

Bradycardia with a heart rate falling to 40 beats per minute or below is the most frequent indication for cardiac resuscitation in the neonate. Ventricular asystole without prior bradycardia is unusual, and ventricular fibrillation is rarely observed except in the terminal stages of advanced heart disease. Thus the question arises as to what heart rate should be tolerated before resuscitation attempts are made when the bradycardia is not caused by ventilatory failure.

The following guidelines assume that pulmonary ventilation is being assisted either by face mask or endotracheal tube and that the heart rate is either inaudible or below 50 beats per minute.

Check for audible heart sounds. The hearing of regular heart sounds, however slow, rules out ventricular fibrillation. Flick the precordium over the midsternum, and listen again (equivalent to the chest "thump" in adults). If the heart rate is still inadequate, immediately start external massage. If two people are present, try to alternate cardiac massage and ventilation (40 seconds of cardiac massage to 20 seconds of ventilation). Examine stat ECG, or attach regular ECG leads to distinguish ventricular asystole (straight line or occasional bizarre QRS complexes), ventricular fibrillation (irregular chaotic line) (Fig. 11-13), and complete heart block (P-wave rate exceds QRS rate, and P-R interval is inconstant) (Fig. 11-10). Precordial compression causes an obvious artifact. If ventricular fibrillation is present, defibrillate with external DC countershock until conversion (usually 10 to 25 watt-seconds). If an acceptable rhythm with evidence of adequate cardiac output does not occur, resume external cardiac massage. After 4 or 5 minutes of cardial arrest and reduced cardiac output during external massage, the blood will certainly be acidotic; sodium bicarbonate should be given intravenously (2 to 6 mEq/kg).

If there has been no response after 5 to

10 minutes of ventilation, external cardiac massage, and alkali therapy, consider the use of pharmacologic agents and cardiac pacing. The pharmacologic agents that may be tried include:

1. Epinephrine–0.2 ml/kg of a 1:10,000 solution, intravenous or intracardiac
2. Isoproterenol–0.1 to 0.4 μgm/kg/min by intravenous infusion or single doses of 1 μgm/kg by intravenous or intracardiac route every 5 minutes
3. Calcium chloride–0.5 to 1 ml of 10% solution administered intravenously or by intracardiac route every 5 minutes
4. Atropine may be indicated if second- or third-degree A-V block is present; intravenous dose–0.01 mg/kg
5. Lidocaine (Xylocaine) may be indicated in the rare instance where ineffective contraction is caused by ventricular arrhythmias that are resistant to DC countershock alone; in infants 0.5 to 2.0 mg/kg may be given immediately before countershock and may be repeated every 10 to 15 minutes

If effective cardiac contraction cannot be restored with one of these agents, it is advisable to pause and determine whether brain damage is irreversible and resusitation should be stopped or whether an attempt at cardiac pacing is warranted.

Cardiac pacing

Major indications for cardiac pacing include bradycardia, cardiac arrest, digitalis intoxication, and complete heart block. The temporary bradycardia associated with the salt-losing crisis of congenital adrenal hyperplasia or any other condition from which it is possible for the infant to recover may warrant pacing. By contrast, a neonate with bradycardia from the terminal stages of HMD or the hypoplastic left heart syndrome would not be a candidate for a pacemaker.

External pacing is rarely effective. Internal transvenous pacemaker catheters may be placed via the external jugular vein and the tip lodged in the trabeculations of the right ventricle or, if the A-V node is functional, in the right atrium. An alternative short-term route is the femoral vein (usually it is not possible to enter the right ventricle from the umbilical vein). The pacing rate should be 100 to 140 beats per minute. Usually a current of 0.5 to 1.0 milliamperes is necessary to obtain a response. Because electrical response is no guarantee of mechanical response, heart sounds and pulses should be checked before it is concluded that the heart is actually propelling blood. The Doppler ultrasound flowmeter is particularly useful for this purpose. If temporary transvenous pacing is successful and the source of the bradycardia is not removed (as in complete A-V block), it will be necessary to implant long-term epicardial or myocardial pacemaker wires.

Because cardiac arrest or bradycardia never occurs without cause, successful resuscitation of the neonate should be followed by a search for heart disease, pulmonary disease, sepsis, and so on.

COMMON CARDIOVASCULAR DISORDERS PRODUCING SERIOUS DISEASE IN THE NEONATE

A classification of the structural disorders more commonly encountered in neonatal practice is offered in the outline below.

A. Transposition of the great arteries
   1. Dextrotransposition
   2. Levotransposition
B. Left heart obstruction
   1. Hypoplastic left heart syndrome
   2. Congenital aortic stenosis
   3. Preductal and juxtaductal coarctation of the aorta
   4. Postductal coarctation
C. Right heart obstruction
   1. Pulmonary atresia or extreme pulmonic stenosis with intact ventricular septum
   2. Pulmonary atresia with open ventricular septum, and severe tetralogy of Fallot
   3. Peripheral pulmonary artery stenosis
   4. Tricuspid atresia with and without transposition
   5. Ebstein's anomaly of the tricuspid valve
D. Lesions that produce common mixing of venous and arterial blood
   1. Truncus arteriosus
   2. Single ventricle
   3. Double-outlet right ventricle without pulmonic stenosis
   4. Total anomalous pulmonary venous return
E. Left-to-right shunts
   1. Patent ductus arteriosus
   2. Ventricular septal defect
   3. Combined patent ductus arteriosus and ventricular septal defect
   4. Common atrioventricular canal
   5. Systemic arteriovenous fistula

F. Myocardial disorders
  1. Myocarditis
  2. Endocardial fibroelastosis
  3. Anomalous left coronary artery
  4. Glycogen storage disease
G. Miscellaneous
  1. Absent pulmonary valve
  2. Tricuspid insufficiency
  3. Cor triatriatum
  4. Dextrocardia

Transposition of the great arteries

Incidence

Transposition accounts for 15% to 30% of neonates undergoing cardiac catheterization and for at least 16% of deaths caused by congenital heart disease at all ages in childhood. The incidence of transposition is between 0.022% and 0.047% of live births (1:2,130 to 1:4,500). Transposition is a common defect, and early recognition is of major importance; hundreds of neonates born with complete transposition of the great arteries have had the defect totally corrected and are leading normal lives. Males outnumber females 2 to 1, and there is some evidence that they have a higher-than-average birth weight.

Pathology

The aorta arises anteriorly and from the venous ventricle, while the pulmonary artery arises posteriorly and from the arterial ventricle. With dextrotransposition (d-transposition) the aortic valve is to the right of the pulmonary valve, whereas with levotransposition (l-transposition) the aortic valve is to the left of the pulmonary valve. There is a well-developed muscular subaortic infundibulum, in contrast to the muscular subpulmonary infundibulum characteristic of the normal heart.

D-transpositions outnumber l-transpositions as a cause for major concern in the newborn period by at least 10 to 1. As a generalization, one can say that d-transposition is a relatively "pure" lesion usually associated only with patent foramen ovale, PDA, and VSD. L-transposition, by contrast, is often associated with dextrocardia, situs inversus, and asplenia when it appears in the newborn period. When it appears in older infants and children, it is usually physiologically "corrected," most commonly by ventricular inversion; unfortunately, there are almost always additional lesions present, such as mitral regurgitation, VSD, and subpulmonic stenosis.

Transposition of the great arteries is sometimes associated with a very large VSD or common ventricle, in which case the fact that the great vessels are transposed becomes of secondary importance.

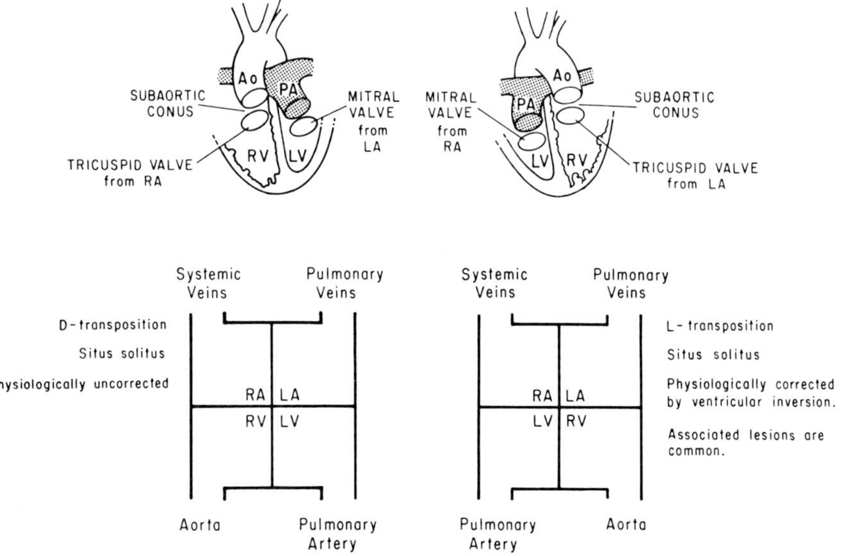

Fig. 11-14. The two commonest types of transposition of the great arteries leading to problems in the neonatal period. In both types the aortic valve is high and anterior and arises from the coarsely trabeculated right (venous) ventricle. D-transposition is the common transposition causing problems in the newborn period.

The association of tricuspid atresia and transposition is not unusual and leads to common mixing at the left atrial level. The adequacy of systemic (aortic) flow then depends on the size of an associated VSD or PDA.

The major emphasis in this section, then, is on the common d-transposition with situs solitus (normal location of the heart and viscera). Brief mention is made of the commonest form of l-transposition—the physiologically corrected (by ventricular inversion) transposition in which the frequently associated VSD and mitral regurgitation may give rise to heart failure in the neonate.

D-transposition of the great arteries

D-transposition with intact ventricular septum and small or absent ductus arteriosus. Neonates with transposition and intact ventricular septum are extremely cyanotic and usually die in the first few days of life as the ductus arteriosus closes. Conversely, if the ductus arteriosus remains open, there is better mixing of venous and arterial circulations, but usually at the expense of pulmonary artery hypertension. If there is only a foramen ovale or ASD, it is necessary for bidirectional shunting to occur at the atrial level; whereas if the duct also is open, a common sequence is for right-to-left shunting to occur at the atrial level and for there to be left-to-right (aorta to pulmonary artery) shunting at the ductal level. The latter situation might seem hemodynamically acceptable; but unfortunately, the ductus is frequently very large, and pulmonary artery pressure is at systemic levels.

Clinical presentation. Cyanosis is present from birth, though the temporary patency of the ductus arteriosus may allow some shunting, and the recognition of cyanosis

A

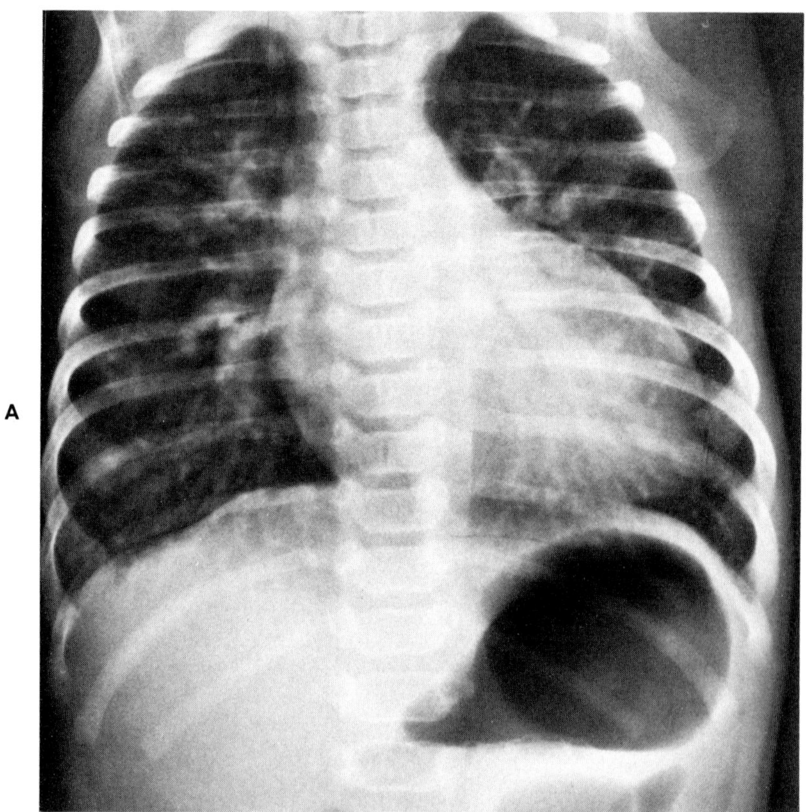

Fig. 11-15. Anteroposterior chest films of two neonates with d-transposition of the great arteries. **A,** Note narrow mediastinum, "egg-on-side" appearance, cardiomegaly, and pulmonary plethora. **B,** Note massive cardiomegaly caused by heart failure.

may be delayed. The breathing rate is characteristically increased to 45 to 80 breaths per minute; there are usually no signs of respiratory distress unless the infant has associated respiratory infection. The peripheral pulses are normal. The cardiac impulse is often normal for the first hours or days but thereafter becomes hyperdynamic. The heart sounds are normal, and frequently there is no cardiac murmur. If a heart murmur is audible, it is likely to be nondescript and grade 3 or less in intensity, probably representing the murmur of a closing ductus. As time passes, the neonate becomes progressively more cyanotic; and when arteriovenous mixing is inadequate over a prolonged period of time, respiratory and metabolic acidosis ensue. Finally, the infant dies from a combination of hypoxemia and acidosis during the first or second week of life. Many die in the first week of life if there is only a patent foramen ovale for exchange of arterial and venous blood.

Diagnosis. Initially the chest roentgenogram may appear normal. However, as time passes, it becomes apparent that the heart is abnormally large and somewhat egg-shaped and that the pulmonary vascular markings are increased (Fig. 11-15). The classical roentgenogram of transposition shows, in addition, a narrow mediastinum when viewed anteroposteriorly and a widened mediastinum when viewed laterally.

There is usually nothing diagnostically helpful in the ECG tracing. Almost always a mild degree of right ventricular hypertrophy is present, similar to that seen in a wide variety of cardiac and pulmonary disease in which the right ventricle is working at systemic pressure.

The arterial oxygen saturation while the infant is breathing room air is usually in the 30% to 70% range, corresponding to a Pa_{O_2} of approximately 15 to 30 mm Hg. The Pa_{CO_2} may remain normal or even decreased for surprising periods of time be-

B

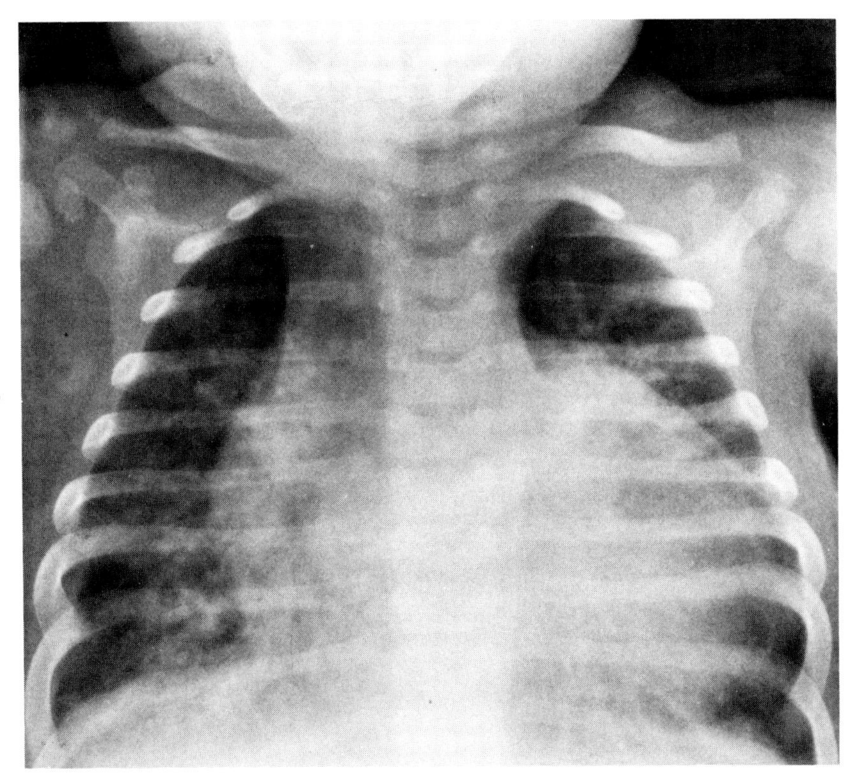

Fig. 11-15, cont'd. For legend see opposite page.

cause of some alveolar hyperventilation. The Pa_{CO_2} usually rises on the second or third day of life to 50 or 60 mm Hg, higher in the very severely hypoxemic baby. Similarly, the arterial pH may remain normal for a time (because of an increase in plasma bicarbonate level), but it inevitably declines in the severely sick infant because of a combination of the accumulation of the products of anaerobic metabolism and the failure of the lungs to eliminate adequate CO_2. Although the total lung blood flow is increased in infants with transposition, the effective pulmonary blood flow (that fraction derived from the systemic venous return) is decreased.

In most infants, 100% O_2 breathing will increase arterial Po_2 by only a few millimeters of mercury (because of the slightly increased O_2 content of pulmonary capillary blood). An occasional infant with transposition, however, shows a much more dramatic response to 100% O_2, with arterial Po_2 increasing from 30 to 70 mm Hg and the infant changing from cyanotic to acyanotic. This change is the result of the effect of oxygen on pulmonary arterioles causing a fall in pulmonary vascular resistance and allowing an existing ductal or ventricular shunt to become exclusively left-to-right, while an existing atrial shunt becomes exclusively right-to-left. The net effect is greater crossover between venous and arterial circuits. In this situation, measurements of arterial O_2 saturation will give the spurious impression of absence of right-to-left shunt; however, measurement of arterial O_2 tension will reveal the true situation—for example, a Pa_{O_2} of only 70 mm Hg versus an expected Pa_{O_2} of at least 300 mm Hg with a normal circulation.

Hemodynamics and angiocardiography. The major problem is lack of communication between pulmonary and systemic circulations after birth. Transposition is of little consequence while the baby is in utero. Infants with transposition are typically large, well-nourished infants and frequently give no cause for concern during the first minutes and hours of life. The deterioration of the infant thereafter corresponds to gradual constriction of the ductus arteriosus. The low Po_2 perfusing this structure appears to lose its vasodilating effect within hours to a day or two after birth. When the ductus arteriosus closes, the infant is totally reliant on a foramen ovale or ASD for the exchange of venous and arterial blood; unless the ASD is large, death will rapidly ensue from hypoxemia,

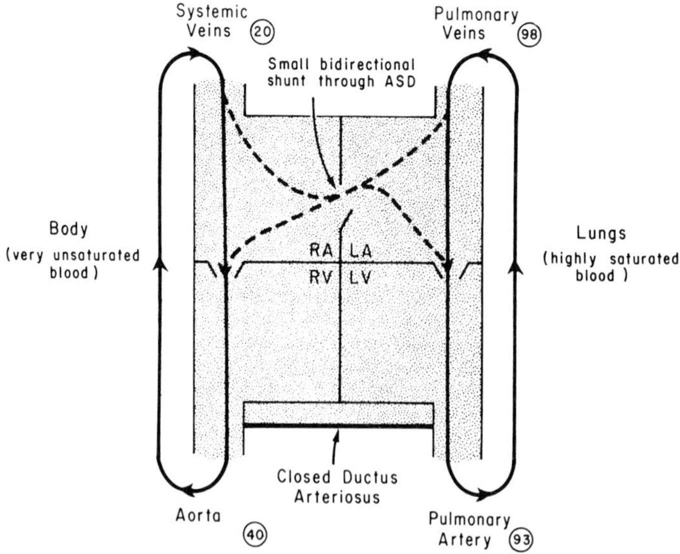

Fig. 11-16. The course of the circulation in d-transposition with intact ventricular septum. Typical oxygen saturations are circled. Small bidirectional shunts of equal magnitude across the atrial septum allow insufficient oxygen to reach the tissues for the maintenance of adequate oxidative metabolism.

hypercapnia, and acidosis (Fig. 11-16).

The major abnormal hemodynamic findings are a right ventricular pressure that is at systemic level and a left ventricular pressure (left ventricle supplies the pulmonary artery) that may be high or low, depending on the pulmonary blood flow and pulmonary vascular resistance (assuming there is no pulmonic stenosis). Aortic oxygen saturation is lower than pulmonary artery saturation; arterial oxygen saturations of about 30% to 40% are not uncommon. The catheter passes easily from the inferior vena cava to the right atrium, right ventricle, and out into the anteriorly placed aorta. In the majority of cases it can also easily be passed across the foramen ovale into the left atrium and left ventricle.

Right ventricular angiography in the lateral projection reveals the high, anterior location of the aortic valve and the presence or absence of a VSD (Fig. 11-17). Left ventricular angiography discloses the posteriorly located pulmonary artery.

Treatment. The advent of balloon septostomy has allowed definitive treatment frequently to commence during the course of cardiac catheterization. The pressure gradient between the left and right atrium is measured; the larger the gradient the smaller the foramen ovale or atrial septal defect. Patients with a demonstrable gradient will benefit from enlargement of the communication, and even those without a gradient may obtain some beneficial effect from balloon septostomy. The exact indications for balloon septostomy are still controversial. Our policy has been to pro-

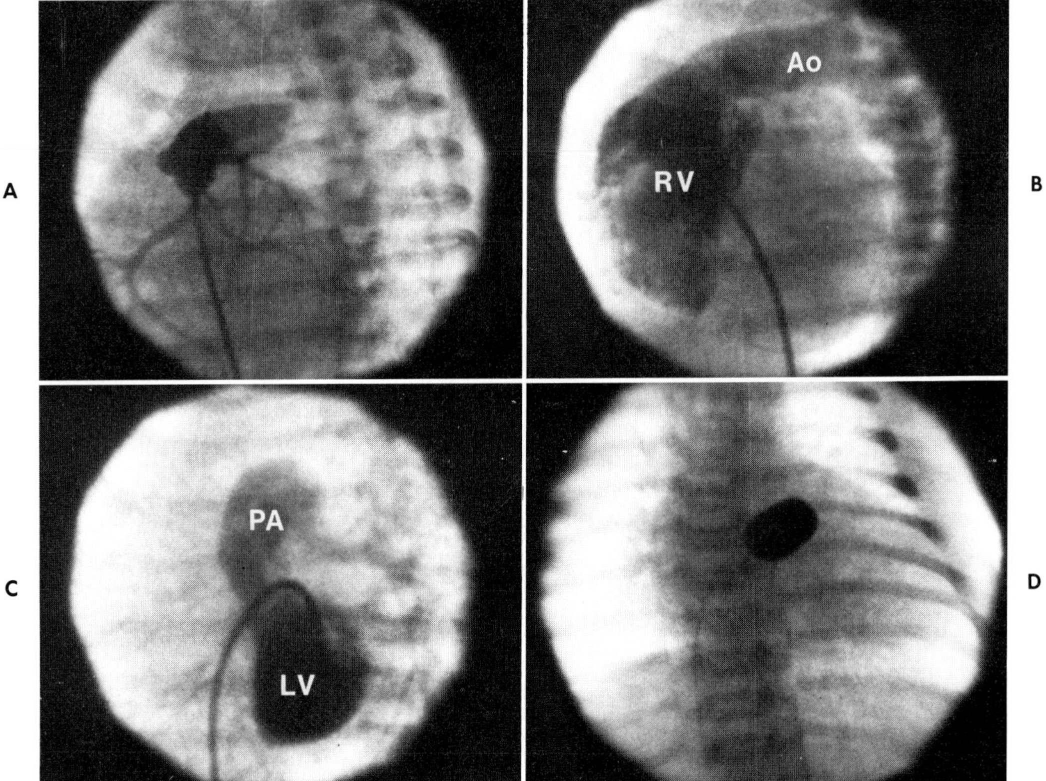

Fig. 11-17. Angiographic appearances in d-transposition. Single frames from cineangiogram. Left anterior oblique position. **A,** Note high, anterior location of aortic valve. The coronary arteries are visible. **B,** Note anterior heavily trabeculated right ventricle (*RV*) giving rise to aorta (*Ao*). **C,** Note smooth-walled left ventricle (*LV*) giving rise to posteriorly located pulmonary artery (*PA*). **D,** Balloon septostomy. The balloon is "jerked" rapidly across the atrial septum, enlarging or tearing the foramen ovale and allowing better mixing of left atrial and right atrial blood. In this frame the balloon is in the left atrium.

ceed with septostomy whether or not a gradient is demonstrable. Opening of the atrial septum by balloon is achieved by placing the tip of a balloon catheter in the left atrium, inflating it with 2 to 3 ml dilute contrast agent, and rapidly pulling it it back across the atrial septum to rupture the thin "membrane" covering the foramen ovale and in some cases to tear the adjacent interatrial septum.

In our experience several results may follow balloon septostomy.

1. Balloon septostomy is dramatically successful in some babies. Arterial O_2 saturation increases from a moribund 40% to a respectable 80%, and the improvement is maintained. The infant survives and can be operated on by total correction (Mustard procedure) at the age of 6 months to 3 years.

2. The balloon septostomy is partially successful. The baby's arterial saturation remains satisfactory for days or weeks, but then increasing cyanosis recurs. A second balloon septostomy after the age of 3 to 4 months is not usually beneficial. The choice is then surgical removal of part of the atrial septum versus total repair by means of the Mustard procedure (essentially switching of the venous return to match the transposed arteries). The choice must depend on the weight of the infant (although total repair is now possible at 3 kg) and the experiences and preferences of the surgeon. Our general approach is atrial septectomy (followed a year or two later by Mustard correction) for those infants under 5 kg or who are under 1 month old or both and primary Mustard correction for those over 5 kg. In cases of doubt a recatheterization to measure pulmonary artery pressure is fully justified, since total correction in a small infant with pulmonary artery pressure of more than 50% systemic pressure carries a higher mortality; for this group atrial septectomy to allow increased oxygen delivery to the tissues and accelerated growth represents a lesser risk.

3. The balloon septostomy may be totally unsuccessful; early atrial septectomy or total correction is desirable.

D-transposition with open ventricular septum. The presence of a moderate or large VSD might appear to be advantageous to the baby with transposed great arteries because of the better mixing of venous and arterial streams. Any small advantage, however, is more than offset by the greater frequency of pulmonary hypertension and heart failure. In addition, surgical correction is more difficult.

Clinical presentation. The symptoms tend to be those of right- and left-sided heart failure rather than severe cyanosis. Neonates with transposition and large VSD frequently appear only mildly cyanotic. The cardiac impulse is hyperdynamic; the signs of heart failure are present; and a loud lower-left sternal border pansystolic murmur suggests a VSD.

Diagnosis. This condition may simulate a large VSD, common ventricle or even truncus arteriosus. On the roentgenogram the heart is seen to be large and the pulmonary vasculature increased. The ECG shows right ventricular hypertrophy.

Hemodynamics. The large interventricular communication necessitates the existence of usually both pulmonary hypertension and greatly increased lung blood flow. The latter leads to a raised left atrial pressure, while the former is associated with the rapid onset of pulmonary vascular obliterative disease. Right and left ventricular pressures are equal. Pulmonary arterial saturation is higher than aortic saturation.

Cardiac catheterization and angiocardiography. The catheter course may proceed from the inferior vena cava to the right atrium, to the right ventricle, and to the aorta or frequently crosses the VSD to enter the posteriorly placed pulmonary artery. The lateral angiocardiogram reveals the VSD.

Treatment. The neonate with transposition, a large VSD, pulmonary hypertension, and increased pulmonary vascular resistance represents one of the most perplexing problems in pediatric cardiology. A seemingly good progress during the neonatal period is at the expense of progressive pulmonary vascular obliterative disease. Neonates with transposition appear to do fairly well yet almost invariably develop rapidly advancing pulmonary vascular resistance. The logical approach appears to be pulmonary artery banding (to reduce distal pulmonary artery hypertension) with or without atrial septectomy, followed by total correction at the earliest possible time. An alternative approach is that of early total correction (in infants under 6 months of age) before pulmonary vascular obliterative disease has advanced too far. A third possible approach is a palliative Mustard operation in infancy followed by VSD closure in early childhood. The results thus far have been disappointing, both because of operative mortality and because of the continued advancement of pulmonary disease.

D-transposition with other anomalies. PDA is common with transposition, and life expectancy is reduced in infants with these conditions when compared with those having similar transposition but without PDA. Pulmonic stenosis is also common, but is usually recognized only in the older infant or child. The site of obstruction is commonly below the pulmonary valve, and it is a progressive lesion. Relief of subpulmonic stenosis is surgically difficult. Recent experience indicates that Mustard correction of venous inflow, leaving the subpulmonic stenosis intact, may be the optimal treatment for infants. If subpulmonic stenosis is severe, an anterior (Waterston) shunt may be indicated.

L-transposition of the great arteries

The presence of a VSD or mitral regurgitation complicating l-transposition (the common form of "corrected" transposition) may lead to heart failure in the newborn period. As in "uncorrected" transposition, pulmonary vascular disease appears to advance at a faster rate than is the case with normally placed great arteries. On occasion, a newborn is encountered with corrected transposition, a VSD, and pulmonary hypertension leading to heart failure. These infants may require pulmonary artery banding to limit pulmonary artery blood flow in an attempt to prevent the progress of pulmonary vascular disease.

Left heart obstruction

Left heart obstructive disease is a frequent cause of death in the neonatal period. The designation left heart obstruction is misleading, since various lesions frequently coexist. The following fairly distinctive entities are the most commonly encountered: (1) hypoplastic left heart syndrome, (2) isolated valvular aortic stenosis, (3) preductal and juxtaductal coarctation of the aorta, and (4) postductal coarctation.

Hypoplastic left heart syndrome

The term hypoplastic left heart syndrome covers a group of left heart defects commonly associated with each other. The major components are mitral valve atresia, underdevelopment of the left ventricle (small cavity), aortic valve atresia, and hypoplasia of the ascending aorta and arch. A clinical diagnosis of the syndrome is often possible, but exact delineation of the anatomy requires angiocardiography. Angiocardiography is important in order to distinguish those cases that have a reasonably normal ascending aorta and arch from those with hypoplasia of these structures. The presence of a good aorta makes palliative surgery possible, whereas with hypoplasia of the aorta (which is usually extreme) surgical help is not practical at the present time. The hypoplastic left heart syndrome has some overlap with the preductal coarctation syndrome; however, we shall consider the latter diagnosis to apply only to those cases with a normal-sized left ventricular cavity and normal ascending aorta.

Clinical presentation. The age at diagnosis ranges from 1 to 21 days. The signs and symptoms are most often those of left heart failure and varying degrees of cyanosis. The typical infant is apathetic and has reduced skin blood flow. Central cyanosis is present, and the arterial pulses are of reduced volume. Doppler measurement of blood pressure commonly indicates a level of about 60/30 mm Hg in all limbs. The infant breathes rapidly, and frequently there are rales. The precordial impulse is slightly overactive unless the neonate is in the final cardiogenic shock phase of his disease. The thrill of an associated VSD may be felt at the lower left sternal border. Auscultation most frequently reveals normal timing of the heart sounds but a pulmonary closure sound of increased intensity. Gallop rhythms are common. The most typical murmur is that of an associated VSD.

Diagnosis. The chest roentgenogram shows that the heart is large, but the contour is not usually diagnostically helpful. If mitral atresia is dominant, the characteristic vascular pattern of pulmonary venous engorgement may be present.

The ECG frequently shows a right ventricular hypertrophy pattern (no doubt accentuated by the small-sized left ventricle). There may be signs of left, right, or biatrial hypertrophy.

The pH is usually normal unless hypoxemia is extreme. The Pa_{CO_2} is normal until left heart failure has produced alveolar transudate and alveolar hypoventilation. Initially, there is little response to oxygen breathing because pulmonary capillary blood is almost completely saturated; however, when left heart failure ensues, the hypoxemia caused by alveolar hypoventilation is abolished, while that caused by right-to-left shunting remains.

Hypoglycemia is frequent, and its recognition and correction improve the chances for survival.

Hemodynamics. The hemodynamics are variable. With mitral atresia it is necessary for blood to flow from left to right across the atrial septum; it then regains the systemic circulation either by way of a VSD or PDA. If aortic atresia is present, a ductal right-to-left shunt is necessary in order to ensure brachiocephalic artery perfusion and, most important, coronary artery perfusion. In aortic atresia, perfusion of the upper half of the body requires the pulmonary artery pressure to be at systemic levels. The poor prognosis is probably most immediately related to inadequate coronary perfusion.

Treatment. Infants with hypoplastic left heart syndrome are frequently hypoglycemic as well as acidotic and may benefit from infusion of glucose and sodium bicarbonate in addition to the usual management of heart failure. If mitral atresia or mitral stenosis is a dominant lesion, balloon atrial septostomy during cardiac catheterization may increase left-to-right shunting at the atrial level and allow the left atrial pressure to fall.

The major defect is usually hypoplasia of the left ventricle, and for this there is no direct therapy. It is, however, possible in those with an adequate-sized ascending aorta to bypass the left ventricle and allow the right ventricle to maintain systemic and pulmonary blood flow. Thus, if the lesions present are mitral and aortic valve atresia together with a hypoplastic left ventricle, a combination of atrial septectomy, anastomosis of the ascending aorta to the right pulmonary artery (Waterston shunt), and distal banding of right and left pulmonary arteries may allow aortic perfusion while protecting the lungs from the harmful effects of pulmonary hypertension.

The major determinant of the effectiveness of palliative surgery is the size of the ascending aorta and proximal arch; unfortunately, these structures are very hypoplastic in the majority of cases. Nevertheless, cardiac catheterization and angiocardiography are warranted in every instance to find the occasional baby who may benefit from palliative surgery.

Congenital aortic stenosis

It is unusual for isolated congenital valvular aortic stenosis to produce symptoms in the neonate. However, the clinical picture is distinctive from that of the hypoplastic left heart syndrome and must be differentiated because of its operability. Isolated congenital aortic stenosis producing serious illness in the neonatal period is practically always valvular, and usually no other cardiac or systemic abnormality is present.

Clinical presentation. Failure of the left heart leads to tachypnea, inappropriate sweating, and pulmonary rales. Right heart failure with liver enlargement follows; but, characteristically, pulmonary symptoms continue to predominate. The infant may have surprisingly normal arterial pulses, but Doppler measurements reveal a pulse pressure of only 25 to 30 mm Hg. A systolic murmur is usually obvious and loudest to the right of the sternum or in the suprasternal notch; an accompanying thrill may or may not be present. A gallop rhythm (presystolic) is common. The second sound is usually single, and an aortic ejection click is frequently heard.

Diagnosis. In contrast to the older child, the infant with critical aortic stenosis almost always has conspicuous left ventricular and left atrial enlargement as shown on a chest roentgenogram. The lung fields appear passively congested.

Severe left ventricular hypertrophy with secondary T-wave changes is apparent in most patients. This characteristic helps to distinguish the condition from the hypoplastic left heart syndrome and also provides an index of severity (secondary T-wave changes indicate critical obstruction).

The combination of an ejection systolic murmur maximal at the upper right sternal border, cardiac enlargement, and an ECG showing severe left ventricular hypertrophy is very suggestive of critical congenital aortic stenosis. Myocarditis usually gives rise to low ECG potentials, while with endocardial fibroelastosis, murmurs are not so obvious. Occasionally, endocardial fibroelastosis with secondary obstruction to left ventricular outflow may closely simulate congenital aortic stenosis. The presence of pathologic Q waves on the ECG favors a diagnosis of anomalous origin of the left coronary artery from the pulmonary artery rather than aortic stenosis.

The neonate with heart failure from aortic stenosis usually has alveolar hypoventilation from alveolar transudate. The Pa_{CO_2} is raised and the Pa_{O_2} lowered. The Pa_{O_2} while the infant is breathing 100% O_2 should increase to above 300 mm Hg unless right-to-left intrapulmonary shunting is occurring through areas of pneumonia or atelectatic lung.

Hemodynamics. Critical aortic stenosis becomes worse with the passage of time, since there is no natural route for bypassing the obstruction (except for unacceptable right-to-left ductal shunting with consequent extreme pulmonary hypertension). It is difficult to measure left ventricular pressure, since the foramen ovale is often functionally sealed by the raised left atrial pressure, and entry through the aortic valve, even when technically possible, is hazardous. Accordingly, if the left ventricle cannot be entered by the foramen ovale route, a transvalvular aortic catheterization should not be attempted, but an aortogram should be performed, with injection of contrast material into the right brachial artery. This angiogram will reveal the caliber of the ascending aorta and an indirect assessment of aortic valve area from the diameter of the stream of unopacified blood coming from the left ventricle. In cases of real doubt, direct transthoracic needle puncture of the left ventricle may be necessary.

Treatment. Surgery for critical aortic

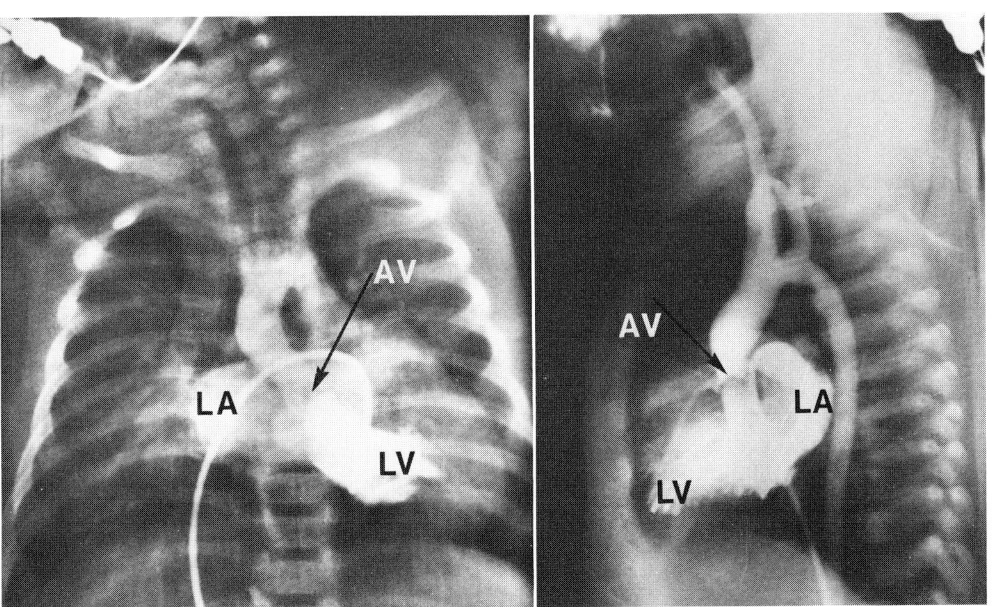

FIG. 11-18. Critical congenital aortic stenosis in infancy. There is considerable cardiac enlargement, and the infant was in clinical heart failure. The catheter tip is in the left ventricle (*LV*). Note marked mitral regurgitation into left atrium (*LA*) and dome deformity of aortic valve (*AV*) with central jet of contrast. The aortic valve gradient was 80 mm Hg.

stenosis in infancy is disappointing when compared with that for severe pulmonic stenosis. Bypass techniques are exceptionally difficult; aortic regurgitation is inevitable, and the neonates who require surgery are among the sickest and poorest anesthetic risks. Notwithstanding the problems, there is an occasional success; and if the infant can be brought through the first critical years, aortic valve replacement for aortic regurgitation later becomes a possibility.

Preductal coarctation of the aorta

The syndrome of preductal coarctation encompasses a wide spectrum of anatomy. The narrow aortic segment may be discrete and located immediately adjacent or just above the entry of the ductus (juxtaductal or discrete preductal), or, as is often the case, the obstructed segment may be long and involve the aortic arch. If the *ascending* aorta is hypoplastic, the condition is usually classified as hypoplastic left heart syndrome. Infants with preductal coarctation almost always have an open ductus so that blood flow to the lower half of the body is from the right ventricle by way of the ductus arteriosus. This would not of itself be dangerous were it not for the fact that right-to-left ductal shunting necessitates extreme pulmonary hypertension and consequent damage to the pulmonary vascular bed. The lungs of the baby with preductal coarctation are faced with a double problem; not only are they subjected to a high vascular pressure, but the flow through them is reduced (the right-to-left ductal shunt acting as a "run-off" for the pulmonary artery).

Clinical presentation. The syndrome is quite common (approximately 4%) in infants having cardiac catheterizations. There is a high incidence of associated defects; PDA is almost always present, and VSD, transposition of the great arteries, and complex lesions are common. Neonates with preductal coarctation usually develop tachypnea and cyanosis in the second or third week of life. It may be possible to recognize differential cyanosis (blue legs, pink arms). The femoral pulses are frequently palpable and may be entirely normal. This characteristic reflects the normal perfusion of the lower limbs via the patent ductus at normal systemic artery pressure. In some neonates the femoral pulses come and go, presumably secondary to variations in the pulmonary artery pressure. Usually there is either normal pulmonary artery pressure and deficient blood flow to the lower half of the body or high pulmonary artery pressure and normal blood flow to the lower half of the body. The latter is more common and preserves adequate kidney perfusion. Eventually, the infant with severe preductal coarctation (and usually associated cardiac anomalies) develops right heart failure. Most of these infants die in the neonatal period.

One may hear the characteristic murmur of a coarctation; and sometimes, if hypoplasia of the arch involves the left but not the right subclavian artery, the right arm blood pressure may be higher. Often the signs of an associated VSD predominate.

Diagnosis. The clinical diagnosis is suggested by a neonate who has a loud pulmonary closure sound, a murmur suggestive of a VSD and signs of left, or left plus right, heart failure. If the baby shows diminished or varying femoral pulses, the diagnosis is strengthened; and if differential cyanosis is observed, it is virtually certain.

The heart is usually slightly enlarged, and the pulmonary arteries appear enlarged (secondary to pulmonary hypertension) on the roentgenogram. The ECG almost always indicates right ventricular hypertrophy.

Typically, the Pa_{CO_2} (blood sampled from the right arm) is 50 to 60 mm Hg, and the Pa_{O_2} is 30 to 40 mm Hg. When blood is sampled from the femoral or umbilical artery, the Pa_{O_2} is further lowered by right-to-left ductal shunting to 15 to 30 mm Hg, while the Pa_{CO_2} is increased only by 2 or 3 mm Hg above that of the right arm sample (because of the small arteriovenous P_{CO_2} difference). This wide difference in Pa_{O_2} between the right arm and leg and the narrow difference in Pa_{CO_2} can be used as a test for right-to-left ductal shunting.

Hemodynamics. Cardiac catheterization of the neonate with uncomplicated preductal coarctation reveals severe right ventricular and pulmonary hypertension. The catheter passes from the pulmonary artery to the descending aorta by way of the usually present PDA. Contrast visualization of the right ventricle discloses filling of the pulmonary artery system and of the descending aorta (via the ductus). Increasing degrees of aortic arch atresia are associated with contrast agent also filling the brachiocephalic arteries, and, in the extreme case of aortic valve hypoplasia, the coronary arteries will fill from the right ventricular injection. However, at this stage the condition is best regarded as hypoplastic left heart syndrome rather than preductal coarctation syndrome.

The left ventricle can usually be entered by the foramen ovale and mitral valve, and opacification of this structure will define the aortic valve, coronary arteries, and aorta up to the point where the contrast agent meets the stream of right ventricle–derived blood. Most characteristically, the brachiocephalic arteries fill from the left ventricle, and the descending aorta fills from the right; but the pattern in each patient is dependent on the aortic arch anatomy and the vascular resistance in the various organs of the body (Fig. 11-19).

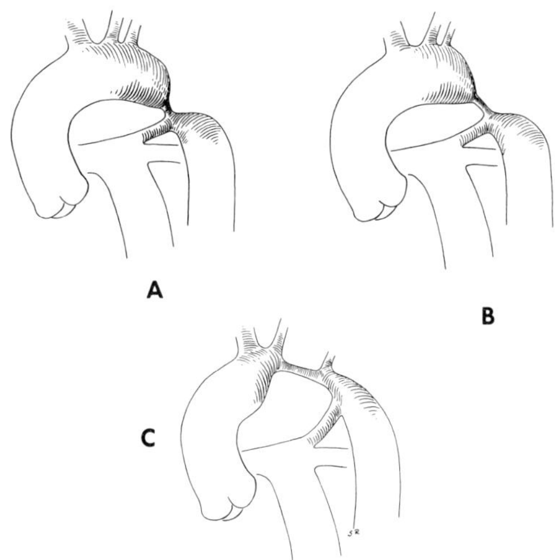

FIG. 11-19. Preductal coarctation of the aorta. Three of the more common variants are: *(A)* juxtaductal localized coarctation, *(B)* preductal long-segment coarctation with hypoplasia of the left subclavian artery, and *(C)* aortic isthmus hypoplasia with hypoplasia of the left brachiocephalic arteries. Many other anatomic variations occur, but the physiology is usually that of a "systemic" right ventricle, whereby the descending aorta receives "venous" blood and the pulmonary artery pressure is usually at systemic levels.

Treatment. Medical treatment of the neonate with preductal coarctation usually results in only temporary improvement. Surgical repair depends on the extent of aortic arch hypoplasia and the presence of associated anomalies. In some cases it is possible to bring down the left subclavian artery and anastomose it directly to the descending aorta (the ductus tissue is usually too friable for this purpose); in others an end-to-end anastomosis or homograft replacement is possible. The ductus is divided. Unfortunately, pulmonary hypertension may remain (especially if there is an associated VSD); however, in others it is completely reversible. Those infants who survive surgery are usually the ones with short-segment juxtaductal coarction.

Postductal coarctation of the aorta (with closed ductus arteriosus)

Isolated postductal aortic coarctation rarely causes problems in the neonatal period. Problems are most commonly encountered when other lesions, especially VSD and PDA, coexist. Infants with simple coarctation of the aorta can usually be brought out of heart failure by medical means; operation can be deferred until the infants are an appropriate age. An infant with absent femoral pulses and heart failure and who is deteriorating requires urgent hemodynamic and angiographic assessment; experience indicates that such infants nearly always have complicating lesions, such as aortic arch hypoplasia, VSD, and so on.

Clinical presentation. The neonate with isolated coarctation of the aorta usually has moderately severe, predominantly left-sided, heart failure. Occasionally, hypertension may be the initial sign. Physical examination reveals the usual signs of heart failure. A diagnosis of coarctation is suggested by a late systolic ejection murmur heard well posteriorly and is made virtually certain by the absence of palpable femoral pulses. In lesser degrees of coarctation or where a good collateral circulation exists, the femoral pulses may be palpable, but there is a time lag between the brachial and the femoral pulse (normally synchronous). The diagnosis can be strengthened by a comparison of arm and leg systolic pressures with the Doppler

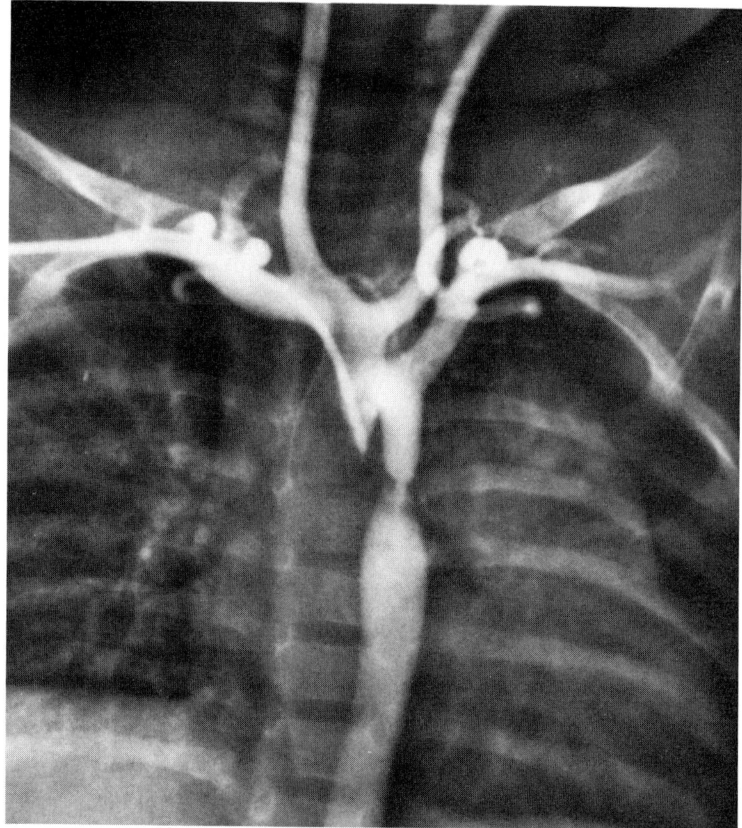

FIG. 11-20. Visualization of isolated aortic coarctation by right brachial artery catheterization.

technique, and in rare instances the coarctation can be visualized by the imprint of prestenotic and poststenotic dilatation on the barium-filled esophagus. Usually there is little doubt about the diagnosis; the only doubt is as to whether other lesions coexist.

Diagnosis. The heart is enlarged, and the lung fields frequently show the appearance of pulmonary venous engorgement. Right ventricular hypertrophy is usual. It is unusual to find left ventricular hypertrophy from isolated aortic coarctation before the infant is 6 months of age. Left-sided heart failure causes an alveolar transudate and impairment of respiratory gas exchange because of alveolar hypoventilation. The breathing of 100% O_2 increases Pa_{O_2} to above 300 mm Hg, but Pa_{CO_2} is unchanged.

Hemodynamics. Frequently there is systemic hypertension above the coarctation; the reason remains unknown. In the presence of heart failure, right heart pressures are slightly elevated. The coarctation may be delineated in several ways: by left ventricular opacification, by right ventricular opacification and subsequent levocardiogram phase, or, if necessary, by right brachial artery injection (Fig. 11-20). If the infant is less than 3 days old, the umbilical artery may be utilized; but use of the femoral artery is ill advised because of the lowered pulse pressure in the vessel. The objective of hemodynamic study is usually not only the delineation of the coarctation but the search for a PDA, VSD, bicuspid aortic valve, hypoplastic aortic arch, and so on.

Treatment. The infant with uncomplicated coarctation usually responds excellently to medical management. Occasionally, a neonate will have a systolic arm blood pressure of 150 mm Hg or higher, and the question arises as to whether antihypertensive treatment is indicated. A trial dose of reserpine (0.07 mg/kg) may be given intramuscularly, and the response may last 24 to 72 hours or longer. Under these circumstances oral administration of reserpine (0.1 mg/day) may be started; however, the latent period before orally administered reserpine starts to act may be 2 to 3 weeks so that further intramuscular doses may be needed. In some cases systemic hypertension is transient, possibly related to the "opening up" of collaterals. Use of other drugs in the treatment of hypertension is discussed on p. 336. The neonate who has hypertension or is given antihypertensive treatment should have his renal function checked at frequent intervals; any suggestion of compromise of renal function should be considered an indication for surgery.

The argument against early surgery in all cases is the high incidence of restenosis and the increased mortality in the neonatal period. However, in the rare instance when surgery for simple coarctation is necessary in the neonatal period, it should be performed, since the surgery for restenosis is as effective as the primary operation.

Right heart obstruction

Classification of obstructive disease of the right side of the heart is somewhat arbitrary. The following are the commoner entities that produce life-threatening illness in the neonatal period: pulmonary atresia with intact ventricular septum, pulmonary atresia with open ventricular septum (pseudotruncus arteriosus, extreme tetralogy of Fallot), tetralogy of Fallot, isolated vavular pulmonic stenosis, multiple peripheral pulmonary arterial stenoses, tricuspid atresia, and Ebstein's anomaly of the tricuspid valve.

Pulmonary atresia or extreme pulmonic stenosis with intact ventricular septum

Pulmonary atresia with intact ventricular septum is relatively common and is probably underestimated, since afflicted infants may die rapidly after birth. The only sources of blood to the lungs are the ductus arteriosus and the bronchial arteries. In most instances the ductus closes on the first, second, or third day of life even though it is being perfused by blood of low oxygen tension. In a few instances the ductus remains patent (perhaps predestined to be a PDA); consequently, older children are occasionally encountered with complete pulmonary atresia and associated ductus arteriosus. The incidence in a series of sick neonates is 9% to 13%. Since the conditions of severe pulmonic stenosis and pulmonary atresia are closely related clinically, hemodynamically, and therapeutically, they are considered here as a single entity. A baby who angiographically appears to have pulmonary atresia, sometimes is found to have a pinhole pulmonary valve orifice at surgery.

Clinical presentation. Neonates with pulmonary atresia show early evidence of distress, presumably corresponding to closure of the ductus arteriosus. Cyanosis is marked. The respirations are characteristically deep, and alveolar ventilation is greatly increased in an unsuccessful attempt to attain physiologic respiratory gas tensions in arterial blood. The infants usually have a good Apgar score, but their color and breathing is noticed to be abnormal a few hours after birth. The cardiac impulse and peripheral pulses are normal, and frequently there is a loud, blowing, systolic murmur at the lower left sternal border, probably representing massive tricuspid regurgitation. A separate continuous murmur of a PDA is frequently heard. The second heart sound is single.

Diagnosis. The most striking finding on the chest roentgenogram is decreased pulmonary vascularity. The heart may be large and often appears egg shaped because of right atrial enlargement; there may be radiologic absence of the main pulmonary artery (Fig. 11-21). Cardiac enlargement is mainly a function of time; the heart may be normal in size during the first hours and days, whereas it is usually greatly enlarged in the occasional infant who survives beyond the neonatal period.

There is a spectrum of right ventricular size so that the ECG may show marked right ventricular hypertrophy in those with a large right ventricular cavity, or it may show left ventricular hypertrophy if the right ventricle is hypoplastic, as is frequently the case. Electrocardiographic evidence of right atrial hypertrophy is usually present.

Increased alveolar ventilation results in

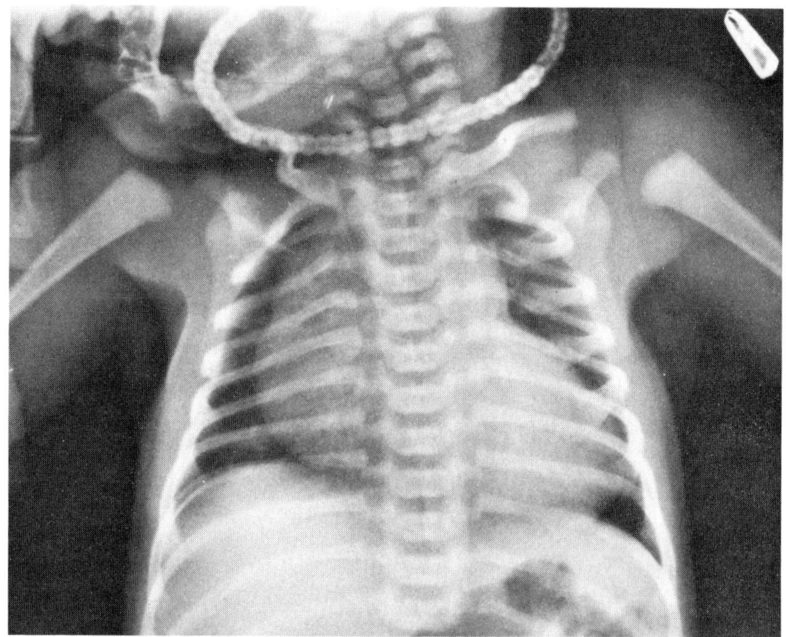

Fig. 11-21. Posteroanterior film of newborn with pulmonary valve atresia and intact ventricular septum. Note large heart and marked decrease in pulmonary vascular markings.

a pulmonary vein P_{CO_2} of about 25 mm Hg and a pulmonary vein P_{O_2} of about 90 mm Hg. The gross right-to-left atrial shunt results in an arterial P_{CO_2} of about 31 mm Hg and a greatly reduced arterial oxygen saturation. There is no response to oxygen breathing. The arterial pH is often surprisingly normal until the infant is too exhausted to continue the high rates of ventilation necessary to maintain a normal Pa_{CO_2}.

Hemodynamics. The hemodynamics of pulmonary atresia and extreme pulmonic stenosis are similar. The right atrial pressure is moderately raised, and the right ventricular pressure is usually in the 70 to 100 mm Hg systolic range (only slightly increased above normal for age). Lack of marked elevation of the right ventricular pressure appears to be caused by the gross tricuspid insufficiency that is often present in infants with pulmonary atresia. Right ventricular angiography is pathognomonic; there is often gross tricuspid regurgitation and either complete absence of pulmonary artery filling or very minor opacification of this structure (Fig. 11-22). The size of the right ventricle can best be assessed angiographically. Many appear hypoplastic, but both the ECG and angiogram can be deceptive in the assessment of the adequacy of the right ventricle as a pumping chamber.

Treatment. The need for therapy is extremely urgent; for many patients immediate thoracic surgical consultation should be obtained. Direct transfer of the baby to the operating room is often indicated. Acidosis should be corrected by sodium bicarbonate; and when necessary, ventilation can be augmented by "bag breathing." If a significant gradient is found to exist between the right and left atria, a balloon septostomy (Rashkind procedure) may allow increased systemic venous return and gain time while preparations are being made for surgery. The outcome of surgery depends to a major extent on the adequacy of the right ventricle. However, in our opinion no neonate should be turned down for surgery because of hypoplastic right ventricle. In those rare infants with an adequate right ventricle and isolated critical valvar pulmonic stenosis, a pulmonary valvotomy (transventricular or transpulmonary-arterial) is dramatically successful. Those infants with right ventricular hypoplasia will often require a right pulmonary

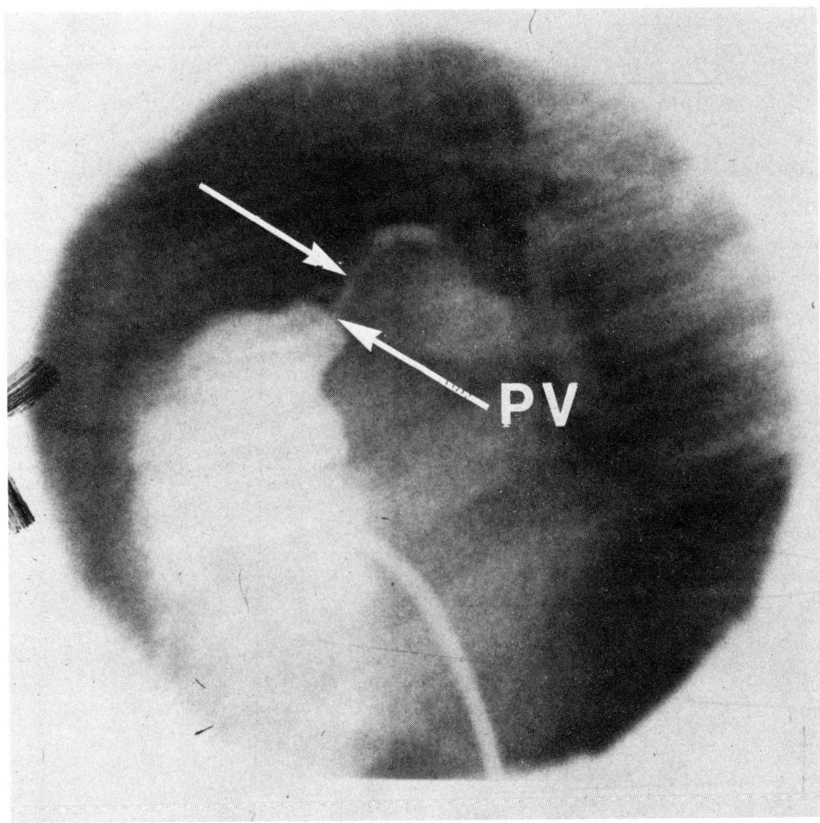

Fig. 11-22. Severe valvar pulmonic stenosis in a 1-day-old infant. Single frame from cineangiogram in lateral projection shows a large anterior right ventricle and a tiny jet of contrast agent (arrow) through the pulmonic valve. Note domelike appearance of valve (*PV*).

artery–to–aorta shunt (Waterston procedure) instead of, or in addition to, relief of right ventricular outflow obstruction. Although mortality is high at the present time, greater alertness and speed at every stage of referral, combined with surgical advances, is steadily improving the prognosis.

Pulmonary atresia with open ventricular septum and severe tetralogy of Fallot

Pulmonary atresia with open ventricular septum may be thought of as the extreme form of tetralogy of Fallot; there is complete obstruction to right ventricular outflow. It has at times been referred to as pseudotruncus arteriosus or type IV truncus arteriosus, since the source of lung blood flow is from the aorta (bronchial arteries). The distinction between severely symptomatic tetralogy of Fallot (that is, continuity between right ventricular outflow tract and pulmonary arteries) and complete pulmonary atresia with open ventricular septum is not usually possible clinically. It is readily made by right ventricular angiography.

Clinical presentation. Infants are cyanotic from birth but usually do not cause concern until a few hours after birth, because temporary patency of the ductus arteriosus allows adequate pulmonary artery blood flow. On the first or second day of life the ductus closes, and the neonate becomes strikingly symptomatic with deep, sighing respirations, increasing central cyanosis, and lethargy. The cardiac impulse is hypodynamic, or one may feel a right parasternal tapping impulse. The second heart sound is single and maximal at the second right interspace (aortic valve closure), and there is frequently an aortic ejection click. There may be no murmur, or, there may be a short ejection murmur of tight infundibular stenosis at the third left interspace.

Diagnosis. The heart is small or normal in size (in contrast to most other cyanotic lesions) and the pulmonary vasculature strikingly diminished. Even on the first day of life the heart may have the characteristic "coeur en sabot" shape of tetralogy (Fig. 11-23). Moderate right atrial and right ventricular hypertrophy are usual but are not diagnostically helpful. Alveolar hyperventilation produces a high pulmonary venous P_{O_2} and low pulmonary venous P_{CO_2}; when pulmonary venous blood is admixed with systemic venous blood (at atrial and ventricular levels), hypoxemia and hypercapnia result in acidosis. In the first hours after birth, surprisingly normal arterial blood gases can be found; but as the infant tires, ventilation falls and acidosis results. There is no response to the breathing of 100% O_2, since hypoxemia is secondary to right-to-left shunting.

Hemodynamics. Diminished pulmonary blood flow leads to diminished left atrial pressure, with consequent right-to-left atrial shunting across the foramen ovale. Blood enters the right ventricle and, in the case of total outflow tract obstruction, leaves to enter the aorta (in systole) and the left ventricle (in diastole). The only source of lung blood flow is via bronchial arteries and in some instances a ductus arteriosus. Clearly, the baby's survival is un-

A

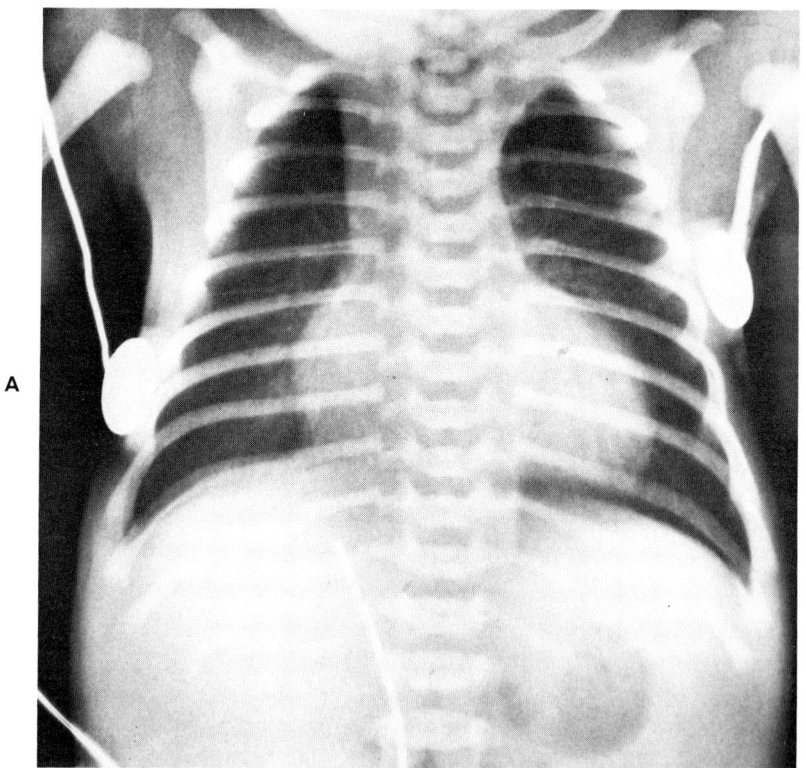

Fig. 11-23. Severe tetralogy of Fallot. **A,** Note normal-sized heart with marked decrease in pulmonary vascular markings. There is a slight "coeur-en-sabot" configuration to the heart. **B,** Right ventricular angiogram in pulmonary atresia with open ventricular septum. Note hypoplastic right ventricle *(RV)*—blind-ending right ventricular infundibulum *(RVI)* and greatly enlarged aorta *(Ao)* receiving right ventricular contents. ***C*** and ***D***, Tetralogy of Fallot with tight discrete infundibular stenosis (arrow) and VSD. The aorta is barely visible, indicating only a small right-to-left shunt at rest. This type of anatomy is often associated with severe life-threatening cyanotic spells. The anatomy is favorable for total correction, since the pulmonary artery *(PA)* is relatively large and the obstruction is discrete.

likely unless bronchial artery flow is excessive or the ductus remains open. Right ventricular systolic pressure is at systemic level, and the catheter usually enters the aorta readily (across the VSD). Diagnosis is confirmed by angiocardiography (Fig. 11-23).

Treatment. A neonate with pulmonary atresia and open ventricular septum considered sick enough to require diagnostic heart catheterization is practically always going to require palliative surgery. Total correction in the neonatal age group has occasionally been attempted but to date appears far more hazardous than is a staged procedure. In most centers, the Waterston procedure (anastomosis of ascending aorta to right pulmonary artery) has supplanted the Blalock and Potts shunt as the first choice for increasing the pulmonary blood flow in the newborn. In selected cases, where an adequate-sized main pulmonary artery exists, a Brock procedure (transventricular "reaming out" of infundibular obstruction) may be preferable. At the time of surgery, the presence and size of the main pulmonary artery are noted, since this structure will be hard to visualize later in the childs life and a knowledge of its size is mandatory before plans are made for total correction in early childhood. The results of palliative surgery for pulmonary atresia with open ventricular septum are disappointing, since there is frequently co-

B

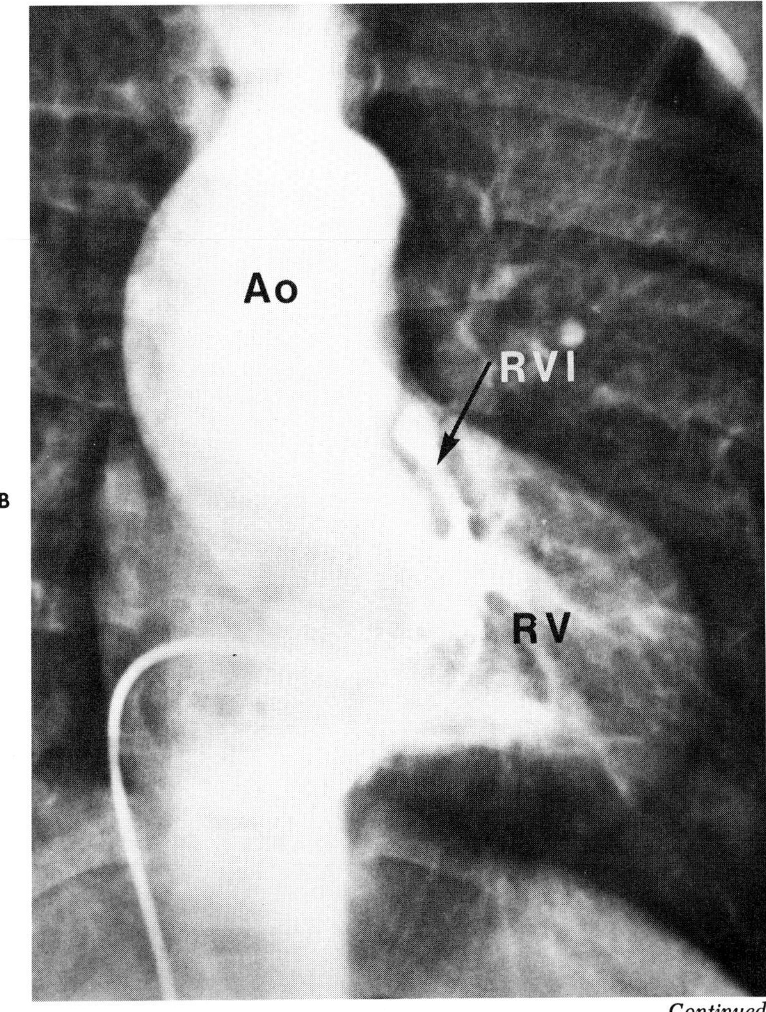

Continued.

Fig. 11-23, cont'd. For legend see opposite page.

existent right ventricular hypoplasia and hypoplasia of the pulmonary arterial system.

Multiple peripheral pulmonary arterial stenoses

The most frequent cause of important pulmonary arterial stenoses giving rise to symptoms in the neonate is intrauterine rubella infection (p. 154). A familial incidence of peripheral pulmonary arterial stenosis also has been recognized, and there is evidence that idiopathic hypercalcemia of infancy is frequently associated with combined pulmonary arterial and supravalvar aortic stenosis. On occasion, peripheral pulmonary artery stenosis is associated with various forms of congenital heart disease, especially tetralogy of Fallot. Cases of cutis laxa (generalized elastolysis), Ehlers-Danlos syndrome, and Takayasu's disease have all been reported in association with peripheral pulmonary arterial stenosis.

Clinical presentation. The symptoms are those of predominant right heart failure unless there is a PDA (as is frequently the case), in which case right-to-left ductal shunting leads to cyanosis. In severe cases, the lungs are underperfused so that there is an increase in pulmonary ventilation similar to that seen in severe tetralogy or pulmonic stenosis. Classically, continuous murmurs are heard in many areas of the chest; however, in many instances only nondescript systolic murmurs are heard. The pulmonary closure sound may be very loud, since although there are peripheral areas of obstruction, central pulmonary arterial pressure is greatly raised.

Diagnosis. The areas of stenosis are associated with poststenotic dilatation (Fig.

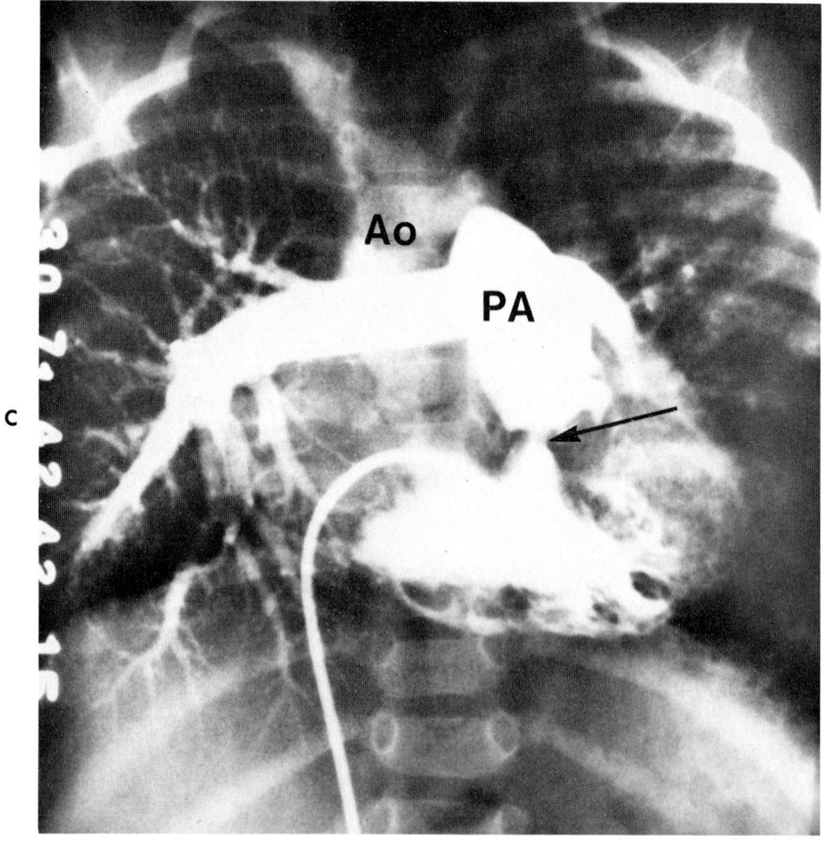

Fig. 11-23, cont'd. For legend see p. 304.

11-24). These may occasionally be visible on the plain film and may give a spurious impression of adequate or even increased vascular markings. The heart is usually small, unless it has dilated from right heart failure. Right ventricular hypertrophy, often of severe degree, is typical. As the child grows and the obstruction becomes relatively more severe, right ventricular hypertrophy increases and is a useful measurement of progress or deterioration. Signs of right atrial hypertrophy are common. Alveolar hyperventilation without right-to-left shunting produces lowered Pa_{CO_2} and increased or normal O_2 saturation. Ductal right-to-left shunts are frequent, in which case cyanosis, unresponsive to 100% O_2 breathing, is present.

Determination of IgM fraction and rubella antibody titer is indicated. If a generalized disorder, such as cutis laxa or Ehlers-Danlos syndrome is suspected, a skin biopsy may be worthwhile. Serum calcium and phosphorus levels should be determined because of their association with hypercalcemia.

Hemodynamics. Very high (200 mm Hg) right ventricular and central pulmonary arterial pressures may be found. Right atrial pressure rises as a consequence of raised right ventricular end-diastolic pressure, and right-to-left shunting through the foramen ovale is common. Definitive diagnosis can be made by observing pressure gradients within the pulmonary arterial system, but pulmonary angiography is essential if

D

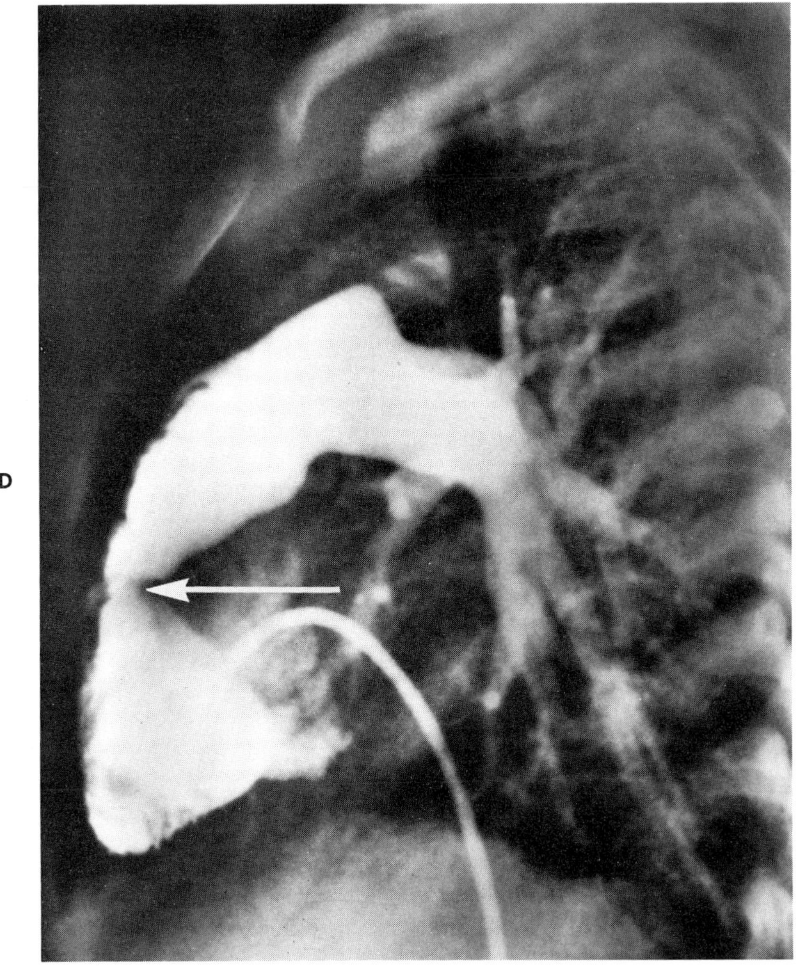

Fig. 11-23, cont'd. For legend see p. 304.

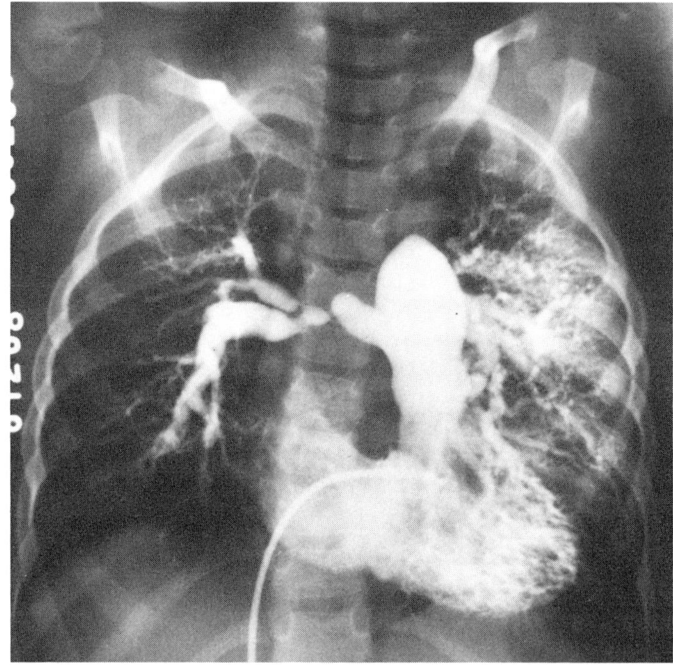

Fig. 11-24. Angiographic appearances in multiple peripheral pulmonary artery stenoses. In this particular case, Ehlers-Danlos syndrome was present, and there were associated abnormalities of systemic arteries. The left lung had been operated upon, but many areas of stenosis remain in the right lung.

surgery is contemplated. Selective angiography defines the exact location and length of stenotic areas and determines the feasibility of corrective surgery.

Treatment. Total correction is rarely possible, since almost invariably the stenotic areas are very numerous. Occasionally, a single stenosis in the main pulmonary artery or a small number of stenoses in primary, secondary, and tertiary divisions can be patchgrafted. Such a patient is illustrated in Fig. 11-24. Although the surgery is time consuming, one advantage is that cardiopulmonary bypass is usually not necessary, since one lung may be operated on while the other serves for gas exchange.

Tricuspid atresia

Atresia of the tricuspid valve may occur with normally placed great arteries; tricuspid atresia without transposition is invariably associated with right ventricular hypoplasia and frequently with pulmonary valve hypoplasia. The presence of a VSD or PDA is necessary for blood to gain access to the pulmonary artery. Because the coexistence of transposed great arteries produces a much different clinical picture from that in patients with normally positioned great arteries, tricuspid atresia and tricuspid atresia with transposed great arteries are considered separately in the following sections.

Tricuspid atresia with ventricular septal defect and normally positioned great arteries

Clinical presentation. Cyanosis is present from birth. Infants with a small VSD have greatly diminished pulmonary blood flow, while those with a large VSD have increased pulmonary blood flow. Diminished lung blood flow is more frequent; and it tends to diminish further with time, since there is evidence that the VSD becomes progressively smaller with growth. A further limitation to pulmonary blood flow is the size of the foramen ovale or atrial septal defect (Fig. 11-25). Pulmonary underperfusion leads to hyperventilation; and the respirations, though not unduly rapid, are increased in tidal volume. The cardiac impulse is quiet; frequently a thrill, caused

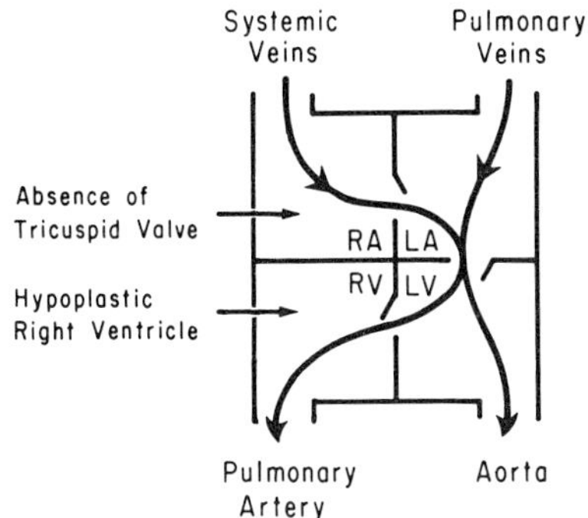

Fig. 11-25. The circulation in tricuspid atresia with patent foramen ovale and VSD.

by a VSD, is present at the lower left sternal border. The arterial pulses are normal. The second sound is frequently single, and a loud grade 4 pansystolic VSD murmur is heard maximally at the fourth left interspace. The clinical findings suggest a VSD, except that the infant is cyanotic.

Diagnosis. A few infants have a characteristic square-shaped heart, but the radiologic appearances are very variable and are influenced by the size of the atrial and ventricular septal defects. In the majority of cases, pulmonary vasculature is obviously diminished (Fig. 11-26). The ECG is of major diagnostic significance. In over 80% of the cases both left axis deviation and left ventricular hypertrophy are present. T-wave inversion in leads V_5 and V_6 is frequent. A typical ECG is shown in Fig. 11-27.

Pulmonary underperfusion and overventilation produce a low P_{CO_2} and high P_{O_2} in pulmonary vein blood. However, since there is almost complete mixing at the left ventricular level, the final arterial blood gas tensions depend largely on the ratio of pulmonary venous to systemic venous return. The pH and Pa_{CO_2} are usually normal, though the Pa_{O_2} is greatly reduced because of the very wide arteriovenous P_{O_2} difference. The breathing of 100% O_2 has almost no effect on arterial P_{O_2}.

Hemodynamics. The diagnosis is usually obvious prior to cardiac catheterization, and the hemodynamics are very characteristic. It is impossible to direct the catheter tip into the right ventricle (ordinarily accomplished without delay). Instead, the catheter passes immediately from the right atrium into the left atrium and can be manipulated into the pulmonary veins and left ventricle. Right atrial angiography reveals the sequence of right atrium, left atrium, left ventricle, and then simultaneous filling of the aorta and pulmonary artery. There may be an unopacified wedge (especially apparent in the frontal projection) corresponding to the hypoplastic right ventricle. On occasion the pulmonary artery can be entered (across a VSD); the pressure is low unless the defect is substantial. The aorta can usually be entered with a flow-guided catheter and is easily visualized by contrast opacification of the left ventricle.

Treatment. There is no definitive correction for tricuspid atresia available at the present time. The limiting factor is the hypoplastic right ventricle. There are, however, various palliative maneuvers. If a gradient is found between the right and left atrial, a balloon septostomy may aid systemic venous return and lower right atrial pressure. Palliative surgery is designed to increase pulmonary blood flow either by means of an ascending aorta-to-right pulmonary artery shunt (Waterston shunt), or in an occasional instance, by a superior vena cava-to-right pulmonary artery shunt (Glenn procedure). The Glenn shunt is rarely indicated in the neonate. It is a more efficient shunt (undiluted venous blood directly into pulmonary artery), but the procedure is technically more difficult to perform and is likely to thrombose postoperatively because of the small caliber of the neonatal vessels involved.

Tricuspid atresia with transposed great arteries. The neonate with transposed great arteries and tricuspid atresia usually has also a large ventricular defect. The problem is not so much hypoxemia as pulmonary overcirculation and pulmonary hypertension. The defect may become apparent on the first day of life or after the neonatal period.

Clinical presentation. Neonates with transposition and tricuspid atresia are cyanotic, but usually not so blue as those without transposition. Respirations are rapid but of small or normal volume, typical for the infant with overperfused lungs. The cardiac impulse is hyperdynamic, and the arterial pulses are normal. If pulmonary overcirculation is marked, the signs

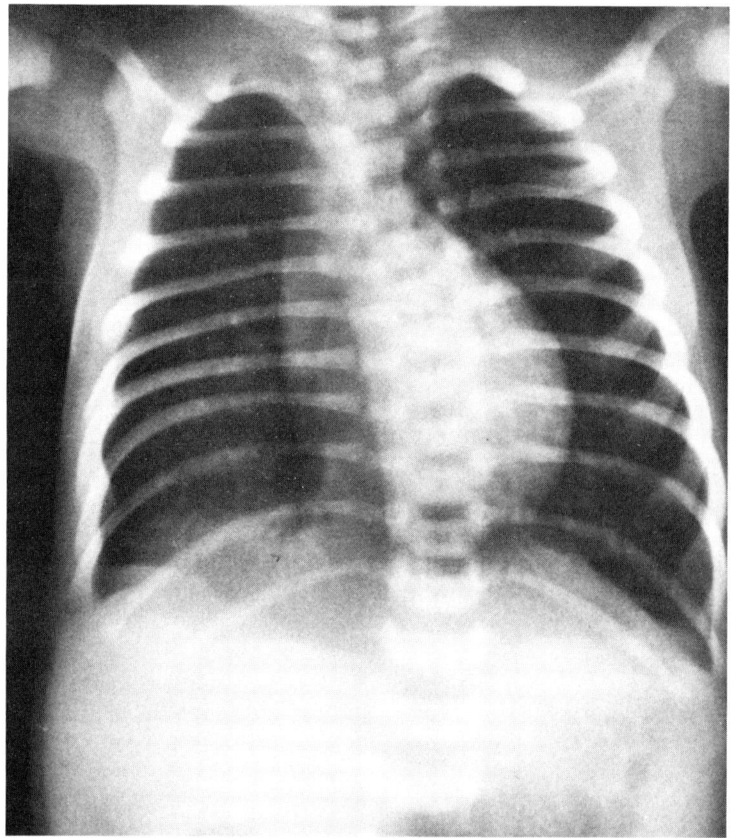

Fig. 11-26. Posteroanterior chest film of a neonate with tricuspid atresia. Note small heart, straight right cardiac border, and decreased pulmonary vascular markings. The plain chest film in tricuspid atresia shows considerable variation in the cardiac contour between patients.

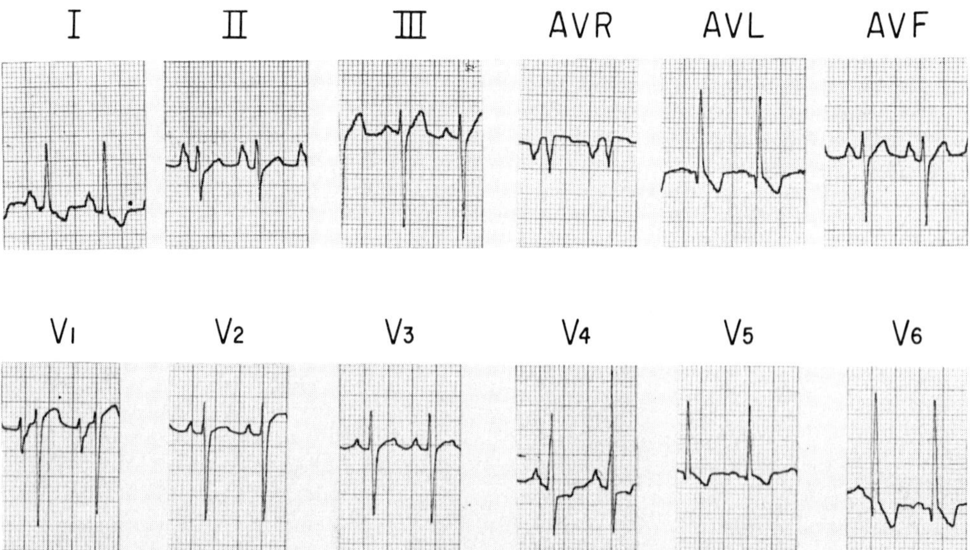

Fig. 11-27. The ECG in tricuspid atresia. Note left axis deviation, right atrial hypertrophy, and left ventricular hypertrophy with "strain" (negative T waves in leads I, V_5 and V_6).

of left-sided heart failure appear, followed by those of right-sided failure. In severe cases there are pulmonary rales, and the infant dies from hypoxemia, hypercapnia, and acidosis.

Diagnosis. The heart is frequently very large and similar to that of uncomplicated transposition. The pulmonary vascular markings are increased. Some infants show the classic left axis deviation and left ventricular hypertrophy of uncomplicated tricuspid atresia. Others display normal axis or right axis deviation. Pa_{CO_2} is usually normal. Pa_{O_2} is decreased and unresponsive to the breathing of 100% O_2. Initially, the arterial pH is normal but when heart failure supervenes and Pa_{CO_2} rises, acidosis develops.

Hemodynamics. The catheter course follows the right atrium, left atrium, left ventricle route. Left ventricular angiography when filmed in the lateral projection reveals the transposed great arteries. The aorta can frequently be entered by passage of the catheter from the left ventricle across a large VSD. Most patients have severe pulmonary hypertension and greatly increased pulmonary blood flow.

Treatment. Tricuspid atresia with transposed great arteries is one of the least rewarding entities to treat. Theoretically, pulmonary artery banding should limit pulmonary blood flow and protect the lungs from developing vascular obliterative changes. In practice, however, the small hemodynamic advantage gained from pulmonary artery banding does not offset the hazards of thoracotomy in a small, sick infant, and the immediate mortality is very high.

Ebstein's anomaly of the tricuspid valve

The tricuspid valve is malformed and is attached partly to the annulus fibrosus and partly to the right ventricular endocardium. The posterior leaflets, which are often grossly malformed and sometimes vestigial or absent, are usually displaced downward. The resulting tricuspid valve is usually both stenotic and incompetent and is displaced deeply into the right ventricular cavity, dividing it into two chambers. The area of the right ventricle proximal to the valve is abnormally thin and sometimes aneurysmal.

Incidence. Ebstein's anomaly is uncommon (about 1 in 50,000 to 1 in 100,000); but its clinical recognition is important, since if it is discovered in the neonatal period, one should be cautious in considering cardiac catheterization because of the risk involved in precipitating an arythmia. Spontaneous improvement in the first months of life is not unusual. Congenital Ebstein's anomaly is often undetected in the neonatal period, and such infants have no symptoms unless there is a bout of PST.

Clinical presentation. The initial symptom in the neonatal period is usually cyanosis. This is caused by right-to-left shunting across a patent foramen ovale or ASD secondary to raised right atrial pressure. Frequently, there is a triple or quadruple rhythm caused by third or fourth heart sounds. A systolic murmur of moderate intensity is heard at the mid or lower left sternal border, and a presystolic murmur is often present. The presence of multiple heart sounds and murmurs when combined with the rapid heart rate of the neonate leads to a confusing auscultatory picture. Ebstein's anomaly is one of the situations in which phonocardiographic analysis may be of great diagnostic help. Though the right atrial pressure may be raised slightly, congestive heart failure is uncommon, since right-to-left shunting limits the elevation of right atrial pressure. Where the foramen ovale is small, however, congestive heart failure may ensue.

Diagnosis. The classic findings are those of gross cardiomegaly with pulmonary undercirculation as shown by a chest roentgenogram. The right atrium accounts for most of the cardiac enlargement. In symptomatic neonates the right atrium is usually enlarged; however, the roentgenogram may closely simulate that of pulmonary stenosis or pulmonary atresia with intact ventricular septum (Fig. 11-28).

Arrythmias are frequent: ectopic beats, PST, atrial flutter, and atrial fibillation are all common; nodal rhythm and A-V dissociation are less common. The Wolff-Parkinson-White syndrome occurs in approximately 9% of cases. Many infants have electrocardiographic evidence of right atrial hypertrophy, and some have prolongation of the P-R interval. Right bundle branch

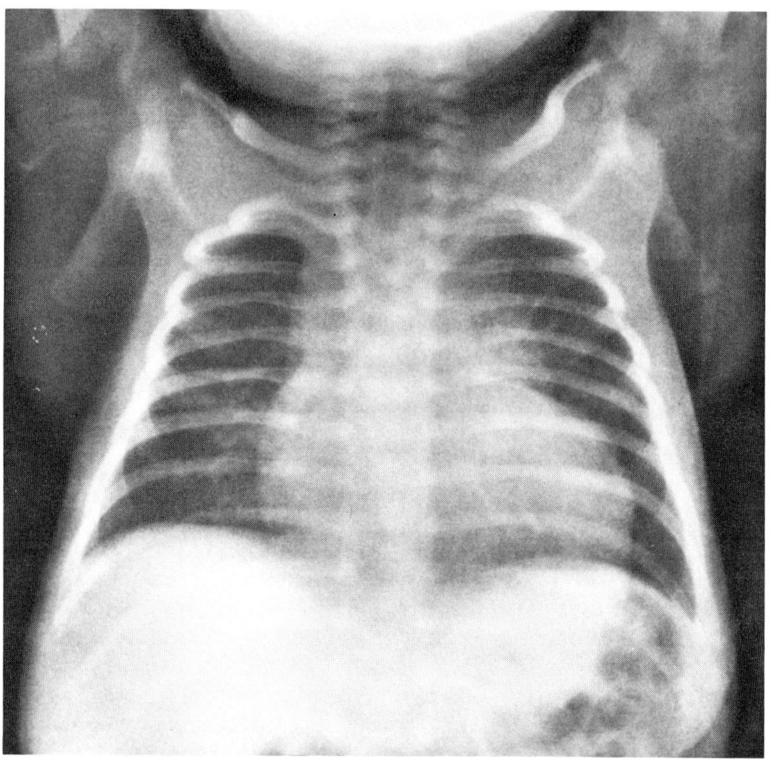

Fig. 11-28. Posteroanterior chest film from a neonate with Ebstein's anomaly of the tricuspid valve. There is cardiomegaly and decreased pulmonary vascular markings.

block is common in older children and though uncommon in the neonate is very suggestive of Ebstein's anomaly.

The symptomatic newborn with Ebstein's anomaly invariably has right-to-left atrial shunting, and the blood gases reflect the situation. The Pa_{CO_2} and pH are normal, but the Pa_{O_2} is low and is not significantly increased by the infant's breathing 100% O_2.

Hemodynamics. It is somtimes possible to make a firm diagnosis of Ebstein's anomaly in the neonate, based on physical signs with characteristic roentgenographic and ECG findings. Unless the neonate is critically sick, hemodynamic study is best deferred, since spontaneous improvement is common and catheterization may precipitate an arrthymia. If the infant's condition is deteriorating, cardiac catheterization is indicated because there are very characteristic findings and surgical treatment is possible. By cardiac catheterization the diagnosis is suggested by a high right atrial pressure, evidence of right-to-left atrial shunting, and difficulty or inability to cross the tricuspid valve. If the tricuspid valve can be crossed, there is a characteristic short ejection phase on the right ventricular pressure tracing; the intracardiac ECG may demonstrate that although the catheter tip is in the right atrium, a right ventricular intracavitary ECG is being recorded (because of the prolapse of the atrium into the ventricle). Angiocardiography is very helpful in disclosing the anatomy of tricuspid valve.

Treatment. Treatment is rarely required in the neonatal period and can be deferred until the child is large enough to undergo replacement of the anomaly with a prosthetic valve or to undergo tricuspid valvuloplasty. If treatment in the neonatal period is essential for survival, the Glenn procedure (anastomosis of superior vena cava to right pulmonary artery) may be of value.

Lesions that produce common mixing of venous and arterial blood

The four most important lesions that produce common mixing of venous and arterial blood are truncus arteriosus, very large VSD or common ventricle, double-outlet right ventricle without pulmonic stenosis, and total anomalous pulmonary venous return. A single atrium produces common mixing but rarely gives rise to serious illness in the neonate. Patients with these lesions tend to have certain features in common: mild cyanosis, a hyperactive cardiac impulse, cardiomegaly with increased pulmonary blood flow, and pulmonary hypertension. The cyanosis may go undetected, since the volume of well-oxygenated pulmonary vein blood exceeds that of the systemic vein blood. The resulting admixed arterial saturation is closer to pulmonary vein levels than it is to systemic vein levels. Frequently, the saturation is 88% to 90%, and cyanosis will be obvious only when the hematocrit value is high.

Persistent truncus arteriosus

Two to 4% of severely sick neonates have this lesion. The recognition of truncus arteriosus, though a relatively uncommon lesion, has become important since the advent of palliative and even corrective surgery.

Pathology. The designation truncus arteriosus implies that only one artery arises from the heart and that this artery (the truncus arteriosus) gives rise to coronary arteries, pulmonary arteries, and the aorta. The truncus arteriosus almost always overrides a large VSD. The fact that the pulmonary arteries are of normal size necessitates the existence of severe pulmonary hypertension or greatly increased pulmonary blood flow; usually both are present. Various anatomic subtypes exist, depending on the exact point of origin of the pulmonary arteries from the truncus arteriosus. The so-called pseudotruncus, or type IV truncus, in the Collett-Edwards classification is now classified as tetralogy of Fallot with pulmonary atresia, the blood supply to the lung being bronchial-arterial rather than pulmonary-arterial.

Clinical presentation. The major problem facing neonates born with a persistent truncus arteriosus is gross pulmonary overperfusion and pulmonary hypertension (usually at systemic artery pressure). In rare instances, the pulmonary arteries are somewhat hypoplastic, allowing near-normal pulmonary blood flow and pulmonary artery pressure.

Neonates with truncus arteriosus appear only *mildly cyanotic;* respirations are rapid but not deep. When left heart failure supervenes, the signs of respiratory distress appear. The cardiac impulse is hyperactive, and the peripheral arterial pulses are bounding. The second heart sound is single and loud; there is commonly a loud, pansystolic murmur of a VSD at the lower left sternal border and on occasion a loud, continuous murmur at the upper left sternal border or an early diastolic murmur of truncal insufficiency. The general picture resembles that of a neonate with a large PDA (a neonate with a large PDA is frequently cyanotic from alveolar hypoventilation secondary to left heart failure).

Diagnosis. The heart size is frequently massive, and the pulmonary vascular markings are very prominent. The sign of "high" origin of the pulmonary artery is not useful in the newborn period. Right ventricular hypertrophy is almost always present, and sometimes there is biventricular hypertrophy. Arterial pH and P_{CO_2} are normal unless the neonate is in heart failure. Pa_{O_2} is low and unresponsive to the infant's breathing of 100% O_2. If heart failure supervenes, that part of the Pa_{O_2} depression caused by hypoventilation is improved by 100% O_2 breathing.

Hemodynamics. There is right ventricular hypertension, and the catheter passes from the right ventricle into the truncus arteriosus. That the pulmonary arteries can usually be entered from the common trunk suggests the diagnosis, which is confirmed by contrast visualization of the truncus arteriosus. The lateral view is useful in defining the exact site of origin of the pulmonary artery (Fig. 11-29).

Treatment. Many neonates respond well to medical measures. However, the response is at the expense of increasing pulmonary vascular resistance. Our policy has been to treat the neonate medically and, then, in consultation with the thoracic team, to make a decision as to whether the baby will grow rapidly enough to allow

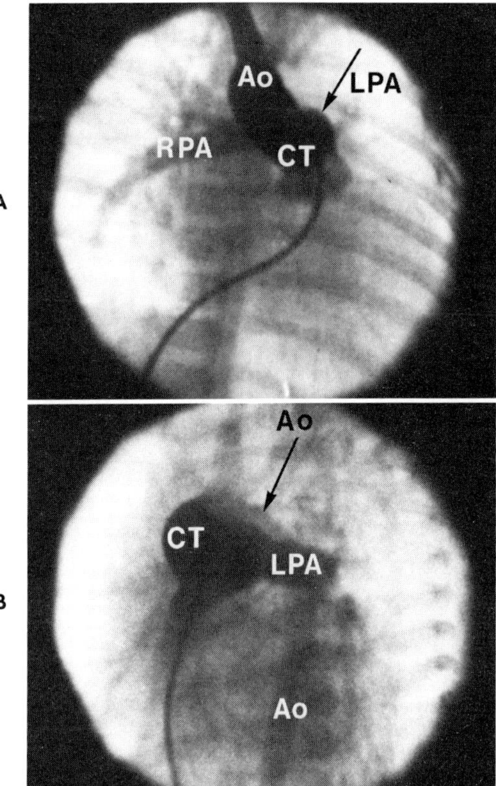

Fig. 11-29. Truncus arteriosus. Single frames taken from cineangiogram. **A,** Anteroposterior projection. Note right *(RPA)* and left *(LPA)* pulmonary arteries arising from the common trunk *(CT)*. Some truncal valve regurgitation is evident. ***B,*** Lateral projection showing the left pulmonary artery arising from the posterior aspect of the trunk. The trunk continues as the aorta *(Ao)*.

a total correction in the first year or two of life. If, as is often the case, the baby gains weight extremely slowly, banding of the pulmonary artery is necessary to lower pulmonary blood flow, reduce distal pulmonary artery pressure, and allow the infant to grow faster. Definitive surgical repair consists essentially of closing the VSD, disconnecting the pulmonary artery from its truncal origin, and joining the pulmonary artery to the edges of the right ventriculotomy by means of a woven Dacron graft or aortic homograft. A prosthetic heart valve is sutured inside the tubular graft, where it functions as a pulmonary valve.

Single ventricle

A single ventricle is very commonly associated with other anomalies: pulmonic stenosis, common atrium, ASD, and endocardial cushion defects. Thirty-five to 40% of neonates with this anomaly die in the first week of life.

Clinical presentation. Mild to moderate cyanosis is present depending on the ratio of pulmonary to systemic blood flow. There is usually no murmur, or there is a nondescript left parasternal systolic murmur. Most infants without pulmonic stenosis have greatly increased pulmonary blood flow so that respirations tend to be rapid. If heart failure ensues, other signs of respiratory distress appear.

Diagnosis. The heart is large, and pulmonary vascularity is increased. Usually the ECG signs of biventricular hypertrophy are present. In the majority of cases normal Q waves are seen.

Hemodynamics. Common mixing occurs at the ventricular level so that arterial saturation is in the 88% to 92% range. If no other lesions are present, there is increased pulmonary blood flow and pulmonary hypertension. The large number of associated lesions makes selective angiography mandatory for detailed diagnosis.

Treatment. Only rarely is operative treatment possible. Banding of the pulmonary artery may be indicated for uncomplicated single ventricle. Infants with associated pulmonic stenosis may do well for many years; those with severe pulmonic stenosis or pulmonary atresia may benefit from an aorta-to-right pulmonary artery shunt.

Double-outlet right ventricle without pulmonic stenosis

Double-outlet right ventricle occurs in 2% to 3% of neonates with congenital heart disease. Unfortunately, the lesion is almost always associated with anomalies of the aortic arch and with VSD. Extracardiac defects are common, and there is an association with trisomy 18 syndrome.

Clinical presentation. Mild cyanosis is present. The obligatory increase in pulmonary artery pressure and pulmonary blood flow rapidly produces tachypnea followed by right-sided heart failure. The outcome is often determined by the degree of

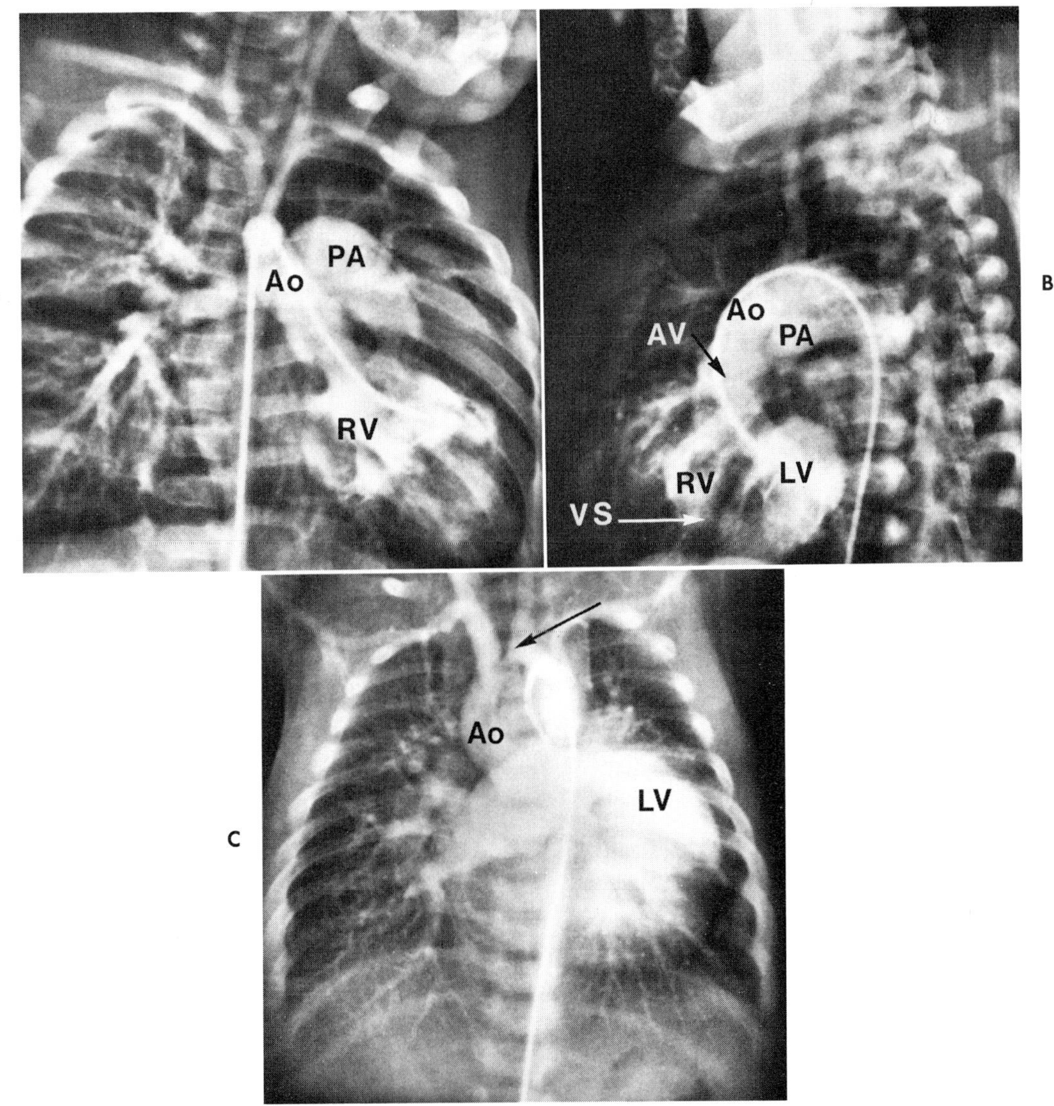

Fig. 11-30. Angiographic appearances in double-outlet right ventricle. Selective streaming from the left ventricle occurs across the VSD into the aorta so that the pulmonary artery fills predominantly from the right ventricle *(RV)* and the aorta from the left ventricle *(RV)*. **A,** Following left ventricular injection, the angiogram shows opacification of the left ventricle, right ventricle, pulmonary artery *(PA)*, and aorta *(Ao)*. **B,** In the lateral projection, the aortic valve *(AV)* is seen to be high, and the ascending aorta proceeds vertically. The two semilunar valves are both anterior to the ventricular septum *(VS)* and are in the same sagittal plane. **C,** Levocardiogram phase following pulmonary artery injection (different infant from that in **A** and **B**). Note left ventricle supplies aorta by way of a VSD. The aortic arch (arrow) is hypoplastic, as is often the case.

hypoplasia of the aortic arch and by the location of the VSD. The murmur of a VSD is usually present.

Diagnosis. Gross cardiomegaly and increased pulmonary vascular markings are characteristic. There is usually combined ventricular hypertrophy. The diagnosis rests on angiographic evidence of the great artery origins. The aortic and pulmonary valves both arise from the right ventricle (anterior ventricle) and at the same level (normally the pulmonary valve is higher) (Fig. 11-30). Frequently there is hypoplasia of the aortic arch.

Treatment. Only rarely is palliative surgery of major value. Infants may benefit from pulmonary artery banding because of the presence of other serious intracardiac and extracardiac anomalies. Double-outlet right ventricle *with* pulmonic stenosis is rarely observed in the neonatal period; the obstruction is often subvalvular in location, and it appears likely that it is an acquired lesion. Complete correction of double-outlet right ventricle with and without pulmonic stenosis has been described, but so far survivors are few.

Total anomalous pulmonary venous return

Total anomalous pulmonary venous return implies the return of all pulmonary venous blood directly or indirectly to the right atrium and requires the presence of an ASD in order that blood may reach the left atrium, left ventricle, and systemic circulation. The lesion is important, since it is frequently surgically correctable. The incidence is 2% to 4%. The lesion appears at all ages in childhood. The singlemost important determinant of the time of presentation appears to be the degree of obstruction to pulmonary venous return. Thus when the pulmonary veins drain below the diaphragm and into the liver, symptoms occur early; whereas when the pulmonary veins drain directly into the right atrium and there is a large ASD, the hemodynamics are very similar to that of an ASD. The mild arterial unsaturation that is present may go unnoticed for many years.

Clinical presentation. Infants with total anomalous pulmonary venous return, who become seriously sick in the newborn period, almost always have a degree of obstruction to the return of pulmonary venous blood. Thus there is increased pulmonary vein pressure, increased pulmonary capillary pressure, and increased pulmonary artery pressure.

There are four main types, according to the mode of entry of the pulmonary veins into the right heart: (1) drainage of pulmonary veins into the right atrium, directly or via the coronary sinus, (2) drainage into the right superior vena cava or azygos vein, (3) drainage into a persistent left superior vena cava, which then empties into the left innominate vein, and (4) drainage of a common pulmonary venous collecting trunk below the diaphragm into the portal vein or ductus venosus. There are a very large number of variations of these four basic types. Neonates with the disease who develop serious symptoms usually have drainage of the anomalous veins below the diaphragm or into the superior vena caval system, with inadequate caliber of the left innominate vein.

Clinically, there is marked tachypnea, and pulmonary rales are heard if pulmonary venous pressure is elevated. Less commonly, the signs of right heart failure develop secondary to raised right atrial pressure. The infants are mildly or moderately cyanotic. A gallop rhythm is frequently present, and there is marked right ventricular overactivity. Commonly, there is no murmur. If present, the murmur often resembles that of an ASD with a midsystolic ejection component at the upper left sternal border and a flow murmur of relative tricuspid stenosis at the lower left sternal border. Frequently, the second heart sound is widely split and fixed with regard to respiration.

Diagnosis. The contours considered characteristic of the condition (figure-of-eight, and so on) are not often seen in the newborn, presumably because insufficient time has elapsed for superior vena caval distension to occur. In the newborn the observation of a small heart with the pattern of pulmonary *venous* congestion is very suggestive of total anomalous pulmonary venous return with obstruction. In those without obstruction but with overwhelming pulmonary blood flow, there is cardiomegaly and an increase in pulmonary *arterial* markings (Fig. 11-31).

The ECG shows moderate right ventricular hypertrophy. There is usually complete reversal of R/S progression in the precordial leads; for example, a dominant R wave in lead V_1 and a dominant S wave in lead V_6. Signs of right atrial hypertrophy are frequent.

The arterial pH and P_{CO_2} are usually normal unless heart failure is present. The Pa_{O_2} is inevitably lowered, though cyanosis may not be clinically apparent (arterial saturation 88% to 92%). The Pa_{O_2} will not exceed 100 mm Hg during oxygen breathing, since hypoxemia is caused by right-to-left shunting.

Hemodynamics. The hemodynamics are extremely variable and are dependent on the presence of obstruction to pulmonary vein return, the adequacy of the ASD, and the presence of additional defects. Typically, right atrial pressure is slightly elevated; and if the anomalous pulmonary collecting trunk can be entered with the catheter (which it frequently can), a rise in pressure can be demonstrated as the catheter advances retrogradely toward the pulmonary capillary bed. The point of entry of pulmonary venous blood into the right heart can frequently be identified by a sudden rise in oxygen saturation. Pulmonary arterial saturation is generally about 2% higher than systemic arterial saturation (because of streaming effects within the right atrium); the degree of pulmonary hypertension is variable, depending on the pulmonary blood flow and pulmonary vein pressure.

Angiography is essential for detailed diagnosis. Ideally, the anomalous pulmonary vein trunk can be carefully opacified; a second choice is opacification of the main pulmonary artery or right ventricle, with filming of the levocardiogram phase (Fig. 11-31). It is important to determine the exact relationship between the collecting trunk and the left atrium if surgery is contemplated. If the infant has not received excessive contrast agent, opacification of

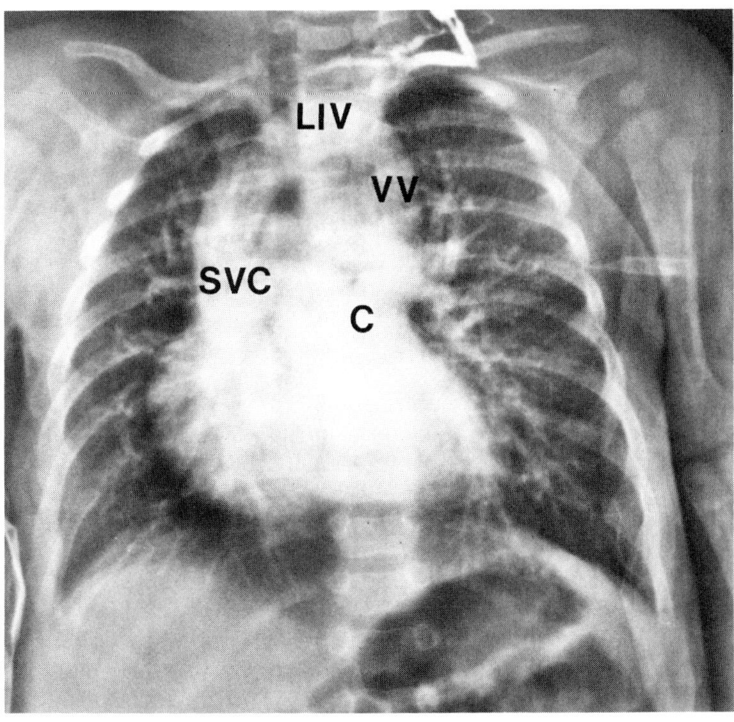

Fig. 11-31. Total anomalous pulmonary venous return. Contrast agent has been injected into a peripheral vein. The levocardiogram phase shows the confluence of pulmonary veins *(C)* ascending via a vertical vein *(VV)* into the left innominate vein *(LIV)* to enter the superior vena cava *(SVC)*.

the left atrium and left ventricle is desirable, since these structures are frequently undersized and may determine the surgical outcome.

Treatment. The presence of a significant gradient across the atrial septum is an indication for a balloon septostomy (Rashkind procedure), and this alone may sometimes decompress the right atrium sufficiently to allow the infant to thrive until weight gain decreases the risk of open-heart surgery. Vigorous treatment of heart failure is indicated; but if the infant is deteriorating, thoracic surgical consultation should be sought and plans made for immediate correction. In the majority of instances the anomalous pulmonary venous collecting trunk runs immediately behind the left atrium so that surgery consists in performing an anastomosis between these two structures.

Prognosis. The mortality is high because the infants are small and frequently very sick, and open-heart surgery may have to be performed under emergency conditions. The mortality in infants is approximately 50% compared with about 18% to 20% in children 2 to 10 years old. The mortality is similar regardless of the anatomy. A major determinant appears to be the adequacy of the left ventricle to handle the additional volume load and avoid pulmonary edema following surgical repair.

Left-to-right shunts

Four types of left-to-right shunts are considered in the following sections: PDA, VSD, combined patent ductus and ventricular septal defects, endocardial cushion (especially common A-V canal), and systemic A-V fistulas. ASDs are present in the newborn period but rarely cause symptoms. Total anomalous pulmonary venous return is considered as a "common-mixing" lesion rather than a left-to-right shunt. Infants with left-to-right shunts have certain clinical characteristics in common. The neonates are acyanotic; the cardiac impulse is hyperactive; and the chest roentgenogram shows cardiac enlargement with an increase in pulmonary vascular markings.

Patent ductus arteriosus

Indirect evidence indicates that the normal human ductus arteriosus undergoes fairly rapid initial constriction during the first few hours after delivery of the baby, followed by a more gradual final functional closure over 1 to 8 days. In premature infants, closure of the ductus may be delayed up until the time of full gestational age and beyond. Thus surgical closure of a PDA is rarely indicated in the premature infant, since spontaneous closure can be anticipated in most instances. Spontaneous closure of the ductus arteriosus occasionally occurs after the neonatal period. The incidence of spontaneous closure is not certain but is well below that of the VSD.

Clinical presentation. In the neonate it is common to hear a soft inconstant systolic murmur at the upper left sternal border in the first 10 hours of life. The closure of the ductus arteriosus is strongly influenced by the Po_2 of the blood perfusing it. However, there are paradoxes; thus the ductus arteriosus remains widely patent in infants with severe HMD but, unfortunately, does not always remain open in infants with pulmonary atresia and hypoxemia, even through arterial and ductal Po_2 may be at fetal levels.

A widely patent ductus arteriosus is an important and fairly frequent cause of serious illness in the neonate. The isolated lesion of PDA is found in 3% of sick neonates. Such neonates may be in serious heart failure and frequently have associated pneumonia. Surgical division or ligation of the ductus is dramatically successful in correcting both heart failure and pneumonia. Neonates with symptomatic ductus arteriosus are tachypneic and later exhibit pulmonary rales and the signs of right heart failure. In advanced left heart failure they are cyanotic from alveolar hypoventilation secondary to airway obstruction. The peripheral pulses are bounding, and the cardiac impulse is hyperdynamic. There is usually no thrill, but a harsh multifrequency systolic murmur is evident at the left sternal border. The murmur resembles that of a VSD but is slightly higher in location and more "grating" in character. The "swishing" continuous murmur heard in some neonates with PDA requires a low pulmonary artery pressure; such infants are rarely in serious trouble in the neonatal period.

Diagnosis. The heart is enlarged, and the

pulmonary vascular markings are increased. The classic contour is that of left ventricular and left atrial enlargement; however, in most cases the cardiomegaly is rather nonspecific. The ECG is almost always abnormal in seriously sick neonates. Both right ventricular hypertrophy and biventricular hypertrophy are seen.

The infant in heart failure from a PDA is frequently hypoxemic from alveolar hypoventilation and may mistakenly be thought to have a right-to-left shunt. The pH is usually normal (compensated respiratory acidosis), the Pa_{CO_2} elevated, and the Pa_{O_2} depressed. Since the depressed Pa_{O_2} is caused by hypoventilation, the breathing of 100% O_2 should result in a level of 300 mm Hg or greater.

Hemodynamics. The diagnosis is easily and rapidly confirmed by right heart catheterization. There is usually right ventricular and pulmonary arterial hypertension, and the catheter readily transverses the patent ductus to enter the descending aorta. There is a step-up in O_2 saturation at the pulmonary artery level, and the degree of left-to-right shunting can be calculated. Frequently, the catheter enters the left atrium across a foramen ovale; the left atrial pressure and left ventricular end-diastolic pressures are raised. When necessary (chiefly to rule out other lesions, such as VSD or aortic arch hypoplasia), left ventricular angiography filmed in the left anterior oblique projection visualizes the ductus and excludes the aforementioned complicating lesions. If doubt exists as to the status of the left ventricle and proximal aorta, it may occasionally be necessary to perform retrograde arterial catheterization using the transfemoral approach or the umbilical artery (if the infant is less than 3 days of age).

Treatment. Medical treatment of heart failure and pneumonia should be pursued vigorously, since the majority of infants with isolated PDA survive the neonatal period, and surgery can be performed electively when the infant reaches age 1 or 2. In a minority, symptoms progress, and ligation of the ductus is indicated. Since the cause of the heart failure and pneumonia are being totally removed by surgery and since the thoracic surgical procedure is rapid, this operation is truly life saving. A neonate may appear to be in irreversible pulmonary edema; yet with careful medical management before surgery and with the operation performed by an experienced surgeon, the infant's recovery is both frequent and rapid.

Ventricular septal defect

Isolated VSD is not a common cause of serious illness in the neonate. This is because of the relatively high pulmonary vascular resistance at birth and the probability (supported by hemodynamic studies) that the normal postnatal fall in pulmonary vascular resistance in those infants with large VSDs may be delayed or slow. The infant destined to develop heart failure from a large isolated VSD typically develops heart failure at 6 weeks to 4 months of age. Nevertheless about 3% of sick neonates will have serious heart failure from an isolated VSD.

VSD is an extremely common lesion in asymptomic newborns and is frequently associated with other congenital heart lesions. A VSD probably is present in at least 1 in every 1,000 newborns. The natural history of isolated VSD has been greatly clarified over recent years, and it is now clear that spontaneous closure can be anticipated in approximately one third, a few closures occurring as late as the fifth decade of life. This realization has greatly influenced management and has resulted in the application of stricter criteria before advising surgical closure in asymptomatic children.

Clinical presentation. The neonate who becomes severely symptomatic from isolated VSD usually has a very large defect and typically develops heart failure in the third or fourth week of life. There is usually common mixing of venous and arterial blood at the ventricular level, resulting in a mildly cyanotic infant. The physical signs of mild cyanosis, an overactive precordium, and a loud pulmonary closure sound are sometimes accompanied by a typical VSD murmur at the lower left sternal border. However, in other neonates, the systemic and pulmonary vascular resistances are almost balanced, and there is little or no murmur. Thus the condition may mimic transposition with VSD, truncus arteriosus, and other "common-mixing" situations.

Diagnosis. The heart is large, but the

contour is usually not diagnostically helpful. The barium swallow may reveal left atrial enlargement. The pulmonary vasculature is increased. Broad-notched P waves indicative of left atrial enlargement are frequent. There may be right or combined ventricular hypertrophy.

The neonate with a large VSD who has severe symptoms usually is cyanotic from a combination of alveolar hypoventilation (alveolar transudate) and right-to-left shunting (at the ventricular level). Typically, there is a mild compensated respiratory acidosis: the Pa_{O_2} is depressed, and only that fraction of the depression caused by alveolar hypoventilation is responsive to the breathing of 100% O_2.

Hemodynamics. The neonate with heart failure from a large VSD has rather different hemodynamics from his older-infant counterpart. The VSD is large, sometimes approaching "single ventricle." In addition, there may be multiple defects, and frequently the muscular part of the septum is involved.

At cardiac catheterization, the venous approach reveals right ventricular and pulmonary arterial hypertension. The increase in O_2 saturation in the right ventricle may be quite small because of near-equaliza-

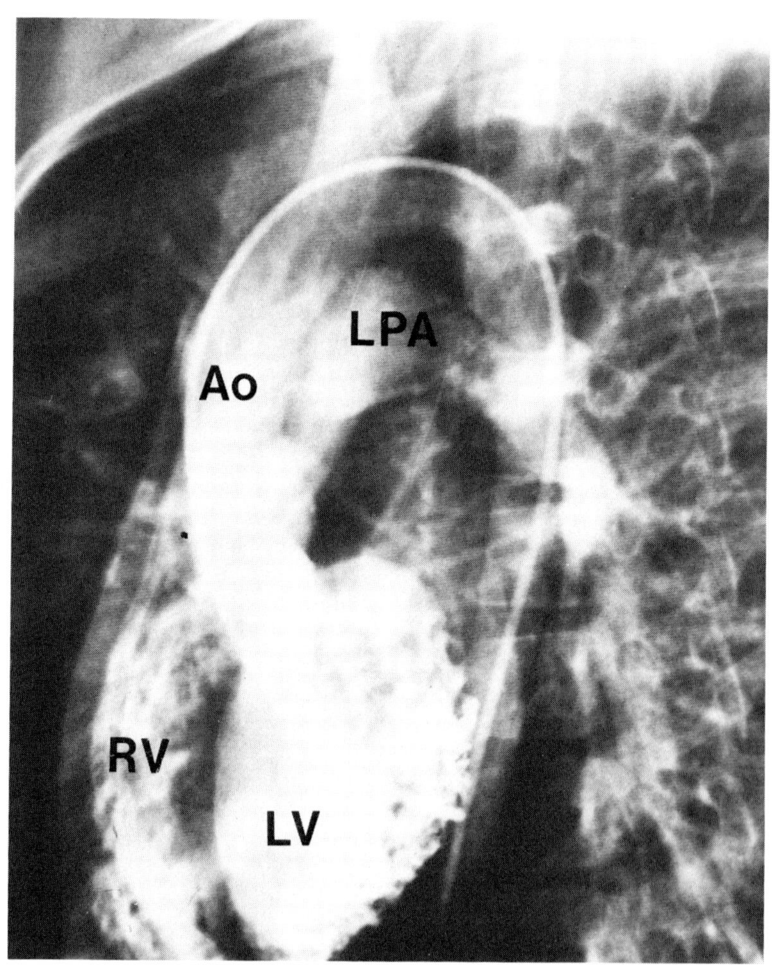

Fig. 11-32. Angiographic appearances of VSD. The catheter is in the left ventricle *(LV)*. Contrast passes through a high VSD into the right ventricle *(RV)* and fills the aorta *(Ao)* and pulmonary artery *(LPA)*.

tion of pulmonary and systemic vascular resistances and ventricular pressures. When the left atrium can be entered, the pressure is usually increased, the degree being proportional to the pulmonary blood flow.

Definitive diagnosis rests on angiocardiography; it is important to know not only the size and location of the VSD but also the existence of other cardiac anomalies. Left ventricular opacification in the lateral or left anterior oblique projection is most useful (Fig. 11-32); but if the left ventricle cannot be entered via the foramen ovale (as is frequently the case), right ventricular angiography can outline the ventricular septum. If there is a right-to-left shunt, the left ventricle and aorta are also visualized. Occasionally, transarterial catheterization may be necessary to visualize the left ventricle.

Treatment. Medical treatment of heart failure is indicated; but if there is not obvious and sustained improvement within 2 or 3 days, serious consideration should be given to early surgical banding of the pulmonary artery. The aim of pulmonary artery banding is not only to relieve the neonate of his immediate problem (heart failure) but to protect the lungs from the long-term effects of increased blood flow and pressure. There is some evidence that neonates who develop heart failure with isolated VSD are particularly likely to have an accelerated onset of pulmonary vascular obliterative disease. This seems especially true of those with left atrial and pulmonary vein hypertension (that is, those who are likely to have pulmonary rales). Since this group of neonates is likely to have large or multiple VSDs, banding and later total repair appears to offer less risk compared with attempts at early one-stage total correction or prolonged medical management with the risks of progressive pulmonary vascular obliterative disease. Small sick infants in intractable heart failure from isolated VSDs can be banded; the hospital mortality is less than 5%, provided intraoperative and postoperative care is optimal.

Combined patent ductus arteriosus and ventricular septal defect

The lesions of PDA and VSD are frequently combined and cause symptomatic disease in the neonate. Either lesion may predominate, though frequently the calculated left-to-right shunts through each are approximately equal.

The physical signs are those of a left ventricular hyperdynamic cardiac impulse, bounding pulses (if the PDA component is substantial), and a systolic thrill and murmur at the third or fourth left interspace. The signs vary somewhat according to which lesion is dominant; it is unusual, however, to hear the typical continuous murmur of a PDA.

The chest roentgenogram discloses a large heart with increased pulmonary vascularity; and the ECG reveals left or combined ventricular hypertrophy except if significant pulmonary hypertension is present, in which case isolated right ventricular hypertrophy may be seen. At cardiac catheterization the ventricular defect is detected by the step-up in oxygen saturation at the right ventricular level, and commonly the catheter crosses the ventricular septum to enter the aorta. When necessary, left ventricular angiography secures the diagnosis. The presence of a PDA is usually demonstrated by catheter passage through it into the descending aorta, and the quantitation of left-to-right shunting is assessed by further increase in oxygen saturation at the pulmonary arterial level. If doubt exists, aortography or left ventriculography is indicated to settle the issue.

It is important to try to determine (by oximetry and angiography) which of the lesions is causing the greater left-to-right shunt. The calculations can be misleading because if a large VSD is present, pulmonary artery pressure may be raised and the ductal shunting reduced (because of a lesser pressure gradient than would exist without the VSD). When both lesions are equally present, division of the ductus usually does not improve the situation. In the case of the neonate in heart failure it seems that the best surgical treatment is division of the ductus, accompanied by banding of the main pulmonary artery, followed by closure of the VSD and unbanding of the pulmonary artery at the appropriate age (usually 1 to 4 years).

Common atrioventricular canal

Common A-V canal is virtually the only type of endocardial cushion defect that causes serious problems in the newborn period. There is a large A-V septal defect of an elliptical configuration, and the aortic leaflet of the mitral valve and the septal leaflet of the tricuspid valve are both cleft. The result is that all four cardiac chambers are in communication, one with another, and additionally there is regurgitation of varying degree through the cleft mitral and tricuspid valves. The association with Down's syndrome is well known; however, neonates without chromosomal anomaly also may have endocardial cushion defects.

Clinical presentation. The severity of the hemodynamic abnormality usually results in symptoms appearing in the first or second week of life. The major important variable is the degree of valvular regurgitation present, especially mitral regurgitation. A few children remain asymptomatic for many years; such children often turn out to have a major atrial component to their lesion, with a small VSD and minimal valvular regurgitation.

Neonates with a common A-V canal tend rapidly to develop tachypnea and liver enlargement. They may be mildly cyanotic from right-to-left shunting. The precordial impulse is hyperdynamic; the pulmonary closure sound is loud. Murmurs are variable. The most frequent finding is a loud pansystolic murmur at the lower left sternal border and a more blowing apical decrescendo pansystolic murmur; the former arises from the VSD, the latter from mitral insufficiency. Frequently, there is a middiastolic apical murmur caused by increased mitral valve diastolic flow.

Diagnosis. The heart is invariably enlarged, and the pulmonary vasculature is increased; but the contour is nonspecific. Left axis deviation is present in the majority of patients and is a most helpful diagnostic finding. Biatrial enlargement and right or combined ventricular hypertrophy are also frequent and depend mainly on whether valvular regurgitation or shunting is hemodynamically dominant. Most infants are in mild heart failure so that a compensated respiratory acidosis with elevated Pa_{CO_2} and normal pH is present. The Pa_{O_2} is depressed from right-to-left shunting and is not responsive to 100% O_2 breathing.

Hemodynamics. Hemodynamic studies of severely symptomatic neonates usually demonstrate raised atrial and right ventricular pressures. The catheter characteristically can be advanced from the right atrium to the left atrium to the left ventricle, and then on withdrawal enters the right ventricle, demonstrating continuity between all four chambers. There is pulmonary artery hypertension and evidence of left-to-right shunting, usually at both the atrial and the ventricular levels. It is important to determine whether the major stepup is at the atrial level or at the ventricular level because of surgical considerations. Mitral and tricuspid valve regurgitation can best be assessed by left and right ventricular angiography.

Treatment. Medical treatment offers the major hope in the neonate. The ultimate aim is to allow the infant to gain sufficient weight for total correction to be attempted. The results of total correction of the common A-V canal have been disappointing because of the gross distortion of normal anatomy, the frequent presence of pulmonary vascular disease, and the risk of postoperative heart block. A small number of infants may benefit from pulmonary artery banding in infancy; these are infants in whom the major shunt is at the ventricular level and A-V valve regurgitation is minimal.

Prognosis. In the series of Stark and associates, 8 of the 13 infants with complete A-V canal survived the operation and are reported well, though most are cyanotic at rest. The child with common A-V canal who fares best following corrective surgery appears to be the one in whom the major shunt is at the atrial level (ostium primum ASD) and in whom the ventricular component is small. Such children are likely to have a near-normal pulmonary artery pressure. The existence of gross mitral or tricuspid valve regurgitation greatly worsens the prognosis both for palliative (pulmonary artery banding) surgery and for total correction.

Systemic arteriovenous fistula

Systemic arteriovenous fistulas are relatively uncommon as a cause of severe illness in the neonate; but their recognition is important because some are treatable, and if they go untreated they may cause death early in the neonatal period. The commonest sites associated with severe heart failure appear to be the brain and the liver. Serious consideration should be given to the possibility of a systemic arteriovenous fistula whenever heart failure of obscure cause occurs in a neonate.

Intracranial arteriovenous fistula. Cerebral malformations involving the great vein of Galen are the most frequent intracranial arteriovenous fistulas. The clinical presentation includes tachypnea, pallor, dyspnea, and cyanosis. Signs of respiratory distress and congestive heart failure may be prominent. A cranial bruit is usually but not invariably heard. Skull measurements and transillumination may be normal. The cardiac impulse is often hyperdynamic and maximal at the lower left sternal border. There may be a systolic regurgitant murmur. The liver edge is usually enlarged below the right costal margin when congestive heart failure occurs.

The chest roentgenogram may show massive cardiac enlargement as well as active and passive pulmonary vascular engorgement. The ECG may suggest right ventricular hypertrophy. Hemodynamic studies may reveal systemic pressures in the pulmonary artery and right ventricle and oxygen saturation as high as 94% in the superior vena cava. Cineangiography with injection of contrast material into the left ventricle shows an intact ventricular septum and normal aortic root. Following opacification of the aortic arch and brachiocephalic vessels, there can be extremely rapid recirculation of the contrast agent so that the jugular veins, superior vena cava, and right atrium become rapidly and densely opacified. The mean left atrial and left ventricular end-diastolic pressures may be elevated, confirming the impression of left ventricular failure. Cerebral angiography establishes the diagnosis (Fig. 11-33).

These infants may respond satisfactorily to medical management. However, most infants with intracranial arteriovenous fistulas deteriorate rapidly. Some have medically irreversible heart failure, while in others CNS symptoms predominate. Surgical clipping of feeding arteries has been successful.

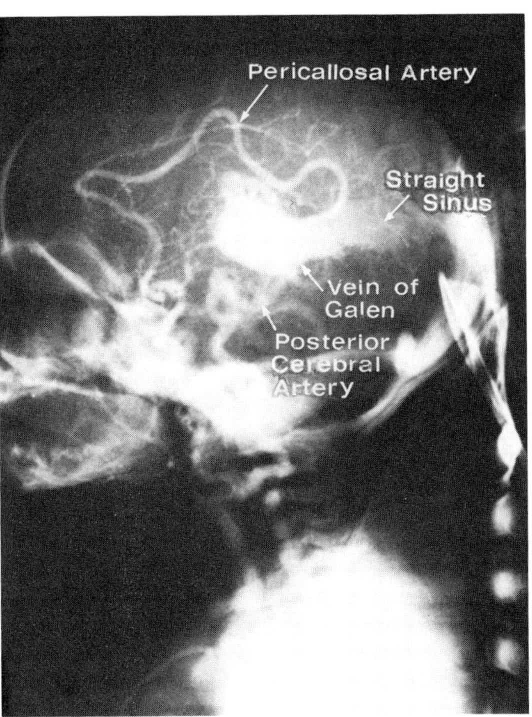

Fig. 11-33. Arteriovenous fistulas; intracranial communication. Right innominate artery injection demonstrates aneurysmal vein of Galen, which is fed directly by the right posterior cerebral artery and an enlarged, tortuous pericallosal artery. A markedly dilated straight sinus is seen draining from the vein of Galen into the transverse sinus.

Giant hemangioma of the liver. Giant hemangioma of the liver may cause heart failure in the newborn period. There is a hyperactive cardiac impulse, gross hepatomegaly, and cardiac failure of obscure origin. Cardiac catheterization reveals highly saturated blood in the inferior vena cava. Berdon and Baker have described a method whereby the blood supply (portal vein or hepatic artery) can be determined by selective angiography, and they have described the successful removal of such a lesion with resolution of heart failure.

Other systemic arteriovenous fistulas. Numerous case reports attest to the many variants that occur and give rise to "high output" heart failure. In many instances they can be surgically corrected. Occasionally a cutaneous hemangioma is large enough to cause death from congestive heart failure in the neonatal period.

Myocardial disorders

The more common conditions giving rise to neonatal heart failure through primary myocardial dysfunction are myocarditis, endocardial fibroelastosis, glycogen storage disease (type II—that is, Pompe's disease), and anomalous origin of the left coronary artery from the pulmonary artery. The latter condition is actually a form of structural cardiovascular disease, but the clinical presentation is frequently that of a myocardiopathy. A large number of rare conditions may produce myocardial dysfunction both as primary disorders (such as tumors of the heart) and as disorders secondary to systemic disease (such as muscular dystrophy). Anomalous left coronary artery, endocardial fibroelastosis, and glycogen storage disease usually appear in infants in the second to sixth month of life. The neonatal series underrepresents the true incidence.

Myocarditis

Neonatal myocarditis may be viral, bacterial, or protozoal *(Toxoplasma gondii)* (p. 148). Viral myocarditis is probably the commonest, though frequently it is not possible to grow any organism from body tissues. The commonest responsible viruses appear to be the coxsackie virus B group and the rubella virus. In addition to the existence of neonatal viral myocarditis the question of the viral cause of congenital malformations has been the subject of much research and speculation. The newborn may have active rubella myocarditis with or without other stigmata of intrauterine rubella infection. Diagnosis is aided by the finding of a high IgM fraction in cord blood and high levels of rubella antibodies. While coxsackievirus infections are often suspected clinically (because of coxsackieviruslike illness in the mother), its presence is frequently difficult to confirm in the newborn. Coxsackievirus myocarditis can occur in epidemic during the neonatal period. The virus is thought to be passed transplacentally.

Septic (bacterial) myocarditis has been rarely encountered since the widespread use of antibiotics. In the past, bacterial myocarditis has been especially associated with pneumonia and diphtheria. *Toxoplasma* may cause myocarditis by direct invasion of the heart by the parasite.

Clinical presentation of viral myocarditis. The neonate with viral myocarditis may appear in a critical state of peripheral circulatory collapse, although in some the onset is more insidious. Frequently there is a history of a viral infection in the mother during the last 2 weeks of pregnancy. Characteristically the infant is normal at birth but rapidly develops the signs and symptoms of heart failure at 3 to 20 days of age. Ausculation usually reveals a gallop rhythm but no murmur. Sometimes the heart sounds are pathologically quiet.

Diagnosis. In the majority the heart is enlarged, and the lungs show the pattern of pulmonary venous congestion. Characteristically the QRS voltages in the standard leads are reduced (Fig. 11-34), and the T waves are frequently inverted or flattened in the left precordial leads.

Although the diagnosis may seem obvious, it is important to rule out septic myocarditis (by blood culture). Any suggestion of anomalous coronary artery (infarct pattern on the ECG or appearance of a mitral regurgitation murmur) may warrant aortography. *Toxoplasmosis* is suggested by abnormal head size, microphthalmia, and chorioretinitis.

Treatment. The mortality from viral myocarditis is very high. Heart failure should be treated and the infant given antibiotics to cover the possibility of septic myocarditis, at least until negative blood cultures are certain. Digitalis should not be given if the infant's heart rate falls below 100 beats per minute. Great attention should be paid to achieving a neutral thermal environment to minimize metabolic needs. The critically sick infant should receive his total nutritional support intravenously. Occasionally, one is confronted with a moribund bradycardic infant as a result of myocarditis. In this situation the use of isoproterenol (0.1 to 0.4 μgm/min/kg or sufficient to raise the heart rate to 120 beats per minute) administered intravenously seems justified.

Endocardial fibroelastosis

Endocardial fibroelastosis occurs both as a primary condition, where the cause is unknown, and as a secondary phenomenon, particularly in association with left heart obstruction. A smooth, glistening, yellowish membrane lines the left ventricle, with

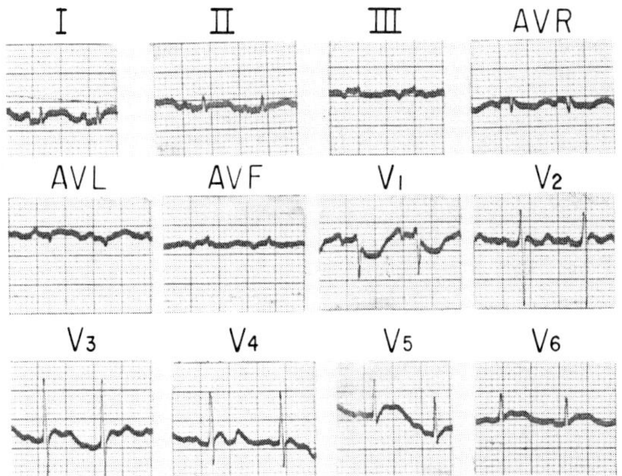

Fig. 11-34. ECG of a baby with proved coxsackievirus myocarditis. At 1 month of age there is low QRS amplitude and S-T depression (V_1). By 2 years of age the cardiogram had returned to normal.

varying degrees of encroachment into the mitral and aortic orifices. The left atrium, and very rarely the right atrium, is occasionally involved. Usually the left ventricle is greatly dilated, but a contracted type of ventricle does occur, especially in the newborn. Theories of causation include genetic determination by an autosomal recessive gene, a form of end-stage myocarditis caused by coxsackievirus or mumps virus, and a theory that the condition may be caused by a primary metabolic defect of cardiac muscle.

Clinical presentation of primary endocardial fibroelastosis. Most infants with endocardial fibroelastosis are referred to diagnostic centers at 2 to 4 months of age with an admission diagnosis of "failure to thrive," heart failure, or cardiomegaly of unknown origin. The history usually reveals that the infant was abnormal during the neonatal period, but the absence of cardiac murmur commonly delays recognition of heart disease.

The symptoms and signs of the primary form of endocardial fibroelastosis are rather characteristic. Infants are undernourished and show evidence of predominantly left heart failure with tachycardia, tachypnea, and inappropriate sweating. The peripheral pulses are normal, and the heart is not hyperdynamic (though it may be large). The heart sounds are normal; some have no murmur, while others have the murmurs of mitral or aortic valve disease.

Diagnosis. There is often gross cardiac dilatation (except the contracted form), and evidence of pulmonary venous congestion is usually present. Marked left ventricular hypertrophy is almost always present. This is manifested not only by the voltage changes but also by secondary T-wave changes (Fig. 11-35). On occasion pathologic Q waves are present.

Differential diagnosis. Endocardial fibroelastosis is usually distinguishable from acute viral myocarditis by the shorter history and by the low-voltage QRS complexes and nonspecific T-wave changes of the latter. Neonates with glycogen storage disease (type II) are hypotonic, have large tongues, and frequently have a positive family history. Skeletal muscle biopsy shows a greatly raised glycogen content in type II glycogen storage disease. The most important differential diagnosis is that of an anomalous left coronary artery arising from the pulmonary artery. This produces a clinical picture and a chest roentgenogram almost identical to those of endocardial fibroelastosis. The diagnosis of anomalous left coronary is strongly suggested by an infarct pattern on the ECG and by the murmur of mitral regurgitation (caused by papillary muscle infarction). Since the anomalous left coronary artery can be surgically treated and mimics endocardial fibroelastosis very closely, it has become our policy to perform an aortogram on every infant with a clinical diagnosis of endocardial fibroelastosis.

Hemodynamics. The left ventricle is large and fails to empty adequately. Left ventricular end-diastolic pressure is raised; and if there is mitral valve involvement, there is frequently a diastolic gradient across the mitral valve, with greatly raised left atrial pressure. Right heart pressures are elevated secondary to left heart pressure elevation. If the patient is undergoing diagnostic studies, it is important to confirm the presence of two normally placed coronary arteries either by left ventricular or aortic root angiography. The cardiac out-put is frequently low and is reflected by a widened arteriovenous oxygen content difference.

Prognosis. The outlook for neonates and infants with the common form of endocardial fibroelastosis (primary form) is unpredictable. Manning and associates re-

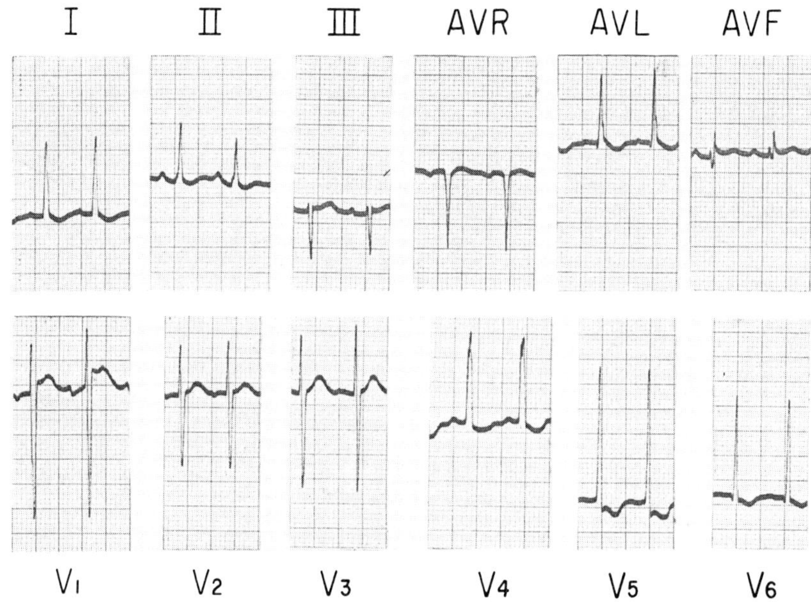

FIG. 11-35. ECG of an infant with endocardial fibroelastosis. All leads are recorded at half standard. There is marked left ventricular hypertrophy with secondary T wave changes (leads I, V_5, and V_6).

ported 31 of 56 infants surviving over 2 years, though many survivors had large hearts and abnormal ECGs. The rapid reversion of the abnormal T waves was a favorable prognostic sign. Since the diagnosis is essentially a pathologic one and it is likely that it is a disease of multifactorial causes, it is extremely difficult to provide parents with a reliable prognosis.

Treatment. There is no specific therapy. Heart failure should be treated and the metabolic needs of the critically sick infant minimized by intravenous feeding and the careful maintenance of thermoneutrality. Digitalis is particularly important, and some infants demonstrate an unusual degree of dependency on digitalis.

Glycogen storage disease

See also p. 429.

The only type of glycogenosis in which the heart is involved to a major extent is type II (Pompe's disease). In this condition there is a defect in the enzyme α 1-4 glucosidase, resulting in the accumulation of glycogen in heart, liver, and skeletal muscle. The disease is usually lethal within the first year.

Clinical presentation. Infants affected with Pompe's disease display a very characteristic clinical picture with failure to thrive, muscular hypotonia, hepatomegaly, and large tongue. Usually there is no cardiac murmur, or there is at most a nondescript systolic murmur that may reflect outflow tract obstruction. Affected infants lay quietly, usually supine and in the hypotonic frog-leg position. The respirations are rapid.

Diagnosis. The heart is large, and the lung fields may show passive pulmonary venous engorgement. A characteristic, but not pathognomonic, ECG has been described. The P-R interval is short; the QRS voltages are much increased; and deep Q waves over the left precordium are frequently seen. In some cases there is T-wave inversion in leads V_5 and V_6. The ECG of a neonate with Pompe's disease is shown in Fig. 11-36.

The diagnosis may be confirmed by the finding of greater than 1.5% glycogen by wet weight in skeletal muscle biopsy; levels of 8% to 10% are not unusual.

Treatment. No definitive treatment is available; the major contribution the pedi-

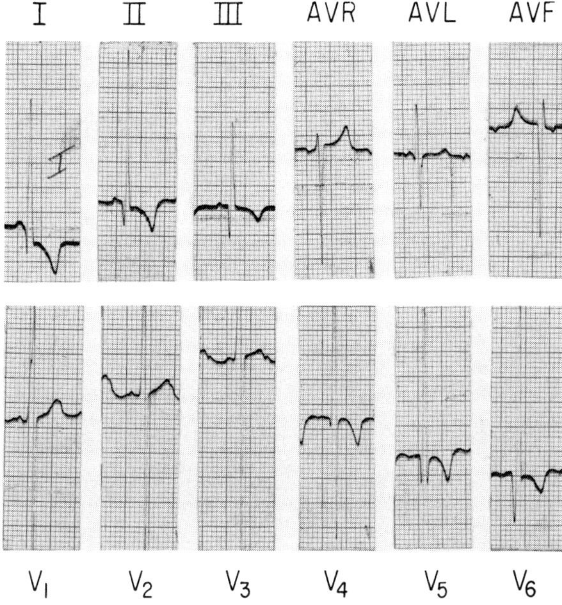

FIG. 11-36. ECG of an infant with type II glycogen storage disease. The P-R interval is short. There is left axis deviation, right ventricular hypertrophy and left ventricular hypertrophy with "strain" (inverted T waves in leads V_5, V_6, and I).

atrician can make is in counseling and alerting the parents to the possibility of diagnosis early in the gestation of future offspring by means of examination of the amniotic fluid for α-glucosidase activity.

Anomalous origin of the left coronary artery from the pulmonary artery

Early recognition of the anomalous left coronary artery is important, since if the condition is untreated the mortality in infancy is high, and both palliative and corrective surgery are available. The incidence is 0.4% to 0.5% of patients with congenital heart disease. The condition is often not recognized in the neonatal period, but symptoms tend to become obvious at age 2 to 4 months. Occasionally the lesion escapes recognition until later childhood or even adult life.

Clinical presentation. The major symptoms are failure to thrive and the manifestations of left ventricular failure. Occasionally, parents will observe episodes that could be interpreted as angina pectoris or coronary occlusion, but in the majority of infants the symptoms differ little from those of endocardial fibroelastosis. There may be no murmur, or the apical systolic murmur of mitral insufficiency may be present. Mitral insufficiency is probably secondary to infarction of the papillary muscles of the mitral valve.

Diagnosis. The heart is characteristically large and empties poorly with each systolic contraction (Fig. 11-37). The most characteristic ECG is that of myocardial infarction (Fig. 11-38). However, in some the appearance is that of ischemia (Fig. 11-39); in a small number only the voltage changes of left ventricular hypertrophy are present.

Hemodynamics. The hemodynamics are greatly influenced by the size and number of anastomoses between the right and left coronary arterial systems and by the pulmonary arterial pressure. Thus infants with many anastomoses and low pulmonary artery pressure have a left-to-right shunt from the aorta to the pulmonary artery by means of the anomalous left coronary artery. This "runoff" into the pulmonary artery compromises coronary capillary–filling pressure and myocardial blood flow to all areas of the heart. Temporary elevation of the pulmonary artery pressure may account for the rarity of diagnosis during the neonatal period. It is important, then, to measure pulmonary artery pressure, assess the degree of left-to-right shunt, and visualize the coronary arterial system. The typical infant shows rapid opacification of the normal right coronary artery, followed by opacification of the anomalous left coronary artery and pulmonary artery (Fig. 11-40).

Treatment. Management is controversial at the present time. Most cardiologists favor medical treatment of the infant with high pulmonary artery pressure, little or no left-to-right shunt, and a stable clinical course. Prolonged survival of these infants is possible, and the anomalous left coronary artery can be anastomosed to the ascending aorta by means of a saphenous vein graft when the child is larger. The sick infant with low pulmonary artery pressure and left-to-right shunting presents a dilemma. Simple ligation of the anomalous coronary artery improves myocardial perfusion but carries a definite mortality. It has been claimed that prolonged medical management can extend the life of these infants to an age at which saphenous vein grafting is feasible. The opposite view favors early ligation in those with left-to-right shunting. Hopefully, infants can survive with or without ligation of the anomalous vessel until saphenous vein autografts or Dacron tube grafts can be placed and prove to be adequate long-term conduits.

Miscellaneous congenital heart conditions

A large number of rare heart lesions may produce symptomatic disease in the neonate. Four of these conditions are men-

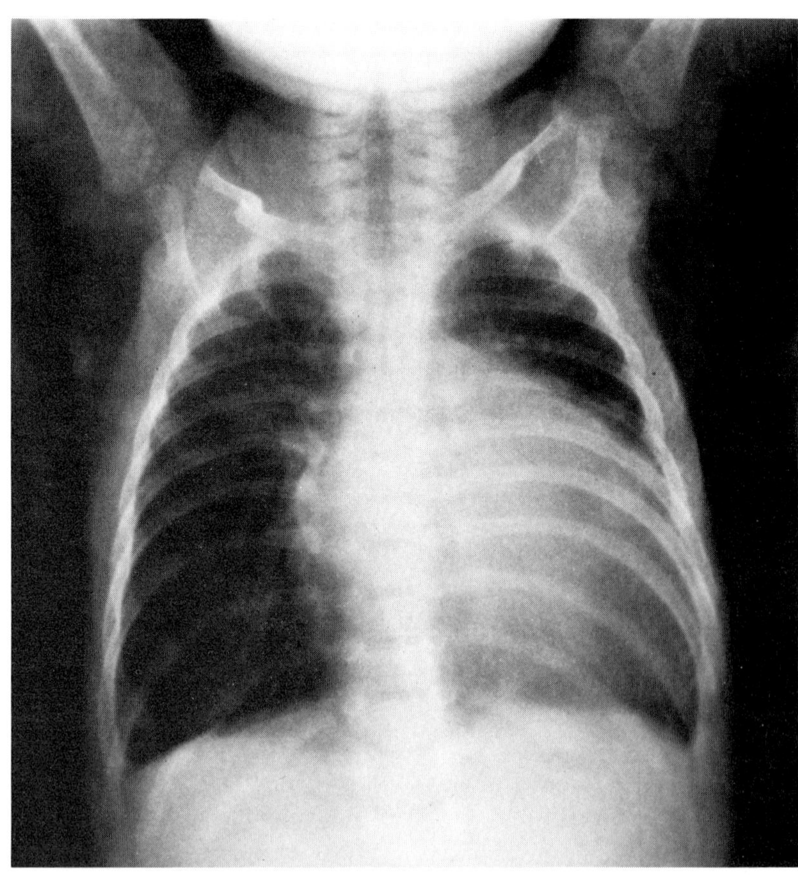

Fig. 11-37. Chest film of an infant with anomalous origin of the left coronary artery from the pulmonary artery. Note extreme cardiomegaly. Fluoroscopically the heart changed very little in volume between systole and diastole.

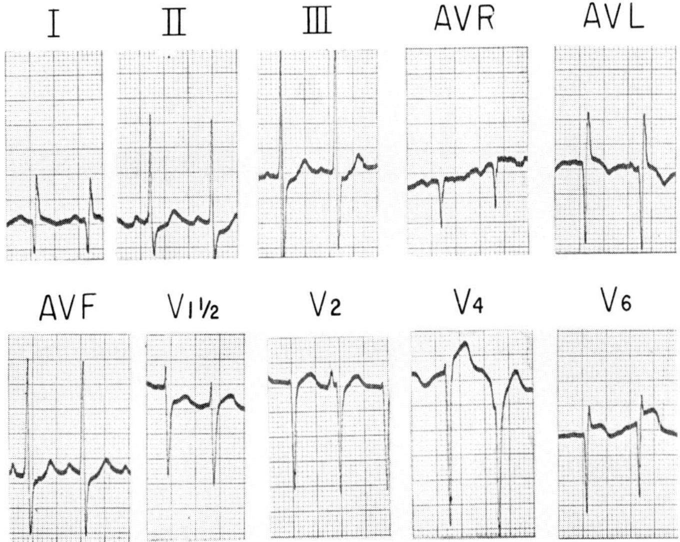

Fig. 11-38. Anomalous origin of the left coronary artery from the pulmonary artery, producing myocardial infarction. Note pathologic Q waves in leads I, AVL, and V_6. At surgery (ligation of anomalous coronary), the apex and posterior wall of the left ventricle showed widespread infarction.

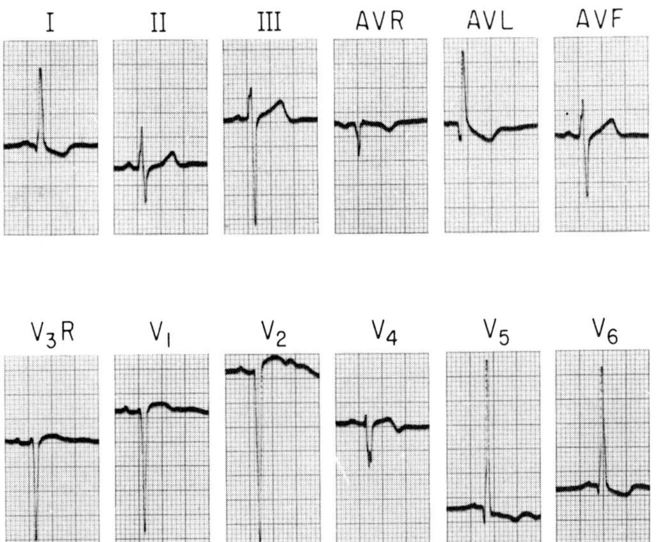

Fig. 11-39. Anomalous origin of the left coronary artery from the pulmonary artery, producing left ventricular hypertrophy with "strain," but no infarction. At surgery (ligation of anomalous coronary) the left ventricle was hypertrophied, but no infarct was found.

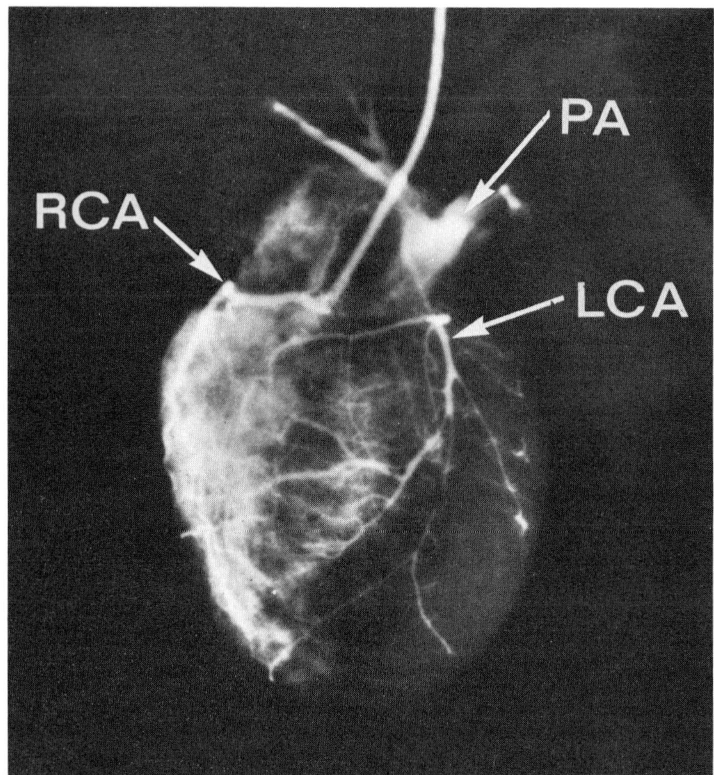

Fig. 11-40. Postmortem coronary arteriogram on an infant with anomalous origin of the left coronary artery. Contrast is injected into the normally placed right coronary artery *(RCA)*. Numerous anastomoses link up the right and left coronary systems. The left coronary artery *(LCA)* is small, and contrast ascends to "run off" into the pulmonary artery *(PA)*. Thus the anomalous coronary artery acts as an arteriovenous fistula and prevents normal perfusion of both the right and left coronary capillary systems.

tioned briefly in the following sections: absence of the pulmonary valve, isolated tricuspid insufficiency, cor triatriatum, and dextrocardia.

Isolated congenital absence of the pulmonary valve

Absence of the pulmonary valve is rare as an isolated anomaly but is found quite frequently in association with tetralogy of Fallot. Diagnosis of the isolated lesion is suggested by a diastolic murmur heard maximally at the second left interspace that is slightly delayed in onset after the pulmonic closure sound. There is an associated systolic murmur because of increased systolic pulmonary valve flow. Pulmonary insufficiency characteristically produces very marked dilatation of the main pulmonary arteries. The diagnosis is confirmed by the absence of a diastolic gradient across the pulmonary valve and by pulmonary artery angiography. The disease has a rather benign course, or the patient dies soon after birth. The poor outcome in some newborns may be because of associated physiologic pulmonary hypertension, causing a significant backward driving force from pulmonary artery to right ventricle and an impairment of adequate right ventricular emptying.

Isolated congenital tricuspid insufficiency

Isolated congenital tricuspid insufficiency is rare and appears to be caused by congenital short chordae tendinae, which prevent closure of apparently adequate valve cusps. The age at death has varied from 5 minutes to 34 years. The diagnosis is suggested by cyanosis (from right-to-left atrial shunting), a loud pansystolic murmur at the lower left sternal border, evidence of grossly raised venous pressure, hepatomegaly, and a large heart with an especially large left atrium. Catheterized neonates have had greatly raised right atrial pressures, and right ventricular angiography has disclosed massive tricuspid regurgitation. Surgical treatment for this condition in the newborn period has been unsuccessful, but the possibility of lowering pulmonary vascular resistance (by increasing inspired oxygen tension or administering vasoactive drugs such as acetylcholine into the pulmonary artery) might allow improved right ventricular emptying.

Cor triatriatum

The division of the left atrium into an inner chamber receiving the pulmonary veins and an outer chamber leading to the mitral valve constitutes cor triatriatum. The communication between the two left atrial chambers is inadequate for the free efflux of pulmonary vein blood so that pulmonary venous pressure rises and the infant dies with the signs of left vetricular failure; failure of the accessory left atrial chamber would be a more accurate description of the hemodynamics.

The condition is rare but important because it is surgically correctable. The first sign is tachypnea, followed by pulmonary rales. Pulmonary hypertension ensues, with a loud pulmonic closure sound. The ECG shows right ventricular hypertrophy. The chest roentgenogram discloses a somewhat enlarged heart with the vascular pattern typical of pulmonary venous engorgement, a lacy pattern throughout the lung fields, often with the Kerley B lines of engorged lymphatics. There is usually no murmur so that the condition mimics primary pulmonary hypertension and a variety of primary respiratory conditions including pulmonary lymphangiectasia and atypical HMD. The condition also mimics other causes of left heart obstruction, especially total anomalous pulmonary venous return with obstruction to pulmonary venous return, pulmonary vein stenosis, and mitral atresia.

Diagnosis is confirmed by cardiac catheterization. There is a discrepancy between pulmonary artery wedge pressure (reflecting the inner chamber) and left atrial pressure. Occasionally the catheter can be passed across the diaphragm connecting the two left atrial chambers, and the gradient can be demonstrated. The anomalous left atrial septum can also be demonstrated angiographically following pulmonary artery contrast agent injection. Surgical relief is possible early in life by excision of the anomalous septum.

Dextrocardia and levocardia with situs inversus

So-called dextroposition of the heart is to be distinguished from true dextrocardia. With dextroposition other pathologic conditions within the chest, such as lung agenesis, congenital lobar emphysema, and diaphragmatic hernia, are responsible for rightward displacement of the heart. In these situations careful appraisal of the lungs and gastrointestinal tract reveals the true nature of the problem. If there is true dextrocardia or true levocardia with situs inversus (that is, no pathologic condition present to cause mediastinal shift), then it is likely that the child will have associated structural congenital heart disease.

Neonates who have either dextrocardia or levocardia with situs inversus account for less than 3% of congenital heart malformations discovered in the newborn period, Dextrocardia with abdominal situs inversus is not infrequently associated with cyanotic cardiac lesions. Neonates with dextrocardia and normally placed viscera or partial situs inversus have a very high incidence of complex cyanotic congenital heart disease, particularly if there is splenic agenesis or polysplenia. Similarly, those with splenic agenesis and levocardia frequently have complex heart disease, whether or not there is abdominal situs inversus.

In management of the neonate with apparent dextrocardia one should consider the following.

1. The possibility of dextroposition caused by movement of the mediastinum secondary to lung agenesis, lobar emphysema, diaphragmatic hernia, and so on should be ruled out. Pulmonary arteriography may be required.
2. An increase in the number of Howell-

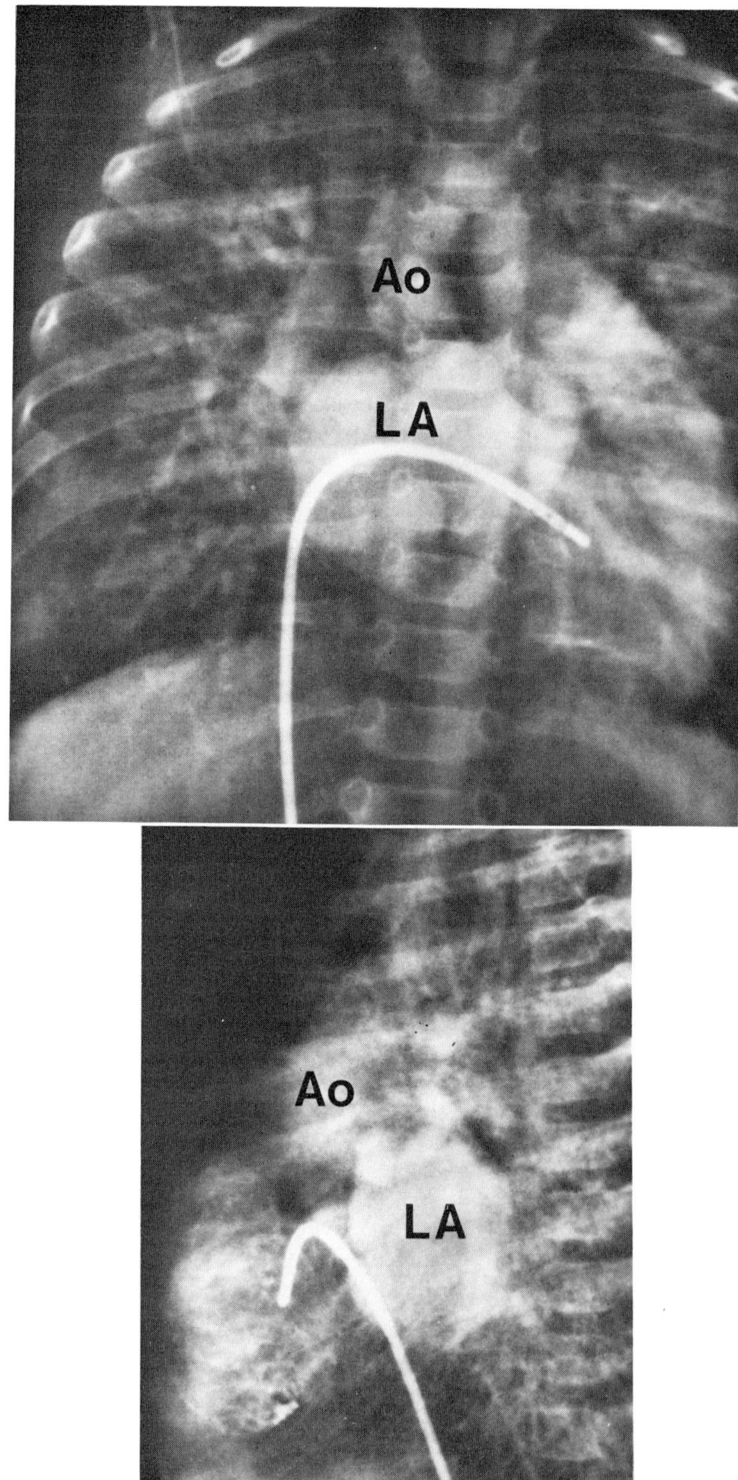

Fig. 11-41. Cor triatriatum in infancy. Catheter tip is in right ventricle. Contrast agent is held up in the left atrium *(LA)*, but the aorta *(Ao)* does opacify. The left ventricle is poorly visualized. Pulmonary artery wedge pressure was 20 mm Hg. At surgery an almost complete web was found in the left atrium and was successfully removed. Cor triatriatum should be considered whenever unexplained pulmonary hypertension is encountered.

Jolly and Heinz bodies and an elevated reticulocyte count suggest splenic agenesis. Splenic agenesis may be confirmed by aortography or by an abnormal spleen scan.
3. An abnormal P axis (such as a negative P wave in lead I) may indicate atrial inversion. It may also be caused by an ectopic atrial pacemaker (sometimes in the left atrium).
4. Cardiac catheterization and angiocardiography are usually necessary for precise chamber localization. The venous atrium and sometimes other chambers are easily reached. However, there is a high incidence of azygos extension of the inferior vena cava, causing a circuitous route. When vein size permits, it is preferable to perform venous catheterization from the right arm. The aorta and systemic ventricle can be conveniently entered by the transfemoral arterial approach.
5. Other congenital defects, especially gastrointestinal and genitourinary tract anomalies, should be looked for.

Treatment. Infants with dextrocardia and levocardia with situs inversus tend to have complex heart disease. This is particularly true if the spleen is absent or rudimentary. If surgical treatment is required, it can usually be only palliative in nature and most often consists of decreasing or increasing pulmonary blood flow by pulmonary artery banding or aortopulmonary shunt.

OTHER CARDIOVASCULAR CONDITIONS

Vascular rings

The precise incidence of symptomatic vascular rings is not known. Out of 6,647 children recorded in the Toronto Heart Registry 0.95% had vascular rings or allied aortic arch anomalies. The overwhelming majority of the estimated 900,000 persons in the United States with an anomalous origin of the right subclavian artery arising from a left descending aorta are asymptomatic and have no positive physical signs. The more important lesions to be considered in the symptomatic newborn are: double aortic arch, right aortic arch with left ligamentum arteriosum, anomalous innominate artery, anomalous origin of the right subclavian artery, and anomalous origin of the left pulmonary artery

Most clinically important vascular rings (for example, double aortic arch and right aortic arch with left ligamentum arteriosum) encircle both the trachea and the esophagus. Some (for example, anomalous origin of the right subclavian artery) give rise to only partial encirclement. The anomalous left pulmonary artery runs between the trachea and esophagus, partially compressing both structures.

Clinical presentation. Neonates with significant constriction usually have respiratory difficulty, often in the first few days of life. Stridor, wheezing, and intercostal retractions all indicate airway obstruction and give rise to hypoventilation, with arterial hypoxemia and hypercapnia when the obstruction is critical. Symptoms related to esophageal compression are usually present and cause aspiration pneumonia. However, it is not usually obvious that the baby has a swallowing difficulty until he takes solid foods. Vascular rings may mimic many other causes of respiratory distress. However, the barium esophagogram is, fortunately, practically always diagnostic.

Diagnosis. Contrast esophagograms should be performed by an experienced radiologist because of the risk of aspiration. Radiologists frequently choose a thin barium mixture, and many prefer to record the swallow on 70-mm or 35-mm cinefluorography for later repeated viewing. Each lesion has rather characteristic features. The double aortic arch produces a constant compression deformity at the level of the aortic arch, with marked posterior indentation and lesser left and right indentations (Fig. 11-42). The features of the right aortic arch with left ligamentum arteriosum are similar, but the indentation on the left side is nonpulsating and sharper (ligamentum arteriosum). The anomalous right subclavian artery produces an oblique or spiral indentation on the posterior esophageal wall, pointing upward and to the right. The anomalous innominate artery arises to the left of the midline and passes in front of the trachea to compress the trachea; the barium swallow is normal. The anomalous left pulmonary artery arises from the main pulmonary trunk just to the

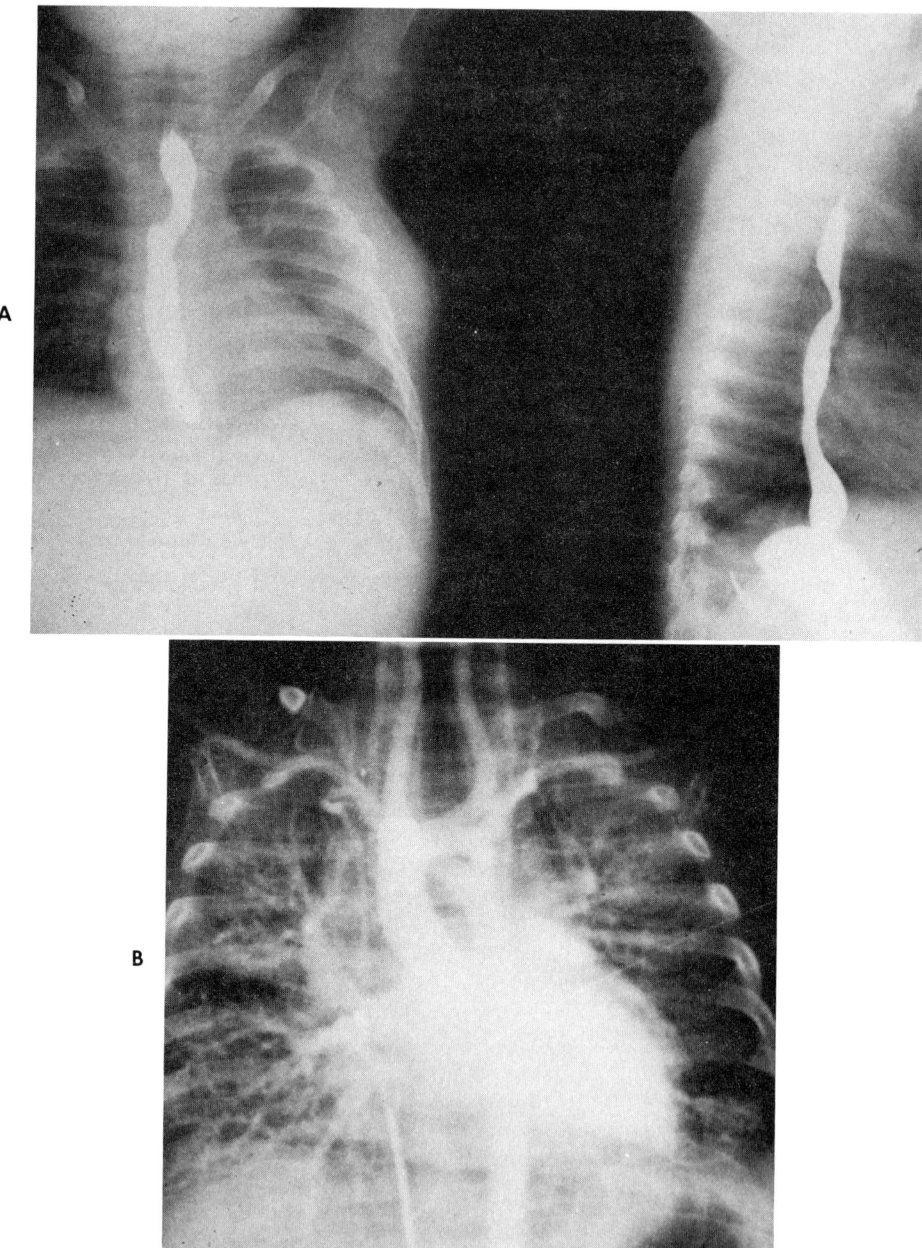

Fig. 11-42. Double aortic arch. **A,** Note imprint of posterior aortic arch on posterior and right aspect of esophagus. **B,** Angiogram discloses double arch. Anterior arch gives rise to left subclavian artery, while the other three brachiocephalic arteries arise from the posterior arch. (Courtesy Dr. John R. Campbell.)

right of the midline. It then proceeds anterior to the esophagus and behind the trachea to compress both structures. An anterior indentation on the esophagus is, therefore, highly suggestive of an anomalous left pulmonary artery (Fig. 11-43). If the trachea shows signs of posterior compression or narrowing, the diagnosis is virtually certain. Frequently the esophagogram is pathognomonic, and no further studies are necessary. In cases of doubt, aortography resolves the issue, though several projections may be necessary. A pulmonary arteriogram usually discloses the anomalous left pulmonary artery. However, a slightly caudally angled anteroposterior projection may be necessary to spatially separate the main and branch pulmonary arteries.

Treatment. Neonates with symptomatic double aortic arch, those with right aortic arch with left ligamentum arteriosum, and those with anomalous left pulmonary artery almost always require surgical correction. Occasionally a neonate with a large retroesophageal right subclavian ar-

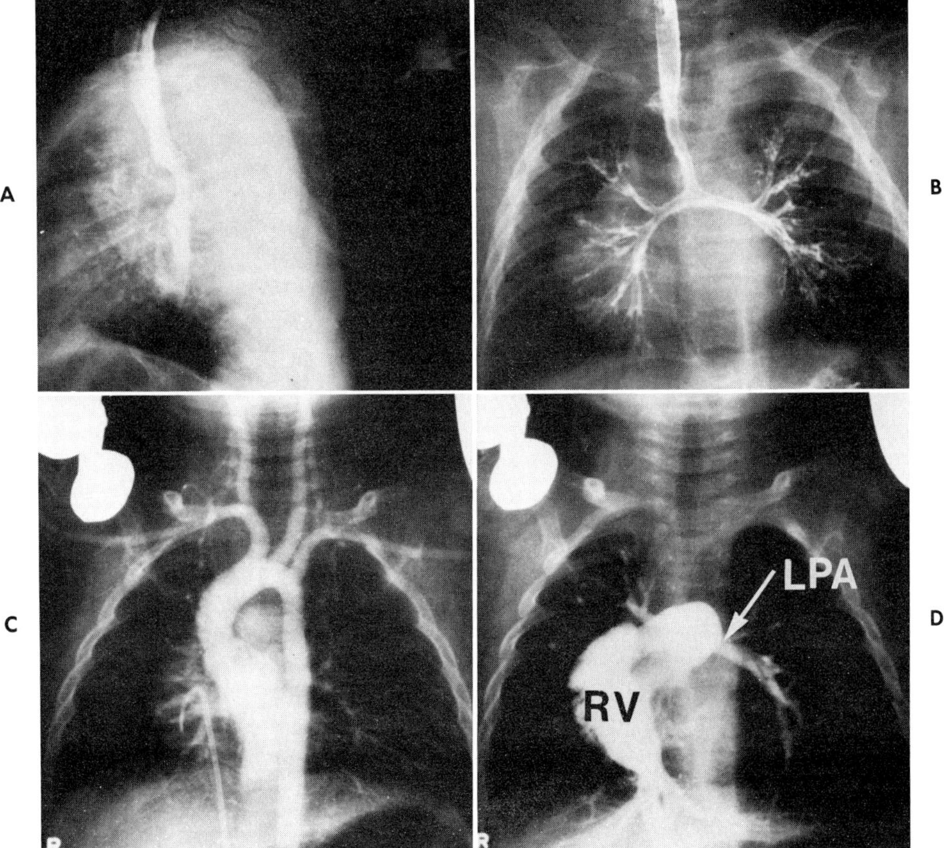

Fig. 11-43. Anomalous left pulmonary artery. The left pulmonary artery proceeds rightward as it leaves the heart. To regain the left lung, it loops leftward between the esophagus and trachea. **A,** Anterior indentation on esophagogram. **B,** Diffuse tracheal narrowing secondary to posterior compression. **C,** Normal levocardiogram. **D,** Right atrial injection. The heart is dextroposed; the right ventricle *(RV)* is in end-systole and has filled an abnormal pulmonary artery (the right ventricle and right atrium are overlapped in this projection). The left pulmonary artery *(LPA)* appears to arise from behind the main pulmonary artery rather than as the usual direct continuation. A more caudally angled anteroposterior projection is necessary to spatially separate the main and branch pulmonary arteries.

tery has respiratory symptoms (usually caused by repeated aspiration pneumonia) sufficiently severe to warrant surgical division of the aberrant vessel. The treatment of the anomalous innominate artery is controversial; it has been suggested that it may occasionally be associated with reflex bouts of apnea. Gross has achieved surgical correction of this anomaly by pulling the vessel forward and attaching it to the sternum. It is, however, a common anomaly and, like the aberrant right subclavian artery, produces no symptoms in the vast majority of patients.

Systemic hypertension

While rarely a true emergency, systemic hypertension in a neonate always requires an explanation and usually treatment. Although antihypertensive treatment may be urgently needed to combat heart failure or minimize the risk of a cerebrovascular accident, the cause must be established even if the hypertension can be successfully controlled with drugs.

Etiology. In the majority of instances systemic hypertension in the neonate is caused by coarctation of the aorta. Nephrogenic hypertension is the next most likely cause. Less likely possibilities include pheochromocytoma, Cushing's syndrome, congenital adrenal hyperplasia, primary hyperaldosteronism, and neuroblastoma (secretion of catecholamines or partial obstruction to the renal artery).

Diagnosis. The accurate estimation of systemic blood pressure and its response to drugs has been much improved by the Doppler reflected ultrasound technique. The blood pressure cuff can be applied to the infant's upper arm, the ultrasound transducer taped over his brachial artery, and repeated measurements made while he is sleeping in an incubator. The blood pressure should be carefully and repeatedly measured in the infant's legs to be sure that isolated coarctation is not present. The leg pressure should be within 20 mm Hg of arm pressure whether measured by the flush or the Doppler method techniques. Brachial and femoral pulses should be felt simultaneously to be sure that they are synchronous.

Examination of the urinary sediment may reveal evidence of underlying acute or chronic renal disease, either of which may be associated with hypertension. Blood should be collected for determination of blood urea nitrogen, creatinine, sodium, potassium, and bicarbonate levels. A 24-hour urine sample can be collected for vanillylmandelic acid, metanephrines, urinary steroid excretion, and, if appropriate, pregnanetriol. A clinical diagnosis of renal disease should be followed by intravenous urography and, if necessary, by renal angiography.

Some nephrologists consider persistent hypertension of unknown cause to be an indication for the estimation of plasma renin activity (to rule out primary hyperaldosteronism) and renal biopsy to rule out the possibility of occult underlying renal disease.

Treatment. The definitive treatment is that of the underlying disease. However, when dangerous hypertension exists, drug therapy is indicated to prevent cerebrovascular complications. The drugs most commonly employed are reserpine and hydralazine hydrochloride. Diazoxide has not yet been approved by the Federal Drug Administration, but there are reports that indicate that it is the simplest and safest mode of therapy in a hypertensive emergency. (A dose of 5 mg/kg body weight, by rapid intravenous injection, has been suggested.) Reserpine may be given intramuscularly at a dose of 0.07 mg/kg body weight. The effect may be transient (4 to 12 hours) but often is quite prolonged (24 to 72 hours). Hydralazine may be given intramuscularly at a dose of 0.2 mg/kg body weight. The effect is variable, and tolerance usually develops; sometimes a dose of up to 2 mg/kg is necessary.

In neonates with coarctation of the aorta, an arm blood pressure of 160/90 mm Hg may be acceptable, since reduction below this level may diminish descending aorta blood flow to a level at which adequate renal perfusion is not maintained.

Cyanotic spells and central nervous system problems

Neonates with cyanotic heart disease, especially those with tetralogy of Fallot or pulmonary atresia with open ventricular septum, may develop cyanotic spells that, if severe, can lead to death. Usually these spells follow crying or bowel movement or occur soon after awakening. They are quite different from the apneic spells of immaturity. Typically, the child becomes progressively more cyanotic and develops deep, sighing respirations. If the condition is unrelieved, acidosis and hypoxemia lead to circulatory and respiratory depression with pallor, flaccidity, bradycardia, and, on occasion, convulsions, cardiac arrest, and death. The underlying heart disease is often surgically treatable, and the occurrence of even minor spells should always lead to hospital admission and usually to surgery.

Treatment. If the spell is mild, the baby should be comforted to stop the crying. Oxygen should be given by face mask if this can be done without further upsetting the infant. If the spell is more severe, with bradycardia or impairment of consciousness, morphine sulfate (0.5 to 1.0 mg/kg body weight) should be administered subcutaneously. If the infant is profoundly depressed and has a very slow heart rate, sodium bicarbonate (2 to 8 mEq/kg over a 2-minute period) should be administered intravenously and external cardiac massage initiated to try to improve the coronary circulation. Ventilation with oxygen (face mask or endotracheal tube) is indicated if respiration is depressed. Most neonates will recover from this latter situation. However, spells of the severe type are always multiple and progressive, unless appropriate surgery to improve pulmonary blood flow is performed. An exception is the infant who is anemic relative to his degree of unsaturation. Thus an infant with an arterial saturation of 70% is anemic if he has a hematocrit value of 40%; sometimes the spells can be completely abolished by treating the anemia, but most often surgery is required.

Phenylephrine has been used to increase bronchial collateral blood flow and propranolol to decrease β-adrenergic activity. It should be emphasized that the occurrence of spells always indicates the need for action, and usually this action is in the form of an aortopulmonary anastomosis (for example, Waterston shunt).

Other CNS emergencies associated with cyanotic heart disease

Brain abscess is very uncommon in infants under 2 years of age but should be considered, especially if the baby has the potential for paradoxical embolism; for example, passage of septic material right to left across the VSD in tetralogy of Fallot.

Cerebral thrombosis is also rare but may occasionally occur with a very high hematocrit value. Immediate treatment consists of venesection 10 to 15 ml/kg, with replacement by 5% dextrose. Anticoagulation with heparin (0.5 mg/kg given intravenously) may be considered.

Anoxic brain damage is far more common in the neonate than is brain abcess or cerebral thrombosis. The hematocrit reading will usually be less than 40% in association with an arterial saturation of less than 60%. Treatment should consist of packed cell transfusion (10 to 20 ml/kg as an exchange transfusion, with an equal quantity of blood removed). Surgery will usually be required to improve pulmonary blood flow and increase arterial O_2 saturation.

Digitalis toxicity

Cardiac glycosides are excreted in an exponential fashion. Digoxin is the most commonly prescribed agent, but ouabain and digitoxin are also used in pediatrics. Toxicity caused by digitoxin is particularly dangerous because of its long biologic half-life (9 days) as compared with that of digoxin (38 hours) and ouabain (22 hours). Ouabain has very little advantage over digoxin. It starts to act slightly faster (3 to 10 minutes as opposed to 5 to 30 minutes for digoxin. However, digoxin is recommended for neonates in need of a cardiac glycoside.

Digitalis toxicity is especially likely if there is a renal disease or hypothyroidism. Certain pathologic states—myocardial disease, hypokalemia, hypomagnesemia, hypercalcemia, anoxia, and alkalosis—sometimes potentiate the action of digitalis and can result in toxicity with "normal" circulating levels of digoxin.

Digitalis toxicity should be differentiated from digitalis effect. *Digitalis effect* consists of slight slowing of the heart rate, prolongation of the P-R interval, shortening of the Q-T interval, a shift of the S-T segment, or a change in the direction of the U wave. These signs merely indicate that digitalis is fixed in the myocardium and do *not* indicate that dosage should be reduced.

Digitalis toxicity in infants and children is mainly manifested by arrhythmias; but vomiting, lethargy, or anorexia sometimes will call attention to digitalis overdose, and with massive digitalis poisoning there may be convulsions, apnea, or sudden death. A digitalis-induced arrhythmia is usually characterized by bradycardia associated with S-A node or A-V node inhibition. A variety of arrhythmias occur: (1) marked sinus arrhythmia with a rate variation greater than 50 beats per minute, (2) sinus arrest with escape beats, (3) A-V nodal rhythm, (4) second-degree A-V block, (5) complete A-V block or A-V dissociation, (6) atrial or ventricular premature beats, bigeminal rhythm, (7) PAT with or without A-V block, and (8) ventricular tachycardia or ventricular fibrillation. Probably the commonest arrhythmias warning of digitalis intoxication are S-A block, second-degree A-V block, or multiple ectopic beats.

Treatments of digitalis toxicity. Treatment of digitalis toxicity involves the following steps.

1. Gastric lavage or emesis is indicated if oral ingestion is recent.
2. Digitalis administration should be stopped and an attempt made to increase the rate of digitalis excretion by fluids given orally or intravenously.
3. The child should be placed in an intensive care unit, and the ECG should be monitored and serum electrolyte levels determined frequently.
4. Correction of any acid-base or electrolyte disturbance should be attempted. If the serum potassium level is low (as after thiazide diuretic administration), potassium chloride (1 gm/10 kg/day) may be given orally. If the situation is urgent, potassium chloride (0.5 mEq/kg) may be given intravenously in not less than 1 hour, as a solution of 40 mEq (3 gm) potassium chloride in 500 ml 5% dextrose. Potassium should be given intravenously only with a physician present and with constant ECG monitoring and frequent serum potassium determinations. McNamara and associates have suggested that potassium should not routinely be administered to patients with digitalis intoxication, because toxic doses of digitalis inhibit the transfer of extracellular potassium into the cell and the resulting high concentration of serum potassium produces myocardial depression.
5. There is a possible source of danger in the misplacement of a decimal point when giving intramuscular doses. If the mistake is realized within a few minutes, it may be possible to drain the site of injection or excise the tissue.
6. Specific arrhythmias require specific treatment. The ease of transvenous pacing even in the newborn has revolutionized the treatment of digitalis poisoning. Slow rates associated with digitalis-induced bradycardia or heart block are common and respond very effectively to temporary insertion of a transvenous endocardial catheter pacemaker and to control of the heart rate by electrical stimulation. Propanolol (0.05 mg to 0.2 mg/kg) may suppress ventricular arrhythmias.
7. Exchange transfusion, hemodialysis, or peritoneal dialysis have not been fully evaluated; but on theoretical grounds they are of limited value, since so much of the digitalis is rapidly fixed in tissues.
8. The use of disodium EDTA to lower the serum calcium level is based upon the synergistic action between calcium and digitalis, but it should probably be used only if other measures fail. A suitable intravenous dose is 15 mg/kg/hr in 5% dextrose in water (maximum dose 60 mg/kg/-day).
9. "Overdrive" pacing to break an arrhythmia, followed by transvenous ventricular pacing at a rate of 140 to 160 beats per minute, should be considered even when the problem is a tachyarrhythmia rather than a bradyarrhythmia.

Pericardial effusion and cardiac tamponade

The term cardiac tamponade or acute cardiac compression denotes an interference with the diastolic filling of the heart and with cardiac contraction because of an increase in intrapericardial pressure. Both pericardial effusion and pericardiac tamponade are rare in the newborn period but are most likely to occur as a complication of septic pericarditis. Stroke output is diminished because the elevated pericardial pressure compresses the right atrium and interferes with the venous inflow from the great veins. A normal cardiac output is temporarily maintained by a compensatory tachycardia, and the blood pressure is at first sustained by peripheral vasoconstriction. At a critical level of intrapericardial pressure (10 to 15 cm of water) there is a sudden reduction in stroke volume and cardiac output, and there is a fall in blood pressure.

Diagnosis. Physical signs include (1) rising venous pressure to 20 cm of water or above (considerably higher than the pressure found in heart failure) leading to liver enlargement and neck vein engorgement, (2) falling arterial pressure with narrowed pulse pressure, (3) usually tachycardia and peripheral vasoconstriction, (4) pulsus paradoxus, a distinct diminution in pulse amplitude by 10 to 20 mm Hg during inspiration, and (5) quiet heart.

The important step is to suspect the diagnosis. Fluoroscopy may reveal a double contour or reduced or absent cardiac pulsations. Angiocardiography is conveniently combined with a recording of central venous pressure and confirms the diagnosis by showing an abnormal gap between the right atrial border and the apparent right cardiac border. Other techniques, such as venous injection of carbon dioxide gas, radioisotope scanning, and reflected ultrasound, have not, in our experience, shown any advantage over right atrial angiography. A further advantage to right atrial angiography is that should the infant turn out not to have a pericardial effusion (as is usually the case), the catheterization may continue in the search for other causes of a large minimally pulsating heart (such as anomalous origin of the left coronary artery from the pulmonary artery and Ebstein's anomaly).

Treatment. Pericardiocentesis may be indicated to confirm the diagnosis, determine the etiologic agent, or relieve the symptoms. The central venous pressure should continue to be monitored as an index of successful treatment. The line may be used for rapid blood replacement, as well as for drug therapy. Pericardiocentesis should be performed under strict sterile conditions with a 3-inch short-bevel 18- or 20-gauge needle to which is attached the V electrocardiographic lead. If the ventricle is touched by the exploring electrode, there is great amplification of existing recorded QRS complexes, or ventricular ectopic beats are provoked. If needle pericardiocentesis is unsuccessful, it is usually because the fluid is too thick for aspiration. In that case, surgical therapy involving pleuropericardial drainage of chronic pericardial effusions or pericardiectomy is indicated.

Bacterial endocarditis

Bacterial endocarditis is very rare in the neonatal period. When it does occur, it is likely to be part of an acute generalized overwhelming septicemia, and the classical signs of subacute endocarditis do not occur. (See p. 129.)

Syndrome complexes

Despite careful attention to the history, physical examination, ECG, and roentgenogram, it is often not possible to make a precise anatomic diagnosis. This is not a reflection of diagnostic inadequacy but is a result of the changing fetal-to-newborn circulation, the presence of heart failure or pulmonary hypertension, and the nonspecificity of some signs. The usual result is that although one may make an intelligent guess at the structural abnormality, one is left with three or four conditions with which the signs are compatible. Certain syndrome complexes emerge, based on the presence or absence of major physical signs. Cardiac catheterization combined with selective angiocardiography is essential for accurate diagnosis except in very rare instances where signs are pathognomonic and the correct treatment is obvious.

The syndrome complexes shown in Table 11-9 are intended only to indicate the more likely possibilities. Hemodynamic and angiocardiographic studies are mandatory in virtually every instance where serious cardiovascular disease is believed to be present.

INDICATIONS FOR CARDIAC CATHETERIZATION AND ANGIOCARDIOGRAPHY

Categorical indications for hemodynamic and angiographic study of the neonate cannot be laid down, but the following are offered as guidelines.

Table 11-9. Syndrome complexes and diagnostic possibilities

Syndrome complex	Possible diagnoses
1. Marked cyanosis; first days of life Increased pulmonary blood flow	Transposition of great arteries Hypoplastic left heart syndrome Preductal coarctation of aorta
2. Cyanosis during first days of life Reduced pulmonary blood flow	Pulmonary atresia with open ventricular septum Pulmonary atresia or extreme pulmonic stenosis with intact ventricular septum Tricuspid atresia Ebsteins' anomaly of tricuspid valve Transposition with pulmonic stenosis
3. Mild cyanosis Increased pulmonary blood flow	Truncus arteriosus Large VSD or common ventricle Total anomalous pulmonary venous return Double-outlet right ventricle and variants Transposition of great arteries with large VSD Common A-V canal
4. Early heart failure, with or without cyanosis secondary to hypoventilation	Arteriovenous fistula (especially cerebral) Severe aortic stenosis, aortic arch hypoplasia, or long-segment aortic coarctation Large PDA Absent pulmonary valve PAT
5. Heart failure at 1 to 4 weeks Insidious onset Murmur present	Large VSD PDA Common A-V canal Postductal coarctation Double-outlet right ventricle Truncus arteriosus
6. Heart failure Large heart Acyanotic No murmur	Primary myocardial disorder Myocarditis Endocardial fibroelastosis Anomalous left coronary artery Glycogen storage disease
7. Heart failure with small or normal-sized heart Roentgenogram of pulmonary venous engorgement	Total anomalous pulmonary venous return with obstruction (for example, drains below diaphragm into liver) Cor triatriatum

Central cyanosis believed to be of cardiovascular origin and persisting for more than a few hours after birth may be an indication. In some patients there may be cause for procrastination, especially if the infant is cold, acidotic, or anemic or has other remediable complications. However, most newborns with obvious cardiovascular central cyanosis become steadily worse and should have a firm diagnosis established at the earliest opportunity.

Heart failure is a less common indication than cyanosis. In general, the earlier the onset the worse the prognosis. Thus in a 1-day-old neonate heart failure believed to be caused by structural cardiovascular disease demands urgent investigation; whereas the 28-day-old neonate has already demonstrated viability, and a more elective approach with a trial of intensive medical treatment may be justified. At 6 weeks to 4 months of age heart failure is more common, and the approach can usually be more elective.

Various *arrhythmias* may be another indication for hemodynamic and angiographic study. Cardiac catheterization may be required for the placement of a temporary transvenous pacemaker in the treatment of complete heart block or digitalis toxicity. The recording of an intracardiac electrogram may occasionally be necessary for the diagnosis of a specific arrhythmia.

Uncertainty of diagnosis might be resolved by cardiac catheterization and angiocardiography. Certain pulmonary diseases may closely mimic heart disease and on occasion diagnostic study is the only way of resolving the issue.

Elucidation of the anatomy of a severe vascular ring causing life-threatening air way obstruction is another indication for hemodynamic and angiographic study.

Other uncommon indications include a suggestion of pericardial tamponade, pulmonary arteriography, and instillation of short-acting pharmacologic compounds directly into the pulmonary artery.

Risk and hazard of cardiac catheterization

The risk of death during or immediately following hemodynamic study is approximately 7%. Many neonates are in critical condition before and during study and in most instances would not survive if investigation and treatment is not undertaken. The major complications occurring during catheterization and leading to death are hypotension and bardycardia, perforation of the heart, arrhythmias, and the hemodynamic effects of contrast agents. Other hazards include the provocation of hypoxic spells, excessive blood loss, obstruction of a semilunar valve orifice or coronary artery by the catheter, acidosis and hypothermia, damage to arteries used in retrograde catheterization, thrombophlebitis, bacteremia, and renal damage probably related to the osmotic effects of contrast agents.

Risks may be minimized by the avoidance of sedative medication in the very sick infant; prompt replacement of excessive blood loss; careful maintenance of body temperature (by use of a water-circulating heating pad under the baby, plus radiant heat if necessary); correction of acidosis by sodium bicarbonate, THAM, or assisted ventilation; use of cardioactive drugs (such as isoproterenol) when indicated; strict aseptic technique; the careful balance of the risks of extensive study against the potential information to be gained (for example, pulmonary artery catheterization is not necessary in a neonate with angiographically obvious tetralogy of Fallot); limiting the use of contrast agent to the minimum amount necessary to establish the diagnosis.

There is literally no neonate with structural heart disease who is too sick to warrant hemodynamic study. The only exception is in patients where improvement with medical management can reasonably be anticipated (as in coexistent sepsis). Occasionally, a neonate has the typical findings of structural heart disease (such as severe tetralogy of Fallot with gross radiologic pulmonary ischemia) and is obviously in need of urgent surgery. Under these circumstances, one may consult one's surgical colleagues and conclude that operation (such as an aortopulmonary shunt) without prior diagnostic study represents the least risk to the baby.

In most instances it is possible to enter all chambers of the heart from the saphenous or superficial femoral vein (because of patency of the foramen ovale). If a retrograde arterial catheterization is necessary, the umbilical artery can often be used in neonates up to 5 days of age and is "disposable." Use of the branchial or femoral artery is, fortunately, rarely necessary in the neonatal period but is sometimes justified when access to the aorta and left ventricle is mandatory.

Care of the neonate after cardiac catheterization

When the neonate returns to the nursery or intensive care unit following cardiac catheterization, he should be treated as an intensive care patient and monitored closely for respirations, heart rate and arrhythmias, blood loss, urine output, blood pressure (Doppler technique), circulatory condition of the limb utilized, "arterialized" capillary pH and Pco_2, and general responsiveness. Deterioration and death can occur in neonates several hours after they have returned from the diagnostic laboratory in seemingly good condition.

TALKING WITH PARENTS

Explanation of the baby's specific condition

Many parents do not understand the spoken anatomic description, and statements such as "hole in the heart" are often misinterpreted. A box diagram of the four heart chambers and two great arteries is readily understood by all and can be kept by the parents when they are called upon to explain the situation to other relatives. An excellent booklet entitled *If Your Child Has a Congenital Heart Defect* is available from local heart associations and from the American Heart Association at 44 East 23rd Street, New York, New York 10010.

The natural history of the lesion should be indicated so that a strong case can be made for or against surgery. The risks of cardiac catheterization of the sick neonate vary from less than 1% for the infant with a straightforward PDA to over 10% for an infant with anoxic bradycardia caused by heart disease. Surgery is even more hazardous, not only because of intraoperative problems but also because of recovery room death on the first days after surgery. Such postoperative deaths are usually caused by respiratory complications (atelectasis, airway obstruction, and intrapulmonary right-to-left shunting).

Genetic counseling

The overall incidence of structural heart disease can be stated as approximately 1%. For parents who already have one effected child, the risk increases to 3% or 4%. These odds are more easily understood if one states that 24 out of 25 times the next child will have a normal heart. If two first-degree relatives are affected or if multiple second-degree relatives are affected, one would be unwise to quote odds, since an unusual heritable tendency has already been demonstrated.

MARTIN H. LEES

BIBLIOGRAPHY

Ainger, L. E., Lawyer, N. G., and Fitch, C. W.: Neonatal rubella myocarditis, Br. Heart J. **28:** 691, 1966.

Anthony, C. L., Crawford, E. W., Morgan, B. C.: Management of cardiac and respiratory arrest in children; a survey of major principles of therapy, Clinical Pediatr. (Phila.) **8:**647, 1969.

Benzing, G., Schubert, W., Hug, G., and Kaplan, S.: Simultaneous hypoglycemia and acute congestive heart failure, Circulation **40:**209, 1969.

Berdon, W. E., and Baker, D. H.: Giant hepatic hemangioma with cardiac failure in the newborn infant; value of high-dosage intravenous urography and umbilical angiography, Radiology **92:**1523, June 1969.

Beuren, A. J., Schulze, C. Eberle, P., Harmjanz, D., and Apitz, J.: The syndrome of supravalvular aortic stenosis, peripheral pulmonary stenosis, mental retardation and similar facial appearance, Am. J. Cardiol. **13:**471, 1964.

Blaufox, M. D.: Systemic arterial hypertension in pediatric practice, Pediatr. Clin. North Am. **18:** 577, 1971.

Burnell, R. J.: Venous pressure in congestive heart failure in infancy, Arch. Dis. Child. **45:**360, June 1970.

Campbell, M.: Causes of malformations of the heart, Brit. Med. J. **2:**895, 1965.

Campbell, M.: Natural history of ventricular septal defect, Br. Heart J. **33:**246, 1971.

Capitanio, M. A., and Kirkpatrick, J. A.: Roentgen examination in the evaluation of the newborn infant with respiratory distress, J. Pediatr. **75:** 896, 1969.

Collett, R. W., and Edwards, J. E.: Persistent truncus arteriosus; classification according to anatomic types, Surg. Clin. North Am. **29:**1245, 1949.

Danilowicz, D., Rudolph, A. M., and Hoffman, J. I. E.: Delayed closure of the ductus arteriosus in premature infants, Pediatrics **37:**74, 1966.

Deely, W. U., Ehlers, K. H., Levin, A. R., and Engle, M. A.: Hypoplastic left heart syndrome; anatomic, physiologic and therapeutic considerations, Am. J. Dis. Child. **121:**168, 1971.

Edwards, J. E., and Burchell, H. B.: Congenital tricuspid atresia; a classification, Med. Clin. North Am. **33:**1177, 1949.

Edwards, J. H.: The epidemiology of congenital malformations. In Second International Conference on Congenital Malformation, New York, 1964, The International Medical Congress, Ltd., p. 297.

Emmanouilides, G. C., Moss, A. J., and Adams, F. H.: The electrogram in normal newborn infants; correlation with hemodynamic observations, J. Pediatr. **67:**578, 1965.

Engle, M. A., Ehlers, K. H., and Frand, M.: Natural history of congenital complete heart block, a cooperative study, Circulation, Supplement III to Vols. 41 and 42, 112, 1970 (Abstract).

Fearon, B., and Shortreed, R.: Tracheobronchial compression by congenital cardiovascular anomalies in children, Ann. Otol. **72:**949, 1963.

Feldman, B. H., and Scott, L. P., III: Aortic stenosis in infancy, Pediatrics **33:**931, 1964.

Finnerty, F. A., Jr., Davidow, M., and Kakaviatos, N.: Hypertensive vascular disease, Am. J. Cardiol. **19:**377, 1967.

Freundlich, E., Engle, M. A., and Goldberg, H. P.: Coarctation of aorta in infancy; analysis of a 10-year experience with medical management, Pediatrics **27:**427, 1961.

Gatti, R. A., Muster, A. J., Cole, R. B.: and Paul, M. H.: Neonatal polycythemia with transient cyanosis and cardiorespiratory abnormalities, J. Pediatr. **69:**1063, 1966.

Gersony, W. M., Duc, G. V., and Sinclair, J. C.: "PFC" syndrome (persistence of the fetal circulation), Circulation, Supplement III to Vols. 39 and 40, 111, October 1969 (Abstract).

Goldring, D., and Wohltmann, H.: Flush method for blood pressure determination in newborn infants, J. Pediatr. **40:**285, 1952.

Gootman, N. L., Scarpelli, E. M., and Rudolph, A. M.: Metabolic acidosis in children with severe cyanotic congenital heart disease, Pediatrics **31:**251, 1963.

Gross, R. E.: The surgery of infancy and childhood, Philadelphia, 1953, W. B. Saunders Co.

Hall, R. J., Nelson, W. P., Blake, H. A., and Geiger, J. P.: Massive pulmonary arteriovenous fistula in the newborn; a correctable form of "cyanotic heart disease," an additional cause of cyanosis with left axis deviation, Circulation **31:** 762, 1965.

Hastreiter, A. R., and Abella, J. B.: The electrocardiogram in the newborn period. I. The normal infant, J. Pediatr. **78:**146, 1971.

Hastreiter, A. R., and Abella, J. B.: The electrocardiogram in the newborn period. II. The infant with disease, J. Pediatr. **78:**346, 1971.

Hernandez, A., Jr., Hartman, A. F., Jr., and Goldring, D.: The Doppler method for indirect measurement of blood pressure in infants, The Society for Pediatric Research, Atlantic City, April 29 to May 2, 1970, p. 151 (Abstract).

Hoffman, J. I. E., and Rudolph, A. M.: The natural history of ventricular septal defects in infancy Am. J. Cardiol. **16:**634, 1965.

Hohn, A. R., Lowe, C. U., Sokal, J. E., and Lambert, E. C.: Cardiac problems in the glycogenoses with specific reference to Pompe's disease, Pediatrics **35**:313, 1965.
Hosier, D. M., and Newton, W. A., Jr.: Serious Coxsackie infection in infants and children, Am. J. Dis. Child. **96**:251, 1958.
Ito, T., Engle, M. A., and Holswade, G. R.: Congenital insufficiency of the pulmonic valve, Pediatrics **28**:712, 1961.
James, T. N.: QT prolongation and sudden death, Modern Concepts of Cardiovasc. Dis. **38**:35, 1969.
Jegier, W. Gibbons, J. E., and Wiglesworth, E. W.: Cor triatriatum—clinical, hemodynamic and pathological studies; surgical correction in early life, Pediatrics **31**:255, 1963.
Johnson, K. G., and Babson, S. G.: Resuscitation of the apneic premature infant, Pediatrics **40**: 99, 1967.
Kitterman, J. A., Edmunds, L. H., Jr., Gregory, G. A., Heymann, M. A., Tooley, W. H., and Rudolph, A. M.: Patent ductus arteriosus in premature infants, N. Engl. J. Med. **287**:473, 1972.
Lambert, E. C., Canent, R. V., and Hohn, A. R.: Congenital cardiac anomalies in the newborn; a review of conditions causing death or severe distress in the first month of life, Pediatrics **37**: 343, 1966.
Lees, M. H., Burnell, R. H., Morgan, C. L., and Ross, B. B.: Ventilation/perfusion relationships in children with heart disease and diminished pulmonary blood flow, Pediatrics **42**:778, 1968.
Lees, M. H., and Jolly, J.: Severe congenital methaemoglobinaemia in an infant, Lancet **2**: 1147, 1957.
Lees, M. H., Menashe, V. D., Sunderland, C. O., Morgan, C. L., and Dawson, P. J.: Ehlers-Danlos syndrome association with multiple pulmonary stenoses and tortuous systemic arteries, J. Pediatr. **75**:1031, 1969.
Lees, M. H., Way, R. C., and Ross, B. B.: Ventilation and respiratory gas transfer of infants with increased pulmonary blood flow, Pediatrics **40**:259, 1967.
Liebman, J. Cullum, L., and Belloc, N. B.: Natural history of transposition of the great arteries; anatomy and birth and death characteristics, Circulation **50**:237, 1969.
Lister, J. W., Cohen, L. S.: Bernstein, W. H., and Samet, P.: Treatment of supraventricular tachycardias by rapid atrial stimulation, Circulation **38**:1044, 1968.
Lown, B., and Kosowsky, B. D.: Artificial cardiac pacemakers, N. Engl. J. Med. **283**:907, 971, 1023, 1970.
Lundsgaard, C., and Van Slyke, D. D.: Cyanosis, Medicine **2**:1, 1923.
Macauley, D.: Acute endocarditis in infancy and early childhood, Am. J. Dis. Child. **88**:715, 1954.
Manning, J. A., Sellers, F. J.: Bynum, R. S., and Keith, J. D.: The medical management of clinical endocardial fibroelastosis, Circulation **29**: 60, 1964.
McNamara, D. G., Brewer, E. J., Jr., and Ferry, G. D.: Accidental poisoning of children with digitalis, N. Engl. J. Med. **271**:1106, 1964.
Mehrizi, A., and Drash, A.: Birth weight of infants with cyanotic and acyanotic congenital malformations of the heart, J. Pediatr. **59**:715, 1961.
Messer, J. V.: Management of emergencies. XIV. Cardiac arrest N. Engl. J. Med. **275**:35, 1966.
Michaelsson, M.: Electrocardiographic studies in the healthy newborn, Acta Pediatr. Scand. **48**: 108, 1959.
Mitchell, S. C., Korones, S. B., and Berendes, H. W.: Congenital heart disease in 56,109 births; incidence and natural history, Circulation **43**:323, 1971.
Morgan, B. C., Bloom, R. S., and Guntheroth, W. G.: Cardiac arrhythmias in premature infants, Pediatrics **35**:658, 1965.
Moss, A. J., Duffie, E. R., Jr., and Emmanouilides, G.: Blood pressure and vasomotor reflexes in the newborn infant, Pediatrics **32**:175, 1963.
Mustard, W. T., Keith, J. D., Trusler, G. A., Fowler, R., and Kidd, L.: The surgical management of transposition of the great vessels, J. Thorac. Cardiovasc. Surg. **48**:953, 1964.
Nadas, A. S.: Pediatric cardiology, ed. 2, Philadelphia, 1963, W. B. Saunders Co.
Nadas, A. S., Daeschner, C. W., Roth, A., and Blumenthal, S. L.: Paroxysmal tachycardia in infants and children, Pediatrics **9**:167, 1952.
Neill, C. A.: Development of the pulmonary veins; with reference to the embryology of anomalies of pulmonary venous return, Pediatrics **18**:880, 1956.
Nora, J. J.: Multifactorial inheritance hypothesis for the etiology of congenital heart diseases; the genetic-environmental interaction, Circulation **38**:604 September 1968.
Nora, J. J., Dodd, P. F., McNamara, D. G., Hattwick, M. A. W., Leachman, R. D., and Cooley, D. A.: Risk to offspring of parents with congenital heart defects, J.A.M.A. **209**:2052, September 29, 1969.
Nora, J. J., McNamara, D. G., Hallman, G. L., Sommerville, J. J., and Cooley, D. A.: Medical and surgical management of anomalous origin of left coronary artery from pulmonary artery, Pediatrics **42**:405, 1968.
Oliver, T. K., Jr., Demis, J. A., and Bates, G. D.: Serial blood-gas tensions and acid-base balance during the first hour of life in human infants, Acta Paediatr. Scand. **50**:346, 1961.
Ongley, P. A.: Heart sounds in total anomalous pulmonary venous return and in Ebstein's anomaly, Circulation **16**:431, 1957.
Rainier-Pope, C. R., Cunningham, R. D., Nadas, A. S., and Crigler, J. F.: Cardiovascular malformation in Turner's syndrome, Pediatrics **33**: 919, 1964.
Rashkind, W. J., and Miller, W. W.: Creation of an atrial septal defect without thoracotomy, a palliative approach to complete transposition of the great arteries, J.A.M.A. **196**:991, 1966.
Roberton, N. R. C., Hallidie-Smith, K. A., and Davis, J. A.: Severe respiratory distress syndrome mimicking cyanotic heart disease in term babies, Lancet **2**:1108, 1967.

Rook, G. D., and Gootman, N.: Pulmonary atresia with intact interventricular septum; operative treatment with survival, Am. Heart J. **81**: 476, 1971.

Rosenberg, H. S., and McNamara, D. G.: Acute myocarditis in infancy and childhood, Progr. in Cardiovasc. Dis. **7**:179, 1964.

Rowe, R. D., and Uchida, I. A.: Cardiac malformation in mongolism; a prospective study of 184 mongoloid children, Am. J. Med. **31**:726, 1961.

Rudolph, A. M.: Complications occurring in infants and children. In Braunwald, E., and Swan, H. J. C., editors: Cooperative study in cardiac catheterization. American Heart association Monograph No. 20, 1968; published as Circulation Supplement III to vols. 37 and 38, May 1968.

Rudolph, A. M., Mesel, E., and Levy, J. M.: Epinephrine in the treatment of cardiac failure due to shunts, Circulation **28**:3, 1963.

Sommerville, R. J., Nora, J. J., Clayton, G. W., and McNamara, D. G.: Adrenal insufficiency mimicking heart disease in infancy, Pediatrics **42**:691, 1968.

Sparrow, A. W., Friedberg, D. Z., and Nadas, A. S.: The use of ethacrynic acid in infants and children with congestive heart failure, Pediatrics **42**:291, 1968.

Stark, J., Aberdeen, E., Waterston, D. J., Bonham-Carter, R. E., and Tynan, M.: Pulmonary artery constriction (banding); report of 146 cases, Surgery **65**:808, May 1969.

Stewart, J. R., Kincaid, O. W.: Edwards, J. E.: An atlas of vascular rings and related malformations of the aortic arch system, Springfield, Ill., 1964, Charles C Thomas, Publisher.

Swiderski, J., Lees, M. H., and Nadas, A. S.: The Wolff-Parkinson-White syndrome in infancy and childhood, Br. Heart J. **24**:561, 1962.

Valdés-Dapena, M., and Miller, W. H.: Pericarditis in the newborn, Pediatrics **16**:673, 1955.

Van Praagh, R., Van Praagh, S., Vlad, P., and Keith, J. D.: Diagnosis of the anatomic types of single or common ventricle, Am. J. Cardiol. **15**:345, 1965.

Walsh, S. Z.: Evolution of the electrocardiogram of healthy premature infants during the first year of life, Acta Paediatr. Scand. Suppl. **145**:1, 1963.

Wigger, H. J., Bransilver, B. R., and Blanc, W. A.: Thromboses due to catheterization in infants and children, J. Pediatr. **76**:1, 1970.

Wood, J. L.: Plethora in the newborn infant associated with cyanosis and convulsions, J. Pediatr. **54**:143, 1959.

Yamauchi, T., and Cayler, G. G.: Ebstein's anomaly in the neonate, Am. J. Dis. Child. **107**:165, 1964.

12 Diseases of the respiratory system

FUNDAMENTAL CONSIDERATIONS

Pulmonary disease in the newborn infant most often develops as a result of failure of adaptation to extrauterine life. This may be caused by factors related to an immature state of development, untoward factors in the immediate antenatal or postnatal environment, or other incompletely understood influences operating in the perinatal period. At birth the infant must establish a lung volume (functional residual capacity) and match ventilation and perfusion as closely as possible to ensure proper blood gas exchange. The infant born prematurely or the infant suffering from asphyxia is frequently confronted with serious obstacles to obtaining these primary goals. Conditions occurring as a result of infection or congenital anomaly are less common. Because of the nature of many pulmonary problems in the neonate and the fact that treatment is most often supportive, a background orientation to certain aspects of pulmonary physiology is a prerequisite to a proper understanding of the disease processes, as well as a rational approach to treatment.

Lung volumes

The lungs may be conceptualized as compartments (Fig. 12-1). The size of the compartments is related to the height, weight, and surface area of the subject. The functional residual capacity (FRC) is most critical in the newborn, since conditions in which it is too small (atelectasis) or too large (emphysema) dominate the spectrum of neonatal lung disease. FRC is the volume of gas in the lungs at end-expiration. FRC is further subdivided into the expiratory reserve volume (ERV) and the residual volume (RV). One of the principal functions of the first breaths is to transform the fluid-filled fetal lung from an airless state to one with an appropriate FRC.

The ability of the lung to maintain a volume of gas at end-expiration depends on two factors. One is the chest wall, which acts as a support for the lungs; the other is the ability of the lung to develop an alveolar lining that can produce zero surface tension at end-expiration and thus act to stabilize an expanded alveoli. Both of these functions are less developed in the premature infant. A normal FRC allows the individual to maintain stable blood gases throughout the respiratory cycle by buffering the effect of large variations in P_{CO_2}, P_{O_2} and pH that occur with inspiration and expiration. In addition, when FRC is too large or too small, pulmonary work and airway resistance are increased and compliance is decreased. In normal infants the FRC usually exceeds 1.0 ml/cm of body length, and all of the gas in the lung at end-expiration is in communication with major airways.

Other lung volumes commonly measured in newborn infants are total lung capacity (TLC), vital capacity (VC), and dead space (V_D). Dead space is more directly related to ventilation-perfusion relationships and is discussed under that heading. The measurement of VC is obtained by stimulating the infant to cry into a spirometer; the volume displaced from maximum expiration to peak inspiration is recorded as VC. Measurement of VC is an excellent screening test in that it provides an overall

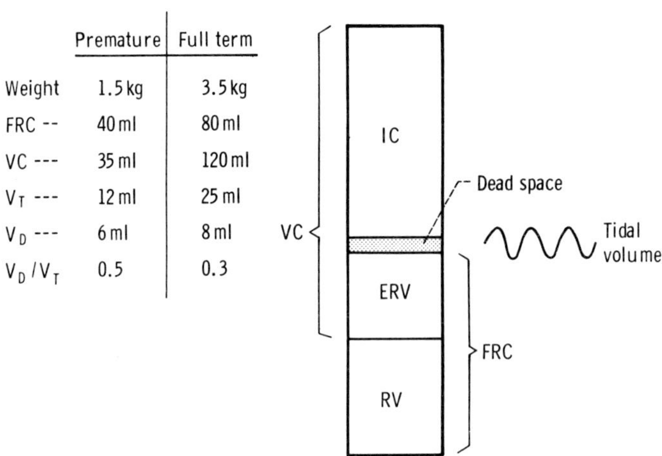

	Premature	Full term
Weight	1.5 kg	3.5 kg
FRC --	40 ml	80 ml
VC ---	35 ml	120 ml
V_T ---	12 ml	25 ml
V_D ---	6 ml	8 ml
V_D/V_T	0.5	0.3

Fig. 12-1. Important subdivisions of lung volume. Representative values are for nondistressed infants.

assessment of lung volume and mechanical factors. VC is directly related to FRC.

The lung surfactant system

The ability of the lung to form an alveolar lining that can produce zero surface tension in alveoli at end-expiration is one of the major factors in the development of FRC. The alveolar wall consists of a continuous layer of cells that are overlaid by a liquid alveolar lining layer, much like a film. Surfactants are the important component of this film. The best-known surfactants are phospholipids; lecithins (dipalmitoyl lecithin) are the phospholipids present in highest concentration. They are the most important, although other pulmonary phospholipids have been identified. Two cell types are recognized in the alveolar wall: type I—thin surface epithelial cells; and type II—large granular cells. Pulmonary phospholipids are produced in type II cells.

The pulmonary surfactant system plays a major role in reducing surface tension in alveoli. Alveoli at end-expiration would be expected to obey LaPlace's law:

$$\text{Pressure} = \frac{2 \text{ Surface tension}}{\text{Radius}}$$

In such a case the inwardly directed force (pressure) increases as the radius of the alveolus decreases; thus, as the alveolus approaches end-expiration the tendency to collapse is minimized in the presence of surfactant. As well as allowing the lung to retain an FRC, a low surface tension balances the effects of capillary hydrostatic pressure and colloid osmotic pressure to keep the alveolus dry. Much of the elastic recoil of the lung at end-inspiration is also caused by the effects of surface tension; at end-inspiration surface tension is high, thus promoting collapse at peak volume.

The surfactants are secreted into the fluid-filled fetal lung. The initiation of air breathing increases the production of surfactants to form an alveolar lining. However, hypoxia, acidosis, and reduced pulmonary blood flow disrupt the production of surfactants. The consequences of disruption of the pulmonary surfactant system are atelectasis and intraalveolar fluid accumulation. Hyaline membrane disease (HMD) is the major clinical condition in which surfactant is deficient.

The time of appearance of surfactants in fetal development is unknown, although normal surface tension has been reported in the lungs of a 200-gm fetus. The ability to produce the phospholipids increases with gestational age; Gluck has demonstrated a marked increase in lecthin:spingomyelin ratio in amniotic fluid samples at 36 weeks' gestation (Chapter 1, pp. 20-21).

Mechanics of the lung

Mechanics of the lung are those factors that are concerned with the bellows function and include compliance of the lungs

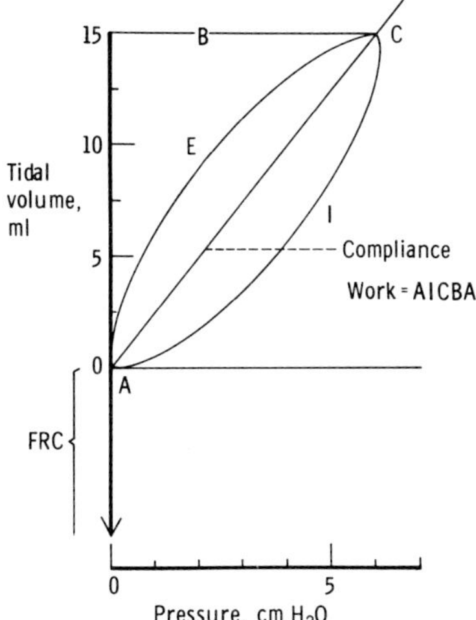

Fig. 12-2. Pressure volume diagram of the lung. Note that inspiration AIC and expiration CEA occur on top of FRC. AC is the compliance line. Pulmonary work is the area AICBA. A tidal volume of 15 ml is produced by a pressure change of −6 cm H_2O.

and thorax, work of breathing, and airway resistance. The mechanical functions of the lung are best understood when viewed in the form of the pressure volume diagram (Fig. 12-2).

Compliance of the lung

Compliance of the lung (C_L) is the relationship of the change in tidal volume (ΔV) to the pressure change that produced it (ΔP) at points of no air flow. It is a measure of the distensibility or stiffness of the lung. Reduced compliance indicates a decreased distensibility of the lung. Compliance is related to FRC and decreases when FRC decreases. Thus a true index of lung stiffness can be best obtained by calculating specific compliance, C_L. In the newborn infant measurements of compliance generally have been made during normal respiration and are thus classified as dynamic compliance measurements. Compliance is determined by the simultaneous measurement of esophageal pressure change and tidal volume. As with most pulmonary functions, compliance depends on the size of the infant. Compliance of both the lung and chest wall have been determined in the living infant. Compliance of the tracheobronchial tree has been measured in postmortem specimens. In general, the chest wall and tracheobronchial tree are more compliant than the lungs. In distressed infants in whom lung compliance is markedly reduced, the compliant chest wall poses a disadvantage in that as the infant attempts to increase negative intrathoracic pressure the chest wall collapses (retractions). The more compliant airway of the smaller infant may predipose him to actual airway collapse during expiration and result in distal gas trapping.

Airway resistance

The flow of air through the nasopharynx, trachea, and bronchi is dependent on the size of the airway, the flow rate, and the resistance imposed by lung tissue. This is total pulmonary resistance, and it is calculated from the formula R (resistance) $= \frac{\text{Flow}}{\Delta P}$. In the infant, air flow is determined by breathing through a pneumotachograph, whose essential element is a fine wire mesh screen. Pressure change that causes the air flow, or ΔP, is determined by intraesophageal catheterization. In the full-term infant, total pulmonary resistance is 29 cm H_2O/liter/sec, approximately six times greater than that in the adult. The major site of airway resistance in the neonate is in the nasopharynx (the resistance caused by the tissues). In the normal infant, airway resistance (resistance that is imposed by the breathing tubes) is approximately 18 to 20 cm H_2O/liter/sec, and viscous resistance (the resistance caused by the tissues) is 8 to 10 cm H_2O/liter/sec. This latter value is also larger than that in adults. Because of the higher resistances that occur in infants, respiratory apparatus that would materially increase airway resistance further must be avoided.

The work of breathing

The work of breathing is a measure of the energy expended in inflating the lungs and moving the chest. In general terms, Work $= 0.6$ P $\times$ V (where P is pressure change and V is volume of air moved). In the normal infant total pulmonary work has been determined to equal an average value of 1,440 gm/cm/min. In an infant with respiratory distress the total pulmonary work may increase as much as six times. This becomes most important when considered in terms of the oxygen cost of breathing. The neonate requires a greater caloric expenditure to breathe than the adult, and the distressed infant requires an even greater caloric expenditure for this function. In the full-term infant the work of breathing is minimal when the infant has a respiratory rate of 30 breaths per minute. Little information is available on the work of breathing in premature infants.

Ventilation-perfusion relationships

For normal gas exchange to occur at the alveolocapillary interface, ventilation and perfusion should be similarly proportioned; that is, ideally 1 ml of alveolar ventilation should be matched with a perfusion of 1 ml to result in a ventilation-perfusion relationship ($\dot{V}_A/\dot{Q}$) equal to 1.0. However, in the healthy adult there are variations in $\dot{V}_A/\dot{Q}$ in different parts of the lung so that the overall $\dot{V}_A/\dot{Q}$ is more nearly 0.8. Measurements with radioactive gases have demonstrated that in the upright state the upper lobes have a $\dot{V}_A/\dot{Q}>1$ (relatively underperfused or overventilated) (Fig. 12-3). When the patient assumes a reclining position, these variations in $\dot{V}_A/\dot{Q}$ are abolished. Direct determination of actual $\dot{V}_A/\dot{Q}$ is difficult and has not been carried out in the newborn. Indirect assessment of the distribution of ventilation and perfusion

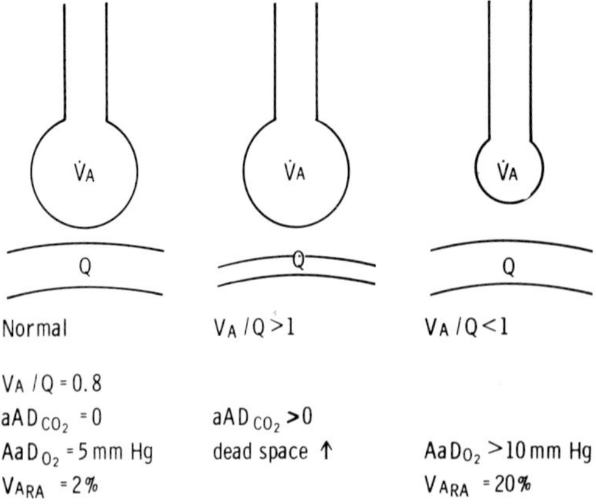

Fig. 12-3. $\dot{V}_A/\dot{Q}$ relationships: $\dot{V}_A$ = alveolar ventilation, $\dot{Q}$ = perfusion; normal $\dot{V}_A/\dot{Q}$—ventilation and perfusion are well matched; $\dot{V}_A/\dot{Q} > 1$—alveoli are underperfused with respect to ventilation and $AaDco_2$ is present; $\dot{V}_A/\dot{Q} < 1$—alveoli are underventilated with respect to perfusion.

and $\dot{V}_A/\dot{Q}$ has been obtained by measurement of alveolar arterial gradients for O_2, CO_2, and nitrogen.

The most common disturbance in ventilation-perfusion relationships in neonates is intrapulmonary shunting, which is a consequence of atelectasis. Areas of the lung in which intrapulmonary shunting occurs are perfused but not ventilated and thus have $\dot{V}_A/\dot{Q} = O$. Areas of gas trapping that are virtually nonventilated but perfused also function essentially as a shunt. The result of intrapulmonary shunts is a decrease in arterial Po_2 similar to what occurs when there is a right-to-left shunt in the heart or through a patent ductus arteriosus (PDA) (Fig. 12-4). Similar arterial unsaturation may occur when the alveoli are well ventilated, but the ventilation is poor with respect to perfusion (for example, asthma or emphysema). A decrease in arterial Po_2 also occurs when a diffusion barrier exists in the transfer of oxygen from alveolus to capillary (such as edema or scar tissue forming a block in the alveolar wall).

It is important to determine which abnormality is causing hypoxia. This is done by measurement of the alveolar-arterial oxygen gradient ($AaDo_2$). With this test an $AaDo_2$ of 5 to 10 mm Hg is usual when a normal subject is breathing air. This degree of venous admixture (VA_{RA}) is caused by venous blood entering pulmonary veins from thebesian veins, bronchial veins, and alveoli that are perfused but not ventilated. In healthy infants 1% to 2% of cardiac output is not exposed to alveolar gas and can be classified as venous admixture.

In disease states venous admixture and $AaDo_2$ may be greater. When this occurs, it must be determined whether the venous admixture is caused by shunting, maldistribution of ventilation, or abnormal diffusion. To distinguish shunting from abnormalities of ventilation and diffusion the infant is given 100% oxygen to breathe for 10 minutes. This results in increasing the alveolar Po_2 to approximately 680 mm Hg. The normal subject increases arterial Po_2 to approximately 650 mm Hg. Infants with diffusion block and maldistribution of ventilation increase Po_2 to similar levels after 10 minutes. When shunting is present, the increase in Po_2 is smaller (Fig. 12-5), and

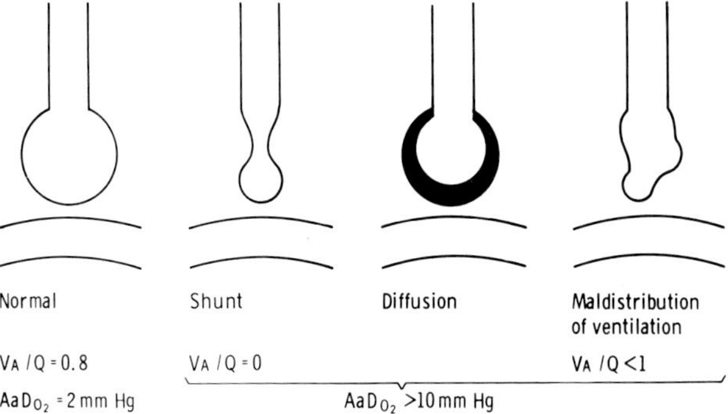

Fig. 12-4. Causes of venous admixture. Normally, venous admixture is small. Abnormal venous admixture is caused by shunt, diffusion, or maldistribution of ventilation. $\dot{V}_A/\dot{Q}$ abnormalities caused by these disturbances are shown.

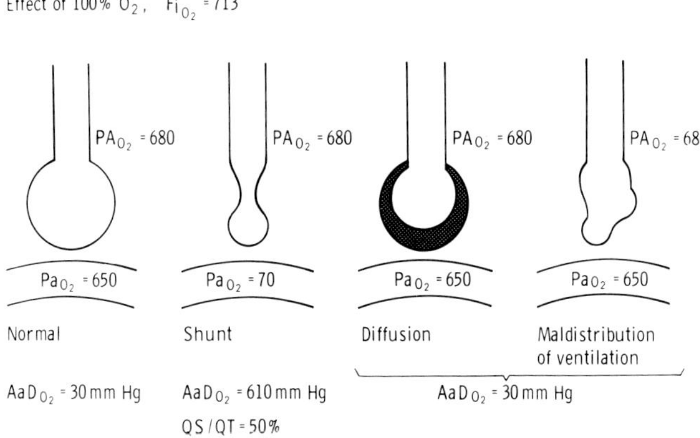

Fig. 12-5. Use of 100% O_2 breathing to differentiate cause of venous admixture. An $AaDo_2$ persists in 100% O_2 only when shunting is present $P_{AO_2} = 680$ mm Hg in alveolar oxygen tension breathing 100% O_2.

the percent of cardiac output not exposed to alveolar gas is large. Localization of the site of shunting depends on the site from which the arterial blood is obtained. For example, if an $AaDo_2$ is present in 100% oxygen and pulmonary venous blood is sampled, then the shunt is in the lungs. If blood is sampled from the umbilical artery and a large $AaDo_2$ is measured in 100% oxygen, then the right-to-left shunt could be anywhere between the alveolus and the artery (for example, lungs, foramen ovale, or PDA).

The presence of maldistribution of ventilation may be evaluated by nitrogen washout and nitrogen gradient determinations. To perform the *nitrogen washout test* the infant inspires 100% oxygen through a low-resistance nose valve. The washout of nitrogen from the lung is recorded breath by breath with a nitrogen analyzer. A semilogarithmic plot of the washout is made. In the normal test, nitrogen washout is smooth and even, and a straight line is recorded. This line signifies that all alveoli ventilate as a single space. When maldistribution of ventilation is present, washout is slow, and more than a single straight line can be drawn, indicating that alveoli are emptying at different rates. This occurs in infants with meconium aspiration or transient neonatal tachypnea who have reduced arterial O_2 tension because of maldistribution of ventilation ($\dot{V}_A/\dot{Q}<1$). A *nitrogen gradient* between blood and alveolar gas is an indication of the presence of alveoli with a low $\dot{V}_A/\dot{Q}$. The arterial-alveolar nitrogen gradient (aAD_{N_2}) is not affected by shunting. In the normal subject an aAD_{N_2} up to 10 mm Hg is present. Infants with meconium aspiration and transient neonatal tachypnea have significantly elevated aAD_{N_2}.

At present it is not possible to accurately evaluate infants for the presence of a diffusion barrier.

Small, nondistressed premature infants, as well as those with HMD, may have a high $\dot{V}_A/\dot{Q}$ from overventilation or underperfusion. The presence of these areas can be identified by measuring the arterial-alveolar carbon dioxide gradient, thus identifying $\dot{V}_A/\dot{Q}>1$. The test is performed by simultaneously sampling arterial blood for P_{CO_2} and end tidal gas for P_{CO_2}. The latter is determined with a rapid-response infrared analyzer. Accurate assessment of end-tidal P_{CO_2} is difficult in rapidly breathing subjects. In normal individuals no aAD_{CO_2} is present. Because of the easy diffusibility of CO_2, the shape of CO_2 dissociation curve, and small a-v CO_2 difference, a large abnormality must exist before an aAD_{CO_2} is recorded. While an aAD_{CO_2} indicates the presence of high $\dot{V}_A/\dot{Q}$, an elevated arterial P_{CO_2} alone may also indicate hypoventilation. In this case both alveolar and blood P_{CO_2} would be equal and elevated.

It is important to realize that the lung of any patient may have areas of both high and low $\dot{V}_A/\dot{Q}$, and if this is the case both a significant AaD_{O_2} and aAD_{CO_2} would be measured.

Dead space (Fig. 12-21)

Dead space is that portion of the tidal volume not involved in gas exchange, and thus it will vary with the presence or absence of areas of high $\dot{V}_A/\dot{Q}$. The dead space is divided into several compartments. Anatomical dead space is the constant airway volume not involved in gas exchange and is made up of the air passages from nares to terminal bronchioles. Alveolar dead space is the volume of gas in alveoli that are well ventilated but underperfused ($\dot{V}_A/\dot{Q}>1$). Physiologic dead space is the sum of anatomical and alveolar dead space. In the normal newborn physiologic dead space is 6 to 8 cc, and smaller values are obtained in premature infants.

The relationship of dead space to tidal volume (V_D/V_T) is physiologically significant. When V_D/V_T is increased over the normal 0.3, an aAD_{CO_2} exists and areas of high $\dot{V}_A/\dot{Q}$ are present. It is also of practical importance to minimize the dead space added by apparatus for assisted ventilation or measurement of lung function in order to avoid rebreathing and accumulation of carbon dioxide.

Measurement of blood gases

The collection of blood for determination of blood gases requires precise technique. The sample must be obtained anaerobically and the measurement made as soon as possible. Preservation of the sample in ice may not be adequate, since the total sample is seldom reduced to the required 0 C. Each nursery caring for sick infants or infants at risk should have an apparatus for measuring blood gases in the immediate vicinity so that samples can be run as soon as they are collected.

Sampling

Anaerobically collected arterial blood is required to accurately assess pH, P_{CO_2} and P_{O_2}. A gas-tight syringe should be used for collection. With practice, radial artery, brachial artery, and temporal artery samples can be obtained without complication. Peripheral arterial sampling is carried out using a No. 23 scalp vein needle set. Most of the plastic tubing is removed and a blunt No. 18 needle inserted in the cut end. When the needle is inserted in the artery, blood flows back, fills the dead space, and then a gas-tight syringe is attached for collection. At the end of the collection all bubbles are immediately removed, and the sample is capped. The umbilical artery is also a useful source of blood for the first few days of extrauterine life. The umbilical artery catheter is most easily inserted soon after birth. A No. 3½ French catheter is used and can be kept from clotting by using the catheter for constant fluid infusions. In infants with respiratory distress the sampling site of blood for P_{O_2} has considerable importance in interpreting the result in terms of pulmonary function and toxicity to the retina. Temporal and right brachial or radial arteries are the best sites for measuring P_{O_2} since they avoid the effects of right-to-left ductal shunt, a common situation in the sick neonate. Umbilical artery Po_2 may not reflect retinal Po_2 when a significant right-to-left ductus shunt exists. Similarly, poor blood flow to an extremity used for sampling may invalidate the usefulness of the determination.

Because of the small difference between arterial and venous pH and Pco_2 free-flowing venous blood can be used to assess these parameters when arterial blood is unobtainable. Similarly, capillary blood obtained from the warmed heel provides a source of blood for measurement of pH and Pco_2. Capillary Po_2 measured in blood from this site is not reliable in sick infants.

Measurement

There are a number of excellent apparatus available for rapid determination of pH, Pco_2, and Po_2 on small samples of blood. Bicarbonate and base excess can be calculated when pH and Pco_2 are known from the Singer-Hastings nomogram or the Siggaard-Andersen nomogram. These nomograms provide graphic solutions to the Henderson-Hasselbalch equation. The hemoglobin level or hematocrit should be determined with each blood gas in order to use the nomogram. Pco_2, Po_2, and pH are temperature dependent; therefore, these tests must be run at the temperature of the patient, or, as is generally done, the sample is measured at 37 C and corrected to the patient's temperature. Tables are available for this purpose. Whole blood pH rises 0.0147 pH units per degree fall of temperature under anaerobic conditions. Corrections must be applied for Po_2 and Pco_2 as well.

Po_2 and Pco_2 can be converted to their respective saturations using Dill's nomogram modified for infants by Edwards and Ross. If the hemoglobin level is determined as well, oxygen and carbon dioxide content can be calculated.

Oxygen transport

Normal oxygen transport depends on many factors other than those related to the pulmonary system. Thus cardiac output, blood volume, hemoglobin concentration, and oxygen affinity of hemoglobin are most important. Attention must be directed to factors that affect both oxygen uptake in the lung and release to the tissues. Considerations of oxygen transport are best appreciated in terms of the oxygen dissociation curve (Fig. 12-6). Tissue uptake will be impaired by factors that shift the position of the curve to the left, such as the presence of large amounts of fetal hemoglobin, pH in the alkalotic range, and a decrease in body temperature. Shift of the curve to the right will facilitate unloading at the tissues. Acidosis and an increase in body temperature will have this effect.

When the affinity of hemoglobin for oxygen is reduced (the oxygen dissociation curve is shifted to the right), oxygen release to the tissues is facilitated. Red blood cells contain organic phosphates, of which the most important is 2,3-disphosphoglycerate (DPG), that reduce O_2 affinity. Fetal deoxyhemoglobin has less affinity for 2,3-DPG than adult deoxyhemoglobin, and this failure to bind 2,3-DPG is a major reason for the leftward shift of the fetal curve (Fig. 12-6). Adult and newborn red blood cells have similar levels of 2,3-DPG. Premature infants on the other hand have decreased amounts of 2,3-DPG. The newborn curve approaches the adult at 4 to 6 months of age.

Red blood cell 2,3-DPG is reduced in shock, acidosis, and in stored blood. The increased affinity of neonatal red blood cells for O_2 in the capillaries of the lungs also implies a decreased ability to release O_2 to the tissues. Whether or not this is an important physiologic deficit is yet to be determined and depends on whether or not there is a "critical Po_2" below which there is minimal O_2 delivery to the tissues and what the dissociation curve actually is at the tissue level.

Other factors affect tissue oxygenation: cardiac output, peripheral vascular resistance, and factors related to oxygen content such as hemoglobin concentration and inspired oxygen concentration. If the tissues require more oxygen, cardiac output is increased and arteriolar resistance is decreased. The limitations of cardiac output in response to tissue oxygen needs in the newborn are not as yet defined. Newborn infants respond to stress by constricting peripheral skin vessels to direct oxygenated blood to vital areas. The level of hemoglobin that must be maintained to ensure adequate oxygenation of tissue is unknown; it

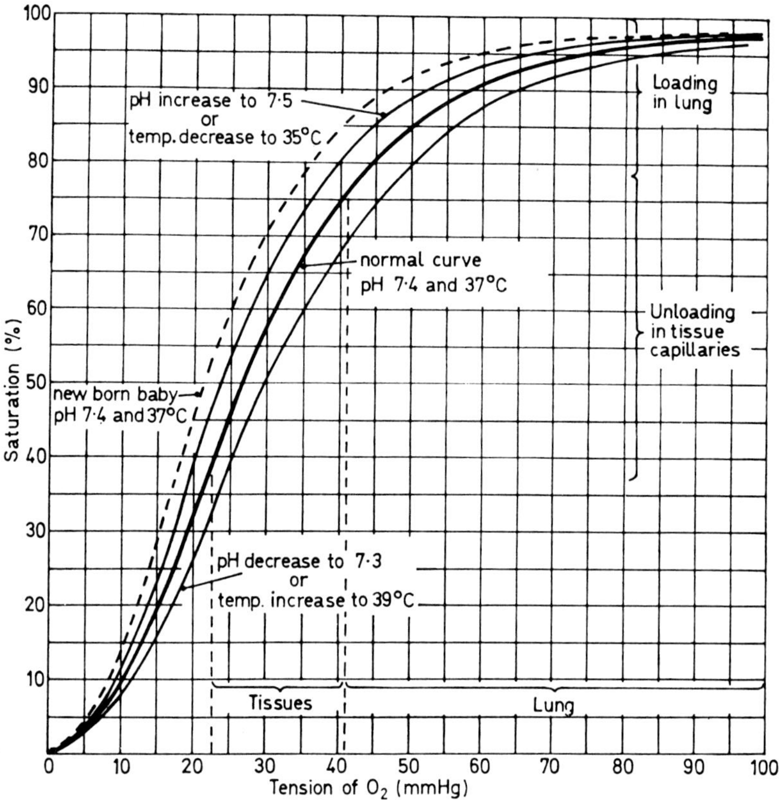

FIG. 12-6. Dissociation curve for oxyhemoglobin, showing effects of various influences on its position. Data compiled by Severinghaus. (From Cotes, J. E.: Lung function, Oxford, 1968, Blackwell Scientific Publications Ltd.)

depends in part upon the infant's ability to increase cardiac ouput.

ADAPTATION OF THE LUNGS TO EXTRAUTERINE LIFE

In a description of the physiologic events that occur during adaptation of the lungs to extrauterine life, the state of the lungs just prior to birth is of vital importance. The pulmonary development of premature infants is less than the full-term infant, and this difference profoundly affects the adaptive process.

Factors in the intrauterine state that will affect extrauterine adaptation

Embryology

The airways develop as an outpouching from the gut. For the first 16 weeks, growth consists mainly of branchings of this tube into the mesenchyme surrounding it. Canalization of the tubes begins at 20 weeks, and then a cuboidal lining appears. Alveoli develop as outpouchings of the bronchioles, beginning at approximately 28 weeks and continuing until term. At 26 to 28 weeks the capillary network arising from the mesenchyme begins to approximate the developing alveoli. Thus for developmental reasons extrauterine life is rarely possible under 28 weeks, and survival improves as alveolocapillary development continues.

Development of the alveolar lining layer

The development of an alveolar lining with surfactants capable of reducing surface tension to zero at end-expiration is extremely important in producing stable alveoli (p. 21).

Fetal lung fluid

The lung contains a large volume of fluid prior to birth that is distinct from amniotic fluid, although under certain conditions there may be intermixing of the two. Fetal pulmonary fluid at term has normal surface tension properties because of the phospholipids in it. Compression by the thorax during labor and delivery, plus the reabsorption by pulmonary capillaries and lymphatics are the major ways in which the fluid is removed prior to and with the onset of breathing. Prominent lymphatics are a feature of the necropsy findings in newborn lungs, reflecting the role they play in absorption of fluid. Infants who fail to rapidly clear lung fluid usually have respiratory distress.

Mechanics of the fetal lung at different gestational ages

Both the distensibility of the lung and its stability improve with increasing gestational age. The fluid-filled lung has an intrapulmonary pressure equal to the intrapleural pressure.

Fetal respiratory movements

Fetal respiratory movements are characteristic of most mammalian fetuses, including man.

Fetal blood gas status

There is little information available on the acid-base and blood gas status of the undisturbed human fetus in utero. It is presumed on the basis of fetal blood obtained at cesarian section, scalp blood samples, and animal studies that the intrauterine arterial Po_2 is in the vicinity of 35 to 40 mm Hg and the pH 7.35 to 7.40.

Attainment of a stable extrauterine state

The establishment of lung function at birth will be directly related to gestational age. Lung fluid must be removed, functional residual capacity established and maintained, and appropriate ventilation-perfusion relationships developed to provide for optimum exchange of gases between the alveolus and blood.

Normal newborn infant

During the passage down the birth canal the thorax of the fetus is subjected to large pressure changes (at least 95 cm H_2O) that compress and decompress the lungs and promote removal of the lung fluid. The fluid itself enhances aeration of the gas-free lung by lowering the pressure required to open alveoli.

First breath. The factor or factors responsible for the first breath are unknown. Multiple stimuli such as exposure to environmental temperature and tactile changes undoubtedly play a role. However, the exact interrelationships of pH, Po_2, and Pco_2 that combine to induce breathing in the human neonate are still to be determined.

The pressure change of the first breath must overcome the effects of viscosity of fluid in the airway, overcome the effects of surface tension, and overcome the effects of tissue resistance. In full-term infants, intraesophageal pressure changes up to −70 cm H_2O have been recorded during the first breath, with a lesser pressure required for subsequent breaths. No information is available about the pressure changes developed by the premature infant.

Establishment of lung function. Roentgenographic studies of the lung indicate that inflation with air occurs immediately with the first breath. FRC is rapidly established, with little change throughout the first week of life. There is some evidence for gas trapping for 2 or 3 days, which may be related to the gradual disappearance of lung fluid during this period.

Both $AaDo_2$ and $aADco_2$ are present for several days after birth, reflecting a degree of mismatching of both ventilation and perfusion. Although there is some evidence of maldistribution of ventilation in the first 2 hours, the $AaDo_2$ is primarily caused by intracardiac and pulmonary R→L shunting. The $aADco_2$ reflects the presence of areas of lung that are poorly perfused.

Premature infant

Adaptation to air breathing at birth in premature infants has not been as well studied as in full-term infants. However, it is reasonable to suppose that the same qualitative changes are present; for example, the first breath requires a relatively high pressure. Further, the presence of a very compliant chest wall must put the infant at a considerable disadvantage during the first breath. In terms of attainment of lung volume, ventilation-perfusion relationships, and acid-base balance, the premature infant is qualitatively the same as the full-term infant, but the quantitative aspects depend on size and maturity. The FRC is smallest in the most immature infants and reflects the presence of atelectasis. Atelectasis is a feature of the lungs of the premature, no doubt related to the state of alveolar development and pulmonary surfactant production. Gas trapping persists longer in the premature infant for reasons not completely understood. Serial studies of ventilation-perfusion relationships by $AaDo_2$, $aADco_2$, and $aADn_2$ gradients are similar to the full-term infant except that the abnormalities are greater and persist for longer periods of time. The smallest infants have the most profound disturbances, and in very immature infants the abnormalities are quantitatively similar to larger infants with HMD. Large $AaDo_2$ and $aADco_2$ are present, reflecting again cardiopulmonary shunting and the presence of alveoli underperfused with respect to ventilation. The shunts are through atelectatic or gas-trapped alveoli and through the foramen ovale and patent ductus arteriosus.

These limitations in the adaption of the nondistressed premature infant to extrauterine life result in low PA_{O_2} (frequently around 40 to 50 mm Hg), slightly elevated PA_{CO_2}, and respiratory acidosis. The changes are secondary to atelectasis and reduce pulmonary perfusion. As the infant grows and matures, FRC increases and ventilation-perfusion relationships normalize; the $AaDo_2$ and $aADco_2$ eventually return to normal. There is evidence to indicate that when atelectasis disappears, alveoli "pop open," with no intervening stage when the alveoli are poorly ventilated. The lung volume and ventilation-perfusion abnormalities in the nondistressed premature are qualitatively similar to those of the infant with HMD.

Control of respiration in the infant

The relative effects of pH, Po_2, and Pco_2 on the initiation of breathing in the newborn infant are poorly understood. Apneic spells in small premature infants may be a reflection of the immaturity of the central nervous system control mechanism or another reflection of pulmonary immaturity, with a confused signal being sent to the central nervous system. Full-term and many premature infants increase minute volume in response to small increases in inspired CO_2 similarly to adults. The small premature infant with apnea and a high arterial Pco_2 seems to be an exception to this observation. Po_2 exerts its control on respiration through action on the chemoreceptors. In adults, hypoxia (10% O_2) invariably stimulates respiration, whereas hyperoxia (100% O_2), by releasing chemoreceptor tone, depresses it. In full-term and premature infants hyperoxia markedly depresses respiration initially, indicating strong chemoreceptor activity, even at birth and in the smallest infants. Hypoxia may have no effect or a depressant effect initially, which may persist. Hypoxic and apneic premature infants do not generally respond to this depressed Po_2 with improved respirations, but may have improved ventilation when exposed to high concentrations of ambient oxygen.

Frequent inspiratory sighs are noted in premature infants. They arise through a deflation reflex that is stimulated by atelectasis. An inflation reflex is also present. It is stimulated by distension of the lung, which results in a decrease in the frequency of inspiratory efforts. The inflation and deflation reflexes are also called the Hering-Breuer reflexes. The paradoxical reflex of Head, which is a gasp produced by sudden inflation of the lungs, is also active in the premature and full-term infant.

Breathing patterns in newborn infants

The irregularity of respiration in newborn infants is readily apparent. A similar pattern of chest movements has been observed in the fetus. The sleeping infant breathes first rapidly, then slowly. The premature infant frequently shifts his breathing pattern from one of regular rhythmicity to a totally disorganized pattern.

Periodic breathing is the characteristic pattern, occurring at some time in most premature infants. The apneic pauses are rarely associated with color change or change in heart rate. The pattern stops and starts for no apparent reason. Prolonged breathing of hypoxic gas mixtures often precipitates the pattern. Increasing the inspired oxygen tension will convert periodic breathing to regular breathing, as will almost any external stimulus. Blood gas measurements carried out in infants with periodic breathing have revealed a mild respiratory alkalosis compared with those infants with regular breathing; this indicates the net result is hyperventilation. There is an increase of 2 to 4 mm Hg PA_{CO_2} during the apneic pause. There is evidence suggesting that the major stimulus to this breathing pattern is in the lung rather than in the respiratory center.

Apnea

Because of its serious implications, the infant with prolonged apneic pauses must be distinguished from the one with periodic breathing. Very small premature infants are most frequently affected, but larger infants with HMD also show this pattern. The pauses most frequently occur from the second to the sixth day of life, but rarely may occur on the first day or after the fourth or fifth week. They occur without known cause or they may be associated with sepsis, HMD, and intracranial hemorrhage. Almost invariably apnea results in bradycardia or cyanosis or both, and some form of stimulation may be necessary to get the infant breathing again. An oxygen-enriched atmosphere can markedly decrease the frequency of bradycardia and cyanosis, although such practice runs the risk of retrolental fibroplasia. In severe cases it may be necessary to provide assisted ventilation with bag and mask for a short time in order to terminate an episode.

Sighs

Frequent inspiratory gasps or sighs are observed in most premature infants and sometimes in the full-term infant. Sighs are thought to be caused by repeated stimulation of deflation receptors in response to a tendency to recurrent atelectasis.

Adaptation of the heart to extrauterine life

While a detailed description of the changes in the cardiovascular system at birth is not within the scope of this chapter, it must be emphasized that the regulation of cardiac output and pulmonary blood flow are closely related to pulmonary adaptation. It is probable that in the distressed infant inability to increase cardiac output may be a limiting factor for survival. Also as pointed out above, the distribution of pulmonary perfusion is equal in importance to the distribution of ventilation.

Summary of process of pulmonary adaptation to extrauterine life

In the normal infant FRC is rapidly established and increases in size as the infant grows; pulmonary gas trapping is a constant feature of the first few days in all neonates. Large areas of the lung are nonventilated and perfused, while other areas are underperfused relative to ventilation. The full-term infant has well-developed chemoreceptor response at birth, and the respiratory center responds with an increased rate of breathing to increased PA_{CO_2}.

The premature infant shows a qualitatively similar pattern. Atelectasis caused by poor chest wall support and lack of pulmonary surfactants may result in persistent gas trapping for weeks because of the tendency to airway collapse. The gas-trapped and atelectatic areas function as large shunts, resulting in an $AaDo_2$ and low arterial Po_2. Areas of underperfusion also exist and may result in elevated Pa_{CO_2}. Periodic breathing and sighs occur frequently and may be a further reflection of small FRC. Chemoreceptor tone is present, but the pattern of responses has not been delineated.

CLINICAL APPROACH TO THE INFANT WITH RESPIRATORY DIFFICULTY

There is rarely any difficulty in determining that a newborn infant has a cardiopulmonary problem, but differentiation between heart and lung pathologic conditions is often a challenge. A careful history is very important. Unfortunately, because of lack of communication between obstetrician and pediatrician, knowledge of the events of the pregnancy, labor, and delivery is frequently unavailable to the physician caring for the infant at the time he most needs it.

Factors in the fetal and maternal history of importance in differential diagnosis of respiratory distress

Transfer of relevant obstetrical information is best accomplished by direct communication between the obstetrician and pediatrician. However, the use of a special delivery form can be very helpful if properly filled out.

Maternal history

Knowledge of the previous medical history of the mother, especially with relation to diabetes mellitus, is of value. Diabetic women have an increased likelihood of delivering an infant with a major abnormality of the heart that can result in respiratory distress. The increased likelihood of HMD in infants of a diabetic mother is mainly related to the fact that these infants are often born prematurely; the problem is encountered infrequently unless the infant is premature. Accurate knowledge of gestational age is important in determining if the infant is prematurely born or small for gestational age. Premature infants have a high incidence of HMD. Infants who are small for dates are more likely to have respiratory distress from meconium aspiration. The postmature infant is also at risk from meconium aspiration. Polyhydramnios in the mother may be indicative of esophageal or upper gastrointestinal atresia; oligohydramnios suggests renal anomalies and pulmonary hypoplasia. Maternal infection with rubella during pregnancy may result in an infant with congenital heart disease and respiratory distress.

Events of labor and delivery

Premature labor and delivery are very important determinants of the development of HMD. A difficult labor with fetal distress may result in an infant with meconium aspiration, pneumothorax, and pneumomediastinum. Asphyxia during labor and delivery may result in respiratory distress, acidosis, and hypoxia. Prolonged rupture of membranes should suggest that respiratory difficulty is caused by intrauterine pneumonia. Infants subjected to instrumentation during resuscitation may have breathing difficulty because of the effects of the trauma. By considering all these factors, the physician can have a reasonable idea of the cause of the respiratory difficulty before any further diagnostic evaluation is undertaken.

Evaluation of the infant with respiratory distress

Observation. Observation is the most important part of the physical examination of the distressed infant. The normal newborn infant and nondistressed premature have a barrel-chested appearance at birth, which disappears over the second and third days. This appearance is most obvious in the premature infant, and its disappearance corresponds to the release of trapped gas. When the chest appears overinflated, both intercostal muscles as well as the diaphragm are used for respiration; when the chest volume decreases, breathing becomes almost entirely abdominal.

The distressed infant may have dyspnea, tachypnea, subcostal and suprasternal retractions, expiratory grunt, pallor, or cyanosis. These signs are usually minimal at the onset but increase in severity as the disease progresses. When disease is severe, prolonged apneic pauses become a prominent feature. When atelectasis is present, as in HMD, the chest cage is collapsed (most obvious in the axilla). A barrel-chested appearance accompanies conditions associated with emphysema such as meconium aspiration or transient neonatal tachypnea.

Physiologic correlates of signs of respiratory distress

Retractions. Retractions are prominent in pulmonary disease in premature infants because of the compliant chest wall. The disease process results in decreased lung compliance, and this coupled with the compliant chest wall places the infant at a considerable disadvantage as he attempts to develop higher intrathoracic pressure changes.

Expiratory grunt. This is usually a feature of the early clinical course and tends to disappear as pulmonary disease worsens. Expiratory grunt is less common in the smallest infants. The cause is unknown. A plausible theory relates it to the effects of the high intrathoracic pressure change of the distressed infant that is transmitted to very compliant airways at the beginning of expiration, with consequent airway collapse. The grunt is then an attempt to keep alveoli open and to empty trapped alveolar air. It is probable that the increased expiratory resistance that occurs with grunting serves to redistribute gas to maintain FRC and Po_2.

Pallor. Pallor is a frequent occurrence in the sickest infants. It is associated with acidosis and is most likely the result of a compensatory mechanism to redistribute peripheral blood to more vital areas. Shock or hypotension may also be associated with pallor.

Cyanosis. In the newborn, cyanosis is invariably a consequence of right-to-left cardiopulmonary shunting. In the early stages of respiratory disease cyanotic infants frequently become pink when high concentrations of oxygen are administered; whereas in right-to-left shunting associated with congenital heart disease, oxygen has little effect. This difference is related to the severity of the shunt in the two conditions. As respiratory disease worsens and shunting increases, one can no longer rely on this maneuver to distinguish heart disease and lung disease. Cyanosis is frequently masked by pallor; if this is the case the tongue is often the best place to look. Acrocyanosis of the hands and feet is common and rarely indicates the presence of a pathologic process; it should not be confused with true central cyanosis.

Cyanosis and a scaphoid abdomen should suggest diaphragmatic hernia. Movement of only the hemithorax and cyanosis may indicate diaphragmatic paralysis.

Auscultation. Auscultation of the chest is seldom as rewarding in the infant as in the older child. Normally, breath sounds are fine and tinkling. Breath sounds in infants are widely transmitted and cannot always be relied on to detect a pathologic condition. In moderate to severe HMD, breath sounds are decreased or absent because of atelectasis.

Examination of the heart is obviously an important assessment of every newborn infant, and the detection of murmurs is important in the differential diagnosis of respiratory distress. A short ejection murmur maximal along the left sternal border, presumably caused by a persistent PDA, may be a normal finding in the first week of life. Frequently, in the recovery phase of HMD a similar murmur is heard, again most probably caused by a PDA. The murmur in this instance may persist for long periods of time and eventually assume the classic to-and-fro or continuous characteristic when pulmonary vascular resistance falls. It is thus important to realize that in the presence of cyanosis and respiratory distress, congenital heart disease is not necessarily present. Distant heart sounds should suggest pneumomediastinum or pericardial effusion. Bowel sounds in the chest signify diaphragmatic hernia.

Percussion of the newborn chest is seldom useful and is best omitted.

Chest roentgenograms. Because of the limitations of physical examination in the newborn, chest roentgenograms should be requested immediately in any infant with respiratory distress. A posterior-anterior projection and lateral film should be obtained, since lesions such as pneumothorax and pneumomediastinum require both views for diagnosis. The roentgenogram is required to rule out difficulties such as pneumothorax or diaphragmatic hernia that may require emergency surgery. Interpretation of chest roentgenograms in newborn infants is difficult because few clinicopathologic correlations have been made. The films are generally highlighted by numerous streaks and linear densities that may represent atelectasis, blood vessels, lymphatics, or infiltrates. Confluent densities that signify pneumonia in the older child may merely reflect the presence of atelectasis in the newborn.

The chest film of a normal full-term or nondistressed premature infant taken in the first day of life may appear overaerated and contain multiple linear streaks. A repeat film several days later frequently shows that the hyperaeration has disappeared. These changes appear to parallel the disappearance of trapped gas.

In specific disease states the plain chest roentgenograms can be most helpful. For pneumothorax, pneumomediastinum, diaphragmatic hernia, and, on occasion, tracheoesophageal fistula, the chest roentgenogram may provide a characteristic picture. Every nursery must have easy access to x-ray facilities. That portable x-ray units are seldom completely satisfactory for assessment of heart size and pulmonary vasculature should not preclude their use.

A typical roentgenogram has been identified for HMD. However, these findings may not always be present in HMD; they may not be present on the initial study, only to appear on a film taken 12 hours later. The typical reticulogranular pattern with air bronchogram is a reflection of the pathologic picture of atelectasis that allows the air-containing bronchi to stand out in relief. If the clinical picture is typical and the x-ray film is not, the physician should avoid repeated studies in an attempt to eventually show the pattern. Repeat roentgenograms of sick infants should be kept to a minimum and only performed when a dramatic change in clinical condition may signify a complication.

Infants who have aspirated meconium may develop a characteristic roentgenographic appearance consisting of hyperaeration and coarse streaking throughout both lung fields. These changes frequently take 12 to 24 hours to develop.

Assessment of heart size and pulmonary vasculature should be part of the examination. Cardiomegaly generally means that congenital heart disease is present. However, transient cardiomegaly may accompany the meconium aspiration syndrome, birth asphyxia, and infants of diabetic mothers. Assessment of pulmonary vasculature in the newborn is complicated by the generally present streaks of atelectasis that make interpretation difficult.

Posterior-anterior and lateral films of the chest, especially magnification films, rarely need supplementation with more sophisticated studies. In tracheoesophageal fistula, iodized oil (Lipiodal) placed in the blind pouch is diagnostic. A barium swallow is usually necessary to identify a vascular ring.

Other studies. Direct laryngoscopy to view the larynx and trachea can be useful to diagnose tracheal or laryngeal malformations but should be performed by those expert in newborn laryngoscopy.

The electrocardiogram. In the instances in which difficulty is encountered in distinguishing cardiac from pulmonary disease the ECG may be very useful (p. 251).

Laboratory methods. Blood gas and acid-base studies are essential for the evaluation and management of all infants with respiratory distress from any cause. The initial blood gas evaluation should occur as soon as possible after the infant's arrival in the nursery area, since it allows the physician to determine how effectively the infant is compensating for the problem, to assess severity, and to plan treatment. Repeated determinations of pH, P_{CO_2}, and P_{O_2} are often necessary for planning continuous treatment and to determine clinical progress. Frequent determinations of hematocrit are important since pulmonary or intracranial hemorrhage or repeated blood gas measurements can result in anemia. Measurements of blood glucose, bilirubin, and electrolytes levels and of serum osmolarity should be readily available. Therapy with glucose and water and with sodium bicarbonate or underlying disease may produce chemical abnormalities so that monitoring of these parameters is essential.

Differentiation of pulmonary disease and cardiac disease. The need to differentiate pulmonary from cardiac disease is more frequently encountered in the full-term infant than in the premature infant. The distinction is important in order to avoid cardiac catheterization in those for whom it is of no value and to use it when indicated. (A more detailed discussion of this problem is presented on p. 259.) Cyanotic congenital heart disease (transposition of great vessels, anomalous pulmonary venous drainage, hypoplastic left heart syndrome, and pulmonary atresia) is occasionally confused with HMD and aspiration syndromes. The infant with congenital heart disease often has a grayish blue pallor, which is only a very late event in the most severely ill infant with HMD. Some infants with severe congenital heart disease do not have heart murmurs. Hepatomegaly may be caused by congestive failure, or the liver may be pushed down by overdistended emphysematous lungs. In HMD the distress is often present from birth; in congenital heart disease distress may not be obvious for 12 to 24 hours.

In congenital heart disease palpation may reveal hyperactivity of the heart beat and an unduly prominent ventricular thrust. If a murmur is present, the diagnosis of heart disease is more likely but not inevitable (p. 249). The breath sounds in HMD may be decreased or absent; in heart disease they are generally well transmitted.

The roentgenogram and laboratory tests may help to distinguish the two problems. In the early stages oxygen administration will raise the arterial P_{O_2} in cyanotic infants, with respiratory disease producing little, if any, rise in Pa_{O_2} in infants with cyanotic congenital heart disease. Respiratory acidosis is an invariable accompaniment of HMD. A low P_{CO_2} is common in heart disease and some cases of aspiration pneumonia. (See p. 371 for full discussion of this problem.)

ABNORMAL STATES

The diagnosis and management of the various types of pulmonary disease is a major concern of those caring for the newborn. The common conditions rarely have a specific therapy; the physician must provide supportive measures based on a knowledge of the normal physiology and pathophysiology. The challenge is to provide appropriate supportive treatment that ensures survival and minimizes morbidity and to use measures that do not in themselves produce complications. (Resuscitation of the newborn infant is discussed in Chapter 2, p. 50.)

Respiratory conditions whose principal pathology is atelectasis

Atelectasis is the principal pathologic lesion in premature infants who die after developing a respiratory distress syndrome. Two clinical patterns are prominent: one is generally agreed to be HMD (or idiopathic respiratory distress syndrome); the other has been referred to by some as chronic pulmonary insufficiency of the very small infant and by others as a variant of HMD.

Chronic pulmonary insufficiency of the very small infant

This clinical syndrome is similar in pathophysiology and pulmonary pathology to HMD. However, the clinical events are distinct enough to consider it as a separate entity.

Clinical presentation. These infants are almost always between 800 and 1,200 gm birth weight (28 to 30 weeks' gestational age). Characteristically, the infant is in good condition for the first day or two after birth, pink in appearance, and has minimal respiratory distress. On physical examination the chest appears overinflated, and the lungs are clear to auscultation. Studies of blood gases and acid-base balance are not remarkable at this stage; temporal arterial Po_2 is 40 to 60 mm Hg, depending on the postnatal age. After 2 to 3 days of apparent stability, the patient's condition begins to deteriorate. Respiratory distress is characterized by frequent prolonged apneic spells in addition to tachypnea and retractions. Cyanosis may occur. Hyperbilirubinemia may be a complication of the prematurity. Blood gases show an increasing respiratory acidosis and hypoxia, which require acid-base correction and administration of increased oxygen concentrations. This deteriorating course may end in death, or there may be a slow, gradual recovery over the ensuing 2 or 3 weeks. Chest volume is visibly decreased when the clinical signs are most severe. Surviving infants require close monitoring and therapy for a prolonged period before stable lung function is attained. In some infants the initial clinical problem fades into the typical clinical and roentgenographic picture of Wilson-Mikity syndrome. If this occurs, tachypnea, retractions, cyanosis, and respiratory acidosis may be present for months.

Pathology and pathophysiology. Extensive atelectasis is a common finding in the lungs of these infants (Fig. 12-7). Hyaline membranes lining alveolar ducts are usually not present. Massive cerebral intraventricular hemorrhage may be an associated lesion in sick small prematures.

The disturbances in pulmonary physiology are qualitatively similar but more severe than those seen in the large nondistressed premature infants. Air trapping may persist to some extent for weeks. FRC is small, reflecting the extensive atelectasis, and frequently becomes smaller as the condition worsens. Lung compliance is very low. There is cardiopulmonary shunting and a low $\dot{V}A/\dot{Q}$ ratio, which result in low arterial Po_2, high Pco_2, and decreased pH. These physiologic abnormalities may persist with less severity long after the infant appears to be improving clinically.

Etiology and pathogenesis. The atelectasis may be the result of inadequate alveolar development and an immature surfactant system. In addition, the immature thoracic cage is very compliant. Then as these systems mature, the infant's condition improves, if supportive oxygen has not irreparably damaged the lungs. The physiologic abnormalities result from atelectasis and poorly distributed pulmonary perfusion.

The limitations of lung function demand that oxygen be provided, but it may cause irreparable damage to the lung. Some investigators think that the entire clinical

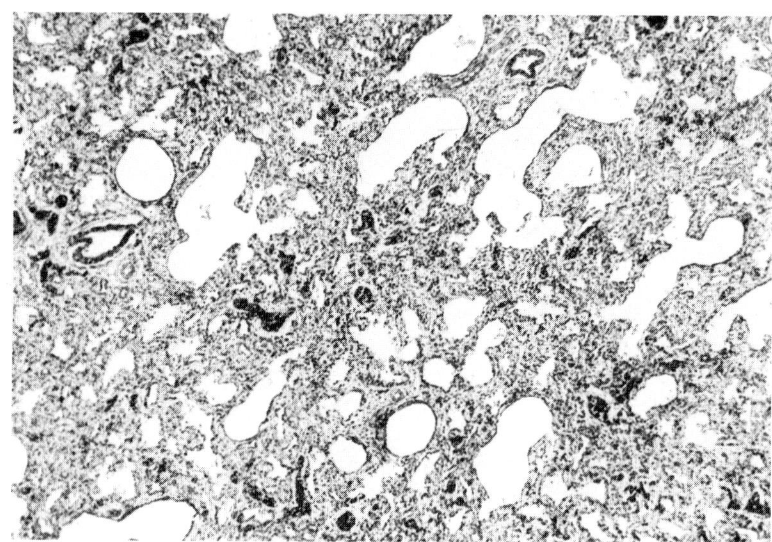

Fig. 12-7. Photomicrograph of the lung of a 780-gm infant who survived 24 hours. Note poor alveolar development.

condition described here is the Wilson-Mikity syndrome and that this condition is the clinical response of the immature lung. Others suggest that Wilson-Mikity syndrome is produced by the toxic effects of oxygen on the immature lung.

Laboratory findings. Blood gas studies reveal respiratory acidosis and low Pa_{O_2}. Constant monitoring of these parameters can be difficult because of the prolonged course and size of the infants. Chest roentgenograms show multiple streaks or occasionally prominent air bronchograms (Fig. 12-8) or may be normal. The findings of Wilson-Mikity syndrome may be present later.

When mechanical ventilation is necessary, careful monitoring of Pa_{O_2} is particularly important in order to avoid retrolental fibroplasia.

Treatment. The details of treatment are essentially the same as for HMD and is considered in that discussion. The aim of therapy is to support cardiopulmonary function until the infant becomes mature enough to support it by himself.

Management of apneic spells. Apneic spells are extremely common in small premature infants. They occur most frequently from the second to the tenth day of life, but may persist in some infants for weeks. The cause of apneic periods is unknown. They should not be confused with the apneic pauses that occur during periodic breathing (p. 354). The duration of apneic spells varies from several seconds to 20 to 30 seconds. When prolonged, cyanosis and bradycardia may be prominent.

Premature infants with the likelihood of apneic spells should have respirations monitored continuously. In the majority of instances, gentle stimulation will result in the resumption of breathing. In severe cases the spell may have to be treated with assisted ventilation with bag and mask.

Hyaline membrane disease (idiopathic respiratory distress syndrome)

HMD is a common condtion of the premature infant and occurs rarely in the full-term infant. The true incidence of HMD has been difficult to determine because a definitive diagnosis can be made only at postmortem examination. Nevertheless, most workers consider HMD to be the major cause of death in premature infants. Avery and Oppenheimer reported a death rate of 3.8% of live premature births between 1,000 and 2,500 gm caused by this condition. In general, the smaller the infant the higher the mortality. A recent review of the New York Hospital covering the years 1968 to mid 1971 shows a mortality of 12% for all newborn premature infants between 1 and 2 kg admitted to the nursery. Some of these

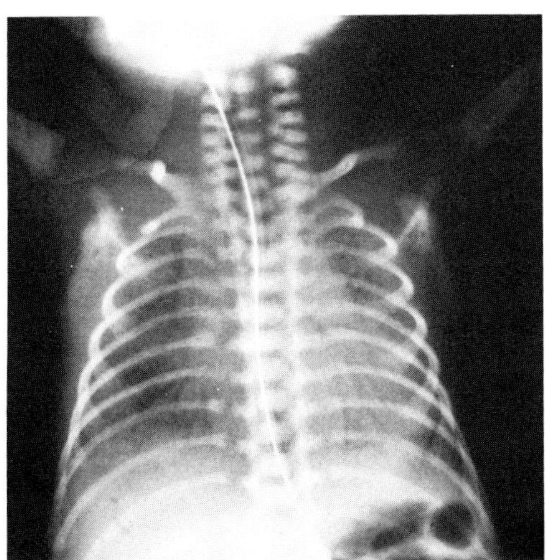

Fig. 12-8. Chest roentgenogram of an infant with chronic pulmonary insufficiency. Note left lower lobe air bronchogram and generalized streak of densities.

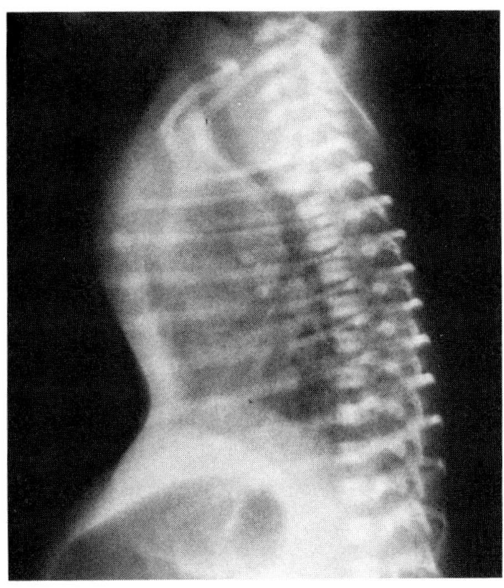

Fig. 12-9. Lateral roentgenogram of thorax, showing collapsed chest typical of HMD, which resulted in low FRC.

infants are transferred from outlying hospitals. A death rate of 16% caused by HMD was recorded at autopsy for this group. The mortality for HMD, defined as all infants with an abnormal chest x-ray film or with autopsy evidence of the disease, was 33%. Another recent analysis of death from the Toronto Hospital for Sick Children, which deals only with transferred infants, reveals a mortality of 33% in infants with HMD. In the United States, 25,000 infants die yearly with this disease.

Clinical presentation. The infants with HMD are usually prematurely born infants with a birth weight between 1,200 and 2,000 gm and a gestational age of 30 to 36 weeks. However, smaller and larger infants are also affected. The infant may be large as a result of maternal diabetes, in which case the disease is not related to maternal diabetes as such, but is caused by the premature delivery that is often necessary because of a deteriorating intrauterine condition.

The disease begins at birth or in the first 6 hours of life. The infant may have suffered prior intrauterine asphyxia, but frequently this cannot be documented. Tachypnea, chest retraction, cyanosis, and expiratory grunting are often present before the infant leaves the delivery room. The clinical course is characterized by a progressive worsening of these symptoms, with a peak severity from 48 to 72 hours, although occasionally maximum severity occurs in less than 12 hours. Infants show a need for increasing oxygen concentrations to abolish cyanosis. The expiratory grunt, so prominent early, diminishes, and prolonged apneic pauses occur. Some infants show pitting edema of the extremities. The volume of the thorax ceases to increase (Fig. 12-9); this is most obvious in the axilla. There is often a striking decrease in breath sounds.

If the infant survives and there are no complications, there is a gradual decrease of clinical signs, associated with a reduced oxygen requirement, and lessening tachypnea and retractions. Clinical recovery is complete in 10 days to 2 weeks.

Laboratory findings. When the infant is first seen, a chest roentgenogram should be obtained. The classic picture of HMD is associated with an air bronchogram and a reticulogranular appearance to the lung fields (Fig. 12-10). Normally, an air bronchogram is noted in the left lower lobe. In HMD it is obvious elsewhere as well, particularly in the upper lobes. Frequently, an initial x-ray film may be normal, only to develop the typical pattern at 12 to 24 hours. It is rare for a infant to succumb and not show an abnormal roentgenogram. Occasionally, a typical clinical course is seen,

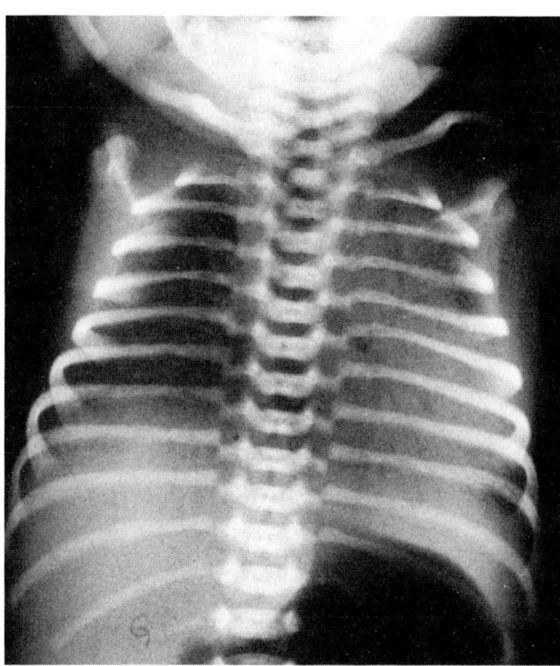

FIG. 12-10. Chest roentgenogram showing characteristic picture of HMD with air bronchogram.

and the x-ray film is normal. This is more common in larger infants. Heart size is normal. Not infrequently a cardiac murmur, ejection or continuous in type and maximal at the base, may be heard during recovery. This murmur is caused by a persistent patency of the ductus arteriosus and may be associated with cardiomegaly and increased vascular markings.

If the infant is depressed at birth, both metabolic and respiratory acidosis may be present. After the initial resuscitation, blood gases may normalize; or if the disease process advances rapidly, increasing respiratory acidosis may develop. If the infant is adequately oxygenated, respiratory acidosis may be the only disturbance of acid-base metabolism. An arterial Po_2 below 40 mm Hg in room air is a constant feature of the disease and indicates the need for oxygen therapy. With recovery, Pa_{O_2} is maintained with lessening amounts of oxygen, and Pco_2 begins to fall toward normal.

FRC falls in the first 3 days and on recovery reaches normal values in most survivors by 15 to 20 days. The compliance is decreased to very low levels in the sickest infants, and airway resistance is normal. The $\dot{V}_A/\dot{Q}$ abnormalities in the acute stage are caused by right-to-left cardiopulmonary shunts (lungs, foramen ovale, ductus arteriosus) causing an $AaDo_2$ that decreases arterial Po_2 and underperfusion (low $\dot{V}_A/\dot{Q}$) causing $aADco_2$ and a high arterial Pco_2. Both of these abnormalities persist long after clinical recovery, indicating persistence of $\dot{V}_A/\dot{Q}$ abnormalities.

The ECG is normal. The hematocrit reading may fall gradually because of repeated blood sampling; a sudden fall may indicate intracranial hemorrhage. Blood electrolytes are usually normal if the infant receives proper fluid and electrolytes. Serum potassium levels may be elevated because of tissue catabolism if sufficient calories are not provided. The serum sodium level may be elevated because of therapy with sodium bicarbonate.

Acute complications. Pneumothorax may occur more commonly in the large premature infant. Presumably this is because he can develop greater intrathoracic pressure changes that can result in rupture of an overdistended alveolus. At autopsy small infants frequently show large intraventricular hemorrhages in the brain. They may be

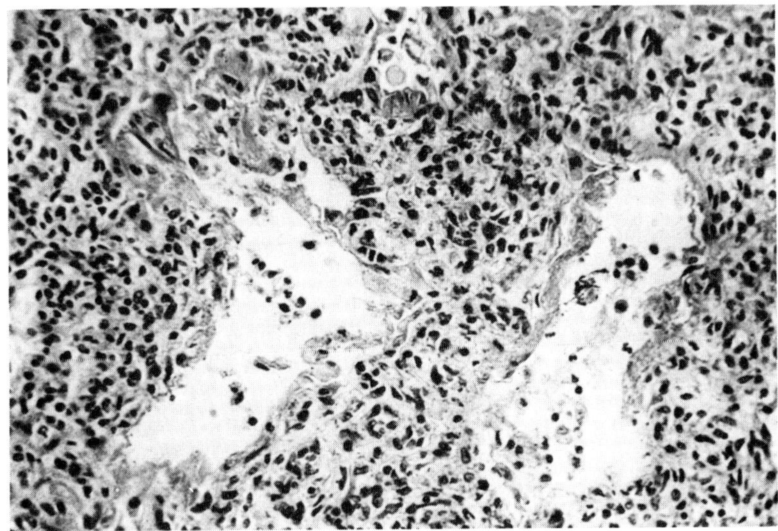

Fig. 12-11. Photomicrograph of lungs of infant with HMD. Note marked atelectasis and hyaline membrane lining and dilated alveolar ducts.

caused by hypoxia or acidosis. Finberg has suggested that very large infusions of sodium bicarbonate may be responsible for intracranial hemorrhages.

Pathology and pathophysiology. Grossly, the lungs of an infant who succumbs to HMD are like liver. Microscopically, the alveoli are atelectatic but interspersed with a few widely dilated alevoli (Fig. 12-11). The hyaline membranes line these dilated areas in the alveoli and are seen also at the bronchiolar-alveolar junction. The bronchiolar epithelium underlying the membranes is destroyed. The membranes themselves consist of necrotic cells and fibrin. On electron microscopy the type II alveolar lining cells show signs of beginning regeneration, even in the infant who succumbs in the first 24 to 36 hours.

The principal abnormality of HMD is atelectasis, and extensive physiologic disturbances are secondary to this lesion. Right-to-left shunts through the lungs, foramen ovale, and ductus arteriosus are constant findings in HMD. The major site of shunting is thought to be through the lung in areas that are nonventilated but perfused. These shunts increase with time, leading to a progressive fall in Po_2, an increase in $AaDo_2$, and a need for increasing oxygen therapy. During recovery, shunts persist for a variable time, although the persistence of a low Po_2 (when the infant appears clinically well) is also caused by other factors (maldistribution of ventilation-diffusion). The progressive increase in $aADco_2$ and Pa_{CO_2} reflects the presence of areas of underperfusion (high $\dot{V}_A/\dot{Q}$.) These areas increase the physiologic dead space and may be secondary to vascular spasm caused by acidosis or hypoxia. The alveoli with high $\dot{V}_A/\dot{Q}$ persist well into the recovery phase. Thus the effects of shunting and underperfusion are low Pa_{O_2} and high Pa_{CO_2}. These major disturbances in blood gases often result in acidosis; respiratory or mixed types are common.

The work of breathing is increased tenfold in the distressed infant. The lungs are stiff, with a very low compliance. Respiratory frequency may approach 100, tidal volume is normal to slightly decreased, and minute volume markedly increased.

Hemodynamic studies have failed to document congestive heart failure. Systemic hypotension is frequently noted and is caused by either depressed cardiac output or decreased peripheral resistance. It is seen in only the sickest infants.

The disturbances in acid-base balance are secondary to altered pulmonary function and depressed cardiac output. Hypoxia if severe (that is, Pa_{O_2} less than 30) will result in the development of lactic acidosis secondary to anaerobic metabolism, but attention to proper oxygenation can minimize this. More severe and protracted respiratory acidosis is secondary to underperfusion (areas of high $\dot{V}A/\dot{Q}$), and it is the acid-base abnormality that causes the greatest disturbance.

Etiology of hyaline membrane disease. The causes of HMD are presently not completely elucidated. Some maintain that the disease is a direct consequence of immaturity of some aspect of pulmonary development; others contend that the infant who develops HMD has been subjected to some insult prior to or during birth that sets off a series of events to produce the disease; while still others contend that both factors are operating. All theories must take into consideration the fact that the disease occurs almost exclusively in premature infants.

Early workers perceived the hyaline membranes as aspirated and inspissated amniotic fluid. The observation by Gitlin and Craig that fibrin was a major constituent of the membranes directed attention to the thought that the membranes may actually have originated from within the infant's own vascular system and appeared in alveoli as a transudate. Various toxic agents, such as hypoxia, hyperoxia, and aspirated gastric contents, have been considered as noxious agents sufficient to damage the pulmonary capillaries and to result in transudation. Congestive left heart failure was suggested as a possible explanation for the transudation, and patency of the ductus arteriosus was proposed as the initial event. The presence of cellular debris in the membranes and the necrosis of cells at the bronchiolar-alveolar junction suggested that the membranes may have originated from the agent that caused this lesion. Aspiration of gastric contents was incriminated in this theory as the event capable of causing this damage. A derangement of coagulation sufficient to cause disseminated intravascular clotting also has been put forth as an explanation for hyaline membranes. Alteration of fibrinolytic activity, with depletion of fibrinolysins, has been suggested as playing a role, although treatment with various fibrinolysins has failed to alter the clinical picture.

Alternatively, the production of atelectasis may be considered the primary event. Pulmonary surfactants have been demonstrated to be decreased in the lungs of infants with HMD. These phospholipids are required for alveolar stability; their absence is viewed as playing a key role in producing atelectasis. Surfactants may be absent because of the immaturity of the cells producing them. This is thought to result in a failure of the biochemical pathway to keep up with the consumption of surfactant during breathing.

Another theory suggests that the surfactant system is destroyed or damaged by some factor—hypoxia, acidosis, pulmonary hypoperfusion—with resultant atelectasis. Hyperoxia and carbon dioxide are also known to interfere with surfactant activity. Attempts to provide supplemental surfactant by aerosolization into the lungs have not produced a significant change in survival.

General management and therapy of hyaline membrane disease and chronic pulmonary insufficiency

The treatment of both HMD and chronic pulmonary insufficiency is supportive and directed toward maintenance of certain normal physiologic parameters while those that are abnormal are corrected.

General supportive measures. The general principles of supportive care for any premature infant must be adhered to. These include minimal disturbance (especially the limitation of repeated and unwarranted chest roentgenograms) and gentle handling. The proper environmental temperature should be maintained by placing the infant in a heated isolette to maintain body temperature between 97.7 and 98.6 F (36.5 and 37 C). Smaller infants require higher environmental temperatures than larger infants. As a general rule oral feedings should be avoided since they tend to tire the infant; calories and fluid should be provided intravenously. For the first 36 to 48 hours 10% glucose and water is infused at the rate of 100 cc/kg/day; this supplies 40 calories/kg/day, a caloric intake sufficient to prevent catabolism. Higher rates may be needed for sick infants. After 48 hours, the fluid may be changed to glucose and one fourth normal saline. By the fourth or fifth day it may be necessary to add potassium if the infant is still receiving an intravenous infusion. Electrolytes should be measured at approximately 3 days of age. Oral feedings by intermittent or continuous gavage can occasionally be given by the third day, but in severe disease oral feedings may have to be delayed for a longer time. When feedings are begun, milk formulas prepared to 30 calories/oz may be indicated in infants in whom caloric intake has been postponed because of severity of the disease; adequate fluid intake is needed to prevent hyperosmolarity. (See p. 118 for discussion of intravenous alimentation.)

Hyperbilirubinemia is frequently excessive in infants with HMD. The danger of kernicterus is increased in these infants because of low albumin levels, hypoxia, and acidosis, which interferes with albumin binding of bilirubin. Prophylactic phototherapy is indicated in infants with this disease when indirect bilirubin levels approach 10 mg/100 ml and may be indicated from the outset in badly bruised and distressed infants (p. 227). Every effort should be made to keep indirect bilirubin levels below 12 to 15 mg/100 ml in infants under 1,500 gm. (See Chapter 10, p. 230, for discussion of indications for phototherapy and exchange transfusion.) Exchange transfusion can be carried out in even the sickest infants if attention is paid to the essentials of newborn care (temperature and so on). Buffering of the blood used for exchange transfusion is not necessary; however, frequent monitoring of blood gases during the procedure is mandatory, and acidosis should be corrected as necessary.

Some workers have recommended monitoring of arterial blood pressure through a catheter in the umbilical artery, because systemic hypotension may occur in the sickest infants. Specific therapy for hypotension should be directed toward correction of acidosis when present and may include blood transfusions.

Antibiotics are not routinely indicated in the infant with HMD. Some workers advise use of prophylactic antibiotics (ampicillin and kanamycin) with indwelling umbilical vessel catheters.

Specific supportive measures

Oxygen therapy. Oxygen is almost always required by infants with HMD. However, overoxygenation (hyperoxia) must be avoided; a Pa_{O_2} of 60 mm Hg should be aimed for. This value is based on the observation that nondistressed premature infants are pink and develop normally with a Pa_{O_2} in this range. Because one of the major defects in oxygenation in HMD is caused by cardiopulmonary shunting, inspired oxygen concentrations up to 100% frequently are necessary to abolish cyanosis and maintain Pa_{O_2}.

The two goals of oxygen therapy are to provide adequate oxygenation and prevent lactic acid accumulation caused by hypoxia and to avoid toxic effects, especially retrolental fibroplasia and pulmonary oxygen toxicity. In order to accomplish all these goals a reliable system of monitoring oxygenation is necessary. Sampling of arterial blood from the temporal artery or right radial artery should provide the best reflection of the Pa_{O_2} of blood perfusing the retina, but it is technically difficult and can only be carried out a few times. A widely accepted alternative method is intermittent monitoring of blood oxygen tension by sampling through an indwelling umbilical arterial catheter (p. 112). However, the technique is associated with complications, and the Pa_{O_2} in this artery may not reflect retinal artery P_{O_2} because of right-to-left shunting at the level of the ductus arteriosus. All methods of monitoring Pa_{O_2} by blood sampling are limited by the fact that Pa_{O_2} varies from minute to minute and that sick infants have frequent apneic spells; it may be difficult to sample often enough to control these problems. Continual observation of an infant's color to detect cyanosis is an important adjunct to frequent measurements of Pa_{O_2} in providing a basis for regular adjustment of ambient oxygen concentrations. Noninvasive monitoring methods, such as ear oximetry, are not adequately developed for these purposes at this time.

The greatest risk from hyperoxia occurs during recovery, when shunting is no longer a major cause of venous admixtures; this period often occurs when umbilical catheters have been removed. The nursing staff should be constantly aware of the hazards of unnecessary oxygen, and infants should be removed from an increased oxygen environment as soon as possible.

Acid-base therapy. The need for therapy

for acid-base disturbances should be determined by evaluation of pH, Pco_2, bicarbonate, and changes in buffer base.

Metabolic acidosis is most often encountered at birth when the infant has required resuscitation. (See p. 57 for emergency treatment in the delivery room of acidosis associated with asphyxia.) Subsequently, metabolic acdiosis may also require correction based on similar calculations. In general, initial alkali therapy is directed at correcting 50% of the measured base deficit.

Respiratory acidosis may require transient or prolonged ventilation therapy. Administration of sodium bicarbonate to infants with respiratory acidosis provides only transient correction at best and may further increase the Pco_2. It is usually not necessary to correct a pH>7.25 resulting from respiratory acidosis unless an infant's condition is unstable or deteriorating. Severe acidosis, respiratory or metabolic, especially when coupled with hypoxia, may result in pulmonary arterial vasoconstriction and ventilation-perfusion abnormalities or may result in arrhythmia and decreased cardiac output or both. In severe respiratory acidosis, alkali therapy should be withheld until assisted ventilation with bag and mask or an endotracheal tube and positive pressure has first been tried. If this fails to improve oxygenation and raise the pH, sodium bicarbonate may be administered in the dosage outlined below in an attempt to relieve arterial vasoconstriction of the pulmonary and coronary circulations. The assisted ventilation should be continued. Alkali therapy should be considered when pH is below 7.30, and repeat blood sampling indicates that it is decreasing and that the infant's condition is worsening.

The dosage of sodium bicarbonate (7.5%) is calculated as follows. While ventilating, measure pH and Pco_2 and determine the bicarbonate concentration (HCO_3^-) from the Siggaard-Andersen nomogram. Then, assuming no further change in Pco_2 with continued ventilation, determine what the HCO_3^- would be from nomogram if pH was compensated to pH 7.35. This difference is the HCO_3^- deficit in mEq/liter. The infant's bicarbonate space is assumed to be 0.6 × total body weight. Then 0.6 × (HCO_3^-) deficit × body weight = (HCO_3^-) deficit in the infant.

Example in a 2-kg infant
pH 7.20, Pco_2 60 mm Hg, HCO_3^- = 23 mEq/liter
Correcting to pH 7.35: HCO_3^- = 32 mEq/liter
HCO_3^- deficit = 11 × 0.6 × 2.0 = 13 mEq/liter (desired correction)

Only one half the calculated dose (that is, 6 mEq) should be given, and the blood gases repeated in 30 minutes. If acidosis is still present, the other half of the calculated dose is given. Frequent monitoring of pH and Pco_2 must be continued while acidosis is being corrected, and repeated measurements are necessary to determine the need for future therapy. Because of the potential for complications from bicarbonate therapy, each dose should be infused over 5 or 10 minutes.

THAM or tris (hydroxymethyl) aminomethane (0.3 M), may be used when hypernatremia or congestive heart failure is present or when the infant has received more than 15 mEq/kg/24 hr of sodium bicarbonate. This drug acts by binding the H^+ ion to form NH_3^+. It has the advantage of not producing CO_2, but the disadvantage of depressing respiration and occasionally causing hypoglycemia and hyperosmolarity.

THAM dosage: Base excess × body weight (kg) × 0.3 = ml 0.3 M THAM

The physician must be aware of the potential hazards of alkali therapy. These are (1) skin sloughs if infiltration occurs, (2) an increase in serum osmolarity that may damage capillaries and brain cells, and (3) a decrease in cerebrospinal fluid pH because the CO_2 produced enters the spinal fluid and causes acidosis before bicarbonate compensation occurs.

Assisted ventilation. The goals of assisted ventilation are (1) to improve oxygenation when breathing an increased O_2 concentration alone is not sufficient to maintain Pa_{O_2}, (2) to reduce Pco_2 and thus correct respiratory acidosis, and (3) to ventilate atelectatic alveoli. This type of therapy is required only in the most severely distressed infants. It is definitely indicated when Pco_2>70 mm Hg and pH<7.20 and when Po_2<40 mm Hg or cyanosis is present in 100% O_2. Limited mask-and-bag–assisted ventilation may be indicated to correct mild respiratory acidosis in the early newborn period.

It is not the purpose here to discuss in detail various respirators that are available (p. 109). In general, respirators that deliver a preset volume, volume respirators, are better adapted to the requirements of small infants than positive pressure respirators. These latter respirators usually require an endotracheal tube. Some neonatalogists prefer a negative pressure respirator because the use of an endotracheal tube can be avoided. However, negative pressure respirators are difficult to use effectively on small infants; no respirator is completely without shortcomings when used for small infants.

Because of the limitations of mechanical respirators, some workers prefer to use a simple anesthesia bag and mask without valves to provide assisted ventilation. This method requires a nurse to stand by the crib and ventilate the infant by hand for long periods of time, sometimes up to 10 days. A tube is placed in the stomach to avoid overdistention. This method has several advantages over the mechanical respirators: it avoids an endotracheal tube; it can be used for short periods of time; it can be used intermittently, for example 20 minutes every hour; it provides for constant observation and assessment of the infant's condition by the nurse performing the ventilation; and it is readily adaptable to the smallest infants. The major drawback is that large numbers of specially trained nurses are required.

Regardless of which method is used, inspired gases should be humidified. Mist aerosols are not indicated in the care of newborn infants.

Elevation of airway pressure. Constant positive airway pressure (CPAP) has been suggested as a specific therapy for HMD. CPAP can be accomplished by positive pressure on the airway or constant negative pressure around the chest. The positive airway pressure reduces the tendency to atelectasis and results in increased Pa_{O_2}. It can be coupled with assisted ventilation. The major problem with this approach is the possibility that pulmonary blood flow may be impeded and result in right heart failure and reduced cardiac output. The consequences of CPAP will need further study before it can be recommended for routine therapy of HMD.

Concept of intensive care. Because of the high degree of technical proficiency required in their management and the appropriate demands on personnel and laboratory facilities, infants with HMD should be treated in intensive care nurseries. The monitoring and therapy outlined here cannot be carried out without a skilled nursing staff, a reliable laboratory, and expert medical supervision. Both morbidity and mortality are reduced when sick infants or infants at high risk are cared for in neonatal intensive care units.

Complications of therapy. Complications that arise during the clinical course of HMD may be directly or indirectly related to therapeutic efforts; some are unavoidable, others can be minimized with greater attention to detail.

Complications of O_2 therapy. Retrolental fibroplasia is an uncommon complication of HMD, principally because it is very difficult to overoxygenate an infant with severe cardiopulmonary shunting. The infant is at greatest risk during recovery. In chronic pulmonary insufficiency, on the other hand, retrolental fibroplasia occurs with greater frequency, because oxygen therapy is required for prolonged periods of time.

It is also highly likely that prolonged periods of breathing gases with high oxygen concentrations can result in damage to the lung. The toxic effects principally involve the capillaries and the alveolar walls. The lesion itself increases the need for oxygen so that a vicious circle is established. The injury can result in the death of the infant, or as is more usual, complete resolution may occur after a period of weeks. Although many infants with apparent pulmonary oxygen toxicity have had respirator therapy as well, the respirator does not appear to be the primary cause of the injury.

The diagnosis of pulmonary oxygen toxicity is usually based on circumstantial evidence. The first indication of its presence is a prolongation of the clinical course of HMD beyond the usual recovery period. The chest roentgenogram shows coarse streaks throughout, with areas of atelectasis and emphysema. Pathologically the lesion is characterized by destruction and proliferation of capillaries and thickening of the alveolar septum. Treatment of this complication is essentially the same as that for HMD.

Complications of indwelling catheters. Indwelling catheters, whether in a peripheral vein or an umbilical vessel, can be a source of septicemia. This complication can be minimized by attention to the details of asepsis during catheter placement and limiting their use to short periods of time. Catheters in the umbilical vein may cause liver necrosis and thrombus formation, most probably because of the hypertonic solutions infused into them. This complication can be minimized by inserting the umbilical venous catheter into the inferior vena cava with x-ray confirmation. Umbilical artery catheters can produce blanching of the legs, obstruction of arterial flow, and thrombosis of renal vessels. These hazards can be reduced considerably when the catheterization is carried out by skilled personnel.

Endotracheal tubes can result in tracheal erosion and infection if nebulization is inadequate and they are left in place for prolonged periods of time. They should be removed immediately when they are no longer necessary.

Other complications consist of skin sloughs caused by infiltration of hypertonic solutions, perforation of the stomach from bag and mask breathing, pneumothorax, pneumomediastinum and pneumoperitoneum, and anemia caused by excessive blood loss. As can be expected, complications are less frequent in nurseries with greater experience in treating sick infants.

Respiratory problems whose principal feature is emphysema

The conditions occurring under this heading are principally, but not exclusively, diseases of full-term infants.

Meconium aspiration

Meconium aspiration is seen almost exclusively in the SGA, full-term, or postmature infant. Infants who develop the disease have been subjected to some intrauterine insult that causes fetal distress with passage of meconium into the amniotic fluid. In utero or with the first breath, the meconium stained fluid is aspirated into the lungs and results in a chemical pneumonitis. Complications of the disease in the form of pneumothorax and pneumomediastinum can threaten the life of the infant, and the physician must be alert to the possibility of these complications.

Pathophysiology. Anoxia is often the cause of fetal distress that results in the passage of meconium. Meconium in the lung results in obstruction and secondary atelectasis. Subsequently, a pneumonitis may occur, on either a chemical or an infectious basis, with the production of additional areas of atelectasis and emphysema throughout the lung. Gas trapping is invariably present. Infants with this condition often have difficulty oxygenating blood because of cardiopulmonary shunting and maldistribution of ventilation. Respiratory acidosis occurs in only the most severely affected infants. Pneumothorax is considered to result from rupture of the emphysematous area into the pleura. Pneumomediastinum occurs when the gas tracks along vascular sheaths and through the interstices back to the mediastinum. Why the lungs of these infants are so susceptible to pneumothorax and pneumomediastinum is not entirely undertood, although it appears to be a direct complication of emphysema.

Clinical presentation. The infant who develops this condition frequently requires resuscitation at birth and may appear depressed from hypoxia (Chapter 2, p. 55). Respiratory distress may develop at once or may not become obvious for several hours after birth. The respiratory distress may be complicated by bizarre neurologic signs related to the initial hypoxic insult. The infants are often meconium stained and usually have tachypnea, frequently up to 100 breaths per minute. The finding of meconium-stained gastric aspirate, finger nails, and skin may be confirmatory. Cyanosis is obvious in the most severely affected infants. Marked overdistention of the chest, a reflection of the emphysema, is prominent. Chest retractions are not a prominent sign. Ausculation may not reveal anything other than poor heart sounds, which are the hallmark of pneumomediastinum. The presence of a pneumothorax may be difficult to detect clinically, so that a chest roentgenogram should be performed if it is suspected. Extreme tachypnea may persist for many days or weeks, although recovery is generally complete in 7 to 10 days and no residual of the pulmonary problem has been reported. Severely affected infants may not survive.

Diagnosis. As with any respiratory problem, close monitoring of blood gases and acid-base balance is mandatory. Arterial Po_2 is generally low. Respiratory and metabolic acidosis may be noted in the immediate newborn period, especially if the infant has required resuscitation. Mild forms of the disease may result in respiratory alkalosis from hyperventilation; respiratory acidosis only occurs in the severely affected infants.

The volume of the lungs is increased with increased anteroposterior diameter and flattening of the diaphragm, reflecting the emphysematous change. Coarse streaks are present throughout both lung fields (Fig. 12-12). Since the pneumonic picture frequently takes time to develop, the typical findings may not be present on the first examination. Frequently, the heart shadow shows a general increase in size, and this may cause some confusion with congenital heart disease. Pneumothorax (Fig. 12-13) and pneumomediastinum may be present (Fig. 12-14, *A* to *C*).

Management and treatment. The general principles of management outlined for HMD apply here. The physician must be constantly alert for the development of pneumothorax and pneumomediastinum (p. 380). Any sudden worsening of the condition should arouse suspicion and is an indication for repeat chest roentgenogram. Blood gas and acid-base monitoring should be carried out as frequently as indicated. Most infants require an increased oxygen environment to abolish cyanosis and maintain an arterial Po_2 of 60 mm Hg. The acid-base disturbances that are present at birth should be corrected. (p. 57). When respiratory acidosis is present, assisted ventilation and alkali therapy may be indicated. Antibiotics (ampicillin and kanamycin) are frequently given to these infants, although some question the need.

Pneumomediastinum rarely causes the infant difficulty, and no treatment is indicated. Pneumothorax, on the other hand, may be so severe, especially when under tension, as to require surgical intervention with removal of air and constant underwater-seal drainage. The decision to treat the pneumothorax must be based on its size and the severity of symptoms. A small pneumothorax may be observed

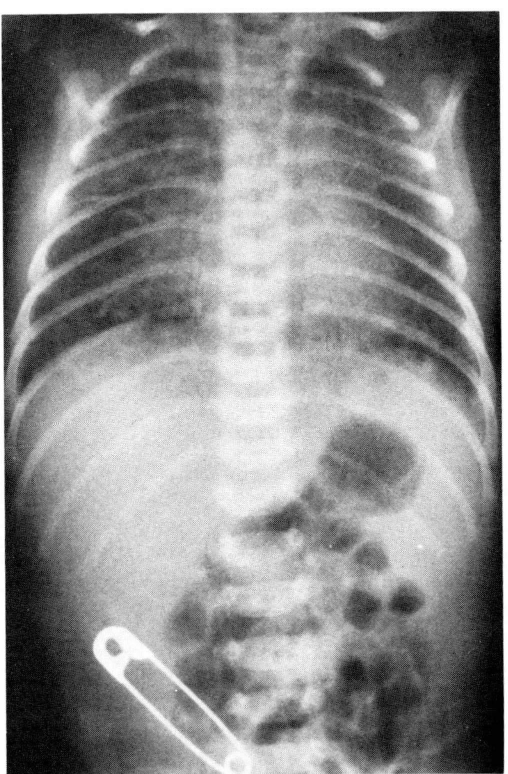

Fig. 12-12. Chest roentgenogram showing multiple linear streaks typical of meconium aspiration pneumonia.

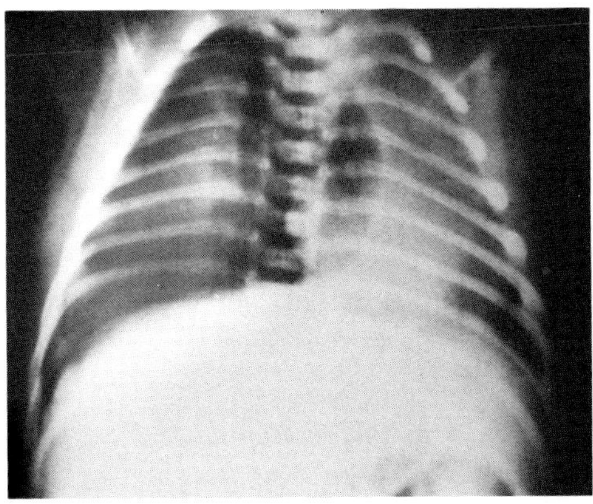

Fig. 12-13. Tension pneumothorax with shift of the heart and mediastinum to the left.

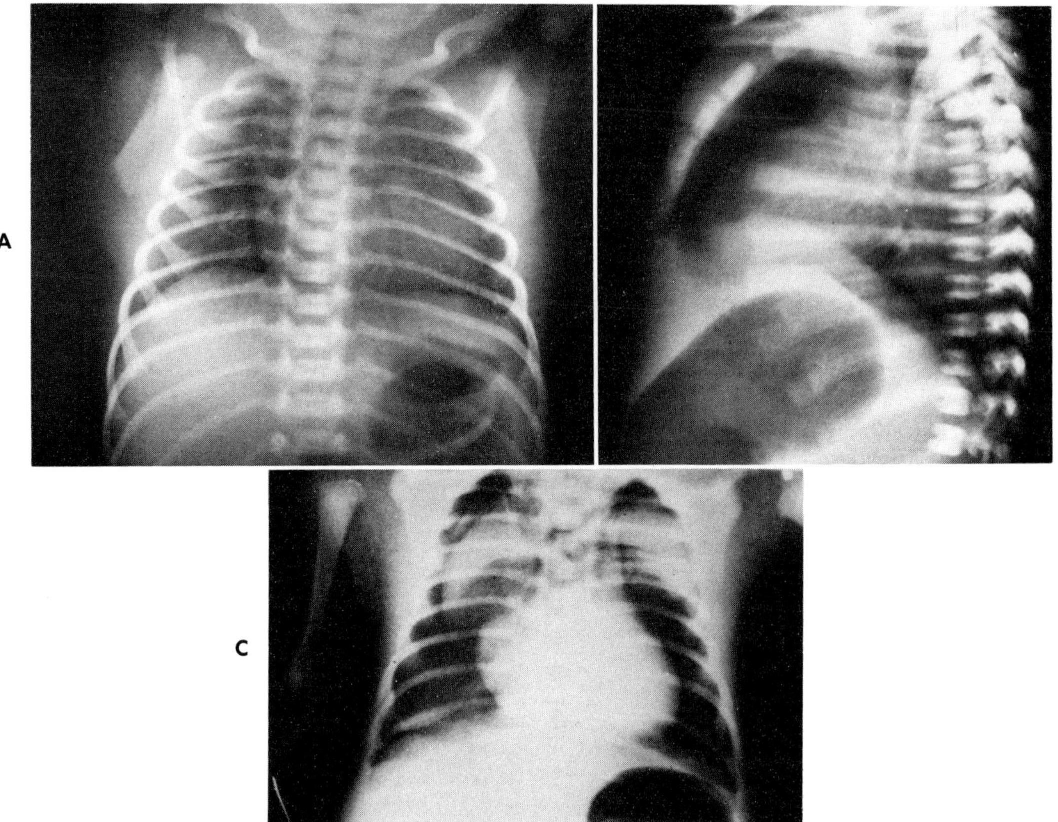

Fig. 12-14. Pneumomediastinum, **A,** indicated by line of hyperlucency along right heart border; **B,** lateral chest radiograph; **C,** air in mediastinum forms a "batwing" appearance.

closely; larger ones require surgical treatment. Tension pneumothorax with mediastinal shift requires immediate treatment. Infants with this complication may appear pale and in shock because of a compromise of cardiac output. An infant with meconium aspiration should be considered at risk to develop pneumothorax; a 50-cc syringe, needle, and stopcock should be placed at the bedside so that emergency treatment may be readily available. If the pneumothorax is small, breathing 100% oxygen will free the blood of nitrogen, creating a gradient for nitrogen between pneumothorax and blood that will promote reabsorption of the pleural air collection.

Transient neonatal tachypnea

Short-lived periods of respiratory difficulty in full-term infants are a frequent occurrence, but it was Avery and her coworkers who first identified the condition as a syndrome. While the infants frequently appear severely ill, the physician and the family can be reassured that prognosis is usually favorable.

Clinical presentation. Infants with transient neonatal tachypnea have a clinical appearance similar in many respects to those with meconium aspiration, except, of course, that they are not meconium stained. Almost all cases involve vigorous full-term infants. Not infrequently, the infants who develop respiratory distress have been delivered by cesarian section, but usually labor and delivery are uneventful. Signs of respiratory distress develop soon after birth. In its mildest form the disease may last only 12 hours, although severe cases last from 5 to 7 days. Signs include marked tachypnea up to 100 breaths per minute, hyperinflation of the chest, and occasionally cyanosis. Grunting occurs early in the course, but subcostal retractions are not

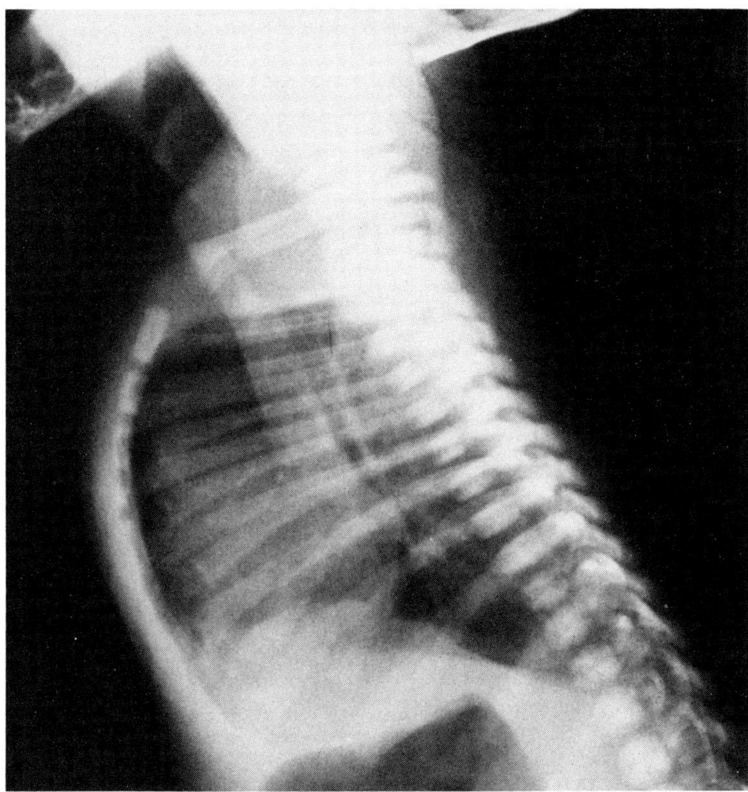

Fig. 12-15. Radiograph of transient neonatal tachypnea. Note flat diaphragms.

seen because the overdistended chest actually prevents it. Bizarre breathing patterns are not infrequent. The infants sometimes breathe in cogwheel patterns and at other times in couplets and triplets. Recovery occurs gradually and is associated with a disappearance of the overdistended chest. A generally favorable outcome can be predicted, although the infants may be extremely ill.

Etiology and pathophysiology. The cause of the condition is unknown. Although clinically similar to mild HMD (type II RDS), it has been suggested that delayed resorption of lung fluid may be etiologic. Arterial Po_2 is low because of shunting and maldistribution of ventilation. Emphysema and gas trapping are prominent. The disease may merely represent an excessive degree of gas trapping. Pa_{CO_2} and pH seldom show acidosis, but respiratory alkalosis is common as a result of hyperventilation.

Chest roentgenogram. The chest roentgenogram reflects the clinical findings. Chest volume is increased with overaeration, increased anteroposterior diameter, and flat diaphragms (Fig. 12-15). Coarse streaks radiating from the hilum of the lungs may be prominent.

Management and treatment. Treatment is supportive. Most infants require only increased oxygen to maintain Pa_{O_2} and abolish cyanosis. Oral feeding should be discontinued to avoid aspiration, and intravenous therapy should be used to provide calories and fluid.

Aspiration pneumonia

Aspiration pneumonia is a rare occurrence in the newborn, except for aspiration of meconium, amniotic fluid, and maternal blood. The appearance of streaks throughout the lung fields on the chest roentgenogram is frequently interpreted as being caused by aspiration, when in fact the streaks actually are caused by primary atelectasis. It was common practice in the United States 10 years ago to delay the oral feeding of all premature infants for several days because of fear that aspiration might result. With skilled nursing the danger of aspiration is less likely and is no longer a valid reason for delaying the feeding of otherwise normal premature infants.

The finding of squamous cells in the airways and alveoli at postmortem examination has been interpreted to substantiate the diagnosis of aspiration of amniotic fluid. However, a similar picture has been seen in infants who died but had no respiratory difficulty, and the fetal lung itself may produce a fluid that from time to time intermixes with amniotic fluid. These considerations may cast doubt on the existence of the clinical state of amniotic fluid aspiration.

Surgically treatable causes of respiratory distress should be ruled out first and supportive therapy provided while attempting to identify the physiologic abnormalities responsible for aspiration. Several conditions require special attention.

1. The contents of the blind pouch in tracheoesophageal fistula may be aspirated and cause severe respiratory embarrassment. Early diagnosis is often suggested by excessive oral secretions. Prompt definitive surgical correction is indicated.

2. When maternal amnionitis is present and the infant exhibits signs of respiratory distress, aspiration of infected amniotic sac contents should be suspected. Appropriate cultures should be obtained and treatment begun with antibiotics as if there were presumptive septicemia (p. 132). Prolonged rupture of membranes, with no signs of disease in the mother or infant, are seldom indications for prophylactic antibiotics in full-term infants born to parents from an adequate socioeconomic setting.

3. Aspiration of maternal blood at delivery is a rare cause of respiratory distress. Treatment is supportive.

4. Bacterial pneumonia, viral pneumonia, and protozoan pneumonia have all been observed in the newborn, although their occurrence is infrequent to rare (pp. 136-138). Because of the difficulty of diagnosing pneumonia and sepsis, the physician should be constantly alert. Infants with primary respiratory disease not caused by infection who develop sudden unexplained worsening of their clinical condition may have developed pneumonia.

Pulmonary hemorrhage

Extensive hemorrhage into alveoli and interstitial tissues is a frequent finding at autopsy, although its presence is rarely suspected by the clinician (Fig. 12-16). Esterly and Oppenheimer report the presence of massive pulmonary hemorrhage in

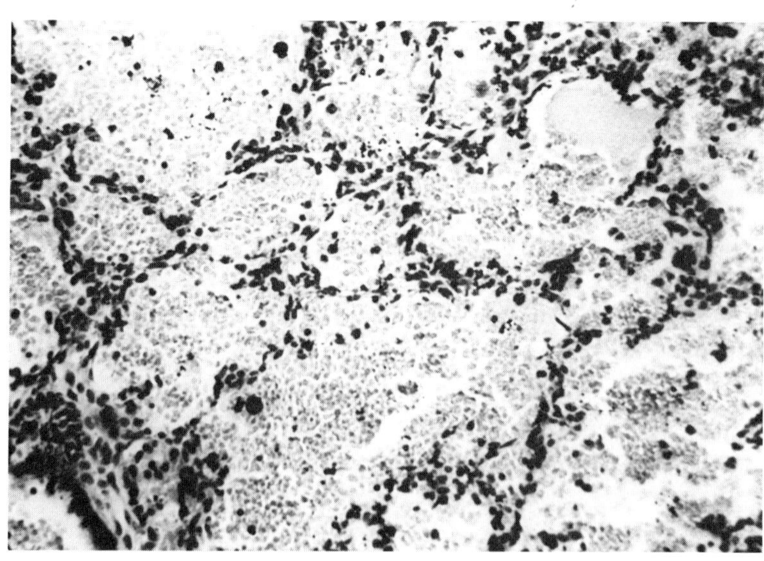

Fig. 12-16. Photomicrograph of the lungs with massive alveolar hemorrhage.

17 (8%) of 758 autopsies. There is debate as to whether this lesion exists as a primary entity or is merely a phenomenon secondary to other pulmonary or systemic disorders in the infant.

The diagnosis of pulmonary hemorrhage should be considered when obvious bleeding is noted arising from the trachea, nose or mouth. More often, the infants who are subsequently proved to have pulmonary hemorrhage are in respiratory difficulty from birth; the clinical course mimics HMD, and no external bleeding is evident.

Because the condition is rarely diagnosed premortem, no specific laboratory findings have been identified. Chest roentgenograms are not diagnostic; they may show a reticulogranular appearance with air bronchograms or coarse streaks of increased density. Pulmonary hemorrhage may be associated with HMD, pneumonia, erythroblastosis fetalis, or congenital heart disease. Occasionally the pulmonary hemorrhage is associated with a generalized bleeding disorder.

Treatment is supportive, with attention to the same details as outlined for HMD (p. 364). Evaluation of defects in the clotting mechanism should be carried out and appropriate therapy given if an abnormality is detected.

The cause and pathogenesis of the disturbance can only be speculated upon. Hypoxia and hyperoxia are commonly mentioned etiologic factors. Most of the infants who succumb and who show pulmonary hemorrhage have had large amounts of oxygen as therapy. Oxygen is certainly capable of damaging pulmonary capillaries. The frequent association of HMD and pulmonary hemorrhage caused Rowe and Avery to speculate that perhaps factors that produced hyaline membranes may also operate to cause pulmonary hemorrhage (that is, high surface forces acting on the open alveoli could result in transudation of blood from the capillaries into the alveoli).

Abnormalities of the airways—trachea and bronchi

The airways may be narrowed or obstructed from within or by pressure from without. Regardless of the cause the compromise of the airway is generally identified by noisy breathing or stridor. When frank obstruction is present, no sound is evident, and the infant will die unless the obstruction is immediately relieved.

Intrinsic lesions of the airways

Choanal atresia. (See also p. 65.) Choanal atresia is a rare condition causing obstruction by either bone or membrane at the junction of the posterior nares and nasopharynx. The obstruction may be complete or partial, and unilateral or bilateral. The condition can occur as an isolated malformation or in association with other abnormalities involving the nasopharynx. There is a distinct familial tendency. Embryologically, the condition occurs when the septum between the nares and foregut fails to disappear.

Since newborn infants tend to be obligatory nose breathers, patients with complete choanal atresia have symptoms soon after birth. Indeed, if the condition is not immediately recognized, the infant may succumb from asphyxia. On the other hand, surprisingly, infants with complete atresia may survive for days with few signs of respiratory difficulty. The diagnosis should be excluded in the delivery room by passing a tube through the posterior nares. The diagnosis is confirmed by placing radiopaque dye in the nares and noting the obstruction on lateral radiograms of the nose (Fig. 12-17). Unilateral obstruction may not be recognized until well after the newborn period.

The treatment of choanal atresia requires great patience and nursing skill. Membranous obstructions can be readily perforated and held open by rubber tubes. Care should be taken to ensure that these tubes do not measurably increase dead space. Repeated dilatation of the nares will be necessary to avoid their closing off. When a bony abnormality is present, surgery may be performed in the neonatal period; if it is delayed, these infants can be taught to breathe through the mouth with the use of an oral airway, which can often be discarded after 2 or 3 weeks. Teaching the infant to suck and breathe through the mouth requires considerable skill on the part of physicians and nurses.

Pierre Robin syndrome. (See also p. 568.) The infant with this syndrome has micrognathia, posterior positioning of the tongue,

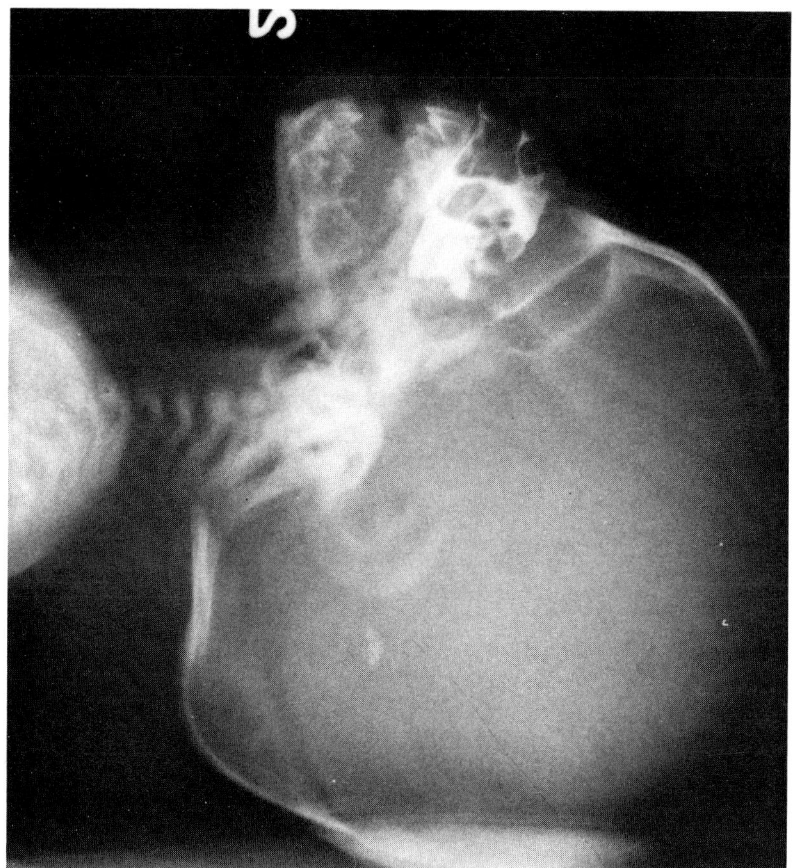

Fig. 12-17. Choanal atresia. Note failure of contrast material to enter nasopharynx.

and frequently a cleft palate. Difficulties arise when the tongue falls backward and interferes with breathing. While some authors recommend suturing the base of the tongue to the inferior alveolar margin to assure patency of the airway, careful nursing care may obviate this. Nursing of the infant in the prone or lateral position is usually successful in avoiding airway obstruction.

Congenital laryngeal stridor (laryngomalacia). Congenital laryngeal stridor is a relatively common condition that is characterized by signs of noisy stridulous breathing, usually within the first or second week after birth. Full-term infants rarely develop the condition while still in the nursery, but return at a later date with typical signs. Premature infants, who spend a longer time in the nursery, frequently are diagnosed prior to discharge.

Although almost always a benign condition, signs of noisy breathing frequently are of great concern to the parents. The stridor is intermittent and may or may not be associated with intermittent severe retractions. The noise is invariably dry in quality and occurs only during inspiration. There is no hoarseness, and the infant's cry is normal. Cyanosis is never present, and the infant thrives in spite of the noisy breathing. The clinical picture described above is so characteristic as to usually preclude the need for any further diagnostic tests. Treatment consists of reassuring the parents that the condition will abate and disappear slowly over the first year of life.

The cause of laryngomalacia is unclear; the clinical picture has been ascribed to floppy epiglottis, redundant aryepiglottic folds, or loose arytenoids. Findings from direct laryngoscopy may be normal or only show inspiratory collapse of the larynx. It is important to differentiate this condition from serious obstructive lesions of the airways. If in doubt, direct laryngoscopy may be necessary; and in some cases contrast studies of the larynx, trachea, and esophagus may be indicated.

Congenital malformations of the larynx and trachea. It is virtually impossible to separate congenital malformations of the larynx from those of the trachea on the basis of clinical presentation alone. The abnormalities result in various degrees of obstruction to inspiration, with signs most often present from birth. When a congenital abnormality of the larynx or trachea is suspected, immediate visualization by a skilled endoscopist is mandatory.

1. Laryngeal webs are usually located in the region of the vocal cords, but they may occur as well in the supraglottic and subglottic areas. The lesion develops as a result of an arrest in development at 7 to 10 weeks of gestation (that is, various degrees of failure of recanalization of the primitive solid tube that eventually forms the larynx). The condition is exceedingly rare.

A complete web should be suspected when at birth the child makes inspiratory gasps and is unable to expand the lungs. Less severe forms are recognized by inspiratory stridor and hoarse cry. If the obstruction is severe, subcostal and suprasternal retractions will be present from birth. Diagnosis is made by direct laryngoscopy. Therapy consists of perforation of the web or tracheostomy.

2. Vocal cord paralysis giving rise to a hoarse cry may be the result of a congenital abnormality or a birth injury to the vagus nerve (p. 80). Direct visualization of the glottic area is necessary for diagnosis.

3. Tracheal stenosis is rare and not usually diagnosed prior to death.

Extrinsic lesions resulting in airway compression

Masses or vascular structures may cause airway narrowing in the newborn infant.

Thyroid enlargement. (See also p. 466.) Benign thyroid goiter in newborn infants may result in tracheal compression; in severe disease, the trachea may be seen only as a fine linear structure on lateral radiographs. The condition has been the result of administration of iodides to the mother as a cough medicine during pregnancy. Careful nursing care can frequently avoid tracheostomy, while specific drug therapy in the form of L-thyroxine is being administered to shrink the gland. The drug should be administered as soon as possible after birth. It produces noticeable relief of the symptoms of airway compression within 48 hours. The degree of airway narrowing should be assessed and the progress followed by lateral radiographs of the neck.

Congenital malformation of the aortic arch and branches. (See also p. 333.) Anomalies of the aortic arch and its branches may form vascular rings around the trachea, bronchi, and esophagus. Depending on the type of lesion present, symptoms and signs may be related to compression of the airways or esophagus or both. Early recognition is important so that corrective surgery may be performed.

The common anomalies are double aortic arch; right aortic arch with the vascular ring formed by a ligamentum arteriosum, anomalous left or right subclavian artery, innominate artery, or left common carotid artery; and anomalous pulmonary artery causing a vascular ring around the bronchus.

Signs and symptoms. Vascular rings may not produce symptoms unless they cause tracheal or esophageal compression; that is, anomalous right subclavian artery may be identified only on an esophagram. Tracheal compression results in noisy breathing, inspiratory or expiratory stridor, and occasional cyanosis. A brassy cough may be present, and the infant may lie with head extended to reduce airway narrowing. Bronchial compression may cause atelectasis or emphysema. The respiratory signs are accentuated with crying, feeding, and neck flexion. Poor feeding and vomiting are associated with esophageal compression.

Diagnosis. The specific diagnosis is made by the impression that aberrant vessels make on the air-filled trachea and barium-filled esophagus. For example, double aortic arch compresses the esophagus from behind and the trachea from the front. An anomalous right subclavian artery arising as the last branch on the aortic arch indents the back of the esophagus obliquely from below, upward and to the right.

Treatment. Surgical correction has been accomplished for all abnormalities of the great vessels. The timing of surgery depends on the severity of symptoms and the presence of complications such as persistent vomiting and aspiration pneumonia.

Tracheotomy in the newborn period. Infants with obstructive lesions of the larynx and trachea may require emergency tracheotomy to save their lives. Although it is important to do a tracheotomy if necessary, great efforts should be made to avoid this type of operation by providing good nursing care and supportive treatment (p. 99). It is frequently difficult to remove a tracheotomy in a newborn infant because of the tendency to tracheomalacia, which frequently occurs after this procedure and leads to tracheal collapse and respiratory obstruction. Some tracheotomies performed in the newborn period have had to be maintained for several years, often long after the original lesion was corrected.

Cysts of the lung. Cystic changes in the lung of the newborn are rare. Caffey did not observe a single patient with cysts of the lung on 7,000 chest roentgenograms of newborn infants. Few reports are available in which the physiologic problems posed by cystic lesions have been thoroughly delineated, but they are presumed to cause clinical difficulty either because of compression of surrounding lung or because of rupture. They are diagnosed from chest roentgenograms of newborn infants taken because of respiratory distress and are of importance because occasionally surgical intervention may be life saving.

There is controversy about the origin of lung cysts, although most authors describe both a congenital type and an acquired type. Both bronchogenic cells and alveolar cells are seen in what are presumed to be congenital cysts and in acquired cysts, so that the microscopic picture cannot be used to differentiate the type of cyst. The presence of cysts in stillborn infants suggests that at least some are of congenital origin. Whatever their origin, cysts in the lung are rarely associated with cystic disease in other organs.

Clinical presentation. Infants with cystic disease in the lung come to the physician's attention because of respiratory distress caused by either overdistention of the cysts or infection. These lesions are in communication with the major air passages, and ball-valve type obstruction may result in overdistention, rupture, and pneumothorax. Signs are nonspecific and consist of dyspnea, tachypnea, subcostal retraction, and cyanosis (when severe). If a pneumothorax occurs, respiratory distress may become severe. Blood gases may show a low Arterial Po_2, but respiratory acidosis is unusual.

Diagnosis. The diagnosis is made by identifying on a chest roentgenogram single or multiple cysts in the lung. They appear as round or oval translucent areas within the pulmonary parenchyma. It is not unusual for cystic disease to be misdiagnosed as diaphragmatic hernia because of its similarity to air-filled bowel. On occasion cysts must also be distinguished from a pneumothorax.

Treatment. Therapy of an infant with cysts of the lung must be expectant, unless infection or pressure signs intervene. In many instances the cysts regress spontaneously (Fig. 12-18). The cysts may also rupture, coalesce, and produce signs of tension with mediastinal shift and severe respiratory embarrassment. In these patients aspiration of air from the cyst may be life saving. In other instances resection of the diseased area of the lung may be necessary if compression of surrounding structures is compromising pulmonary function.

Cystic adenomatoid malformation of the lung is a rare type of congenital cystic lung lesion occurring in the newborn period. The condition has been noted in all lobes of the lung, although it is generally confined to a single lobe. The cysts are multiple and lined by epithelium similar to the bronchial lining so that they appear to represent bronchial overgrowth. Alveolar ducts are rarely seen. An association between this condition and generalized edema or hydrops has been noted. Hydramnios is often present as well.

Symptoms and signs of this lesion are similar to those for other cysts. They communicate with major airways so that infection and ball-valve obstruction both occur. Compression of surrounding lung produces

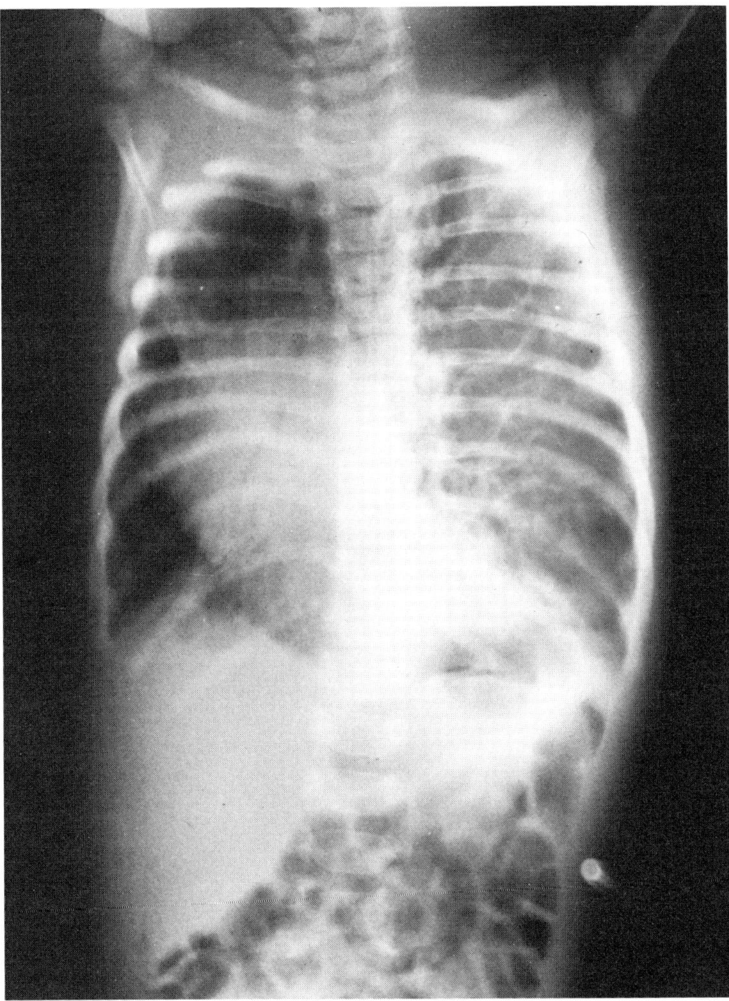

Fig. 12-18. Multiple cystic areas of the left lung. Cysts cleared spontaneously over 2 months, although spontaneous rupture resulted in severe respiratory distress requiring aspiration and underwater seal drainage. The child had no residual pulmonary difficulty.

respiratory distress. Treatment is expectant, but signs of compression may dictate removal of the diseased lung. It is difficult to exclude bilateral disease in an infant at the time initial surgery is required, so that long-term prognosis must be guarded until this point is clarified.

Acquired cysts. Single or multiple pneumatoceles caused by staphylococcal pneumonia are a frequent cause of a cystic appearance in the lung. While these pneumatoceles are large and may persist for months, they generally disappear and rarely cause any respiratory embarrassment.

Cysts, presumably acquired in origin, are a common radiographic finding in the Wilson-Mikity syndrome and bronchopulmonary dysplasia. These lesions, while appearing cystic, are actually areas of emphysema scattered throughout the lung. With healing the cystic-appearing emphysematous lesions disappear.

Congenital lobar emphysema. Although frequently mentioned in a differential diagnosis of neonatal respiratory distress, congenital lobar emphysema is rarely recognized. Emphysema presumably occurs as a result of partial obstruction of the airway occurring on expiration. Intraluminal lesions, such as infection or tumors, or extraluminal lesions causing compression from without can result in lobar emphysema. In addition, airway collapse because of overly compliant airways is a possible cause of emphysema. All these circumstances act to produce a ball-valve effect, allowing entry of air during inspiration but preventing egress during expiration.

Signs produced by lobar emphysema are caused by compression of surrounding lung or by mediastinal shift. Diagnosis is suggested on radiographic examination by finding a radiolucent lobe, often producing compression of surrounding lung and a mediastinal shift.

While lobar emphysema appears to be a well-recognized clinical entity, its cause is rarely found even when the lobe is removed. If the child is in acute distress, bronchoscopy should be performed to attempt to determine a causative lesion. Immediate surgery and excision of the lobe may be life saving when cyanosis and respiratory distress are present. In conditions where symptoms and signs are minimal, expectant observation is recommended.

Although large follow-up studies of the effects of lobectomy performed in the newborn period are not available, initially the infants appear to tolerate the procedure well. Careful postoperative follow-up is necessary because of the incidence of pneumothorax and other complications.

Aplasia and hypoplasia of the lungs

Aplasia

In true aplasia the lung is absent, and there are no remnants of bronchi or pulmonary artery radicles. The left lung is most often affected. The mediastinum is shifted to the affected side, and the normal lung may herniate and partially fill the abnormal side. In this case, the remaining lung may appear emphysematous. Vertebral anomalies such as hemivertebrae have been associated with pulmonary aplasia.

Asymmetry of the chest may not always be present. Furthermore, breath sounds may appear normal, even on the affected side, because of sounds originating from the herniated lung. On the other hand, the diagnosis may be suspected because of shift of the cardiac apex and deviation of the trachea to the affected side. In some patients fluid may fill the thoracic cavity.

The roentgenogram of the chest shows opaqueness of the involved hemithorax. The heart and mediastinum are shifted to the affected side. The affected hemithorax is decreased in volume.

Survival is related to the presence or absence of other anomalies.

Pulmonary hypoplasia

Partial pulmonary hypoplasia may be apparent as a primary abnormality or secondary to another lesion restricting lung growth. In the former case, the chest roentgenogram shows opacity of the lung in the affected area with normally aerated lung surrounding it. Bronchograms show that part of the bronchial tree is present. The condition may be associated with absence of the pulmonary artery on the affected side.

Hypoplastic lungs are associated with diaphragmatic hernia. It is presumed that the presence of bowel in the thoracic cavity restricts lung growth and results in hypoplasia. Hypoplasia of the lungs is associated with renal agenesis or Potter's syndrome.

Congenital pulmonary lymphangiectasis

Congenital pulmonary lymphangiectasis, a rare condition, also must be considered in the differential diagnosis of neonatal respiratory distress. Infants reported to have pulmonary lymphangiectasis are usually full term. Respiratory distress begins soon after birth, and the condition is universally lethal. The roentgenographic appearance shows generalized haziness and on occasion a reticulogranular appearance, and air bronchograms similar to HMD are noted. Bilateral pleural effusions have been noted in some patients.

At autopsy the lungs are bulky, with pronounced lobulation caused by the distended subpleural lymphatic network. Subpleural lymphatic cysts filled with clear serous fluid are prominent. On microscopic examination lungs are honeycombed with irregular-shaped cysts. There is a marked increase in the fibrous tissue of the interlobular septa.

The position of the cysts along the normal distribution of the lymphatics indicates their origin. The malformations may be caused by an arrest of lymphatic growth as the surrounding lung continues to develop or by failure of isolated lymphatic spaces to be linked with the main drainage channels. The condition should be differentiated, pathologically, from interstitial emphysema. In congenital pulmonary lymphangiectasis the cysts are confined to the lungs. Other major anomalies occur in over half of the cases.

Wilson-Mikity syndrome

In 1959 Wilson and Mikity reported five cases of a new type of respiratory distress syndrome in premature infants. The clinical course was characterized by gradual development of dyspnea and cyanosis and a tendency to develop cor pulmonale in some cases. The most characteristic feature of the syndrome was the chest roentgenograms, which showed coarse, reticular infiltrations, overexpansion, and a multicystic appearance. In those infants who died, the lungs showed alveolar septal fibrosis and an infiltration of mononuclear cells. In some of the infants there was a tendency for the pulmonary disease to resolve. There have been a moderate number of case reports and papers since the original description. Attempts to determine the cause of the condition have been unsuccessful. In some patients pulmonary oxygen toxicity has been implicated. The similarity of chest roentgenograms of this syndrome and that of bronchopulmonary dysplasia suggests that they may have a similar developmental cause.

Clinical presentation. Infants with Wilson-Mikity syndrome are usually of very low birth weight and are prematurely born. The cases reported in full-term infants have most often been associated with meconium aspiration. There is still uncertainty about the clinical course of Wilson-Mikity disease, because one must rely on nonspecific changes in the chest roentgenogram to make the diagnosis. Since the affected infants are immature, they have frequently required oxygen therapy early in life. Most small premature infants demonstrate an abnormal chest roentgenogram in the form of increased reticular markings, and this is not necessarily a sign of impending Wilson-Mikity disease.

Infants who develop the condition may have respiratory distress starting soon after birth, others may not become obviously distressed until 1 or 2 weeks later. Respiratory difficulty in the form of dyspnea, tachypnea, chest wall retractions, and cyanosis is characteristic. This difficulty may persist for weeks and months and necessitate the institution of oxygen therapy or continuance of it if oxygen was necessary initially. Coughing and rarely wheezing may also be present. Rales are rare in most neonatal respiratory difficulty, but are a common feature of Wilson-Mikity disease. The chest roentgenogram changes from the early nonspecific reticular pattern to a specific picture characterized by cystic changes and coarsening of the reticular markings. Infants who recover show a gradual lessening of symptoms over a period of months, and eventually the chest roentgenograms become normal. Other infants may develop progressive respiratory failure and are unable to survive. A small number of infants develop signs of cor pulmonale with cardiomegaly, right ventricular hypertrophy, and congestive heart failure. A long-term follow-up of two such infants with cor pulmonale and high pulmonary vascular resistance revealed that the disease may eventually resolve at 2 to 3 years of age. Infants with this severe form may have an increased number of lower respiratory tract infections in the first year of life.

Roentgenographic appearance. Three stages in the development of the roentgenographic appearance of Wilson-Mikity disease have been described.

1. The *acute stage* consists of a bilateral diffuse reticulonodular or reticular pattern with small, round lucent foci, producing a bubbly appearance (Fig. 12-19).
2. The *intermediate stage* appears in weeks or months, with coarse streaks radiating from the hilus and persistence of hyperaeration and disappearance of focal lucent areas.
3. In the *clearing stage* roentgenographic abnormalities disappear in 4 to 11 months.

Pathophysiology. Infants with Wilson-Mikity disease have marked oxygen dependency caused by right-to-left cardiopulmonary shunting and maldistribution of ventilation. These physiologic studies reflect the pathologic changes of atelectasis and emphysema. Retention of carbon dioxide caused by underperfusion of alveoli

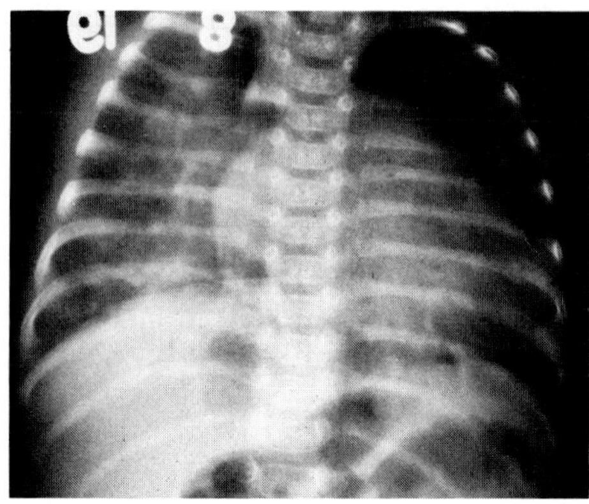

Fig. 12-19. Typical changes of Wilson-Mikity disease on the right. Increased density on the left is caused by technique only.

(high $\dot{V}_A/\dot{Q}$ areas) is common and results in respiratory acidosis. Compliance of the lungs is decreased, and airway resistance is increased. Infants who develop cor pulmonale have increased pulmonary vascular resistance not responsive to oxygen breathing. The electrocardiogram in these patients shows marked right ventricular hypertrophy. Cardiac catheterization in severe cases has frequently demonstrated a small left-to-right ductus arteriosus shunt.

Grossly the lungs have a hobnailed appearance with cystic areas in the parenchyma and thickened fibrous septa. Microscopically, the lungs show alveolar wall thickening, proliferation of capillaries, and infiltration of mononuclear cells. Infants with cor pulmonale show evidence of destruction of capillaries and arterioles.

Treatment. Treatment of Wilson-Mikity disease is supportive. Close monitoring of blood gases and acid-base balance is often necessary for months. Oxygen must be provided to overcome cyanosis. Acid-base disturbances must be corrected by buffers and assisted ventilation. Antibiotics are contraindicated because of dangers of developing resistant organisms. Therapy with digitalis and diuretics is necessary when cor pulmonale develops. Great patience is required on the part of the medical personnel and parents in treating these infants.

Bronchopulmonary dysplasia

In 1967 Northway and associates reported a number of infants who developed pulmonary disease following respirator therapy and therapy for HMD. The condition is similar in most respects, clinically, radiologically, and pathologically, to Wilson-Mikity syndrome. In addition, the proliferative lesions produced in monkeys as a result of chronic exposure to oxygen are similar in many respects to the lesions of bronchopulmonary dysplasia and Wilson-Mikity disease. Lesions have not been reproduced in animals treated only with respirator therapy.

Clinical presentation. Infants severely ill with HMD who have received oxygen therapy in high concentrations for prolonged periods of time and who may have had assisted ventilation may develop this condition. The physician should first be alerted when respiratory distress in a patient with HMD fails to abate in the usual 10 days to 2 weeks. The infants continue to require high oxygen concentrations for weeks and months to maintain an arterial Po_2 over 40 mm Hg. Tachypnea, dyspnea, and retractions persist. The chest roentgenogram, which had previously shown the typical reticular granular pattern and air bronchogram of HMD, now changes to show coarse streaking and focal areas of emphysema (cystic appearance), which are strikingly similar to Wilson-Mikity disease. Respiratory acidosis may be present. Therapy is supportive. Close monitoring of blood gases and acid-base balance and provision of oxygen are important supportive measures. Recovery begins when the requirement for oxygen lessens over a period of months as healing takes place. One infant in our nursery was weaned from oxygen after 5 months.

Diseases of the pleura and mediastinum

Pneumothorax and pneumomediastinum

The early recognition and specific treatment of pneumothorax in the newborn infant is critical in reducing the significant mortality that occurs from this disorder. Pneumomediastinum, while less commonly a cause of death, is very often associated with pneumothorax.

Early diagnosis and treatment depends on a high index of suspicion plus a knowledge of the disease states that are likely to produce the condition. These disease states include:

1. Spontaneous pneumothorax or pneu-

momediastinum with no underlying causative agent.
2. Meconium aspiration.
3. A history of intrauterine distress, difficult delivery, and vigorous resuscitation (p. 63). It is not clear to what extent the resuscitative maneuvers themselves cause the condition, but obviously careless or inept resuscitation can produce pneumothorax and pneumomediastinum.
4. A complication of HMD. It occurs most often in infants of birth weights over 2,000 gm.
5. A complication of assisted ventilation especially with positive pressure or volume mechanical respirators.

Any infant with a history of the above conditions is a candidate for pneumothorax or pneumomediastinum or both. A sudden dramatic change in the clinical condition should suggest the diagnosis. Pneumothorax may be unilateral or bilateral. In infants it is rare for mediastinal air to track into the neck and produce crepitus.

Etiology and pathogenesis. Pneumothorax and pneumomediastinum are the result of alveolar rupture. Air tracks through the interstitial tissue along the vessels and into the mediastinum or pleura or both. Many cases of pneumothorax and pneumomediastinum are thought to occur at birth. The first breaths require large pressure changes, often as high as 100 cm of water. If this high pressure is developed to expand lung units that are not yet open, the units already open may be subjected to large pressure changes and rupture. In the case of meconium aspiration it is theorized that a ball-valve obstruction occurs. In this situation alveolar rupture would appear to be almost unavoidable. In HMD, especially in larger infants, high pressure changes are directed toward the few alveoli that are still expanded, and sometimes rupture occurs.

Clinical presentation

Pneumothorax. Infants with this condition most often have respiratory distress characterized by dyspnea, tachypnea, and cyanosis. If the disease is unilateral and uncomplicated, there may be asymmetry of the chest movement, and the cardiac apex may be shifted toward the side of the pneumothorax. In tension pneumothorax the cardiac apex is pushed away from the affected side. Breath sounds may be decreased or absent, but this is not a reliable sign. If a tension pneumothorax exists, signs of shock may be present because of compression of the great veins and decreased cardiac output. If meconium aspiration is associated, a hyperinflated chest is common.

Pneumomediastinum. Pneumomediastinum frequently escapes detection because of a paucity of clinical signs. Overdistention of chest suggests the lesion; distant or absent heart sounds are stronger evidence. Subcutaneous emphysema is unusual in newborn infants.

Diagnosis. The diagnosis is made on the basis of posteroanterior and lateral roentgenograms of the chest, which should be taken of infants in whom there is a strong possibility of pneumothorax and pneumomediastinum and of every infant with respiratory distress. Chest roentgenograms should be taken as an emergency procedure because of the potential rapid progression of the disease. A single posteroanterior film with the infant recumbent frequently will not reveal the diagnosis. Lobar emphysema or a large lung cyst may be confused with pneumothorax. These lesions have lung markings in the hyperlucent areas, whereas they are absent in the area of lung collapse. The edge of the collapsed lung can be seen to stand out in relief against the pneumothorax. Shift of the mediastinal structures away from the pneumothorax should be looked for as a sign of tension pneumothorax (Fig. 12-13).

Pneumomediastinum is evident on the posteroanterior film as an area of hyperlucency around the heart border (Fig. 12-14, *A*). On lateral films it is apparent as an hyperlucent area between the sternum and heart border (Fig. 12-14, *B*). On occasion, the thymus appears outlined by air in a "batwing" appearance (Fig. 12-14, *C*). A generalized emphysematous appearance may be present in other parts of the lung.

The Pa_{O_2} is normal or, in severe cases, low, with or without respiratory acidosis.

Treatment. No treatment is necessary for a pneumomediastinum. A small pneumothorax with minimal respiratory distress requires only careful observation. Breathing of 100% oxygen for an hour may accelerate the disappearance of the air. The administration of 100% oxygen clears the blood of nitrogen and establishes a nitrogen pressure gradient from the air collection to the blood that results in acceleration of absorption of the air into the surrounding capillaries. Moderate to large pneumothoraces that are asymptomatic, those producing significant distress, or a tension pneumothorax should be treated as an emergency. Needle aspiration of the air may be life saving but usually should not be regarded as definitive therapy; a chest tube should be inserted and attached to underwater-seal drainage. When the air stops bubbling in the water-seal the leak has stopped and the tube may be clamped. The tube may be removed in 24 hours after clamping if there is no reaccumulation of pleural air. Oxygen also should be administered, since its advantage in accelerating the absorption of air is usually greater than the risk of retinal or pulmonary toxicity.

Chylothorax and pleural effusions

Pleural effusions are exceedingly rare in the newborn. They occur in association with hydrops fetalis, as part of generalized anasarca, and in staphylococcal pneumonia. Thoracentesis may be indicated to identify an infectious agent or to relieve respiratory distress or to do both.

Chylothorax is a rare cause of pleural effusion in the newborn infant. The condition is first recognized from chest radiographs taken to diagnose respiratory distress. Unilateral diminished breath sounds may suggest the diagnosis. The definitive diagnosis is made by thoracentesis, which early in life (prior to a substantial milk intake) may yield only serous fluid. Once the infant is on a fat intake diet the fluid becomes cloudy and can be shown to have a high fat and protein content. The cause of chylothorax is unknown; it is presumably related to a disturbance of the thoracic duct.

A single thoracentesis may result in permanent resolution of a chylothorax. However, prolonged drainage may be necessary, and this therapy may result in severe malnutrition unless adequate protein and calories are provided. The condition is associated with a mortality of 25%. Thoracentesis also may be necessary to relieve respiratory distress.

Cysts and tumors of the mediastinum

Cysts and tumors of the mediastinum are rare in the newborn infant. The commonest mediastinal cysts are dermoids and teratomas. They rarely produce symptoms in the newborn period. They are situated in the anterior mediastinum and may contain teeth and skeletal structures. Ganglioneuromas occur in the posterior mediastinum.

Anlage of the trachea and esophagus may produce mediastinal cysts lined with primitive respiratory or gastrointestinal epithelium. They are called bronchogenic or gastrogenic cysts. Cysts may be present in the posterior mediastinum as remnants of incomplete dorsal enteric fistulas. If present, they are usually associated with vertebral body abnormalities.

Cystic hygromas that appear in the mediastinum do so by extension from a similar lesion in the neck. The tumors consist of lymphatic vessels and are cystic in nature.

In general, surgical excision is the treatment of choice for cysts and tumors of the mediastinum. If there is no respiratory distress, emergency treatment is not necessary.

Defects of the diaphragm

A knowledge of the embryology of the diaphragm is necessary for an understanding of the clinical conditions that are associated with defects in the diaphragm. The diaphragm arises from four sources that appear at varying times throughout embryonic life. The transverse septum is the first part to appear, and although it initially serves to separate the heart and the diaphragm, it eventually becomes part of the pericardial sac. Pleural canals posterior to the transverse septum connect the thoracic and abdominal cavities. The canals gradually become obliterated by outgrowths from the posterior and lateral wall. These outgrowths are the pleuroperitoneal folds. The diaphragm is formed by a fusion of these folds plus a small part of the primary mesentery. The fusion is generally complete by the eighth week. Somewhat later, a narrow ridge of muscle is formed around the posterolateral margin by muscle from the body wall.

Diaphragmatic hernia. A diaphragmatic hernia is the result of failure of the pleuroperitoneal folds to fuse completely. This failure is more common on the left than the right side and can, rarely, be bilateral. In the area where the pleuroperitoneal folds fail to develop the peritoneum and pleura are absent and allow a communication between the thoracic and abdominal cavities. If the defect is on the right, the intestine and part of the right lobe of the liver are in the thorax. When the defect is on the left, the stomach, spleen, left lobe of the liver, and intestine may be in the chest. The amount of abdominal viscera in the thorax depends on the size of the defect. Since the defects are in the posterior part of the diaphragm, the heart is pushed anteriorly, and the lungs are compressed as well. This compression results in bilateral hypoplasia of the lungs, more severe on the side of the hernia.

Clinical presentation. The typical patient is a full-term infant who has great difficulty initiating breathing (p. 66). The infant's general appearance is normal, although the abdomen may appear scaphoid because its contents are in the chest. Inability to expand the affected side with respiration is noted. Rarely, bowel sounds heard in the chest can reinforce the clinical impression.

Diagnosis. The diagnosis should be suspected in a full-term infant who has gasping respirations at birth. It is confirmed by a chest radiograph taken as an emergency procedure (Fig. 12-20). Loops of bowel are visible on the side of the hernia. The mediastinal structures are displaced to the opposite side; the lung on the affected side is compressed, while the lung on the opposite side is emphysematous.

Treatment. Early diagnosis is usually essential for successful surgical treatment. Severely affected children are often hypoxic and have respiratory and metabolic acidosis, which must be corrected before surgery is attempted. When the diagnosis is made in these infants, endotracheal intubation should be carried out and assisted ventilation applied. Assisted ventilation with bag and mask should be avoided since

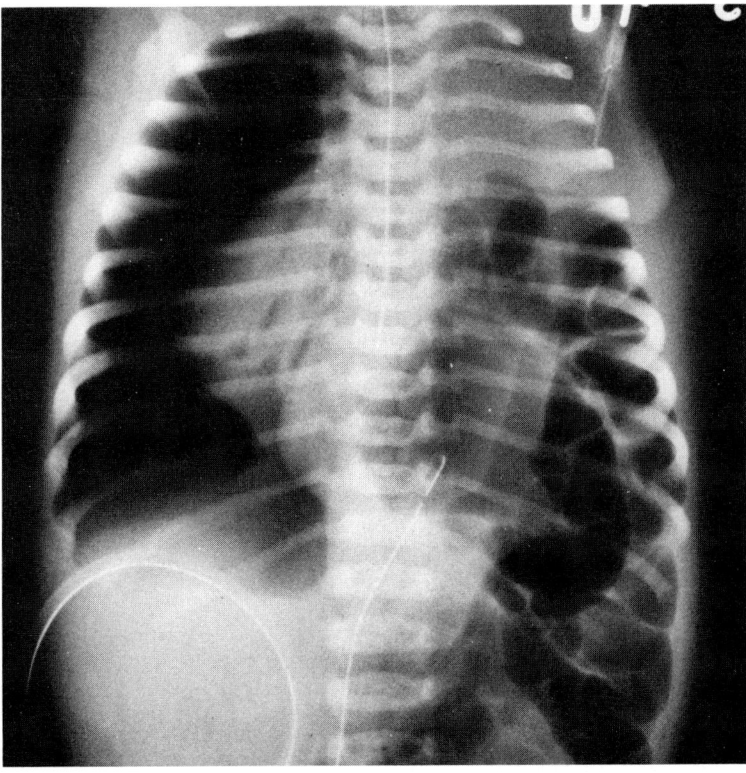

Fig. 12-20. Diaphragmatic hernia on the left. Note similarity to patient with multiple pulmonary cysts.

it may cause overdistension of the loops of intestines in the thorax, resulting in a further compromise of lung function. Some mild to moderately affected infants may not require intubation, assisted ventilation, and emergency surgery. Surgical treatment consists of removing the bowel from the chest and closing the defect if there is sufficient tissue. Even if this is accomplished, the infant may not survive, because the hypoplastic lung may cause severe ventilation-perfusion imbalance. Some workers have suggested that the hypoplastic lung should be removed to avoid this complication. Ladd and Gross, on the other hand, have reported a large number of infants in which successful repair of the diaphragmatic defect has been carried out.

Other sites of herniation. Although rarely obvious in the newborn period, intestinal herniation through the esophageal hiatus, Morgagni's foramen, or Bochdalek's canal occurs. Small defects in closure of the pleuroperitoneal folds may result in hernias as well. Small defective areas of the diaphragm closed by only pleura and peritoneum may serve as a hernial sac, producing localized eventrations.

Eventration of the diaphragm occurs when one leaf of diaphragm balloons up and encroaches on the chest cavity. This may result from paralysis of the diaphragm or defective musculature.

Tracheoesophageal fistula

Tracheoesophageal fistula is considered here because it may produce respiratory symptoms in the newborn period (p. 389). The condition occurs in approximately 1 in 3,000 births and is frequently associated with other major anomalies. There are several morphologic types of lesions; the most common is a combination esophageal atresia, with a communication between the lower segment of the esophagus and the trachea.

Clinical presentation. The presence of maternal polyhydramnios should alert the physician to a diagnosis of esophageal atresia with tracheoesophageal fistula. An attempt should be made to pass a catheter into the stomach; failure to do so can be diagnostic, but one can be misled if the catheter curls up or gets tangled during passage. The first sign of esophageal atresia is the presence of excessive oral secretions associated with frequent gagging and choking. The infant often will choke and gag on the first feeding. Aspiration of the secretions into the lungs results in respiratory distress.

Diagnosis. The definitive diagnosis can be made by a chest roentgenogram in which the air and a curled-up catheter in the esophageal pouch delineates the lesion. Radiopaque media (diatrizoate) may be instilled into the blind pouch to further identify it, but this material should be removed as soon as the diagnosis is made in order to avoid aspiration into the lungs (Fig. 12-21).

The rare H-type fistula without atresia often presents a difficult diagnostic problem that is seldom resolved in the newborn period. The history of infants with this condition is one of coughing with feedings, failure to thrive, repeated aspiration pneumonia, and upper abdominal distention. The diagnosis is made by roentgenographic contrast studies in which the contrast material is made to enter the trachea by placing the child in the head-down position. The fistula may be visualized on bronchoscopy as well.

Treatment. Surgical closure of the fistula and anastomosis of the ends of the esophagus, if there is sufficient tissue available,

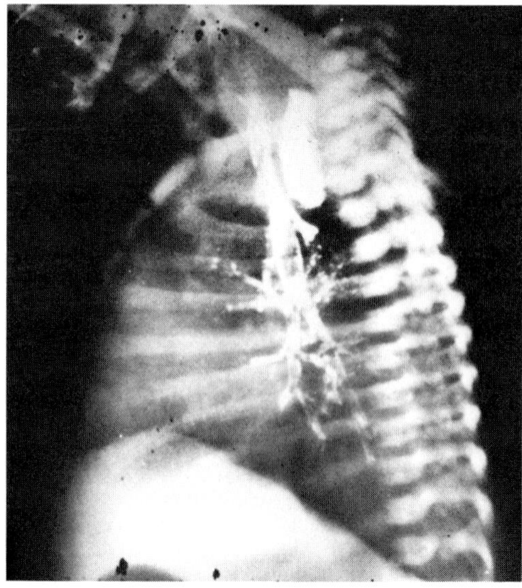

Fig. 12-21. Lateral roentgenogram showing esophageal atresia and tracheo-esophageal fistula.

should be performed as soon as the diagnosis is made. This can be done in the majority of the patients with atresia and distal tracheoesophageal fistula. If it is not possible to anastomose the ends of the esophagus, then the fistula is simply closed, a gastrostomy is done for feeding, and constant suction is applied to the blind pouch to avoid aspiration. Closure is done at a later date. It is imperative that the source for aspiration be removed as soon as possible after birth. Therefore, upon discovery of lesion, suction is applied immediately to the blind pouch while the infant awaits surgery.

PETER A. M. AULD

BIBLIOGRAPHY

Adams, F. H., Fujiwara, T., and Rowshan, G.: The nature and origin of fluid in the fetal lamb, J. Pediatr. **63**:881, 1963.

Auld, P. A. M.: Oxygen therapy for premature infants, J. Pediatr. **78**:705, 1971.

Avery, M. E.: The lung and its disorders in the newborn infant, ed. 2, Philadelphia, 1968, W. B. Saunders Co.

Avery, M. E., Gatewood, O. B., and Brumley, G.: Transient tachypnea of the newborn, Am. J. Dis. Child. **111**:380, 1966.

Avery, M. E., and Mead, J.: Surface properties in relation to atelectasis and hyaline membrane disease, Am. J. Dis. Child. **97**:517, 1959.

Brumley, G. W.: The critically ill child. XIV. Respiratory distress syndrome, Pediatrics **47**:758, 1971.

Burnard, E. D., Grattan-Smith, P., Picton-Warlow, C. G., and Grauaug, A.: Pulmonary insufficiency in prematurity, Aust. Pediatr. J. **1**:12, 1965.

Chu, J., Clements, J. A., Cotton, E. K., Klaus, M. H., Sweet, A. Y., and Tooley, W. H.: Neonatal pulmonary ischemia, Pediatrics **40** (Suppl.): 709, 1967.

Gitlin, D., and Craig, J. M.: Nature of the hyaline membrane in asphyxia of the newborn, Pediatrics **17**:64, 1956.

Karlberg, P.: Physiology of prematurity. In Lanman, J. T., editor: Transcription of the Second Macy Conference, New York, 1957, The Josiah Macy Foundation.

Krauss, A. N., and Auld, P. A. M.: Pulmonary gas trapping in premature infants, Pediatr. Res. **5**: 10, 1971.

Murdock, A. I., Kedd, B. S. L., Llewellyn, M. A., Reid, M. McC., and Swyer, P. R.: Intrapulmonary venous admixture in the respiratory distress syndrome, Biol. Neonat. **15**:1, 1970.

Nelson, N. M.: On the etiology of hyaline membrane disease, Pediatr. Clin. North Am. **17**:943, 1970.

Nelson, N. M., Prod'hom, L. S., Cherry, R. B., Lipsitz, P. J., and Smith, C. A.: Pulmonary function in the newborn infant; the alveolar-arterial gradient, J. Appl. Physiol. **18**:534, 1963.

Rudolph, A. M., Drorbaugh, J. E., Auld, P. A. M., Rudolph, A. J., Nadas, A. S., Smith, C. A., and Hubbell, J. P.: Studies on the circulation in the neonatal period; the circulation in the respiratory distress syndrome, Pediatrics **27**:551, 1961.

Scarpelli, E. M.: The surfactant system of the lung, Philadelphia, 1968, Lea & Febiger.

Swyer, P. R.: An assessment of artificial respiration in the newborn; problems of neonatal intensive care units, Columbus, Ohio, 1969, Fifty-ninth Ross Conference on Pediatric Research.

Thibeault, D. W., Grossman, H., Hagstrom, J. W. C., and Auld, P. A. M.: Radiologic findings in the lungs of premature infants, J. Pediatr. **74**: 1, 1969.

Thibeault, D. W., Poblete, E., and Auld, P. A. M.: Alveolar-arterial O_2 and CO_2 differences and their relation to lung volume in the newborn, Pediatrics **41**:574, 1968.

Usher, R.: The respiratory distress syndrome of prematurity; clinical and therapeutic aspects, Pediatr. Clin. North Am. **8**:525, 1961.

Wilson, M. G., and Mikity, V. G.: A new form of respiratory disease in premature infants, Am. J. Dis. Child. **99**:489, 1960.

13 Diseases of the gastrointestinal tract

MOTILITY ASPECTS OF THE INFANT GASTROINTESTINAL SYSTEM

Ingestion—normal intake apparatus

Sucking and swallowing

Integration of breathing, sucking, and swallowing is coordinated by a special mechanism that is present in normal babies weighing more than 1,500 gm at birth and that usually persists to about 6 months of age. Small bursts of three to four consecutive sucks occur in the neonate, and more efficient groupings of 10 to 30 occur after several days of life. The nipple (natural or artificial) is grasped between the tongue and hard palate. Withdrawal of the tongue from the palate produces suction and apposition leads to compression, the two alternate processes causing milk to be passed from the nipple to the mouth cavity. Breathing is possible during the sucking process because the airway is open and the oral cavity is separated from the pharynx by the posterior part of the tongue, which is elevated with initiation of each suck. This action serves not only to maintain separation of mouth and pharynx but also forces the contents of the posterior pharynx into the esophagus. With the onset of swallowing, the epiglottis closes the entry to the larynx, and the muscles of the soft palate occlude the connection with the nose, interrupting airway continuity. A variable amount of the air that is present in the posterior pharynx as the act of swallowing is initiated is propelled to the stomach by the bolus of food.

Infants under 3 months of age are clumsy with attempts to move semisolid material from front to back in their mouths. For this reason, efforts to administer foods prior to this age sometimes meet with failure. Despite the fact that motility records demonstrate uncoordinated esophageal peristaltic activity in the first days of life, babies clinically have little difficulty passing swallowed milk to their stomachs. The motility pattern rapidly becomes coordinated in most infants, but uncoordinated patterns and swallowing difficulties may persist for some time during the early weeks in brain-damaged children.

Gastric motility

Precise data are not available for the capacity and emptying characteristics of the infant's stomach. A number of factors such as the state of health, degree of hunger at the time of study, type of meal fed, the timing and volumes of feedings, and psychic stresses all play roles. The pylorus of the newborn opens immediately as feedings reach it, and air usually traverses the pylorus within minutes of birth. Infants fed in upright positions or on their right sides discharge liquid or solid materials from their stomachs more quickly and are less likely to pass air to the duodenum than do those fed in other positions.

Studies of emptying time of the stomach in low birth weight infants fed aqueous or milk mixtures with barium show wide variations but generally demonstrate complete emptying of aqueous mixtures by 5 hours and of milk by 7 to 8 hours. Emptying is markedly delayed by the presence of fat in a meal, especially saturated fatty acids. Large milk curds or chunks of solid food also delay opening of the pylorus. Emptying is retarded when the stomach contains increased amounts of mucus or when the muscular tone of the organ is lax, conditions normally present in low birth weight infants and induced in larger infants by fever, infection, and states of malnutrition. Factors contributing to early emptying are larger volume feedings, increased carbohydrate content, greater degree of denaturation or fragmentation of protein particles, and coldness of food. Relatively isosmotic materials pass through the pylorus more readily than extremely hypotonic or hypertonic foods.

Intestinal motility—the connection between intake and outgo

Transit time through the intestines has not been adequately measured in neonates and has been measured only in a limited number of older infants. Techniques have been relatively crude (feeding of colored markers, manometry, and x-ray film studies), and the resultant reports show wide variations. The small intestinal transport time of a barium meal varies from ½ to 6 hours in patients less than 1 year old. Contrast roentgenograms of the small intestine in infants below 1 year of age differ from those of older children and adults in that the material progresses more slowly, appears in clumps, and does not usually show the feathery appearance caused by the intestinal mucosa. The differences are usually attributed to the increased secretion of mucus in early life.

Two types of motility occur in the large intestine. Closely approximated segments may simultaneously be engaged in different types of resting activity, involving mixing of contents and exchanging of fluid, electrolytes, and nutriments. At other times these patterns disappear, and coordinated propulsive motility supervenes to push the colonic contents toward the anus. Such mass coordinated movements occur during feeding (gastrocolic reflex). When boli reach the rectum they generally induce immediate relaxation and accommodation, slowly followed by patterns associated with fluid absorption.

Defecation—normal outgo

Passage of material from the upper esophagus to the lower colon is entirely under autonomic control, but defecation is a voluntary act. Normal individuals do not defecate involuntarily. Material projected into the rectum distends that organ. If the volume is appreciable or if the process occurs when there is a particularly resistant state of rectal muscular tone, receptors in the lower rectal mucosa are activated to set up the reflex urge to defecate. The more vigorous the colonic peristalsis and the less distensible the rectum, the more urgency results. In the neonate initiation of the gastrocolic reflex usually propels sufficient material into the rectum to induce a bowel movement.

Net transmural flux of fluids and electrolytes at any level of the gastrointestinal tract varies with the state of hydration of the individual, the osmolality of gastrointestinal contents, the nature of the luminal solutes, the tonus of the intestinal musculature, the state of health, and so on. Intestinal contents remain relatively fluid until they reach distal colon. The rectum and sigmoid are the areas for final desiccation, and the consistency of the stool that is passed is determined largely by the length of time during which material is retained and by the water-resorbing capacity of these organs. In the neonate, the reduced capacity to retain material in the rectum results in more frequent passage of stools of smaller volume and of increased water content.

The initial discharges are of *meconium*, a dark brownish green, semisolid material. It is the residue of bile and embryonic intestinal secretions, which are high in nitrogenous and mucopolysaccharide content, to which have been added squamous epithelial cells and hair that have been swallowed in utero. Normal meconium contains representative amounts of the amylolytic, tryptic, and lipolytic secretions from the pancreas. Bacterial contributions are present. Meconium is usually passed four to six times a day for the first 2 or 3 days. When the flora becomes well established, the appearance changes to that of normal feces.

The *stools of healthy breast-fed infants* are usually pale to yellow, but they may often be green. The consistency is normally pasty to loose, with a slightly sour odor and acid reaction (between 4.5 and 5.1). Since the acidity is caused by carbon dioxide as well as by organic acids, loss of the former accounts for the reaction becoming less acid on standing. The number of stools passed by breast-fed infants in the early weeks varies from two to six daily. The total quantity passed in one day usually ranges from 30 to 45 gm.

The *stools of an infant fed cow's milk* are usually firmer, with paler color and a somewhat more unpleasant odor. The reaction tends to be more alkaline, ranging between pH 4.6 and 8.3. Undigested masses in the stool may take the form of bean-sized lumps composed of coagulated casein or of small, yellowish white fatty curds. The former are of no clinical significance; the latter may indicate that the infant is not completely digesting fats. Infants fed cow's milk tend to have fewer stools than do breast-fed infants.

Variations in stool color occur during infancy that are not seen in later childhood. Bilirubin in the bile is less completely reduced to stercobilin by infants, partly because of the relatively higher content of swallowed air in their tracts and partly because of the flora induced by a milk diet. A variable amount of bilirubin is excreted as such, frequently in identifiable crystalline form. Since bilirubin is readily oxidized in air to the green biliverdin, one often sees a yellow stool become green on standing. A pale stool in an infant does not necessarily mean that bile pigment is absent; it may be caused by the fact that nearly all of the pigment exists as the colorless stercobilin. These stools darken on standing and may thus be easily distinguished from acholic stools. Red stools and diapers from the presence of *B. serratio* must be distinguished from those with streaks of blood caused by small anal fissures in constipated infants or from those with flecks of blood and mucus sometimes present with diarrhea.

CLINICAL DISTURBANCES ASSOCIATED WITH DISORDERED MOTILITY

Disturbances of intake—vomiting

Vomiting occurs in neonates for a variety of reasons. Distinction is sometimes made between regurgitation (bringing up of a mouthful or two of food with little effort or distress) and vomiting (virtual emptying of the stomach) in order to evaluate the seriousness of the cause. However, the volume that is vomited is usually a less reliable indicator of the seriousness of disease than is its persistence and recurrence. The stomach is normally atonic and distended during vomiting; the holdup of the column of food is in the duodenum beyond the pylorus. The expelling force is supplied by strong contractions of the abdominal musculature and diaphragm. Only in those rare instances in which there is obstruction at the pylorus does vomiting originate from the stomach, in which case vigorous reverse peristaltic contractions provide the expelling force.

Vomiting in the newborn that is caused by irritating material swallowed during the birth process may be benign and self-limited. An intracranial pathologic condition, septicemia, and metabolic abnormalities, particularly those associated with chronic acidosis, usually result in persistent and projectile vomiting by the neonate. Obstructive vomiting is common with congenital anomalies of the gastrointestinal tract. Generally, the higher the level of obstruction the earlier symptoms appear. Polyhydramnios in the mother or discovery of a single umbilical artery at delivery should alert the physician to an increased likelihood of one of these conditions. Bile-stained or fecal vomiting virtually always indicates gastrointestinal obstruction. Presence of blood in the first 72 hours of life requires determination of the type of hemoglobin by alkaline denaturation (Apt test) to indicate whether it is probably of maternal or of infant origin.

Functional vomiting or regurgitation

Overdistention of the stomach by swallowed air or by ingestion of too large a volume of milk or by both is especially common as a cause of vomiting in young infants. In these instances, other evidences of disease are absent, and vomiting occurs effortlessly within minutes of feeding, often after the child is moved or during the burping process. Some air swallowing is normal, but excessive amounts of gastric air occur in breast-fed infants when the supply of milk is small or when the nipple is retracted and in bottle-fed infants with use of a nipple with inadequate aperture or with failure to keep the neck of the bottle filled with milk during feeding. In both breast- and bottle-fed babies it may be the result of prolonged feeding times. A mother's mistaken belief that the infant's cry of discomfort (often from distention by milk or air) is caused by hunger may lead to too frequent offering of excessive quantities of milk. These infants usually do not indicate that they are satiated but respond to stimulation by the breast or bottle by suckling, even if this ultimately aggravates their discomfort.

Regurgitation caused by excessive air swallowing can be prevented by limiting the sucking periods to approximately 20 minutes, by encouraging prolonged intervals (about 4 hours) between feedings, by feeding the infant in the semierect position to maintain the air bubble at the cardiac end of the stomach, and by burping (patiently holding the infant upright over the shoulder for a few minutes while patting him gently on the back until belching occurs) at least once in the middle and also following the feeding. Rarely, persistent cases of functional vomiting necessitate thickening of liquid feedings with addition of 2 tablespoonsful of infant cereal to an 8-oz bottle of milk to induce better gastric retention, or changeover to formulas containing a vegetable oil source to promote more rapid stomach emptying. Even if vomiting persists, vegetable oil milks result in less malodorous vomitus. Sedation and antispasmodics are usually ineffective since they simply increase the degree of atonicity of the stomach.

Systemic illness and vomiting

Unlike the hungry babies with functional regurgitation, those infants in whom vomiting results from parenteral infection or systemic disease may have an impaired desire for food. In neonates this may occur from airway obstruction, even with mild upper respiratory tract infections. Vomiting associated with infections usually has no clear-cut relationship to feeding and may be delayed for some hours after a meal. Severe projectile vomiting with such vigorous (anterograde) gastric peristalsis as to suggest pyloric stenosis may occur in neonates with infections of the urinary tract.

Projectile vomiting is common in infants with organic nervous system diseases. In newborns, this results particularly from increased intracranial pressure with birth trauma and hemorrhage, or with meningitis. Vomiting is very frequent in infants with adrenocortical insufficiency associated with congenital adrenal hyperplasia. Infants with severe metabolic acidosis from diabetes, renal tubular disease, lactic or isovaleric acidemias and with congenital galactosemia also may vomit excessively. Drugs such as digitalis, sulfonamides, broad-spectrum antibiotics, acetylsalicylic acid, and various anesthetic agents may induce vomiting.

Congenital lesions

Vomiting and regurgitation may arise from congenital disturbances in esophageal motility. *Chalasia,* or an abnormally relaxed cardiac orifice, is one such very rare problem. Ingested material may be demonstrated via fluoroscopy to be refluxed effortlessly after passage to the stomach. The condition is self-limited and disappears within a few months after birth unless it is complicated by associated pyloric obstruction, hiatal hernia, or severe peptic esophagitis and acid reflux. If the condition is uncomplicated, the usual treatment is constant maintenance of the infant in a semiupright position and thickening of feedings with cereal to render the mixture more difficult to regurgitate. Surgical repair of hiatus hernia or severe pyloric obstruction may be necessary if chalasia is complicated by their influences. The opposite condition, *achalasia,* a disease in which degeneration of neuronal elements of the esophagus induces distal spasm and difficulty with deglutition, has not been reported in neonates.

A variety of congenital malformations of the esophagus are encountered, including diverticula, fistulous communications, stenoses, atresias, duplications, and congenital shortening. In addition, the effects on the esophagus of congenital vascular rings may also lead to disturbances of deglutition.

The most common esophageal anomaly is *atresia with tracheoesophageal fistula* (p. 384). Most frequently, the upper part of the esophagus terminates in a blind pouch, and the lower part communicates with the trachea or with a primary bronchus at or near the bifurcation. Less commonly, the atresia exists without a fistula, or the fistula is connected to the upper pouch. The infant constantly drools because of inability to swallow even saliva; attempts to feed result in prompt regurgitation. Coughing and choking attacks with cyanosis result from the inevitable aspiration of food and saliva. Pneumonia and atelectasis result from repeated aspirations in all forms of esophageal atresia and, in addition, from regurgitation of gastric juice into the lung via the fistula when it is connected to the lower segment. The existence of atresia should be suspected in the presence of any of the above signs or symptoms in a newborn infant. It atresia is present, the tip of a soft rubber catheter passed via the mouth will fail to pass beyond the bottom of the blind pouch or will double back and reappear in the pharynx. It is not necessary to confirm the configuration of the rubber tube with a radiocontrast agent, especially since overfilling results in aspiration, which should be avoided because these agents are irritants in the lungs. Demonstration of air in the upper gastrointestinal tract in the presence of the atresia confirms the presence of tracheoesophageal communication with the lower segment; in the absence of fistula or when it is connected to the upper pouch, the stomach and intestines contain no gas and the abdomen is scaphoid. Prompt diagnosis is vital, since survival is dependent on early surgical division of the fistula and suitable correction of the esophageal discontinuity. Without surgical treatment and careful attention to preoperative and postoperative hydration and adequate therapy for pulmonary complications the outlook is hopeless, the infant seldom surviving beyond the seventh day of life. Presence of other major anomalies or of low birth weight decreases the chances of survival.

A rare lesion is the H-type fistula without atresia. The periodic bouts of coughing, choking, and aspiration pneumonia associated with this lesion may not appear in the first month of life. The swallowing mechanism is normal. Surgical closure of the fistula is mandatory when diagnosed.

Stenosis of the esophagus, which virtually always is restricted to the lower third segment, may be severe enough in the neonatal period to simulate atresia. If the infant is unable to tolerate normal milk feedings, it may be necessary to provide a gastrostomy for many months until more definitive studies indicate whether repeated dilatations or surgical correction is required.

Congenital duplication of the esophagus is a rare anomaly that, though it may occur at any level, is also seen most often in the lower portion. It usually does not manifest itself in the neonatal period. Symptoms are either caused by compression of the esophageal lumen with resultant dysphagia or by hemorrhage from erosions in the duplication. A similar mechanism of compression of the main lumen results from presence of an abnormal vascular ring surrounding both esophagus and trachea (p. 333). In this condition, unless the stricture imposed by the encircling vessels is extremely tight, symptoms usually are delayed until solid foods are taken. Deglutition is characteristically associated less with vomiting than with symptoms of tracheal compression; that is, cough and cyanosis. Surgical correction is necessary both for duplications and for vascular rings.

Neonatal vomiting in *hiatal hernia* is similar to that seen in chalasia, and maintenance of the infant in the semiupright posture is often the only treatment needed to prevent the emesis. The hernia may become smaller or even disappear with postural therapy alone. However, if the associated reflux of acid gastric juice persists for a time, peptic esophagitis may develop. The ulceration and hemorrhage from the esophagus that follow are important causes of hematemesis in the young infant. A short esophagus of congenital origin may produce hiatal hernia by drawing the stomach into the chest, or cicatrization secondary to peptic esophagitis from persistent congenital hiatal hernia may lead to a shortened esophagus. If the hernia is repaired early, before the scarring of advanced esophagitis produces permanent shortening, the esophagus always stretches easily to permit replacement of the cardia below the diaphragm. The diagnosis of esophageal hiatal hernia may be made by esophagram, preferably with cinefluorography. Demonstration of reflux from stomach to esophagus is an essential part of the diagnosis. Since most of these hernias are of the sliding type and many are small, they may not appear on all films; multiple films or repeated examinations may be necessary.

If postural therapy does not relieve vomiting or if hematemesis or obstruction caused by spasm or early stricture occurs, transthoracic repair of the hernia should be undertaken promptly. This operation is associated with an extremely low mortality and morbidity, even in the newborn period. Esophageal dilations are usually not effective for cure and carry a real danger of perforation. They further tend to delay definitive repair until the inflammatory and cicatrical changes are no longer reversible. When this happens, simple repair of the hernia will not effect a cure.

Congenital hypertrophic pyloric stenosis

Congenital hypertrophic pyloric stenosis is a relatively common condition characterized by persistent vomiting, constipation, weight loss, marked visible gastric peristalsis, and usually a pyloric mass. Although seen in early infancy, it is seldom symptomatic in the first 2 weeks of life, and only in exceptional instances do symptoms appear in the first few days after birth. Four of five cases occur in male infants, more commonly in firstborn children. There is some evidence for a genetic factor, since the disease occurs in successive generations of the same family; when one identical twin is affected the other is also usually affected, while the same is not true of nonidentical twins. Many cases are reported from North America, England, and northern Europe, whereas reports are scanty from Latin America and Africa.

Pathogenesis and pathology. Although hypertrophied pyloric muscle has been described in autopsies of stillborn infants, indicating inception of the process before birth, the usual onset of symptoms at about 2 weeks of age suggests a postnatal onset. The pyloric tumor consists of a hard, whitish mass about 2 cm long and about 1.5 cm in diameter, with lumen so narrow that they barely admit a fine probe or permit water to be forced through the stenosed canal. On section the circular layer of muscle is thickened and elongated, and the lower end of the pylorus may project into the duodenal lumen. The hypertrophied smooth muscle cells contain a large amount of glycogen.

Clinical presentation. Symptoms characteristically appear between the second and third weeks of life, rarely in the first few days, but they may be delayed for up to 12 weeks. Delay is especially seen in premature infants. Typically, symptoms begin in an infant who has been thriving and eating well; he commences vomiting without evident cause. Vomiting characteristically changes from occasional to repeated episodes and becomes more forceful and projectile within a day or two from onset. The contents of the stomach shoot out, usually immediately after feeding. Nursing is avidly resumed after vomiting. In a number of patients unconjugated hyperbilirubinemia has been observed after persistent vomiting commenced. The cause is uncertain, although the condition is called stasis hyperbilirubinemia.

The vomitus is not bile stained, since the obstruction is proximal to the ampulla of Vater, but it may become coffee-ground in appearance as a consequence of gastritis or peptic ulceration. Most patients vomit regularly after every feeding, while others may retain two or three feedings in succession. The quantity of vomiting may exceed the feeding just taken, indicating considerable gastric retention. The infant may suffer from dehydration, with dry and inelastic skin and scanty urine. Excessive vomiting of gastric juice leads to alkalosis, hypochloremia, hypokalemia, and occasionally tetany. Constipation results from the reduced volume of food traversing the intestinal tract, although some infants pass frequent small stools consisting mostly of bile-stained mucus. Subcutaneous fat is depleted more than muscle, with the progressive weight loss, and some babies present a particularly muscular appearance despite small size. Once fat loss is excessive, heat control is impaired, and infants with persistently subnormal temperatures must be considered in critical condition.

The epigastrium is protuberant, while the lower half of the abdomen is usually scaphoid. The characteristic gastric peristaltic waves usually appear spontaneously immediately following feeding. If they do not, they may usually be elicited by gentle friction or by tapping of the epigastrium. The wave begins as a ball-like prominence in the left upper quadrant and progresses slowly to the right, preceded by a trough. Waves appear sequentially for a while and then slow down, usually to become reversed in direction just prior to vomiting. Palpation for the pyloric tumor requires considerable patience and is facilitated if the infant's stomach is empty, usually just after vomiting, and a pacifier is used to relax the abdominal muscles. Examination should be performed with the infant lying on a firm surface. The hardened pylorus is usually located just lateral to the right rectus muscle, about 3 to 5 cm below the costal margin. Careful observation of the course of the peristaltic waves will aid the examiner in finding it. The tumor is virtually always palpable, depending on the thoroughness, patience, and experience of the examiner, although it may be obscured or displaced by an enlarged stomach or liver.

Diagnosis. The postnatal onset, almost uninterrupted progression of symptoms, absence of bile in the vomitus, presence of visible gastric peristaltic waves, and a palpable pyloric mass establish the diagnosis. Suction by catheter of a large gastric residue of food and secretions is also virtually pathognomonic, and this residue may persist even after vomiting or fasting for many hours. In atypical cases and in those infants where the tumor cannot be palpated with certainty, roentgen examination may be necessary. Plain film usually shows the large gas-filled stomach, and studies with contrast material reveal an elongated and narrowed pyloric canal with delayed opening. The base of the duodenal bulb is frequently indented and tipped superiorly.

Pyloric stenosis is occasionally confused with conditions causing increased intracranial pressure because of the projectile vomiting or with vomiting associated with improper feeding or with parenteral infection. However, persistence of vomiting after feedings administered by experienced nurses and continuation of good appetite in the absence of signs of central nervous system disease or of evidence of infection serve to rule out these differential possibilities. Congenital duodenal obstruction may simulate the symptoms and signs of pyloric stenosis. In these cases, symptoms usually appear earlier after birth, and the vomitus contains bile, except in the rare instances of supraampullary obstruction.

Treatment. In the United States the treatment of choice is the Fredet-Ramstedt operation, in which the pyloric mass is incised along its longitudinal axis and the hypertrophied muscle layers are split along the entire length of the tumor down to the submucosa, without opening the lumen of the stomach. Surgical mortality is less than 1%, and symptoms are almost immediately relieved. The low operative risk has been achieved by preoperative correction of dehydration and metabolic derangements. Parenteral fluids are given postoperatively until oral intake is adequate. Surgeons vary in their timing of initial oral feedings, some offering oral intake at 3 to 6 hours, others giving nothing for the first day. Usually, initial feedings are 30 ml of 5% glucose water, repeated at 3- to 4-hour intervals. Following three or four such feedings, half-strength milk formula is begun at 30 ml per feeding and is gradually increased as tolerated. The infant is held semiupright for all feedings, after which he is placed flat in his crib, lying on one side or the other. Vitamins are withheld during the immediate postoperative period but are usually resumed by the fifth postoperative day. Vomiting may occur during the initial postoperative days. Complications such as perforation of the duodenum at the time of operation, persistent obstruction caused by incomplete separation of the circular muscle, intestinal obstruction caused by postoperative adhesions, and dehiscence of the abdominal wound are rare. Most patients resume weight gain rapidly and may be discharged from the hospital within 3 to 7 days after the operation.

In a limited number of patients with less marked symptoms and a less relentless weight loss, medical treatment may be attempted with the hope that the pylorus will ultimately relax spontaneously if normal nutrition is maintained. Feedings are thickened and concentrated to improve their retention in the stomach. If a feeding is vomited, better retention may follow refeeding. Antispasmodics are reported to be helpful, but they exert less effect on the pylorospasm than they induce gastric distention and cut down on the hyperperistalsis, thus improving retention. Atropine methylnitrate (Eumydrin) in aqueous (1:10,000) or alcoholic (0.6%) solution is applied drop by drop to the base of the infant's tongue where it is absorbed locally. The drug is given 15 to 20 minutes before each feeding, starting with doses of about 0.05 mg and working up quickly to amounts of about 0.3 mg, the dosage being adjusted to the individual patient. Some patients have improved with administration only once daily or when the drug was discontinued after only a week or two of therapy. Thus, the optimal length of time that treatment should be continued is not known.

Eumydrin, though less toxic than atropine itself, produces similar side effects, which include mydriasis, flushing, dry mouth, and fever. These symptoms subside with omission of the next dose. Abdominal distention from gastric atony or paralytic ileus may supervene in spite of improvement in the vomiting and is an ominous sign, in the face of which the drug must be discontinued. Comparable success has been reported with the use of methscopolamine nitrate (Skopyl, Skopolate), a pharmacologically related drug whose toxicity is somewhat less pronounced than that of atropine and its derivatives.

Disturbances of continuity—small intestinal obstructive lesions

In early fetal life the mucosa lining the developing gut cavity proliferates and occludes the lumen. For a long time it was believed that deficiencies in the subsequent recanalization process explained *congenital stenoses* and *atresias*. While this mechanism may account for some fore and hind gut abnormalities, the embryonic area that develops into the connection between the intake and outgo regions (the midgut) has not been proved to develop the solid embryonic stage, and a strong body of evidence indicates that lesions of this segment probably arise from compromise of the fetal circulation to the part. *Intrauterine volvulus, vascular occlusions, intussusceptions, herniations,* and *bowel strangulations* lead to infarction, and the resulting gangrenous loop of intestine is ultimately resorbed. The only evidence of this fetal accident may be an atretic segment connecting two patent areas. In some cases evidence of intrauterine peritonitis may be seen. In others the demonstration of bile, of squames from the vernix caseosa, or of lanugo in the material found in segments distal to the interruptions or in the meconium testifies to the fact that the bowel was functioning and patent from end to end prior to the development of atresia.

Symptoms of disturbed continuity may also follow from extrinsic pressure on the gastrointestinal tract. Such congenital lesions as *cysts, diverticula,* and *duplications* may become obstructing when they become distended with secretions or trapped intestinal contents and impinge on the main tract. The same effect results from the constricting effects of *encircling blood vessels, annular pancreas,* or *mesenteric bands.*

Although milder lesions may delay their appearances until later in childhood, the symptoms of major disturbances of gastrointestinal continuity usually occur in the early neonatal period. The higher and more complete the obstruction, the earlier symptoms appear. The objective signs are similar to those in older individuals; for example, the relation of the site of an obstructing lesion to the biliary outflow will determine whether vomitus contains bile. Since the newborn is in the process of aerating his gastrointestinal tract, barium swallows are rarely necessary, the position of air giving just as much information. If one must use barium, its introduction via enema is usually far more helpful than via swallow. Another important difference between the neonate and older individuals lies in the regularity with which newborns with atresias as low as the terminal ileum will pass meconium. Presence or absence of stools may be used with only some degree of reliability as an indicator of obstruction after the initial passages of meconium are over.

Duodenal obstruction of the newborn is easily diagnosed by the "double bubble" radiologic sign, which shows air and fluid in the stomach, and a similar arrangement in a hugely dilated duodenum, with absence of air beyond. Most of the time the obstructive level is distal to the ampulla of Vater, and the vomitus contains bile. This picture of complete obstruction most frequently is caused by *atresia of the duo-*

denum by a mucosal diaphragm. Vomiting begins within a few hours of birth. The upper abdomen may or may not appear distended, depending on the degree of emptying from vomiting, but the lower abdomen is always scaphoid. *Stenosis* is less frequently encountered than atresia. Variable degrees of obstructive symptoms are present with this lesion, depending on the severity of the narrowing. Duodenal atresia and stenosis are reported to have a high coincidence with Down's syndrome. Surgical management of stenosis and atresia is by duodenojejunostomy or duodenoduodenostomy.

Complete obstruction may also result from tight extrinsic constriction by an *annular pancreas* or *mesenteric band,* although these lesions are more frequently incomplete and in some instances may not be symptomatic in the first month of life. Operative division of the pancreatic ring is usually avoided because of the frequency of occurrence of pancreatitis, pancreatic fistula, or other types of inflammation that may lead to a secondary inflammatory obstruction. The preferred management is the same as that for atresia. Peritoneal bands connecting an incompletely rotated cecum in the left upper quadrant to the peritoneum in the right upper quadrant may also cross over and obstruct the duodenum. The picture with this lesion is usually one of incomplete obstruction, and diagnosis is often missed with barium swallow. Contrast enema study that demonstrates the incomplete rotation of the colon often provides the clue to the correct diagnosis. Surgical lysis of the bands, with correction of the malrotation, is the operation of choice.

Congenital atresias of portions of the small intestine lying between the duodenum and lower ileum are not common. Duplications of this region of small intestine are somewhat more frequent, but they are usually not symptomatic in the neonatal period.

Ileal atresia and *meconium ileus* tend to simulate each other. Positive diagnosis of the latter condition is aided by knowledge of cystic fibrosis of the pancreas in previous siblings and by the radiographic granular appearance of viscid meconium with tiny air bubbles, as opposed to the more characteristic larger air fluid levels of obstruction by atresia. In both conditions the entire abdomen is distended. Vomiting is persistent and becomes fecal if it is allowed to continue long enough. The management of both conditions is surgical, with attempts to irrigate the inspissated meconium using acetylcysteine solution in meconium ileus. Meconium ileus may be complicated by ileal atresia arising from an intrauterine vascular accident often associated with perforation of the bowel that had been obstructed by the inspissated material.

Meconium peritonitis of the newborn results from intrauterine rupture of the intestine, frequently proximal to an obstructive mechanism with resultant spillage of its contents into the peritoneal cavity. The perforation is usually resealed by the time of birth, but symptoms of the underlying intestinal obstruction continue. In such infants the roentgenograms reveal calcification in areas of the abdomen where there are no gas-filled loops or in the scrotum. Surgery is indicated unless there are no signs and symptoms of the predisposing obstructive condition requiring correction.

Disturbances in outgo—defecating difficulties

In the commonest form of *constipation of infants* there is no defect in peristalsis of material to the rectum. Excessive drying of rectal contents is associated with less frequent or difficult evacuations. The tendency is constitutional and hereditary, as evidenced by frequent strong family histories, by greater concordance among monozygotic than dizygotic twins, and by the fact that some infants display extreme constipation from the first days of life, even though they are ingesting formulas identical to those that do not evoke this symptom in the vast majority. Cow's milk, with its higher content of casein and calcium salts, leads to bowel movements that are firmer and less frequent than those of breast-fed infants.

Infants who strain and pass small stools should have digital examinations of their rectums, and if the finger can be introduced, any tightness that is encountered is probably caused by muscle spasm rather than by a rare sphincteric anomaly. In addition, finding of stool in the rectum virtually rules out organic or neurogenic obstructions above this level. The objective of treatment of constipation in the neonate is to soften the consistency of the feces in such a way that they can be passed readily. This may most easily be accomplished by increasing the concentration or changing the type of carbohydrate in the formula. Lactose appears to be slightly more laxative than cane sugar. Substitution of certain carbohydrate preparations such as honey, molasses (dark cane syrup is preferable to light), brown sugar, and malt soup extract is effective. Malt dextrin preparations as such exert no laxative effect, but their addition to formulas increases the carbohydrate load, thus permitting more undigested sugar to pass to the colon where its fermentation by bacteria leads to stool softening.

Congenital aganglionosis

Constipation in infants rarely may result from disturbances in propulsion of material into the lower colon caused by hypothyroidism, diabetes, or neuromuscular disorders. However, a more frequently occurring anomaly that causes constipation by interfering with peristalsis in the colon is *congenital aganglionosis (Hirschsprung's disease).* Intestinal aganglionosis may manifest itself in the newborn as intestinal obstruction, with vomiting a prominent symptom. Plain films of the abdomen show numerous dilated loops of intestine, and it is extremely difficult to be certain whether the distended loops represent colon or small intestine in the infant. A carefully performed barium enema may be helpful. If diagnostic, it will show a narrow rectum and sigmoid and dilated proximal colon. Otherwise the enema may lead to the discharge of inspissated meconium and yield temporary relief. Failure to evacuate barium adequately after examination should alert the radiologist to the correct diagnosis, even in the absence of the typical transition zone. If the infant's clinical condition permits and there is doubt about diagnosis, a rectal biopsy should be done. Simple rectal suction biopsy has become popular in obviating the need for general anesthesia. This technique is useful only if ganglia are demonstrated in the muscularis submucosae; absence of ganglia from tissue secured by this technic should not be considered diagnostic of Hirschsprung's disease, since such biopsy specimens may be too small and too superficial. Manometric diagnostic studies that are sometimes useful in older children are inappropriate in the infant.

In the acutely ill and distended infant with aganglionic megacolon, emergency correction of fluid and electrolyte deficits and of any existing hypoproteinemia is mandatory. Following restoration of reasonable homeostatic balance the patient is provided with an emergency colostomy in a segment in which normal ganglia have been identified on pathologic review of frozen sections. No infant in whom the diagnosis is established should knowingly be permitted to go without such temporary surgery until definitive repair becomes possible, usually not before 6 months of age. While occasional small enemas of isotonic solutions may be used for brief periods of temporizing with surgical treatment, it is dangerous to the infant to carry this course out over many months, the most important possible complication being the development of *pseudomembranous enterocolitis.* Its precise cause and treatment are unknown, but once developed it represents a persistent problem with extremely grave prognosis in the majority of patients.

Diagnostic contrast enemas, especially with gastrografin, may dislodge a large *meconium plug* from the tranverse or more distal colon to explain and relieve symptoms of intestinal obstruction in some neonates. In some instances the intestinal atony of these infants is associated with depression of nervous system activity from one of the various causes that affect newborns. In rare cases, the meconium plug will prove to be associated with Hirschsprung's disease. Most babies with the meconium plug syndrome have no underlying disease and remain perfectly well thereafter.

Imperforate anus

A variety of lesions, ranging from a web at the anus to complex deformities, which present some of the most vexing and discouraging problems in management, are usually all lumped together and classified as *imperforate anus.* Together, these malformations of the anus and rectum are among the most common of congenital anomalies, occurring about once in every 5,000 births. A most important diagnostic feature is the relationship of the termination of the bowel, even as a fistula, to the puborectalis sling of the levator ani musculature, since the higher anomalies imply much greater incidences of associated urologic and vertebral malformations with increased mortality and morbidity and poorer surgical results. In the instances where the termination of the bowel has passed through the puborectalis sling, a better functional result may generally be anticipated following surgery.

Diagnosis. The diagnosis can usually be made soon after birth by careful examination of the perineum. The normal anal site may be imperforate, but the anal dimple sharply defined. In others it may be less evident, and instead a prominent ectopic opening of the bowel may be seen in the perineum, or stool may be observed coming from such a fistulous connection to the vagina, urethra, or bladder. Nearly all of the females with higher levels of rectal agenesis have a fistula communicating with the perineum or the vagina but not with the urinary tract. A fistula to the perineum or the urinary tract (usually urethral, rarely vesical) may be found in 70% of the males.

So-called upside-down roentgenograms, in which the baby is held inverted while the anal dimple is marked with a radiopaque material to the level of the termination of the bowel, is a technique that has many pitfalls. Delay in air traversing to the farthest patent point of the bowel and wide variations in the apparent terminal open point within the same patient, depending on the state of contraction of the perineal and pelvic musculature, lead to considerable misinformation. It is important to evaluate roentgenograms for the possibilities of accompanying vertebral and urologic abnormalities. Abnormalities of the lumbosacral spine occur in over 50% of infants with high anomalies, and the accompanying neurologic defects may significantly lessen the likelihood of a well-functioning bowel after correction in these infants. In addition, the incidence of associated urologic abnormalities may exceed 70% among patients with abnormalities of the lower spine. Early intravenous pyelography should be performed in all babies with imperforate anus.

Treatment. Definitive treatment varies with the type of anomaly present. The imperforate anal membrane, which becomes apparent soon after birth, as a very thin bulging membrane that looks dark because of the meconium lying just behind it, is treated either by making a cruciate incision through the membrane or by excising it. This is followed by daily anal dilations with catheters or with the finger. The parents are instructed in the technique so that these dilations may usually be continued several times a week for 3 to 6 months. The frequency is gradually decreased as the stricture softens and the anus remains supple.

With longer segments of rectal agenesis the surgical treatment may be more complicated. Generally, infants with anomalies in which the bowel has come through the puborectalis sling of the levator ani muscle may have definitive surgery in the neonatal period, followed by daily dilations. Those babies with higher anomalies should have a preliminary divided sigmoid colostomy performed in the newborn period. This procedure protects the genitourinary tract by ensuring that fecal contamination will not continue and allows more leisurely and thorough study of the various involved anomalies. This course offers greater possibilities of successful definitive attempts at correction of the bowel difficulties and separation of fistula or an abdominoperineal procedure at 9 to 12 months of age.

BIOCHEMICAL ASPECTS OF THE DIGESTIVE SYSTEM

Nutritional, digestive, and absorptive factors

Carbohydrates

The quantities of saliva and of salivary amylase have been demonstrated to be small for some weeks after birth. Pancreatic amylase is also deficient in the newborn, and it does not reach full activity until 4 to 6 months of age. Amylolytic activity, which splits starch and glycogen primarily to maltose, with a lesser amount of isomaltose, begins in the mouth of the infant. Despite the limitations in secretions among neonates, digestion of starch is adequate within wide ranges of intake, even in low birth weight infants. The electrolyte levels of saliva are hypotonic to serum throughout the life span, but they are less diluted in the neonatal period than later in life. No clinical importance has been ascribed to this variation.

Specific disaccharidases that are located in the outer cell layer of epithelium of the intestinal villi hydrolyze either of the naturally occurring disaccharides, lactose and sucrose, or the maltose and isomaltose, which result from amylolytic activity on polysaccharides. At least four individual alpha-glycosidases are present that are capable of digesting maltose. Two of these, in addition, are able to split sucrose, and one is able to hydrolyze isomaltose. Two beta-glycosidases capable of hydrolyzing lactose are described, one concentrated in the brush border and the other in the cytoplasm of the muocsal cells. Although there are variations in rate of fetal development, all of the alpha-glycosidase activities reach adult values by 6 to 7 months of fetal life. The beta-glycosidases (lactases) develop more slowly and reach normal levels of activity only at the end of gestation. Despite this fact, the act of birth stimulates their maturation and babies born prematurely usually display decreased lactase activity only for the first 3 days of life.

Lactose is the natural carbohydrate of mammalian milks and is generally bound to the protein. In a number of commercial formula preparations, sugar is added to raise the carbohydrate content from the normal 3.5% level of cow's milk toward the 7.0% found in human milk. In many, the added sugar is lactose, although a few preparations are supplemented with dextrose, maltose, or dextrins. In most normal infants who are breast fed or fed cow's milk to which lactose has been added, some of the disaccharide reaches the colon undigested, and softer stools result from bacterial fermentation of the excess disaccharide. In the formulas that do not have intact mammalian milk protein as a base (soybean, casein digest, or meat base formulas), the added disaccharide is usually sucrose, although varying amounts of dextrose, maltose, and dextrins are used in a few.

The monosaccharides glucose and galactose are absorbed against a concentration gradient by an active transport mechanism that is energy dependent, while fructose absorption is of such a lower order that it is believed to simply result from passive diffusion. The absorption of monosaccharides facilitates absorption of water and sodium (solvent drag). Normally, even low birth weight infants are able to digest and absorb carbohydrates within wide ranges of feedings. Maintenance of adequate neonatal serum glucose concentrations and the avoidance of symptomatic hypoglycemia is facilitated to some extent by early feeding of low birth weight infants, especially those suffering from intrauterine malnutrition.

Protein

Protein requirements for the first months of life in full-term infants have been approximated from the assumption that their needs are correctly indicated by the amounts that would be available if they were breast fed; that is 2.0 to 2.5 mg/kg/day. For low birth weight infants the requirements have been shown to be closer to 4.0 gm/kg/day. The major protein components of mammalian milks are casein and the various lactalbumins and lactoglobulins of the whey fraction.

Although coagulation of casein is an important gastric function that is usually attributed to renin, this enzyme has not been shown to be present in the human infant, though it is demonstrable in newborn calf gastric juice. Gastric pepsin and acidity also aids in milk curdling, the solubility of casein being minimal at its isoelectric point (pH 4.7). Volume and acidity of gastric secretion are at adult levels in newborn infants. However, the ability to secrete acid is impaired for a number of weeks beyond the first days of life, especially among infants of low birth weight or in malnourished children of higher weights. This poor acid output limits peptic digestion, which is effective only at a pH below 3.0. Nevertheless, some gastric proteolysis does occur because of two factors. Plasma pepsinogen levels of the first weeks of life are higher than later in infancy, presumably because of stimulation by supplemental maternal corticosteroids. The enzyme cathepsin is also present in newborn gastric juice, and it is effective over a wider range of pH (2.0 to 5.0) than is pepsin. Nevertheless, most of the infant's protein hydrolysis is accomplished by the peptidases of pancreatic juice, which are secreted in inactive zymogen forms and activated by enterokinase from the duodenal mucosa. The active pancreatic peptidases include trypsin, chymotrypsin, and the carboxypeptidases. Proteolytic activity is normally easily demonstrable even in young low birth weight infants, and defects of protein hyrolysis are virtually confined to situations in which flow of pancreatic secretions is impaired. The rare failure of precursor forms of the peptidases to be activated because of a *congenital enterokinase deficiency* may simulate conditions in which secretions are excluded from the duodenum. Hydrolysis of proteins to amino acids in the digestive lumen is virtually complete, and absorption occurs in the upper small intestine, probably by an active transport mechanism.

Fat

Fat exerts at least three important influences in the infant diet. It is a factor in satiety; it is the vehicle for naturally occurring fat-soluble vitamins and essential fatty acids; and it represents the high energy component. Fat digestion and absorption are impaired to a limited extent in the neonatal period among full-term infants. Most full-term infants digest and absorb between 80% to 90% of the saturated animal fats in their diets and are able to absorb more than 90% of the unsaturated fatty acids. Low birth weight infants are less able to absorb animal fat from their diets than the full-term infant; their ability improves only with growth and time. However, unsaturated fatty acids are better absorbed and are usually utilized in their feedings.

Emulsification of fat results from mechanical activity of the stomach. Pancreatic lipase hydrolyzes triglycerides to diglycerides, monoglycerides, free fatty acids, and glycerol. These end-products form polar complexes with bile salts (micelles) to facilitate solubilization and absorption by the upper small intestinal mucosa. Once the lipid digest products have been absorbed, the bile salts that enter into this carrier process pass down the lumen to the ileum for reabsorption and recirculation via excretion in the bile (the enterohepatic circulation). The absorbed fatty acids and glycerol are resynthesized to triglycerides within the intestinal mucosal cells, are invested with a lipoprotein membrane, and then pass via the lacteals into the lymphatic system as chylomicrons.

Triglycerides of fatty acids below 10 carbons (short and medium chain) may be able to be absorbed intact and pass directly into the portal circulation. Preparations of infant formulas using this fat source are not currently important in the feeding of normal full-term infants. Their use has been advocated by some for low birth weight infants, since they are virtually quantitatively absorbed. However, experience with these preparations is still somewhat limited, and their practical value and potential hazards have not been evaluated.

Fluid and caloric needs

Although the minimal daily water requirement necessary to protect a full-term infant from dehydration is 75 to 90 ml/kg, the usual feeding regimens used exceed these levels with a wide margin. In the low birth weight infant, the requirements for fluid are even higher and are tied to caloric needs, the water requirements imposed by renal immaturity, greater growth needs, and so on. The recommended levels range from 130 to 150 ml/kg/day.

Caloric needs in the early weeks of life have been evaluated relatively precisely for low birth weight infants; calculated growth needs are included in the allowances. For full-term, normal-weight infants the emphasis has been on the caloric intake that might be available if the infant was breast fed. However, in both instances the calculations come out to similar average values, 120 calories/kg/day.

Specific feeding regimens

It is readily apparent from the available information on intestinal motility and on digestive and absorptive abilities of the normal full-term infant that he will thrive on a variety of regimens, with wide latitude for personal preferences. Preparation of the infant formula from unmodified or evaporated cow's milk with addition of carbohydrates and water or with the use of the premixed commercially filled preparations all satisfy the requirements of the infant for the various dietary constituents outlined. Obviously, since neonates do not readily handle solid food in a physiologic manner, there is no need to supplement milk feedings in the first month of life. Many pediatricians do so in the mistaken belief that solids offer more satisfaction and produce happier babies. The evidence that this is so is not very well substantiated.

The need of low birth weight infants to quickly resume rates of gain comparable to the rates attained in utero and the limitations imposed on their gastric capacities and digestive functions by small size and immaturity provide less latitude for safety than for full-term infants; there is need for a more carefully worked out program of feeding.

Feedings should be started early, at 3 to 6 hours of age if the infant's condition permits. The first two feedings are of clear fluid, and if tolerated they are followed by a schedule of formula feedings every 3 hours. The initial amounts of clear fluid and formula follow from empiric allowances for different birth weights: below 1,000 gm, 2 to 4 ml; 1,000 to 1,499 gm, 4 to 8 ml; 1,500 to 1,999 gm, 8 to 15 ml; and 2,000 to 2,500 gm, 15 to 20 ml. The standard formula that meets their special needs contains 120 calories, 4.0 gm cow's milk protein, 5.2 gm corn oil fat, and 14.5 gm carbohydrate per 150 ml. The formula is increased daily or every other day by 1 or 2 ml per feeding in accordance with the infant's ability, until a total intake of 150 to 160 ml/kg/day is attained. The formulas are maintained in this range as the infant continues to gain weight, though the program of feeding for each baby must be individualized within the general scheme.

For infants below 1,650 gm birth weight who may not have a well coordinated sucking and swallowing reflex, it may be safest to initiate feedings by intermittent gavage or through an indwelling nasogastric tube. Once the infants reach the point at which they gag on the tubes, or for those above 1,650 gm birth weight, feedings are given by bottle with a special soft rubber "premature" nipple.

GASTROINTESTINAL DISTURBANCES OF WATER, ELECTROLYTE, AND NUTRITIONAL METABOLISM

Diarrhea—general considerations

The significance of the passage of loose stools by an infant less than 1 month of age is not as easy to interpret as that in an older child. Infants with excessive degrees of rectal spasm that does not permit colonic contents to reach the lower colon easily for drying out may experience explosive stools from passage of flatus and trapped contents. Such stools, if not excessive, do not lead to dehydration or to other difficulties, but the children are often overtreated by their physicians who may be more influenced by the appearance of the stools than by the behavior of the baby. One must therefore be careful to evaluate the particular clinical situation and not simply switch from formula to formula in effort to treat loose stools.

Most serious for the welfare of the infant with true diarrhea are the resultant disturbances in water and electrolyte metabolism. Stool losses of water in severe cases of diarrhea may range from 250 to 500 ml or more per day—from 10 to 15 times the normal—and the electrolyte deficits may also approach a loss that is 10 times above normal. As the number of loose stools rises, colonic resorption of sodium and chloride is interfered with, and the stools contain progressively increasing concentrations of these ions. Thus deficits in mild diarrhea are mainly of water; and as the condition becomes more severe, the importance of electrolyte losses becomes increasingly greater. The loss of water and electrolytes in the stools is promptly reflected by a reduction of blood volume and of interstitial fluid volume. When a deficit of water predominates, hyperelectrolytemia may develop if the physician treats the condition by feeding the infant fluids with high concentrations of electrolytes, such as skim milk, to compensate for the diarrhea. Hypoelectrolytemia is exacerbated chiefly by frequent intake of fluids low in electrolytes, with concomitant increasing diarrheal losses.

The program of small, frequent feedings of clear fluids, which is useful in vomiting but is too often mistakenly prescribed for diarrhea, induces multiple gastrocolic reflexes and bowel movements. The aim of therapy must, therefore, be to maintain fluid intake, while at the same time lowering the number and volume of stools. Widely separated large dilute oral feedings tend to accomplish this, and it is more advisable to reduce stool electrolyte losses in this manner than to attempt to compensate for them by feedings of the electrolyte mixtures, which tend to produce hyperelectrolytemia. The total volume of fluid intake should not be allowed to fall below 150 ml/kg/day. Isotonic solutions of glucose may be encouraged, either as a substitute for or as an addition to milk. If milk is given, simple dilution of the regular formula is usually adequate treatment. Lowering of its fat content is believed by many to serve to abort the course of mild diarrhea. However, skim milk should be avoided entirely or diluted to half strength to avoid the problem of hyperelectrolytemia.

Oral feedings may also be instituted after an initial hydration period among hospitalized infants receiving parenteral fluids. The feedings should be viewed simply as a source of calories and nutriment, with the expectation that they may increase losses of fluid and electrolytes by their effects on the colon. Use of combined oral feedings and parenteral fluid and electrolyte regimens has been successfully employed in a number of instances of protracted infantile diarrhea. Parenteral therapy can be relaxed only in the combined oral-intravenous treatment when it is clear that sufficient fluids are being absorbed from the oral intake. Such combined oral nutrition with prolonged parenteral fluid therapy forestalls inanition and obviates the need to consider parenteral (central venous) alimentation (p. 113), which may be difficult to carry out successfully in the presence of infection (diarrhea) in this age group. This form of combined alimentation may be more useful in noninfected patients.

The cause of *acute infantile diarrhea* (p. 138) often remains obscure. Viruses of both enteric and systemic varieties undoubtedly contribute to pathogenesis in many instances. Not infrequently, the source of difficulty lies in gastrointestinal reaction to septicemia or to a primary infection in another system such as the genitourinary or respiratory tract. Increasingly, evidence is being accumulated that neonatal diarrhea is in large measure caused by infection with enteropathogenic strains of *E. coli.* This is especially true of premature infants. The organism has been shown to exert its effect primarily by a choleralike toxin that disrupts salt and water absorption in the colon. Oral administration of neomycin sulfate solution in the dose of 100 mg/kg/day or colistin sulfate at doses of 10 to 15 mg/kg/day, each drug divided into three or four doses, for 4 to 5 days is the treatment of choice. More recent evidence that *E. coli* invades the intestinal epithelium and may extend to other organs via the circulatory system suggests that the neonate who does not respond readily to oral treatment of his diarrhea with these nonabsorbable agents requires simultaneous systemic therapy with antimicrobial agents.

Neonatal necrotizing enterocolitis

A particularly virulent and lethal type of acute diarrhea among neonates is necrotizing enterocolitis. This condition is particularly prevalent among low birth weight infants and may account for as much as 2% of admissions to intensive care nurseries for newborns. The cause is unknown, but mesenteric vascular ischemia and hypoxia of the intestinal mucosa have been suggested for the probable pathogenesis.

Clinical presentation. Infants with this syndrome are initially difficult to distinguish clinically from neonates with other types of diarrhea. They are lethargic, irritable, become distended, have difficulty in maintaining their body temperatures, eat poorly, and vomit. The clues that help distinguish this entity from other types of diarrhea are difficulty with aeration at birth, increased apneic episodes, and blood in the stools. *Pneumatosis intestinales,* or presence of air in the submucosa or subserosal surfaces of the colon, is virtually always present and is pathognomonic. Increased air in the bowel lumen or in the peritoneum (indicating perforation of gangrenous bowel) is seen but is not a specific sign of necrotizing enterocolitis. Barium examination is not necessary for demonstration of any of the roentgenogram findings associated with the condition, and if carried out, these studies may lead to perforation.

Treatment. Once the condition is suspected, infants should have intermittent or continuous gastric suction with discontinuation of oral feedings. Systemic antibiotic therapy, usually a combination of penicillin and kanamycin, is instituted, as is parenteral fluid therapy. Repeated plain and upright roentgenograms of the abdomen are obtained every 6 to 12 hours to follow the progress of the infant. In some, the picture will regress after 48 to 72 hours. However, mortality is above 50% in most series, and there is an increasing tendency to approach the situation aggressively. Among patients who exhibit clinical signs of deterioration after institution of medical management, surgery is advised even in the absence of signs of perforation. Resection and primary anastomosis are carried out for localized lesions; in more extensive cases resection and exteriorization with ileostomy or colostomy is indicated. The extensive nature of the surgical procedure in many instances dictates a prolonged period of parenteral alimentation to ensure survival of the infant.

Malabsorption and chronic diarrhea

The presence of a malabsorptive condition and distinction of chronic from acute diarrhea are often difficult to establish in the neonatal period. A major concomitant of malabsorption in an infant is the symptom of failure to thrive. Sufficient time has usually not elapsed for the neonate to establish a clear-cut pattern of deviation from expected growth. This is especially true of the problems associated with steatorrhea. On the other hand, the extreme vulnerability of young infants to the effects of fluid and electrolyte losses may suggest over a few days during a bout of diarrhea that weight loss is from failure to absorb nutriments, when in fact the fluctuations may be related only to changes in body water. An additional confusing feature results in some of the malabsorptive conditions that will not clearly manifest themselves during the first month of life, since offending foods may not yet have been introduced into the diet in sufficient amounts and with sufficient regularity to manifest a consistent deleterious effect. This is especially true of gluten-sensitive enteropathy, which is therefore omitted from discussion below.

Defects in fat digestion and absorption

Abnormalities of utilization of dietary fat that affect the neonate may be based on disorders of lipolysis, of mucosal cell transport, or of lymphatic transport of fat. In some instances, the precise locus of the defect is not clear, as in the steatorrhea associated with low birth weight.

Infants with lipolytic defects may, unlike those with absorptive deficiencies, demonstrate oil droplets in their stools. The most frequently encountered disorder of lipolysis in neonates results from pancreatic insufficiency associated with *cystic fibrosis of the pancreas. Isolated lipase deficiency* has also been described in rare infants.

Among patients with *impaired hepatic function* or with *biliary obstruction,* critical micellar levels of conjugated bile salts may not be attained in the duodenum; and although lipolysis is normal, solubilization of the split products will be defective. *Bacterial overgrowth* from bowel stasis may result in deconjugation of the bile salts and thus produce the defect. Bacterial overgrowth is encountered with malrotations or with multiple small intestinal strictures, jejunal diverticula and duplications, or neurogenic deficits. Other factors that may limit the size of the available bile salt pool are disturbances in the enterohepatic circulation, which, in the neonate, is restricted to excessive loss of distal small intestine following surgery for a congenital problem.

Hypobetalipoproteinemia is a rare hereditary disease in which synthesis of this protein moiety is impaired. Abnormalities of the central nervous system and eyes appear at a much later age in these patients. The malabsorptive defects and the red blood cell membrane deficiencies that produce the thorny spiculated cells from which the secondary name of *acanthocytosis* is derived may be present in the neonate. However, the presence of acanthocytes may occur in normal newborns. Malabsorption results from inability to invest the absorbed and reconstituted triglycerides with a β-lipoprotein envelope, thus limiting chylomicron formation and impeding lipid transport via the lymphatics. Pileup of lipids in the mucosal cells is easily demonstrated on examination of a peroral biopsy specimen. Treatment results in decrease of steatorrhea and in improved nutrition and consists of changeover to a low fat milk or to one that contains medium chain triglycerides.

Mechanical obstruction to lymphatic flow away from the intestinal mucosa results in dilation of the villous lacteals and steatorrhea from exudation of fat, which is also accompanied by protein loss. Lymphatic obstruction does not usually make itself apparent in the neonatal period, but congenital obstruction abnormalities of the mucosal lacteals alone *(congenital lymphangiectasia)* or in combination with widespread anomalies of the lymphatic system *(Milroy's disease)* may appear in the newborn period, usually with generalized edema from hypoproteinemia. Diagnosis is made from a characteristic peroral mucosal biopsy in which the dilated lacteals occupy a prominent position in the lamina propria of the villus. As with hypobetalipoproteinemia, administration of low-fat milk or of milk containing medium chain triglycerides reduces protein loss and steatorrhea in these patients. In the rare instance in which lymphangiectasia can be demonstrated by roentgenographic examination to be confined to a limited extent of the intestine, surgical excision of the affected region may afford a cure.

Defects in carbohydrate digestion and absorption

A *congenital inability actively to absorb either glucose or galactose* is inherited as an autosomal recessive disease, affecting transport mechanisms of both intestine and kidney. Ingestion of glucose or galactose by these infants leads to profuse watery diarrhea, but these monosaccharides are metabolized normally following intravenous infusions, though the decreased urinary resorptive ability commonly leads to glucosuria. Mucosal morphologic characteristics of intestinal cells are normal, and the basic defect appears to be in the inability of the microvilli to bind either of the monosaccharides. Fructose is absorbed normally in this disease, and it is used as the source of carbohydrates in the diet.

Transient malabsorption of monosaccharides may also appear in infants who have suffered episodes of acute gastroenteritis. For several weeks to months after an acute illness, such infants may not tolerate any feeding with more than 1% to 2% carbohydrates.

Sucrose-isomaltose malabsorption is caused by congenital deficiencies of both intestinal sucrase and isomaltase and is inherited as in autosomal recessive disorder. Since the first month after birth is a period in which most infants ingest either breast milk or formulas that contain lactose, clinical manifestations of the defect do not appear until later when sucrose- or starch-containing foods are added to their diets. However, if the infant is fed a proprietary formula containing sucrose, clinical signs may be manifested in the early neonatal period.

Congenital lactose malabsorption is a rare disease, with few documented cases in the neonatal period. Because of the difficulty in diagnosing the entity precisely, its exact incidence and mode of inheritance have not been determined. Patients with the defect who are breast fed or fed cow's milk formulas suffer from diarrhea and failure to thrive. The liquid, frothy diarrhea results in part from fermentation and in part from the osmotic effect of the abnormal amounts of low molecular weight acids (principally lactic) that are being excreted. Stool pH is consequently low, and reducing substance is demonstrable in the stool. Changeover to a milk substitute in which lactose is absent results in clearing of the symptoms.

The morphologic characteristics of the small intestine are normal by light microscopy and activities of all disaccharidases other than those specifically involved in the condition and of the various other digestive enzymes are within normal ranges.

Acquired disaccharidase deficiencies may appear in any disorder in which intestinal cells are damaged, and the most important cause in the neonate would be infectious diarrhea. Although this condition differs from the congenital deficiencies in that all of the disaccharidases are affected, lactase is most vulnerable and the most likely to result in clinical symptoms, since this enzyme is normally lowest in activity as compared with sucrase and maltase. Mucosal injury in neonates may require longer periods for repair than would adult mucosa, so that depressed activities of intestinal disaccharidases (lactase) that result from such infections might persist for longer periods of time. Oral administration of neomycin in infantile diarrhea may further depress lactase activity by an unknown mechanism.

Infants with secondary lactase insufficiency may vomit in addition to having diarrhea, and the mechanism for this complaint is not clear. It has been suggested that the cause is specific toxicity of lactosemia or that it results from delayed gastric emptying or from a reflex response to distention of the lower colon by gas and fluid. Initially, infants may be able to compensate for losses imposed by the diarrhea and vomiting, but after a short period of time they become lethargic, irritable, and anorexic. If the disorder is unrecognized and significant dehydration, acidosis, and mucosal damage are allowed to continue over a period of weeks, irreversible damage to the small intestine may ensue that would lead to steatorrhea, protein-losing enteropathy, intractable and unrelenting diarrhea, and finally may cause the infant to succumb in a severely malnourished state with a pathologic picture resembling that of necrotizing enterocolitis.

Screening procedures for patients suspected of disaccharidase deficiency include examination of fresh stools or of rectal swabs for acidity and reducing substances. One must be certain that the patient has been ingesting the carbohydrate to which he is intolerant, otherwise the expected changes in the stool may not be detected. Disaccharide and monosaccharide tolerance tests, in which flat curves are generally relied on in screening for the condition, have limitations in the neonate. The usual delay in emptying time of the stomach of young infants may result in a misleading very slow rise in blood glucose after feeding an otherwise tolerated sugar. Also, feeding of an adequate dose (usually 2.0 to 2.5 gm disaccharide per kg body weight) to cause the normal increase in blood glucose concentration of greater than 25 mg/100 ml within 1 hour as indication of significant hydrolysis usually produces severe abdominal cramps and watery diarrhea within 2 to 6 hours following ingestion of the test substance in deficient individuals. This effect may be especially injurious in a sick infant, since simultaneous administration of balanced intravenous fluids that would be protective to his circulatory and extracellular fluid systems cannot easily be given during the test, because they may interfere with the interpretations. Biopsies of the mucosa of the small bowel and direct assay of the disaccharidases are the best methods of correctly diagnosing the disorder. If biopsies are taken from the duodenum or jejunum that has been damaged, the activities of the enzymes are decreased. If the ratios of activities such as sucrase:lactase or isomaltase:lactase are used, the interpretations may be made with greater validity.

Treatment consists of withdrawing the offending sugar or sugars from the diet. Infants with glucose-galactose malabsorption must only take fructose in their diets. Newborn infants with lactose malabsorption must be fed formula that does not contain lactose; they will grow and develop if they are fed soybean, meat base, or other formula in which sucrose, glucose, or maltose has been substituted for lactose.

Defects in protein digestion and absorption

Congenital deficiency of pancreatic exocrine secretion results in an assimilatory defect caused by incomplete splitting of protein. This lesion is restricted almost exclusively in the neonate to cystic fibrosis of the pancreas. A small number of infants with isolated pancreatic deficiencies have been described. These babies have metaphyseal dysostosis and bone marrow insufficiencies that result in neutropenia, anemia, and thrombocytopenia. Postmortem examination of the pancreas in this condition reveals extensive replacement with fat; hence the alternative name of *congenital lipomatosis of the pancreas.*

Infants with isolated *congenital deficiencies of trypsinogen* have been reported. These patients may be identical to those with the congenital defect in secretion of the intestinal enzyme enterokinase. Activation of trypsin from trypsinogen is autocatalytic, but production of the necessary initial small amounts of active trypsin results from the action of enterokinase on trypsinogen. Infants with *enterokinase deficiency* behave clinically as if pancreatic elaboration of trypsinogen was impaired, and they respond favorably to pancreatic extract supplementation. That the salutory effects of such extracts lies in activation of the patient's own normal trypsinogen can, however, be demonstrated in vitro by addition of either trypsin or enterokinase to duodenal fluid from an affected infant. Intestinal morphologic characteristics on examination of peroral biopsy is normal. The most frequent symptoms are hypoproteinemia, anemia, and failure to thrive because of decreased protein digestion. Correction of the deficit in protein digestion may be compensated for either with use of hydrolyzed protein feedings or with supplementation of feedings with pancreatic extracts.

Problems with cow's milk ingestion

In addition to the rare instances of congenital lactase deficiency, ingestion of cow's milk may occasionally be associated with marked intolerance to the protein during the first weeks. Severe vomiting or profound rectal bleeding and diarrhea simulating ulcerative colitis may be encountered. In these infants, examination of the mucosa by sigmoidoscopy reveals friability and multiple bleeding points. Following biopsy, microscopic examination of the specimen shows an inflammatory process with infiltration of the submucosa by plasma cells and eosinophils. Withdrawal of cow's milk leads to complete clearing. In a patient in whom we observed congenital steatorrhea related to the ingestion of cow's milk β-lactoglobulin there was severe diarrhea in the newborn period. This condition ultimately spontaneously improved.

MISCELLANEOUS SYMPTOMATIC PROBLEMS OF THE GASTROINTESTINAL TRACT

Gastrointestinal bleeding

Although *hematemesis* is not uncommon in the newborn period, the blood may not originate from the infant. Blood that was swallowed during the birth process may be vomited as long as 72 hours after birth. Maternal blood may be distinguished from infant's blood by the alkali denaturation test. Vomited blood of infant origin need not always come from the stomach in newborn infants. Trauma to the nasopharynx from vigorous suctioning may lead to swallowing (and then vomiting) of blood. True gastric hemorrhage may arise from ulcers that occur with anoxemia, septicemia, and hemorrhagic disease of the newborn. Erosion of esophageal mucosa by regurgitated gastric juice with hiatus hernia of the stomach may also result in bleeding in the newborn period.

Breast-fed infants may draw blood from a fissure or ulcer in the mother's nipple, and in some instances alarmingly large amounts of blood may be vomited although the children appear quite well. Examination of the mother will generally reveal the source of the trouble. It may sometimes be noted that vomiting of blood follows nursing from one breast and not from the other.

If swallowed blood or active gastric bleeding is promptly vomited, the emesis may be bright red. Because of the high gastric acidity of the first few days of life, if blood remains in the stomach for any length of time it turns dark brown to black, resembling coffee grounds. Stools from babies with upper gastrointestinal tract bleeding invariably contain blood. If there has been passage of more than 10 to 30 ml of blood in the average weight newborn, the stool will be tarry in appearance. With lesser amounts, only chemical tests show its presence. Symptoms of shock may be present and will depend upon the amount and rapidity of blood loss. It is always important to examine the infant's nose and pharynx, as well as the nipples of the mother of a breast-fed baby, before assuming that upper gastrointestinal tract bleeding is gastric in origin.

The infant with gastrointestinal hemorrhage must be kept quiet, and one must sometimes restrain the enthusiastic pursuit of a specific diagnosis in the best interests of the baby. Hematocrit readings must be followed frequently and regularly to evaluate continuing losses of blood and the pulse carefully watched for signs of collapse, in which cases immediate transfusion is urgently indicated. Supportive transfusions with whole blood to replace cells and blood volume are prescribed as indicated from serial hematocrit values and the condition of the infant. During the early period of doubt with respect to specific diagnosis, frequent small formula feedings may be given infants. There are no known causes of hematemesis in neonates for which feedings are contraindicated, as there might be in patients with esophageal varices. Parenteral fluids are given as indicated.

Hematochezia, or the appearance of gross blood in the stool, is usually associated with bleeding from the lower intestines. Melena, or tarry stool, indicates presence of blood from the upper gastrointestinal tract that has been altered by secretions as it passed to the rectum. However, massive gastric bleeding may be followed by recognizable red blood in the stool, while slow oozing of blood from the lower ileum may occasionally result only in tarry stools. Acute rectal bleeding in the first days of life is usually associated with upper gastrointestinal sources. One important exception is from direct rectal trauma caused by passage of a thermometer, tube, or finger. Later during the first month of life hematochezia may herald the onset of milk-induced colitis or of necrotizing enterocolitis. Occasionally, a bleeding diathesis in the neonate will initially manifest itself in this manner (p. 205). In rare instances congenital abnormalities such as hemangioma of the colon or Meckel's diverticulum may be seen with massive fresh rectal hemorrhage prior to the end of the first month of life. Fissures and rectal polyps in ano are not as common as causes of rectal bleeding in the neonate as they are later in infancy and childhood, but they do occasionally occur.

Peptic ulcer and gastric perforation

Acute infantile peptic ulcers occur with equal frequency in the stomach and duodenum. The newborn is particularly vulnerable during the first 48 hours of life because of increased gastric acidity and parietal cell mass during a period when he is more likely to suffer hypoxia and stress. The most frequent symptoms are severe gastrointestinal bleeding, acute distension, and perforation. Morbidity is compounded by the underlying illness.

Except in the low birth weight infant, in whom stress and hypoxia may persist beyond the first few days of life, peptic ulceration is rare beyond this period of neonatal life. However, severe peptic ulcer disease associated with the *Zollinger-Ellison syndrome* may rarely appear in the neonate. In this condition non–beta cell islet adenomas secrete a gastrinlike material, and patients suffer marked gastric hypersecretion that leads to severe watery diarrhea and steatorrhea, which complicates the problem. The ulcers are usually single, located in the duodenum, and are intractable, with symptoms usually resistant to medical therapy. Severe bleeding is treated with blood volume replacement.

In infants with acute ulcers, surgical procedures are restricted only to emergency complications such as perforation and obstruction. Plication of the ulcer is usually adequate treatment. The rare infants with ulcerogenic tumor syndromes must be carefully explored and the tumors removed; total gastrectomy has been reported to be the operation of choice for direct treatment of the ulcer in this group. Infants and children with resected stomachs have been shown to thrive under proper careful dietary management.

Spontaneous perforation or rupture of the stomach occurs among seriously ill neonates, especially of low birth weight, when anoxia and respiratory distress occur in the first few days of life. Increasing abdominal distention is the prominent symptom. Upright roentgenograms of the abdomen usually demonstrate considerable quantities of free air in the peritoneal cavity and establish the diagnosis of a perforated viscus. The situation is a surgical emergency, and abdominal exploration for closure of the perforation should be carried out as soon as possible. Prior to and following surgery infants must be supported with oxygen and systemically administered antibiotics.

Appendicitis and peritonitis

Appendicitis is extremely rare in the neonate. Its cause is unknown, but it has been suggested that distal obstruction and back pressure from the colon or that generalized infection or septicemia lead to necrosis and inflammation of the appendix. The lesion is especially difficult to diagnose in the neonate. Radiographic examination for fecaliths, needle aspirations of the peritoneal cavity, and other techniques have been advocated by some for diagnosis. However, the lesion is rare; one's index of suspicion is usually low; and the symptoms of frequently associated conditions such as septicemia and a respiratory or gastrointestinal infection tend to obscure the diagnosis. Even the authors who champion a particular diagnostic maneuver present among their data an incidence of at least 80% of patients with perforations of the appendix, indicating late diagnosis. The condition must, therefore, be regarded as one that is diagnosed mainly after perforation has occurred and peritonitis has developed.

Peritonitis in the neonate is of three varieties. Most frequent is the bacterial infection that follows perforation of a viscus or spread of infection from septicemia or gastroenteritis. As with the other surgical problems of the neonatal gastrointestinal tract, the signs of peritonitis and of the underlying disease are superimposed on each other. Rigidity and spasm of the abdominal wall musculature do not readily occur. Demonstration of free fluid by shifting dullness or demonstration of extraintestinal fluid or air by roentgenogram examination is the closest one may come to pathognomonic signs. The most important cornerstones of therapy are initially to support the infant as one would any sick newborn; that is, with appropriate intravenous fluids, oxygen if necessary, warmth, and so on (p. 99). A second feature of treatment consists of appropriate antibiotic therapy for the infection. Exploration after the patient is in reasonably good condition to withstand laparotomy is necessary for identification and repair of the site of perforation that has led to the peritonitis.

The second form of neonatal peritonitis occurs only prior to birth and is a sterile, foreign body reaction from leakage of noninfected meconium into the peritoneal cavity. Perforation may also occur within the first hours of postnatal life, before the meconium has become contaminated by bacteria to fit this diagnostic category. The perforation occurs proximal to the site of an obstruction, usually from a congenital abnormality, volvulus, or meconium ileus. Infants with this lesion are usually born with severe abdominal distension, which may cause difficulty with delivery. The infants are usually quite ill from birth, with respiratory distress, difficulty with temperature regulation, and evidence of pressure on return venous flow from the lower extremities and scrotal area, with edema of these parts. Radiographic study reveals a ground glass type of opacity of the abdomen, with scattered bits of calcified material from antepartum peritoneal reaction to spilled meconium, and only in the rarer sterile perforations that occur in the first few hours after birth is free air demonstrable. On occasion, the precipitating obstructive site and the site of tear may spontaneously be healed by the time of birth, and nothing further need be done. Usually, however, the infant requires surgical exploration such as that for infected peritonitis acquired from perforation at a later age.

Prognosis among infants with neonatal peritonitis is grave, whether infection is present or not. Few series report a survival approaching 50%. The difficulty possibly is attributed to the severity of the underlying causative lesions and to the poor outcome associated with treatment of these lesions.

The third form of peritonitis encountered in neonates is not truly peritonitis but *ascites,* involving accumulation of a major body fluid in the peritoneal cavity unrelated to a perforation of the gastrointestinal tract. The two fluids most frequently encountered are bile and chyle. Both types of ascites usually do not manifest themselves during the first month of life. Bile peritonitis results from rupture of a bile duct or of the liver. Acholic stools are part of the picture, although jaundice is disproportionately mild because of the absence of significant regurgitation. Treatment consists of laparotomy and drainage and definitive reconstruction of the biliary tree to correct the tear and obstruction. In the case of *chylous ascites* demonstration of the precise site of tear and treatment is much more difficult. Surgery is usually avoided because of the uncertain results.

MURRAY DAVIDSON

BIBLIOGRAPHY

Ames, M. D.: Gastric acidity in the first ten days of life of the prematurely born baby, Am. J. Dis. Child. **100**:252, 1960.

Ardran, G. M.: A cineradiographic study of breast feeding, Br. J. Radiol. **31**:156, 1958.

Astley, R., and Carre, I. J.: Gastro-oesophageal incompetence in children, Radiology **62**:351, 1954.

Berdon, W. E., and others: The radiologic evaluation of imperforate anus; an approach correlated with current surgical concepts, Radiology **90**:466, 1968.

Berenberg, W., and Neuhauser, E. B. D.: Cardio-esophageal relaxation (chalasia) as a cause of vomiting in infants, Pediatrics **5**:414, 1950.

Bill, A. H., Jr., and Chapman, N. D.: The enterocolitis of Hirschsprung's disease; its natural history and treatment, Am. J. Surg. **103**:70, 1962.

Collins, J. R.: Small intestinal mucosal damage with villous atrophy—a review of the literature, Am. J. Clin. Pathol. **44**:36, 1965.

Davidson, M.: Disaccharide intolerance, Pediatr. Clin. North Am. **14**:93, 1967.

Davidson, M.: Congenital aganglionosis. In Code, C. F., editor: Handbook of physiology—alimentary canal, Washington, D. C., 1968, Am. Physiol. Soc., chap. 134, p. 2783.

Donovan, E J., and Santulli, T. V.: Gastric and duodenal ulcers in infancy and in childhood, Am. J. Dis. Child. **69**:176, 1945.

Drucker, M. M., Polliack, A., Yeiven, R., and Sacks, T. G.: Immunofluorescent demonstration of enteropathogenic *Escherichia coli* in tissues of infants dying with enteritis, Pediatrics **46**: 855, 1970.

Dykstra, G., Sieber, W. K., and Kiesewetter, W. B.: Intestinal atresia and stenosis of the jejunum and ileum, Surgery **64**:661, 1968.

Filler, R. M., Randolph, J. G., and Gross, R. E.: Esophageal hiatus hernia in infants and children, J. Thorac. Cardiovasc. Surg. **47**:551, 1964.

Fraser, G. C., and Berry, C.: Mortality in neonatal Hirschsprung's disease; with particular reference to enterocolitis, J. Pediatr. Surg. **2**:205, 1967.

Gryboski, J. D.: The swallowing mechanism of the neonate. I. Esophageal and gastric motility, Pediatrics **35**:445, 1965.

Herbst, J. J., Sunshine, P., and Kretchmer, N.: Intestinal malabsorption in infancy and childhood, Adv. Pediatr. **16**:11, 1969.

Hood, J. H.: Effect of position on amount and distribution of gas in the intestinal tract of infants and young children, Lancet **2**:107, 1964.

Jeffries, G. H., Chapman, A., and Sleisenger, M. H.: Low-fat diet in intestinal lymphangiectasia; its effect on albumin metabolism, N. Engl. J. Med. **270**:761, 1964.

Lamy, M., Frezal, J., Polonovski, J., Druez, G., and Rey, J.: Congenital absence of beta-lipoproteins, Pediatrics **31**:277, 1963.

Linkner, L. M., and Benson, C. D.: Spontaneous perforation of the stomach in the newborn; analysis of thirteen cases, Am. J. Surg. **149**: 525, 1959.

Louw, J. H.: Jejunoileal atresia and stenosis, J. Pediatr. Surg. **1**:8, 1966.

Mellin, G. W., Santulli, T. V., and Altman, H. S.: Congenital pyloric stenosis, J. Pediatr. **66**:649, 1965.

Santulli, T. V.: Meconium ileus. In Mustard, W. T., and others, editors: Pediatric surgery, ed. 2, Chicago, 1969, Year Book Medical Publishers, p. 983.

Santulli, T. V.: Meconium ileus.: In Mustard, W. T., and others, editors: Pediatric surgery, Chicago, 1969, Year Book Medical Publishers.

Spencer, R.: Gastrointestinal hemorrhage in infancy and childhood; 476 cases, Surgery **55**: 718, 1964.

Stevenson, J. K., Oliver, T. K., Jr., Graham, C. B., Bell, R. S., and Gould, V. E.: Aggressive treatment of neonatal necrotizing enterocolitis; 38 patients with 25 survivors, J. Pediatr. Surg. **6**: 28, 1971.

Swenson, O., and Grana, L.: Long term results of surgical treatment of imperforate anus, Dis. Colon Rectum **5**:13, 1962.

Vasko, J. S., and Tapper, R. I.: The surgical significance of chylous ascites, Arch. Surg. **95**:355, 1967.

Wayson, E. E., Garnjobst, W., Chandler, J. J., and Peterson, C. G.: Esophageal atresia with tracheoesophageal fistula; lesions of a quarter century's experience, Am. J. Surg. **110**:162, 1965.

14 Inborn disorders of intermediary metabolism

This chapter limits itself to those diseases that have clinical manifestations in the neonatal period and to those that lack clinical manifestations for which therapy in the neonatal period has been advised. In recognizing inborn errors of metabolism in the neonatal period, the most important clinical finding is the presence of a similar disorder in a sibling; metabolic disease in this period has few specific signs. The most common manifestation is probably failure to thrive, but suspicion should be raised by any of the following: hypoglycemia, prolonged, unexplained jaundice, metabolic acidosis, persistent vomiting, seizures, depression of the central nervous system, or acetonuria.

Without doubt, a substantial number of infants with lethal metabolic disorders die undiagnosed within the first few days of life. In such cases determination of plasma amino acids and organic acids, together with careful postmortem examination, can be of substantial benefit in genetic counseling.

Once a diagnosis is established in a surviving infant, there are four general approaches to appropriate management.

1. No specific management may be indicated in the absence of clear information as to the efficacy of any specific therapy.
2. The intake of the metabolite that accumulates in the disorder should be reduced. Present evidence suggests that this approach is beneficial in phenylketonuria, but completely acceptable objective evidence is lacking for this therapy in any disorder. Furthermore, adequate levels of the normal product of a blocked reaction may be dependent, in part, upon elevation of the precursor metabolite.
3. The intake of the normal metabolite that is not produced because of the metabolic error should be increased. This approach has produced chemical remission in orotic aciduria. Its clinical efficacy is not established beyond reasonable doubt in any disorder.
4. Large amounts of whatever cofactor is altered or lacking in the impaired reaction should be given. This form of therapy has produced chemical remission in some cases of methylmalonic acidemia and homocystinuria. The clinical efficacy and safety of this approach have not been established.

When one is faced with the question of managing such an infant with a disorder of intermediary metabolism it is worthwhile to discuss the problem directly with an investigator studying the disease.

DISORDERS OF AMINO ACID METABOLISM

Disorders of the metabolism of phenylalanine and tyrosine

Phenylketonuria

Phenylketonuria is caused by an inborn defect in the hydoxylation of phenylalanine to form tyrosine. Although some individuals with this entity are clinically normal, severe motor and mental retardation usually occurs. There is substantial evidence that a diet low in phenylalanine instituted within the neonatal period significantly improves the outlook for normal intellectual development in an infant with phenylketonuria.

Etiology and pathogenesis. There is little doubt that the primary defect in phenylketonuria is marked reduction in the activity of phenylalanine hydroxylase (Fig. 14-1). However, the mechanism by which clinical disease is produced is unknown.

All evidence to date indicates that phenylalanine catabolism normally proceeds through the synthesis of tyrosine (Fig. 14-1). Both of these amino acids are nutritionally essential; neither can be synthesized de novo. Phenylalanine in the diet reduces the requirement for tyrosine. Since the hydroxylation of phenylalanine is irreversible, phenylalanine cannot be synthesized from tyrosine. The irreversible nature of phenylalanine hydroxylation has some significance in the interpretation of laboratory data. Defects in the metabolism of tyrosine have no direct effect on the level of phenylalanine in plasma; individuals with hereditary tyrosinosis characteristically exhibit normal plasma levels of phenylalanine. Therefore, an elevation of plasma phenylalanine occurring under normal dietary conditions indicates an impairment in phenylalanine hydroxylation. The degradation of tyrosine is initiated in the liver by tyrosine transaminase, an enzyme that also catalyzes the transamination of phenylalanine and tryptophan. In the experimental animal any of these three aromatic amino acids is capable of inducing increased activity of tyrosine transaminase. It seems likely that these aromatic amino acids share other enzymatic activities in vivo, some of which may be involved in the synthesis of neurally active substances.

The development of the catabolic pathway for phenylalanine and tyrosine occurs in very late fetal life, with the result that the majority of premature infants exhibit elevations of plasma tyrosine and phenylalanine in the neonatal period. A much smaller percentage of full-term infants do so. These elevations are temporary, persisting for days to weeks only, but can be reversed by the administration of ascorbic acid, which is known to activate p-hydroxyphenyl pyruvic acid oxidase in vitro and to abolish the tyrosyluria observed in patients with scurvy. Since ascorbic acid has no known action with respect to either phenylalanine hydroxylase or tyrosine transaminase, its mode of action in reducing plasma phenylalanine and tyrosine in the neonate remains in part obscure.

Fig. 14-1 illustrates diagrammatically the metabolism of phenylalanine and tyrosine and some of the secondary effects that have been suggested as important in the production of clinical manifestations. The experimental evidence for these secondary defects is still inconclusive. Effects that are not specifically related to these metabolic pathways have been noted in phenylketonuric infants; these include failure of normal my-

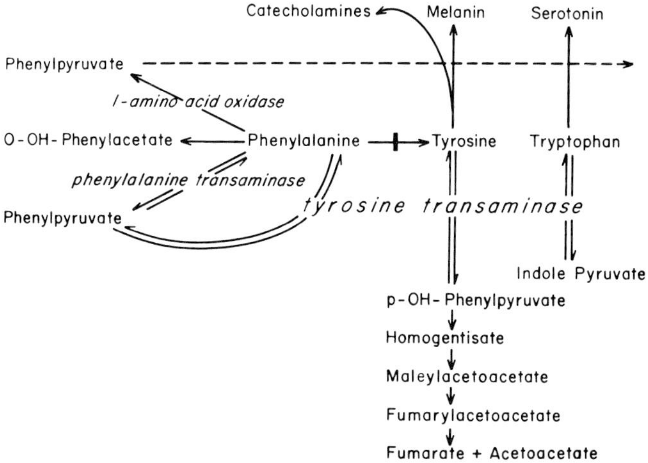

FIG. 14-1. Schematic representation of the metabolism of phenylalanine, tyrosine, and tryptophan. Solid crossbar indicates the metabolic block demonstrated in phenylketonuria, while broken crossbars indicate postulated secondary metabolic blocks.

elinization and a general depression of the levels of plasma amino acids other than phenylalanine.

Clinical features. The majority of phenylketonuric infants show no clinical manifestations during the neonatal period. In a number of cases vomiting has been prominent in the first weeks of life. A few patients have shown unusual irritability. The mousy odor of phenylacetic acid should be present soon after birth, but early recognition of this sign has not been noted in reported cases. Eczema and seizures, when present, generally occur after the first month of life.

Laboratory findings. By definition, the hallmark of phenylketonuria is the presence of phenylpyruvic acid in the urine. While this acid is present in the urine of all older, untreated patients, it is not present in the urine of the newborn phenylketonuric infant. At birth the plasma level of phenylalanine in the affected infant is similar to that of his mother. As the infant's intake of phenylalanine is established in early neonatal life, plasma phenylalanine rises. In older subjects, phenylpyruvic acid is not excreted in urine until plasma phenylalanine is 12 to 18 mg/100 ml. However, in the neonate phenylpyruvic acid may not appear in the urine for several weeks, even though plasma phenylalanine is greater than 20 mg/100 ml. Therefore, the ferric chloride test for this substance is of extremely limited value in the early diagnosis of phenylketonuria. Ortho-hydroxyphenylacetic acid appears in the urine in abnormal amounts earlier than does phenylpyruvic acid but is considerably more difficult to determine than phenylpyruvic acid. In any case neither compound is an abnormal metabolite. Abnormalities in their excretion are simply reflections of substantial elevation in tissue phenylalanine.

Diagnosis. The diagnosis of phenylketonuria in the early neonatal period depends on direct determination of plasma phenylalanine. The interpretation of the value obtained is complicated by the variation in activity of the enzymes involved in the catabolism of phenylalanine and tyrosine in the neonatal period. Elevations in plasma phenylalanine with accompanying elevations in plasma tyrosine are not indicative of phenylketonuria but of a relative impairment in the metabolism of both phenolic amino acids. If plasma tyrosine is normal or low, a persistent elevation of plasma phenylalanine to levels of 30 mg/100 ml or more is usually diagnostic of phenylketonuria, regardless of the presence or absence of phenylpyruvic acid in the urine. Persistent elevation of plasma phenylalanine to levels less than 15 mg/100 ml, associated with low or normal tyrosine, indicates either heterozygosity for phenylketonuria or some hyperphenylalaninemic state other than phenylketonuria. Patients whose plasma levels of phenylalanine fall between 15 and 30 mg/100 ml constitute a serious problem in diagnosis and management. Each must be given careful individual attention. It appears that the risk of ultimate mental retardation is limited almost exclusively to that group of patients whose plasma phenylalanine is greater than 20 mg/100 ml. It is, therefore, generally agreed that restriction of dietary phenylalanine is indicated when plasma phenylalanine is 20 mg/100 ml or more. On arbitrary grounds, we feel that specific phenylalanine restriction is also indicated when plasma phenylalanine is 15 to 20 mg/100 ml and phenylpyruvic acid is excreted in the urine. We do not believe that treatment is absolutely indicated if plasma phenylalanine is less than 20 mg/100 ml and the urine does not contain phenylpyruvic acid. This opinion is based on the assumption that the ability to maintain plasma phenylalanine at levels less than 20 mg/100 ml without excreting phenylpyruvic acid is indicative of substantial ability to synthesize tyrosine from phenylalanine. In individual cases it may be necessary to measure the amounts of phenylalanine, phenyllactic acid, ortho-hydroxyphenylacetic acid, and phenylacetylglutamine excreted in the urine before arriving at a final decision regarding an infant's ability to hydroxylate phenylalanine.

Guidelines regarding diagnosis and therapy in phenylketonuria are summarized in the outline below.

DIAGNOSIS OF PHENYLKETONURIA

A. Treatment group
   1. Plasma phenylalanine $\geqq$ 20 mg/100 ml; plasma tyrosine normal or low
   2. Plasma phenylalanine $\geqq$ 15 mg/100 ml; less than 20 mg/100 ml plasma tyrosine;

low or normal phenylpyruvic acid present in the urine

B. Careful follow-up without treatment indicated
   1. Plasma phenylalanine $\geqq$ 5 mg/100 ml but $<$ 20 mg/100 ml*; plasma tyrosine normal; no phenylpyruvic acid in the urine

C. Transient tyrosinemia of the neonate: plasma phenylalanine and tyrosine elevated above normal but both reduced by administration of ascorbic acid (25 mg/day × 3 days)

Genetics. The available evidence shows conclusively that classical phenylketonuria is an autosomal recessive disease. In some instances both parents of an affected child can be shown to be different from the normal population with regard to phenylalanine metabolism. However, the total population of individuals with persistent hyperphenylalaninemia does not appear to be clinically homogenous, and indirect assessments by phenylalanine tolerance tests or by determinations of fasting plasma phenylalanine do not discriminate completely between phenylketonuric infants and carriers on the one hand and between carriers and normal individuals on the other.

Treatment. The evidence regarding diet therapy in phenylketonuria strongly suggests that restriction of phenylalanine intake is beneficial to some patients and also that overrestriction of dietary phenylalanine is seriously detrimental to all patients. The objective of therapy as currently practiced is to reduce plasma phenylalanine to a level that allows normal intellectual development in the patient while giving amounts of dietary phenylalanine adequate to ensure against phenylalanine deficiency.

Snyderman and Holt have established that the usual requirement for phenylalanine in the neonatal period is 60 to 80 mg/kg/day. Infants diagnosed as having treatable hyperphenylalaninemia are therefore given a low-phenylalanine formula (3 mg phenylalanine per ounce of prepared formula) together with enough cow's milk (50 mg phenylalanine per ounce) to provide 70 mg phenylalanine per kg per day. Plasma phenylalanine is monitored and dietary phenylalanine adjusted to achieve an appropriate level of phenylalanine in plasma. Most workers in this field believe that adequate growth cannot be achieved unless plasma phenylalanine is allowed to remain several mg/100 ml above the normal fasting level. Our clinic strives to maintain plasma phenylalanine at approximately 10 mg/100 ml with consistently negative reactions to ferric chloride tests in the urine.

Solid food is added at appropriate intervals, according to a diet plan such as that offered by a manufacturer of low-phenylalanine formula (for example, Mead-Johnson & Co., Evansville, Ind.).

The hazards of a treatment program for phenylketonuria cannot be overemphasized. Points of particular concern are given in the following sections.

Accuracy of diagnosis. The criteria given above are appropriate for a single point in time only. Apparent phenylalanine tolerance, as manifested by plasma phenylalanine levels, may change markedly with time. Borderline cases, not selected for treatment, should be followed closely. Those subjected to treatment should be assessed periodically for accuracy of diagnosis. For this latter purpose, we prefer a trial of unlimited phenylalanine intake to an abrupt test of phenylalanine tolerance.

Overtreatment—phenylalanine deficiency. Rouse has documented the hazards of prolonged inappropriate restriction of phenylalanine in the diet of infants not having phenylketonuria. Hanley and coworkers suggested that their rather disappointing results in dietary treatment may have been, in part, the result of unrecognized phenylalanine deficiency. In young infants, both phenylalanine requirement and phenylalanine intake may fluctuate widely over brief periods of time under ideal conditions. Stress, such as infection, accentuates such fluctuations. It is therefore necessary to monitor plasma phenylalanine at very frequent intervals. The following schedule is suggested.

0 to 6 months: 2× weekly
6 months to 1 year: 1× weekly
1 year to 18 months: 2× monthly
18 months until cessation of therapy: 1× monthly

*When plasma phenylalanine is greater than 15 mg/100 ml but less than 20 mg/100 ml, it is advisable to reduce protein intake to 1.5 to 2.0 gm/kg/day in order to reduce plasma phenylalanine to levels allowing relatively infrequent determinations of plasma phenylalanine.

The analyses must be promptly done, and the results promptly applied to management.

Growth. Data on the growth pattern of treated phenylketonuric infants is scanty. However, it appears that many appropriately treated patients do not grow normally. The distinction between impairment of growth caused by phenylalanine deficiency and that caused by the effects of a largely synthetic diet is sometimes difficult to make.

Tyrosinosis, acute tyrosinosis, chronic tyrosinemia, and hypermethioninemia

Tyrosinosis. Tyrosinosis is a very rare entity in which plasma tyrosine is strikingly elevated and in which there is marked tyrosyluria without clinical manifestations clearly referable to disordered metabolism. In one case impairment in the transamination of tyrosine was demonstrated (Fig. 14-1).

Acute tyrosinosis, chronic tyrosinemia, and hypermethioninemia. These terms are applied to a heterogeneous group of disorders in which it now seems likely that no primary defect in tyrosine or methionine metabolism exists. The clinical manifestations are predominantly those of acute and chronic liver disease, renal tubular disorders, and impairment of central nervous system development.

Etiology and pathogenesis. A number of infants seen within the first year of life, primarily with manifestations of severe hepatic dysfunction, have been shown to have striking elevations of plasma tyrosine or methionine or both. Enzymatic deficiencies in the metabolic pathways for these amino acids have been clearly documented in these infants. However, in some instances the condition has proved to be self-limited and the clinical course compatible with neonatal hepatitis. On the other hand, some of these infants have shown only partial recovery, with persistence of low-grade liver disease and disorders of renal tubular function, associated with chronic elevation of plasma tyrosine. Familial incidence compatible with autosomal recessive inheritance has been documented in the latter group. Cases of chronic disease have been reported in which acute disease was never present. Since hereditary fructose intolerance has also been shown to produce the clinical and laboratory findings of acute tyrosinosis, it is entirely possible that a genotype having no primary effect on the metabolism of tyrosine can produce the manifestations of acute tyrosinosis and chronic tyrosinemia.

Clinical manifestations. The manifestations of this syndrome in the neonatal period are largely those of acute hepatic dysfunction. Listlessness, vomiting, diarrhea, abdominal enlargement with hepatomegaly, splenomegaly, and the development of ascites are prominent clinical features. Bleeding disorders are common, and coma may evolve in the course of this disorder. Mortality is high in the neonatal period.

It is readily apparent that the manifestations described above are similar to those of hereditary fructose intolerance, galactosemia, and neonatal septicemia, all of which enter into the differential diagnosis of this condition.

Laboratory manifestations. Moderate to striking elevations of plasma tyrosine or methionine or both are present. In acute tyrosinosis, tyrosyluria is a constant finding. Hyperphenylalaninemia and elevation of other plasma amino acids may be seen. Hypoglycemia, hypophosphatemia, and galactosuria have been noted. The results of usual tests of hepatic function are grossly abnormal. Anemia, thrombocytopenia, and leukopenia are common.

Treatment. Some patients with acute tyrosinosis have responded favorably to a diet restricted in tyrosine and phenylalanine. Plasma levels of tyrosine have predictably fallen under this treatment, but clinical response has been less uniform. It seems likely that the amount and type of carbohydrate in the diet is as important as the amino acid composition, but studies to date do not allow a clear recommendation as to carbohydrate feeding. Given the mortality of the condition, it is probably wise both to employ low-phenylalanine, low-tyrosine feedings and to alter the carbohydrate source for affected infants (for example, from sucrose to lactose or from lactose to sucrose).

Prognosis. The disorder may be fatal early, enter a chronic phase, or remit completely, the result probably dependent upon both cause and management.

Genetics. As indicated earlier, a genetic basis for some forms of this disorder has been clearly established.

Alcaptonuria

Alcaptonuria, a disorder of the oxidation of homogentisic acid (Fig. 14-1), leads to the excretion of large amounts of homogentisic acid in the urine. The only manifestation of the disorder in the neonatal period is the darkening of diapers on standing. This reaction is the basis for the diagnostic test in which sodium hydroxide is added to freshly voided urine or dropped onto a freshly wet diaper. The production of a blackish brown color is almost immediate and is virtually diagnostic of alcaptonuria. Plasma tyrosine and phenylalanine are normal in alcaptonuria.

While a low-phenylalanine, low-tyrosine diet has been recommended in this condition in order to prevent the deposition of melaninlike by-products in joint cartilage, there is little justification for the imposition of such an abnormal diet in children with this disorder.

Alcaptonuria is inherited as an autosomal recessive disease.

Homocystinuria

Homocystinuria is a disorder of the metabolism of sulphur-containing amino acids that is associated with a progressive clinical syndrome involving the lens of the eye, the skin, and the blood vessels.

Etiology and pathogenesis. The fundamental defect in homocystinuria is marked reduction of activity of cystathionine synthetase. This defect leads to the accumulation in blood and urine of homocystine and, to a variable extent, of methionine. The synthesis of cystine is also impaired.

There is evidence to suggest that homocysteic acid derived from homocystine in this disorder is a causative factor in the development of the fibrous vascular lesions seen in this disorder and that homocystine itself by activating Hageman factor is directly involved in the production of thromboses. It has been suggested that faulty development of the suspensory ligaments of the lens is related to disordered homocystine metabolism. The cause of the intellectual impairment seen variably in these patients and of the psychiatric difficulties noted in families with homocystinuria is as yet unknown. The extent to which these phenomena are related to vascular thrombosis is as yet undetermined.

Clinical manifestations. Infants with homocystinuria are normal at birth and remain so throughout the neonatal period. The clinical manifestations of homocystinuria are those of a progressive disorder; the most characteristic manifestation is ectopia lentis, which commonly appears between 2½ and 3½ years of age. Many affected individuals develop constitutional features of Marfan's syndrome, malar flush, and livedo reticularis of the lower extremities. Roughly half of the patients have intellectual deficits. Thrombotic episodes involving both small and large veins and arteries are a constant threat to the older cystinuric individual.

The characteristic laboratory manifestation of homocystinuria is the presence of homocystine in the urine. This substance can be readily detected by the cyanide nitroprusside test for compounds containing -SS or -SH groups. Confirmation of the diagnosis is best obtained by column chromotography of amino acids from plasma or urine. The amount of free homocystine in homocystinuric plasma is relatively small. Since homocystine reacts readily with plasma protein, the diagnosis can be missed if plasma samples are allowed to stand for long periods of time prior to analysis.

Treatment. Dietary treatment of homocystinuric infants from birth has been recommended strongly by several authors. A few cases so treated have been clinically normal on follow-up for several years. The interpretation of these results is complicated by the variability in progression of this disorder. While no clinically normal adults with homocystinuria have been observed, the degree of clinical involvement in the first few years of life shows substantial variation. Several modes of therapy are available. A significant number of homocystinuric infants have shown reversion of their biochemical abnormalities when treated with large doses of pyridoxine. While this would seem to be the ideal therapy for the affected neonate, there is inadequate information as to its safety. Various regimes also have been suggested for supplementing the diet with cystine or cystathionine or both and for reducing the requirement for cystathionine synthesis by reducing dietary methionine. These have been discussed at length by Gerittsen and Waisman.

Genetics. Homocystinuria is inherited as an autosomal recessive disorder.

Nonketotic hyperglycinemia

Nonketotic hyperglycinemia is a familial disorder of glycine metabolism in which profound dysfunction of the nervous system is noted shortly after birth. Roughly a third of the reported patients have died within the first 2 weeks of life, and the remainder have exhibited severe motor and mental retardation.

Etiology and pathogenesis. Of the many pathways of glycine metabolism noted in Fig. 14-2, only glycine cleavage is known to be affected in nonketotic hyperglycinemia, and this appears to be the primary phenomenon in the pathogenesis of this disorder. The mechanism through which the profound clinical effects of the disease are produced is unknown. Elevation in plasma glycine is not known to be harmful in itself. Although a disturbance in glycine cleavage could lead to reduced levels of serine and hence to impaired gluconeogenesis, neither low plasma serine nor hypoglycemia has been noted in this disorder. Reduction in the one carbon pool through reduced synthesis of methyl tetrahydrofolic acid might be operative in producing the clinical disease, but there is at present no evidence to suggest that this is the case. Plasma levels of methionine are normal in patients with this disorder.

Clinical manifestations. Almost all patients with this disorder show serious abnormalities within the first few days of life. Poor feeding, lethargy, and hypotonia progressing to coma and apnea have been noted regularly. Seizures, both myoclonic and generalized, have also been seen. Physical examination reveals lack of responsiveness, hypotonia, and diminished Moro and deep tendon reflexes.

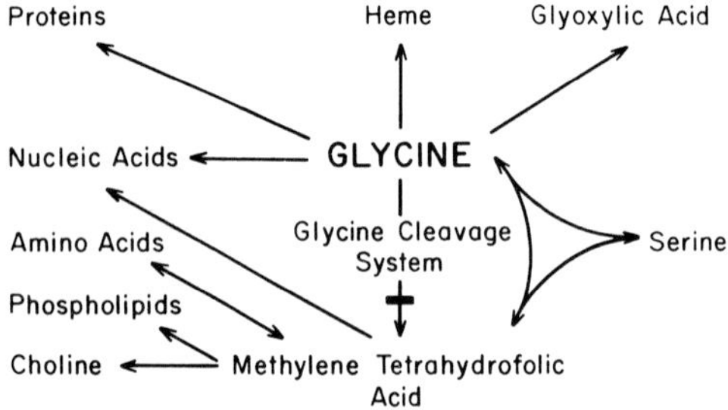

Fig. 14-2. Schematic representation of the metabolism of glycine. Crossbar indicates the metabolic block in nonketotic hyperglycinemia.

Laboratory findings. The only consistent laboratory findings are elevation of plasma glycine (two- to twenty-fold) together with increased urinary glycine. Ketosis is notably absent. Respiratory acidosis has been prominent in severely affected patients. Although two patients showed lower than expected plasma bicarbonate levels in the presence of elevated Pco_2, no metabolic component of their acidosis was identified.

Treatment. No form of treatment has been effective in this disorder. Dietary control of plasma glycine has been achieved in some patients. In addition, both methionine and sodium benzoate, administered orally, have been shown to reduce plasma glycine in affected subjects.

Genetics. Data available from the limited number of patients reported strongly supports an autosomal recessive inheritance of the disease.

Histidinemia

Histidinemia is a disorder of the catabolism of histidine caused by lack of histidase activity. It is characterized by the excretion of imidazolepyruvic acid, which gives positive reactions to ferric chloride and 2,4-dinitrophenylhydrazine tests on urine samples, similar to the reactions obtained in phenylketonuria. Plasma histidine is generally four to ten times normal.

While there may be considerable genetic heterogeneity in histidinemia, there is no clear evidence at present that it is a harmful condition. There are no neonatal manifestations other than the laboratory findings noted above. Although dietary therapy has been proposed for affected neonates, it cannot be recommended at this time.

Disorders of the urea cycle

The disorders of the urea cycle (Fig. 14-3) form a more or less homogeneous entity whose predominant manifestation is clinical hyperammonemia—periodic vomiting with lethargy progressing to coma. When any of these disorders appears symptomatically within the neonatal period, it is very likely that the defect is lethal and that central nervous dysfunction will be progressive and unresponsive to therapy.

Etiology and pathogenesis. Since urea is the principal form in which ammonia nitrogen is fixed for excretion, it is readily apparent that a serious impairment of urea synthesis could lead to an accumulation in tissue of free and highly toxic ammonia. However, most of the patients with disorders of the urea cycle have been found to produce normal amounts of urea in spite of lowered activities of one or more of the urea cycle enzymes. Therefore, the precise mechanism by which hyperammonemia is produced is as yet unknown. It is presumed that surviving patients have deficient but not absent activity of the affected enzymes and that reduction in activity to the point of effective absence is highly lethal, leading to death in utero or early in the neonatal period. This latter form of these disorders has been termed malignant hyperammonemia.

Clinical manifestations. The onset of clinical disease may occur soon after birth, with seizures and intractable coma. Respiratory symptoms are common, and death usually occurs within the first 10 days to 2 weeks. Terminal massive pulmonary hemorrhage has been noted. In other patients the onset of symptoms has been related to increasing protein intake. Vomiting, with the development of lethargy even to the point of coma, followed by remission as protein intake decreases, is the usual clinical picture.

Since all of the disorders of the urea cycle produce similar clinical manifestations in older patients, it may be presumed that each of these, given a sufficiently marked reduction in enzyme activity, is capable of producing the malignant neonatal form of the disorder. To date four of these disorders have been recognized in the neonatal period. There are no specific physical findings other than the *trichorrexis nodosa* seen in patients with argininosuccinicaciduria.

Laboratory findings. The cardinal laboratory finding is elevation of postprandial blood ammonia, usually to levels in excess of 300 μg/100 ml of whole blood. Specific diagnosis requires laboratory differentiation of the disease entities that produce hyperammonemia. When liver tissue is required for diagnosis, it is suggested that percutaneous needle biopsy be employed, since operative biopsy has been followed by lethal crises in two patients.

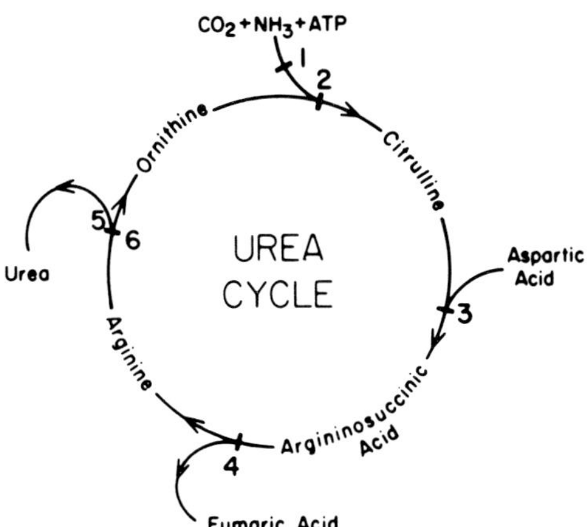

Fig. 14-3. Numbers denote enzymes whose function is impaired in the various errors of urea synthesis: *1*, carbamyl phosphate synthetase; *2*, ornithine carbamyl transferase; *3*, argininosuccinic acid synthetase; *4*, argininosuccinic acid lyase; *5*, arginase, primary defect; and *6*, arginase, secondary defect caused by elevated levels of lysine.

Carbamylphosphate synthetase deficiency (Fig. 14-3). Three patients with deficiency of carbamylphosphate synthetase and apparently adequate activity of other urea cycle enzymes have been reported. One of these had a complex disorder without documented hyperammonemia, while another had clinical and chemical ammonia intoxication within the neonatal period. The latter patient had in addition hyperglycinemia, intermittent neutropenia, and ketoacidosis. Since a sibling had a similar clinical illness, it is presumed that the disorder was inherited. The diagnosis is made by enzyme assay of liver tissue.

Sex-linked hyperammonemia: ornithine carbamyltransferase deficiency (Fig. 14-3). Ornithine carbamyltransferase deficiency is unique among these disorders in that all evidence to date suggests sex-linked inheritance. The majority of patients recognized thus far have been females, with reduced but not absent enzyme activity. Mother-to-daughter transmission has been demonstrated. Affected males have shown either a variant enzyme or absence of enzyme activity. Absence of enzyme activity is lethal within the first week of life in affected males.

Surviving patients with ornithine carbamyltransferase deficiency generally show elevations in plasma and urinary glutamine and alanine. Some have excreted large amounts of orotic acid, apparently synthesized in response to diminished utilization of carbamylphosphate for citrulline synthesis. Diagnosis is made by enzyme assay of liver tissue.

Citrullinemia (Fig. 14-3). One patient with citrullinemia has been recognized in the neonatal period. She was normal for the first 3 days of life, then showed hypertonia, seizures, and progressive diminution in consciousness. Death occurred on the seventh day of life. Diagnosis may be made by analysis of plasma and urinary amino acids, with or without enzyme assay.

Argininosuccinicaciduria (Fig. 14-3). Unique among these disorders is the peculiarly friable hair seen even within the neonatal period in infants with argininosuccinicaciduria. Inheritance in argininosuccinicaciduria appears to be of the autosomal recessive type. Definitive diagnosis may be established by finding large amounts of argininosuccinic acid in the urine or by enzyme assay.

Arginase deficiency (Fig. 14-3). Arginase deficiency has only recently been recognized. There has been no known instance of neonatal presentation. Diagnosis is made by enzyme assay.

Lysine intolerance with hyperammonemia (Fig. 14-2). A single instance of this disorder has been recorded, without neonatal manifestations. It is postulated in this disease that an impairment in lysine catabolism results in elevated tissue levels of lysine that competitively inhibit the hydrolysis of arginine by arginase.

Treatment. The treatment of choice for disorders of the urea cycle is reduction of dietary protein to the lowest level compatible with acceptable growth. While the usual allowance of dietary protein for optimal growth in the newborn infant is approximately 2.5 gm/kg/day, infants with disorders of nitrogen catabolism may do well on much less dietary protein. Therefore, it is best to begin by eliminating protein from the diet to obtain the optimal neurologic state, then add protein in increments of 0.25 to 0.5 gm/kg/day until the best balance between neurologic state and growth is achieved. These increases should not be made more frequently than every fourth day.

In infants whose metabolic defect reduces the synthesis of arginine, arginine (or citrulline if citrulline synthesis is impaired) should be added to the diet. No clear recommendation as to dosage can be made, but 0.5 mol/kg/day is suggested as a starting point. Citrulline can be given as the neutral amino acid, while arginine must be administered as the acid salt (for example, arginine hydrochloride). It is preferable to employ the salt of a metabolizable organic acid. If the acid hydrochloride is administered, it should be given with equimolar amounts of sodium bicarbonate.

Prognosis. Prognosis is related, in part, to age at onset of symptoms; infants with late onset of symptoms have a better outlook. The prognosis concerning intellectual development must be guarded.

DISORDERS OF THE METABOLISM OF ORGANIC ACIDS

In disorders of the metabolism of organic acids, failure of catabolism of one or more organic acids results in their excretion in the urine. Since the organic acids are strongly acidic (in contrast to the amino acids), a large burden is imposed on the renal buffering system. As a result, the organic acidurias are characterized by metabolic acidosis, which can be manifest constantly or occur intermittently in a series of recurrent crises (Fig. 14-4).

Maple syrup urine disease

Maple syrup urine disease, or branched chain aminoaciduria, is the result of an impairment in the decarboxylation of the keto acid derivatives of the three branched chain amino acids: leucine, isoleucine, and valine. Profound depression of the central nervous system and death early in life occur in the vast majority of untreated patients.

Etiology and pathogenesis. The transamination of the branched chain amino acids occurs normally in maple syrup urine dis-

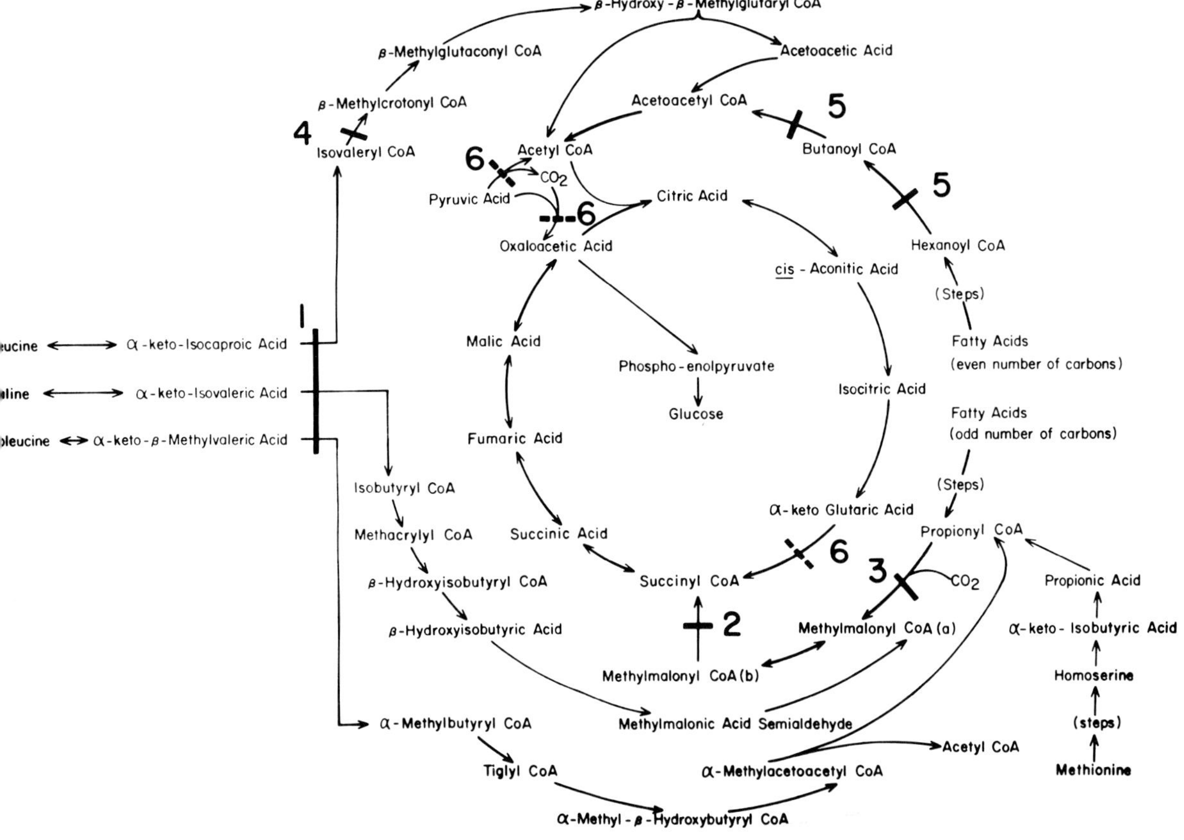

Fig. 14-4. Schematic diagram of the metabolism of organic acids. Solid bars denote metabolic blocks for which convincing evidence exists. Broken bars indicate postulated metabolic blocks. *1,* Maple syrup urine disease; *2,* methylmalonic acidemia; *3,* propionic acidemia, ketotic hyperglycinemia; *4,* isovaleric acidemia; *5,* hexanoic/butanoic aciduria; and *6,* congenital lactic acidosis.

ease, but the keto acids produced by transamination are not oxidized normally. Since the transamination reaction is freely reversible, accumulation of these keto acids leads to a corresponding increase in the levels of the branched chain amino acids. The clinical manifestations of the disease are correlated with elevations in plasma leucine and α-ketoisocaproic acid, but not with accumulations of isoleucine, valine, and their keto acid analogues. The metabolic acidosis observed in this disease is only in part explained by the excretory load of organic acid. The mechanism by which the profound disturbance of the central nervous system is produced remains unknown. On postmortem examination the brains of affected infants exhibit defective myelination and spongy degeneration of the white matter. Although hypoglycemia and excessive glycogen deposition in the liver have been noted in these patients, presumably as a result of excessive stimulation of insulin release by leucine, the central nervous system manifestations cannot be explained solely on the basis of hypoglycemia.

Clinical manifestations. Affected infants appear normal at birth. The onset of clinical manifestations generally occurs very early, most patients exhibiting profound illness within the first week. Initially there may be rapid, shallow respirations, followed shortly by profound alteration in consciousness. The affected infant appears apathetic and characteristically develops alternating hypertonia and hypotonia, accompanied by brief tonic seizures. The odor of maple syrup is usually detected at the time of clinical illness, but has occasionally not been noted in fatally affected infants. The untreated disease is rapidly progressive, death occurring within the neonatal period generally from respiratory failure, with or without complicating bronchopneumonia.

Laboratory manifestations. The presence of α-keto organic acids in the urine, as detected by the 2,4-dinitrophenylhydrazine test, is characteristic of the untreated disease and strongly suggests the diagnosis in infants whose clinical presentation is compatible with the disorder. The diagnosis is confirmed by finding striking elevations of leucine, isoleucine, and valine levels in plasma. These amino acids are also excreted in the urine in abnormal amounts. Alloisoleucine, an enantiomer of isoleucine, is also present in plasma. This amino acid was erroneously identified as methionine in early descriptions of the disorder.

Metabolic acidosis is probably characteristic of the untreated disease, though most reports do not emphasize this aspect of maple syrup urine disease.

Hypoglycemia usually occurs.

Treatment. Restriction of dietary leucine, isoleucine, and valine has been employed with some degree of success. Dietary treatment requires frequent monitoring of plasma leucine, isoleucine, and valine in order to provide sufficient amounts of these essential amino acids for growth and development while avoiding the severely deleterious effects of excessive administration. Crises with central nervous system dysfunction and metabolic acidosis are associated not only with dietary indiscretion, but also with infections and other forms of stress. Dietary therapy must be continued for life.

Crises have been treated successfully by peritoneal dialysis. This therapy has also been suggested for neonates who have become severely affected prior to the institution of dietary therapy.

A thiamine-responsive form of the disease has been described.

Prognosis. Even with early institution of therapy the prognosis for both life and normal intellectual development must be guarded. An intermittent form of the disease has been reported in which typical crises occur in children who are otherwise clinically normal. The metabolic defect appears to be similar to, but less severe than, that found in the classic form of the disease. The relationship of the intermittent variety to clinical disease in the neonate has not been elucidated.

Genetics. The disease shows autosomal recessive inheritance.

Propionic acidemia, ketotic hyperglycinemia, methylmalonic acidemia

Proprionic acidema, ketotic hyperglycinemia, and methylmalonic acidemia result from impairment of the metabolism of propionic acid. Clinical disease in the neonatal period is common.

Etiology and pathogenesis. Propionic acid normally undergoes a series of reactions resulting in the synthesis of succinic acid and allowing its ultimate participation in the tricarboxylic acid cycle (Figs. 14-4 and 14-5). As shown in Fig. 14-5, the initial reactions require two enzymes and two cofactors, coenzyme A and biotin, and result in the formation of methylmalonyl CoA. Isomerization of methylmalonyl CoA yields succinyl CoA. Since this pathway is employed for the catabolism of ketogenic amino acids, its integrity is of considerable metabolic importance. In both propionic acidemia and ketotic hyperglycinemia, marked reductions in the activity of propionyl carboxylase have been demonstrated. Two varieties of methylmalonic acidemia have been documented, one in which activity of methylmalonyl CoA mutase is reduced, and another in which there is impairment in the synthesis of the active vitamin B_{12} cofactor. A third disorder has been proposed recently in which isomerization of methylanalonyl CoA is impaired. Differences among these disorders have been noted. The level of propionic acid in plasma and urine in ketotic hyperglycinemia, while elevated, is of an order of magnitude less than that seen in proprionic acidemia. The administration of leucine precipitates ketosis in ketotic hyperglycinemia but not in methylmalonic acidemia. Excessive methylmalonic acid is not produced in either propionic acidemia or ketoic hyperglycinemia. However, similarities far outnumber the differences. Patients with any

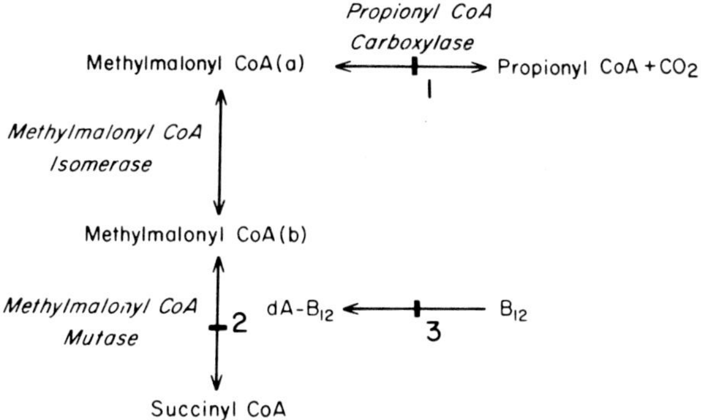

FIG. 14-5. Metabolism of propionyl CoA, with proved inborn errors indicated by crossbars. *1,* Propionic acidemia, ketotic hyperglycinemia; *2,* B_{12}-resistant methylmalonic acidemia; and *3,* B_{12}-sensitive methylmalonic acidemia.

of these disorders are intolerant of methionine, isoleucine, valine, and threonine. Ketoacidosis occurs as a prominent feature of each, as does the excretion of unusual, long-chained ketones. Intermittent neutropenia is a feature of each, as is hyperglycinemia. Hyperammonemia may be noted in early infancy in these patients.

Clinical manifestations. Lethargy and vomiting within the first week of life have been described in a number of affected infants. Hyperpnea, caused by metabolic acidosis, has been the initial sign in others. When the disease manifests itself within the neonatal period, progressive depression of consciousness, ultimately ending in coma and death, has been common. There is generally profound hypotonia. Seizures are not characteristic of these disorders.

In some infants the onset has been more gradual, manifestations including failure to thrive, recurrent ketoacidosis, and the periodic vomiting and lethargy characteristic of hyperammonemia in early life.

Laboratory findings. The most prominent laboratory finding is profound metabolic acidosis, with elevation of plasma undetermined anions. Ketoacidosis occurs even in the neonatal period. In a few patients the dominant laboratory finding has been hyperammonemia. Hyperglycinemia is the most constant abnormality of plasma amino acids, but, during crises, elevation of other plasma amino acids, particularly the branched chain amino acids, is regularly noted. While determination of the levels of methylmalonic acid and of propionic acid in plasma and urine serves to categorize patients, diagnosis ultimately rests upon determination of the specific enzyme defect in white blood cells or liver.

Intermittent neutropenia and thrombocytopenia have been described repeatedly in these patients. Hypoglycemia has been observed on occasion.

Treatment. Restriction of protein intake to the least amount compatible with normal growth and development is indicated in these patients. In some instances specific restriction of isoleucine, valine, threonine, and methionine (leucine also, in ketotic hyperglycinemia) may be efficacious. (See disorders of the urea cycle, p. 414.)

In methylmalonic acidemia caused by failure of synthesis of active vitamin B_{12}, the administration of massive doses of vitamin B_{12} may cause resolution of the clinical manifestations. Therapeutically significant responses to other cofactors have not been reported.

Prognosis. In general, patients with these disorders do poorly, even under optimal medical management. Death during an exacerbation of the disease is common, and survivors generally show some intellectual impairment. A few patients have responded well to diets restricted in protein.

Genetics. The limited data available strongly favor an autosomal recessive mode of inheritance.

Congenital lactic acidosis

Lactic acidosis results from tissue hypoxia and as a complication of apparently unrelated disorders affecting metabolism. There are also syndromes in infancy in which lactic acidosis is the dominant feature.

The metabolic fate of lactate is essentially that of pyruvate. If either the thiamine-dependent decarboxylation or the biotin-dependent carboxylation of pyruvate were impaired, it would be expected that both alanine and lactate, with which pyruvate is in equilibrium, would accumulate in tissues (Fig. 14-4).

While the etiologic possibilities for congenital lactic acidosis seem to be limited to the enzymes and cofactors involved in the two primary reactions of pyruvic acid, it must be kept in mind that pyruvic acid can be overproduced by excessive glycolysis as in type I glycogenosis. In addition, both the decarboxylation and carboxylation of pyruvate are largely mitochondrial functions and therefore require the maintenance of a normal mitochondrial environment.

No comprehensive biochemical explanation of the congenital lactic acidoses is available. Congenital lactic acidosis can appear in the neonatal period, and the disorders involved can be divided as follows.

Hypoglycemic congenital lactic acidosis

Fructose-1-6-diphosphatase deficiency. Fructose-1-6-diphosphatase catalyzes a critical step in the reversal of the glycolytic pathway. Deficiency of the enzyme is associated not only with hypoglycemia but also with overproduction of pyruvic and lactic acids and alanine.

Clinical manifestations. Limited information on the neonatal presentation suggests that hyperpnea, poor feeding, vomiting, and depression of the central nervous system predominate as manifestations. The liver is characteristically enlarged.

Laboratory findings. In addition to lactic acidosis and hypoglycemia, there is characteristically ketosis. The liver shows fatty infiltration and may, in addition, have increased glycogen. Fructose-1-6-diphosphatase activity in the liver is markedly reduced or absent.

Treatment. Correction of lactic acidosis should be carried out as indicated for normoglycemic congenital lactic acidosis. Correction of hypoglycemia by glucose infusion is indicated. Restricted dietary protein and avoidance of fructose are probably wise, though unproved. In older children with fructose-1-6-diphosphatase deficiency, folic acid therapy has been reported to increase enzyme activity and ameliorate symptoms.

Prognosis. For infants with neonatal disease, the prognosis must be guarded.

Genetics. Autosomal recessive inheritance is probable.

Low Km-pyruvate carboxylase deficiency. A single infant with this disorder has been described. Neonatal manifestations included hypoglycemic seizures and metabolic acidosis with elevations in plasma lactate, pyruvate, and alanine. The acidosis responded dramatically to therapeutic doses of thiamine HCl, presumably through enhancement of the decarboxylation of pyruvate.

Normoglycemic congenital lactic acidosis

Normoglycemic congenital lactic acidosis is a syndrome that includes chronic, exacerbating, and remitting lactic acidosis, profound depression of the central nervous system, and seizures, which may be tetanic in type.

Etiology and pathogenesis. Some patients with congenital lactic acidosis fall into a spectrum that includes Leigh's disease, a progressive encephalopathy whose pathologic anatomy is similar to that seen in experimental thiamine deficiency. Efforts have therefore been made to identify a deficiency of pyruvate decarboxylation in these disorders. While there is substantial indirect evidence to support this concept, analysis of enzymatic activities in a single patient with Leigh's disease showed deficient total pyruvate carboxylase activity and normal decarboxylase activity.

Clinical manifestations. The most sriking clinical manifestation is hyperpnea. Most affected infants have been somewhat obese and profoundly hypotonic, but a few have been cachetic and hypertonic. Seizures that appear to be tetanic are common. The infant appears unaware of his surroundings even when the acidosis has been corrected, and lack of vision has been noted frequently. Episodes of severe acidosis tend to appear without known precipitating cause, last several days, and subside spontaneously.

Laboratory findings. Lactic and pyruvic

acids are generally increased in plasma to some extent at all times, marked elevations occurring during acidotic crises. The levels of other organic acids, particularly ketoglutaric and citric acids, have been variable in both plasma and urine. While the acidosis is characteristically a pure metabolic acidosis, a respiratory component is sometimes seen, thought to be related to spasm of the upper airway caused by alteration in plasma ionized calcium and magnesium. Plasma alanine may be modestly elevated. Hypoglycemia does not occur.

Treatment. Very large amounts of sodium bicarbonate may be required to control acidosis (20 mEq/kg/day). Methylene blue has been used to increase the ratio of pyruvic acid to lactic acid, thus increasing renal organic acid clearance. Therapy with sodium lactate is obviously contraindicated. Transfusions with blood containing citrate have been followed by exacerbations of the acidosis.

Cofactor therapy (lipoic acid 0.7 mg, thiamine 60 mg, and pantothenic acid 30 mg, given intramuscularly three times weekly) has been also suggested in this disorder. Biotin (1.0 mg administered intramuscularly) has been used in a single patient, without proved effect. Thiamine derivatives have appeared to be superior to thiamine itself in the therapy of Leigh's disease.

Prognosis. Even though patients with normoglycemic congenital lactic acidosis form an apparently heterogeneous group, the prognosis for almost all of them is poor, most dying in infancy during acidotic crises.

Motor and mental development has generally been severely impaired during the period of survival. An occasional patient has shown progressive spontaneous improvement. Therapy has not appeared to alter the overall course of any patient.

Genetics. In families with more than one involved sibling, autosomal recessive inheritance of the disease is indicated.

Sweaty feet syndromes: hexanoic/butanoic aciduria, isovaleric acidemia (3-methyl butanoic acidemia)

Hexanoic/butanoic aciduria

Sidbury reported three infants in one sibship and a fourth unrelated infant, all of whom died in the neonatal period of intractable metabolic acidosis and septicemia. Extracts of urine from two of these patients contained large amounts of hexanoic and butanoic acids. Since these compounds could not be demonstrated in the urine of control infants, it was postulated that the acids were excreted as a result of lack of activity of the green acyl dehydrogenase, which initiates the oxidation of hexanoyl CoA and butanoyl CoA (Fig. 14-4).

All four infants smelled like sweaty feet.

Reevaluation of the frozen urine of one of these patients by more recently developed techniques indicates that the infant actually suffered from isovaleric acidemia. Since the metabolic products of the latter disease are easily confused with butanoic and hexanoic acids in the chromatographic system employed by Sidbury, the existence of hexanoic/butanoic aciduria has been questioned.

Isovaleric acidemia

Several instances of an inborn error in leucine metabolism associated with isovaleric acidemia have been reported, generally in older children. Neonatal death associated with intractable isovaleric acidosis, seizures, and respiratory failure has been reported, symptoms beginning on the second day of life. Affected individuals have the cheesy or sweaty feet odor characteristic of short chain fatty acids.

Failure of oxidation of isovaleric acid (Fig. 14-4), a metabolite in the pathway for leucine catabolism, has been demonstrated in older patients with this disorder.

In addition to measures directed toward correction of the metabolic acidosis, a diet low in protein or specifically restricted in leucine content seems to be indicated.

Succinyl-CoA: 3-ketoacid CoA-transferase deficiency

A single infant with this enzyme deficiency and ketoacidosis in early neonatal life has been reported. The infant died at 6½ months of age in spite of vigorous management.

Beta-methyl crotonylglycinuria

Two instances of this disorder have been described, both associated with disease in early life. One patient had clinical Werdnig-Hoffman disease, perhaps unrelated to the otherwise subclinical aciduria. The other patient had striking metabolic acidosis, dramatically responsive to biotin therapy.

DISORDERS OF MONOSACCHARIDE METABOLISM

Neonatal diabetes mellitus

Carbohydrate intolerance to an extent requiring insulin therapy has been noted with some frequency in the neonatal period. The disorder may be temporary or permanent.

Etiology and pathogenesis. As in the case of diabetes in later life, the cause of diabetes mellitus in the neonate is unknown. No consistent abnormalities of pancreatic tissue have been noted in autopsy material from infants with this disorder. Plasma insulin levels have not shown a consistent pattern in the few subjects in whom these measurements have been made.

There is some association between the development of diabetes mellitus in the neonatal period and the following: postmaturity and low birth weight, neonatal hypoglycemia, and steroid therapy early in the neonatal period.

Clinical manifestations. The age of patients at detection of this disorder has varied from 4 to 44 days. The most prominent manifestations have been weight loss and dehydration in association with polyuria. Characteristically, the affected infant maintains a good oral intake and does not become comatose. The vast majority probably have some degree of metabolic acidosis, but severe ketonuria is not the rule.

Laboratory manifestations. In the excellent review of this disorder by Gentz and Cornblath, blood sugar was noted to range from 245 to 2,300 mg/100 ml in affected infants. Hypernatremia was common, and ketonuria was variable, but metabolic acidosis was detected in most subjects whose acid-base status was evaluated.

Treatment. All patients with this disorder require careful attention to fluid and electrolyte balance. The dose of insulin required to achieve carbohydrate homeostasis varies markedly from patient to patient and from day to day in individual patients. Except for the very severely ill infant, insulin therapy should be gradually instituted. Initially, one-half unit of regular insulin per kg of body weight should be administered, and the blood sugar monitored for 12 hours in order to assess the insulin sensitivity of the patient. It is not always possible to establish a regime of management that employs a single injection of insulin each day. For many patients coverage with regular insulin on the basis of degree of glycosuria is optimal management for the first several months of life. Dietary allowances of protein and carbohydrate should be liberal. Since the risk of insulin-induced hypoglycemia with secondary brain damage is high in the early months of life, it is best not to attempt to achieve aglycosuria.

Prognosis. Gentz and Cornblath found that 30 of 50 patients with neonatal diabetes had temporary disorders requiring treatment for a mean period of 65 days. For those neonates with permanent diabetes there is no indication that prognosis is worse than it is for individuals who develop diabetes later in life.

Genetics. There is a relatively high incidence of diabetes mellitus in the families of affected infants, but no clearly definable inheritance pattern for the disorder.

Disorders of galactose metabolism

Galactokinase deficiency

Deficient activity of galactokinase results in disordered metabolism of galactose and in the development of cataracts.

Etiology and pathogenesis. The initial step in the metabolism of dietary galactose is the phosphorylation of galactose, a reaction catalyzed by galactokinase. When this reaction is impaired, ingested galactose is either excreted in the urine or metabolized by unusual pathways. Marked reduction in activity of galactokinase thus results in postprandial galactosuria and in the production of galactitol by enzymatic reduction of galactose. There is substantial evidence to suggest that galactitol, acting as a nondiffusible osmotic agent within the lens of the eye, causes swelling of the lens fibers and ultimate distortion of the architecture of the lens. In addition, the reduction of galactose to galactitol drains the lens of compounds that are able to act as hydrogen donors in the stabilization of sulfhydryl-containing proteins. The instability of affected proteins, coupled with the osmotic effects of galactose, ultimately leads to cataract formation.

Clinical manifestations. In individuals homozygous for galactokinase deficiency, cataract formation occurs early in life and has been noted within the neonatal period. Cataract formation in the third and fourth decades of life has been reported in individuals apparently heterozygous for this disorder. Dysfunction of liver and kidney are not seen in galactokinase deficiency, nor is hypoglucosemia produced by galactose ingestion.

Laboratory findings. The diagnosis is established by demonstration of reduction of activity of galactokinase in red blood cells. Measurement of galactose in blood and urine in the postprandial state can be employed as a screening procedure. Increased urinary galactitol is a more constant finding in this disorder than is either galactosuria or galactosemia.

Treatment. Elimination of galactose from the diet is the treatment of choice. Resorption of cataracts has been reported in some individuals so treated. It appears that galactose restriction should be lifelong in this disorder.

Prognosis. The prognosis for general health is excellent, the only morbidity associated with this condition being visual impairment caused by cataracts.

Galactosemia

Galactosemia is a hereditary disorder of the metabolism of galactose-1-phosphate that is analogous to hereditary fructose intolerance, in which manifestations of renal disease and liver dysfunction follow the ingestion of galactose. Cataracts and some degree of mental retardation are also features of galactosemia.

Etiology and pathogenesis. The biochemical lesion in galactosemia is lack of activity of galactose-1-phosphate uridyltransferase. This impairment of function leads to the accumulation within cells of galactose-1-phosphate; galactose accumulates both intracellularly and extracellularly. Cataract formation presumably occurs by the mechanism proposed for the development of cataracts in patients with galactokinase deficiency. The disorders of hepatic and renal function appear to be well correlated with the intracellular levels of galactose-1-phosphate. As in the case of hereditary fructose intolerance, hypoglucosemia occurs promptly upon the administration of galactose, and renal function can be shown to be impaired during the course of a galactose tolerance test. While galactose-1-phosphate is known to inhibit phosphoglucomutase in vitro, the precise mechanism by which hypoglucosemia occurs is not completely understood. The cerebral, renal, and hepatic lesions of galactosemia have not been satisfactorily explained.

Clinical manifestations. Infants with galactosemia are physically normal at birth, although their birth weights may be somewhat lower than those of unaffected siblings. Clinical manifestations may be fulminant, death occurring within the first few days of life or may be delayed until some weeks after birth. Vomiting and diarrhea, hepatosplenomegaly, and jaundice, frequently associated with anemia, are the cardinal manifestations. Renal tubular acidosis may occur. Cataracts are usually but not invariably present in the neonatal period. The clinical manifestations that occur early within the neonatal period are strikingly similar to those of neonatal septicemia, and in a number of instances the coexistence of these two entities has been demonstrated. In those infants whose disease has a more insidious onset, clinical manifestations may be predominantly those of failure to thrive associated with hepatomegaly. The major clinical risk to life is progressive liver dysfunction complicated by cirrhosis.

Laboratory findings. The diagnosis of galactosemia is made by finding absence or near absence of activity of galactose-1-phosphate uridyltransferase in red blood cell hemolysates. Some genetic variants of the disorder have been described in which the activity of the enzyme is reduced or unusually unstable. Therefore, in some instances it may be necessary to obtain clarification of the diagnosis by measurement of red blood cell galactose-1-phosphate. The normal value for RBC galactose-1-phosphate is less than 1 mg/gm of hemoglobin. Untreated galactosemia is always accompanied by marked elevation in RBC galactose-1-phosphate. This determination is also useful in monitoring dietary therapy, most clinics restricting galactose to the extent necessary to maintain RBC galactose-1-phosphate at 4 mg/gm of hemoglobin.

Measurement of blood and urinary galactose has some value in screening but cannot be depended upon to exclude the diagnosis of galactosemia in an infant who is so ill as to have little intake of galactose.

The galactose tolerance test has no place in the diagnosis of neonatal galactosemia. It is potentially dangerous and offers no advantage over the assay of RBC galactose-1-phosphate uridyltransferase and measurement of RBC galactose-1-phosphate.

Treatment. Prompt and progressive improvement follows the elimination of galactose from the affected infant's diet. Non-lactose-containing formulas, such as Nutramigen and Prosobee, may be used for this purpose. The very ill neonate may require vigorous supportive therapy, including transfusion and antibiotics for infection, in addition to elimination of dietary galactose. The appropriate duration of dietary treatment is not precisely known. It appears that the risk of severe liver and renal damage and of cataracts is limited to infancy and that tolerance for dietary galactose increases with age.

If the diagnosis of galactosemia is suspected in a very ill neonate, the proper course of action is to institute a galactose-free diet, obtaining blood for enzymatic evaluation whenever this is feasible. The elimination of galactose from the diet does not invalidate the enzyme assay, irrespective of the duration of elimination of dietary galactose.

Prognosis. The mortality for symptomatic galactosemia in the neonatal period is approximately 20%. This is thought to be related to delay in the institution of therapy but may be related, in part, to concomitant severe bacterial infection. For patients successfully treated in the neonatal period the prognosis for general health is good. Appropriate treatment is generally associated with complete resolution of the hepatic and renal lesions and occasionally even of cataracts. Cataract formation does not progress following the institution of therapy.

The relationship between dietary therapy and its time of initiation on the one hand and intellectual and psychic function on the other is not clear. There is an inverse relationship between the age at onset of therapy and intellectual achievement. However, some galactosemic infants recognized at birth and treated promptly have shown inadequate intellectual development when compared with their siblings. Furthermore, there is a high incidence of behavioral and learning disorders in the population of galactosemic infants, whether treated or untreated.

Genetics. Galactosemia is inherited as an autosomal recessive disease. Since there is considerable heterogeneity within the population of galactosemic individuals, precise genetic evaluation of the parents of the galactosemic infant is advisable.

Disorders of fructose metabolism

Deficiency of fructose kinase; essential fructosuria

Deficiency of fructose kinase, an asymptomatic disorder that results in fructosuria after the ingestion of fructose by affected subjects, is caused by an inborn deficiency in the enzymatic phosphorylation of fructose. It has no apparent clinical significance.

Hereditary fructose intolerance

Hereditary fructose intolerance is a serious disorder of carbohydrate metabolism; the ingestion of fructose produces hypoglycemia, abdominal pain, vomiting, and severe liver and kidney dysfunction.

Etiology and pathogenesis. In hereditary fructose intolerance, there is a marked decrease in the activity of fructose-1-phosphate aldolase and usually a reduction in the activity of fructose-1, 6-diphosphate aldolase. Since the two enzymatic activities are closely related chemically, it appears possible that the disorder is related to an abnormality in a single protein. In affected subjects the ratio of fructose-1-phosphate aldolase to fructose-1, 6-diphosphate aldolase is almost always found to be greater than 2.0, whereas the normal ratio of these activities is less than 2.0.

In response to fructose ingestion or infusion, patients exhibit a variable rise in blood fructose and a prompt and striking fall in blood glucose. Plasma inorganic phosphate falls, while magnesium rises somewhat. Serum glutamic oxaloacetic transaminase (SGOT) and serum glutamic pyruvic transaminase (SGPT) also rise upon the ingestion of fructose, and there is a marked increase in the excretion of amino acids.

The precise mechanism for the development of these findings is not entirely understood, though they are generally considered to be related to the impairment in the metabolism of phosphorylated hexose. The hypoglycemia does not respond to glucagon.

Clinical manifestations. Affected infants are normal at birth. Clinical manifestations occur only when the infants receive formulas containing fructose or sucrose. When such formulas are fed, vomiting, sometimes accompanied by diarrhea, promptly develops. There may be postprandial seizures. With continued ingestion of fructose, evidence of liver dysfunction appears, with hepatomegaly, jaundice of the obstructive type, and bleeding. At the same time, renal function is impaired, a substantial number of patients developing renal tubular acidosis. If fructose is not eliminated from the diet, progressive deterioration and death may occur within the neonatal period.

Affected infants who survive the early months of life develop a striking aversion to fructose.

Laboratory findings. Definitive evidence of this disorder is reduction in the level of activity of fructose-1-phosphate aldolase, together with elevation of the ratio of fructose-1-phosphate aldolase to fructose-1, 6-diphosphate aldolase in liver tissue obtained by biopsy. An alternative method of diagnosis requiring less elaborate clinical facilities is provided by the fructose tolerance test. Fructose, 0.5 gm/kg body weight, is injected intravenously over a few minutes. In the presence of hereditary fructose intolerance there is a striking reduction in blood glucose and plasma phosphate levels. If the question of hereditary fructose intolerance arises in the neonate, fructose should be eliminated from the diet as a therapeutic trial. Definitive tests may be delayed for a year or two if the fructose-free diet proves efficacious.

Elevations of plasma tyrosine and methionine have been noted in an infant with hereditary fructose intolerance.

In addition to evidence of impaired renal acidification, urinary abnormalities in hereditary fructose intolerance include generalized aminoaciduria, tyrosyluria, intermittent fructosuria, and occasionally galactosuria.

Treatment. The acute manifestations of fructose intolerance are ameliorated by the infusion of glucose. Definitive management is the elimination of fructose from the diet. Supportive measures may be necessary for acutely ill infants. In the management of these patients it is well to remember that orally administered medications sweetened with sucrose are definitely contraindicated.

Prognosis. For those patients who survive early infancy the prognosis is excellent. The vast majority of affected adults show no clinical disease but retain a rigid aversion to dietary fructose. Interestingly, dental caries are virtually absent in persons with hereditary fructose intolerance.

Genetics. In general, family histories of hereditary fructose intolerance are compatible with autosomal recessive transmission. However, the disorder appears to have shown dominant inheritance in several families.

GLYCOGENOSES

Glycogenoses (Table 14-1 and Fig. 14-6) can be made somewhat less bewildering to the clinician if the disorders are divided into three groups that reflect the clinical diseases associated with each disorder: (1) disorders that directly affect glucose homeostasis (types I, III, VI, and VIII), (2) disorders that affect primarily general hepatic function without directly involving glucose homeostasis (type IV), and (3) disorders that primarily affect neuromuscular function. For the physician caring for newborn infants a further simplification can be made by considering those disorders that can be expected to have clinical manifestations during the neonatal period. All the disorders that affect glucose homeostasis fall into this category (types I, III, VI, and VIII). Of the disorders that primarily affect neuromuscular function, only type II has neonatal manifestations. Since this disease is a disorder of lysosomal function, it is further discussed in the section on lysosomal storage disorders. In the third group, which contains only type IV,

TABLE 14-1. Glycogenoses

Cori type	Eponym	Deficient enzyme	Affected tissue
I	von Gierke	Glucose-6-phosphatase	Liver Kidney Gastrointestinal tract
II	Pompe	Acid maltase	All tissues
III	Forbes	Debrancher	Liver, HBC, WBC Muscle variably
IV	Andersen	Brancher	All tissues
V	McArdle	Muscle phosphorylase	Muscle
VI	Hers	Liver phosphorylase	Liver, WBC
VII	Tarui	Muscle phosphofructokinase	Muscle, ?RBC
VIII	Hug and Schubert	Phosphorylase kinase	Liver, WBC, all other tissues

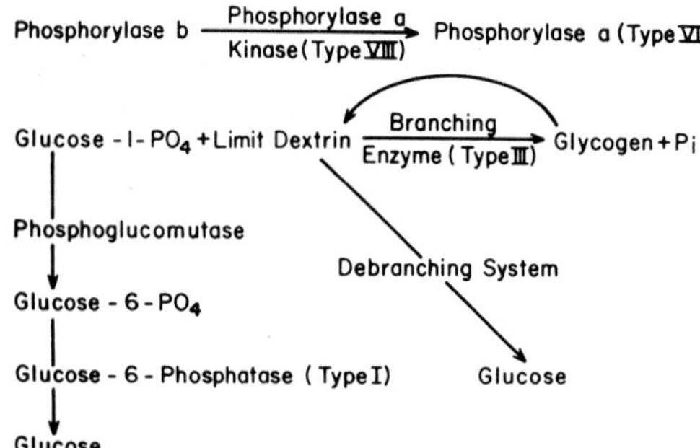

FIG. 14-6. Reactions impaired in the principal types of hepatomegalic glycogenosis. The Cori classification of the disease produced is indicated parenthetically.

there is no neonatal clinical manifestation; the disease is manifest as hepatomegaly at several months of age, followed by progressive cirrhosis, hepatic dysfunction, and death within the first few years of life.

Disorders affecting glucose homeostasis

Etiology and pathogenesis. The variation in both clinical and chemical manifestations in each of the disorders affecting glucose homeostasis is so great that only liver biopsy can definitively exclude the diagnosis. Theoretically, the enzyme deficiency in each of these disorders should affect the release of free glucose from glycogen in the liver (Fig. 14-6). In each disorder the response of blood glucose to the administration of glucagon or epinephrine (both glycogenolytic agents) may be blunted. In type III glycogenosis, which is caused by deficiency of the debrancher system, blood glucose may rise more upon administration of these agents immediately after meals than it does upon their administration after prolonged fasting. This finding is to be anticipated if prolonged fasting depletes outer chains of glycogen. The degree of fasting hypoglycemia varies somewhat with the disorder, being generally more severe in type I than in type III and more severe in type III than in types VI and VIII. Ketosis is much less prominent in type I glycogenosis than in the other types. It must be noted that these differences are only guidelines and cannot be used for positive identification of any of these disorders.

Since type I glycogenosis leads to the accumulation of glucose-6-phosphate, it is to be expected that excessive glycolysis, which results in the production of lactic acid in quantity, would be part of the chemical disorder associated with type I disease. Plasma lactate levels in glucose-6-phosphatase deficiency are generally elevated, and symptomatic lactic acidosis occurs with some regularity. The other types of glycogenosis are less prone to lactic acid accumulation. Similarly, elevations in the levels of plasma uric acid, associated with elevated levels of plasma lactic acid, are more common in type I disease but are not confined to it.

Clinical manifestations. The most prominent clinical feature of these forms of glycogenosis is hepatomegaly. In the neonatal period splenomegaly is not present. Affected infants may have no symptoms, but feeding difficulties and vomiting have been noted, accompanied less commonly by hypoglycemic seizures. Jaundice has occurred with some frequency. Ketoacidosis within the neonatal period has been reported.

Laboratory findings. Hypoglycemia, frequently asymptomatic, with failure of a normal response to glucagon and epinephrine, is often found in these disorders. Ketosis, hyperlipidemia, and elevation of plasma lactic acid may also be noted.

In general, the glycogen content of RBC is normal in type I glycogenosis and elevated in types III, VI, and VIII. In type III, RBC glycogen is excessively branched, reflecting the debranching deficiency.

Definitive diagnosis rests upon the demonstration of the particular enzyme defect involved in the disorder. All cases should be evaluated for each of the enzymes, both for assessment of prognosis and for genetic counselling. The enzyme deficiency in type III can be demonstrated in red and white blood cells. Deficient phosphorylase in type VI disease can be defined in WBC preparations free of platelets. Phosphorylase kinase deficiency (type VIII disease) can be demonstrated in crude WBC preparations. Glucose-6-phosphatase deficiency in type I disease can be demonstrated in the liver, kidney, and gastrointestinal tract; liver obtained by percutaneous biopsy is the universally recommended tissue for such analysis. Although spontaneous bleeding disorders are uncommon in these diseases in the neonatal period, coagulation defects are noted with some regularity in screening tests prior to liver biopsy. Such disorders should be corrected prior to biopsy.

Treatment. Treatment of glycogenosis in the neonatal period is directed primarily toward correcting hypoglycemia. It is advisable to give frequent small feedings (intervals of 2 to 4 hours) containing glucose as the sole carbohydrate source. Ketoacidosis, if present and severe, should be treated by intravenous administration of fluids. Milder degrees of acidosis in clinically stable patients can be managed by the addition of relatively small amounts of sodium bicarbonate to the oral feedings.

Diazoxide and zinc glucagon are not recommended. Some older patients with intractable hypoglycemia have responded favorably to portal-systemic transposition.

Hyperlipidemia with xanthomatosis is seen in some patients with these disorders and has been reported to respond favorably to the substitution of medium chain triglycerides for the ordinary fat in the diet.

Hyperuricemia, if present, can be corrected by administration of allopurinol.

Prognosis. Prognosis depends in large part on the nature of the enzyme defect. Patients with type I glycogenosis have a relatively poor prognosis, with continued severe symptoms and shortened life span. Disorders of debranching and phosphorolysis, on the other hand, tend to show clinical remission with the passage of time, although the enzymatic defect persists; severely symptomatic infants may become clinically normal adults.

Genetics. With the exception of phosphorylase kinase deficiency (type VIII), these disorders show autosomal recessive inheritance. Phosphorylase kinase deficiency is inherited as a sex-linked, partially recessive disorder; affected females show a relatively mild clinical disorder consistent with their hemizygous state.

DISORDERS OF LIPID METABOLISM

Hyperlipoproteinemia

In recent years evidence has accumulated that links premature atherosclerotic cardiovascular disease to inborn errors of lipid metabolism (Table 14-2). Although xanthomata may appear in the neonatal period in these diseases, the life-threaten-

TABLE 14-2. Hyperlipidemia

Fredrickson type	Plasma triglycerides	Cholesterol	Xanthomata	Synonym
I	Increased (milky plasma)	Increased	Present	Familial hyperchylomicronemia
II	Slightly increased (clear plasma)	Increased	Present	Familial hypercholesterolemia
III	Normal	Normal	Absent	"Floating beta" disorder
IV	Normal	Normal	Absent	Familial endogenous hyperlipemia
V	Normal	Normal	Absent	Familial endogenous and exogenous hyperlipemia

ing cardiovascular manifestations do not appear for years to decades after birth. In some instances even the abnormalities of plasma lipids, which appear to be genetically determined, are not manifest during childhood. The demonstration that dietary manipulation, with or without the addition of drugs such as cholestyramine and clofibrate, can cause the plasma lipids of some diseased subjects to return to normal or near normal levels has led to an interest in the prevention of the clinical manifestations of these disorders by similar therapy instituted early in infancy.

Type I hyperlipoproteinemia

Type I hyperlipoproteinemia, a rare disorder, is a result of the failure of release of lipoprotein lipase activity in response to the ingestion of fat. This failure leads to the accumulation in plasma of large numbers of chylomicrons, giving the plasma a "cream of tomato soup" appearance. The hyperlipoproteinemia is accompanied by hypercholesterolemia and in many cases by the development of xanthomata. Although this disease is not a lysosomal storage disorder, hepatosplenomegaly with infiltration by foam cells is common in early childhood. Affected individuals develop episodes of abdominal pain that are sometimes associated with evidence of pancreatitis. Premature cardiovascular disease of the atherosclerotic type is apparently not a feature of this disorder.

The lactescence of plasma develops quite soon after the dietary intake of fat is established, and xanthomata have been reported within the neonatal period. Elimination of fat from the diet causes prompt remission in the hyperlipemia.

Diets containing adequate amounts of essential fatty acids and medium chain triglycerides rather than the usual dietary fat may be of benefit to patients with this disorder. No systematic trial of this management has been made nor is any likely considering the rarity of the condition. Type I hyperlipoproteinemia is inherited as an autosomal recessive disease, heterozygous individuals having no abnormality detectable by present methods.

Type II hyperlipoproteinemia

Type II hyperlipoproteinemia, or familial hypercholesterolemia, is a genetic disorder that has clinical manifestations in both heterozygous and homozygous individuals. While the pathogenesis of type II hyperlipoproteinemia has not been completely elucidated, delay in the removal of cholesterol from plasma has been demonstrated in affected individuals.

Clinical manifestations in the neonatal period are not common, but xanthomata have been noted at birth. Hypercholesterolemia is present in cord blood in a large number of affected subjects. Individuals homozygous for this disease characteristically exhibit plasma cholesterol levels in excess of 500 mg/100 ml, while heterozygous individuals have elevated but lower levels. Hypertriglyceridemia, though present, is not striking, and fasting plasma is clear.

Homozygous subjects have an extremely high mortality from atherosclerotic cardiovascular disease in the first 3 decades of life. The prognosis for the heterozygous state is somewhat better, though these individuals are subject to premature atherosclerotic cardiovascular disease. Dietary manipulation and the use of cholestyramine and clofibrate have not been notably successful in the treatment of homozygous type II hyperlipoproteinemia. Some benefit may be derived from these measures in the heterozygous condition. In infants found by screening procedures to have type II disease, it seems best to employ a diet as low in cholesterol as feasible, though the efficacy of such a measure has yet to be established. Neither the efficacy nor the safety of cholestyramine and clofibrate in early life has been established.

The other types of hyperlipoproteinemia have neither clinical manifestations nor detectable laboratory abnormalities in the neonatal period.

Congenital lipodystrophy

Congenital lipodystrophy is a rare disorder, characterized by the absence of fat deposits in skin and viscera.

Etiology and pathogenesis. Present evidence indicates that lipids are readily synthesized in congenital lipodystrophy, but that storage of lipids is impaired. It has been postulated that a primary hypothalmic abnormality leads to the secretion of a fat-mobilizing pituitary hormone related to growth hormone. This mechanism would account for the muscular and skeletal overgrowth seen in this disorder and, at least in part, for the diabetes mellitus, which characteristically occurs after some years.

Clinical findings. Affected infants are long and thin at birth, already exhibiting an absence of subcutaneous fat. The face is typically wrinkled. Hepatomegaly, which is always present in later life, is not a prominent finding in neonates. No disability has been attributed to the disorder in early life.

Laboratory findings. There may be no laboratory abnormality in the affected neonate, hyperlipemia and glucose intolerance developing only with time. Hypoglycemia has been noted early in the course of one patient.

Treatment. There is no specific treatment for this disorder, although the hyperlipemia generally responds to a low-fat diet.

Prognosis. Prognosis for life and general health are good during the early years. The disorder is disfiguring, and in about half the patients is associated with mental deficiency. Acanthosis nigricans is characteristic of later stages, as is diabetes mellitus with its accompanying microangiopathy. Fatty infiltration of the liver, accompanied by fibrosis, is invariably present in the fully developed disorder, and liver dysfunction may result.

Genetics. The current evidence strongly suggests autosomal recessive inheritance.

DISORDERS OF LYSOSOMAL STORAGE

A large number of new storage diseases have been described and defined by recently developed, precise laboratory techniques. The older, largely clinical literature is in the process of reexamination in the light of this recent work. Thus it is inevitable that some classic descriptions will be found to apply, not to the disease named by their authors, but to more recently defined entities. The present review of these diseases attempts to extract from the current literature those entities that can clearly be recognized in the neonatal period.

An increasing number of storage diseases are being classified as disorders of lysosomal function. The lysosome is an intracellular organelle whose role is the isolation of molecules from the cytosol and the degradation of these molecules. Under the electron microscope the lysosome is seen as a cytoplasmic membrane enclosing various cellular constituents. It is characterized by its high acid phosphatase activity.

Hers has suggested the following criteria for disorders of lysosomal function: (1) the disease is characterized by storage of material within lysosomes; (2) the stored material can be degraded by a mixture of normal lysomal enzymes; and (3) an enzymatic activity necessary for this degradation is absent from affected tissues.

Table 14-3 lists proved lysosomal diseases and those diseases that, in my opinion, may ultimately be shown to be disorders of lysosomal function. It is likely that all of the lysosomal storage diseases can be recognized before or shortly after birth by appropriate laboratory studies. The present discussion concerns itself with those diseases that have significant clinical manifestations in the neonatal period. It must be borne in mind that all the storage diseases are progressive; clinical manifestations appear when accumulated material has grossly distorted morphologic characteristics or function or both. Factors such as the normal rate of turnover of the stored material, the degree of deficiency of the enzymes involved, and the degree of awareness of the observer determine the time of initial manifestation.

Amino acid storage diseases

Cystine storage disease, more commonly referred to as the De Toni-Fanconi syndrome, probably does not produce clinical disease within the first month of life, though it may be diagnosed in the neonatal period by appropriate laboratory studies. An infant having evidence of gross renal tubular dysfunction in this period of life should be investigated for primary renal tubular disease, galactosemia, hereditary fructose intolerance, and glucose-6-phosphatase deficiency.

Polysaccharide storage disease

Type II glycogen storage disease

Pompe's disease, type II glycogen storage disease, has been observed to produce clinical abnormalities from birth, although this observation is not necessary for the diagnosis.

Etiology and pathogenesis. Pompe's dis-

TABLE 14-3. Lysosomal storage diseases

Eponym	Major stored material	Clinical involvement		Membranous cytoplasmic bodies identified	M.C.B. have acid phosphatase	Enzyme incriminated
		Visceral	Neuromuscular			
Amino acid storage diseases						
De Toni-Fanconi syndrome	Cystine	Yes	No	Yes	No	?
Polysaccharide storage diseases						
Pompe's disease	Glycogen	±	Yes	Yes	Yes	Acid maltase
Neutral lipid storage diseases						
Wolman's disease	Cholesterol Triglycerides	Yes	No	Yes	Yes	Acid lipase
Cholesterol ester storage disease	Cholesterol ester Triglycerides	Yes	No	Yes	?	
Mucopolysaccharide storage diseases						
Hurler's syndrome	Dermatan SO_4 Heparan SO_4	Yes	Yes	Yes	?	α-iduronidase
Hunter's syndrome	Dermatan SO_4 Heparan SO_4	Yes	Yes	Yes	?	Sulfoiduronate Sulfatase
Sanfilippo's syndrome						
A	Heparin SO_4	Yes	Yes	Yes	?	Heparin sulfate sulfatase
B	Heparan SO_4	Yes	Yes	Yes	?	-acetylglucosaminidase
Morquio's syndrome	Keratan SO_4	Yes	No (?)	Yes	?	?
Scheie syndrome	Dermatan SO_4 Heparin SO_4	Yes	±	?	?	α-iduronidase
Maroteaux-Lamy syndrome	Dermatan SO_4	Yes	±	?	?	?
Complex lipid storage diseases						
Farber's disease	Ceramide	Yes	Yes	?	?	?
Fabry's disease	Galactosyl galactosyl glucosyl ceramide	Yes	Yes	Yes	Yes	Ceramide trihexosidase
Lactacyl ceramide storage disease	Galactosyl glucosyl ceramide	Yes	Yes	Yes (?)	?	Ceramide dihexosidase
Gaucher's disease						
1 (adult)	Glucosyl ceramide	Yes	No	Yes	Yes	Glucocerebrosidase

2 (infantile)	Glucosyl ceramide	Yes	Yes	—	—	Glucocerebrosidase
3 (juvenile)	Glucosyl ceramide	Yes	Yes	Yes	?	Galatocerebroside
Krabbe's disease	Galactosyl ceramide	No	Yes	Yes	?	β-galactosidase
Tay-Sachs disease	Ganglioside G_{M2}	No	Yes	Yes	Yes	Hexoseaminidase A
Sandhof's disease	Ganglioside G_{M2}	Yes	Yes	?	?	Hexoseaminidase A and B
Niemann-Pick disease						
A	Sphingomyelin	Yes	Yes	Yes	Yes	Sphingomyelinase
B	Sphingomyelin	Yes	No	Yes	Yes	Sphingomyelinase
C	Sphingomyelin	Yes	Yes	?	?	?
D	Sphingomyelin	Yes	Yes	?	?	?
E	Sphingomyelin	Yes	Yes	?	?	?
MLD (late infantile)*	Sulfatide	No	Yes	Yes	Yes	Arylsulfatase A
MLD (adult)*	Sulfatide	No	Yes	?	?	Arylsulfatase A
Mucolipid storage disease						
MLD*	Sulfatide					Multiple sulfatase deficiency
Variant	Mucopolysaccharide	Yes	Yes	Yes	?	Multiple sulfatase deficiency
G_{M1} gangliosidosis	Ganglioside Mucopolysaccharide	Yes	Yes	Yes	Yes (?)	β-Galactosidase
I-cell disease	?	Yes	Yes	Yes	?	?
Gal+ disease	(?) Glycoprotein	Yes	Yes	?	?	?
Fucosidosis	Mucopolysaccharide containing fucose	Yes	Yes	Yes	Yes (?)	α-Fucosidase
Mannosidosis	Mucopolysaccharide containing mannose	Yes	Yes	?	?	α-Mannosidase
Unclassified storage diseases						
Stiff skin syndrome	?	Yes	No	?	?	?
β-Glucuronidase deficiency	Chonaroitin-4-SO_4 Chonaroitin-6-SO_4	Yes	?	?	?	β-Glucuronidase

*MLD, metachromatic leukodystropy.

ease is the prototype for diseases of lysosomal function. The causative biochemical lesion is absence of activity of a lysosomal hydrolytic enzyme, acid maltase (acid α-glucosidase). The cytoplasmic enzymes of glycogen synthesis and degradation—those responsible for the maintenance of glucose homeostasis—are present in normal amounts and function normally. However, two factors prevent hydrolysis of glycogen engulfed by lysosomes. The first is the absence of the hydrolytic enzyme that normally accomplishes the function. The second is that the glycogenolytic enzymes of cytoplasm cannot catalyze this hydrolysis in the hostile lysosomal environment. For reasons as yet obscure the devastating effects of the disease occur in the neuromuscular system, even though lysosomal accumulation of glycogen can be demonstrated in many other tissues, including liver and kidney. Mechanical distortion of cellular architecture has been incriminated in the malfunction of nerve and muscle.

Clinical features. Clinical manifestations can appear at any time during the first few months of life. The single most constant finding is profound muscular hypotonia, with diminution of reflexes but without loss of muscle mass. The muscles are firm to the touch. Cardiac failure as a result of myocardial involvement in the disease is very common as the initial complaint. Cardiomegaly is massive, and no murmur suggesting a congenital malformation is present. Hepatomegaly, when present, is probably related to congestive heart failure. Alertness is unaffected. The initial response to cardiotonic measures is generally good, but the overall course of the disease is one of relentless progression. Death is usually the result of respiratory failure, with or without complicating bronchopneumonia.

Laboratory studies. Results of all tests of hepatic glycogen release are normal, as is the structure of the glycogen stored by these patients. The ECG characteristically shows very large QRS deflections, a shortened P-R interval, and a leftward axis. The electromyogram shows typical and virtually diagnostic myotonic discharges. Nerve conduction is slowed.

Confirmation of the diagnosis may be made by demonstration of typical lysosomal inclusions of glycogen in white blood cells, liver, or muscle. Enzymatic confirmation may also be obtained using these tissues, though some patients with Pompe's disease with normal levels of acid maltase in white blood cells have been reported.

Treatment. Attempts have been made to treat such patients by infusing an appropriate enzyme mixture obtained from cultures of *Aspergillus niger*. Beneficial effects have been noted in serial electron micrographs of material obtained by liver biopsy, but no substantial clinical benefit has been shown. Therapy at this time is only supportive.

Prognosis. In general, patients with cardiac involvement as a primary manifestation die within the first year of life, while those whose clinical disease does not involve the myocardium may survive several years.

Genetics. Evidence suggests an autosomal recessive inheritance, though there is some preponderance of males among the reported patients.

Neutral lipidoses

Wolman's disease

Wolman's disease is a disorder of the storage of cholesterol and triglycerides, involving viscera much more than the central nervous system and leading to death within the first few months of life.

Etiology and pathogenesis. The absence of an acid lipase activity (E600-resistant acid esterase) leads to the accumulation of cholesterol and triglycerides within intracellular membranous cytoplasmic bodies throughout the body. The liver, spleen, adrenal glands, and gastrointestinal tract are most prominently involved. The nervous system shows definable but less striking abnormalities.

Clinical manifestations. Infants with Wolman's disease show failure to thrive from birth. Vomiting and diarrhea are prominent manifestations, as is progressive abdominal distention with hepatosplenomegaly of massive proportions. The infants show progressive inanition, with maintenance of apparently normal alertness until very late in the course of the disease.

Laboratory manifestations. The most important diagnostic sign is the presence of enlarged calcified adrenal glands on the abdominal x-ray film. Vacuolated leukocytes are prominent in peripheral blood smears, and foam cells in the bone marrow are characteristic. The diagnosis is established by the demonstration of abnormal accumulation of triglycerides and cholesterol in biopsy tissue; the liver is the preferred organ for biopsy. Confirmation by assay of acid lipase activity is useful and may become an essential diagnostic technique.

Treatment. Although several agents known to influence cholesterol metabolism have been used to treat this disorder, no success has been reported. Because of the involvement of adrenal cortex, replacement therapy with adrenal steroids may be indicated. Such therapy has not altered the course of the disease.

Prognosis. The prognosis is uniformly poor, death usually occurring within the first 6 months.

Genetics. Analysis of the few reported cases indicates an autosomal recessive inheritance.

Mucopolysaccharidoses

It is likely that none of the mucopolysaccharidoses listed in Table 14-3 can be recognized clinically in the neonatal period. Congenital cases reported in previous years are now generally felt to be examples of more profound lysosomal dysfunction, currently classified as mucolipidoses. If a reasonable means of treating patients with mucopolysaccharidosis becomes generally available, laboratory recognition of the disorder at birth will assume much greater importance.

Complex lipidoses

Farber's disease

Farber's disease is an infantile disorder of ceramide storage that is characterized by the accumulation of this material in granulomatous lesions, which involve the skin, subcutaneous tissues, joints, larynx, liver, and the central nervous system. It is generally lethal within the first 2 years of life.

Etiology and pathogenesis. The biochemical basis of Farber's disease has yet to be defined. It is known that ceramide accumulates in foam cells in many tissues in this disorder and that these foam cells accumulate within granulomas, which appear to evolve into the hyaline fibrotic masses characteristic of the disease. The inflammatory character of Farber's disease is unique among the storage diseases.

Clinical manifestations. Painful swelling of multiple joints, hoarseness, and stridor may appear at any time during the first few weeks of life. Palpable nodules develop in skin and subcutaneous tissue, particularly over the joints. Hepatomegaly and deterioration of central nervous system function, with the evolution of retinal cherry-red spots, form the remainder of the fully developed disease.

Laboratory manifestations. X-ray examination reveals generalized demineralization of bone, destruction of normal joint relationships, erosion of bones at the articular surfaces, and soft tissue calcification. Routine laboratory studies are not helpful in making the diagnosis, though occasional lipid-laden cells may be found in the bone marrow. Microscopic examination of a nodule obtained by biopsy is the best means presently available to confirm the clinical diagnosis.

Treatment. No specific treatment is available.

Prognosis. The prognosis is uniformly poor, death characteristically occurring within the first 2 years.

Genetics. The disease has occurred in siblings and in both males and females.

Gaucher's disease; malignant infantile form

The malignant infantile form of Gaucher's disease is caused by the widespread storage of glucosyl cerebroside in brain, liver, spleen, and other tissues. It is a progressive disorder, with severe central nervous system dysfunction and death generally occurring within the first year of life.

Etiology and pathogenesis. The fundamental biochemical lesion in malignant infantile Gaucher's disease is marked reduction in the activity of glucosyl cerebrosidase. The consequent accumulation of glucosyl cerebroside is considered to be responsible for the clinical findings, though the pathogenetic mechanisms have not been elucidated. There is some degree of neuronal loss on pathologic examination of the brain.

Clinical features. The clinical features of

the disease can develop at any time within the first few months of life. Feeding difficulties, vomiting, hepatosplenomegaly, and muscular hypertonia are found in various combinations. Cough and respiratory difficulty are also common. Deterioration of central nervous system function is characteristic with the evolution of a vegetative state. Retinal cherry-red spots do not develop.

Laboratory findings. The serum acid phosphatase is elevated to a striking degree. Absolute confirmation of the diagnosis requires demonstration of the enzymatic deficiency in leukocytes or tissue or both obtained by biopsy. Microscopic examination of bone marrow and of other tissues generally reveals cellular characteristics specific enough to establish the diagnosis.

Treatment. Treatment is supportive.

Genetics. Gaucher's disease is inherited as an autosomal recessive disorder.

Gaucher's disease; chronic nonneuropathic form

While the chronic nonneuropathic form of Gaucher's disease is seldom recognized in the early months and years of life, it seems likely that the visceral manifestations noted in malignant Gaucher's disease in early life are in fact present at similar ages in the nonneuropathic disease. The striking differences are the normal neural function and much better prognosis of the nonneuropathic disease.

Ganglioside storage diseases

Tay-Sachs disease

Tay-Sachs disease is a progressive infantile disease of neurologic function, characterized by regression of development, blindness, spasticity, and ultimate fatality. It exhibits no characteristic clinical manifestations outside the nervous system.

Etiology and pathogenesis. Tay-Sachs disease is the result of a deficiency of activity of a hexoseaminidase A, which is necessary for the degradation of ganglioside G_{M2}. While the accumulation of ganglioside G_{M2} is probably generalized in a chemical sense, clinically significant accumulation is limited to the nervous system, and predominantly to the gray matter of the central nervous system. The precise mechanism by which clinical disease occurs is unknown. Infants dying very early have shrunken brains showing enlarged lateral ventricles and gliosis; those dying late in the disease have enlarged brains, with small ventricles, the result of progressive storage of ganglioside.

Clinical manifestations. The onset of clinical manifestations is generally within the first 8 months of life, but onset prior to 3 months of age is unusual. There is gradual deterioration of cortical function. The most characteristic clinical manifestation is hyperacusis, a striking extensor response to sharp sounds. Lack of normal awareness, poor muscle tone, and spasticity are also frequently noted. The retinal cherry-red spots, which eventually develop in nearly all patients with Tay-Sachs disease, are not present in the neonatal period. Seizures, which may be myoclonic, focal, or generalized, have occurred in the neonatal period, but are unusual early in the course of the disease.

Laboratory studies. The absence of hexoseaminidase A activity in any of several tissues, including white blood cells, liver, and skin fibroblasts, is diagnostic of Tay-Sachs disease. Reduction in the activity of fructose-1-phosphate aldolase in the red blood cells has been documented, but the measurement of this activity cannot be considered a substitute for the assay of hexoseaminidase A.

Therapy. No specific therapy is available.

Prognosis. The course is relentlessly progressive, death generally occurring 13 to 30 months after the onset of clinical manifestations.

Genetics. The inheritance is autosomal recessive.

Niemann-Pick disease; type A

Infantile Niemann-Pick disease is a progressive disease associated with the storage of sphingomyelin in nervous system and viscera.

Etiology and pathogenesis. Severe deficiency of sphingomyelinase in all tissues leads to the intracellular accumulation of sphingomyelin within membranous cytoplasmic bodies. The predominant clinical effects are in the nervous system.

Clinical manifestations. Niemann-Pick

disease is usually recognized after the neonatal period. Persistent neonatal jaundice and hepatosplenomegaly have been noted retrospectively in a number of patients. The retinal cherry-red spots develop quite early in many cases, but are not reliably present within the neonatal period. Neurologic deterioration usually occurs after the neonatal period.

Laboratory manifestations. Vacuolated leukocytes may be observed in blood smears, and Niemann-Pick cells (lipid-laden macrophages) can be seen in the bone marrow. The level of plasma acid phosphatase is occasionally elevated. Specific diagnosis depends upon the demonstration of sphingomyelin accumulation and of markedly reduced activity of sphingomyelinase in tissue obtained by biopsy or in tissue cultures of skin fibroblasts or bone marrow. The enzymatic defect has also been demonstrated in peripheral leukocytes.

Therapy. No specific therapy is available.

Prognosis. The disorder exhibits autosomal recessive inheritance. A preponderance of reported cases have occurred in Jews, but no racial or ethnic group appears to be spared.

Niemann-Pick disease; type B

Type B Niemann-Pick disease is different from type A disease only in that the nervous system is spared in type B disease. Visceral manifestations are similar in the two disorders, but the prognosis is better in type B disease; the course resembles that of chronic Gaucher's disease.

Mucolipidoses

Generalized gangliosidosis

Generalized gangliosidosis is a disorder combining the morphologic features of Hurler's syndrome with a clinical course similar to that of the infantile cerebral lipidoses.

Etiology and pathogenesis. Ganglioside G_{M1} is the major storage material, but there is also storage of mucopolysaccharide. Assays of lysosomal enzymes have revealed marked deficiency of activity of β-galactosidases A, B, C, and D.

Clinical manifestations. It seems likely that cases reported as neonatal or congenital Hurler's syndrome represent instances of generalized gangliosidosis. The Hurler's facies, hepatosplenomegaly, and bony defects of dysostosis multiplex may be seen at birth or very shortly thereafter. Developmental retardation is manifest very early, and there is profound failure to thrive. Macular cherry-red spots appear in approximately 50% of cases.

Laboratory findings. The excretion of mucopolysaccharides in the urine is normal. However 10% to 80% of leukocytes contain Reilly bodies, and bone marrow examination reveals finely vacuolated histiocytic cells. Similar evidence of storage is seen in biopsy material from various tissues, particularly the liver. Definitive diagnosis requires demonstration of marked deficiency in galactosidases A, B, and C.

Treatment. There is no specific treatment.

Prognosis. The prognosis is uniformly bad. Death usually occurs prior to 2 years of age as a result of pulmonary complications.

Genetics. Autosomal recessive inheritance occurs.

I-cell disease

I-cell disease is a recently described disorder of lysosomal storage that has not been well characterized chemically.

Etiology and pathogenesis. An unusual material accumulates in cultured fibroblast. The unidentified inclusions are sufficiently distinctive to separate this entity from other storage disorders.

Clinical manifestations. Affected infants have low birth weights and subsequent growth failure. These infants are quiet from birth and show severe developmental retardation early in life. Clinical manifestations have not been recognized within the neonatal period to date. There is no significant hepatosplenomegaly, and the corneas are clear.

Laboratory manifestations. The excretion of mucopolysaccharide in the urine is normal. No inclusions are seen in leukocytes. The diagnosis is established by finding typical inclusions within cultured fibroblasts.

Treatment. No specific treatment is known for I-cell disease. The prognosis is poor.

Mannosidosis

Mannosidosis is a recently described storage disease in which hepatosplenomegaly, skeletal changes, central nervous system dysfunction, and marmoration of skin appear within weeks after birth.

The absence of acid α-mannosidase has been demonstrated. Vacuolated lymphocytes and polymorphonuclear inclusions are seen in the bone marrow.

There is no specific treatment, and the prognosis is poor.

Uncategorized storage disorders

Stiff skin syndrome

Four patients have been described who have stiff skin and limitation of joint mobility; clinical manifestations have been noted in the newborn period. Histologic changes in the skin suggest mucopolysaccharide storage.

Beta-glucuronidase deficiency

An infant with this disorder had clear signs of a Hurler-like mucopolysaccharidosis without corneal clouding when first examined at 7 weeks of age. The urine showed excessive excretion of chondroitin-4-sulfate and chondroitin-6-sulfate.

JOHN F. NICHOLSON

BIBLIOGRAPHY

GENERAL

Stanbury, J. B., Wyngaarden, J. B., and Frederickson, D. S., editors: The metabolic basis of inherited disease, New York, 1972, McGraw-Hill Book Co. Most of the disorders covered in this chapter are discussed exhaustively in this encyclopedic work.

PHENYLKETONURIA

Hackney, I. M., Hanley, W. B., Davidson, W., and Linsao, L.: Phenylketonuria; mental development, behavior, and termination of low phenylalanine diet, J. Pediatr. **72**:646, 1968.

Kang, E. S., Sollee, N. D., and Gerald, P. S.: Results of treatment and termination of the diet in phenylketonuria (PKU), Pediatrics **46**:881, 1970.

Kennedy, J. L., Wertelecki, W., Gates, L., Sperry, B. P., and Cass, V. M.: The early treatment of phenylketonuria, Am. J. Dis. Child. **113**:16, 1967.

Knox, W. E.: Phenylketonuria. In Stanbury, J. B., Wyngaarden, J. B., and Frederickson, D. S., editors: The metabolic basis of inherited disease, New York, 1972, McGraw-Hill Book Co., p. 266.

Rouse, B. M.: Phenylalanine deficiency syndrome, J. Pediatr. **69**:246, 1966.

Snyderman, S. E., Pratt, E. L., Cheung, M. W., Norton, P., and Holt, L. E.: The phenylalanine requirement of the normal infant, J. Nutr. **56**: 253, 1955.

TYROSINOSIS, ACUTE TYROSINOSIS, CHRONIC TYROSINEMIA

Gaull, G. E., Rassin, D. K., Solomon, G. E., Harris, R. C., and Sturman, J. A.: Biochemical observations on so-called hereditary tyrosinosis, Pediatr. Res. **4**:337, 1970.

Grant, D. B., Alexander, F. W., and Seakins, J. W. T.: Abnormal tyrosine metabolism in hereditary fructose intolerance, Acta Paediatr. Scand. **59**:432, 1970.

La Du, B. N., and Gjessing, L. R.: Tyrosinosis and tyrosinemia. In Stanbury, J. B., Wyngaarden, J. B., and Frederickson, D. S., editors: The metabolic basis of inherited disease, New York, 1972, McGraw-Hill Book Co., p. 296.

Scriver, C. R., Larochelle, J., and Silverberg, M.: Hereditary tyrosinemia and tyrosyluria in a French Canadian geographic isolate, Am. J. Dis. Child. **113**:41, 1967.

Yu, J. S., Walker-Smith, J. A., and Burnard, E. D.: Neonatal hepatitis in premature infants simulating hereditary tyrosinosis, Arch. Dis. Child. **46**:306, 1971.

DISORDERS OF THE UREA CYCLE

Shih, V. E., and Efron, M. L.: Urea cycle disorders. In Stanbury, J. B., Wyngaarden, J. B., and Frederickson, D. S., editors: The metabolic basis of inherited disease, New York, 1972, McGraw-Hill Book Co., p. 370.

CITRULLINEMIA

van der Zee, S. P. M., Trijbels, J. M. F., Monnens, L. A. H., Hommes, F. A., and Schretlen, E. D. A. M.: Citrullinemia with rapidly fatal neonatal course, Arch. Dis. Child. **46**:847, 1971.

MAPLE SYRUP URINE DISEASE

Dancis, J., and Levitz, M.: Abnormalities of branched-chain amino acid metabolism (hypervalinemia, branched-chain ketonuria, maple syrup urine disease), isovaleric acidemia. In Stanbury, J. B., Wyngaarden, J. B., and Frederickson, D. S., editors: The metabolic basis of inherited disease, New York, 1972, McGraw-Hill Book Co., p. 426.

Goodman, S. I., Pollack, S., Miles, B., and O'Brien, D.: The treatment of maple syrup urine disease, J. Pediatr. **75**:485, 1969.

Sallan, S. E., and Cottom, D.: Peritoneal dialysis in maple syrup urine disease, Lancet **2**:1423, 1969.

Scriver, C. R., Clow, C. L., Mackenzie, S., and Oelyin, E.: Thiamine-responsive maple-syrup-urine disease, Lancet **2**:310, 1971.

Snyderman, S. E.: The therapy of maple syrup urine disease, Am. J. Dis. Child. **113**:68, 1967.

PROPIONIC ACIDEMIA

Gompertz, D., Storrs, C. N., Bav, D. C. K., Peters, T. J., and Hughes, E. A.: Localization of enzymatic defect in propionic acidemia, Lancet **1**: 1140, 1970.

Rosenberg, L. E.: Disorders of propionate, methylmalonate, and vitamin B_{12} metabolism. In Stanbury, J. B., Wyngaarden, J. B., and Frederickson, D. S., editors: The metabolic basis of inherited disease, New York, 1972, McGraw-Hill Book Co., p. 440.

HOMOCYSTINURIA

Gerritsen, T., and Waisman, H. A.: Homocystinuria. In Stanbury, J. B., Wyngaarden, J. B., and Frederickson, D. S., editors: The metabolic basis of inherited disease, New York, 1972, McGraw-Hill Book Co., p. 404.

Hagberg, B., and Hambraeces, L.: Some aspects of the diagnosis and treatment of homosystinuria, Dev. Med. Child. Neurol. **10**:470, 1968.

Schimke, R. N.: Low-methionine diet treatment of homocystinuria, Ann. Intern. Med. **70**:642, 1969.

HISTIDINEMIA

Neville, G. R., Bentovim, A., Clayton, B. E., and Sheperd, J.: Histidinaemia—study of relation between clinical and biological findings in 7 subjects, Arch. Dis. Child. **47**:190, 1972.

Thalhammer, O., Schreibenreiter, S., and Pantlitschko, M.: Histidinemia; detection by routine newborn screening and biochemical observations on three unrelated cases, Z. Kinderheilkd. **109**:279, 1971.

CONGENITAL LACTIC ACIDOSIS

Brunette, M. G., Delvin, E., Hazel, B., and Scriver, C. R.: Thiamine responsive lactic acidosis in a patient with deficient low-Km pyruvate carboxylase activity in liver, Pediatrics **50**:702, 1972.

Gautier, E.: Lactic acidosis in infancy, Helv. Med. Acta **35**:423, 1970.

Greene, H. L., Schubert, W. K., and Hug, G.: Chronic lactic acidosis of infancy, J. Pediatr. **76**: 853, 1970.

Greene, H. L., Stifel, F. B., and Herman, R. H.: Ketotic hypoglycemia due to hepatic fructose-1, 6-diphosphatase deficiency, Am. J. Dis. Child. **124**:415, 1972.

Hartmann, A. F., Sr., Wohltmann, H. J., Parkerson, M. L., and Wesley, M. E.: Lactate metabolism; studies of a child with serious congenital deviation, J. Pediatr. **61**:165, 1962.

Lie, S. O., Loken, A. C., Stromme, J. H., and Aagenaes, O.: Fatal congenital lactic acidosis in two siblings. I. Clinical and pathological findings, Acta Paediatr. Scand. **60**:129, 1971.

THE SWEATY FEET SYNDROMES: HEXANOIC/BUTANOIC ACIDURIA AND ISOVALERIC ACIDEMIA

Ando, T., Nyhau, W. L., Bachmann, C., Rasmussen, K., Scott, R., and Smith, E. K.: Isovaleric acidemia; identification of isovalerate, isovalerylglycine and 3-hydroxyisovalerate in urine of a patient previously reported as having butyric and hepanoic acidemia, J. Pediatr. **82**:243, 1973.

Newman, C. G. H., Wilson, B. D. R., Callaghan, P., and Young, L.: Neonatal death associated with isovaleric acidemia, Lancet **2**:439, 1967.

Pagliara, A. S., Karl, I. E., Keating, J. P., Brown, B. I., and Kipnis, D. M.: Hepatic fructose-1, 6-diphosphatase deficiency, J. Clin. Invest. **51**: 2115, 1972.

Sidbury, J. B., Jr., Smith, E. K., and Harlan, W.: An inborn error of short-chain fatty acid metabolism; the odor of sweaty feet syndrome, J. Pediatr. **70**:8, 1967.

Tildon, J. T., and Cornblath, M.: Succinyl-CoA: 3-CoA: 3-ketoacid CoA-transferase deficiency, J. Clin. Invest. **51**:493, 1972.

NEONATAL DIABETES MELLITUS

Gentz, J. C. H., and Cornblath, M.: Transient diabetes in the newborn, Adv. Pediatr. **16**:345, 1969.

DISORDERS OF GALACTOSE METABOLISM

Kelly, S.: Septicemia in galactosemia, J.A.M.A. **216**:330, 1971.

Komrower, G. M., and Lee, D. H.: Long-term follow-up of galactosemia, Arch. Dis. Child. **45**: 367, 1970.

Monteleone, J. A., Buetler, E., Monteleone, P. L., Utz, C. L., and Casey, E. C.: Cataracts, galactosuria and hypergalactosemia due to galactokinase deficiency in a child, Am. J. Med. **50**:403, 1971.

Segal, S.: Disorders of galactose metabolism. In Stanbury, J. B., Wyngaarden, J. B., and Fredrickson, D. S., editors: The metabolic basis of inherited disease, New York, 1972, McGraw-Hill Book Co., p. 174.

DISORDERS OF THE METABOLISM OF FRUCTOSE

Froesch, E. R.: Essential fructosuria and hereditary fructose intolerance. In Stanbury, J. B., Wyngaarden, J. B., and Fredrickson, D. S., editors: The metabolic basis of inherited disease, New York, 1972, McGraw-Hill Book Co., p. 131.

Levin, B., Snodgrass, G. J. A. I., Burgess, E. A., and Dobbs, R. H.: Fructosaemia; observations in seven cases, Am. J. Med. **45**:826, 1968.

GLYCOGENOSIS

Fernandez, J., and Pikaar, N. A.: Ketosis in hepatic glycogenosis, Arch. Dis. Child. **47**:41, 1972.

Howell, R. R.: The glycogen storage diseases. In Stanbury, J. B., Wyngaarden, J. B., and Fredrickson, D. S., editors: The metabolic basis of inherited disease, New York, 1972, McGraw-Hill Book Co., p. 149.

Spencer-Peet, J., Norman, M. E., Lake, B. D., McNamara, J. M., and Patrick, A. D.: Hepatic glycogen storage disease, Q. J. Med. **40**:95, 1971.

DISORDERS OF LIPID METABOLISM

Fredrickson, D. S., and Levy, R. I.: Familial hyperlipoproteinemia. In Stanbury, J. B., Wyngaarden, J. B., and Fredrickson, D. S., editors: The metabolic basis of inherited disease, New York, 1972, McGraw-Hill Book Co., p. 545.

Seip, M.: Generalized lipodystrophy, Ergeb. Inn. Med. Kinderheilkd. **31**:59, 1971.

DISORDERS OF LYSOSOMAL STORAGE

Clement, D. H., and Godman, G. C.: Glycogen disease resembling mongolism, cretinism, and amyotonia congenita, J. Pediatr. **36**:11, 1950.

Di Ferrante, N., Nichols, B. L., Donnelly, P. V., Neri, G., Hrgovcic, R., and Bergland, R. K.: Induced degradation of glycosaminoglycans in Hurler's and Hunter's syndromes by plasma infusions, Proc. Natl. Acad. Sci. U.S.A. **58**:303, 1971.

Esterly, N. B., and McKusick, V. A.: Stiff skin syndrome, Pediatrics **47**:360, 1971.

Fredrickson, D. S., and Sloan, H. R.: Glucosyl ceramide lipidoses; Gaucher's disease. In Stanbury, J. B., Wyngaarden, J. B., and Fredrickson, D. S., editors: The metabolic basis of inherited disease, New York, 1972, McGraw-Hill Book Co., p. 730.

Fredrickson, D. S., and Sloan, H. R.: G_{M2} gangliosidoses; Tay-Sachs disease. In Stanbury, J. B., Wyngaarden, J. B., and Fredrickson, D. S., editors: The metabolic basis of inherited disease, New York, 1972, McGraw-Hill Book Co., p. 615.

Fredrickson, D. S., and Sloan, H. R.: Sphingomyelin lipidoses; Niemann-Pick disease. In Stanbury, J. B., Wyngaarden, J. B., and Fredrickson, D. S., editors: The metabolic basis of inherited disease, New York, 1972, McGraw-Hill Book Co., p. 783.

Hers, H. G.: Inborn lysosomal diseases, Gastroenterology **48**:625, 1965.

Hug, G., and Schubert, W. K.: Lysosomes in type II glycogenosis; changes during administration of extract from *Aspergillus niger,* J. Cell Biol. **35**:C1, 1967.

Lake, B. D., and Patrick, A. D.: Wolman's disease; deficiency of E600-resistant acid esterase activity with storage of lipids in lysosomes, J. Pediatr. **76**:262, 1970.

Moser, H. W., Prensky, A. L., Wolfe, N. J., and Rosman, N. P.: Farber's lipograngulomatosis, Am. J. Med. **47**:869, 1969.

Rosenstein, B.: Glycogen storage disease of the heart in a newborn infant, J. Pediatr. **65**:126, 1964.

Schneider, J. A., Wong, J., and Seegmiller, J. E.: The early diagnosis of cystinosis, J. Pediatr. **74**: 114, 1969.

Spranger, J. W., and Wiedeman, H. R.: The genetic mucolipidoses, diagnosis and differential diagnosis, Humangenetik **9**:113, 1970.

Wolman, M., Sterk, V. V., Gatt, S.. and Frenkel, M.: Primary familial xanthomatosis with involvement and calcification of the adrenals, Pediatrics **28**:742, 1961.

BETA-METHYL CHROTONYLGLYCINURIA

Gompertz, D., Draffan, G. H., Watts, J. L., and Hull, D.: Biotin-responsive beta-methylcrotonylglycinuria, Lancet **2**:22, 1971.

UNCLASSIFIED STORAGE DISEASES

Sly, W. S., Quinton, B. A., McAlister, W. H., and Rimoin, D. L.: Beta glucuronidase deficiency; report of clinical, radiologic and biochemical features of a new mucopolysaccharidosis, J. Pediatr. **82**:249, 1973.

15 Metabolic and endocrine disturbances

HYPOGLYCEMIA

Neonatal hypoglycemia is not a specific diagnosis; rather it is a laboratory finding that reflects a breakdown in the mechanisms that govern carbohydrate homeostasis. It is a significant cause of morbidity and mortality that can be prevented in many infants when promptly diagnosed and properly treated. Though knowledge of carbohydrate metabolism is extensive, the exact pathophysiology of neonatal hypoglycemia is not well understood. In recent years metabolic differences between the fetus, newborn, older infant, and child have been delineated.

Fetus

Carbohydrate is the principal energy source of the fetus. As pregnancy progresses, liver, heart, and muscle glycogen stores increase and are several times above normal adult values at term. Originally, glucose was thought to diffuse only passively across the placenta, but it now appears that active transport of facilitated diffusion is involved. Fetal scalp blood studies prior to labor and umbilical vein samples at vaginal hysterotomy prior to therapeutic abortion have demonstrated that the fetal blood glucose level is approximately one half the maternal level. In general, the human fetal glucose levels parallel the maternal glucose values. Though insulin is present in the fetal pancreas early in gestation, neither its role nor the role of the pituitary-adrenal system in the regulation of fetal blood glucose levels is clearly delineated.

Newborn

After birth the newborn infant must immediately provide the energy for temperature regulation, respiration, and muscle activity. Studies of respiratory quotients (RQ) in the first days of life indicate that carbohydrate is still the major energy source. Chemical analysis of the carbohydrate content of the human liver before and after birth supports the conclusion that glycogen stores provide the early postnatal energy supply.

The blood glucose level is maintained by a sensitive balance between hepatic carbohydrate metabolism and release of glucose and peripheral uptake and utilization of glucose. The hepatic release of glucose is dependent on adequate glycogen stores and response to glucagon, while the peripheral utilization and uptake of glucose are dependent on insulin, pH, temperature, and muscle activity. Imbalances in these factors result in neonatal hypoglycemia.

The full-term infant has adequate glycogen stores, but the premature infant has not had sufficient time to accumulate stores and is particularly vulnerable to hypoglycemia; the SGA infant who has had recurrent anoxia in utero and has depleted his carbohydrate stores in utero is also at high risk. Insulin levels in the first several days of life are generally lower than at 1 week of life; decreased glucose disappearance rates after intravenous glucose tolerance tests and the failure of leucine and tolbutamide to produce significant hypoglycemia suggest that the newborn is unable to secrete large amounts of insulin. Grasso has shown that infusion of amino acids produces marked increases in insulin secretion and suggests that the primary role of insulin in the neonate may be anabolic; that is, to stimulate the utilization of amino acids for protein synthesis.

Contrary to the findings in normal newborns, infants with symptomatic hypoglycemia have increased glucose disappearance rates, suggesting increased peripheral utilization or increased uptake by the brain. Babies who are SGA tend to have higher rates of oxygen consumption in the first 12 hours of life. Sinclair has suggested that the metabolic requirements of a brain that is disproportionately large in relation to body weight may account for the high oxygen consumption rates; the requirements of this brain for carbohydrate may exceed the liver's glycogen stores. Other factors operating in this group of infants are low cortisol production rates, possibly increased insulin levels, and a decreased epinephrine release in response to hypoglycemia.

Infants with erythroblastosis fetalis have had hyperinsulinism evoked as the cause for the well-documented association with hypoglycemia. A proposed mechanism for the hyperinsulinism is the destruction of insulin by glutathione released by rapid hemolysis of red blood cells. Both the full-term and preterm infant produce adequate levels of catecholamines and epinephrine. Growth hormone levels are generally high in both full-term and premature infants in the first days of life, and studies have documented increased levels of growth hormone in response to hypoglycemia in both groups.

From the moment of birth an array of factors are brought into play that affect carbohydrate homeostasis and that may tip the metabolic balance sufficiently to produce hypoglycemia. Excessive chilling in the delivery room, birth asphyxia, and delay in establishing feeding are examples of such factors that may have no significant effect in a normal full-term infant but that may lead to hypoglycemia in a premature or SGA infant.

Definition. An infant is hypoglycemic when his blood glucose level is significantly lower than the established mean for a similar population of infants. Full-term infants maintain their blood glucose levels above 30 mg/100 ml during the first 72 hours of life, while premature infants maintain levels above 20 mg/100 ml. Values below these levels constitute neonatal hypoglycemia. The incidence of hypoglycemia for all weight groups is approximately 2 to 3 per 1,000 live births, but it is higher in premature infants and infants whose intrauterine weight gain has been less than normal for gestational age. As many as 50% of the infants of diabetic mothers may become hypoglycemic. The outline below lists the causes of hypoglycemia in the newborn. Several of these entities are discussed in detail elsewhere (Chapter 14, p. 408).

CAUSES OF HYPOGLYCEMIA

I. Decreased hepatic glucose output
  A. Decreased glycogen stores
    1. Prematurity
    2. In-utero malnutrition
    3. Starvation
    4. Severe hypothermia
    5. Liver disease
  B. Defect in hepatic glucose formation or release
    1. Glycogen storage disease (type I)
    2. Galactosemia
    3. Fructose intolerance (hereditary)
    4. Adrenal insufficiency
II. Increased peripheral utilization of glucose
  A. Pancreatic islet cell adenoma
  B. Pancreatic islet cell hyperplasia
    1. Infants of diabetic mothers
    2. Erythroblastosis
    3. Beckwith's syndrome
    4. Tyrosinemia
  C. Hyperinsulin states
    1. Maternal tolbutamide ingestion
    2. Maple syrup urine disease
    3. Sudden discontinuation of hypertonic glucose infusion
III. Idiopathic hypoglycemias
  A. Cyanotic congenital heart disease and congestive failure
  B. Central nervous system disease
  C. Ketotic hypoglycemia
  D. Idiopathic hypoglycemia

Clinical presentation. Because many of the symptoms of hypoglycemia also occur with other illnesses (infections, central nervous system anomalies, hypocalcemia, birth asphyxia), the exact incidence of symptomatic hypoglycemia is unknown. Below is a list of symptoms reported in neonatal symptomatic hypoglycemia. The onset of symptoms varies from several hours of life to a week after birth. Because these signs may result from many causes, it is important to determine if they disappear with the simultaneous administration of glucose and the return of blood sugar to normal levels. If the symptoms do not clear, other diagnosis must be excluded. Hypocalcemia and hypomagnesemia have also been associated with hypoglycemia.

SYMPTOMS REPORTED IN NEONATAL SYMPTOMATIC HYPOGLYCEMIA

Tremors
Cyanosis
Convulsions
Apnea or irregular respirations or both
Lethargy
Peculiar cry, high pitched or weak
Hypotonia
Poor feeding
Abnormal eye movements

Treatment. After birth, infants who are likely to develop hypoglycemia should be monitored on a regular schedule with Dextrostix and intermittent determination of the blood glucose level. The blood glucose level should be measured at the time of birth when possible or at least within 1 hour of birth. Subsequent measurements should be taken every 1 to 2 hours for the first 6 to 8 hours and every 4 to 6 hours until 24 hours after birth. Well infants who are normoglycemic but are at risk (outline on p. 440) should receive oral or gavage feeding with 10% to 20% glucose water or formula started at 2 to 3 hours of age and continued at 2-hour intervals for 24 to 48 hours. If early oral feedings are contraindicated, peripheral infusion of 5% to 10% glucose should be started until the blood glucose is stabilized within the normal range and the infant is tolerating enteral feedings. Below are listed the sequential steps in the management of infants who are at risk of developing hypoglycemia and who, despite proper monitoring, become hypoglycemic.

After documentation of hypoglycemia, 1 to 2 ml/kg of 50% glucose diluted with equal volumes of sterile water are infused rapidly through a peripheral vein. The umbilical vessels should not be routinely used for this injection because of the hypertonicity of the solution. Following the infusion of this 25% glucose solution, a peripheral infusion of a 10% to 15% glucose solution should be started and maintained until the blood glucose level has been normal for 24 to 48 hours. At this point a gradual tapering of the infusion over 2 to 3 days is started simultaneously with initiation of successful enteral feedings.

MANAGEMENT OF POTENTIALLY HYPOGLYCEMIC INFANTS

1. Identification of infants at risk (p. 440)
2. Monitoring infants at risk (Dextrostix, Blood Sugars)
3. Early feedings when possible or peripheral infusions of 5% to 10% glucose solutions or both
4. If hypoglycemia develops, 50% glucose solution by peripheral vein: 1 to 2 ml/kg body weight diluted with equal amounts of water, followed by continuous infusion of 10% to 15% glucose solution for 24 to 48 hrs; gradual tapering of intravenous glucose controlled by serial blood glucose over 3 to 4 days.
5. Hydrocortisone (2.5 mg/kg/12 hr) or prednisone (1 mg/kg/day) for resistant hypoglycemia

If peripheral infusion of a 15% to 20% glucose solution fails to maintain normal blood concentrations and to eliminate symptoms, hydrocortisone (2.5 mg/kg/12 hours) or prednisone (1 mg/kg/day) should be administered. The value of epinephrine, fructose, glucogen, and diazoxide has not been established, and these drugs are, therefore, contraindicated for the treatment of hypoglycemia. Recurrence of hypoglycemia is relatively rare after adequate initial treatment. Hypocalcemia and hypomagnesemia should be treated when diagnosed (p. 445 and p. 449).

Prognosis. Prognosis for life is good in the absence of potentially lethal congenital anomalies; the outlook for normal intellectual functioning must be guarded, since prolonged and severe hypoglycemia may be associated with neurologic sequelae and death. Symptomatic infants with hypoglycemia, particularly low birth weight infants and large infants of overtly diabetic mothers, have a worse prognosis for subsequent normal intellectual development than asymptomatic infants.

Infants of diabetic mothers

With the improved management of diabetes, an increased number of diabetic patients reach childbearing age and are able to reproduce. In addition, certain women develop abnormalities of carbohydrate metabolism during pregnancy that are characterized as gestation diabetes. This state may presage later adult diabetes. In all pregnant diabetic women, regardless of their class, there is an increased incidence of maternal and fetal complications; the diabetic state creates an intrauterine environment that is unfavorable for the developing fetus. The infants of diabetic mothers may share certain morphologic characteristics. In addition to the distinctive physical characteristics of macrosomia (discussed later), these infants have a high incidence of hydramnios and intrauterine death after the thirty-sixth week of gestation and high neonatal morbidity and mortality. Poor control of maternal diabetes with recurrent ketoacidosis is associated with significant fetal wastage. Despite vigorous medical management, there is also an increased perinatal mortality as the severity of diabetes increases. Even with mild gestational diabetes, there is an increased incidence of fetal and neonatal morbidity.

Pathophysiology. The pathophysiology of this intrauterine metabolic disorder is poorly understood. If the mother is a class D or more severe diabetic, the maternal vascular changes may be associated with a small placenta and a SGA infant. More commonly, both placental and infant weight are increased. Maternal plasma lactogenic hormone levels, villous surface area, and DNA are increased proportionately with placental weight; infant organ weights, except the brain, are also increased. The infants of diabetic mothers present a picture of functional hyperinsulinism, and postmortem studies demonstrate hyperplasia of the pancreatic islets and their beta cells. There is uncertainty as to whether the insulin activity in infants of diabetic mothers is increased. Although fetal hyperinsulinism has been postulated as the cause of macrosomia and neonatal hypoglycemia, it does not explain the large size of infants of prediabetic mothers. The cushingoid, plethoric appearance of the diabetic infant is not associated with elevation of serum 17-hydroxycorticoid levels as one would anticipate if there were increased secretion of fetal or maternal corticotropin. Body composition studies have shown an increase in total body fat rather than an increased content of fluid and electrolytes. Total body water, particularly extracellular water, is decreased.

Clinical presentation. The infants of diabetic and prediabetic mothers often bear a striking resemblance to one another. They are large, plump infants with puffy, plethoric faces. It should be noted that these infants may also be normal or low birth weight and of full-term or preterm gestational age, particularly when there is maternal vascular disease. In well-controlled diabetics, Pedersen has demonstrated that the macrosomia can be minimized or prevented. The infants tend to be lethargic or jittery or both during the first several days of life and may have any of the clinical signs of hypoglycemia (see list on p. 441). The early onset of signs is more likely to be related to hypoglycemia, and the later onset of similar signs related to hypocalcemia or hypomagnesemia or both; these abnormalities may also be seen together. Hyperbilirubinemia is often noted in these infants and is most likely related to their immaturity.

Many infants are tachypneic during the first 3 to 5 days of life. This may be a transient sign of hypoglycemia, hypothermia, polycythemia, or cerebral edema from birth asphyxia; the tachypnea may also represent the early stages of HMD. There is an increased incidence of renal vein thrombosis, and this diagnosis should be suspected in the presence of a flank mass and hematuria (p. 509). The frequency of congenital anomalies is increased, particularly when there is polyhydramnios.

The subsequent incidence of diabetes mellitus in infants of diabetic mothers is higher than that in the general population. There is also evidence that the macrosomic infant is likely to be obese in later childhood and adult life. Evidence is conflicting about whether there is a slightly increased risk of impaired intellectual development for these infants unrelated to the occurrence of hypoglycemia.

Treatment. Management of these infants should be initiated before birth by frequent prenatal evaluation of all pregnant women with overt or gestational diabetes and by delivering their infants in hospitals where expert obstetrical and pediatric care is continuously available. Since there is no predictable relationship between the clinical course of the infant and the severity of maternal disease, all of the infants of diabetic mothers, regardless of size, should initially receive intensive observation and care. Asymptomatic infants should have their blood glucose levels determined within 1 hour of birth and then every 1 to 2 hours for the first 6 to 8 hours after birth; if well and normoglycemic, oral or gavage feedings with 10% to 20% glucose water or milk formula should be started at 2 to 3 hours of age and continued at 2-hour intervals. If there is any question about an infant's ability to tolerate oral feeding, the feedings should be discontinued and 10% to 15% intravenous glucose initiated by peripheral intravenous infusion. Blood glucose values under 30 mg/100 ml should be treated, even in asymptomatic infants, with intravenous infusions of glucose sufficient to keep the blood levels well above this level. A single intramuscular injection of glucagon (300 μg/kg), in addition to the administration of glucose, has been proposed but is not generally accepted for treatment of well, asymptomatic, large, hypoglycemic infants. The management of hypoglycemia in sick or symptomatic infants with the immediate infusion of glucose and of refractory hypoglycemia with infusion of glucose and steroids is discussed in the section on hypoglycemia (p. 441). Hypocalcemia should be treated with the intravenous infusion of calcium gluconate and the discontinuation of formulas with a high phosphate content (see treatment of tetany, p. 448). Hypomagnesemia may require intramuscular magnesium therapy as well as correction of coexistent hypocalcemia. The management of the respiratory distress syndrome is discussed on p. 360.

JOHN M. DRISCOLL, Jr.
RICHARD E. BEHRMAN

BIBLIOGRAPHY

Baird, J. D., and Farquhar, J. W.: Insulin-secreting capacity in newborn infants of normal and diabetic women, Lancet 1:71, 1962.

Beard, A., Cornblath, M., Gentz, J., Rellum, M., Person, B., Zeiterstrom, R., and Haworth, J. C.: Neonatal hypoglycemia; a discussion, J. Pediatr. 79:314, 1971.

Cornblath, M., and Schwartz, R.: Disorder of carbohydrate metabolism in infancy, Philadelphia, 1966, W. B. Saunders Co.

Farquhar, J. W.: The influence of maternal diabetes on fetus and child. In Gairdner, D., and Hull, D., editors: Recent advances in pediatrics, ed. 3, Boston, 1965, Little, Brown and Co.

Grasso, S., Messina, A., and Saprite, N.: Serum insulin response to glucose and amino acids in the premature infant, Lancet 2:755, 1968.

King, K. C., Adams, P. A. J., Clemente, G. A., and others: Infants with diabetic mothers; attenuated glucose uptake without hyperinsulinemia during continuous glucose infusion, Pediatrics 44:381, 1969.

Pederson, J.: The pregnant diabetic and her newborn; problems and management, Baltimore, 1967, The Williams & Wilkins Co.

Sinclair, J. C., and Silverman, W.: Intrauterine growth in active tissue mass of the human fetus, with particular reference to the undergrown baby, Pediatrics 38:48, 1966.

ABNORMALITIES OF CALCIUM AND MAGNESIUM METABOLISM

Calcium metabolism

Calcium represents the fifth most common organic element in the body and is involved in numerous physiologic functions. At birth, 90% of the total body calcium is present in bone and serves primarily a mechanical function. This mineralized deposit also serves as a reservoir of calcium, magnesium, phosphorus, and carbonate that can be made available to body fluids. Approximately 1% of the total body calcium is in solution in body fluids. During the neonatal period samples from cord blood have demonstrated an average serum calcium concentration of 10.5 mg/100 ml. Within a few days, the total serum calcium level decreases to a value that is characteristic for older children and adults; that is, 9.5 mg/100 ml. Of the plasma calcium 45.5% is protein bound, primarily to albumin. This protein binding is pH dependent, and a decrease in albumin binding occurs with a more acid pH. Changes in the serum albumin concentrations proportionately affect the total serum calcium concentration. The major portion of the plasma calcium is free or ionized calcium, and this represents the physiologically active component of the total serum calcium. Changes in this fraction bring about changes in neuromuscular irritability and numerous other biologic processes. In addition, certain plasma constituents affect the concentration of ionized calcium. An increase in serum bicarbonate, phosphate, citrate, and other organic anions causes a decrease in the ionized calcium, with a subsequent increase in the bound calcium. Therefore, the ionized calcium may be low in certain pathologic conditions, while the total plasma calcium concentration is normal or even increased. Because of the clinical significance of ionized calcium in biologic mechanisms and the inadequacy of present techniques for measuring this fraction, the McLean-Hastings nomogram is frequently employed to determine the value of the ionized calcium when the total serum protein and total plasma calcium values are known. However, recent work by Brown and others has demonstrated that this nomogram cannot be relied upon as a precise indicator of the serum ionized calcium in the neonatal period.

Calcium homeostasis in the fetus is primarily dependent on maternal regulatory factors, and the fetus plays an entirely passive role under normal circumstances. Wide variations in maternal nutrition have little effect on the fetal calcium, phosphorus, and skeletal growth, since the active transport of calcium and phosphorus across the placenta is almost entirely at the expense of maternal stores. Factors determining calcium homeostasis in the adult become operational in the immediate neonatal period. Calcium absorption occurs primarily in the small intestine by an active transport mechanism and to a lesser extent by simple diffusion. Absorption of calcium is dependent upon certain factors:

1. Diet—a dietary intake deficient in calcium increases the efficiency of calcium absorption, and, within limits, the percent of calcium absorbed decreases as the calcium content of the diet increases.
2. Age—in the neonate, with a rapidly growing skeletal mass, the efficiency of the transport of calcium across the intestinal mucosa is increased.
3. Vitamin D—this vitamin enhances the absorption of calcium across the intestine.
4. Intestinal pH—a low intestinal pH enhances calcium solubility and secondarily facilitates its absorption.
5. Hormones—parathyroid hormones (discussed later) enhance intestinal absorption of calcium, while the glucocorticoids inhibit calcium transport.

The principal route of calcium excretion is the kidney. Urinary calcium concentration is dependent upon:

1. Diet—urinary calcium increases exponentially with calcium consumption. An increase in the oral intake of phosphorus interferes with calcium absorption and secondarily leads to a reduction in urinary calcium excretion.
2. Serum calcium levels—when the serum calcium falls to hypocalcemic levels, the efficiency of calcium reabsorption in the proximal tubules can rise to 100%.
3. Hormones—parathyroid hormones reduce urinary calcium by increasing its tubular reabsorption. Administration of large quantities of cortisone and other glucocorticoids increases urinary calcium.

The bulk of the *inorganic phosphate* in the body is found in the skeleton in intimate association with calcium in the inorganic mineral phase of bone. Phosphorus is more widely distributed in the body than calcium, and greater fluctuations in the blood phosphorus levels occur than in the serum calcium levels. These fluctuations appear to be age related, and immediately after birth the serum phosphorus concentration begins to increase from its initial level of 5.5 mg/100 ml and reaches levels of 7 to 8 mg/100 ml within the first week of life. The absorption of phosphorus is primarily at the level of the small intestine via an active transport mechanism. Phosphorus absorption is dependent upon:

1. Diet—the efficiency of phosphate absorption is increased as phosphorus intake diminishes. The absorption of phosphate may be inhibited by excessive dietary intake of calcium, strontium, aluminum, and magnesium.
2. Hormones—parathyroid hormones stimulate phosphate absorption in the small intestine.

The excretion of phosphorus is primarily by the kidney. During the immediate neonatal period, urinary phosphate excretion is low, and data suggest that most of the filtered phosphate is reabsorbed. This decreased clearance of phosphate is presumably secondary to the relatively low glomerular filtration rate characteristic of the neonatal period. Nevertheless, renal excretion of phosphorus does depend to some degree on:

1. Diet—urinary excretion of phosphate is proportional to dietary intake.
2. Hormones—phosphate excretion is increased by parathyroid hormones.

However, as will be discussed later, the parathyroids are hypoactive during the first week of life and have little effect on phosphate reabsorption in the kidney. Growth hormones and glucocorticoids decrease phosphate excretion.

Two principal sources of *vitamin D* are available to the newborn infant. One source is through dietary ingestion of preformed vitamin D present naturally in foods or added by the manufacturer. A second source of vitamin D is available through the bioconversion of vitamin D precursors found in the skin. Vitamin D is thought to have two major biologic roles relevant to calcium and phosphorus metabolism. It is necessary for the adequate intestinal absorption of calcium. The mechanism for this absorption appears to be related to a vitamin D-directed synthesis of a calcium-binding protein in the intestinal mucosa. Although vitamin D has little effect on bone reabsorption, it is an essential cofactor of parathyroid hormone and is necessary for the action of this hormone on bone metabolism. Vitamin D requirements during the neonatal period are not well defined. The recommended dose of 400 IU of vitamin D per day provides a wide enough margin of safety to allow for individual variation in requirements.

Parathyroid hormone is normally synthesized in the parathyroid gland. The ionized fraction of the blood calcium is the important determinant of hormone secretion. The parathyroid glands respond to hypocalcemic stimulation with increased synthesis and release of hormone, and the biosynthesis is terminated under normal conditions by a negative feedback mechanism. Parathyroid hormone affects the transport of calcium and other ions in bone, kidney, and the gastrointestinal tract. The main effect of parathyroid hormone is on bone metabolism where it promotes an increased rate of release of calcium from bone into the blood, presumably by affecting the metabolism of bone osteocytes. Parathyroid hormone also has an effect on ion transport in the renal tubules where it inhibits the tubular reabsorption of phosphate and increases the renal excretion of sodium and potassium. To a lesser extent, parathyroid hormone promotes tubular reabsorption of calcium and magnesium. The gastrointestinal effects of parathyroid hormone are related to its ability to promote intestinal absorption of calcium.

Studies with human parathyroid explants have demonstrated that the parathyroids are functional by the twelfth week of gestation. Disturbances of maternal parathyroid function substantiate this intrauterine potential since such disturbances evoke appropriate responses in the fetal glands. During normal pregnancy the fetal parathyroid glands remain inactive since the calcium and phosphorus concentrations in the fetal circulation are maintained by the maternal parathyroid hormone and renal function. The increased levels of parathyroid hormone characteristic of pregnancy are capable of transplacental passage and suppression of the fetal parathyroid gland. The cause of this hyperparathyroidism of pregnancy has not been adequately explained but does not seem to be a secondary response to the demands of the growing fetus on maternal calcium stores. It may be caused by an end-organ resistance to the normal action of this hormone. This gestational hyperparathyroidism may be an explanation for the transient hypoparathyroidism that is demonstrated in the neonate during the first few days of life.

Thyrocalcitonin is a recently described polypeptide secreted by the parafollicular cells of the thyroid gland in response to elevated serum calcium levels. The hypocalcemic effect of this hormone seems to be related to its inhibition of bone reabsorption. The relationship of this important hormone to neonatal calcium and phosphorus metabolism has not yet been delineated.

Hypocalcemia

Neonatal hypocalcemia does not describe a single clinical entity, but a group of related disorders. No agreement exists as to what level of calcium constitutes hypocalcemia; this is particularly difficult to determine because the serum levels of this element vary with gestational age. For clinical purposes neonatal hypocalcemia is defined here as a total serum calcium concentration of less than 7.5 mg/100 ml.

The clinical signs and symptoms of neonatal hypocalcemia are varied and, to some degree, are related to the level of maturation of the central nervous system. During the immediate neonatal period, the signs and symptoms of hypocalcemia are subtle and may include seizures, irritability, lethargy, apnea, vomiting, and cardiovascular aberrations. In the older infant, initial signs and symptoms may include seizures, tetany, stridor, carpopedal spasms, Chvostek's and Trousseau's signs, hypertonia, edema, and disturbances of cardiac rhythm. Since none of these signs and symptoms are specific for hypocalcemia, the clinician must remain suspicious and obtain immediate laboratory confirmation to establish the diagnosis. The administration of calcium with subsequent abatement of symptoms is not sufficient for diagnosis, since calcium acts in a nonspecific manner to decrease neuromuscular irritability.

Hypocalcemia in infants of diabetic mothers. These infants have a high incidence of neonatal hypocalcemia, 25% to 50%, even when such factors as gestational age and perinatal complications are considered. The severity of the neonatal hypocalcemia correlates with the severity of the maternal diabetes. The cause of this hypocalcemia has not been fully explained. Recent observations of maternal serum calcium and phosphorus levels by Tsang and others suggest that the gestational hyperparathyroidism in maternal diabetics may be of a greater order of magnitude than in nondiabetic controls. The hypercalcemia in these mothers may lead to a greater suppression of fetal parathyroid function than in control infants, and this may be the major factor in the pathogenesis of neonatal hypocalcemia in infants of diabetic mothers. More definitive conclusions must await parathyroid hormone assays in this patient population. It should be kept in mind that infants of diabetic mothers are also more susceptible to other conditions that predispose to neonatal hypocalcemia, such as prematurity and perinatal complications.

Hypocalcemia in low birth weight infants. The association between neonatal hypocalcemia and low birth weight has been appreciated for many years. The incidence of hypocalcemia in this heterogeneous patient population is not well defined, since early studies failed to consider gestational age and, therefore, did not discriminate between the SGA and AGA low birth weight neonate. Tsang's studies demonstrated that low gestational age (32 weeks or less) was associated with hypocalcemia and that birth weight as such had a poor correlation. The mechanism of hypocalcemia in the premature infant seems to depend on several interrelated factors. These infants generally have a decreased oral intake during the first few days of life, and, as a result, the amount of calcium available for intestinal absorption is limited. In addition, and perhaps more important, diminished oral intake limits the number of calories available to these infants, necessitating breakdown of endogenous nutrients (body fat and protein) to maintain caloric requirements. This tissue breakdown results in the liberation of phosphate, which is poorly excreted by the premature because of immature renal function. The resulting hyperphosphatemia may lead to hypocalcemia. The incidence of hypocalcemia in the low birth weight infant can be diminished by early feedings and provision of adequate calories.

Hypocalcemia in traumatic labor and delivery. The incidence of hypocalcemia in the neonate is increased following complicated labor or delivery or both, even when factors such as gestational age are excluded. The explanation for this hypocalcemia is speculative. These infants have a characteristic hyperphosphatemia and hypocalcemia immediately following delivery when compared with age-matched controls. The serum changes in calcium and inorganic phosphate may be related to increased tissue breakdown or impaired placental transport of calcium and phosphate. However, most investigators hypothesize that the hyperphosphatemia represents a response to maternal or fetal adrenal gland activity or to both. During normal pregnancy, the maternal levels of 17-hydroxycorticoids are higher than those in nonpregnant women, and these levels increase further during labor. Cortisol can cross the placenta. Increased secretion of adrenocorticoids during a stressful labor and delivery may increase serum levels of inorganic phosphate and at the same time further inhibit the already compromised renal clearance of phosphate.

Hypocalcemia and congestive heart failure. Calcium plays a major role in the metabolism of the myocardium, and characteristic electrocardiographic changes are common in hypocalcemic states (p. 254). Serious cardiovascular abnormality caused by a deficiency in calcium has been reported rarely, probably because tetany occurs early and responds to appropriate treatment with calcium. Troughton and others recently reported six neonates with congestive heart failure for which no cause could be found apart from the low serum calcium level. Three of these infants had tetany, and all six patients responded to intravenous calcium therapy. Some investigators doubt the existence of this entity as a separate and distinct syndrome of neonatal hypocalcemia.

Classic neonatal tetany. In contrast to the clinical entities described above, classic tetany of the newborn usually begins after oral feedings have been started and characteristically occurs between the fifth and tenth day of life. Once feedings have been initiated, changes in the concentration of calcium and inorganic phosphate in the serum are influenced by the kind of milk the baby consumes. Gittleman and, more recently, Oppé and others measured serum calcium and inorganic phosphate in a large group of infants during the immediate neonatal period. In infants who received cow's milk formulas, the mean serum concentration of calcium fell, whereas the mean serum inorganic phosphate concentration rose. Infants who received breast milk had no significant change in the serum calcium concentration, whereas the mean serum inorganic phosphate concentration decreased. These differences in serum calcium and inorganic phosphate levels are not wholly attributable to the calcium and phosphate concentration of the milk products but, more important, are related to the calcium-to-phosphorus ratio of the solution. Infants fed cow's milk formula consume more calcium and phosphorus than do breast-fed infants, but the higher phosphate intake is associated with an increased gastrointestinal absorption of this element and a resultant hyperphosphatemia. Limitations in neonatal parathyroid and renal function compromise the infant's ability to respond to such a phosphate load, and tetany results. With the advent of artificial formulas that simulate breast milk, the incidence of classic neonatal tetany has decreased.

Parathyroid-induced hypocalcemia (maternal hyperparathyroidism). Maternal parathyroid disease induces transient functional changes in the neonate after delivery. Tetany, lasting several weeks, has been described in infants of hyperparathyroid mothers. It is not known whether the neonatal hypocalcemia is secondary to suppression of fetal parathyroid activity by elevated maternal calcium or to excess parathyroid hormone. Both calcium and parathyroid hormone readily cross the placenta and are capable of suppressing fetal parathyroid activity. Conversely, hyperparathyroidism has been reported in the offspring of a hypoparathyroid mother by Aceto and others. It is therefore important to examine maternal serum for calcium and inorganic phosphate in all cases of neonatal hypocalcemia.

Congenital absence of the parathyroid glands. Congenital absence of the parathyroid glands usually is associated with other congenital anomalies involving ectodermal defects, cardiovascular abnormalities, and thyroid dysfunction. A group of children have been described with absent parathyroid glands and thymus tissue (DiGeorge syndrome). This syndrome has been explained by defective development of structures arising from the third and fourth pharyngeal pouches. Such children have hypocalcemia in the first few days of life and demonstrate defective development of cell-mediated immunity. They are therefore susceptible to infections, primarily viral and fungal, which eventually lead to their death. Recent success with thymus transplants has been encouraging.

Congenital hypoparathyroidism. Peden reviewed seven patients with congenital hypoparathyroidism and added two additional patients. The youngest was 5 days old, and all of these infants exhibited tetany and seizures, hypocalcemia, and hyperphosphatemia. There is characteristically no evidence suggesting secondary hypoparathyroidism or pseudohypoparathyroidism; all children tested have had normal renal response to parathyroid hormone. Most reported patients have been male, suggesting a sex-linked pattern of inheritance.

Vitamin D deficiency rickets in the newborn. *Congenital rickets* is rare in Western civilization. Wide variations in maternal nutrition generally have little or no demonstrable effect on fetal skeletal development. However, congenital rickets secondary to maternal malnutrition and semistarvation continues to be recorded by workers in the Far East. Tetany and seizures are common features in these patients, and signs of scurvy are invariably present. Coutinho and others recently described two cases of congenital rickets in which the abnormality in calcium and phosphorus metabolism was associated with a previously unsuspected malabsorption syndrome in the mother.

Neonatal rickets is also uncommon in most patient populations, since milk preparations are usually fortified with vitamin D. While requirements of this vitamin have not been established for the newborn, it appears that the recommended 400 IU/day (available in 1 quart) provide a wide enough margin of safety to allow for individual variation. However, it is important to remember that the premature, SGA, and sick newborn may consume only limited amounts of formula and therefore be deficient in vitamin D intake and thus susceptible to rickets. It is recommended that these patients receive a daily vitamin D supplement containing 400 IU.

Treatment of hypocalcemia. Symptoms usually respond promptly to the intravenous administration of calcium salts. Initially 10% calcium gluconate is administered intravenously at a rate of less than 1 ml/min. A continuous electrocardiographic tracing should be available during intravenous calcium administration, and the drug should be discontinued at the first sign of bradycardia. After the acute stage, calcium should be given by mouth as chloride, 1 gm every 8 hours mixed in formula, or given by nasogastric tube. Treatment with this salt should not be continued for more than 48 hours, because calcium chloride can induce metabolic acidosis. Calcium gluconate or lactate is later substituted in a dose of 3 or 4 gm/day in three divided doses for a 4-week period. Calcium salts should be used with caution in children receiving digitalis, since the calcium ion may potentiate the effects of this drug.

Idiopathic hypercalcemia

Idiopathic hypercalcemia is a poorly defined clinical syndrome characterized by elevated serum calcium levels, without evidence of exposure to known toxic quantities of vitamin D and without evidence for hyperparathyroidism or neoplasia. The increased incidence of this disease in Great Britain during World War II, associated with increased ingestion of vitamin D by infants in the form of fortified milk products plus cod liver oil and other vitamin D concentrates, suggested that the disorder represented a form of vitamin D toxicity. However, certain features of this syndrome such as low birth weight, mental retardation, elfin faces, and cardiovascular abnormalities (p. 306) suggested that the disorder had its origin during intrauterine life. The clinical syndrome may represent an unusual susceptibility to the toxic effects of vitamin D on some fetuses. Treatment is initially directed at correction of the hypercalcemic state by discontinuing all vitamin D ingestion and by providing a diet low in calcium and a short course of steroid medication. Once the hypercalcemia is corrected, a normal diet with minimal vitamin D content may be resumed. Unfortunately, the somatic aberrations of this syndrome are not reversible.

Magnesium metabolism

Magnesium is the fourth most common cation in the body and the second most abundant intracellular cation; it is involved in numerous physiologic functions. Approximately half of the total body magnesium is present in bone, while the remainder is equally divided between muscle and nonmuscular soft tissue. The total serum magnesium concentration in the neonatal period ranges between 1.5 and 2.0 mg/100 ml. Approximately one third of the serum magnesium is protein bound, while the remainder is free or ionized. The ionized magnesium concentration may be estimated by using a nomogram when the total serum protein and total serum magnesium values are known. However, the clinical significance of the ionized magnesium levels is unknown.

During pregnancy, magnesium homeostasis is primarily dependent upon maternal regulatory factors. The fetal levels of serum magnesium exceed maternal values, and this has been explained on the basis of an active transport mechanism across the placenta. Elevation in maternal magnesium concentration results in corresponding increases in fetal levels. However, in deficiency states during pregnancy, the maternal magnesium levels are maintained at the expense of the fetus.

After birth, magnesium absorption occurs primarily in the small intestine by an active transport mechanism and to a lesser extent by passive diffusion. *Intestinal absorption* of magnesium is dependent upon several factors:

1. Diet—the percentage of magnesium absorbed depends upon the total magnesium intake. Increased consumption of calcium and phosphorus interferes with magnesium transport across the intestinal mucosa.
2. Age—in the neonate the efficiency of magnesium transport across the intestines is increased.
3. Vitamin D—this vitamin, in large doses, interferes with magnesium absorption.

The principal route of *magnesium excretion* is the kidney, and urinary magnesium concentration is dependent upon:

1. Diet—in magnesium deficiency states renal excretion of magnesium is markedly reduced.
2. Serum magnesium level—with higher serum magnesium levels there is greater urinary magnesium excretion.
3. Age—magnesium excretion is decreased in the neonate, presumably because of the decreased glomerular filtration rate characteristic of the neonatal period.
4. Hormones—hyperaldosteronism and hyperthyroidism result in increased urinary excretion of magnesium. Parathyroid hormone decreases the urinary excretion of this element.

Hypomagnesemia

Neonatal hypomagnesemia does not describe a single clinical entity, but a group of related disorders that have in common a low serum magnesium level. The clinical signs and symptoms of neonatal magnesium deficiency are nonspecific and may mimic the clinical findings previously described for hypocalcemia. In the immediate neonatal period, the clinical picture includes neuromuscular hyperexcitability, muscle twitching, and seizure activity. The older child may have tetany, ataxia, vertigo, muscle weakness, tremors, depression, or psychotic behavior. Since magnesium deficiency may be clinically indistinguishable from hypocalcemia, the ECG may be a helpful adjunct in distinguishing between these two syndromes. Depression of the S-T segments and inversion of the T waves in the precordial leads of the ECG occur in magnesium deficiency. The two syndromes can be definitely distinguished only by measurements of the serum content of each of these elements. A serum magnesium value below 1.5 mg/100 ml is diagnostic for hypomagnesemia.

Hypomagnesemia secondary to maternal hyperparathyroidism. Neonatal hypomagnesemia may occur in the offspring of hyperparathyroid mothers. Several infants have been reported in whom the hypocalcemia and hyperphosphatemia responded to calcium therapy, while the neurologic abnormalities and depressed magnesium level responded only to magnesium supplements. Familial hypoparathyroidism is associated with depressed levels of serum magnesium, presumably secondary to the hyperphosphatemia and deposition of magnesium phosphate in tissue stores.

Hypomagnesemia secondary to maternal magnesium deficiency. Neonatal hypomagnesemia has been reported in one infant born to a mother with chronic hypomagnesemia secondary to celiac disease of 16 years' duration. In experimental animals magnesium deficiency during pregnancy is associated with neonatal hypomagnesemia.

Hypomagnesemia secondary to magnesium malabsorption. A group of male infants have been reported who experienced neurologic abnormalities in the neonatal period that were attributable to hypomagnesemia without hypocalcemia. Balance studies in these infants documented specific malabsorption of magnesium. All symptoms responded to magnesium supplements, which were required throughout infancy. Infants undergoing surgical manipulation of the gastrointestinal tract are likewise susceptible to magnesium deficiency, presumably because of interference with magnesium absorption in the proximal jejunum.

Hypomagnesemia in infants of diabetic mothers. Infants of diabetic mothers may develop neonatal hypomagnesemia. In addition to depressed serum magnesium levels, such children frequently demonstrate hypocalcemia and hyperphosphatemia. The calcium and phosphorus abnormalities invariably respond to calcium therapy, but magnesium supplements may be necessary for cessation of neurologic abnormalities.

Hypomagnesemia secondary to miscellaneous causes. Exchange transfusions performed with acid-citrate blood may result in postexchange hypomagnesemia. Magnesium depletion of a severe degree has been documented in protein-calorie malnutrition, following intensive diuretic therapy, hyperthyroidism, and hyperaldosteronism. However, hypomagnesemia as a complication of these clinical conditions has not been documented in the neonatal period.

Treatment of hypomagnesemia. Hypomagnesemia is treated with magnesium salts given orally or parenterally or both. The suggested initial treatment for hypomagnesemia consists of 0.5 ml of 50% magnesium sulfate given intramuscularly. If the dose is given intravenously, it should be infused cautiously over a 10-minute period, with electrocardiographic monitoring to detect acute cardiovascular disturbances such as prolongation of atrioventricular conduction. The dose of magnesium may be repeated every 8 hours, depending on the clinical course of the infant. Maintenance doses, if necessary, may be given orally in the form of sulfate, lactate, chloride, or citrate. Assuming a normal intestinal absorption, the therapeutic dose is approximately 0.25 ml/kg of 50% magnesium sulfate. This should be diluted to a 10% concentration. In malabsorptive states, 1.25 ml/kg of a 50% magnesium sulfate solution diluted appropriately is required and should be continued for an indefinite period of time.

Hypermagnesemia

Magnesium sulfate continues to be used in the management of toxemia of pregnancy. Unfortunately, magnesium administered to the mother crosses the placenta and may result in markedly elevated magnesium levels in the neonate. Affected infants usually manifest evidence of depressed respirations and profound muscle weakness. Conservative management of these newborn infants by maintaining ventilation and fluid and electrolyte balance will generally result in a marked clinical improvement by 24 to 36 hours of age.

WILLIAM SPECK

BIBLIOGRAPHY

Aceto, T., and others: Intrauterine hyperparathyroidism; a complication of untreated maternal hypoparathyroidism, J. Clin. Endocrinol. Metab. **26**:487, 1966.

Brown, D. M., and others: Serum ionized calcium in newborn infants, Pediatrics **49**:341, 1972.

Coutinho, M., and others: Maternal malabsorption presenting as congenital rickets, Lancet **1**: 1049, 1968.

Cushard, W. G., and others: Physiologic hyperparathyroidism in pregnancy, J. Clin. Endocrinol. Metab. **34**:767, 1972.

Gittleman, I. F., and others: Influence of diet on the occurrence of hyperphosphatemia and hypocalcemia in the newborn infant, Pediatrics **8**: 778, 1951.

Oppé, T. E., and others: Calcium and phosphorus levels in healthy newborn infants given various types of milk, Lancet **1**:1045, 1968.

Peden, V. H.: True idiopathic hypoparathyroidism as a sex linked recessive trait, Am. J. Hum. Genet. **12**:323, 1960.

Stromme, J. H., Nesbakken, R., Normann, T., and others: Familial hypomagnesemia, Acta Paediatr. Scand. **58**:433, 1969.

Troughton, O., and others: Heart failure and neonatal hypocalcemia, Br. Med. J. **4**:76, 1972.

Tsang, R. C., and Oh, W.: Neonatal hypocalcemia in low birth weight infants, Pediatrics **45**:773, 1970.

Tsang, R. C., and others: Hypocalcemia in infants of diabetic mothers, J. Pediatr. **80**:384, 1972.

Wacker, W. E. C., and Paris, A. F.: Magnesium metabolism, N. Engl. J. Med. **278**:658, 712, 772, 1968.

INFANTS OF ADDICTED MOTHERS

The increasing use of drugs in our society has produced a unique problem in newborn infants of addicted mothers. Its magnitude is unknown, but it is estimated that the incidence of addicted infants has increased in recent years from 1 out of 200 deliveries to 1 out of 50 deliveries in some large urban hospitals. In addition, in the 1960s the incidence was largely confined to urban populations, but now many suburban communities face similar problems. Though heroin is the most common agent, addiction to methadone, cocaine, barbiturates, and amphetamines has also increased.

The addicted mother and her fetus are exposed to a broad spectrum of medical and obstetrical complications. The pregnant addict has an increased incidence of fetal wastage and seldom receives adequate antenatal care; in most studies, the number of antepartum visits has averaged one to two per gestation. To support her habit, the addicted mother turns to prostitution and thereby exposes her fetus to the risk of venereal disease. Other obstetrical problems commonly associated with addiction include prematurity, toxemia, abruptio placentae, premature rupture of membranes, and breech presentations. In most series, approximately 50% of infants born to addicted mothers have birth weights less than 2,500 gm; 40% of that group are full-term infants who are SGA and the remainder are premature infants, some of whom will also be SGA. Despite the increased incidence of prematurity, few of these infants develop the idiopathic respiratory distress syndrome or jaundice so commonly associated with prematurity. Animal experiments have shown that while heroin does not induce surfactant, it does produce increased hepatic bilirubin glucuronyl transferase activity. There is no statistically significant incidence of congenital anomalies, despite some evidence of chromosomal breakage in addicted populations.

Clinical presentation. After delivery, the number of infants who will become symptomatic is related to the duration of the mother's habit, the severity of her habit, and the timing of her last dose in relation to her delivery. The higher the mother's dose, the longer her addiction, and the closer her last dose was to delivery, the more likely her infant is to develop withdrawal symptoms. Approximately 70% of infants born to heroin addicts will become symptomatic, with 60% of them developing their symptoms within the first 24 hours of life; the remainder generally display signs within 4 days of birth. When the onset of symptoms occurs after the first 24 hours, the need for treatment is more likely. Rarely, symptoms may be delayed until 7 to 10 days of life.

Below is a list of the signs and symptoms most frequently observed in infants of addicted mothers. The tremors, hyperactivity, and flailing movements of these infants frequently produce abrasions of the face, knees, and knuckles. The characteristic prolonged, persistent, high-pitched cry readily identifies the affected infant in the nursery. Despite ravenous appetites, these infants frequently feed poorly, with subsequent poor weight gain. Less commonly, affected infants have excessive tearing, increased salivation, and sneezing. Some infants have developed tachypnea, probably of central origin, with a concomitant respiratory alkalosis. Diarrhea, through an infrequent problem, may be the most difficult symptom to control.

SIGNS AND SYMPTOMS OF INFANTS OF ADDICTED MOTHERS

Tremors
Irritability
Seizures
Poor feeding or vomiting or both
Hypertonicity
High-pitched cry
Sneezing
Fever
Diarrhea; dehydration
Stuffy nose

Diagnosis. Because most symptoms are easily controlled with therapy and since delays in diagnosis are associated with increased morbidity and mortality, nursery staffs must be familiar with symptoms of withdrawal to facilitate early diagnosis. A problem in the differential diagnosis of the addicted infant is the separation of the hyperactive, tremulous infant from others with actual seizure disorders; an electroencephalogram may be helpful. Hypoglycemia and hypocalcemia commonly are seen clinically as tremors and must be excluded in all infants undergoing withdrawal. The poor feeder and the infant with diarrhea should be evaluated for sepsis. Because of the increased incidence of venereal disease in addicted mothers, all infants should be routinely screened for congenital syphilis and gonococcal ophthalmia. A careful maternal history should identify the infant with neonatal hyperthyroidism. Congenital pneumonia and aspiration syndromes also must be considered in tachypneic infants.

When there is any question of a baby's having withdrawal symptoms, a thorough history must be obtained from the mother. Contrary to general belief, most addicted mothers are genuinely concerned about their infants and will frankly discuss their habits to assure better care for the infant. Mothers and infants should be reported to the appropriate social agency to mobilize all the assistance possible for the involved family. Routine screening of the infant's urine for morphine derivatives or dilutants commonly mixed with heroin may readily identify the occasional infant whose mother refuses to admit her habit. Other facts in the maternal history that may identify the addicted mother include a history of thrombophlebitis, multiple skin infections or hepatitis, a resistance to analgesia during labor, or a rush to leave the hospital after delivery.

Treatment. Not all infants who become symptomatic require treatment, but in most large series 75% of such infants have been treated. Many drugs have been used to treat addicted infants, but phenobarbital (5 to 8 mg/kg/day) is the most commonly used agent. Effective but limited experience has been reported with paregoric USP (3 to 6 drops every 3 to 4 hours), chlorpromazine hydrochloride (Thorazine) (2.2 mg/kg/day), diazepam (Valium) (1 to 2 mg every 8 hours), and methadone (0.3 to 0.4 mg/kg/day). Infants with diarrhea as part of their withdrawal syndrome will often require both paregoric and parenteral fluids to control their symptoms. The duration of required treatment may range from 7 to 40 days. Generally, once symptoms have been controlled, therapy should be maintained at that level for 2 to 4 days and then gradually tapered. With recurrence of symptoms, dosage should be increased to the previously effective level for several days before tapering a second time. In Zelson's series, 22.5% were treated less than 10 days, 49.5% for 10 to 20 days, and 28% for 28 to 40 days.

Methadone and phenobarbital addiction

Different neonatal withdrawal symptoms have been described for infants addicted to phenobarbital and methadone. Infants delivered to mothers addicted to phenobarbital or to mothers being treated medically with other barbiturates have withdrawal symptoms similar to heroin-addicted infants. But the barbiturate-addicted infants are usually full-term and AGA. They have later onset of symptoms (4 to 7 days) and longer duration of signs. Infants of medically treated mothers appear to have milder symptoms lasting for shorter periods than infants of addicted mothers. Barbiturate-addicted infants usually respond well to treatment with phenobarbital (5 mg/kg/day).

From the obstetrical viewpoint, mothers in methadone treatment programs receive better antenatal care than mothers who are heroin addicts. However, despite earlier reports suggesting milder withdrawal symptoms in infants of methadone-treated mothers, more recent evidence suggests a higher incidence of symptoms, more severe signs of withdrawal, and a longer duration of symptoms. Birth weights and Apgar scores are similar to those of heroin-addicted infants. All infants are treated initially with phenobarbital (5 to 8 mg/kg/day), but occasionally infants require methadone to control symptoms. No longitudinal studies on infants who have received methadone are available.

Prognosis. Prior to treatment of withdrawal, infant mortality ranged from 17% to 90%; but with the advent of therapy, mortality has been lowered to the range of 3% to 34%. No long-term follow-up studies are available on the ultimate outcome for these infants. However, there is recent, disquieting evidence that maternal addiction may have adverse effects on behavioral development in these infants. With proper identification of the infant at risk and early treatment, death should be an infrequent occurrence.

JOHN M. DRISCOLL, Jr.

BIBLIOGRAPHY

Desmond, M. M., Schwanecke, R. P., Wilson, G. S., Yasunaga, S., and Burgdorff, I.: Maternal barbiturate utilization and neonatal withdrawal symptomatology, J. Pediatr. **80**:190, 1972.

Nathenson, G., Golden, G. S., and Litt, I. F.: Diazepam in the management of the neonatal narcotics withdawal syndrome, Pediatrics **48**:523, 1971.

Perlmutter, J. F.: Drug addiction in pregnant women, Am. J. Obstet. Gynecol. **79**:569, 1967.

Rajegowda, B. K., Glass, L., Evans, H. E., Maso, G., Swartz, D. P., and LeBlanc, W.: Methadone withdrawal in newborn infants, J. Pediatr. **81**:532, 1972.

Zelson, C., Rubio, E., and Wasserman, E.: Neonatal narcotic addiction; 10 year observation, Pediatrics **48**:178, 1971.

THYROID

Thyroid disorders of neonates must be considered in the light of many physiologic factors that influence the fetal and neonatal thyroid function. These include embryogenesis of thyroid, action of thyroid hormones, synthesis and transport of these hormones, regulatory mechanisms of thyroid function, fetal-maternal relationships, and the dynamic alteration of thyroid function with birth. These physiologic aspects, many of which are unique to neonates, are important in understanding the pathophysiology of neonatal thyroid disorders, in approaching diagnosis, in interpreting laboratory data, in treating the infant, and in assigning prognosis.

Embryogenesis of thyroid

The major portion of human thyroid originates from the median anlage, which arises from the pharyngeal floor and is identifiable in the 17-day-old embryo. Initially, the median anlage is in close contact with the endothelial tubes of the embryonic heart. Following the descent of the heart, the rapidly growing median thyroid is progressively pulled caudally until it reaches its definitive level in front of the second to sixth tracheal ring. Some investigators have suggested that the descent of the heart influences the downward movement of thyroid, probably because of its topographic contact. Usually the median anlage grows caudally so that no lumen is left in the tract of its descent. Ectopic thyroid and persistent thyroglossal duct or cyst are the results of abnormalities of the thyroid descent. The lateral parts of the descending median anlage expand to form the thyroid lobes and the isthmus.

The second anlage of the thyroid is composed of a pair of ultimobranchial bodies arising from caudal extension of the fourth pharyngeal pouch. This anlage is initially connected to the pharynx by the ductus pharyngobranchialis IV (late seventh week). Subsequently the pharyngeal connection is lost and the ductal lumen becomes obliterated. The ultimobranchial bodies are incorporated into the expanding lateral lobes of the median anlage. The contribution of ultimobranchial bodies to the ultimate thyroid tissue is small, and its differentiation appears to require the influence of median anlage. There is a growing body of evidence to suggest that the cells arising from ultimobranchial bodies are identifiable as parafollicular cells or C-cells in mammals and that these cells are the source of thyrocalcitonin. However, confirmation of these observations in man is still lacking.

By the latter part of the tenth week the histiogenesis of the thyroid is virtually complete, although the follicles do not contain colloid. A single layer of epithelial cells surrounds the follicular lumen. Thyroxine has been detected in the serum of a 78-day-old fetus. Thus, the fetal thyroid contributes to the fetal requirement of thyroidal hormones by the beginning of the second trimester. The pituitary regulatory mechanism of the fetal thyroid may begin to operate at this stage, as evidenced by the detection of thyroid-stimulating hormone (TSH) in the same fetal blood.

Physiologic action of thyroid hormones

The principal function of the thyroid is to synthesize, store, and release the classic thyroid hormones, thyroxine (T_4) and triiodothyronine (T_3), into the circulation. T_3 has one less iodine atom than T_4 and is more potent than T_4 in its physiologic action; this is caused by its greater speed of action rather than a qualitative difference in its metabolic effects. Therefore, physiologic action of these two hormones need not be considered separately.

One of the principal actions of T_4 is to stimulate the rate of cellular oxidation in a large variety of tissues, leading to increased oxygen consumption, liberation of carbon dioxide, and production of heat. Changes in the basal metabolic rate (BMR) in hypothyroidism and hyperthyroidism, of course, are well known. This action of T_4, in turn, may be mediated through increased microsomal protein synthesis. Clinically the calorigenic action of T_4 affects the circulation by increasing the heart rate, stroke volume, and cardiac output. The pulse pressure is widened mainly by a decrease in the diastolic pressure and by some elevation in the systolic pressure. Circulation time is shortened. In hypothyroidism the ECG may show decreased voltage of all complexes, prolongation of the P-R interval, and depression or inversion of the T wave. The effect on the ECG, however, may be secondary to myxedema of the myocardium.

Thyroxine affects protein metabolism. There is a negative nitrogen balance in hyperthyroidism, unless the patient is protected by adequate caloric intake to cover the increased energy requirement. In severe hypothyroidism, deposition of a mucoprotein containing hyaluronic acid occurs in extracellular myxedematous fluid.

Thyroxine influences the incorporation of creatine into the phosphocreatine cycle. In hypothyroidism, there appears to be an excessive storage of creatine, and in hyperthyroidism, the urinary excretion of creatine is increased. However, the total excretion of creatine and creatinine is not affected by T_4. Thus, T_4 changes the urinary creatine and creatinine ratio; creatine accounts for 10% to 30% in the normal child, 0% to 10% in hypothyroidism, and 25% to 65% in hyperthyroidism.

The effect of T_4 on lipid metabolism can be seen by an elevated serum cholesterol level in hypothyroidism, except in infants. The total neutral fats, fatty acids, and phospholipids of the serum are also increased in hypothyroidism.

Thyroxine also affects the metabolism of carbohydrates, calcium, vitamins, and water and the liver function. The rate of glucose absorption and use is increased by T_4. In hypothyroidism, hypercalcemia may occur, the serum carotene level may be high, and the glucuronic acid conjugation mechanism of the liver may be impaired. Retention of water in the extracellular compartment occurs in hypothyroidism, producing the myxedematous fluid. In hyperthyroidism, on the other hand, increased calcium excretion in the urine and feces may lead to demineralization of the bones.

Another principal action of T_4 and T_3 is their effect on growth and development. Thyroidectomy in neonatal monkeys results in defective growth and development of the brain; and in untreated cretinism, mental retardation often ensues. The degree of mental retardation in cretinism is related to the severity and duration of the hypothyroid state of the infant whose brain is growing. The brain is more susceptible to lack of the thyroid hormones during its rapid growth and development, while defective growth and permanent damage do not occur if hypothyroidism begins after morphologic maturation of the brain is completed.

Other aspects of growth and development also require thyroid hormones. When hypothyroidism occurs in childhood, dental eruption, linear growth, and skeletal maturation are retarded. The retardation of skeletal maturation results in immature skeletal proportions and immature facial contours and contributes to the characteristic body configuration of hypothyroidism, which is different from that seen in stunted growth caused by isolated growth hormone deficiency. Ossification of cartilage is also disturbed in hypothyroidism. This produces the characteristic picture of epiphyseal dysgenesis in x-ray films of the ossifying epiphyseal centers.

Thyroxine also affects the peripheral nerves. In hypothyroidism, the relaxation phase of the ankle and knee jerk reflexes is prolonged. In hyperthyroidism, sympathetic and autonomic response may be exaggerated.

In addition to the classic thyroid hormones, T_4 and T_3, a calcium-lowering principle is found in the thyroid gland. This principle has been named thyrocalcitonin or calcitonin. Although thyrocalcitonin has hypocalcemic and hypophosphatemic actions when administered to man, its physiologic role is not yet understood. Thyroidectomy does not lead to hypercalcemia.

Synthesis, release, transport, and utilization of thyroid hormones

The biologically active thyroid hormones, L-thyroxine (T_4) and 3,5,3′-triiodothyronine (T_3) are iodinated amino acids. Their synthesis occurs exclusively within the follicular cells.

Iodine is supplied to the body mainly through dietary intake. However, it can be absorbed readily from the skin and lungs. Thus, application of iodine-containing ointment or lotion to the skin can result in misleadingly high protein-bound iodine (PBI) levels. Although some organic iodine compounds, including T_4 and T_3, can be absorbed unchanged from the gastrointestinal tract, most are reduced and absorbed as ionic iodide. Generally, one fourth to one third of ingested iodide is taken up by the thyroid, which constitutes the basis for ^{131}I uptake studies. This iodide-trapping mechanism involves an active transport process, an iodide pump that is dependent on oxidative phosphorylation. The iodide pump is present both at the basal and apical surfaces of follicular cells, the former serving to concentrate iodide into the cells from the extracellular space and the latter serving to pump iodide into the follicular lumen as a secondary reservoir. The mechanism is capable of maintaining the intrathyroidal iodide concentration some 20-fold to 100-fold higher than that of serum. In one type of goitrous cretinism there is a defect in this iodide transport mechanism.

Immediately upon entering the follicular cells, iodide is oxidized to an active form for iodination of thyroglobulin, probably by a peroxidase enzyme system. Thyroglobulin, a glycoprotein, is snythesized by the ribosomes of the follicular cells and is then secreted into the follicular lumen. Almost all of the iodine taken up by the thyroid is rapidly incorporated into the 3-position and the 5-position of the many tyrosyl residues of thyroglobulin to form monoiodotyrosine (MIT) and diiodotyrosine (DIT). Once iodide is organically bound to the tyrosyl residues, it can no longer be released readily from the thyroid. Defects in the iodide organification can be seen in two types of goitrous cretinism.

Synthesis of T_3 requires coupling between MIT and DIT molecules, accompanied by elimination of an alanine residue. Thyroxine is formed by coupling between two molecules of DIT. These reactions appear to occur within the structure of thyroglobulin and involve oxidative processes. Several patients with goitrous hypothyroidism caused by a coupling defect have been described.

Secretion of T_4 and T_3 into the circulation requires liberation of these moieties from the peptide bonds. Thyroglobulin molecules pass from the lumen of the follicles into the follicular cells where proteolysis takes place. Congenital hypothyroidism may occur as a result of abnormal proteolysis of thyroglobulin. Of the approximately 125 tyrosyl residues in the thyroglobulin, only 10 or so form iodothyronines, while another 20 consists of MIT and DIT. Following proteolysis of thyroglobulin, the freed MIT and DIT are deiodinated by the iodotyrosine deiodinase, and the liberated iodide is reused by the thyroid for iodination. A defective deiodination mechanism of free iodotyrosines results in wastage and depletion of iodine from release of these molecules into the circulation and subsequent excretion into the urine and thus brings about goitrous cretinism.

Thyroxine and T_3 secreted into the circulation are transported by loosely attaching, through noncovalent bonds, to the plasma proteins. Three proteins play a role in the transport system. Over 75% of T_4 is normally bound to thyroxine-binding globulin (TBG). The second carrier protein is the T_4-binding prealbumin (TBPA); only about 15% of T_4 is bound to TBPA. The third protein is the serum albumin, which usually carries less than 10% of the circulating T_4. Whereas T_4 binds with all three proteins, T_3 binds only with TBG and albumin, and its intensity of binding is considerably less than that of T_4. The protein-bound thyroid hormones are biologically inactive and are in equilibrium with active nonprotein-bound hormones. If the capacity of TBG is increased, a rise in the concentration of total hormone will follow, and the concentration of free hormone will be maintained at the normal level.

The exact mechanism by which free T_4 exerts its biologic effect is not known. Recent studies suggest that a significant proportion of T_4 undergoes peripheral deiodination to produce T_3. It has been speculated that T_3 may be the active form of iodothyronines at the cellular level. Catabolism of iodothyronines involves further deiodination, deamination, decarboxylation, and conjugation.

Regulatory mechanism of thyroid function

The major control mechanism of thyroid function is the hypothalamic-pituitary-thyroid axis with its negative feedback mechanism. The basophilic cells of the anterior pituitary gland produce and store thyrotropin (TSH), which is a glycoprotein capable of rapidly increasing the intrathyroidal cyclic adenosine-3′,5′-monophosphate (AMP). It causes increased uptake of iodine by the thyroid, accelerates virtually all steps of iodothyronine synthesis and release, and increases the size and vascularity of the thyroid gland. It has been suggested that these changes may be mediated by the increase in cyclic AMP. The secretion and the plasma level of TSH is inversely related to the levels of free (nonprotein-bound) thyroid hormones. The inhibitory feedback action of free iodothyronines involves a direct action of these hormones on the pituitary gland without involving the hypothalamus. Thus the secretion of TSH is directly regulated through an intrinsic mechanism of the pituitary gland that is sensitive to the levels of free iodothyronines. On the other hand, the hypothalamus does influence the TSH secretion. The hypothalamus secretes a neurohumoral factor, the thyrotropin-releasing factor (TRF), which stimulates the release of TSH by the pituitary gland. The hypothalamus regulates the set point of feedback control as a thermostat through TRF. This control can be seen in neonates whose circulating T_4 becomes rapidly elevated when exposed to a cold environment.

In addition to the hypothalamic-pituitary regulation, the thyroid is responsive to an intrinsic autoregulatory mechanism, the intrathyroidal iodide, which compensates for the fluctuation in dietary iodine intake. Glucocorticoids also appear to inhibit the thyroid function. However, clinically significant hypothyroidism rarely, if ever, occurs following prolonged administration of large amounts of glucocorticoids or ACTH.

Commonly used chemical thyroid function tests

Protein-bound iodine (PBI)

In the PBI test, serum or plasma proteins are precipitated, organic iodine is converted to iodide, and the total iodide is quantitated. Usually T_4 accounts for 80% to 90% of the PBI. Since this test measures the total iodide, it is influenced not only by the T_4 level but also by the levels of inorganic iodine, organic iodine (including MIT and DIT), and iodothyronine-binding proteins. Administration of T_3 results in a fall of PBI; it suppresses the endogenous T_4 secretion, and it contributes little to the serum iodine since it is administered in small quantities because of its much greater biologic activity compared with T_4. The availability of T_4-binding sites on TBG also affects the PBI. Diphenylhydantoin (Dilantin) competes with T_4 at the TBG-binding sites, while diphenylhydantoin and salicylates displace T_4 from the TBPA-binding sites. Thus these drugs are capable of depressing the PBI value.

Butanol-extractable iodine (BEI)

In this method, serum is acidified, and protein-bound T_4 is extracted with butanol. Some iodinated proteins are insoluble in butanol and thus eliminated. The extract is then washed to remove inorganic iodide, MIT, and DIT. The iodine content in the butanol extract is measured as in the PBI. Most of the exogenous forms of organic iodine, however, are soluble in butanol and hence give rise to a falsely elevated PBI. Changes in the iodothyronine-binding proteins of the plasma also affect the BEI determination as they do the PBI. The consistent difference between PBI and BEI has been observed. This difference consists of butanol-insoluble iodine (BII) and represents hormonally inactive iodoproteins, commonly of thyroid origin. In normal serum, BII accounts for 10% to 25% of the total organic iodine. BII is often increased in goitrous cretinism because of inborn errors of thyroxine synthesis, hyperthyroidism, and thyroiditis.

T_4-column

The most commonly used procedure employs an anion-exchange resin to separate the protein-bound T_4 from other organic and inorganic iodine in serum or plasma. The eluted fraction containing T_4 obtained from this chromatographic step is subjected to quantitative iodide determination. This iodide content is referred to as thyroxine-iodine (T_4-I). The difference between T_4-I measured by this method and PBI is about equal to BII. Although iodotyrosines and most of the inorganic and organic iodines do not interfere with T_4-I determination, organic iodine is not completely eliminated. Nevertheless, this method is superior in its specificity to that of BEI. Changes in the T_4-binding capacity of the plasma proteins affect T_4-I measured by this method as in the PBI and BEI. Inorganic iodine, which crosses the placental barrier, administered in a large dose can falsely elevate T_4-I through nonspecific iodination of plasma proteins. Iodine contamination also occurs from iodinated dyes used as x-ray contrast media. Iiophenoxic acid (Teridax), formerly used for gallbladder series, has been shown to cross the placenta and interfere with T_4 determination for many years.

T_4 by competitive protein binding (Murphy-Pattee test)

The Murphy-Pattee method of assessing T_4-I does not depend on iodine determination. The method involves reacting a crude extract of the patient's T_4 with standardized human TBG saturated with radioactive T_4. The T_4 in the extract competitively displaces the radioactive T_4 from TBG in proportional amounts. The bound and the newly freed radioactive T_4 is separated, and the radioactivity in each fraction is measured. Comparison of these measurements against a standard curve permits the patient's T_4 level to be expressed in terms of μg of T_4-I per 100 ml. The value obtained by the Murphy-Pattee method is identical to that obtained by the T_4-column assay in the absence of an interfering substance. The nature of the competitive protein-binding assay eliminates the interference by exogenous iodinated substances. However, interference by changes in T_4-binding capacity of the plasma proteins, including the competitive displacement of endogenous T_4 from the binding proteins by diphenylhydantoin, salicylates, and T_3, can be predicted to affect the Murphy-Pattee test. The normal values in the neonatal period range from 8.2 to 16.6 mg T_4 per 100 ml.

Free thyroxine

The four methods described above largely measure the biologically inactive protein-bound T_4. In contrast, the minute amounts of free T_4 (FT_4) in the serum cannot be determined by conventional analytic technique. The method of estimating the FT_4 depends on the fact that the level of FT_4 is governed by an equilibrium between the levels of binding proteins, protein-bound T_4, and FT_4, following the law of mass action. FT_4 does not depend on the T_4-binding capacity as such, since a change in such capacity will soon be compensated by a concordant change in the amount of T_4 released from the thyroid. To estimate the FT_4, serum is equilibrated with a tracer dose of radioactive T_4, which apportions itself between free and bound forms in the same ratio as that of the endogenous hormone. The dialyzable fraction of the labeled serum contains the radioactive FT_4 in amounts proportional to the endogenous FT_4. The concentration of FT_4 in the serum is calculated as the product of the total T_4-I and the dialyzable fraction. In normal serum, FT_4 averages about 2 $m\mu g$/100 ml.

Assessment of thyroxine-binding protein saturation

T_3-resin uptake. A tracer dose of radioactive T_3, which competes for the binding sites with the endogenous hormones, is added to the serum. When the specimen is passed through resin, the unbound radioactive T_3 is absorbed on the resin and can be measured by a radioassay. The amount of radioactive T_3 taken up by the resin is inversely proportional to the unsaturated T_4-binding capacity of the plasma proteins. The normal range, in the neonate, is 66% to 114% of the standard.

TBG test. Since the major portion of plasma T_4 is bound to TBG, measurement of the binding capacity of TBG gives a good approximation of T_4-binding protein capacity. In this method, the serum is equilibrated with a large excess of radioactive T_4. By relating the proportion of radioactive T_4 in the TBG area to the T_4-I, it is possible to estimate the TBG values in terms of μg of T_4-binding capacity per 100 ml of serum. The binding capacity of TBG is increased by estrogens and, therefore, in pregnancy and neonates. It may be increased in acute hepatitis and in a genetic disorder (p. 468). It is decreased by administration of androgens or glucocorticoids. In the nephrotic syndrome, chronic hepatic disease, and a sex-linked genetic disorder, it is also decreased. Diphenylhydantoin competes with the T_4-binding sites of TBG and gives a falsely low value. In all these circumstances T_3-resin uptake is inversely related to the TBG test. T_3-resin uptake is increased by administration of salicylates, since this drug competes with T_4 at the TBPA-binding sites.

Thyroid function; fetal-maternal relationship

Thyroxine is detectable in the fetal serum by the twelfth week of gestation. Thereafter, both the total T_4-I and FT_4 increase linearly in relation to the gestational age. At term, the T_4-I reaches a level of 12.6 ± 4.0 (S.D.) μg/100 ml in the umbilical cord serum, which is 10% to 20% lower than the corresponding value in maternal serum. The FT_4 in the cord blood is equal to or higher than in the maternal blood. TSH is also present in the 12-week-old fetus and rapidly rises thereafter, paralleling the increasing levels of FT_4. It does not correlate with levels of fetal T_4-I or the maternal FT_4. The TSH level is higher in the fetus than in the mother, and at term the fetal value is more than twice that found in the mother. This suggests that fetal TSH regulates fetal thyroid function.

Thyroxine-binding proteins also can be detected in the 12-week-old fetus. During early fetal life, T_4 seems to be bound mainly to the TBPA and albumin. The fetal concentration of TBG increases rapidly and by midgestation reaches a level close to that of a full-term infant. During early gestation the rise of fetal TBG parallels the increase in T_4-I, and the proportion of T_4 bound to TBG similarly increases during this period. The binding capacity of TBG in premature and full-term infants is close to 1½ times that of the normal adult but is lower than that of the mother. The high level of TBG in the neonate is caused by a transplacental transfer of estrogens from the mother and, to a large extent, accounts for the high PBI or T_4-I values in these infants. The level of TBPA is low in both newborn and maternal sera. The TBPA probably plays a minor role after midgestation.

The ability of fetal and newborn thyroids to take up iodine is much greater than that of the adult. This observation and the relatively high FT_4 in serum from the umbilical cord suggest that the thyroid function at birth in the full-term infant is in a hyperactive state. Shortly after birth a transient but marked hyperactivity occurs in the thyroid function. Within the first minutes of life an acute release of TSH occurs; this reaches a peak level between 15 and 30 minutes after delivery and then falls slowly over the following 72 hours. There is evidence that this acute rise of TSH may be stimulated by the drop in body temperature of the fetus with birth.

The levels of PBI, T_4-I, T_3-resin uptake, and FT_4 increase progressively during the first hours of extrauterine life, reaching a peak by about 48 hours of age. Thereafter, the levels remain comparable to the hyperthyroid range for adults during the ensuing 2 weeks. For example, during the first 1 to 3 days, PBI may be as high as 16.8 μg per 100 ml, and FT_4 13.2 mμg/100 ml. These changes are not accompanied by a change in TBG or TBPA levels and are caused by the marked increase in the serum TSH concentration. The level of PBI gradually falls after the first 2 weeks of life until the child reaches puberty. During this period PBI and T_4-I concentrations are age and sex dependent. At 1 months of age the mean PBI level is 6.3 μg/100 ml in the male and 6.7 μg/100 ml in the female, with 5% and 95% limits of 4.7 to 7.9 and 5.1 to 8.3 μg/100 ml for the respective sex.

Iodine kinetics in infants and children are also different from those in the adult. The thyroid weighs about 2 gm at birth, which is about one tenth of the adult weight. The 24-hour ^{131}I uptake by the thyroid is similar to that of the adult after the first month of age. Thus, the concentration of ^{131}I per gm of thyroid tissue in the infant is greater than that in the adult. The thyroid of the infant is more susceptible to damage by radiation. The T_4 turnover rate is also higher in infants and children than in the adult. This accounts for the greater thyroid hormone requirement in children per unit of body weight.

In considering the fetal-maternal relationship, the placenta is of major importance. Recently a thyrotropic substance, human chorionic placental thyrotropin (HCT), was discovered. The role of HCT in the fetal thyroid function, however, has not been established. TSH does not cross the placental barrier. The placenta is almost completely impermeable to T_4 during the early stage of pregnancy, and at term the T_4 transport across the placenta is slow and limited. Thus the fetus during the first trimester either does not require T_4 for its growth and development or is totally dependent on small amounts of maternal T_4. During the later stages of gestation, the fetus is largely dependent on his own T_4 production. The maternal T_4, at best, can only supplement the fetal supply.

Iodides can cross the placenta readily. Iodides or iodine when given in a large quantity produce a transient inhibition of

T_4 synthesis by diminishing the iodination process, probably through its effect on thyroidal autoregulation. Thus, in rare instances, iodine given to the mother in large amounts has produced goiter in the offspring.

Other clinically important compounds that can affect the fetal thyroid function by crossing the placenta from mother to fetus are the antithyroid compounds (goitrogens) and the long-acting thyroid stimulator (LATS). The former include perchlorates and thionamide compounds such as thiourea, thiouracil, propylthiouracil, methimazole, and carbimazole. Transplacental transfer of these drugs can result in fetal goiter with or without hypothyroidism. LATS, a substance with certain characteristics of globulin, is produced in Graves' disease and stimulates the thyroid function in a manner similar to that of TSH. Transfer of LATS across the placenta into the fetus can result in neonatal thyrotoxicosis.

Congenital hypothyroidism (cretinism)

Congenital hypothyroidism, or cretinism, is a deficiency of the thyroid believed to have been present at or before birth. Cretinism must be diagnosed promptly because delay in treatment can lead to irreversible brain damage. Yet the overt signs of hypothyroidism are rarely present at birth, and abnormalities of thyroid function may be overlooked during the neonatal period. The dynamic changes in thyroid function following birth, the elevated levels of TBG in neonates, and the sudden deprivation of maternal T_4, however inefficient its transplacental transfer may be, all contribute to the obscurity. Thus recognition of cretinism requires considerable judgment in the interpretation of laboratory data.

Etiology and pathophysiology. The etiologic classification of congenital hypothyroidism is shown in the outline below. The term sporadic cretinism applies to all forms of primary congenital hypothyroidism, except those caused by dietary iodine deficiency and those caused by inborn errors of hormone synthesis or metabolism.

CLASSIFICATION OF CONGENITAL HYPOTHYROIDISM

- I. Primary hypothyroidism
  - A. Defective embryogenesis of thyroid
    - 1. Agenesis (athyreosis)
    - 2. Dysgenesis
      - a. Thyroid remnant in normal location
      - b. Maldescent
  - B. Inborn error of hormone synthesis or metabolism (familial cretinism)
    - 1. Iodide-trapping defect
    - 2. Iodide organification defect
      - a. Without deafness
      - b. With deafness (Pendred's syndrome)
    - 3. Coupling defect of iodotyrosines
    - 4. Deiodination defect
      - a. Generalized
      - b. Limited to thyroid gland
      - c. Limited to peripheral tissues
    - 5. Defect of thyroglobulin
    - 6. Goiter with calcification
    - 7. Peripheral tissue unresponsiveness to thyroid hormone(?)
    - 8. Unresponsiveness of thyroid to TSH(?)
  - C. Goitrous cretinism caused by maternal ingestion of goitrogens
  - D. Iodine deficiency (endemic goiter)
- II. Secondary hypothyroidism

In contrast to the clearcut preponderance of thyroid disorders in females over males during childhood and adult life, there is no sex difference in the incidence of congenital hypothyroidism.

The relative incidence of each type of cretinism varies widely in different geographic locations. In the nongoitrous regions, defective embryogenesis of the thyroid accounts for 70% to 85% of all cretinism. Failure in the anatomic development of the thyroid gland may be complete or partial. Although it was believed that complete absence of a functioning thyroid (athyreosis), or agenesis of the thyroid, was the principal cause of cretinism, wider use of radioiodine scintillation scanning with better spectrometry in recent years has detected residual thyroid tissue in the normal position or in ectopic areas in 60% to 80% of infants and children with hypothyroid. Ectopic thyroid is usually composed of a remnant of undescended thyroid tissue (cryptothyroid) and is situated in the midline. The undescended thyroid is located in the base of the tongue in about one half of the cases, between the tongue and the hyoid bone in about one fourth, and between the hyoid bone and normal location in the remaining cases. The ectopic tissue is often capable of undergoing compensatory hypertrophy when the hormone production becomes inadequate and may be found as a midline mass. The cause of defective embryogenesis of the thyroid is unknown.

Dysgenesis of the thyroid can occasionally be a familial condition. Destruction of the fetal thyroid by maternal thyroid antibodies acquired transplacentally has been suggested as a possible etiologic factor in some instances of sporadic athyreotic cretinism.

Genetically determined errors of T_4 synthesis or metabolism involve a deficiency of one or more enzymes necessary at various stages of the biosynthetic and metabolic pathway. Impaired hormonal secretion results in hypersecretion of TSH, usually leading to compensatory hyperplasia of the thyroid. Hence, familial cretinism is often referred to as goitrous cretinism. Hypothyroidism or goiter or both may or may not be present in the newborn and infant, depending on the degree and time of onset of hormonal deficiency. Family members of a goitrous cretin often are found to have less severe defects manifested by goiter without associated hypothyroidism. The exact enzyme defect in some goitrous cretins, including those assumed to result from defects in the coupling mechanism and thyroglobulin synthesis, is still open to question.

Cretins caused by a defect in the trapping of iodide can be confused with infants with athyreosis because of the lack of administered radioiodine to concentrate in the neck. However, a goiter is present in these patients, and the saliva fails to concentrate radioiodine.

There are two types of defects in the organification of iodide: one in which iodide peroxidase is deficient and another in which an iodide transferase is lacking. The former is generally associated with more severe hypothyroidism. The latter is called *Pendred's syndrome* and is associated with congenital deafness and usually a small euthyroid goiter. Genetic studies of Pendred's syndrome indicate that it is an autosomal recessive trait.

In the coupling defect of iodotyrosines, T_4 and T_3 are decreased, and MIT and DIT are increased in both the serum and thyroid gland. In patients with deiodination defects, there is a rapid turnover of thyroid iodine and wastage of iodotyrosines into the urine. The defect may be generalized, or it may be limited to intrathyroid or peripheral deiodination.

A defect in thyroglobulin synthesis was postulated in patients who had abnormal iodoproteins in their sera. Other unusual types of familial cretinism include a large kindred with goiter characterized by extensive intrathyroid calcification. The transmission pattern in this family suggested an autosomal dominant trait. A family with possible inability of the peripheral tissue to respond to T_4 has been reported. The affected members of this family had deaf-mutism, goiter, delayed bone maturation, and elevated levels of PBI. A possible unresponsiveness of the thyroid to TSH was postulated in a boy who had congenital hypothyroidism without a goiter, low PBI, normal ^{131}I uptake, and elevated levels of serum TSH.

Maternal ingestion of antithyroid drugs, especially the thionamides and potassium perchlorate, can cause neonatal goitrous hypothyroidism. Although the correlation between the dose of drug and the incidence of neonatal goiter is poor, prolonged administration of large doses of these drugs increases the risk of goitrous cretinism. Administration of inorganic iodides to the mother in large amounts, usually for treatment of various respiratory disorders, can also produce a large congenital goiter filled with colloid (Fig. 15-1). Radioiodine treatment given to pregnant women during the second trimester has resulted in hypothyroidism in the offspring. The hypothyroidism was not obvious at birth in most instances.

Endemic goiter occurs in large land areas where dietary iodine is deficient. However, the incidence of goiter in neonates is relatively low in these areas, and many individuals living in the same environment do not develop goiter. These observations suggest that there may be other factors superimposed on iodine deficiency.

Secondary hypothyroidism is rare in neonates but not uncommon in older children. Pituitary aplasia, when present, is usually associated with anencephaly or other severe malformation of the brain. Patients who have aplasia of the pituitary, with or without malformation of the brain, rarely survive beyond the neonatal period.

Clinical presentation. Even in the athyreotic cretins the classic clinical features of cretinism are usually absent at birth

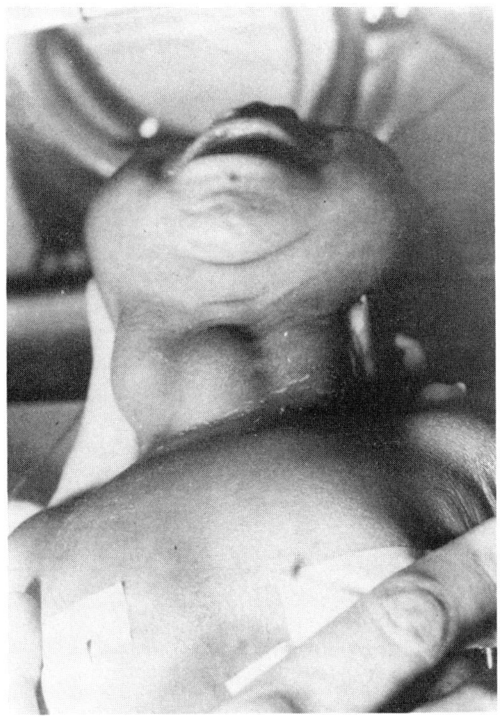

Fig. 15-1. Iodine-induced goiter in a neonate. The lateral bulging of the neck is caused by enlarged lateral lobes of the thyroid.

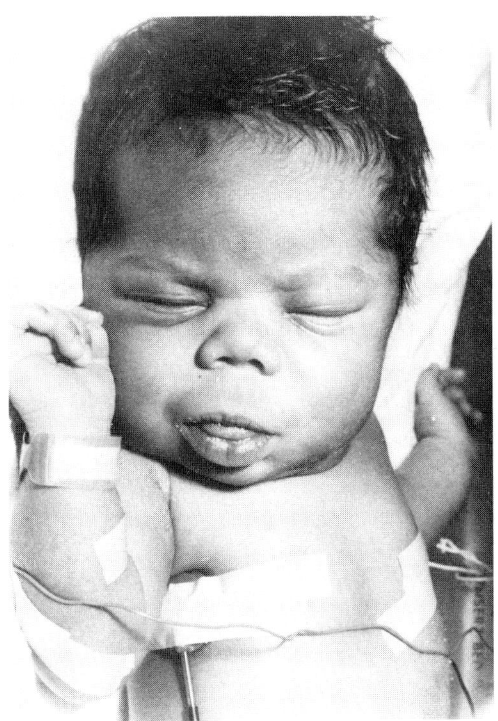

Fig. 15-2. Typical facial features of cretinism.

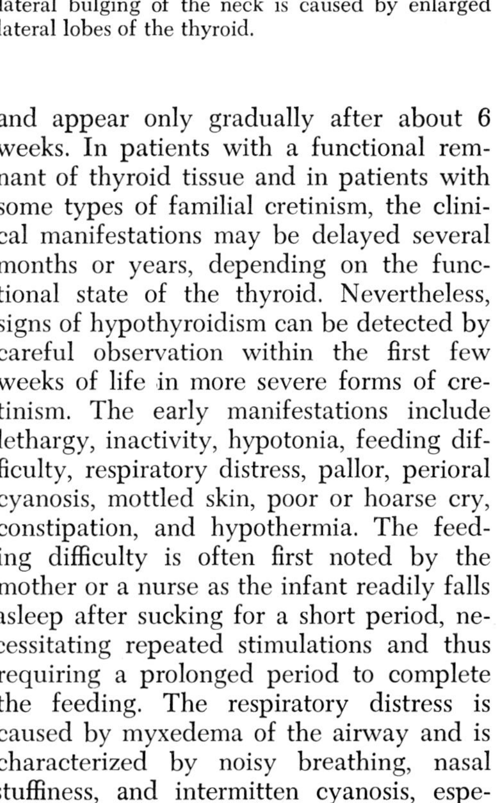

and appear only gradually after about 6 weeks. In patients with a functional remnant of thyroid tissue and in patients with some types of familial cretinism, the clinical manifestations may be delayed several months or years, depending on the functional state of the thyroid. Nevertheless, signs of hypothyroidism can be detected by careful observation within the first few weeks of life in more severe forms of cretinism. The early manifestations include lethargy, inactivity, hypotonia, feeding difficulty, respiratory distress, pallor, perioral cyanosis, mottled skin, poor or hoarse cry, constipation, and hypothermia. The feeding difficulty is often first noted by the mother or a nurse as the infant readily falls asleep after sucking for a short period, necessitating repeated stimulations and thus requiring a prolonged period to complete the feeding. The respiratory distress is caused by myxedema of the airway and is characterized by noisy breathing, nasal stuffiness, and intermitten cyanosis, especially in the perioral area. These respiratory symptoms may lead one to suspect congenital anomalies of the airway or congenital heart disease. After the first 2 weeks of life, prolonged physiologic jaundice may be an indication of hypothyroidism. The jaundice may appear to be further prolonged when carotenemia is superimposed after feeding a diet high in carotene.

The classic features of cretinism usually occur after about 6 weeks of life (Fig. 15-2). These include: the typical facies characterized by depressed nasal bridge, relatively narrow forehead and puffy eyelids, thick, dry, and cold skin, coarse hair, which may appear long and abundant, and large tongue; abdominal distension; umbilical hernia; hyporeflexia; bradycardia; hypotension with widened pulse pressure; and anemia.

Lingual thyroid can be seen in occasional infants and children as a discrete round mass at the base of the tongue, especially when it is hypertrophied from endogenous TSH stimulation (Fig. 15-3). The base of the tongue must be firmly depressed to

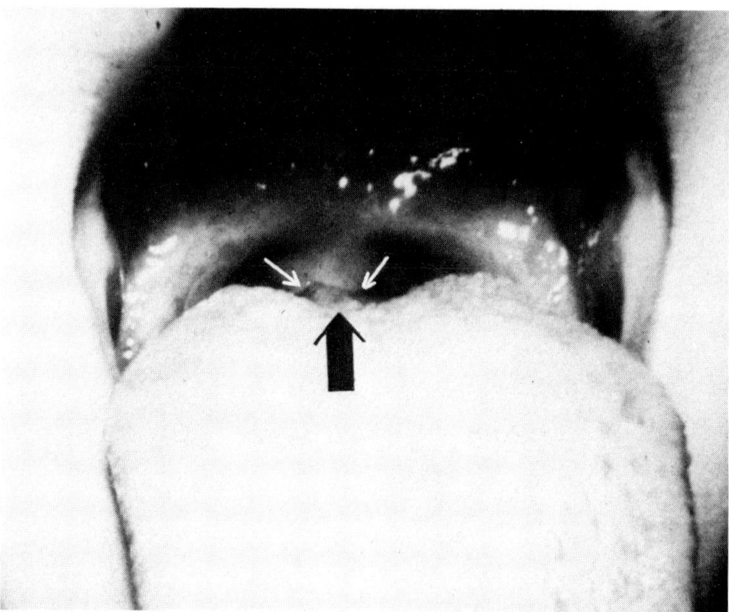

Fig. 15-3. Visualization of a lingual thyroid.

visualize this mass. In some instances, sublingual thyroid is palpable as a round midline mass deep under the mandible.

Neonatal goiters may be extremely large, asymmetrical, and grotesque, and may be confused with a hygroma or other type of mass (Fig. 15-1). Alternatively, the goiter may be quite small and escape notice on a cursory examination.

Diagnosis. There is no single test by which a diagnosis of cretinism can be established. When the diagnosis is suspected, several appropriate thyroid function tests should be employed. Commonly used chemical tests and the normal values found in the neonates have been described above. It is advisable to assess both the T_4 level and the saturation of T_4-binding proteins. The results of these tests must be interpreted in combination and in light of the infant's age and the clinical evidence for hypothyroidism.

Retardation of bone maturation is present in about half of the cretins at birth and when detected should help in establishing the diagnosis. Thus the assessment of bone age is particularly useful in the newborn. However, it should be noted that roentgenographic examination of the hand and wrist, which is most commonly used in estimating bone age, is almost totally useless during the neonatal period since the first ossification center, the hamate, does not appear in the normal infant until 3 to 4 months of age. Retardation of bone maturation in neonates is best assessed by x-ray examination of the knee and the foot. The ossification centers of the calcaneus and talus appear at about the twenty-sixth to twenty-eighth week of gestation, and the distal femor at about the thirty-fourth to thirty-sixth week of intrauterine life. The absence of the distal femoral epiphyses in a newborn weighing 3,000 gm or more or the absence of the distal femoral and proximal tibial epiphyses in an infant weighing 2,500 to 3,000 gm at birth suggests intrauterine thyroid hormone deficiency.

Ossification of the cartilages of the epiphyses is also disturbed in hypothyroidism. Normally, ossification begins from the center of the cartilage and extends peripherally in an orderly manner. In hypothyroidism, calcification of epiphyseal centers starts from multiple irregular foci scattered in the developing cartilage. The irregular calcification pattern appears in the roentgenogram as stippled or fragmented ossification centers and is referred to as epiphyseal dysgenesis (Fig. 15-4). This finding is highly characteristic of hypothyroidism and provides a strong clue for the diagno-

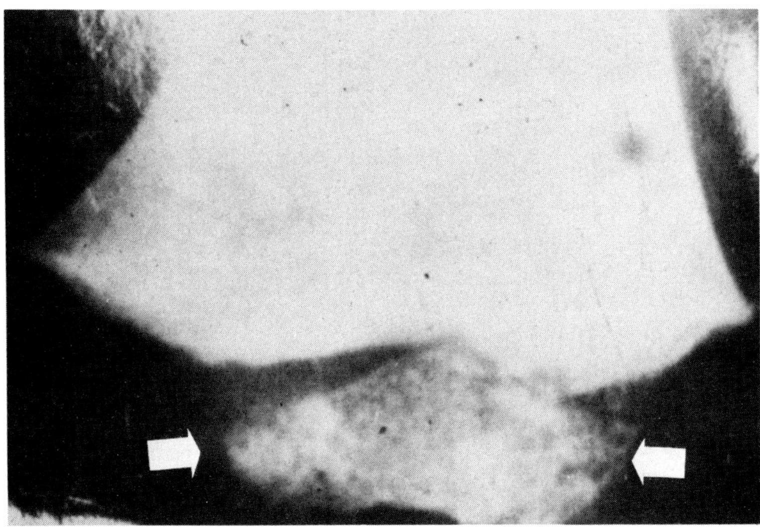

Fig. 15-4. Epiphyseal dysgenesis of the distal femoral center.

sis. A roentgenographic examination of the knee and the foot is useful in detecting epiphyseal dysgenesis during the neonatal period. Abnormal changes occur in the epiphyseal cartilage secondary to thyroid hormone deficiency prior to calcification so that even after the hypothyroidism is treated, the characteristic pattern of calcification, epiphyseal dysgenesis, may appear in all centers, which normally would have calcified during the period of deficiency.

A goiter and tracheal compression by an enlarged thyroid may be visualized by roentgenographic examination of the neck.

An estimate of visceral myxedema may be made by detecting a low votlage of all complexes in the ECG and EEG. A roentgenogram of the chest may also reveal the presence of cardiomegaly, reflecting myxedema of the heart.

Measurements of the serum cholesterol levels and the BMR are not reliable diagnostic aids in the assessment of thyroid function during the neonatal period. Tests that utilize in vivo administration of radioiodine or technetium-99m (technetium shares with iodide the same active transport mechanism into the thyroid) are unnecessary for the diagnosis of many cretins. However, a radioiodine uptake test can be used to confirm the presence of an agenetic or dysgenetic thyroid. The thyroid 24-hour uptake of radioiodine is variable during the first several weeks and may exceed 90% during the first week of life. A 24-hour uptake of less than 2% is highly suggestive of thyroid agenesis, and if the uptake is less than 10%, presence of a dysgenetic thyroid can be suspected. An ectopic thyroid is usually not detected by the radioiodine uptake test because of the relatively small aperture of the counter used for such a study. In neonates, radioiodine should be administered through a nasogastric tube, and the tube should then be flushed with water in order to avoid any loss of the tracer. To detect an undescended thyroid, a scintillation scan of the pharyngeal area and the neck may be obtained after administration of radioiodine.

The presence of a defective iodine-trapping mechanism can be suspected in goitrous cretins when the thyroid fails to concentrate radioiodine within 2 to 4 hours after oral administration of the tracer. The defect can be demonstrated by comparing the radioiodine concentrations in simultaneously obtained samples of the saliva and plasma 1 to 2 hours after the administration of the tracer. In the normal individual the salivary concentration is about tenfold greater than that in the plasma, whereas the salivary glands of patients fail to concentrate radioiodine.

In patients with an iodide organification defect, the iodide taken up by the thyroid is readily released from the gland. When the thyroid uptake of radioiodine is measured at 2, 4, 6, and 24 hours after oral administration of radioiodine in these patients, the uptake may be normal or elevated during the earlier hours. However, the uptake rapidly declines within 24 hours. In normal individuals, on the other hand, the thyroid uptake of radioiodine gradually increases during the first 4 to 6 hours and remains at a plateau level of 15% to 30% of the administered dose at the end of 24 hours. When rapid organification of inorganic iodide fails to take place in the thyroid, an anion such as perchlorate can competitively inhibit the iodine accumulation, and there is a net loss of iodide from the gland. This property of perchlorate is utilized in the perchlorate discharge test. This test involves measuring the 2-hour thyroid uptake of radioiodine and then administering soduim or potassium perchlorate orally in amounts of 10 mg/kg of body weight. One to two hours thereafter, the thyroid uptake is remeasured. If the uptake decreases by more than 10% to 15% of the initial value, the presence of a defect in normal organification of iodide is suggested.

Differentiation among other types of familial cretinism is more difficult and often technically impossible to achieve during infancy. The studies required for the differential diagnosis usually involve administration of radioactive substances in doses greater than considered safe for infants. Thus, in most instances, patients should be treated for a few years and a definitive study undertaken at a later date. However, secretion of abnormal iodoproteins into the circulation, as would occur in the coupling defect of iodotyrosines, can be suspected when the BII is elevated.

The diagnosis of cretinism caused by maternal ingestion of goitrogens is usually established from the history and is confirmed by its self-limiting course. The reactions to the perchlorate discharge test are positive in both iodine-induced goiter and following administration of antithyroid drugs.

In cretinism caused by iodine deficiency, the radioiodine uptake is elevated.

Differential diagnosis. Errors of diagnosis of cretinism usually result from a failure to suspect the condition or from diagnosing other disorders as hypothyroidism. These errors commonly arise from basing the diagnosis on a few suggestive clinical features and misinterpreting the laboratory data.

During the early neonatal period, respiratory difficulty, pallor, and cyanosis in cretinism must be differentiated from other common causes of respiratory distress and from congenital heart disease. Lethargy, inactivity, hypotonia, and feeding difficulty may be mistaken for manifestations of brain damage from a variety of causes. The prolonged jaundice in cretinism must not be confused with icterus caused by hemolytic anemia, septicemia, or hepatic disease. The coarse facial features, macroglossia, and dry skin of cretinism can mislead one to suspect Hurler's syndrome, chondrodystrophy, or mongolism. In rare instances hypothyroidism has been found in patients with mongolism. A large goiter must not be confused with a hygroma, cyst, or tumor of the neck. A lingual thyroid, when visible or obstructing the airway, has been mistaken for a tumor of the pharyngeal area. Although epiphyseal dysgenesis may resemble osteochondritis deformans in its roentgenographic appearance, the latter does not occur during the neonatal period.

Treatment. All hypothyroid infants, with or without goiter, should be rendered euthyroid as promptly as possible by a substitution therapy. Neonates with a euthyroid goiter should be regarded as being in a state of impending hypothyroidism and, in most instances, should be treated. Desiccated thyroid, sodium-L-thyroxine, or triiodothyronine can be used for treatment. Desiccated thyroid has the advantages of being inexpensive and maintaining the PBI or T_4-I values within the normal range when the patient is rendered euthyroid. Desiccated thyroid has an estimated plasma half-life of 6.9 days in the adult; and its latent period, the interval between administration of the drug and the onset of its effect, is longer than T_3. Sodium-L-thyroxine is better standardized for its potency than desiccated thyroid but will result in elevated PBI and T_4-I values when the patient is euthyroid. PBI values of 10 to 14 μg/100 ml have been reported in adequate substitution therapy. T_3 has an estimated plasma half-life of 1.3 to 2.5 days and a shorter latent period than desiccated thyroid. Administration of T_3 results in a depression of the PBI and T_4-I. When the patient is adequately treated with T_3, the PBI may range from 2 to 3 μg/100 ml or less. Sixty-five mg (1 grain) of desiccated thyroid is the equivalent of 100 μg of L-thyroxine and 35 μg of T_3.

In treating infants with severe myxedema, possible complications should be kept in mind. Cardiac insufficiency from overtaxing the myxedematous heart by too rapid a mobilization of the myxedema fluid into the circulation is well known in the adult. This complication is avoided by administering a small dose of thyroid hormone at first and gradually increasing the dosage. The infant, however, generally tolerates a rapid restoration to euthyroid state better than the adult, and some authors have advocated a prompt restoration of the PBI or T_4 to a normal value. It is our opinion that thyroid hormone should be increased judiciously when evidence of severe myxedema, particularly of the heart, is present. Aspiration of food is another complication of cretins; it may occur after therapy has been started, when the infants begin to feed more vigorously. It results from an impairment in swallowing, caused by myxedema of the pharyngeal area, compounded by increased appetite as the euthyroid state is restored. Therefore, when myxedema is severe, the infant should be fed carefully and slowly by an expert nurse during the early phase of treatment.

There are different views on the exact mode of treatment of severe cretinism. Initially the patient may be given orally 8 mg of desiccated thyroid per day; after 1 week the dose is increased to 16 mg; at 2 weeks, to 32 mg; at 3 weeks, to 48 mg; at 4 weeks, to 65 mg; and thereafter this dose is maintained during the first 2 years of life. This or a similar schedule of treatment has been used successfully by a large number of physicians over a period of many years. Alternatively, because of the more rapid action and shorter half-life of T_3, others prefer to use this drug in treatment of infants with hypothyroidism. The patient is started on 5 μg T_3 per day administered orally; after 7 days, the dose is increased to 10 μg; thereafter, the dose is increased by 5 μg every 4 to 5 days until the dosage reaches 25 μg per day; then T_3 is discontinued, and the patient is placed on the maintenance dose of desiccated thyroid of 65 mg/day so that the PBI can be restored to the normal range for future reference.

Restoration of milder hypothyroidism to an euthyroid state can be accomplished more rapidly. Patients with an euthyroid goiter may be placed on a maintenance dose of thyroid hormone immediately.

Until hypothyroidism is corrected, the infant should be kept under careful observation, and the cardiovascular function should be monitored. Clinical observation should be supplemented by following the growth curve, the maturation of the bones, and the PBI or T_4-I. All cretins, except those caused by maternal ingestion of goitrogens and by iodine deficiency, require lifetime substitution therapy.

Goitrous cretinism caused by maternal ingestion of goitrogens is a self-limiting condition. The blocking effect of antithyroid drugs usually disappears after several days following birth. Therefore, if the goiter is small and the patient is euthyroid, no treatment is required. If the patient is hypothyroid, however, or if the goiter is large, it is safer to treat the infant for several weeks or months. The antithyroid agents are secreted in breast milk. Shrinkage of the goiter may be hastened by substitution therapy, and the treatment can be withdrawn after the thyroid returns to normal size. Occasionally, the goiter may be huge, and asphyxia may occur in the neonate from a goiter that encircles the trachea. This complication is most commonly seen in iodide-induced goiter and constitutes a medical emergency. The asphyxia is best treated by surgical splitting of the isthmus.

Endemic cretins should be given substitution therapy for an indefinite period, unless iodine prophylaxis can be assured in the specific geographic location.

Prognosis. Shortly after adequate substitution therapy is instituted, all clinical manifestations of hypothyroidism will disappear, and accelerated linear growth will occur if growth was retarded prior to the treatment. After a period of "catch-up" growth, an optimal rate of growth will be maintained. Goiter or hypetrophied ectopic thyroid will gradually shrink in size when the patient is properly treated. The coarse hair is gradually lost and is replaced by finer, normal hair over a period of several months. After a latent period of a few months, a marked acceleration in bone maturation (catch-up) will occur, and thereafter the osseous development should parallel the chronologic age. When hypothyroidism is treated with a slightly excessive dosage of thyroid hormones for a prolonged period, the bone maturation may gradually exceed the chronologic age, even though the patient may fail to show overt signs of hyperthyroidism or have clearly elevated levels of PBI. With substitution therapy, epiphyseal dysgenesis will appear in centers that failed to calcify while the patient was hypothyroid, and then the calcification will coalesce to form a normal epiphysis.

While the prognosis in cretins for physical recovery is good, the prognosis for normal mental and neurologic performance is uncertain and less favorable. The eventual IQ of severe cretins is inversely related to the duration of thyroid hormone deficiency. Irreversible brain damage can occur from fetal hypothyroidism as well as from postnatal hormone deficiency. Therefore the prognosis of a cretin for mental development should be guarded, even if the treatment is initiated soon after birth. It is our impression that the mental ability of neonates with marked delay in the bone maturation is likely to be worse than that in those with mild or no retardation in bone age. Mental and neurologic competence of cretins is also related to the severity of hypothyroidism. However, even mild cretins, treated promptly after birth, may have impairment of arithmetical ability, speech, or fine motor coordination in later life.

Goiters

The majority of neonatal goiters result from maternal ingestion of goitrogens. Prominent goiter is only occasionally the manifestation of familial goitrous cretinism. These goiters have been described above. It should be noted that most euthyroid goiters of newborns are brought about by compensatory hypertrophy of the thyroid and thus are potentially indicative of impending hypothyroidism. Therefore, these goiters should be treated appropriately.

Congenital neoplasms of the thyroid rarely occur. They include Hürthle cell tumor and adenocarcinoma. We have also encountered a teratoma of the thyroid in a newborn that was suggested by calcification within the thyroid. Neoplasm can be suspected when a nodular goiter is present. Radioidine scintiscan reveals a cold nodular area corresponding to the location of the neoplasm where uptake of radioiodine is lacking. A diagnosis of neoplasm should be confirmed by a biopsy.

Thyrotoxicosis

Etiology and pathophysiology. Neonatal thyrotoxicosis may occur in infants born to mothers either with active Graves' disease or with a history of Graves' disease. The available evidence suggests that LATS, transferred across the placenta from the mother to the fetus, underlies the pathogenesis of neonatal thyrotoxicosis. LATS has been detected in the sera of most neonates with hyperthyroidism and in the sera of their mothers. The relatively low incidence of neonatal thyrotoxicosis is probably caused by the infrequent occurrence of pregnancy in thyrotoxic women, the prevalence of spontaneous abortion in such women, and the low incidence of high titers of LATS in the blood of thyrotoxic women who are pregnant. LATS is an abnormal thyrotropic substance that can be detected in the sera of about 40% of adults with Graves' disease. LATS has also been found in neonatal hyperthyroidism. The serum half-life of LATS is similar to that of gamma globulins, approximately 20 days, judging from its rate of disappearance in neonates with thyrotoxicosis.

Clinical presentation. When neonatal thyrotoxicosis occurs in the infant born to a mother with untreated active Graves' disease, the clinical manifestations of hyperthyroidism may become apparent within the first 24 hours of life. Irritability, excessive movements, tremor, flushing of the cheeks, sweating, increased appetite, weight loss or lack of weight gain, supraventricular tachycardia, goiter, and exophthalmus may be observed. Although a goiter is inevitably present in neonatal thyrotoxicosis, its size varies considerably; it may be small and escape notice on a cursory examination, or it may be large enough to cause tracheal compression. Further, the goiter may increase in size during the early neonatal period. Exophthalmos is usually mild when present. Hepatosplenomegaly, thrombocytopenia, and hypoprothrombinemia have been reported in isolated instances. In severe neonatal thyrotoxicosis, hyperthermia, arryhthmias, and cardiac failure may occur; and if the condition is untreated, death may ensue.

The course of the syndrome is self-limited because of the gradual depletion of transplacentally acquired LATS. The signs and symptoms subside spontaneously after 3 to 12 weeks, depending on the severity of the disease, which in turn is probably related to the titer of LATS in the plasma of the neonate. Goiter, however, may persist for some time after all signs of hyperthyroidism disappear. The thyroid gradually returns to normal size.

In the infant born to a mother who received antithyroid medications for treatment of Graves' disease during the latter part of pregnancy, the onset of clinical manifestations may be modified by transplacental acquisition of the antithyroid agent as well as LATS. At birth, the infant may be euthyroid or even hypothyroid, and the presence of a goiter may be the only abnormal feature. Since the plasma half-life of antithyroid agents is considerably shorter than that of LATS, the typical manifestations of neonatal thyrotoxicosis may appear several days after birth. If the infant is born in a hyopthyroid state, a period of euthyroidism may follow within a few days, and thyrotoxicosis may not occur until 5 to 7 days after birth.

Diagnosis and differential diagnosis. A maternal history of Graves' disease, before or during pregnancy, is of utmost importance in the diagnosis of neonatal thyrotoxicosis. Information concerning the treatment of maternal hyperthyroidism also must be obtained. The infant should be examined repeatedly for signs of thyrotoxicosis, and the neck should be palpated carefully to detect a goiter. Determinations of PBI, T_4-I, or FT_4 should be obtained, together with an assessment of T_4-binding protein saturation. The data should be interpreted in relation to the clinical features and age of the neonate, as already described. The determination of radioiodine uptake by the thyroid is of little value during the neonatal period. LATS can be determined by a bioassay in sera of the mother, umbilical cord, and infant. A high titer of LATS in these specimens will strongly support the diagnosis of neonatal thyrotoxicosis. Serial determinations of LATS in the neonate are helpful in considering the duration of treatment.

In the euthyroid or hypothyroid neonate born to a mother who received antithyroid medication during the latter part of pregnancy, it is virtually impossible to predict whether or not thyrotoxicosis will ensue. Therefore, serial examinations of the infant must be undertaken during the first 10 days of life.

Although neonatal thyrotoxicosis can be confused with various neurologic disorders, congenital heart disease, or sepsis, a positive maternal history of Graves' disease and the presence of a goiter should readily alert one to the correct diagnosis.

Treatment. The treatment of thyrotoxicosis in a neonate is similar to that in an older child and involves the use of antithyroid drugs. Because of the self-limiting course of the disease, however, treatment should be terminated after 1 to 3 months, and care should be exercised not to induce hypothyroidism with excessive medication. Iodine (Lugol's solution), propylthiouracil, and methimazole are commonly used. Lugol's solution can be given in doses of one drop 3 times daily. It should be remembered that while iodine rapidly inhibits the release of thyroxine from the thyroid, its effect tends to disappear after several weeks. Propylthiouracil has been used extensively. It is given orally in amounts of 10 mg/kg/day in 3 divided doses at 8-hour intervals. Methimazole is given in amounts of 1 mg/kg/day in 3 divided doses. It should be noted that circulating thyroxine has a probable half-life of 6.9 days, and therefore little or no clinical response to antithyroid drugs can be expected during the first few days of therapy.

Most signs and symptoms, including the cardiovascular manifestations, of hyperthyroidism are closely related to increased adrenergic response. Antiadrenergic agents, therefore, can alleviate many of the untoward manifestations of thyrotoxicosis. In contrast to antithyroid drugs, these agents can rapidly diminsh the severity of thyrotoxicity, and their effects are evident within a few hours. Thus reserpine, together with propylthiouracil, may be used in the treatment of severe neonatal thyrotoxicosis. Reserpine is given orally in amounts of 0.02 mg/kg/day in 2 or more divided doses. The amount may be increased up to 0.05 mg/kg/day if necessary, provided no adverse effect is observed. The use of reserpine usually obviates the need to use sedatives. In neonates, untoward effects of reserpine use may occur even at recommended dosages. Thus the infant's clinical condition and vital signs must be closely monitored.

Digitalization may be necessary in neonates with cardiac failure. Under these circumstances reserpine may be contraindicated or must be used with extreme caution. A large goiter compressing the trachea and resulting in asphyxia must be treated surgically by splitting the isthmus.

The euthyroid or hypothyroid infant born to a mother who received antithyroid medications during the pregnancy should be managed as described in the section on congenital hypothyroidism. Since these neonates may or may not develop thyrotoxicosis, they should be kept under close observation. If the infant has already received thyroid hormone, it should be discontinued as soon as thyrotoxic manifestations occur, and appropriate management of hyperthyroidism must be initiated. A mother who is receiving an antithyroid medication should not be allowed to breast feed the infant, since these agents are secreted into the milk.

Prognosis. Neonatal thyrotoxicosis carries a high mortality of about 25% if it is not recognized and treated properly. However, the syndrome is usually self-limiting in duration, and no sequelae have been recognized. A goiter may resolve slowly over a period of several months. Premature closure of all cranial sutures occasionally occurs in older infants and in young children with hyperthyroidism. Although this complication has not been reported in neonatal thyrotoxicosis, it is probably advisable to obtain a roentgenogram of the skull at 6 to 12 months of age.

Familial abnormalities of thyroxine-binding globulin

Genetic disorders resulting in either increased or decreased levels of TBG have been reported. Affected individuals are healthy and asymptomatic, since a change in the level of TBG does not lead to an alteration of the FT_4 level. The disorders are usually discovered fortuitously by studying the PBI or T_4-I, which reveals unexpectedly high or low values. The only clinical significance of these conditions, therefore, lies in the fact that abnormal PBI or T_4-I levels may lead to erroneous diagnosis.

Decreased TBG

In several families, affected males had no detectable TBG, whereas presumably heterozygous females were found to have low but detectable levels of TBG. Moreover, there was no male-to-male transmission of the trait. A female member in one of these families had no detectable TBG and a sex chromosome constitution of XO. These observations are consistent with the "inactive X" theory of Lyon and with the fixed differentiation of X chromosome behavior. Thus, in these families, the trait appeared to be transmitted as an X chromosome–linked gene. In another family, however, a deficiency of TBG was found in three males and three females of two generations. The mode of transmission in this family suggested an autosomal dominant trait.

Increased TBG

Studies in two families with increased TBG suggested that the trait may be inherited as an autosomal dominant gene. On the other hand, in another family, affected males transmitted the trait to female but not to male offspring, suggesting that the trait may be X chromosome linked.

The conflicting reports on the mode of inheritance of both the decreased and the increased TBG traits are difficult to reconcile at present. Since the TBG levels are estimated from its binding capacity of T_4, the reported increased TBG may merely reflect an elevated binding capacity of the protein without a quantitative increase in the amount of circulating TBG. Thus the level of TBG may be controlled by more than one gene, one of which could be a regulator gene.

AKIRA MORISHIMA

BIBLIOGRAPHY

Andersen, H. J.: Hypothyroidism; nongoitrous hypothyroidism. In Gardner, L. I., editor: Endocrine and genetic diseases of childhood, Philadelphia, 1969, W. B. Saunders Co.

Bongiovanni, A. M., Eberlein, W. R., Thomas, P. Z., and Anderson, W. B.: Sporadic goiter of the newborn, J. Clin. Endocrinol. Metab. **16:** 146, 1956.

Braverman, L. E., Ingbar, S. H., and Sterling, K.: Conversion of thyroxine (T_4) to triiodothyronine (T_3) in athyreotic human subjects, J. Clin. Invest. **49:**855, 1970.

Czernichow, P., Greenberg, A. H., Tyson, J., and Blizzard, R. M.: Thyroid function studies in paired maternal-cord sera and sequential observations of thyrotropic hormone release during the first 72 hours of life, Pediatr. Res. **5:**53, 1971.

Fisher, D. A., Oddie, T. H., and Burroughs, J. C.: Thyroidal radioiodine uptake rate measurement in infants, Am. J. Dis. Child. **103:**738, 1962.

Fisher, D. A., and Odell, W. D.: Acute release of thyrotropin in the newborn, J. Clin. Invest. **48:** 1670, 1969.

Fisher, D. A., Odell, W. D., Hobel, C. J., and Garza, R.: Thyroid function in the term fetus, Pediatrics **44:**526, 1969.

Florsheim, W. H., Dowling, J. T., Meister, L., and Bodfish, R. E.: Familial elevation of serum thyroxine-binding capacity, J. Clin. Endocrinol. Metab. **22:**735, 1962.

French, F. S., and Van Wyk, J. J.: Fetal hypothyroidism, J. Pediatr. **64:**589, 1964.

Green, H. G., Gareis, F. J., Shepard, T. H., and Kelley, V. C.: Cretinism associated with maternal sodium iodide I^{131} therapy during pregnancy, Am. J. Dis. Child. **122:**247, 1971.

Greenberg, A. H., Czernichow, P., Reba, R. C., Tyson, J., and Blizzard, R. M.: Observations on the maturation of thyroid function in early fetal life, J. Clin. Invest. **49:**1790, 1970.

Grumbach, M. M., and Werner, S. C.: Transfer of thyroid hormone across the human placenta at term, J. Clin. Endocrinol. Metab. **16:**1392, 1956.

Hirsch, P. F., Voekel, E. F., and Munson, P. L.: Thyrocalcitonin; hypocalcemic hypophosphatemic principle of the thyroid gland, Science **146:**412, 1964.

Little, G., Meador, C. K., Cunningham, R., and Pittman, J. A.: "Cryptothyroidism," the major cause of sporadic "athyreotic" cretinism, J. Clin. Endocrinol. Metab. **25:**1529, 1965.

Marshall, J. S., Levy, R. P., and Steinberg, A. G.: Human thyroxine-binding globulin deficiency; a genetic study, N. Engl. J. Med. **274:**1469, 1966.

Marrow, W. J.: Hürthle cell tumor of the thyroid gland in an infant, Arch. Pathol. **40:**387, 1945.

McKenzie, J. M.: Neonatal Grave's disease, J. Clin. Endocrinol., Metab. **24:**660, 1964.

McKenzie, J. M.: Humoral factor in the pathogenesis of Grave's disease, Physiol. Rev. **48:**252, 1968.

Parker, R. H., and Beierwaltes, W. H.: Thyroid antibodies during pregnancy and in the newborn, J. Clin. Endocrinol. Metab. **21:**792, 1961.

Perry, R. E., Hodgman, J. E., and Starr, P.: Maternal, cord, and serial venous blood; protein-bound iodine, thyroid-binding globulin, thyroid-binding albumin, and prealbumin values in premature infants, Pediatrics **35:**759, 1965.

Rogers, W. M.: Normal and anomalous development of the thyroid; normal development. In Werner, S. C., and Ingbar, S. H., editors: The thyroid, ed. 3, Section 22, New York, 1971, Harper & Row, Publishers.

Sokoloff, L., Roberts, P. A., Januska, M., and Klein, J. E.: Mechanisms of stimulation of protein synthesis by thyroid hormones in vitro, Proc. Nat. Acad. Sci. U.S.A. **60:**652, 1968.

Stanbury, J. B., Rocmans, P., Buhler, U. K., and Ochi, Y.: Congenital hypothyroidism with impaired thyroid response to thyrotropin, N. Engl. J. Med. **279:**1132, 1968.

Stanbury, J. B., Wyngaarden, J. B., and Fredrickson, D. S.: The metabolic basis of inherited disease, ed. 2, New York, 1966, McGraw-Hill Book Co.

Stevens, G. A., and Waite, W. W.: Nodular goiter of the new-born with subsequent adenocarcinoma, J.A.M.A. **110:**803, 1938.

Sunshine, P., Kusumoto, H., and Kriss, J. P.: Survival time of circulating long-acting thyroid stimlator in neonatal thyrotoxocosis; implications for diagnosis and therapy of the disorder, Pediatrics **36:**869, 1965.

Wayne, E. J., Koutras, D. A., and Alexander, W. D.: Clinical aspects of iodine metabolism, Oxford, 1964, Blackwell Scientific Publications Ltd.

Weinstein, I. B., and Kitchin, F. D.: Genetic factors in thyroid disease. In Werner, S. C., and Ingbar, S. H., editors: The thyroid, ed. 3, section 26, New York, 1971, Harper & Row, Publishers.

ADRENALS AND REPRODUCTIVE SYSTEM

Abnormalities of sexual differentiation

An infant born with incomplete or abnormal external genital development precluding immediate sex assignment should be treated as a medical emergency. Each day that the family must await a pronouncement of the baby's "true" sex reinforces their doubts and fantasies. This is further complicated by misinformation provided by well-meaning nursery personnel, house officers, laboratory technicians, and so on.

The nosology of the congenital abnormalities of sexual differentiation is complex and too cumbersome for clinical application. The purpose of this section is to provide the pediatrician and his team of special advisors (surgeon, geneticist, endocrinologist, psychiatrist) with a simplified approach for determination of the least troublesome sex of rearing. It is of great importance that diagnostic studies be performed during the first 2 to 3 weeks of life and irrevocable sex assignment made following their conclusion. This will allow the parents to send birth announcements with a minimum of embarrassment. There is no excuse for later change of sex in a child who has been studied thoroughly during infancy.

Normal sex determination and differentiation

Phenotypic sex is determined by an interrelated sequence of cytogenetic, embryologic, and endocrinologic events. Human zygotes have, in addition to 23 pairs of autosomes, at least one X chromosome. Although absence of a second sex chromosome is not lethal, normal gonadal development will not take place without it. Regardless of the number of X chromosomes, the presence of a Y will usually guarantee the formation of a testis in the developing fetus. True hermaphroditism is the only condition where testicular tissue is present with the apparent absence of a Y chromosome. With a sex chromosome complement of two or more X chromosomes without a Y, there usually will be ovarian differentiation of the bipotential fetal gonad.

Undifferentiated gonads first appear in the 4-week-old embryo as thickened portions of the coelomic epithelium, the genital ridges. Primitive germ cells migrate to the genital ridges from the endoderm of the gut. Primary sex cords also arise from the coelomic epithelium and are arranged in the cortical portion of the gonad.

Testicular differentiation occurs between the thirty-fifth and forty-fifth days, when the primary sex cords and germ cells migrate into a central medullary portion of the gonad and provide a framework for germ cell dispersion. The cortical portion disappears rapidly. The sex cords eventually form the seminiferous tubules and Sertoli's cells. The Leydig cells are derived from the mesenchyme and are destined to become hormonally active.

Ovarian differentiation occurs much later than testicular. The first follicles appear at 18 to 20 weeks. Proliferation of the germinal epithelium of the cortex of the primitive gonad produces the sex cords; the medulla all but disappears.

Our understanding of the mechanisms of gential differentiation is based largely upon the elegant experiments of Alfred Jost. Gonads were surgically removed at various stages of development of the fetal rabbit. The external and internal genital structures were examined at term. All males gonadectomized prior to the nineteenth day of gestation were grossly indistinguishable from female rabbits. Moreover, the internal genital ducts had developed into uterus and oviducts. If castration was postponed several days, the mature animals would have normal male internal genitalia but the external appearance remained female. Removal of the fetal testis at an even later date resulted in normal differentiation of both the external and internal genital structures. Female rabbits developed normally for their sex in spite of early removal of the ovaries.

It is generally accepted that the fetal testis elaborates a chemically unidentified inducer substance that promotes regression of the müllerian duct system and stimulation of the wolffian ducts. This effect appears to be a local phenomenon. When only one normal testis is present, wolffian duct structures (vas deferans and epididymis) develop on the ipsilateral side, but müllerian duct derivatives (uterus and oviduct) evolve on the contralateral side. Later in gestation the fetal testis secretes androgen (probably testosterone and androstenedione), which is responsible for normal masculinization of the external genitalia. Fetal androgen, regardless of its source (testis, adrenal, exogenous), will produce fusion of the genital folds to form a phallic urethra, fusion of the genital swellings to form a scrotum, and stimulation of the genital tubercle to produce an elongated penis. An abnormality of the external genitalia at birth should alert the clinician to the possibility of a failure of the androgen function of the fetal testis in a male or a source of extragonadal androgen in the female.

The infant with ambiguous external genitalia at birth

When an infant is born with an abnormality of the external genitalia that does not allow sex assignment, several things must be done immediately.

1. Do not circumcise.

2. Instruct parents that incomplete genital development does not allow for immediate accurate sex assignment, but correct sex of the infant will be determined by a series of laboratory studies.
3. Obtain a buccal mucosal smear for nuclear sex chromatin determination. A leukocyte culture for karyotype preparation may also be begun at this time. The Y chromosome fluorescence test (see below) may also be valuable.

If the scheme in Fig 15-5 is followed, an accurate diagnosis of the cause of the genital abnormality can usually be made during the first 2 weeks of life, allowing for permanent sex assignment. The physician must determine if congenital adrenal hyperplasia (CAH) is present and treat it appropriately to prevent continuing virilization of a female who is potentially fertile. In the absence of CAH or female pseudohermaphroditism secondary to maternal hormone administration, sex of rearing will depend largely upon the anatomy of the external genitalia and the feasibility of reconstructive surgery. Since sex assignment is usually possible without direct visualization of the internal genital structures, exploratory laparotomy is not urgent in the young infant with genital ambiguity. This procedure, when necessary for exact diagnosis and removal of inappropriate organs,

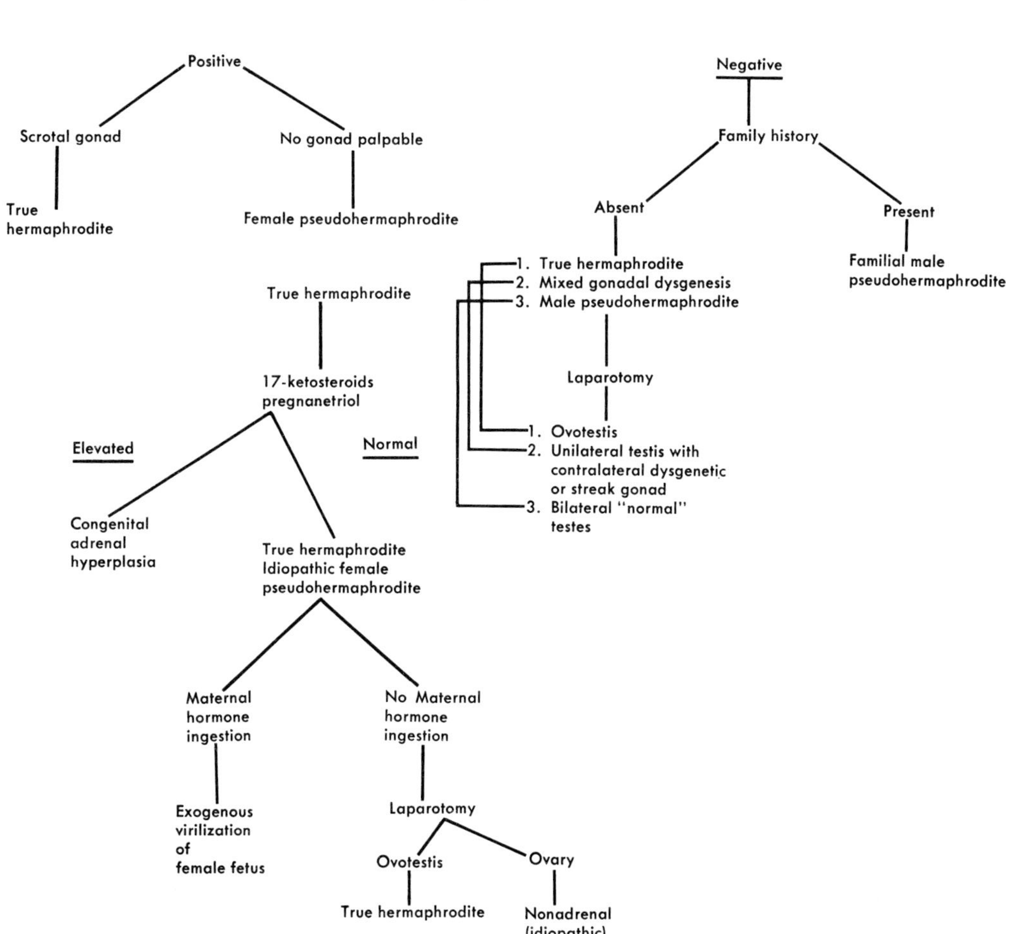

Fig. 15-5. Flow diagram for differential diagnosis of infants with genital ambiguity.

should be postponed several months until it is certain that the infant has no additional congenital abnormalities that would increase the risk of elective surgery.

Chromatin-positive infants with genital ambiguity

The nuclear chromatin pattern in an infant with genital abnormality at birth places the patient into one of two major categories (Fig. 15-5). The proportion of cells with a demonstrable sex chromatin mass (Barr body) may be markedly reduced during the first 48 hours of life in the normal XX individual. Since false negative sex chromatin patterns are more apt to occur the first 2 days of life, all chromatin-negative smears should be repeated after the third day The occurrence of sex chromatin in excess of 25% of cells from buccal mucosa indicates the presence of at least two X chromosomes. Recently it has been shown that following treatment of interphase cells with quinicrine, a fluorescent area is easily demonstrated in nuclei representing the Y chromosome. Thus by cytogenetic techniques it is now possible to predict the sex chromosome complement without cell culture and karyotype analysis (Fig. 15-6). Confirmation of the sex chromosome constitution by leukocyte culture and karyotype preparation should be accomplished whenever possible.

Congenital adrenal hyperplasia. The importance of early diagnosis of CAH, an autosomal recessive inborn error of steroid metabolism, cannot be overemphasized. In addition to a 30% to 40% chance of a severe salt-losing state progressing to shock, the untreated infant will gradually display growth acceleration and progressive virilization. Early recognition, accurate diagnosis, proper sex assignment, and medical therapy will guarantee normal growth and development and future reproductive function since normal gonads are present.

Pathophysiology. The several biochemivariations of CAH have one basic defect in common, inability to synthesize cortisol in sufficient quantity. Fig. 15-7 outlines the three major steroid synthetic pathways in the adrenal gland: glucocorticoid, mineralocorticoid, and androgen.

Congenital adrenal hyperplasia is most commonly associated with a deficiency of the *21-hydroxylase* enzyme. The resulting diminished cortisol production provokes ACTH hypersecretion by the pituitary gland, adrenal enlargement, and an overabundance of precursor steroids proximal to the 21-hydroxylation reaction. These include relatively inert C-21 steroids such as 17-hydroxyprogesterone and virilizing C-19 androgens such as testosterone and androstenedione. The latter are responsible for the virilization of the external genitalia of an affected female fetus. They have no effect on the internal genital structures nor upon the male external anatomy.

Approximately a third of individuals with 21-hydroxylase deficiency are unable to produce adequate amounts of aldosterone for normal sodium and potassium homeostasis. As a consequence, they develop clinical signs and symptoms of severe hyponatremia, hyperkalemia, and dehydration soon after the first week of life. It is uncertain whether the etiologic difference between salt losers and non–salt losers is the degree of 21-hydroxylase deficiency or the absence of two separate enzyme systems closely linked genetically.

In the rare hypertensive variant of CAH there is a deficiency in *11-hydroxylase* activity. This too results in cortisol deficiency with resultant ACTH overproduction, but in this case there is a buildup of 11-deoxysteroids such as deoxycorticosterone (DOC), a potent sodium- and water-retaining mineralocorticoid. Expansion of the extracellular fluid volume causes arterial hypertension. The presence of large amounts of compound S in urine or plasma or both is virtually pathognomonic of this form of CAH (Fig. 15-7). The mechanism for virilization of the female fetus is identical to that in the 21-hydroxylase variety.

Deficiency of a more primitive enzyme, *3β-hydroxysteroid dehydrogenase,* affects the production of glucocorticoids, mineralocorticoids, and both adrenal and gonadal androgens. As a result, females with this disease have not been as severely virilized as in the other forms. In the male, normal masculinization of the external genitalia is incomplete (hypospadias, cleft scrotum), a characteristic that suggests the disorder sooner than in the other types of CAH. Addisonian crisis generally occurs in either sex during the second week of life. Urinary

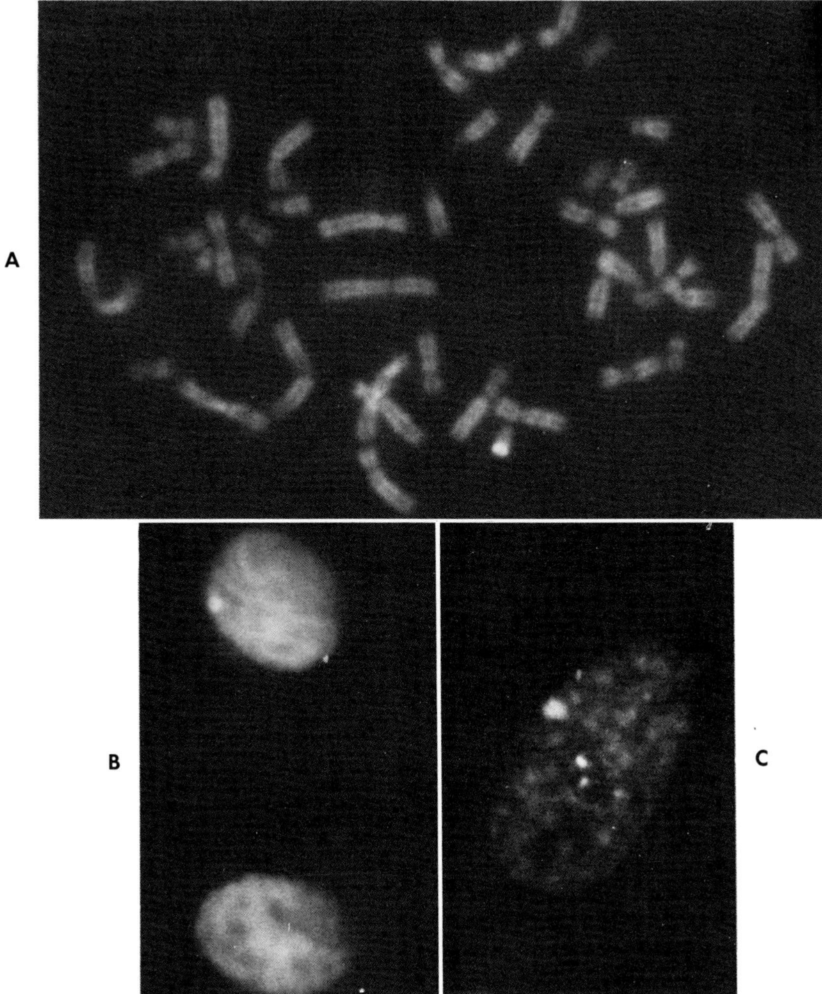

Fig. 15-6. A, Mitotic metaphase cell following quinacrine treatment showing fluorescence of Y chromosome (lower central). **B,** Buccal mucosal cells. Fluorescent Y body seen in upper cell. **C,** Y body in fibroblast. (Courtesy Herman Wyandt, Division of Medical Genetics, Child Development and Rehabilitation Center, University of Oregon Medical School.)

steroid characterization reveals a preponderance of Δ^5, 3β-hydroxysteroid metabolites such as dehydroepiandrosterone sulfate, 17-hydroxypregnenolone, and pregnanetriol. This form of adrenal hyperplasia is associated with a high mortality during the first year of life in spite of replacement therapy; the reason for this remains obscure.

In *congenital lipoid hyperplasia* of the adrenal (Prader syndrome), there is virtual standstill of steroid synthesis. It is postulated that there is a block at the 20,22 desmolase step in the conversion of cholesterol to pregnenolone. Clinically, this syndrome behaves like the 3β-hydroxysteroid dehydrogenase deficiency; there is severe salt wasting and uniform fatality.

A block in steroid *17-hydroxylation* also has been described. All affected individuals have been phenotypically female as a result of inability to produce sex hormones as well as cortisol. Excessve mineralocorticoid is produced, causing systemic hypertension. Since there is no abnormality in the external genitalia, this defect is not recognized at birth.

In all the above types of adrenal hyper-

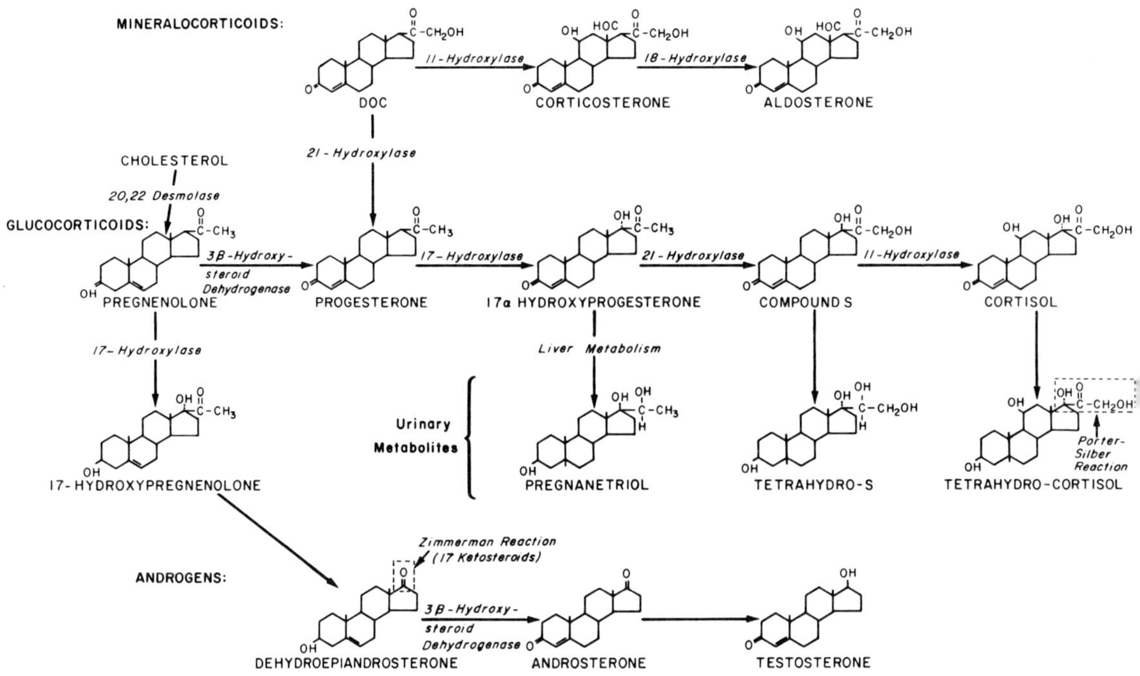

MINERALOCORTICOIDS:
DOC — 11-Hydroxylase → CORTICOSTERONE — 18-Hydroxylase → ALDOSTERONE
21-Hydroxylase
CHOLESTEROL
20,22 Desmolase
GLUCOCORTICOIDS:
PREGNENOLONE — 3β-Hydroxy-steroid Dehydrogenase → PROGESTERONE — 17-Hydroxylase → 17α HYDROXYPROGESTERONE — 21-Hydroxylase → COMPOUND S — 11-Hydroxylase → CORTISOL
17-Hydroxylase
17-HYDROXYPREGNENOLONE
Liver Metabolism
Urinary Metabolites
PREGNANETRIOL
TETRAHYDRO-S
TETRAHYDRO-CORTISOL
Porter-Silber Reaction
ANDROGENS:
Zimmerman Reaction (17 Ketosteroids)
DEHYDROEPIANDROSTERONE — 3β-Hydroxy-steroid Dehydrogenase → ANDROSTERONE → TESTOSTERONE

Fig. 15-7. Biosynthetic pathways for cortisol, mineralocorticoids, and androgens.

plasia except 17-hydroxylase deficiency, the female fetus is exposed to excessive amounts of virilizing hormones. This produces a common urethral and vaginal opening (urogenital sinus), labioscrotal fusion, and hypertrophy of the clitoris. The urethra on rare occasions is sufficiently elongated through complete fusion of the labia to empty on the shaft or tip of the phallus. In the male with CAH, there is insufficient additional androgen to produce penile enlargement at birth. In the 3β-hydroxysteroid dehydrogenase defect, third-degree hypospadias and cryptorchidism are generally present.

Clinical manifestations. In the genetic female, genital ambiguity at birth arouses clinical suspicion (Fig. 15-8). If the disease is known to have occurred in older siblings, the obstetrician and pediatrician should be alerted to the possibility of recurrence. All forms of CAH behave as simple autosomal recessives; that is, there is a 1 to 4 chance of carrier parents having an affected child. The same type repeats itself; that is, if one child is a salt loser, all affected siblings will be salt losers. There is no reliable way to detect the heterozygote. Prenatal diagnosis

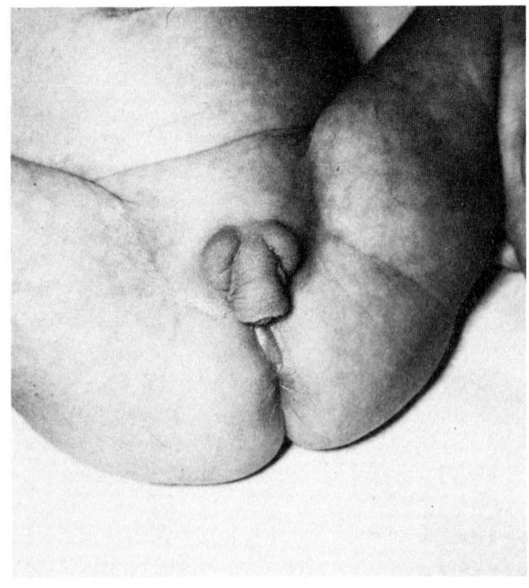

Fig. 15-8. Genitalia of female infant with 21-hydroxylase deficiency congenital adrenal hyperplasia.

through steroid measurement of amniotic fluid has been reported, but the analytic methods are difficult and are available in few centers.

Some female newborns are virilized to a sufficient degree to prompt erroneous male sex assignment and performance of circumcision (Fig. 15-9). Figure 15-8 shows a typical female pseudohermaphrodite with 21-hydroxylase deficiency. Pigmentation of the labioscrotal folds (Fig. 15-9) sometimes occurs, particularly in salt losers. The abnormality is not suspected in affected males at birth, except in the rare cases of 3β-hydroxysteroid dehydrogenase deficiency in which cryptorchidism and hypospadias are present (Fig. 15-10).

If the infant is a *salt-loser,* symptomatic hyponatremia and hyperkalemia will develop during the second week of life. Vomiting is the most frequent symptom and may be associated with refusal of feedings, diarrhea, weight loss, lethargy, and dehydration. The vomiting is frequently projectile, and a diagnosis of hypertrophic pyloric stenosis should be considered, especially in the male. An infant who continues to vomit following pyloroplasty should have urinary steroid determinations made. If the diagnosis of CAH is delayed, the infant may become dangerously hyponatremic and hypovolemic, with progression to irreversible shock. This is more apt to occur in the male whose normal external genitalia do not provoke suspicion at birth. Pigmentation of the scrotum in a male, with vomiting and hyponatremia, suggests CAH with salt wasting. In the male who does not waste salt, the diagnosis is generally delayed until rapid growth and progressive virilization occurs during early childhood.

Diagnosis. Congenital adrenal hyperplasia must be ruled out in any infant with genital ambiguity and presence of nuclear sex chromatin, normal male genitalia with salt loss, and normal male genitalia and a sibling with proved CAH.

Table 15-1 outlines the diagnostic features of the major varieties of the disease. Chromatographic separation and quantitation of individual urinary and plasma steroid metabolites, although desirable, are not essential for diagnosis. Methods for measurement of plasma 17-ketosteroid and corticosteroid concentrations are available but are sometimes difficult to interpret during early infancy because of lack of standardization and presence of interfering substances in blood. Determination of plasma

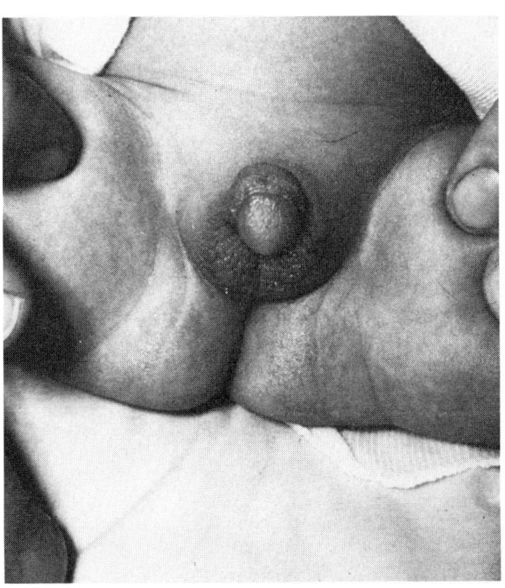

Fig. 15-9. Female infant with 21-hydroxylase deficiency congenital adrenal hyperplasia. Note circumcision and pigmentation of labioscrotal folds.

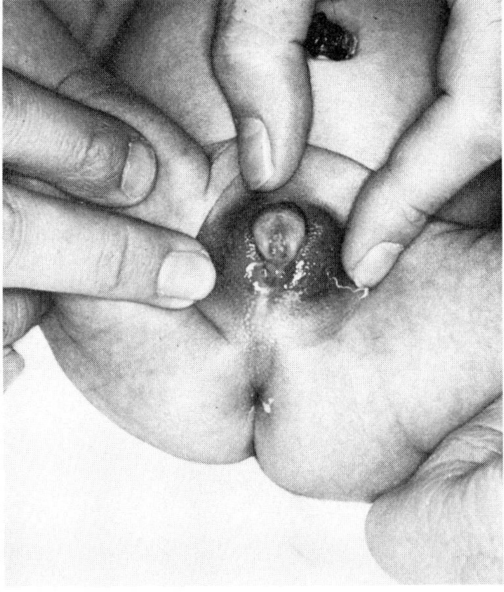

Fig. 15-10. Male infant with 3 β-hydroxysteroid dehydrogenase defect form of congenital adrenal hyperplasia. Note hypospadias and cryptorchidism.

Table 15-1. Distinguishing characteristics of various types of congenital adrenal hyperplasia

Defect	3β-Hydroxysteroid dehydrogenase		17-Hydroxylase		21-Hydroxylase		11-Hydroxylase	
Genotype	Female	Male	Female	Male	Female	Male	Female	Male
Genital abnormality	Clitoral hypertrophy, mild labial fusion	Hypospadias, cryptorchidism	Normal	Female	Female pseudo-hermaphrodite	Normal	Female pseudo-hermaphrodite	Normal
Salt loss	Severe		Absent		Variable		Absent	
Hypertension	Absent		Severe		Absent		Present	
Pigmentation	Present		Absent		In salt loser		Absent	
17-Ketosteroids	Elevated		Diminished		Elevated		Elevated	
Pregnanetriol	Absent		Absent		Elevated		Slightly elevated	
Urinary 17-hydroxycorticoids (Porter-Silber)	Greatly diminished		Absent		Diminished		Elevated (because of Compound S	
17-Ketogenic steroids	Diminished		Absent		Elevated (because of pregnanetriol)		Elevated (Compound S and pregnanetriol)	
Urinary estrogens	Elevated		Absent		Elevated		Elevated	
Virilization	??		Absent		Present		Present	

pregnanetriol and 17-hydroxyprogesterone is valuable but currently available only in specialized steroid research laboratories.

The 24-hour urinary *17-ketosteroid* excretion is elevated in all forms of virilizing CAH, except in the lipoid type. During the first week of life, it is impossible to determine what portion of the infant's total urinary 17-ketosteroids is a reflection of transplacental transport of maternal steroid metabolites. Thus the values for normal infants during the first week of life may be as high as those for infants with CAH. It is safe to assume that the total urinary 17-ketosteroid excretion normally falls to less than 1 mg/24 hr by the end of the second week of life. It is prudent to obtain sequential urinary 17-ketosteroid measurements during the second week of life. If this falls to less than 1 mg/24 hr, CAH may be excluded. A rising value is suggestive, although a falling one does not necessarily rule out the diagnosis of CAH. If the initial measurements are not diagnostic, it is necessary to repeat them after several days have elapsed.

The presence of detectable quantities of *pregnanetriol* in urine or plasma after the first week of life is virtually diagnostic of CAH. Unfortunately, in some patients *pregnanetriol* does not appear until the end of the first month of life. This may be caused by relative deficiency of 3β-hydroxysteroid dehydrogenase in all infants early in life, preventing the conversion of pregnenolone to progesterone. Seventeen-hydroxyprogesterone is produced in excess in both the 21- and the 11-hydroxylase defects; it is converted in the liver to pregnanetriol and conjugated with glucuronide for urinary excretion. Reliable pregnanetriol determination is available through several commercial laboratories. The estimation of urinary cortisol metabolites, the *17-hydroxycorticoids,* is not of great value in the diagnosis of CAH in the newborn period.

One must be aware of the technique employed for measurement for proper interpretation of results. The Porter-Silber method involves enzymatic hydrolysis of glucuronides, solvent extraction of polar steroids, and color production with phenylhydrazine. All extracted compounds with a dihydroxyacetone moiety (Fig. 15-7) will form the yellow Porter-Silber chromogen; for example, tetrahydro-F, tetrahydro-E, and tetrahydro-S, the principle metabolite in the hypertensive form of CAH. Thus, the 17-hydroxycorticoids tend to be low in 21-hydroxylase deficiency and somewhat elevated in 11-hydroxylase deficiency when the Porter-Silber method is employed. The majority of hospital clinical laboratories prefer to measure the urinary 17-ketogenic steroids. Those compounds possessing a 17α-hydroxyl group and a 20-ketone or hydroxyl group are measured by this method. This includes all the known metabolites of cortisol, plus pregnanetriol. Occasionally, a diagnosis of CAH is excluded on the basis of normal or elevated urinary 17-hydroxycorticoids determined by the ketogenic steroid method, because the clinician does not realize he has actually measured pregnanetriol.

Clinical suspicion of the 3β-hydroxysteroid dehydrogenase defect warrants measurement of individual C-19 and C-21 steroids. Large amount of Δ^5, 3β-hydroxysteroid conjugates such as dehydroepiandrosterone and Δ^5 pregnanetriol sulfates are characteristic of this form of the disease; Δ^4, 3-ketosteroids are diminished.

While the infant is in the process of diagnostic studies, it is important to monitor serum and urinary electrolytes. This will allow detection of a falling serum sodium level and excessive urinary salt loss prior to development of serious electrolyte imbalance.

Although elevation of the urinary 17-ketosteroids and pregnanetriol during the first month of life is generally accepted as sufficient evidence for a diagnosis of CAH, it is common practice to perform a suppression test in order to exclude the existence of an adrenal tumor. A convenient method is to administer intramuscularly 25 mg of cortisone acetate daily for 1 week, after which the urinary steroid measurements are repeated. Tumor is ruled out if the 17-ketosteroid and pregnanetriol values fall to normal.

Treatment

Glucocorticoid therapy. The object of treatment is to provide sufficient steroid to replace the cortisol deficit, inhibiting ACTH release by the pituitary gland and preventing progressive virilization. Administration of excessive steroid will produce growth inhibition as well as iatrogenic Cushing's syndrome. Children with the salt-losing variety are frequently short in stature; this characteristic may have a genetic basis or may be a consequence of overzealous steroid administration. Cortisone acetate administered intramuscularly is preferred for initial suppression prior to orally administered replacement therapy; 25 mg administered intramuscularly once daily is sufficient. Following 7 to 10 days of intramuscularly administered cortisone, a 24-hour urine specimen should be collected and 17-ketosteroids and pregnanetriol measured. If both of these values fall to normal or nearly so, adrenal hyperplasia is present, and one should proceed with maintenance therapy.

Some prefer the use of injectable cortisol preparations; however, this is rarely necessary, except when the patient is unable to take oral medication. It is not advisable to employ the newer synthetic steroid analogues, which are designed to avoid some of the very properties that are beneficial to individuals with CAH. Cortisone and hydrocortisone are the preparations of choice. A palatable liquid preparation of hydrocortisone cyclopentylpropionate (Cortef fluid) is available that permits accurate estimation of dosage for small infants and avoids dividing and crushing bitter tablets. Precise doses may be measured with a calibrated medicine dropper or a 2-ml disposable syringe. A suitable starting dose is 8 to 14 mg/day in divided doses, depending upon the size of the infant. Some authorities stress the importance of mimicking the physiologic diurnal variation in cortisol secretion by giving one half of the daily dose in the morning, one fourth in the afternoon, and the remainder at midnight. The maintenance requirement will increase with growth and should be titrated on the basis of urinary steroid values and clinical assessment of the patient. By 1 year of age most patients require 20 to 25 mg of cortisol per day. During periods of stress (infection, trauma, surgery) it is advisable to double the cortisol dose temporarily. If the oral route is not feasible because of vomiting, cortisone acetate may be administered intramuscularly once daily in an amount equal to the customary daily oral dose. It is crucial that steroid administration not be stopped under any circumstance.

Mineralocorticoid therapy. In the salt loser, glucocorticoid therapy alone is insufficient to maintain satisfactory sodium and water balance. In the face of severe sodium depletion, dehydration, and incipient shock, it is advisable to use an injectable form of deoxycorticosterone acetate (DOCA). DOCA in sesame oil, 2 to 4 mg/day, is commonly used for its depot effect. It may be administered at 12- to 24-hour intervals, depending upon the response as measured by the serum sodium and potassium concentrations. As the former approaches a normal value, the DOCA requirement will decrease, particularly when cortisol is replenished. DOCA and salt supplementation may be employed in a hyponatremic infant while studies are in progress without fear of alteration of diagnostic urinary steroid values. This will allow withholding of glucocorticoids until initial 24-hour urine samples are collected while simultaneously correcting the electrolyte imbalance.

After the initial treatment and attainment of normal serum sodium and potassium concentrations, daily injections of DOCA are no longer necessary. The potent mineralocorticoid, 9 α-fluorohydrocortisone (Florinef), is of limited value in young infants. The proper dose is approximately one eighth to one fourth of a very small, 0.1 mg tablet, which is difficult to divide. Subcutaneous implantation of DOCA pellets produce a satisfactory degree of sodium retention for 9 to 10 months. This is occasionally complicated by local infection, pellet rejection, and breakage. The most convenient and perhaps safest approach to mineralocorticoid therapy is the monthly injection of a long-acting ester of DOC such as desoxycorticosterone (percorten) pivalate. The parents may be instructed in injection technique, or it may be administered by a visiting nurse or in the physician's office. The latter is preferable initially since it allows the pediatrician to observe the infant more closely during the early "brittle" months.

Regardless of the mode of therapy selected, the parents should be instructed to observe their infant for edema, sudden weight gain, and thirst, indicating excessive sodium retention. If this occurs, especially if the infant is found to be hypertensive, salt should be restricted and mineralocorticoid withheld until diuresis occurs and a normal serum sodium level is achieved. A lower dosage of DOC-ester should then be administered at monthly intervals. The usual safe and effective dose of desoxycorticosterone pivalate is 25 mg/month (1 ml). Occasionally mineralocorticoid-induced hypertension will precipitate cardiac decompensation and persist for several weeks after withholding salt and hormone. Cortisol should not be restricted in the case of mineralocorticoid overdosage.

Sodium supplementation. Mineralocorticoid administration is of little value to the salt loser unless he is offered adequate sodium. To ensure this, additional sodium chloride may be added to the infant's formula or to supplemental fluids if the infant is breast fed; 1 to 2 gm/day is generally sufficient in the small infant. A 10% sodium chloride solution is easily prepared at home by dissolving 2 level teaspoons of table salt in a 4-ounce bottle of boiled water. Two to four teaspoons (0.5 gm/teaspoon) of the solution may be added to the daily batch of formula or may be given in small aliquots of formula or fruit juice in the breast-fed baby. Although salt craving may be present in a sodium-depleted infant, he is unable to communicate this as does the older child.

Treatment of acute adrenal insufficiency. Frequently infants with the salt-losing varieties of CAH, particularly males, have signs of hypovolemic shock and circulatory collapse. Adrenal insufficiency should be suspected if there is hyponatremia and hyperkalemia. Mineralcorticoid deficiency produces excessive loss of extracellular sodium and water. Reabsorption of potassium by the renal tubule is increased, K^+ leaves the cells, and hyperkalemia ensues, in spite of normal or diminished total body potassium. It is important to withhold potassium-containing fluids until the serum level falls to near normal.

If the infant is hypotensive, it is advisable to administer fluids rapidly (20 cc/kg body weight) to expand the vascular volume. Ten percent glucose in 0.9% sodium chloride is the only maintenance solution necessary for infusion during the first 24 hours. A quantity sufficient to raise the serum sodium level to normal should be infused in addition to 2 to 3 mEq of Na^+ per kg body weight per day to compensate for continual losses. Sodium requirements should be calculated on the basis of total body water; replacement based on the extracellular compartment is frequently inadequate. In general, 90 to 100 ml of isotonic saline per kg body weight per day provides for both sodium losses and maintenance. In the extremely ill infant with profound hyponatremia (below 120 mEq/liter), hypertonic sodium chloride (3% to 5%) may be used in an amount calculated to raise the serum sodium level 7 to 8 mEq/liter in the first 2 hours of treatment. Serum sodium and potassium levels should be measured several times daily in infants receiving large amounts of sodium.

Sympathomimetics are sometimes required for maintenance of normal blood pressure and peripheral circulation. Norepinephrine, 1 mg in 250 ml of solution, may be administered simultaneously with an electrolyte solution via a Y connector at a rate sufficient to maintain a normal blood pressure.

If cardiac toxicity from hypercalcemia is manifest by peaked T and U waves on the ECG, calcium gluconate should be given intravenously, slowly, 1 ml/kg body weight over a 5-minute interval or until reversal of these abnormalities is achieved. Cation exchange resins administered either by mouth or by retention enema are useful in the emergency treatment of hyperkalemia. A 30% solution of sodium polystyrene sulfonate (Kayexalate) in a dose of 5 gm/kg is sufficient. If used rectally, the resin should be suspended in 20% sorbitol to prevent impaction.

Corrective surgery. The proper timing and technique for correction of the genital abnormalities of females born with CAH remain controversial issues. With early diagnosis and steroid replacement, the clitoris may regress significantly in size and become partially obscured by the labia majora. If it appears that persistent clitoral enlargement will be a source of embarrassment to the child, surgical correction should be attempted between 1 and 2 years of age. A procedure whereby the clitoris is freed and placed beneath the mons pubis (clitoral recession) is often preferred to clitorectomy. Separation of labioscrotal fusion may be performed during early infancy or later in childhood. Exploratory laparotomy in suspected or proved cases of CAH is not indicated.

True hermaphroditism. A true hermaphrodite possesses both ovarian and testicular tissue. The condition is not noticed in many of these infants because of their resemblance to normal males with hypospadias and cryptorchidism (Fig. 15-11). A disorder of sexual differentiation is not suspected until an ovotestis is discovered during hernia repair or when gynecomastia with or without cyclic bleeding through the urethra begins at puberty. A nuclear sex chromatin determination should be performed on all infants with hypospadias and unilateral or bilateral undescended gonads. If true hermaphroditism is present, the buccal smear will be chromatin positive in a majority of instances in spite of predominantly male external characteristics.

Although lateralization is possible (that is, a testis on one side and an ovary on the opposite), it is more common to find either bilateral ovotestes or one ovotestis with a contralateral normal-appearing ovary or testis. The latter variant is the least common, but when present the testis is usually descended. Ovarian tissue is virtually never completely descended into the scrotum. Ovotestes may either be abdominal or in the groin, usually associated with an inguinal hernia.

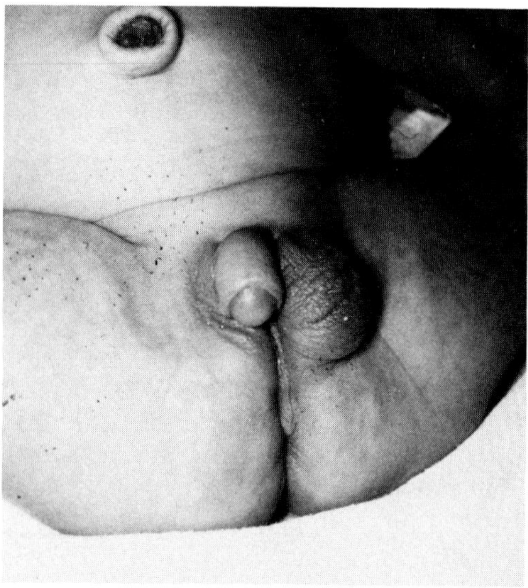

Fig. 15-11. True hermaphrodite with scrotal testis and abdominal ovotestis.

Cytogenetic studies indicate that the great majority of true hermaphrodites have normal female karyotypes, 46/XX. A few mosaics have been reported, such as XX/XY and XX/XXY. The paradox of testicular tissue in the absence of a discernible Y chromosome has been attributed to the presence of genes originating from a Y that have been translocated or have crossed over with an X chromosome. It is possible that a small portion of Y translocates to the X during meiotic pairing.

The internal genital duct structures conform to the theories of sexual differentiation of Jost as described above. On the side where a testis is present, there is usually a vas deferens; a tube will accompany an ovary. There is generally some degree of uterine development regardless of gonadal structure. With an ovotestis there is a tube and sometimes a vas. The external genitalia appear male in the majority of patients, and consequently most patients are reared as males with hypospadias and with bifid scrotum or cryptorchidism or both. There is little correlation between the degree of external masculinization and the amount of testicular tissue present. Moreover, the testis of the true hermaphrodite is unable to elaborate sufficient inducer to inhibit müllerian duct development.

Assignment of sex should be based mainly upon the anatomy of the external genitalia. With good phallic development and complete labioscrotal fusion, male gender is more appropriate. To avoid pubertal gynecomastia and cyclic bleeding through the urethra, the gonads should be removed and prosthetic testes placed into the scrotum when technically possible.

Iatrogenic female pseudohermaphroditism. The chromatin-positive infant with genital ambiguity who has normal or falling urinary 17-ketosteroid and pregnanetriol excretion rates may suffer the consequences of maternal androgen or progestin therapy during pregnancy. The degree of clitoral hypertrophy, corpus spongiosum formation, labioscrotal fusion, and urethral elongation depends upon the type, amount, and period of maternal hormone administration. Occasionally, the mother is unaware that she has taken a hormonal preparation and states that she "took shots" to save her pregnancy or took special vitamins for leg cramps. It is therefore necessary to ascertain from the mother's physician exactly what preparations were given during pregnancy.

Although the most common offenders have been the synthetic orally administered progestins, including contraceptive preparations, virilization of the female fetus has occurred with testosterone, androstenediol, stilbestrol, and progesterone. Complete masculinization with phallic urethra has been produced by testosterone administration with preparations used for osteoporosis, leg cramps, and other symptoms of pregnancy.

The external genitalia are rarely sufficiently masculinized to warrant an erroneous male sex assignment. Since the internal genital structures and ovaries are intact, allowing normal reproductive potential, there is no justification for male birth registration. Progressive virilization obviously does not occur. Progestational steroids rarely produce hypertrophy of the corpus spongiosum of the clitoris.

There is no explanation why only a small fraction of females born to mothers given progestins are partially virilized at birth. Differences in placental transport, fetal metabolism, and sensitivity of end-organs have been postulated. The more recently available compounds have had a safer record compared with ethinyltestosterone (Pranone) and 17 α-ethinyl-19-nortestosterone (Norlutin).

Rarely, a virilizing tumor of the ovary (arrhenoblastoma) will produce sufficient androgen to masculinize a female fetus.

The diagnosis of iatrogenic female pseudohermaphroditism should be made only after CAH is excluded with appropriate steroid measurements. Surgical exploration of the pelvis is unnecessary, but correction of the genital abnormality should be undertaken prior to 2 years of age. In many cases the degree of virilization is insufficient to justify repair.

Idiopathic female pseudohermaphroditism. Occasionally, a partially masculinized female is born to a mother who has taken neither progestins nor androgens during pregnancy. Urinary steroid determinations are normal. Many infants in this category have congenital anomalies of other systems. Absence of the palpebral fissures, defects of the ocular globes, cleft palate, imperforate anus, and cardiac and renal defects have occurred with clitoral hypertrophy and complete labioscrotal fusion. This has been referred to as the cryptophthalmos syndrome and is inherited by an autosomal recessive mechanism. Affected males appear to have normal genitalia.

When there is no clear history of maternal hormone ingestion, idiopathic female pseudohermaphroditism is difficult to distinguish from true hermaphroditism with undescended gonads. It therefore becomes necessary to perform exploratory surgery to distinguish these conditions. If frozen section reveals ovotestis, the gonads should be removed; normal-appearing ovaries should remain in the pelvis since they may function normally at puberty.

Chromatin-negative infants

A chromatin-negative buccal mucosal smear in a newborn with genital abnormality usually indicates the presence of one X chromosome with a normal or partially deleted Y. Rarely, a chromatin-negative infant with clitoral enlargement will prove to have 44 autosomes plus XO, but will display physical stigmata of Turner's syndrome, such as webbed neck, peripheral lymphedema, highly arched palate, aortic coarctation, and so on. The fluorescent Y body (Fig. 15-6) is helpful in distinguishing XY from XO.

A chromatin-negative smear does not always exclude a diagnosis of CAH. The rare 3β-hydroxysteroid dehydrogenase defect (p. 472) precludes normal masculinization of a male fetus because of inability to synthesize testicular androgen. Thus it is good practice to measure urinary steroid excretion in any infant with genital ambiguity, regardless of the sex chromatin pattern.

Male pseudohermaphroditism. A wide spectrum of genital abnormality occurs in male pseudohermaphroditism. Sex assignment usually depends upon the degree of penile development. By definition, both gonads resemble normal testes microscopically, with well-developed seminiferous tubules and Leydig cells. In one form, the external genitalia are entirely female, and an abnormality is not suspected at birth. The diagnosis is made later when a testis is found in an inguinal hernia or when there is failure of sexual hair development and amenorrhea at puberty (syndrome of testicular feminization).

The male pseudohermaphrodite with genital ambiguity generally has undescended testes, although occasionally one or both may be palpable in the inguinal canals. A small hypospadiac phallus with an orifice at its base or posteriorly in a scrotal cleft should suggest the condition at birth (Fig. 15-12).

The anatomy of the internal duct structures is variable. With deficiency of the fetal testicular inducer, the uterus, tubes, and vagina will be fully developed. If the inducer function of the testis is preserved, there is a blind vaginal pouch without cervix and vasa deferentia internally.

Male pseudohermaphroditism may be familial. The syndrome of testicular feminization is transmitted through a sex-linked recessive or sex-limited autosomal dominant mode of inheritance. Since affected individuals are sterile, it is impossible to determine which of these mechanisms is operative. The presence of normal-appearing testes and genetic transmittance suggests a biochemical defect. In testicular feminization the affected individual appears unable to convert testosterone to biologically active dihydrotestosterone. Thus there is no masculinization of the fetal external genitalia, and sexual hair does not appear at puberty. The presence of a vas and the absence of uterus and tubes indicates that fetal testicular inducer is produced normally. Occasionally, infants with testicular feminization are recognized at birth because of clitoral enlargement. Affected siblings will also have genital ambiguity, and the term *partial testicular feminization* or *Reifenstein's syndrome* has been applied to this condition. Although testicular feminization is clearly familial, this is not so with other forms of male pseudohermaphroditism. One type with ambiguous or predominantly male external genitalia may show normal androgen function at puberty and sometimes occurs in siblings.

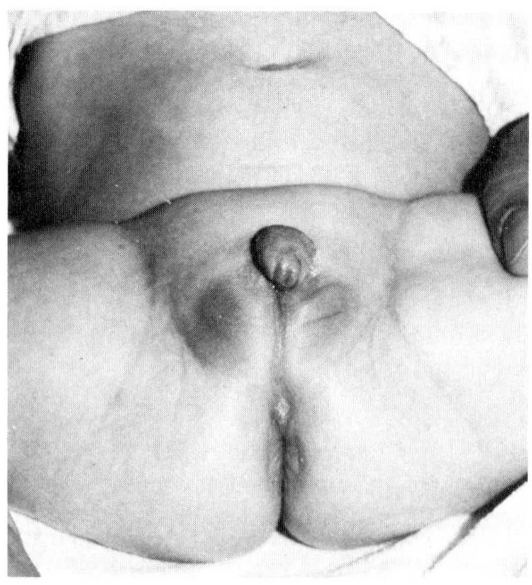

Fig. 15-12. Male pseudohermaphrodite.

Gross abnormalities of the chromosomes are unusual in male pseudohermaphroditism with bilaterally normal appearing testes, but XO/XY mosaicism has been reported in several instances.

It is impossible to predict from the appearance of the external or internal genital structures or karyotype whether a child will masculinize, feminize, or remain undeveloped at puberty. For this reason and because of the increased risk of gonadal neoplasm, it is suggested that abdominal testes be removed at the time of diagnostic laparotomy. Prosthetic testes can be placed in the scrotum when the child is older and appropriate hormone replacement therapy begun during the early adolescent years.

Sex of rearing should be based more upon the appearance of the perineum than such factors as genotype, gonadal histology, or internal genital duct structures. The majority are best reared as females. With gonadectomy, clitoral recession, and separation of labial fusion, the child will adopt an appropriate feminine psychosexual orientation. She should be able to enjoy normal sexual relations as an adult. At early puberty it becomes necessary to administer estrogen and progesterone cyclically to promote breast development and menses. When there is a well-developed hypospadiac phallus with corpus spongiosum, complete labioscrotal fusion, and palpable gonads, a male sex assignment is justifiable.

The tragedy of male assignment in an infant with scant erectile penile tissue and severe hypospadias is encountered all too frequently. Many become inadequate, frustrated adult males with little benefit from systemic or local testosterone therapy. Surgical construction of an artificial vagina is no more difficult than reconstructing a penis and is more functional.

In rare chromatin-negative XY infants with genital ambiguity, no gonads are found when exploratory surgery is performed; both müllerian and wolffian duct derivatives are present. These patients are listed as male pseudohermaphrodites in spite of the absence of testicular tissue. Testes may have been present during fetal life but later degenerated for unknown reasons.

Mixed gonadal dysgenesis. Another group of chromatin-negative infants with genital ambiguity are found to have unilateral testicular development with contralateral fibrous streaks in place of a gonad or no gonad at all. These individuals are human examples of Jost's rabbit experiments. The normal-appearing testis is generally accompanied by a vas deferans and an epididymis. Beside the dysgenetic gonad or streak is a fallopian tube and unicornuate uterus. The müllerian duct remnants may appear with the gonad in an inguinal hernia sac.

The anatomy of the external genitalia varies with the degree of masculinization afforded by the fetal testicular androgen. Those with mild hypospadias and unilateral cryptorchidism at birth have been raised as males. When the phallus is little more than an enlarged clitoris and there is posterior labial fusion, female gender is more practical.

Sex chromosome abnormalities occur in this group of patients with much greater frequency than in other categories. XY/XO mosaicism is the most common karyotypic abnormality reported. Others have had XO/XXXY, XYY, XO/XY_iy,* Xy. These represent sporadic nondisjunctional abnormalities without familial occurrences.

Sex assignment should be based primarily upon the adequacy of the phallus. Withdrawal bleeding will usually occur with cyclic estrogen replacement therapy during puberty because of the presence of endometrial tissue.

*Y_i, isochromosome long arm of Y; y, partially deleted Y.

Miscellaneous genital abnormalities

Cryptorchidism. Bilateral or unilateral undescented testis is present in 2.7% of newborn males at term. The incidence increases with decreasing gestational age. Scorer found that 57% of testes not in the scrotum at birth had fully descended by 1 month of age and 80% by 1 year. Of those remaining undescended after 1 year, the majority are in the inguinal canal. In cases where there is accompanying hypospadias, bifid scrotum, or small phallus, urinary steroid determinations and cytogenetic studies are warranted.

Microphallus. This abnormality is fortunately rare and usually accompanied by an empty, poorly developed scrotum. The penis in the normal, full-term male extends 2 to 3 cm from the pubis. Occasionally, a mother will express concern over her son's small penis. In most instances, the phallus is normal in size, but the shaft is embedded in the pubic fat pad. Cytogenetic, radiographic, and urinary steroid studies should be performed to exclude CAH with complete labioscrotal fusion and phallic urethra.

In true microphallus, a plastic procedure will usually be necessary after maximum phallic growth is attained. Androgen administration is of little value because of the absence of a corpus cavernosum. Infants born with complete *absence of the penis* should be reared as girls with later construction of an artificial vagina. This defect is frequently accompanied by other lethal anomalies.

Ectopic scrotum is generally unilateral and accompanies other anomalies such as imperforate anus, sacrococcygeal teratoma, and lipoma of the buttock. A normal testis may be descended into the abnormally placed scrotal sac (Fig. 15-13).

Imperforate hymen or *vaginal atresia* are usually discovered at puberty, but sometimes will cause hydrometrocolpos during the early weeks of life. Secretory activity of the glands of the cervix is provoked by maternally derived sex hormones. The retained mucoid material may cause abdominal mass, vaginal distension, and urethral obstruction. Diagnosis is made by abdominal or rectal palpation of a pelvic mass and visualization of a bulging hymenal membrane between the separated labia majora. Incision of the membrane and evacua-

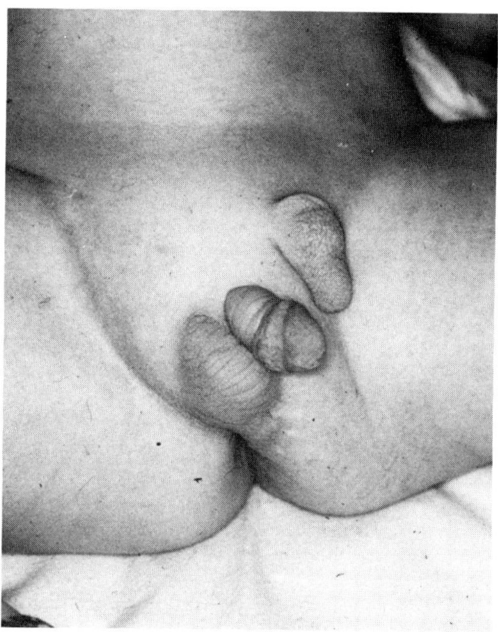

Fig. 15-13. Ectopic scrotum and testis in infant with gluteal lipoma.

tion of the fluid is all that is necessary to relieve the obstruction. A *transverse vaginal septum* may be present at the junction of the müllerian duct epithelium and the urogenital sinus. It is asymptomatic at birth unless it produces obstruction and hydrometrocolpos.

Adhesion of opposing mucosal surfaces of the infant's labia majora is a frequent source of concern to parent and pediatrician. Manual separation of synechiae has been the traditional pediatric approach to this problem. Recurrence is common following the tearing of adhesions, even with the use of local therapy with estrogen cream. There is little evidence that labial adhesion predisposes the infant to either urinary retention or infection or both. Treatment is not indicated unless dysuria or perineal discomfort seems to be caused by urinary pooling behind the adherent labia.

Counseling parents of infants with abnormalities of sexual differentiation

Regardless of anatomic, genetic, or endocrinologic diagnosis, if the external genitalia are appropriate for the assigned sex of the infant, the parents should have little difficulty in adjusting to the problem. The more inappropriate the genitalia seem to the parents, the greater is the likelihood of development of confusion regarding their infant's "real" sex. Psychosexual orientation in the human is more dependent upon parental attitude and behavior toward the child than upon hormonal or anatomic factors.

Once the medical team reaches a firm decision, the suggested sex of rearing should be reported to the parents, enabling them to distribute appropriate birth announcements. It is of great help to utilize anatomic diagrams in order to provide the parents with a clear concept of the infant's abnormalities. It is useful to allow the grandparents to attend a conference with the parents, since they will undoubtedly assist to some degree in the baby's care and should be apprised of the genital abnormality. If the parents are young, the grandparents will frequently suspect that the doctors have withheld information from them. In general, it is best to be honest and thorough, but in some instances (for example, true hermaphroditism) it is more humane to withhold certain details. The parents of a male pseudohermaphrodite reared as a female need not be told that testes are present but that the gonadal structures are incompletely formed and may not be functional in later life. They may be told that the incomplete gonads should be removed because of predisposition to malignancy and the possibility of masculinization at puberty.

In cases where sex assignment cannot be made at birth, the parents should be instructed to postpone distribution of birth announcements until studies have been completed. Circumcision is always contraindicated in newborns with any degree of genital abnormality and certainly when there is uncertainty regarding sex. Most authorities agree that surgical procedures of the external genitalia should be performed prior to 2 years of age in order to minimize problems of sexual identity.

HARVEY D. KLEVIT

BIBLIOGRAPHY

Jost, A.: Recherches sur la differenciation sexvelle de l'embryon de Lapin, Arch. Anat. Micro. et Morphol. Exper. **36**:151, 1947.

Lyon, M. F.: Gene action in the X-chromosome of the mouse (Mus Musculus L), Nature **190**: 372, 1961.

16 Diseases of the kidney and urinary tract

RENAL FUNCTION AND ITS MORPHOLOGIC CORRELATES

During intrauterine life the function of the nephric system is minimal. The task of maintaining the homeostasis of the fetus is fulfilled by the placenta, as evidenced by the absence at birth of abnormalities in fluid and electrolyte balance in newborns with bilateral renal agenesis. Formation and excretion of urine are essential, however, for the maintenance of an adequate amount of amniotic fluid. Moreover, urine formation plays a role in the embryogenesis of the urinary system.

At birth, the kidneys have a combined weight of about 25 gm, compared with 40 gm at 3 months of age and 300 gm in the adult. They often demonstrate persistence of a fetal lobular structure; and because of the laxity of the abdominal wall, they are readily palpable. A cut section of the superficial renal cortex appears thin, whereas the juxtamedullary and medullary areas are relatively well developed. These characteristics correspond to the more advanced state of development reached by the deeper (more central) parts of the kidney and reflect the centrifugal pattern that characterizes the growth of this organ. Despite its small size and the thin cortex, the kidney of the full-term newborn infant contains its full complement of nephrons (800,000 to 1,000,000 per kidney). According to Potter and Thierstein, formation of new glomeruli ceases in the normal fetus when the fetus's length reaches 46 to 49 cm and its weight reaches 2,100 to 2,500 gm. The diameter of the glomerulus in the newborn is about half of the adult, and the length of the tubule is no more than one tenth. This relative predominance of glomerular tissue over tubular tissue is considered to influence the functional pattern of the kidney during infancy.

The most important distinctive physiologic feature of the newborn kidney is its relatively low level of function. The uncorrected rate of glomerular filtration in the newborn is around 4 ml/min, or about 35 ml/min/1.73 m^2. This can be compared with the glomerular filtration of 125 ml/min/1.73 m^2 of the average adult male and explains why the newborn is unable to dispose rapidly and efficiently of excess water and solute. Since the process of growth results in a high degree of anabolism of substances such as nitrogen, potassium, sodium, calcium, phosphorus, and water, the excretory burden of the kidney is minimized.

An important characteristic of the newborn kidney is the more advanced maturation of the juxtamedullary nephrons. These nephrons, which are endowed with long loops of Henle, have a great capacity to reabsorb sodium and water and are principally responsible for the concentration of urine. The fact that the newborn is unable to reach levels of urine osmolarity in excess of 700 mOsm/liter, compared with 1,300 mOsm/liter in the older child, is only in small part the result of morphologic immaturity. The main reason is the limited availability of urea, which constitutes about half the total osmolality of the renal medullary interstitium in the mature kidney. The almost complete anabolism of protein, which characterizes the healthy newborn, results in relatively little urea for excretion. If protein is provided in sufficient amounts, within 2 or 3 months the kidney reaches a concentrating ability that approaches that of the mature organ.

Another peculiarity of the kidney during early extrauterine life is the high degree of both anatomical and functional heterogeneity of its component units, the nephrons. For example, an elevenfold difference in tubular length has been found among the nephrons of the same kidney. The glomeruli, on the other hand, show a much smaller degree of variation. The physiologic consequence of this feature is an expanded range of transport capacity of different nephrons. This can be observed when the serum concentration of a substance actively transported by the kidney, such as bicarbonate, is progressively increased and its reabsorption is plotted as a function of the amount filtered. The blood concentration of the substance necessary to saturate the transport capacity of all nephrons, relative to the blood concentration at which the substance first appears in urine (indicating saturation of nephrons with the lowest transport capacity), is much greater than that in the adult.

Morphologic studies have also pointed out the fact that the ratio between glomerular diameter and tubular volume is higher in the infant than later in life. This high ratio is considered to result in a higher capacity of the kidney to filter than to reabsorb or to secrete, and it probably explains why the newborn excretes in the urine a higher fraction of the filtered load of substances such as amino acids, phosphate, and bicarbonate. The practical impact is greater for bicarbonate than for any of the other substances. The concentration of bicarbonate in blood is controlled by its renal threshold. This mechanism allows bicarbonate to remain in the blood only as long as its concentration is below a certain level. Above this level (the renal threshold), filtered bicarbonate is incompletely reabsorbed, and thus some is excreted in the urine. If the threshold is low, as it is in the newborn, the concentration of bicarbonate in serum, and therefore the buffering capacity of the blood, is maintained at a low level. This is a major factor contributing to the tendency to acidosis in the newborn period, especially in premature infants. Also responsible for this phenomenon are an increased production of organic acids and, during the first few days of life, the inability of the kidney to establish a steep gradient of H^+ and, as a consequence, to excrete strongly acid urine. The low phosphate intake that is prevalent at this early age contributes to a low rate of excretion of titratable acid. If phosphate is added to the diet, a significant increase in urinary titratable acid ensues. Finally, ammoniogenesis also is diminished during the first few weeks of life, even under conditions of stress such as administration of ammonium or calcium chloride. The response of the kidney to acid loading becomes comparable to that of the adult by the end of the first month of life.

In summary, the immature kidney is characterized by a generally low functional capacity, a relatively better-developed juxtamedullary than cortical area, nephronic heterogeneity, and glomerular preponderance. The low rate of glomerular filtration limits the ability of the kidney to dispose rapidly of a fluid or solute load. The even greater limitations in tubular reabsorption may result in inappropriate loss in urine of substances present in the glomerular filtrate, such as glucose, amino acids, bicarbonate, and phosphate. Although none of these limitations has a detrimental effect in a healthy neonate, they restrict the capacity of the newborn to respond under conditions of stress. It is under these latter circumstances that the vulnerability of the neonate becomes evident.

REACTION OF THE IMMATURE KIDNEY TO INJURY

Suppuration, ischemic necrosis, and hemorrhage are lesions common to all tissues and all ages, but the tissue reaction of the newborn seems to incorporate a greater proliferative or regenerative component than that in the adult. In the kidney, epithelial cells undergo dedifferentiation and apparent multiplication to form distinctive glomerular and tubular forms that mimic a fetal appearance. Such epithelial patterns can result from both regressive transformation and failure of differentiation; and while commonly seen in dysplastic kidneys, they do not in themselves signify a developmental anomaly, nor do they constitute evidence of an underlying congenital abnormality in an otherwise diseased kidney. These epithelial abnormalities, both glomerular and tubular, often coexist with involutional changes. In glomeruli, for example, both epithelial changes and hyalinization are part of a process common enough to be regarded as normal. We have come to expect that as many as 10% of glomeruli will show histologic evidence of glomerular sclerosis and obsolescence, although we do not understand either the pathogenesis or the significance of the finding. Such structures are found in increased numbers as a consequence of renal necrosis, ischemic damage, and urinary tract obstruction. There is also increased severity of glomerular sclerosis in premature infants and in those with congenital heart disease.

Glomerular sclerosis is frequently accompanied by glomerular cyst formation; variable tubular atrophy and tubular cyst formation also may be present. In autosomal trisomy syndromes D and E, sclerotic glomeruli, incorporating both primitive and cystic changes, are often found in the peripheral cortex. Grossly, cystic glomeruli of the peripheral cortex are found in Jeune's asphyxiating dystrophy, Zellweger's cerebrohepatorenal syndrome, and Schwartz-Jampel's syndrome.

Cyst formation seems to be a common response of the fetal or neonatal kidney to severe forms of injury. In addition to glomerular cysts, tubular cysts commonly develop as a response to urinary tract obstruction. Cysts are found at the ampullary ends of collecting tubules in association with lower urinary tract obstruction, perhaps because hydrostatic pressure is easily transmitted along the relatively short and straight collecting ducts and tubules. The relationship between these lesions and what has been described as glomerular cystic disease remains unresolved. It is not known if these are truly abnormalities of renal organogenesis or acquired changes of formed nephrons secondary to undefined, nephrotoxic metabolic abnormalities.

Another important aspect of the reaction of immature kidneys to injury is the effect on subsequent renal growth. Inflammatory parenchymal disease beginning very early in life may lead to very small, end-stage kidneys, probably because subsequent growth and development are impaired by extensive epithelial damage, fibrosis, and vascular changes. In localized or unilateral diseases, on the other hand, the uninvolved parenchyma is capable of considerable compensatory hypertrophy. This may relate to the fact that compensatory hypertrophy in early life, like normal renal growth in early life, has been demonstrated experimentally to incorporate rapid, cellular proliferation (hyperplasia), whereas compensatory growth in older animals is associated predominantly with increase in cell size (hypertrophy). All changes, even in newborns, take place in the existing nephrons, and no new ones are formed.

INVESTIGATION FOR RENAL DISEASE

Clinical evaluation of the kidneys must include assessment of both morphologic status and functional capacity.

Morphologic evaluation

Gross morphologic characteristics can be investigated by a variety of radiographic and radioisotopic methods. *A plane film of the abdomen* often delineates the edge of the kidney, providing information concerning renal size and shape. In the neonate, a small kidney almost always reflects a developmental abnormality rather than the effects of acquired disease. An irregular contour may be indicative of scarring following vascular obstruction or infection. This should be differentiated from fetal lobulation, which often persists into extrauterine life.

Intravenous urography is the most widely used and the most valuable method of radiologic investigation of the kidney. The usual dose of 50% diatrizoate (Hypaque) sodium given to a child is 1 ml/kg body weight, but for the infant a dose of 3 ml/kg (up to a total of 20 ml) is used. For evaluation of a mass in the neonate, as much as 5 ml/kg may be given. Since 50% diatrizoate has an osmolarity of 1,600 mOsm/liter and a sodium concentration of 50 mEq/liter, the material should be used with caution in dehydrated infants and in those with cardiac failure or renal insufficiency. Films taken shortly after the injection of contrast material reveal a "bodygram" effect from opacification of the vascular space. As a consequence, organs or other masses that are highly vascular are opaque, whereas cysts and other avascular structures appear translucent, but surrounded by a dark shadow. Since the renal parenchyma is visualized during the same phase, the resulting nephrogram can be used for measurement of kidney size and cortical thickness. Subsequent films permit visualization of the entire urinary tract and serve to define the status of the calyceal systems, pelves, ureters, and bladder.

Voiding cystourethrography should be considered an essential part of the radiologic examination whenever obstructive uropathy is suspected or urinary tract infection has been documented. A 12% to 15% solution of a water soluble contrast medium is instilled into the bladder through a proper size catheter lubricated with an antibiotic ointment (a No. 5 feeding tube is adequate for the newborn). The catheter is removed when complete filling of the bladder is evidenced by leakage around the tube. Fluoroscopic observation of the urethra during voiding and of the bladder and lower ureters toward the end of voiding is done.

Aortography and selective renal angiography are used in the differential diagnosis of abdominal masses, although their role is still controversial. The inferior vena cavagram may be of great help in the diagnosis of renal vein thrombosis. The diagnosis of Wilms' tumor usually can be confirmed by an intravenous urogram, most of these tumors having a distinctive vascular pattern. Since some are avascular, however, an angiogram may not help in the differentiation from an abscess. Angiography is of value in the diagnosis of vascular anomalies, such as segmental hypoplasia and arterial obstruction.

Radioisotopic methods such as the renal scan and the renogram are gaining increasing popularity as their diagnostic role is better defined. Both of these methods have the advantage of requiring much lower irradiation than the usual x-ray techniques. The renal scan is of value in locating anomalous kidneys, determining kidney size, and demonstrating renal and other abdominal masses. In the infant the renogram is used mainly in the investigation of urinary tract obstruction.

The microscopic morphologic characteristics of the kidney can be investigated by examining tissue obtained by *needle biopsy*. This procedure is now used extensively in the diagnosis of parenchymal renal disease; in expert hands the associated risks are minimal. Although indications for performing a renal biopsy in the newborn are limited, it is an extremely valuable procedure in appropriate patients.

Functional evaluation

Assessment of the ability of the kidneys to fulfill their role of maintenance of body homeostasis requires an array of tests directed toward a number of specific aspects of renal function.

Examination of a *freshly voided specimen of urine* provides immediate, invaluable information regarding the condition of the kidney. Although the neonate excretes a higher fraction of filtered protein in urine than does the older child, the concentration usually does not exceed 5 to 10 mg/100 ml of urine; as a consequence, protein is not detected by conventional methods of testing, such as Albustix or 10% sulfosalicylic acid. The claim made in the past that the urine of the newborn contains significant amounts of protein was based on testing with trichloroacetic acid, which gave false positive results by reacting with urates.

Microscopic examination of the sediment obtained by centrifugation of a 10-ml aliquot of urine for 5 minutes should reveal less than 2 to 3 white blood cells (WBC) per high-power field, usually no red blood cells (RBC), and no casts or bacteria. Abnormal numbers of leukocytes are usually interpreted as indicative of infection. It should be realized, however, that leukocyturia occurs in many noninfectious conditions as well, including obstructive uropathy and a number of types of glomerulonephritis. More than a few cellular casts in the urinary sediment are suggestive of renal parenchymal disease; RBC casts are considered the hallmark of glomerulonephritis.

The *Addis count* provides quantitative information on the rate of excretion in the urine of cells, casts, and protein. In addition, it can serve as a test of concentrating ability if appropriate restriction of fluid intake is imposed prior to and during the collection period. Since an accurately timed collection is essential for this determination, the test is difficult to perform in the infant. Moreover, data from which the range of normal can be established are extremely limited. Up to 100,000 WBC and 75,000 RBC are considered normal. Detection of casts is unusual in the absence of disease. The amount of protein should not exceed 5 to 10 mg/12 hr. After an overnight thirst older children normally have concentrated urine of at least 900 mOsm/liter. After the first few days of life an osmolality of 700 or more is expected in infants' urine.

Since the elimination from the blood of certain substances, such as *urea* and *creatinine,* depends on the rate of glomerular filtration, their *plasma concentrations* serve as indicators of the level of renal function. However, the relationship between their concentrations in plasma and glomerular filtration rate (GFR) is described by a hyperbola, so that until renal function is severely impaired, the increases in plasma urea and creatinine concentrations are relatively small, and their concentrations may still fall within the normal range. Furthermore, it must be recognized that the concentration of these substances in healthy infants is much lower than it is in older children. A creatinine concentration of 0.6 mg/100 ml, for instance, which is well within what is generally accepted to be the normal range for older children and adults, might represent a 100% increase over normal in a newborn and signify, therefore, a 50% reduction in GFR. Technical difficulties in measuring creatinine accurately in concentrations below 0.5 mg/100 ml further complicate interpretation of the results. Finally, the concentration of urea in plasma is markedly affected by the intake and rate of anabolism of protein.

A better estimate of the functional capacity of the kidney is given by measurement of GFR by one of a variety of *clearance methods.* The renal clearance is the amount of plasma that would need to be totally cleared of a particular substance by the kidney per unit of time to account for its rate of excretion in urine. The mathematical expression is $C = \frac{U \times V}{P}$ in which C = renal clearance, U = concentration in urine of the substance under study, V = volume of urine per unit of time, and P = concentration in plasma of the substance under study. Conventionally, clearances are expressed as ml/min/1.73 m^2 of body surface area. If a substance is freely filterable through the glomerular membrane, is physiologically inert, and is neither reabsorbed nor secreted, its clearance is equal to GFR. Inulin, a polymer of fructose, is such a substance. Its clearance remains the best determinant of GFR. However, since a continuous infusion of inulin must be given in order to maintain an adequate blood concentration during the test and since the measurement of inulin involves a tedious chemical procedure, the clearance of inulin is not measured routinely. Nevertheless, with this method, GFR has been shown to be 25 to 30 ml/min/1.73 m^2 during the first few days of life and about 50 ml/min/1.73 m^2 by the end of the first month. It must be emphasized, however, that individual variation and variability related to the method make interpretation of isolated results rather difficult unless they are clearly abnormal.

In order to obviate the need for continuous infusion, the clearance of some substances normally present in blood may be used to estimate GFR. The most commonly used are urea and creatinine. The advantage of the urea clearance is the high concentration of urea in blood and urine and the ease of its chemical determination. The disadvantage is the dependence of its excretion on the rate of urine flow, since urea is variably reabsorbed during passage through the nephron. Nevertheless, at moderate rates of urine flow (2 to 6 ml/min/1.73 m^2) approximately 60% of filtered urea is excreted in the urine, and thus the clearance of urea represents approximately 60% of the actual GFR.

The main advantage of the creatinine clearance is its independence of rate of urine flow. However, the low concentration of creatinine in plasma in infants and young children makes the laboratory method difficult and inaccurate. Since creatinine is excreted by tubular secretion as well as by glomerular filtration, its clearance may overestimate true GFR. Nevertheless, the clearance of creatinine remains the best and most widely used method for measurement of GFR under usual clinical circumstances.

Recent progress in the mathematical analysis of multicompartmental models has made possible the use of plasma disappearance curves for the calculation of GFR. Substances excreted by glomerular filtration that can be labelled with isotopes, such as ^{125}I-Iothalamate sodium and ^{51}Cr-EDTA, currently are employed with much success. This method obviates the need for continuous infusion and timed urine collections, which are so difficult to achieve in infants and small children. The amount of radioactivity provided by a single procedure is negligible.

Many clinical situations require assessment of *renal acidifying mechanisms*. This is done by a determination of urinary pH and rates of excretion of titratable acid and ammonium during spontaneous metabolic acidosis or after administration of ammonium chloride and by performance of a bicarbonate titration. These are highly specialized tests and therefore are not detailed here. It is of importance to note, however, that after the first few days of life healthy infants are able to achieve a urinary pH as low as 5.0. In the presence of acidemia, higher values cannot be considered normal.

PRESENTING SIGNS AND SYMPTOMS

It is characteristic of the seriously ill newborn to have nonspecific signs of his disease, such as fever, irritability, poor feeding, and failure to thrive. In such infants disease of the kidneys and urinary tract must be considered in the differential diagnosis. Nevertheless, certain signs point directly toward urinary tract disease, and these are discussed in this section.

Disorders of micturition

Ninety-two percent of healthy infants pass urine within the first 24 hours after birth, and 99% have done so by 48 hours. Often, however, the first micturition takes place in the delivery room and passes unnoticed. In the rare instance in which the newborn does not urinate within 72 hours, serious consideration should be given to the possibility of bilateral renal agenesis (p. 494), urinary tract obstruction (p. 499), or a renovascular accident (p. 508). Of these possibilities, the most important to diagnose is obstructive uropathy, since it is amendable to surgical correction.

Abnormalities in the volume of urine passed by the newborn each 24 hours are practically impossible to assess unless special attention is directed to the urinary system. The frequency of micturition varies from 2 to 6 times during the first and second days of life and from 5 to 25 times per 24 hours subsequently. The daily urinary volume is 30 to 60 ml during the first and second day, 100 to 300 ml during the following week, and between 200 and 400 for the rest of the first month.

Oliguria (urinary output below 15 to 20 ml/kg/24 hr) most often is a consequence of dehydration. Oliguria or anuria can also result from malformation, renal vascular accident, or urinary tract obstruction. Oliguria of prerenal origin, as in association with diarrheal disease, maternal diabetes, or respiratory distress syndrome, usually can be identified by the high solute content of the urine; whereas in oliguria of the true renal insufficiency, urinary osmolality is low. Urinary retention can mimic anuria of renal origin. This can result from neurologic abnormalities, such as meningitis or disturbances in the innervation of the bladder (for example, meningomyelocele), or from obstruction secondary to phimosis, posterior urethral valves, balanoposthitis, or vulvovaginitis. Palpation of the urinary bladder, which is easy to perform during the newborn period, and, if necessary bladder catheterization establish the diagnosis.

Polyuria is most often the result of a defect in concentrating capacity, secondary to medullary abnormalities in renal dysplasia (p. 495), to renal hypoplasia (p. 496), or to nephrophthisis or medullary cystic disease (p. 497). It is seen also in association with lack of antidiuretic hormone or nephrogenic diabetes insipidus (p. 504).

Proteinuria

It is generally accepted that small amounts of protein ordinarily pass through the semipermeable glomerular basement membrane. Although the concentration of these proteins in the proximal tubular fluid probably does not exceed 1 to 2 mg/100 ml, it can account for a significant loss of protein through the urinary tract (up to

3.5 gm/24 hr with a GFR of 120 ml/min). Under normal circumstances more than 95% of this protein is reabsorbed in the proximal tubule, and some (such as insulin and beta-2-macroglobulin) may be metabolized by the kidney. The remainder of the nephron apparently is also able to reabsorb protein, allowing only very small amounts to appear in the final urine. The protein content of the normal urine has been estimated to range as high as 10 to 25 mg/24 hr in children. In 1967 de Luna and Hullet reported a mean urinary excretion in newborns of 45 mg/24 hr. However, we rarely find more than trace proteinuria in random urines from newborn infants.

The usual semiquantitative methods of measurement do not detect concentrations of protein below 5 to 10 mg/100 ml; as a consequence significant amounts of protein can pass unnoticed under conditions of diuresis. This makes mandatory quantitative determination of protein excretion in 12- or 24-hour urine collections whenever renal disease is suspected. Documentation of proteinuria is only the first step in the diagnosis of kidney disease, however, since practically any form of injury, whether glomerular or tubular, can result in an increase in the excretion of protein. Furthermore, nonrenal disorders, such as cardiac insufficiency, venous obstruction, pulmonary edema, head injury, and fever, may be accompanied by transient proteinuria. Attempts have been made recently to use the molecular size of the urinary proteins (protein selectivity or selectivity index) as an indicator of the nature and severity of the underlying lesion and to determine prognosis. The basic assumption is that the more serious the lesion, the larger the molecules that are able to pass through the glomerular membrane. However, since there is a high degree of variability in the selectivity index obtained in various clinical and pathologic disease entities, the assumption is of little diagnostic value in any given patient.

Hematuria

Blood can enter the urine at any point of the urinary system from the kidney to the urethra. In the normal newborn, the excretion of RBC in urine does not exceed 100 per minute or 75,000 per 12 hours. Red urine usually indicates hematuria, but it may also be caused by the presence of bile pigments, porphyrins, urate, or hemoglobin. The differential diagnosis between hemoglobinuria and hematuria is easy to make if the urine is examined soon after collection. With standing, RBC may hemolyze, especially in hypotonic urine, and no longer appear as formed elements.

When hematuria is diagnosed, its origin must be determined. Extraurinary sources, such as the vagina, must be excluded. The next step is to determine if the RBC originate from the upper or the lower urinary tract. In some cases the history and clinical findings offer a clearcut answer. Examination of a freshly voided urine specimen to detect the presence of RBC or other types of casts is extremely helpful, the presence of casts being pathognomonic of parenchymal renal disease. Sometimes more complex methods of examination, such as intravenous urography, cystourethrography, cytoscopy, and renal arteriography or venography, may be necesasry to establish the diagnosis. Hematuria in the newborn may result from a renal vascular accident (p. 508), corticol and medullary necrosis (p. 509), neoplasia (p. 511), obstructive uropathy (p. 499), infection (p. 506), nephritis (p. 500), or coagulopathy (p. 509).

Pyuria

Pyuria is the presence of an abnormal number of WBC in the urine. The dividing line between normal and abnormal is uncertain. We do not expect to find more than 2 to 3 WBC per high-power field in a centrifuged specimen of urine. In a recent study (Littlewood, 1971) bag specimens of well-mixed, uncentrifuged urine obtained from 600 newborns on the sixth or seventh day of life contained 5 or less WBC per mm^3 in 98% of boys but in only 56% of girls. The percentage in girls increased to 94 when a clean-catch technique was used, suggesting perineal contamination of the bag specimens. The most common cause of pyuria is urinary tract infection (p. 506). Increased rates of excretion of WBC also can accompany nephritis (p. 500) and nephrosis (p. 501) and can be indicative of any type of inflammatory process within the urinary tract.

Edema

Accumulation of fluid in the interstitial space is a common manifestation of renal disease. It can be the consequence of a decrease in the colloid osmotic pressure of the plasma proteins, as in the nephrotic syndrome, or of a marked decrease in GFR, as in the various nephritides and congenital malformations. Almost invariably, the pathophysiologic mechanism is complex involving, in addition to physical factors, hypersecretion of aldosterone and, possibly, inhibition of a natriuretic hormone. At an early stage the retention of fluid can be detected only by repeated, accurate measurements of weight. Later, swelling becomes obvious. It is generally stated that the edema of renal disease involves primarily the face and is soft, whitish, and painless. None of the characteristics, however, is specific.

Ascites is the intraabdominal accumulation of fluid. It can occur in the nephrotic syndrome, in which case the fluid has the character of an exudate with a protein content that usually does not exceed 500 mg/100 ml. A more common cause of ascites in the newborn is obstruction of the lower urinary tract, particularly in association with posterior urethral valves. At least 50 cases have been described in the literature, although this is a rather unusual complication of urinary tract obstruction. The ascitic fluid apparently represents urine that has leaked through a ruptured pelvis or calyx. The differential diagnosis includes chylous ascites, ascites caused by syphilis, hepatobiliary obstruction, ruptured intraabdominal cyst, meconium peritonitis, and bile ascites.

Edema is occasionally found in premature babies during the first few days of life. This has been shown to be the result of shifts of fluid between body water compartments. So-called *late edema* develops among some newborns with birth weights below 1,300 gm and short gestational age. The accumulation of fluid seems to correspond to the thirty-fifth to thirty-sixth week of gestational age. No other gross abnormalities are found in these babies, and the edema usually is transtitory. Studies performed in infants with late edema and healthy controls have not detected significant differences in external water and electrolyte balances. A difference was observed, however, in the distribution of fluids between various body compartments, with the extracellular compartment being larger than normal in the edematous babies. The cause of this condition remains obscure, although some of these cases have been shown to be associated with vitamin E deficiency and anemia. Unusual causes of edema in the newborn include primary lymphedema (Milroy's disease), congenital lymphedema with gonadal dysgenesis, the syndrome of inappropriate antidiuretic hormone secretion, hyperaldosteronism, congenital analbuminemia, severe protein deficiency, protein-losing gastroenteropathy, scleredema, syphilis, erythroblastosis fetalis, and hereditary angioneurotic edema. The differential diagnosis also should include maternal diabetes.

Abdominal masses

Examination of the abdomen by palpation usually can be performed easily during the first 48 hours of extrauterine life because of the laxity of the abdominal muscles. The kidneys of the newborn are in a lower position than they are later in life, the right usually being lower than the left. The technique of examination is described in detail in a recent study of 10,000 infants (Mussels and others, 1971). Anomalies were suspected in 71 infants and confirmed by intravenous pyelography in 55. The most common anomaly was a horseshoe-shaped or fused kidney, which occurred in 16 infants. Conditions accounting for an apparently large kidney are hydronephrosis (p. 499), Wilms' tumor (p. 511), thrombosis of the renal vein (p. 509), and cystic disease (p. 497). The possibility of an adrenal hemorrhage also should be kept in mind. A smooth mass is more likely to be the result of hydronephrosis or renal vein thrombosis, whereas an irregular surface suggests malformation or cystic disease. An intravenous pyelogram or a renal scintiscan often suggests the diagnosis, although the differential diagnosis may be difficult. A renal venocavagram may be necessary when renal vein thrombosis is considered.

RENAL INSUFFICIENCY AND RENAL FAILURE

Inadequacy of renal function may be a consequence of any of the developmental anomalies, may arise from prerenal factors such as dehydration and shock, or may be the result of acquired disease of the kidneys. The recognition and treatment of renal insufficiency is discussed in this section without regard to the nature of the specific underlying cause.

Diagnosis. Renal insufficiency is often suspected on the basis of oliguria or anuria, or may be detected from biochemical examination of the blood. Urinary output less than 15 to 20 ml/kg/24 hr in the newborn (beyond the first few days of life) is indicative of oliguria. It is vital to determine if the cause of oliguria or anuria is *prerenal* (that is, caused by inadequacy of the blood supply to the kidney), *postrenal* (that is, urine being formed but not voided, because of obstructive uropathy or a neurogenic bladder), or *true renal failure* (that is, malfunction of the kidneys caused by intrinsic disease, whether congenital or acquired). This differentiation usually is simple. In some instances, extensive radiologic or urologic investigation may be required to demonstrate the cause of postrenal failure. In order to rule out prerenal failure, the adequacy of the circulation must be assessed. If insufficiency of the vascular volume is suspected, the response to administration of fluid may be helpful. For this purpose, isotonic saline in a dose of 15 to 20 ml/kg body weight or mannitol (0.5 to 1.0 gr/kg) can be given intravenously. A prompt increase in urinary output suggests that additional fluids may be needed. If there is no response, care must be taken to avoid administration of excessive amounts of fluids in order to "force" a diuresis.

Treatment. Treatment of renal insufficiency in the neonate is similar to treatment of the older child. Consideration must be given to maintenance of the balance of water, electrolytes, and hydrogen ions, and at the same time to provision of as near optimal nutrition as possible. Acute renal insufficiency is treated by providing a fluid intake equal to insensible water loss (25 to 40 ml/kg/24 hr) plus urinary output. In the anuric or severely oliguric patient, solute requiring urinary excretion is not given. In addition to withholding potassium, it may be necessary to reduce dangerously high plasma levels. When the concentration in plasma exceeds 6 mEq/liter, Kayexalate, a Na^+/K^+ exchange resin, can be given (by enema) in a starting dose of 0.5 to 1.5 gm/kg body weight. This is repeated as needed. Moderate or severe degrees of acidemia are treated by administration of sodium bicarbonate. Peritoneal dialysis may be indicated in the infant with total renal failure lasting more than 7 to 10 days or when severe metabolic disturbances cannot be managed with medical treatment alone.

In infants with chronic renal insufficiency, special attention must be paid to provision of adequate nutrition. Mild to moderate degrees of renal insufficiency usually can be managed by utilizing humanized milk (such as PM 60-40) as the sole source of nutrition. The usual dose of supplemental vitamins should be given.

With lesser degrees of function, other specific therapy may be required. Normal levels of pH and bicarbonate in the blood should be maintained by administration of sodium bicarbonate. The dose is adjusted to the patient, starting with 1 to 2 mEq/kg/day, and increasing as needed. Concentrations of calcium and inorganic phosphate in the blood should be measured frequently. Young infants fed low-phosphate diets usually do not develop hyperphosphatemia until they reach advanced stages of renal failure. In such cases, phosphate-binding gels (such as aluminum hydroxide gel [Amphojel]) can be administered, although they are usually poorly tolerated. A dose of 50 to 150 mg/kg/day given orally is customary. If the plasma calcium level falls significantly below normal, supplemental calcium (such as glubionate calcium [Neo-Calglucon]) is given in a dose of 10 to 20 mg (of elemental calcium) per kg body weight per day. If these measures are not successful in maintaining normal blood levels of calcium, pharmacologic doses of vitamin D should be prescribed, starting with a dosage of 10,000 units per day. Care must be taken to avoid too vigorous therapy and induction of hypercalcemia. The serum calcium × phosphate product should not be allowed to exceed 70.

In infants with severe uremia, vomiting may be a most troublesome symptom. Treatment with one of the phenothiazine drugs may be helpful.

Hypertension in infants is treated as in older children. Every effort should be made to maintain normal levels of blood pressure. Treatment is usually initiated with reserpine (0.01 to 0.02 mg/kg/day) or hydralazine hydrochloride (1 to 2 mg/kg/day in four divided doses) or both. If these drugs are not successful, guanethidine sulfate can be added (0.2 to 0.3 mg/kg/day as a single dose).

Infants who cannot be maintained in a satisfactory metabolic state by dietary and medical therapy alone are candidates for dialysis. Peritoneal dialysis can be used for short periods of time but probably is inadvisable if prolonged treatment is anticipated. Hemodialysis, although technically difficult, has been done in infants. Candidates for such therapy should be referred to appropriate centers.

Finally, renal transplantation must be considered for infants with irreversible renal failure. This has not been a successful procedure in the neonate; but as experience is gained and technical problems are solved, it is likely that this form of treatment ultimately will be available for even the smallest infants.

MALFORMATIONS

Renal maldevelopment

Clinical manifestations of renal maldevelopment in the newborn provide few clues to specific anatomic or etiologic diagnoses. Renal enlargement is at times detectable on abdominal palpation and occasionally causes abdominal distention. The contrary, an inability to palpate the kidney, may be an indication of renal hypoplasia. Oliguria is less apparent than anuria, and abnormalities of micturition may pass undetected unless particularly looked for. Under normal circumstances the newborn urinates within 48 hours of birth. Unusual delay or difficulty in passing urine is reason for evaluating the renal status of the baby. Less specific abnormalities include poor feeding, fussiness, vomiting, dehydration, and persistent respiratory difficulty. A high degree of suspicion is required to establish the diagnosis within the first days of life, and clinical examination should include urinalysis, blood chemical determinations, and excretory urography. Urologic examination may be necessary to evaluate abnormalities of the lower urinary tract. Therapy tends to be supportive rather than curative.

Certain lesions will be lethal because of irremediable parenchymal malformation and because of severe urinary tract obstruction, which is often associated with renal dysplasia. Less severe degrees of malformation lead to partial functional impairment with few differentiating features. The objective of prompt clinical recognition is to arrest and to prevent continuing deterioration, and particularly to identify those cases amenable to surgical intervention.

Abnormalities of renal development considered in this section include (1) agenesis, the lack of renal embryogenesis, (2) dysplasia, indicating an altered embryogenesis and abnormal differentiation of metanephric structures, and (3) polycystic disease, a diffuse cystic alteration of the kidney without evidence of other maldevelopment. In renal agenesis, one or both kidneys are lacking. The diagnosis of dysplasia, on the other hand, rests on microscopic evaluation and on the finding of abnormally differentiated metanephric structures. Such abnormalities may affect all or part of a kidney, and examples of dysplasia encompass both extremely small, rudimentary kidneys and greatly enlarged kidneys. Some types are markedly cystic, but they must be differentiated from polycystic disease, despite diffuse or total involvement. Polycystic disease, as defined here, differs clinically and morphologically from cystic dysplasia; this discussion follows the classification of Elkin and Bernstein, which is based on clinical, morphologic, radiographic, and genetic observations.

Bilateral renal agenesis, the complete absence of both kidneys, is a common malformation, occurring in approximately 1 out of 4,000 deliveries. This condition is accompanied by certain characteristic external abnormalities, including an abnormal facies with a wizened look, known as Potter's facies (Fig. 16-1). The ears are low set, often with folded helices; the chin is small, and the nose seems to be turned down at the tip. A skin crease characteristically curves around the inner canthus of the eye and runs laterally over the cheek. The legs commonly are bowed, and the feet frequently are clubbed. These abnormalities and vernix nodules (amnion nodosum) of the placental membranes have been attributed to oligohydramnios, a state

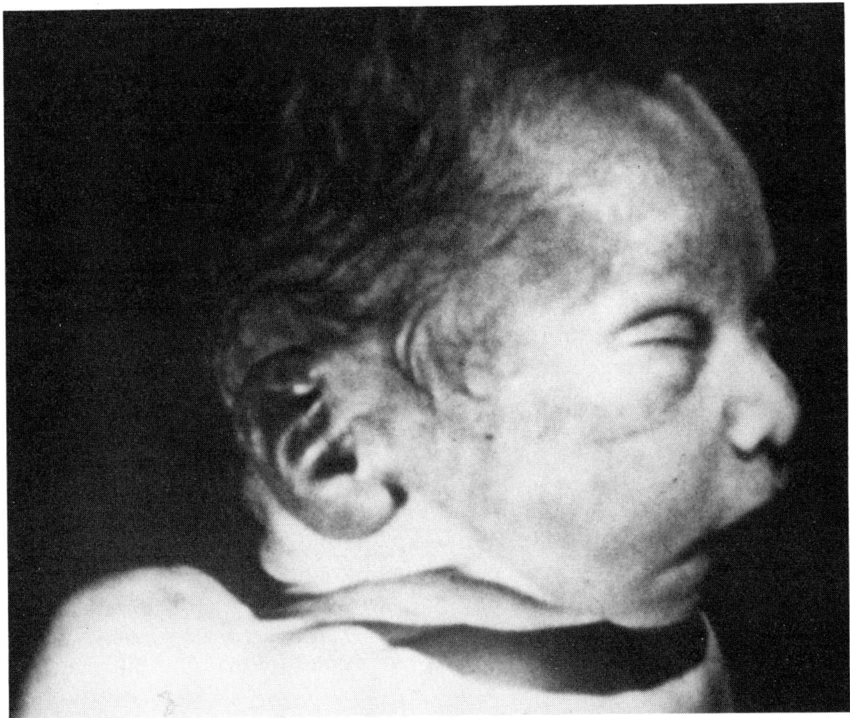

FIG. 16-1. Potter's facies. Characteristic are epicanthal folds, hypertelorism, low-set ears, mongoloid slant of the eyes, crease below the lower lip, and receded chin.

common to several malformations in which fetal urination is absent or markedly diminished.

Most cases are sporadic; a few familial instances have been noted. Chromosomal studies have shown normal karotypes. Males are affected considerably more often than females. Infants with bilateral renal agenesis are commonly born prematurely, and their birth weights also indicate intrauterine growth retardation. Breech deliveries are, therefore, common. A large number of affected infants, perhaps 40%, are stillborn, and most of the others die shortly after birth. A major postnatal problem is severe respiratory distress, secondary to accompanying pulmonary maldevelopment. Occasionally infants surviving for several days appear to have died of renal failure.

One of the most important accompanying visceral malformations is pulmonary hypoplasia. The lungs weigh as little as half the expected amount and often appear to be underdeveloped histologically. Other frequent internal abnormalities include anal, duodenal, and esophageal atresia; colonic agenesis and Meckel's diverticulum also have been found. The internal genitalia derived from the paramesonephric duct are usually defective or lacking: vas deferens and seminal vesicle in the male, and uterus and upper vagina in the female. The absence of one umbilical artery is often observed during examination of the umbilical cord and is confirmed at necropsy. Malformations of the caudal region of the fetus have been described with some frequency, and sirenomelic monsters characteristically have renal agenesis.

Unilateral agenesis becomes a problem in newborn infants only in the event of injury to the other kidney.

Renal dysplasia, a condition of abnormal metanephric differentiation, is also a relatively frequent problem in the newborn. Severe bilateral dysplasia, like agenesis, is associated with oligohydramnios, Potter's facies, and death from renal insufficiency within the first few days of life. Histopathologic studies of the kidney reveal two common anatomic forms of dysplasia: (1) aplastic kidneys, which are extremely small, sometimes barely recognizable buttons of tissue, and (2) multicystic kidneys, which are enlarged and grossly cystic. The two conditions are structurally similar, except for the cysts, and form the two ends of a spectrum of parenchymal malformation. Cyst formation is variable, and the two conditions cannot always be sharply separated. Multicystic dysplasia is the most common form of cystic renal disease in the newborn, and bilateral multicystic dysplasia has in our experience been more common than polycystic disease. The condition is only rarely familial; it has been described in chromosome abnormalities.

The essential anatomic features are structural disorganization and histologic evidence of altered metanephric differentiation in the form of metaplastic cartilage and of abnormal ductal and nephronic elements. Corticomedullary differentiation is poor, although clusters of primitive ducts representing rudimentary medullary tissue are related to adjacent caps of poorly developed nephrons representing rudimentary cortex. Cysts arise as terminal dilatations of collecting tubules (Fig. 16-2). Simple renal hypoplasia, without evidence of parenchymal maldevelopment, is seldom severe enough to cause renal insufficiency during the neonatal period. Oligonephronic hypoplasia, which also becomes clinically apparent in older children, is characterized by a decreased number but markedly increased size of glomeruli.

Renal dysplasia is commonly associated with other anomalies of the urinary tract, with an incidence approximating 90%. Multicystic kidneys have in our experience been invariably associated with ureteral atresia and pyelocalyceal occlusion. The state of the ureter in renal aplasia has been more variable, partly because of the difficulty in drawing a sharp line between aplasia and less severe degrees of malformation. Consequently, descriptions of ureteral stenosis, ureteral ectopy, and ureteral dilatation are not uncommon in reports of renal aplasia. With bilateral aplastic or multicystic kidneys, abnormalities of the lower urinary tract such as small bladders and constricted or occluded urethras, may reflect the lack of urine production. Malformations of other systems, particularly cardiovascular and alimentary, are common. The incidence of imperforate anus, for example, is 15% to 20%; that of aortic coarctation, 20% to 25%. In other words, the frequency of renal involvement in newborns with multiple malformations is high.

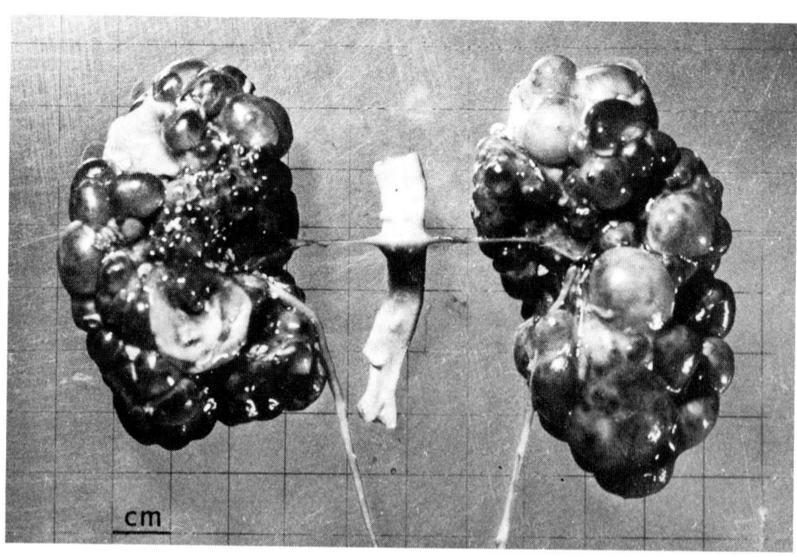

Fig. 16-2. Bilateral multicystic dysplasia in a newborn infant. The kidneys are enlarged and irregularly cystic, and the usual reniform configuration is barely apparent. Both ureters are atretic, and the renal arteries are extremely small. This condition is a cause of total renal nonfunction.

Both aplastic and multicystic kidneys can be unilateral. Unilateral aplasia is asymptomatic, and its disclosure in newborns is usually incidental to the study of some other condition. The differential diagnosis of unilateral nonvisualization includes agenesis and severe hypoplasia. The enlarged, unilateral multicystic kidney, on the other hand, frequently appears as a flank mass, most often on the left side and more often in males. Enlargement is usually moderate, although cystic kidneys can weigh several hundred grams and cause fetal dystocia. Excretory urograms disclose nonopacification, and endoscopic examination may reveal absence of the ureteral orifice or nonpatency of the ureter. The lesion seems to be relatively innocuous, there being only rare reports of hypertension, but nephrectomy is the usual mode of therapy. The prognosis in very young infants is uncertain, principally because of a one-third incidence of contralateral hypoplasia or hydronephrosis. A careful assessment is therefore mandatory to identify abnormalities correctable by reconstructive surgery. The lesion of multicystic dysplasia is not, however, a progressive disease to which the other kidney will eventually succumb. The contralateral kidney in dysplasia is often hypertrophied and seems to be unduly susceptible to infection and lithiasis in older individuals.

Bilaterally aplastic and multicystic kidneys are, as indicated above, incapable of function and are, therefore, lesions of newborns. An uncommon form of severe cystic dysplasia has been observed in newborns also suffering from cerebral malformation. This lesion resembles polycystic disease in that the kidneys are enlarged and spongy; they retain a reniform configuration, and the pelves and ureters are patent. Histologic examination discloses large numbers of cystic collecting tubules with little metanephric differentiation. A similar lesion is seen in newborns with Meckel's syndrome of cerebral malformation with encephalocele, eye anomalies, cleft palate, congenital heart disease, polydactyly, and other anomalies. Less severe degrees of parenchymal maldevelopment with patent urinary tracts, lesions retaining limited capacity to function, have different clinical and pathologic implications because they can excrete urine and can concentrate contrast media to some degree. Cortical dysplasia has been observed in association with Jeune's asphyxiating dystrophy. Other lesions in syndromes of multiple malformations such as trisomy D and cerebrohepatorenal syndromes, are postmortem findings without clinical significance for the newborn.

Infantile polycystic disease appears in newborns as bilaterally enlarged, diffusely spongy kidneys. Pathologic studies have shown dilatation of collecting tubules and relatively little fibrosis. Polycystic disease is differentiated from cystic dysplasia by the preservation of renal shape and landmarks and by the absence of dysplastic microscopic elements (Fig. 16-3). Microdissection has also shown that the principal site of dilatation is in the collecting tubules. Portions of nephrons, including glomeruli, are variably dilated, and medullary collecting ducts are characteristically ectatic. Characteristic polycystic changes are present also in the liver and occasionally in other organs.

Many affected infants are stillborn, and the majority of those born alive die within the first few days of life. The condition can be diagnosed clinically in infants with Potter's facies, abdominal enlargement, and a history of oligohydramnios. Abdominal distention has at times been severe enough to cause fetal dystocia. Respiratory distress and congestive heart failure are common. ECGs show left ventricular hypertrophy and left ventricular strain. Other infants have less severe renal insufficiency and survive the neonatal period; they probably have the same disease. Excretory urography discloses delayed concentration of dye, a mottled nephrogram, and retention of contrast medium in small cysts (Fig. 16-4); retrograde pyelography sometimes demonstrates pyelotubular back flow and medullary tubular ectasia.

Variation in clinical expression and in anatomic findings seems to be related to the natural history and progression of a single disease, although it has also been suggested that infantile polycystic disease consists of several age-related entities with somewhat differing morphologic characteristics and clinical expression. Infants surviving the neonatal period suffer from gradually increasing renal insufficiency and hy-

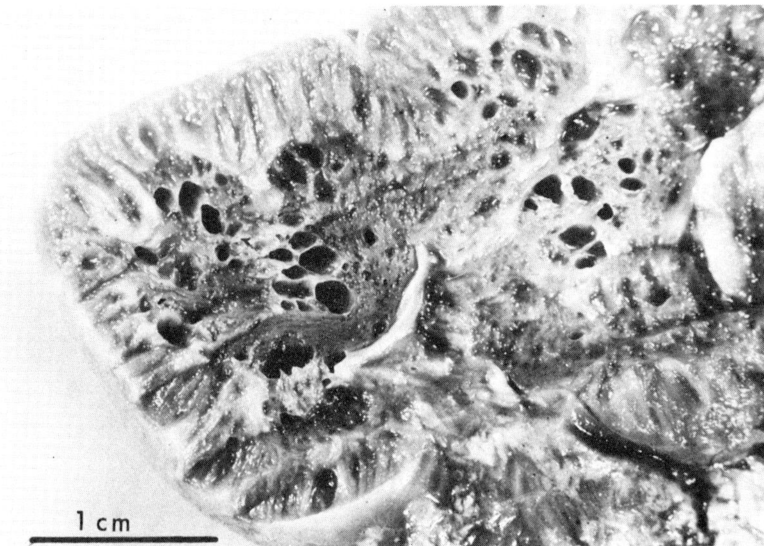

Fig. 16-3. Infantile polycystic disease in a newborn, showing the preservation of lobar structure and cortical-medullary differentiation. The cortex is thickened and spongy, and the medullary pyramids contain grossly apparent cysts; the latter are sometimes visible radiographically. (From Elkin, M., and Bernstein, J.: Clin. Radiol. **20**:68, 1969.)

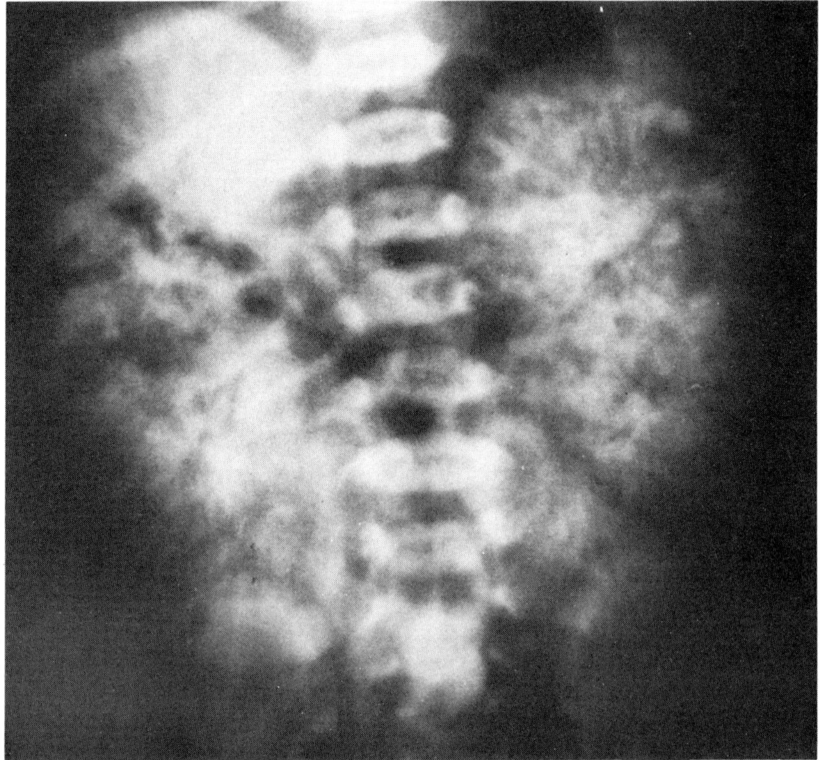

Fig. 16-4. Radiologic presentation of infantile polycystic disease. The irregular renal contour is caused by the presence of cysts.

pertension. Older children also develop hepatic fibrosis and portal hypertension, which we have regarded as part of the clinical spectrum of infantile polycystic disease. Genetic studies indicate transmission as an autosomal recessive trait. The disease appears as a sporadic malformation or in more than one sibling of a single generation, and it bears no genetic relationship to polycystic disease of the adult type. Examples of the adult type of polycystic disease in newborns are rare and may be difficult to recognize in the absence of a positive family history; they differ morphologically from infantile polycystic disease. For want of a better term, we must speak, therefore, of adult polycystic disease in the newborn. Since the adult type of polycystic disease is transmitted as an autosomal dominant trait, the differentiation of the two conditions carries some implications for genetic counseling.

Urinary tract obstruction

Urinary obstruction in the fetus is a cause of renal parenchymal maldevelopment. An example is the condition known as *ectopic ureterocele.* The kidney and ureter are duplicated, and one of the ureters drains abnormally in the trigone or bladder neck, commonly terminating in an intravesical cyst. The obstructed segment of kidney is usually dysplastic; the normally draining segment is normally developed. On occasion, the kidney associated with ureteral or ureteropelvic occlusion is normally formed and merely hydronephrotic. We have, in such instances, theorized that the obstructive ureteral lesion was acquired relatively late in gestation, perhaps shortly before birth. Many of these specimens are only moderately hydronephrotic, despite complete ureteral obstruction, suggesting a course of short duration. *Hydronephrosis* occurs also without obvious anatomic obstruction, most often as a bilateral lesion, and when unilateral more often on the left. Many cases are in premature infants, and most are in male infants. The cause of the ureteral lesion or of isolated hydronephrosis remains speculative. A renal mass may be palpable on abdominal examination. The differential diagnosis of neonatal unilateral hydronephrosis includes ureteropelvic obstruction, ureteral ectopy, ureterocele, and ureteral and renal duplication. Diagnosis rests on excretory and retrograde urography and urologic examination; reconstructive surgery may be beneficial.

Lower urinary tract obstruction is more common in the newborn and is almost exclusively an affliction of males. The most frequent cause is valvular obstruction of the posterior urethra; other obstructive lesions with similar effects of varying severity are urethral atresia, cysts of the verumontanum, and urethral diverticula. So-called bladder neck obstruction is a disease of older children. Clinical findings of outlet obstruction early in life relate to urinary retention. Mild degrees of obstruction may go undetected for years, and severe obstruction results, of course, in vesical dilatation, hydroureter, and hydronephrosis. Respiratory distress, abdominal distention, vomiting, and poor feeding are frequent complaints. Fetal ascites has also been described in obstructive uropathy. *Urethral obstruction* is occasionally associated with aplasia or absence of the abdominal musculature, the "prune-belly" syndrome (Fig. 16-5).

Bilateral flank masses and a midline suprapubic mass in male infants are evidence of bladder neck or urethral obstruction, despite a common clinical inclination to think

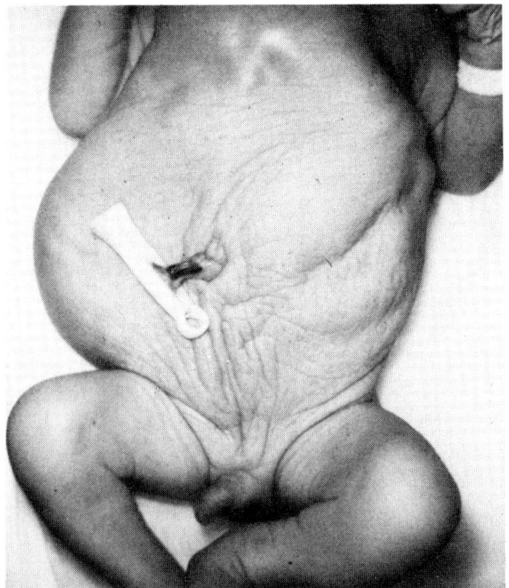

Fig. 16-5. Prune-belly syndrome. Note the distended, flabby abdomen wrinkled like a dried prune.

first of cystic kidneys. Poor urinary stream, dribbling, and other abnormalities in micturition are apparent quite early in life; and there may be complete obstruction, with failure to pass urine at birth. Roentgenographic studies show the obstruction usually as a dilated prostatic urethra ending abruptly at cusp-like valves. The bladder is heavily trabeculated; there is evidence of secondary hypertrophy; and ureteral reflux is common. Infection readily gains a foothold, particularly after instrumentation. Obstructing valves are most often exaggerations of the two mucosal folds that are normally continuous with the lower end of the verumontanum. Supraverumontanal folds and mucosal diaphragms are less common. Obstruction results not just from coaptation of the folds, but also from a narrow, stenotic orifice between them. Ureteral dilatation and tortuosity need not be symmetrical, and hydronephrosis is often only moderate. Infants with an obstruction severe enough to be apparent in the newborn period frequently have associated renal parenchymal maldevelopment, presumably resulting from the effect in utero of obstruction on the developing kidney. Renal dysplasia is much less often associated with milder degrees of obstruction apparent later in life. Removing the urethral obstruction is only part of the treatment. Ureteral dilatation and tortuosity are secondary causes of obstruction, frequently requiring drainage of the upper urinary tract. Infection must be treated vigorously to prevent continuing renal damage, but the impairment imposed by parenchymal malformation cannot be reversed.

The condition known as the *prune-belly syndrome,* or *congenital absence of the abdominal musculature,* has been a subject of considerable fascination. The newborn male infant has a distended, flabby abdomen, which is creased like a dried prune (Fig. 16-5). Female infants are seldom affected, less than 5% of cases. The condition is rarely familial, and no cytogenetic abnormality has been detected. Failure of testicular descent is a characteristic finding. Other congenital malformations may also be present. The ureters are dilated and tortuous, and the kidneys are hydronephrotic and often dysplastic, suggesting to some that a generalized developmental defect of abdominal parietes and mesenchyme is responsible for the entire syndrome. The bladder is large, dilated, and hypertrophied, indicating, on the other hand, that infravesical obstruction might be a common denominator. Certainly, aplasia or agenesis of the abdominal musculature has been seen in association with urethral atresia, urethral diverticulum, and posterior urethral valves. The bladder, however, is not trabeculated, despite its large capacity, and complete emptying can often be observed radiographically. The posterior urethra, also characteristically dilated, tapers at the membranous urethra; but evidence of increased resistance is lacking. Compelling evidence for a primary embryologic defect of the bladder and ureters remains to be found. Prognosis is related to the degree of obstruction, the extent of associated renal dysplasia, and the control of infection. Reconstructive surgery has been of limited help, and vigorous antibacterial therapy may be the main factor in prolonging survival. Drainage of the upper tract may be necessary to control infection and prevent continuing damage to kidneys that are frequently dysplastic.

Other abnormalities of the newborn, such as exstrophy of the bladder, epispadias, and neurogenic bladder caused by meningomyelocele are problems in urogolic management requiring careful control of infection.

NEPHRITIS

Neonatal nephritis occurs infrequently. Its principal cause today is congenital syphilis, a disease of resurgent clinical importance. Cytomegalic inclusion disease is also associated with nephritis, and the tubules contain characteristic enlarged inclusion-bearing cells. Although congenital systemic infection with cytomegalovirus, herpesvirus, rubella virus, or *toxoplasma* organisms also can cause an interstitial nephritis with tubular lesions, these usually are portmortem findings of small clinical importance. Significant forms of renal inflammation in the newborn include chronic glomerulonephritis in the congenital nephrotic syndrome (p. 501), and bacterial pyelonephritis (p. 506). Hereditary nephritis also may have its onset in the first month of life. Many clinical descriptions of neonatal nephritis, particularly those in the older literature, are difficult to evaluate. Acute glomerulonephritis in the newborn does not seem to have been documented by contemporary standards, and some examples of hemorrhagic nephritis are undoubtedly cases of renal cortical necrosis.

Congenital *luetic nephritis* causes a nephrotic syndrome in newborns and young infants. Other infants have the clinical appearance of hemorrhagic nephritis, with hematuria, cylindruria, and moderate azotemia, accompanied by less severe proteinuria. Histologic studies have shown a proliferative glomerulonephritis accompanied by prominent cortical infiltrates of plasmacytes and lymphocytes. The interstitial nephritis is a strong clue to the diagnosis in renal biopsies. The clinical diagnosis usually rests on demonstrating other stigmata of syphilis and positive reactions to serologic tests. Antibiotic therapy is usually effective in treating the lesion and in reversing the nephrotic syndrome, although therapeutic failure with penicillin in high dosage recently has been reported.

Chronic glomerulonephritis has been described in several necropsy studies. The patients were severely ill newborns, and in at least one report a rapidly progressing anemia suggested a hemolytic-uremic syndrome. Studies of renal function have been lacking, however, and it is presumed that the infants suffered from renal insufficiency. Some infants have been edematous, and the lesion has been associated with the nephrotic syndrome. The glomeruli were diminished by sclerosis and hyalinization, and severe epithelial proliferation and crescent formation were present in the remainder. Tubular atrophy and cast formation, interstitial inflammation, fibrosis, and vascular sclerosis complete the picture. The lesion must be differentiated from *congenital glomerulosclerosis,* a process of glomerular involution and hyalinization that takes place in many or perhaps all newborns. The number of sclerotic glomeruli found incidentally in newborns dying of other diseases, without renal symptoms, has been as high as 20%, though a figure of 5% to 10% is more usual. These glomerular changes may be associated with slight focal tubular atrophy; more extensive changes reflect some other disease.

THE NEPHROTIC SYNDROME

The characteristic features of the nephrotic syndrome—proteinuria, hypoproteinemia, hyperlipidemia, and edema—are rarely encountered during neonatal life. When present, they are usually the expression of the congenital nephrotic syndrome, a familial disease with an autosomal recessive type of inheritance.

Congenital nephrotic syndrome

The majority of the cases of congenital nephrotic syndrome have originated from Finland, where at least 130 families have been identified. Some 24 families, comprising 40 children, have been reported from the United States, and many other questionable cases have been described in the American literature. The onset of the disease occurs during intrauterine life, as evidenced by large and abnormal placentas, qualitative similarity between protein content of the amniotic fluid and fetal urine, delivery of SGA and premature babies in about 90% of the cases, faulty intrauterine calcification of the bones, erythroblastosis, and polycythemia (probably reflecting intrauterine anoxia). About 95% of the cases become manifest during the first 8 weeks of life, most of the children showing proteinuria from the very first day. Pallor, mottling of the skin, cyanosis, and respiratory distress are accompanying symptoms. Protein electrophoresis shows low levels of albumin and IgG, and high-levels of alpha globulin, mostly alpha-1-macroglobulin.

The pathologic findings vary in severity from minimal glomerular changes to proliferation and mesangial thickening, to complete hyalinization of the glomerular tufts in infants who live long enough for such lesions to develop. A higher proportion than normal of morphologically immature glomeruli also is characteristic; nephrogenesis is delayed and proceeds at a slow rate. Marked dilatation of the proximal tubules often is encountered and has been referred to, inappropriately, as microcystic disease (Fig. 16-6). This finding initially was interpreted as representing evidence that the primary basis of the disease is an intrinsic defect in the development of the renal tubular structures. The absence of these changes in the early phases of the disease, however, makes it more likely that

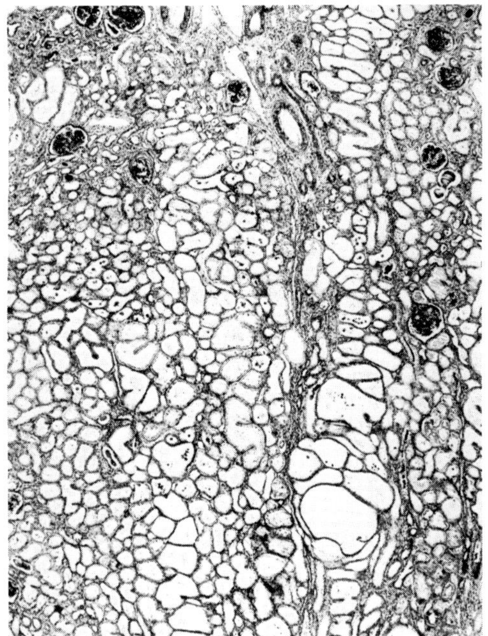

Fig. 16-6. Congenital nephrotic syndrome. Microscopic examination discloses sclerotic and proliferative changes in the glomeruli. The collecting tubules, particularly those near the corticomedullary junction, are dilated to microcystic proportions. (PAS stain; ×40.)

they are secondary to the glomerular abnormalities.

The cause of the disease is unknown. Toxic factors such as mercury and phenol, infectious agents such as *E. coli* and *Toxoplasma,* and drugs such as corticosteroids have been considered, but never documented. An immunologic process has been incriminated in the pathogenesis. Skin transplanted from infants born with this disease to their mothers undergoes accelerated rejection, suggesting intrauterine sensitization to the fetus. However, this could be the consequence of fetal-maternal transfusion resulting from placental damage. In nine patients with the congenital nephrotic syndrome, gamma globulin and complement were demonstrated by immunofluorescent techniques in renal tissue obtained by biopsy or autopsy. These results have been challenged by Hoyer and associates (1967) and more recently by Rapola and Savilahti.

The condition is resistant to all forms of therapy. Approximately 75% of the patients succumb, most to infection, during the first 6 months of life. Isolated patients with a longer natural survival have been reported, in one child to almost 4 years of age. Recent attempts have been made to perform dialysis and transplants in these children.

Other forms of the nephrotic syndrome

Congenital syphilis, renal vein thrombosis, and cytomegalic inclusion disease are among the recognized entities associated with a nephrotic syndrome in early life. A heterogeneous group of patients has been included under the name atypical familial nephrosis.

Congenital syphilis accounts for an increasing number of newborns with the nephrotic syndrome. The clinical presentation and the morphologic changes in the kidney are described in the section on nephritis (p. 500). Important differences from congenital nephrosis, which must be considered in the differential diagnosis, are the high levels of IgG in the serum (in contrast to the low levels encountered in congenital nephrosis) and the good response to antibiotic therapy.

Renal vein thrombosis can be the cause or the consequence of a nephrotic syndrome. Only the second circumstance applies to the newborn. The symptoms and the approach to therapy are described elsewhere (p. 509).

Cytomegalic infection has been associated with a nephrotic syndrome in at least five patients. The inclusion bodies have been isolated from the salivary glands in one case, from the kidneys in two, and from other organs in the remaining two. None of these patients manifested symptoms of cytomegalic disease, such as jaundice, petechiae or central nervous system disturbance.

Atypical familial nephrotic syndrome includes children with the nephrotic syndrome who are within the age range of congenital nephrosis, but show a benign course, and children who have the onset of the disease late in life, but show changes characteristic of the congenital type of nephrosis. No such case has been described in Finland. Many children with this syndrome are offspring of related parents; some of them are identical twins; and in all families more than one sibling has shown signs of disease.

ANOMALIES OF RENAL TUBULAR FUNCTION

Dysfunction of the renal tubule can result from a primary defect in the transport ability of the renal tubular membrane or can be secondary to a systemic disorder or disease. Primary defects include conditions such as renal glucosuria, renal tubular acidosis, renal phosphaturia, and the renal aminoacidurias. The latter group includes, among others, cystinosis, glycogen storage disease, Wilson's disease, galactosemia, heavy metal poisoning, hyperglobulinemia, and idiopathic and secondary hypercalcemia. The causes of the majority of these anomalies of renal tubular transport are unknown; some are inherited, a few are self-limited, many are inconsequential, some have a serious impact on growth and development, and some are amendable to therapy. It should be apparent that this is a heterogeneous group of conditions that have as their common denominator one or more disturbances in the function of the renal tubule.

Cystinuria, Hartnup disease, familial iminoglycinuria, hereditary glycinuria, glucoglycinuria, and congenital lysinuria, although present from birth, usually become symptomatic beyond the newborn period. The same is true for tubular disorders, such as hereditary hypophosphatemia (familial vitamin D–resistant rickets), pseudohypoparathyroidism, and most forms of the de Toni-Fanconi syndrome, including cystinosis (see Chapter 2, p. 429). The reason for listing them is the availability of screening tests for these anomalies that makes possible their early recognition and treatment. Only some of the major syndromes particularly pertinent to the newborn period are discussed here.

Renal glycosuria

Under normal circumstances glucose does not appear in the urine unless its concentration in blood reaches a level that is about twice normal. In patients with renal glycosuria the renal threshold for this substance is diminished, and glucose is excreted in the urine at normal or slightly elevated blood concentrations. Depending on the level of the threshold, glucose is found in the urine either consistently or only after a load, such as following a meal rich in carbohydrates. Two forms of renal glycosuria are described. In one of them (type A) the defect involves a depression in both the threshold and the maximal capacity to reabsorb glucose (TmG). The other variety (type B) is characterized by a low threshold and a normal TmG. This differentiation, even if real, has only theoretical significance, since the blood level at which TmG is observed is far removed from the threshold. As a consequence, the magnitude of the glucosuria relates little to the level of the TmG. No definite evidence exists regarding a defect in the intestinal transport of glucose in patients with renal glycosuria, although such an association has been documented in the familial glucose-galactose malabsorption syndrome.

The defect in renal glycosuria is present from birth and may account for otherwise unexplained episodes of hypoglycemia. The inheritance in the majority of patients is autosomal dominant, although an autosomal recessive mode of transmission also has been described. Results of examination of the renal tubular structures by light microscopy are normal; alterations in the mitochondria have been found on electron micrographs. No therapy is necessary other then recognition of the condition, avoidance of confusion with diabetes mellitus, and provision of a normal intake of carbohydrates.

The aminoacidurias

The amino acids normally present in the glomerular filtrate are actively reabsorbed, almost quantitatively, in the proximal tubule. The quantity that escapes reabsorption can be detected in the urine by paper or column chromatography. The excretory pattern varies with age, both quantitatively and qualitatively. Brodehl and Gellissen, in a study performed in normal full-term infants ranging in age between 16 days and 4 months, were able to demonstrate a relatively high fractional excretion of threonine, serine, proline, glycine, and alanine, suggesting immaturity of only certain transport mechanisms.

An abnormal excretion of amino acids in

urine can result from (1) an increase in the filtered load that exceeds the reabsorptive capacity of the tubule, (2) competition of two or more amino acids for the same transport site, or (3) a selective or a generalized defect of the transport system. Characteristically, in the renal aminoacidurias plasma concentrations are normal. The identification of specific sites for the transport of amino acids was accomplished during the past decade mainly by studies of patients with isolated defects. Five pathways have been described. The first system carries dibasic amino acids (lysine, arginine, and ornithine) and is defective in a condition known as *hyperdibasic-aciduria.* In *cystinuria,* in addition to these amino acids, excessive amounts of cystine are excreted. The second transport mechanism is responsible for reabsorption of the acidic amino acids (glutamic and aspartic acids). No human defect corresponding to this site has been identified. The third pathway transports imino acids (proline and hydroxyproline) and glycine, and is defective in *familial iminoglycinuria.* The remainder of the neutral amino acids share a common transport site, as evidenced by the fact that they are all excreted in excess in *Hartnup disease.* Studies of patients with *β-alaninemia* have served to define the fifth transport system, that for the β-amino compounds, such as β-alanine, β-isobutyric acid, and taurine.

Cystinosis

Cystinosis, inherited as an autosomal recessive trait, is characterized by accumulation of cystine in the lysosomal fraction of the cells (p. 429). Plasma cystine levels are normal. The symptoms result from involvement of several organ systems. The infantile form, which is the most severe, has been detected as early as the first month of life by the presence of aminoaciduria in apparently normal siblings of affected children. Thirst, vomiting, diarrhea, dehydration, unexplained fever, and failure to thrive usually become evident much later in infancy. If the child does not die of infection, acidosis, or hypokalemia, renal insufficiency ultimately occurs.

A reliable method of making a positive diagnosis is the determination of the cystine content of peripheral leukocytes, which is markedly elevated (up to 100-fold normal). Treatment is symptomatic. Reports published after a relatively short period of observation in a few patients who have undergone renal transplantation indicate deposition of cystine in the renal interstitium and not in the tubular cells as is characteristic of cystinosis.

Oculocerebrorenal dystrophy (Lowe's syndrome)

Lowe's syndrome is characterized by multiple tubular dysfunctions, mental retardation, and severe congenital ocular anomalies. The condition is transmitted by a sex-linked recessive gene; all but four of the affected subjects reported were males. These exceptions probably represent a different entity. The age at onset varies from the first few months to late childhood. Cataracts, frequently coexisting with glaucoma, are prominent features. The involvement of the nervous system is manifested by severe mental retardation, muscular hypotony, and tendinous areflexia. Cryptorchidism is common. The renal disorder is characterized by proteinuria, aminoaciduria, and sometimes glycosuria. Therapy is symptomatic. Prognosis depends on the severity of the mental retardation.

Pseudohypoaldosteronism

Pseudohypoaldosteronism results from unresponsiveness of the renal tubule to aldosterone. The consequence is abnormal loss of sodium, hyponatremia, and hyperkalemia. The mode of inheritance seems to be sex linked. The symptoms (anorexia, vomiting, failure to thrive) appear 2 or 3 weeks after birth. Differentiation from the salt-losing form of adrenal hyperplasia is made by appropriate investigation of steroid metabolism. In pseudohypoaldosteronism the excretion of 17-ketosteroids and 17-hydroxysteroids is normal, whereas the excretion of aldosterone is very high. Treatment is urgent and consists of administration of large quantities of sodium chloride. The need for salt supplementation seems to diminish with age.

Nephrogenic diabetes insipidus

Nephrogenic diabetes insipidus is characterized by insensitivity of the renal tubule to vasopressin. The homozygotes are male, suggesting a sex-linked mode of inheritance. Symptoms appear shortly after birth; dehydration, unexplained fever, and failure to thrive are prominent. Polyuria and polydipsia are usually detected only later. A significant delay in psychomotor development often develops, apparently caused by chronic dehydration.

The pathogenesis is unknown. Differential diagnosis should include ADH-lack diabetes insipidus, bilateral renal hypoplasia, hydronephrosis, medullary cystic disease, or familial nephrophthisis. Laboratory tests reveal hyperelectrolytemia with dilute urine. Vasopressin is ineffective. A water deprivation test should be avoided.

The prognosis is good if the diagnosis is made early in life. Therapy consists of administration of sufficient fluids to maintain normal hydration. In infants the need for water can be minimized by giving a solute-poor milk. Thiazide diuretics have been shown to be effective in decreasing urinary volume and improving concentrating ability, although their mechanism of action remains unclear.

Renal tubular acidosis

Renal tubular acidosis (RTA) is a defect in the reabsorption of bicarbonate or secretion of hydrogen ion that is not related to a decrease in GFR. RTA has two main forms: the *proximal* type, resulting from the inability of the kidney to maintain a normal threshold for bicarbonate, and the *distal* type, resulting from the inability of the kidney to establish an adequate gradient of secretion of hydrogen ion.

Proximal renal tubular acidosis

Proximal RTA can appear as an isolated defect or coexist with other proximal tubular anomalies, as in the de Toni-Fanconi syndrome (p. 503) or oculocerebrorenal syndrome (p. 504). The primary form is characterized clinically by failure to thrive and chemically by hyperchloremic acidosis. The great majority of patients are males.

A transient form of proximal RTA has been observed in newborns who have acute infections. This is also self-limited but can account for transitory, "unexplained" metabolic acidosis.

Diagnosis. The diagnosis is made by demonstration of a low renal threshold for bicarbonate and a normal renal acidifying capacity. The former is determined by a study of bicarbonate reabsorption during continuous infusion of increasing amounts of bicarbonate. It should be kept in mind that there is normal variation in threshold with age. The infant has a bicarbonate threshold of 20 to 22 millimoles per liter, whereas in the adult the threshold is 24 to 26 millimoles. The ability of the kidney to acidify the urine is tested by adminstration of an acid load (ammonium chloride) and a test of the pH of the urine. Although during the first few days of life the newborn may not be able to lower urinary pH below 6.5 or 6.0, beyond this period urinary pH should reach a value of at least 5.0.

Etiology. The exact nature of the defect is unknown. As a rule, children with primary proximal RTA do not have a defect in urinary concentration or show evidence of rickets, urolithiasis, or nephrocalcinosis.

Treatment. Therapy consists of administration of sodium citrate or bicarbonate, usually in amounts exceeding 5 mEq/kg/day. The solution should be administered at frequent intervals, since it will leak into the urine shortly after being administered when bicarbonate concentration in blood exceeds the threshold. The condition is self-limited; most patients wtih primary RTA recover following 2 to 3 years of therapy.

Distal renal tubular acidosis. Distal RTA is a persistent defect in urinary acidification that usually occurs in isolated cases but may be inherited as an autosomal dominant trait. The condition affects females predominantly and tends to become overt after the age of 2 years. However, the onset often can be traced to the first months of life by the history of vomiting, anorexia, polyuria, dehydration, and failure to thrive. Beyond infancy, polyuria, growth retardation, nephrocalcinosis, and interstitial nephritis are the prevailing features. Rickets or osteomalacia, commonly encountered in adults with distal RTA, occur rarely in children.

Etiology. The nature of the defect that prevents the kidney from establishing an adequate gradient of hydrogen ion between peritubular blood and tubular fluid is not known. Evidence that the defect is intrinsic to the renal tubular epithelium is provided by the normal behavior of the transplanted kidney in 15 patients with distal RTA.

Diagnosis. The diagnosis is made by observation of a urinary pH consistently above 6.5 or 7.0, despite spontaneous or induced metabolic acidosis.

Treatment. Therapy consists of administration of sodium bicarbonate, usually in amounts of 1 to 3 mEq/kg/day. Some patients may require supplemental potassium as well. The dose is adjusted to maintain blood pH and bicarbonate within normal limits, to ensure a maximal opportunity for normal growth. In addition, therapy is directed toward prevention of nephrocalcinosis, requiring that the dose be sufficient to keep the excretion of calcium in urine below 2 mg/kg/24 hr.

Prognosis. Although primary distal RTA is a permanent defect, when it is correctly treated the prognosis in terms of growth and prevention of renal insufficiency is good.

INFECTION OF THE URINARY TRACT

See also Chapter 8, p. 139.

Asymptomatic bacteriuria has been found in less than 1% of apparently healthy full-term infants, with equal frequency in males and females. By contrast, studies in premature infants have demonstrated bacteriuria, confirmed by suprapubic puncture, in 2% to 5%.

Diagnostic methods. A variety of methods are available for collection of urine from the newborn for urinalysis and bacteriologic examination. As in older subjects, measures must be taken to avoid cellular and bacterial contamination. The simplest method involves careful cleansing of the external genitalia with soap and water, thorough rinsing to ensure removal of all soap residue, and application of a *sterile plastic bag.* Lincoln and Winberg have suggested that irrigation of the preputial folds of male infants is important to prevent gross contamination of the urine specimen, although in our experience this has not been found to be necessary. After application of the bag, the baby is checked every 10 to 15 minutes so that the bag can be removed shortly after urination has occurred. If a stool is passed or if the bag has been in place for more than 1 hour, the bag is removed, the baby is cleansed again, and a fresh bag is affixed.

Catheterization of the bladder is difficult to perform in the neonate because of the normally occurring phimosis of the male and the obscure position of the urtheral orifice in the female. It is now generally recommended that if a "bag" specimen is inadequate, a urine specimen should be obtained by suprapubic puncture of the bladder rather than by bladder catheterization.

Suprapubic aspiration of urine from the bladder is easily performed in the infant. A 24- or 25-gauge, 1-inch needle is used. The needle is directed perpendicular to the skin, in the midline, 1 inch above the symphysis. In 10% or 15% of attemps no specimen will be obtained, because insufficient urine is present in the bladder. Minimal degrees of hematuria are observed transiently in some infants and should be of no concern.

There are insufficient data on what level of bacterial concentration in a clear-voided, or "bag," urine represents the statistical dividing line between contamination and true bacteriuria in infants. Most workers have viewed counts in excess of 10^4 per ml with suspicion, requiring that repeated examinations consistently demonstrate equal or greater numbers of the same organism to confirm the diagnosis. We have had the experience, however, of finding the same organism in concentrations of 10^4 or 10^5 per ml on two or three consecutive "bag" examinations, only to find sterile urine from a suprapubic aspirate. Initial screening, therefore, should be performed on "bag" urine; those with bacterial counts in excess of 10^4 per ml should be repeated, and those found again to be in excess of 10^4 should be examined by suprapubic aspiration. Examination of urine collected by the bag technique will reveal no bacterial growth or less than 10^4 organisms per ml in 70% to 90% of cases, thus excluding these infants from further consideration. Infants with bacterial counts above 10^4 are candidates for repeat examination, although with this method even counts above 10^5 most often prove to be caused by contamination.

It is assumed that any bacterial growth in urine obtained by suprapubic aspiration represents true bacteriuria, thus obviating the need for quantitation. Nevertheless, since most infected urine contains bacteria in excess of 10^5 or even 10^6 per ml, quantitation of bacteria in suprapubic aspirates can be helpful in that concentrations below 10^4 or 10^3 must be viewed as possibly representing contamination, despite the technique of collection. The great majority of cultures from infected infants reveals one organism; mixed cultures, therefore, are also suggestive of contamination.

In the infant about to be treated with antibiotics, urine should be collected by suprapubic aspiration rather than by the bag technique, since the former technique yields the most reliable results; once antibiotic therapy is initiated there is no further opportunity to distinguish between true and false positive reactions. If the clinical circumstances permit repeated examination of the urine prior to institution of antibiotic therapy, the simpler bag technique is acceptable, since positive reactions can then be confirmed or refuted by examination of a suprapubic aspirate.

Much consideration has been given to the significance of pyuria in establishing the diagnosis of urinary infection. Unfortunately, it is difficult to determine what amount of leukocyturia is to be considered normal in the newborn. Houston found 76% of noninfected infants and children to have 0 to 10 leukocytes per mm^3 of urine, with another 20% falling within the range 11 to 50. Lincoln and Winberg concluded on the basis of a survey of 500 newborn infants that normal males should have less than 25 and normal females less than 50 WBC per mm^3 in clean-catch urine specimens. In contrast, Littlewood found less than 5 leukocytes per mm^3 in clean-catch urine specimens in 97% of male and 94% of female infants, suggesting that the higher figures found by other investigators represented contamination. However, Gower and associates reported that the presence of even more than 10 WBC per mm^3 in suprapubic aspirates was usually not associated with a positive culture.

As in subjects of all ages, there is a strong association between pyuria and bacteriuria in infants. Nevertheless, most infants with pyuria, or more properly leukocyturia, do not have bacteriuria; and, conversely, significant bacteriuria can occur in the absence of pyuria. Therefore, the final diagnosis of urinary infection in the neonate lies in the demonstration of bacteriuria, as has been well established in patients in older age groups.

Etiology. The spectrum of organisms that has been cultured from the urine of infants is similar to that from the urine of older children and adults with urinary tract infection. *E. coli* predominates, but *Aerobacter-Klebsiella, Pseudomonas,* coliform bacteria, *Proteus,* and enterococci are encountered more frequently in infants than in older children (see p. 139).

Pathogenesis. It is well established that the majority of urinary tract infections in older infants and children, as well as in adults, represent ascending infections; that is, entry of organisms through the urethra, migration into the bladder, and then in certain instances extension to the kidneys. Information concerning the route of entry in neonates is not available. Infants found on routine screening to have significant bacteriuria may well have a simple cystitis, which represents a pathogenesis similar to that observed in older subjects. It is generally accepted, although proof is lacking that at least some if not all instances of pyelonephritis that occur in the newborn in the absence of urologic malformation represent instances of blood-borne infection, with organisms lodging in the kidney during the course of bacteremia (see p. 140). Many infants with pyelonephritis, diagnosed during life or after death, do have associated septicemia. It is difficult to determine, however, whether the septicemia preceded or occurred as a consequence of the pyelonephritis.

In the majority of neonates with urinary tract infection, urologic-radiologic examination reveals structurally normal kidneys and collecting systems. This finding is in striking contrast to infants diagnosed as having urinary tract infection during the remainder of the first year of life, in whom the prevalence of urologic malformation has been reported to be as high as 50% or 80%.

Pathology. Postmortem studies of acute pyelonephritis have shown pus-containing tubules and ductules, interstitial edema progressing to fibrosis, and interstitial cellular infiltrates. Proliferative glomerular changes, seen occasionally, have been regarded as reactive. The lesion seems to be capable of complete resolution, unless suppuration and fibrosis supervene. Chronic and recurrent pyelonephritis, commonly associated with hydronephrosis, is accompanied by fibrosis, tubular atrophy, and glomerular sclerosis. Changes once regarded as localized nephronic malformations predisposing the infant to infection seem on reevaluation to be secondary sclerotic vascular changes; they are common and are often associated with hypertension.

Clinical features. The majority of infants with urinary infection are asymptomatic; however, even in the sick infant there may be little clinical evidence to suggest infection of the urinary tract. The low incidence of asymptomatic bacteriuria in healthy full-term infants suggests that routine screening in this age group is not a profitable undertaking. In contrast, the infant with any evidence of illness is an excellent candidate for otherwise silent urinary infection; accordingly, he should be examined appropriately. Screening of apparently healthy premature infants has detected significant bacteriuria in 2% to 5%, with some reports showing the incidence to be considerably higher than this. The significance of this finding is not known, but it appears that repeated screening of premature infants during their stay in the nursery is worthwhile.

Although surveys of asymptomatic infants have revealed an equal incidence of bacteriuria in males and females, frank pyelonephritis has been reported to occur three to four times more commonly in males. Neonates with pyelonephritis may exhibit relatively little evidence of serious infection, or they may appear as toxic, septic, desperately ill infants. A peculiar syndrome of pyelonephritis, hepatomegaly, hemolytic anemia, and jaundice (direct- and indirect-reacting bilirubin) has been described in several reports. Other features include poor feeding, lethargy, irritability, occasional vomiting and diarrhea, and azotemia. Hemolysis may be severe enough to require transfusion. The pathogenesis of this syndrome is unknown. The organisms most commonly cultured are the low-numbered serotypes of *E. coli*, especially 04:H5. As in presumptive septicemia (p. 132), treatment is urgent and cannot await the results of cultures. The response to antibiotic therapy usually is prompt, with a return of the blood urea to normal, resolution of hepatomegaly, clearing of jaundice, and cessation of hemolysis.

Treatment. See p. 140 for discussion of specific therapy.

Although urologic malformations in infants with infection of the urinary tract are not encountered commonly, as mentioned above, treatment should be followed by urologic investigation, including intravenous urogram and voiding cystourethrogram. Of utmost importance is the long-term follow-up, with repeated examination of the urine for possible recurrence of infection.

VASCULAR DISORDERS OF THE KIDNEY

The broad category of circulatory disturbances of the kidney includes arterial occlusion, venous thrombosis, cortical necrosis, medullary necrosis, and tubular necrosis. These lesions undoubtedly constitute the most common group of acquired renal diseases in the newborn. All of them are believed to be related to obstruction or diversion of renal blood flow, and the ensuing renal necrosis relates in part to the extent, type, and location of the circulatory abnormality. The degree of renal injury is, however, quite variable; renal vein thrombosis, for example, is associated with complete cortical infarction in one case and inconsequential alteration in another.

The clinical triad of renal enlargement, hematuria, and azotemia applies to almost the entire group of disorders of the kidney. The clinical identification of a specific condition or anatomic lesion is seldom possible. In general, therapy tends to be conservative, principally in maintaining adequate hydration. Anticoagulation may be indicated, but its merits have not been universally established. Peritoneal dialysis has been used in newborns infrequently, although its practicability has been demonstrated in somewhat larger infants. Hemodialysis also may be employed; the technical and practical details are beyond the scope of this discussion. Surgical intervention, formerly advocated as an emergency procedure in the treatment of unilateral renal vein thrombosis, seems to be declining in urgency and popularity.

Arterial occlusion, an uncommon lesion, is usually acute and most often in our experience, the result of thromboembolism. The embolus has usually originated from a thrombus arising in the ductus arteriosus after birth. The ensuing renal infarction can be unilateral or bilateral, and total or segmental, depending on the number and distribution of emboli. The renal arteries may also be obstructed by an aortic thrombus, developing either as the result of embolization or as a local thrombotic consequence of umbilical artery catheterization. Renal infarction can result in an enlarged kidney and either anuria or oliguria and hematuria. There may be vomiting and abdominal tenderness. The blood urea nitrogen level becomes variably elevated. An important consequence of unilateral or segmental arterial occlusion is subsequent renal atrophy with hypertension. Hypertension may be transient, but persistent elevation necessitates a nephrectomy. The capacity of the kidney to recover functionally is impossible to predict in the early stages, and there seems to be little justification for early nephrectomy to prevent progression or spread of thrombi and infarction.

Thrombosis of the renal veins is considerably more common, although its frequency may have declined in recent years. Approximately half of over 300 reported cases have been in infants under 2 months of age. The most important factor in its pathogenesis may be dehydration, a mechanism that can account for cases of both antenatal and postnatal thrombosis. Other factors in newborns include relative polycythemia, relatively low renal blood flow and blood pressure, anoxia, and birth injury. Babies born to diabetic mothers seem to be particularly susceptible, perhaps as the result of glycosuria, polyuria, and dehydration, or perhaps as the result of extravascular fluid shifts, hypovolemia, and effective dehydration. The intrauterine origin of the lesion has been amply demonstrated. We have observed organizing venous thrombi in a newborn with anencephaly, another condition that may be associated with polyuria and intrauterine dehydration. Renal vein thrombosis also complicates diarrhea of the newborn.

The vascular lesion occurs with or without renal infarction, the latter a consequence perhaps of rapid, extensive occlusion of large veins. Venous infarction can result in considerable renal enlargement and anuria or oligohematuria. Thrombocytopenia is a frequent finding, suggesting intravascular consumption. Vomiting, lethargy, anorexia, fever, shock, and associated findings may be related to the initiating causes as much as to the renal lesion. Excretory urography usually discloses nonopacification or slight, diffuse opacification. A venogram may demonstrate vena caval thrombosis. As a later phenomenon, the thrombi, undergoing calcification, are occasionally visible radiographically as radially oriented markings. The thrombi involve the smaller, intrarenal veins, a factor militating against surgical thrombectomy.

The lesion can be unilateral or bilateral, the former occurring perhaps slightly more frequently. Prompt nephrectomy has in the past been advocated in the treatment of unilateral disease to prevent rapid progression and death. However, conservative therapy, developed in relation to bilateral venous thrombosis, has been extended to unilateral involvement. Such measures include rehydration and anticoagulation; reports of survivors indicate some success. Heparin therapy (p. 210) for anticoagulation is potentially dangerous because of bleeding, and its routine effectiveness has not as yet been demonstrated. The late hazards of conservative management are renal atrophy and possible hypertension. Renal vein thrombosis is rarely a cause of the nephrotic syndrome in early infancy. The lesion, once established, seems to carry a poor prognosis, perhaps because of the underlying factors. Recent improvements in neonatal care, particularly in fluid therapy (p. 118), may be effective in reducing the severity of the condition once started in utero and in lowering its incidence after birth.

Cortical and medullary necrosis are appropriately considered together, since the two overlap clinically and often coexist pathologically. They were infrequently reported in the older literature, and there was a tendency to regard cortical necrosis as a variant or phase of renal vein thrombosis. Cortical necrosis is an entity separate from venous thrombosis, with different pathologic features and pathogenetic mechanisms. Both cortical nercosis and medullary necrosis in newborns have been associated with severe anemia or asphyxia. Blood loss in anemic shock has been attributed to twin-twin transfusion, fetal-maternal transfusion, uteroplacental hemorrhage, and severe hemolytic disease. Asphyxial shock is commonly associated with maternal toxemia, and advanced cortical necrosis has been seen in stillborn infants. It has been argued that in hemorrhagic and asphyxial shock renal cortical perfusion is diminished to the point of ischemic tissue necrosis, a mechanism similar to that producing tubular necrosis. Of current interest is the observation of cortical necrosis in some newborns suffering from disseminated intravascular coagulation. Thrombi are not found in major vessels, but the finding of small, scattered arteriolar, venular, and glomerular thrombi has been interpreted as suggesting intravascular coagulation. Cortical necrosis also occurs in association with sepsis, diarrhea, and dehydration. Medullary necrosis in infants with congenital heart disease has been related to the toxicity of large doses of angiographic contrast medium.

The clinical findings are nonspecific: renal enlargement, anuria or oliguria, and hematuria. An accompanying thrombocyto-

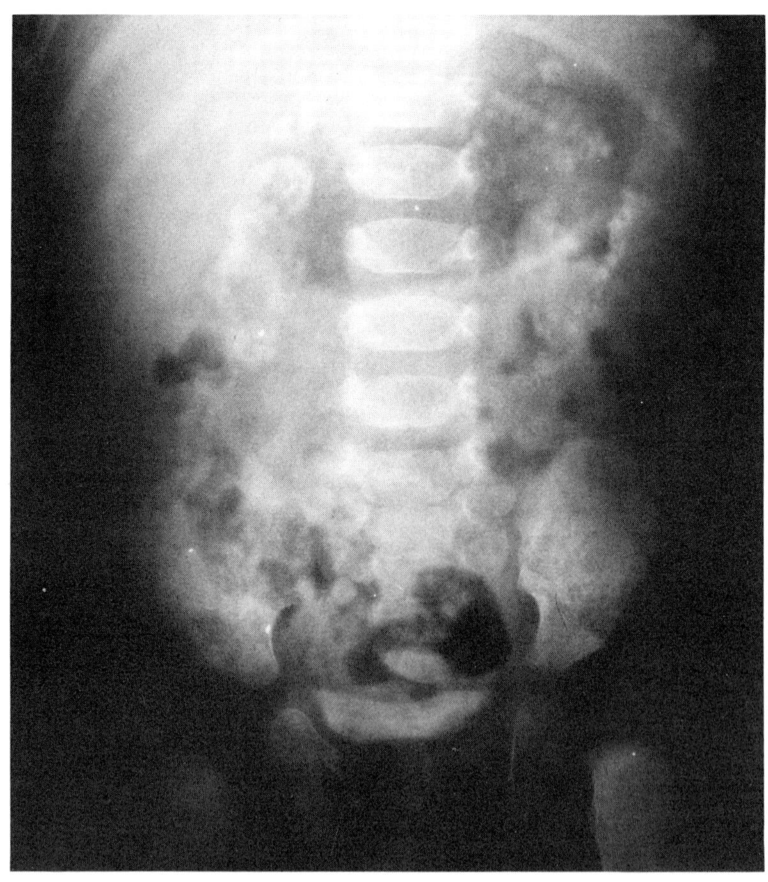

Fig. 16-7. Healing renal cortical necrosis at 9 weeks of age. An intravenous pyelogram at 10 minutes showing a faint nephrogram and faint opacification of the left renal pelvis and bladder. Bilateral renal cortical and adrenal calcification are evident. (From Leonidas, J. C., Berdon, W. E., and Gribetz, D.: J. Pediatr. **79**:623, 1971.)

penia may be evidence of intravascular consumption. Both cortical and medullary necrosis are usually bilateral, but involvement may be patchy or focal. The lesion is a bland, coagulative, ischemic necrosis. Medullary necrosis is commonly hemorrhagic and accompanied by variable cortical involvement. Both conditions are accompanied by focal necrosis in other organs: the liver, adrenal gland, intestines, and the brain. The prognosis is related to the underlying causes as well as to the severity of the renal lesion. As the result of improved supportive care and improved handling of renal failure, relatively long survivals have been described. Necrotic cortical tissue undergoes calcification, producing within weeks a characteristic pattern of bilateral, symmetrical cortical calcification. There may be poor renal visualization by excretory urography because of cortical damage and impaired function. Medullary necrosis may be recognized radiographically by a deformed pyelocalyceal system with evidence of papillary necrosis and cavitation (Fig. 16-7).

The clinical differentiation of these two conditions from renal vein thrombosis may be very difficult, but in all three the clinical management is similar, Conservative therapy calls for careful control of fluids, judicious use of anticoagulation, and treatment of renal failure. Percutaneous renal biopsy may be of value in judging the severity of cortical damage. Prolonged survival may be complicated by severe hypertension. Sparing of juxtamedullary nephrons through collateral circulation in the inner cortex may account for relatively good tubular function despite severe glomerular insufficiency in surviving infants.

Transient and mild oliguria and azotemia have been observed in asphyxiated infants; urinary output is often diminished in newborns with the respiratory distress syndrome. Functional studies have shown depressed GFRs and urea clearances, diminished excretion of creatinine, and impaired dilution and acidification. Increased numbers of cells and casts are found in the urine sediment. *Tubular lesions* in postmortem material are, however, uncommon, and there has been poor correlation between clinical and pathologic findings. Fatty infiltration and necrosis of tubular epithelial cells have been described and attributed to perinatal asphyxia. The observations suggest that functional impairment results from poor cortical perfusion and that tubular injury is a reflection of cortical ischemia rather than the cause of functional impairment.

TUMORS OF THE KIDNEY

Renal tumors in newborns are not common, despite the frequency of Wilms' tumors throughout childhood. Although they account perhaps for 20% of all malignant tumors in childhood, only 3% to 4% of Wilms' tumors have occurred in fetuses and newborns. Renal cell carcinoma is uncommon in childhood and is unknown in the newborn. Renal lymphomas and teratoma in the newborn are medical rarities. In general, renal tumors occurring in early infancy offer a considerably better outlook than do those in later childhood. Apart from the apparently better response of such tumors to the therapeutic measures, the difference may also be because of the occurrence in young infants of relatively benign variants. In newborns, for example, approximately one half of nephromas are nonmetastasizing fibromyomatous tumors or so-called hamartomas. The other half are more typical Wilms' tumors.

Clinical presentation. In newborns, as in older infants, the initial finding is usually that of abdominal swelling or a palpable mass, often detected by the parents. In infants with Wilms' tumor there may be a history of vomiting and fever, and laboratory examination may disclose hematuria and an elevated erythrocyte sedimentation rate. Older infants frequently have hypertension, but its incidence in newborns is not known.

Wilms' tumors have been associated with several nonrenal malformations, among them congential aniridia and hemihypertrophy. The former is believed to be genetically determined, and the latter is a malformation present at birth. Either of these findings in a newborn should alert the clinician to the risk of a subsequent Wilms' tumor, although we are not aware of renal tumors having been found in newborns. Hemihypertrophy has also been associated with adrenal and hepatic tumors, visceral hemangiomas, and pigmented nevi. Other defects associated with aniridia are cataracts, microcephaly, mental retardation, growth retardation, misshapen ears, and cryptorchidism. Another syndrome includes male pseudohermaphroditism with occasional agonadism, glomerulonephritis with nephrotic syndrome, renal failure and hypertension, and Wilms' tumor. The genital abnormalities are present at birth; the tumors apparently develop later. These interesting associations may provide a link between teratogenic factors and the development of certain tumors; the association of Wilms' tumor with fused kidneys, for example, seems to be unduly high. At the moment, the value in recognizing these syndromes—congenital aniridia, hemihypertrophy, or pseudohermaphroditism—lies in early detection of associated malignancy.

Pathology. Wilms' tumors are composed of mesenchymal or nephroblastic cells with variable differentiation into smooth muscle, striated muscle, cartilage, tubules, and glomeruli. Epithelial components are immature, often resembling nephrogenic elements of the fetal cortex. The tumor commonly seems to be discrete, compressing the adjacent kidney tissue into a relatively fibrous capsule. True encapsulation is lacking, however, and the tumor invades the adjacent kidney, renal veins, and adjacent organs. Metastases are principally hematogenous: lungs, liver, bones, and the other kidney. Fibromyomas, on the other hand, are composed of interlacing bundles of spindle cells; they resemble leiomyomas, and differentiation to smooth muscle can be demonstrated. Islands of tubules and glomeruli may represent entrapped kidney, for the tumor is indeed locally invasive, or they may be foci of metanephric differentiation. Wilms' tumor and the fibromyoma are both believed to arise from metanephric blastema.

Diagnosis. The differential diagnosis of an abdominal mass in the newborn includes neuroblastoma, retroperitoneal tumors and cysts, splenomegaly, hepatic tumors, ovarian cysts and tumors, intestinal duplications, and several renal abnormalilites. Radiography is important in localizing the lesion to the kidney, in excluding hydronephrosis and polycystic disease, and in identifying ectopic, fused, and solitary kidneys. Excretory urography in Wilms' tumor commonly shows flattening and distortion of the pyelocalyceal system, a finding common to all intrarenal masses. Excretion of contrast medium may, however, be so impaired by infiltrating tumor or by secondary vascular obstruction that at times roentgenograms show only a nonfunctioning renal mass. Arteriography can be of additional help in identifying and localizing the tumor. Wilms' tumor usually contain a characteristic abnormal vasculature in the form of fine, nodular vessels. The neovascularity is not specific, however, having been found also in some fibromyomas. The fibromyomatous tumors tend to be less vascular. During the nephrographic phase of the arteriogram the denser renal tissue is seen to be displaced by the tumor. Occasional Wilms' tumors are avascular, perhaps because of hemorrhagic or cystic degeneration, and differentiation from cystic lesions may then be difficult. A solitary and localized tumorous lesion such as the benign multilocular cyst, which some have regarded as a nephroblastic hamartoma, may be very difficult to differentiate from an avascular Wilms' tumor. Renal angiography is also of value in defining the extent of neoplastic involvement and in evaluating the contralateral kidney prior to surgery.

Bilaterality in Wilms' tumor (all ages) occurs in approximately 4%; its frequency in newborns is obscured by other developmental abnormalities. Wilms' tumors may also coexist with other renal abnormalities, including cystic disease, duplication, fusion, and ectopia, thus complicating radiologic interpretation. Wilms' tumors, also have occurred with greater than expected frequency in horseshoe-shaped and solitary kidneys.

Treatment. Definitive therapy should be instituted promptly after the diagnosis has been confirmed. The presence of a localized intrarenal mass necessitates surgical exploration. Primary treatment is nephrectomy. Therapeutic regimens currently do not include routine preoperative irradiation; combined chemotherapy and radiotherapy are used postoperatively in cases of Wilms' tumor. The benign mesenchymal tumors require no additional postoperative therapy.

Prognosis. The prognosis in neonatal

Wilms' tumor is good, although precise figures are lacking. The survival of all infants younger than 1 year may be 70% to 80%. Collins' hypothesis that the growth rate of a congenital tumor remains constant may be helpful in evaluating prognosis: The recurrence will take no longer than the original tumor to reach a clinically recognizable size. If this hypothesis is true, newborns are at risk of recurrence for only another 10 months, and the infant who remains free of recurrence during his first year of life is likely to be permanently cured. Clinical staging might be of greater help in determining outcome; tumors confined to the kidney have an excellent prognosis, but progressively poorer results can be anticipated with tumors extending at the time of nephrectomy into the renal fossa and vessels and beyond.

ADRIAN SPITZER
JAY BERNSTEIN
CHESTER M. EDELMAN, Jr.

BIBLIOGRAPHY

RENAL FUNCTION AND ITS MORPHOLOGIC CORRELATES

Bain, A. D., and Scott, J. S.: Renal agenesis and severe urinary dysplasia; A review of 50 cases with particular reference to associated anomalies, Brit. Med. J. **1**:841, 1960.

Brodehl, J., and Gellison, K.: Endogenous renal transport of free amino-acids in infancy and childhood, Pediatrics **42**:395, 1968.

Dean, R. F. A., and McCance, R. A.: Inulin, diodone, creatinine and urea clearances in newborn infants, J. Physiol. (Lond.) **106**:431, 1947.

Edelmann, C. M., Jr., Barnett, H. L., and Troupkou, V.: Renal concentrating mechanism in newborn infants; effect of dietary protein and water content, role of urea and responsiveness to antidiuretic hormone, J. Clin. Invest. **39**: 1062, 1960.

Fetterman, G. H., Shuplock, N. A., Philipp, F. J., and Gregg, H. S.: The growth and maturation of human glomeruli and proximal convolutions from term to adulthood; studies by microdissection, Pediatrics **35**:601, 1965.

Hatemi, N., and McCance, R. A.: Renal aspects of acid base control in the newly born. III. Response to acidifying drugs, Acta Paediatr. Scand. **50**:603, 1961.

McCance, R. A.: The maintenance of stability in the newly born. I. Chemical exchange, Arch. Dis. Child. **34**:459, 1959.

McCance, R. A., and von Finck, M. A.: The titrable acidity, pH, ammonia and phosphates in the urines of very young infants, Arch. Dis. Child. **22**:200, 1947.

McCance, R. A., and Widdowson, E. M.: Renal function before birth, Proc. Roy. Soc. Lond. (B) **141**:488, 1953.

Potter, E. L., and Thierstein, S. T.: Glomerular development in the kidney as an index of fetal maturity, J. Pediatr. **22**:695, 1943.

REACTION OF THE IMMATURE KIDNEY TO INJURY

Bernstein, J.: Developmental abnormalities of the renal parenchyma; renal hypoplasia and dysplasia. In Sommers, S. C., editor: Pathology annual 1968, New York, 1968, Appleton-Century-Crofts, chap. 3.

Bernstein, J., and Meyer, R.: Congenital abnormalities of the urinary system. II. Renal cortical and medullary necrosis, J. Pediatr. **59**:657, 1961.

Emery, J. L., and Macdonald, M. S.: Involuting and scarred glomeruli in the kidneys of infants, Am. J. Pathol. **36**:713, 1960.

Kanasawa, M., Moller, J., Good, R. A., and Vernier, R. L.: Dwarfed kidneys in children; the classification, etiology, and significance of bilateral small kidneys in 11 children, Am. J. Dis. Child. **109**:130, 1965.

Malt, R. A.: Compensatory growth of the kidney, N. Engl. J. Med. **280**:1446, 1969.

Osathanondh, V., and Potter, E. L.: Pathogenesis of polycystic kidneys; type 4 due to urethral obstruction, Arch. Pathol. (Chicago) **77**:502, 1964.

FUNCTIONAL EVALUATION

Goldman, H. S., and Freeman, L. M.: Radiographic and radioisotopic methods of evaluation of the kidneys and urinary tract, Pediatr. Clin. North Am. **18**:409, 1971.

Kassirer, J. P.: Clinical evaluation of kidney function; glomerular function, N. Engl. J. Med. **285**: 385, 1971.

DISORDERS OF MICTURITION

Lattimer, J. K., Uson, A. C., and Melicow, M. M.: Urologic emergencies in newborn infants, Pediatrics **29**:310, 1962.

Lawson, J. S., and Hewstone, A. S.: Microscopic appearance of urine in newborn period, Arch. Dis. Child. **39**:287, 1964.

Sherry, S. N., and Kramer, I.: The time of passage of the first stool and first urine by the newborn infant, J. Pediatr. **46**:158, 1955.

PROTEINURIA

deLuna, M. B., and Hullet, W. H.: Urinary protein excretion in healthy infants, children and adults, Proc. Am. Soc. Nephrol. **16**:16, 1967.

Peterson, P. A., Evrin, P., and Berggard, I.: Differentiation of glomerular, tubular, and normal proteinuria; determinations of urinary excretion of beta-2-macroglobulin, albumin and total protein, J. Clin. Invest. **48**:1189, 1969.

HEMATURIA

Angella, J. J., Prieto, E. N., and Fogel, B. J.: Hemoglobinuria associated with hemolytic disease of the newborn infant, J. Pediatr. **71**:530, 1967.

PYURIA

Gruickshand, G., and Edmond, E.: "Clean catch" urines in the newborn; bacteriology and cell excretion patterns in first week of life, Br. Med. J. 4:705, 1967.

Lincoln, K., and Winberg, J.: Studies of urinary tract infection in infancy and childhood. III. Quantitative estimation of cellular excretion in unselected neonates, Acta Paediatr. Scand. 53: 447, 1964.

Littlewood, J. M.: White cells and bacteria in voided urine of healthy newborns, Arch. Dis. Child. 46:167, 1971.

EDEMA

Cywes, S., Wynne, J. M., and Louw, J. H.: Urinary ascites in newborn; with a report of two cases, J. Pediatr. Surg. 3:350, 1968.

Fisher, D. A.: Obscure and unusual edema, Pediatrics 37:506, 1966.

Kagan, B. M., and Felix, N. S.: Edema of infancy Pediatr. Clin. North Am. 2:391, 1955.

MacLaurin, J. C.: Changes in body water distribution during the first two weeks of life, Arch. Dis. Child. 41:286, 1966.

Wu, P. Y. K., Oh, W., Lubetkin, A., and Metcoff, J.: "Late edema" in low birth weight infants, Pediatrics 41:67, 1968.

ABDOMINAL MASSES

Longio, L. A., and Martin, L. W.: Abdominal masses in the newborn infant, Pediatrics 21:596, 1958.

Mussels, M., Gaudry, C. L., and Bason, W. M.: Renal anomalies in the newborn found by deep palpation, Pediatrics 47:97, 1971.

RENAL INSUFFICIENCY AND RENAL FAILURE

Barratt, T. M.: Renal failure in the first year of life, Br. Med. Bull. 27:115, 1971.

Dobrin, R. S., Larsen, C. D., and Holliday, M. A: The critically ill child; acute renal failure, Pediatrics 48:286, 1971.

Fine, R. N., Stiles, Q., DePalma, J. R., and Donnell, G. N.: Hemodialysis in infants under 1 year of age for acute poisoning, Am. J. Dis. Child. 116:657, 1968.

Holliday, M. A., Potter, D. E., and Dobris, R. S.: Treatment of renal failure in children, Pediatr. Clin. North Am. 18:613, 1971.

Manley, G. L., and Gollipp, J. J.: Renal failure in the newborn; treatment with peritoneal dialysis, Am. J. Dis. Child. 115:107, 1968.

MALFORMATIONS

Bernstein, J.: Developmental abnormalities of the renal parenchyma; renal hypoplasia and dysplasia. In Sommers, S. C., editor: Pathology annual 1968, New York, 1968, Appleton-Century-Crofts, chap. 3.

Bernstein, J.: Heritable cystic disorders of the kidney; the mythology of polycystic disease, Pediatr. Clin. North Am. 18:435, 1971.

Burke, E. C., Shin, M. H., and Kelalis, P. P.: Prune-belly syndrome; clinical findings and survival, Am. J. Dis. Child. 117:668, 1969.

Davidson, W. M., and Ross, G. I. M.: Bilateral absence of the kidneys and related congenital anomalies, J. Pathol. 68:459, 1954.

Elkin, M., and Bernstein, J.: Cystic diseases of the kidney, radiological and pathological considerations, Clin. Radiol. 20:65, 1969.

Goldston, A. S., and others: Neonatal polycystic kidney with brain defect, Am. J. Dis. Child. 106:484, 1963.

Javadpour, N., Chelouhy, E., Moncada, L., Rosenthal, I. M., and Bush, I. M.: Hypertension in a child caused by a multicystic kidney, J. Urol. 104:918, 1970.

Lieberman, E., Salinas-Madrigal, L., Gwinn, J. L., Brennan, L. P., Fine, F. N., and Landing, B. H.: Infantile polycystic disease of the kidneys and liver; clinical, pathological and radiological correlations and comparison with congenital hepatic fibrosis, Medicine (Baltimore) 50:277, 1971.

Lundin, P. M., and Olow, I.: Polycystc kidneys in newborns, infants, and children; a clinical and pathological study, Acta Paediatr. 50:185, 1961.

North, A. F., Jr., Eldredge, D. M., and Tapley, W. B.: Abdominal distention at birth; due to ascites associated with obstructive uropathy, Am. J. Dis. Child. 111:613, 1966.

Passarage, E., and Sutherland, J. M.: Potter's syndrome; chromosome analysis of 3 cases with Potter's syndrome or related syndromes, Am. J. Dis. Child. 109:80, 1965.

Potter, E. L.: Bilateral absence of ureters and kidneys; a report of 50 cases, Obstet. Gynecol. 25: 3, 1965.

Rattner, W. H., Meyer, R., and Bernstein, J.: Congenital abnormalities of the urinary system. IV. Valvular obstruction of the posterior urethra, J. Pediatr. 63:84, 1963.

Rubenstein, M., Meyer, R., and Bernstein, J.: Congenital abnormalities of the urinary system. I. A postmortem survey of developmental anomalies and acquired congenital lesions in a children's hospital, J. Pediatr. 58:356, 1961.

NEPHRITIS

Claireaux, A. E., and Pearson, M. G.: Chronic nephritis in a newborn infant, Arch. Dis. Child. 30:366, 1955.

Collins, R. D.: Chronic glomerulonephritis in a newborn child, Am. J. Dis. Child. 87:478, 1954.

Taitz, L S., Isaacson, C., and Stein, H.: Acute nephritis associated with congenital syphilis, Br. Med. J. 2:152, 1961.

NEPHROTIC SYNDROME

Farquhar, M. G., Vernier, R. L., and Good, R. A: Studies on familial nephrosis. II. Glomerular changes observed with the electron microscope, Am. J. Pathol. 33:791, 1957.

Feinerman, B., Burke, E. C., and Bahn, R. C.: The nephrotic syndrome associated with renal vein thrombosis, J. Pediatr. 51:385, 1957.

Fetterman, G. H., and Feldman, J. D.: Congenital anomalies of renal tubules in a case of "infantile nephrosis," Am. J. Dis. Child. **100**:319, 1960.

Hoyer, J. R., Michael, A. F., Good, R. A., and Vernier, R. L.: The nephrotic syndrome of infancy; clinical, morphologic studies of four infants, Pediatrics **40**:233, 1967.

Kouvalainen, K.: Immunological studies on the congenital nephrotic syndrome, Am. J. Dis. Child. **104**:554, 1962.

McDonald, R., Wiggelinkhuisen, J., and Kaschula, R. O. C.: The nephrotic syndrome in very young infants, Am. J. Dis. Child. **122**:507, 1971.

Medearis, D. N: Cytomegalic inclusion disease; an analysis of the clinical features based on the literature and six additional cases, Pediatrics **19**: 467, 1957

Norio, R.: Heredity in the congenital nephrotic syndrome; a genetic study of 57 Finnish families with a review of reported cases, Ann. Paediatr. Fenn. **12**(Suppl. 27):1, 1966.

Papaioannou, A. C., Asrow, G. G., and Schuckmell, N. H.: Nephrotic syndrome in early infancy as a manifestation of congenital syphilis, Pediatrics **27**:636, 1961.

Rapola, J., and Savilahti, E.: Immunofluorescent and morphological studies in congenital nephrotic syndrome, Acta Paediatr. Scand. **60**:253, 1971.

Scully, J. P., and Yanazaki, J. N.: Congenital syphilitic nephrosis successfully treated with penicillin, Am. J. Dis. Child. **77**:652, 1949.

Walker, C. H. M., Wershing, J. M., Simons, S. L., Holmes, J. H., Sitprija, V, and O'Brien, D.: Hemodialysis in infantile nephrotic syndrome, Am. J. Dis. Child. **106**:479, 1963.

RENAL GLYCOSURIA

Elsas, L. J., Hillman, R. E., Patterson, J. H., and Rosenberg, L. E.: Renal and intestinal hexose transport in familial glucose-galactose malabsorption, J. Clin. Invest. **49**:576, 1970.

Monasterio, G., Oliver, J., Muiesan, G., Pardelli, G., Marrinozzi, V., and MacDowell, M.: Renal diabetes as a congential tubular dysplasia, Am. J. Med. **37**:44, 1964.

AMINOACIDURIAS

Brodehl, J., and Gellissen, K.: Endogenous renal transport of free amino acids in infancy and childhood, Pediatrics **42**:395, 1968.

Chisolm, J. J., Jr., and Harrison, H. E.: Aminoaciduria, Pediatr. Clin. North Am. **7**:333, 1960.

Chisolm, J. J., Jr., and Harrison, H. E.: Aminoaciduria in vitamin D deficiency states, in premature infants and older infants with rickets, J. Pediatr. **60**:206, 1962.

Pruzanksy, W.: Cystinuria and cystine urolithiasis in childhood, Acta Paediatr. Scand. **55**:97, 1966.

Rosenberg, L. E., Durant, J. L., and Elsas, L. J.: Familial iminoglycinuria; an inborn error of renal tubular transport, N. Engl. J. Med. **278**: 1407, 1968.

Whelan, D. T, and Scriver, G R: Hyperdibasic-aminoaciduria; an inherited disorder of amino acid transport, Pediatr. Res. **2**:525, 1968.

CYSTINOSIS

Cramhall, J. C., Lietman, P. S., Schneider, J. A., and Seegmiller, J. E.: Cystinosis; plasma cystine and cysteine concentrations and the effect of D-penicillamine and dietary treatment, Am. J. Med. **44**:330, 1968.

Seegmiller, J. E., Friedman, T., Harrison, H. E., Wong, V., and Schneider, J. A.: Cystinosis, Ann. Intern. Med. **68**:883, 1968.

Serp, M., Steen-Johnsen, J., Vellan, J. E., and Gjessing, L. R.: Dietary treatment of cystinosis, Acta Paediatr. Scand. **57**:409, 1968.

Worthen, H. G.: Growth failure due to diseases of the proximal tubule, J. Pediatr. **57**:14, 1960.

PSEUDOHYPOALDOSTERONISM

Cheek, D. B., and Perry, J. N.: A salt wasting syndrome in infancy, Arch. Dis. Child. **33**:252, 1958.

Donnell, G. N., Litman, N., and Roldan, M.: Pseudohypoadrenalcorticism; renal sodium loss, hyponatremia, and hyperkalemia due to renal tubular insensitivity to mineralocorticoid, Am. J. Dis. Child. **97**:813, 1959.

NEPHROGENIC DIABETES INSIPIDUS

Friss-Hansen, P., Skadhauge, E., and Zetterström, R.: Fluid and electrolyte metabolism in nephrogenic diabetes insipidus, Acta Paediatr. Scand. Suppl. **146**:57, 1963.

Gautier, P. E., and Sympkiss, M.: The management of nephrogenic diabetes insipidus in early life, Acta Paediatr. Scand. **46**:354, 1957.

Schotland, M. G., Grumbach, M. M., and Strauss, J.: The effect of chlorothiazides in nephrogenic diabetes insipidus, Pediatrics **31**:741, 1963.

RENAL TUBULAR ACIDOSIS

Morris, R. C.: Renal tubular acidosis; mehanisms, classification and implications, N. Engl. J. Med. **281**:1405, 1969.

Rodriguez-Soriano, J., and Edelmann, C. M., Jr.: Renal tubular acidosis, Ann. Rev. Med. **20**:363, 1969.

INFECTION OF THE URINARY TRACT

Edelmann, C. M., Jr., Ogwo, J., and Fine, B. P.: The prevalence of bacteriuria in full-term and premature newborn infants, Pediatrics. In press.

Gower, P. E., Husband, P., Coleman, J. C., and Snodgrass, G. J. A. I.: Urinary infection in two selected neonatal populations, Arch. Dis. Child. **45**:259, 1970.

Houston, I. B.: Pus cell and bacterial counts in the diagnosis of urinary tract infections in childhood, Arch. Dis. Child. **38**:600, 1963.

Lincoln, K., and Winberg, J.: Studies of urinary tract infections in infancy and childhood. II. Quantitative estimation of bacteriuria in unselected neonates with special reference to the occurrence of asymptomatic infections, Acta Paediatr. Scand. **53**:307, 1964.

Lincoln, K., and Winberg, J.: Studies of urinary tract infections in infancy and childhood. III. Quantitative estimation of celular excretion in unselected neonates, Acta Paediatr. Scand. **53:** 447, 1964.

Littlewood, J. M.: White cells and bacteria in voided urine of healthy newborns, Arch. Dis. Child. **46**:167, 1971.

Newman, C. G. H., O'Neill, P., and Parker, A.: Pyuria in infancy and the role of suprapubic aspiration of urine in diagnosis of infections of the urinary tract, Br. Med. J. **2**:277, 1967.

Seeler, R. A., and Hahn, K.: Jaundice in urinary tract infection in infancy, Am. J. Dis. Child. **118**:553, 1969.

VASCULAR DISORDERS OF THE KIDNEY

Belman, A. B., Susmano, D. F., Burden, J. J., and Kaplan, G. W.: Nonoperative treatment of unilateral renal vein thrombosis in the newborn, J.A.M.A. **211**:1165, 1970.

Bernstein, J., and Meyer, R.: Congenital abnormalities of the urinary system. II. Renal cortical and medullary necrosis, J. Pediatr. **59**:657, 1961.

Brough, A. J., and Zuelzer, W. W.: Renal vascular disease, Pediatr. Clin. North Am. **11**:533, 1964.

Groshong, T. D., Taylor, A. A., Nolph, K. D., Esterly, J., and Maher, J. F.: Renal function following cortical necrosis in childhood, J. Pediatr. **79**:267, 1971.

Gruskin, A. B., Oetliker, O. H., Wolfish, N. W., Gootman, N. L., Bernstein, J., and Edelmann, C. M., Jr.: Effects of angiography on renal function and histology in infants and piglets, J. Pediatr. **76**:42, 1970.

Leonidas, J. C., Berdon, W. E., and Gribetz, D.: Bilateral renal cortical necrosis in the newborn infant; roentgenographic diagnosis, J. Pediatr. **79**:623, 1971.

Takeuchi, A., and Benirschke, K.: Renal venous thrombosis of the newborn and its relation to maternal diabetes, Biol. Neonate **3**:237, 1961.

TUMORS OF THE KIDNEY

Bolande, R. P., Brough, A. J., and Izant, R. J., Jr.: Congenital mesoblastic nephroma of infancy; a report of eight cases and the relationship of Wilms' tumor, Pediatrics **40**:272, 1967.

Collins, V. P.: The treatment of Wilm's tumor, Cancer **11**:89, 1958.

Drash, A., Sherman, F., Hartmann, W. H., and Blizzard, R. M.: A syndrome of male pseudohermaphroditis, Wilms' tumor, hypertension, and degenerative renal disease, J. Pediatr. **76**:585, 1970.

Favara, B. E., Johnson, W., and Ito, J.: Renal tumors in the neonatal period, Cancer **22**:845, 1968.

Fleming, I. E., and Johnson, W. W.: Clinical and pathologic staging as a guide in the management of Wilms' tumor, Cancer **26**:660, 1970.

Miller, R. W., Fraumeni, J. F., Jr., and Manning, M. D.: Association of Wilms' tumor with aniridia, hemihypertrophy and other congenital malformations, N. Engl. J. Med. **270**:922, 1964.

Poole, C. A., and Viamonte, M., Jr.: Unusual renal masses in pediatric age group, Am. J. Roentgenol. **109**:368, 1970.

17 Central nervous system disturbances*

NEUROLOGIC SCREENING EXAMINATION OF THE HEALTHY NEWBORN

The neurologic examination of the newborn is a neglected area of neonatology as well as of neurology in general. For many physicians the neurologic examination consists only of determining that the Moro reflex is present and symmetrical, that the baby moves all of his extremities, and that the red reflex is present on funduscopic examination. At the other extreme from this inadequate examination stands the excellent and detailed work of neonatologists such as Thomas, Prechtl, and Illingworth, who have designed complex examinations beyond the scope and interest of most pediatricians.

A middle ground is necessary if the neurologic examination of the newborn performed by most pediatricians is to fulfill its purposes. First, it should detect conditions such as meningitis, seizures, hemorrhage, and metabolic disorders that require acute intervention to prevent permanent damage to the nervous system. Second, it should facilitate an accurate prognosis in infants where peripheral damage is documented, as in brachial plexus injuries or meningomyeloceles, and an accurate diagnosis and prognosis of central nervous system (CNS) damage.

The newborn nervous system

The nervous system of the full-term newborn is in a state of rapid development and differentiation. Dendrites are continuing to sprout from neurons and are forming interneuronal connections. Myelination of the CNS is still far from complete, and myelination of the peripheral nervous system (PNS) is just beginning. The physiology of neural membranes in the newborn indicates that the ion pumps are less efficient and the membranes more leaky than they will be with later development. Even cerebral metabolism of the newborn is different from that of the older child. The newborn is far more resistant to anoxia and seems able to utilize ketone bodies as well as anaerobic glycolysis as energy sources far better than the older infant. It is not surprising, therefore, that one is able to obtain little evidence of cortical functioning in the normal newborn. Indeed, the neurologic examination of the anencephalic infant is virtually normal.

Subcortical and brainstem functions, however, are at a higher stage of development morphologically and physiologically. Consequently, the neurologic examination of the newborn is primarily an examination of subcortical structures. Detailed testing of these structures, which include midbrain, brainstem, spinal cord, and peripheral modalities, is possible. Cortical influences on these subcortical structures are doubtless present but are difficult to document. Cortical damage may occasionally be manifested in terms of asymmetries of the peripheral responses.

Detailed testing of the subcortical structures is time consuming but need not be part of the routine examination of every newborn. However, a screening examination is warranted in every infant. A brief

*This work was supported in part by The Child Neurology Training Grant, No. NS5663, and The John A. Hartford Foundation, Inc.

screening examination is outlined in Table 17-1. The mechanics of performing this examination are explained below. When abnormalities are found during the screening examination, they may be confirmed and tested by a detailed neurologic examination.

Comments on the neurologic examination

History

See also p. 11.

Three major aspects of the history are important: the parental history, the obstetrical history, and the infant's neonatal history. Information acquired before the newborn becomes ill will often enable the anticipation and prevention of many problems. The parental history should include the age of the parents, race, and familial diseases, as well as a history of hypertension or diabetes in the mother. The obstetrical history should include parity, bleeding or infections during pregnancy, and a history of previous pregnancies, with detailed results of the outcome and the health of all previous siblings. This latter information, often missing from obstetrical histories, may assist in the prediction of perinatal problems of a biochemical or genetic nature. The infant's history should include details of labor in the mother and its duration, drugs given and their timing, the mode of delivery, and a description of the placenta and of the number of umbilical vessels. Knowledge of the Apgar score at 1 and 5 minutes and the methods of resuscitation of the infant may be crucial. A detailed history of the nursery course and of each examination may be important to the infant who is later found to be abnormal. Of particular relevance are cyanotic spells, apneic episodes, jitteriness and abnormal movements, jaundice, feeding, and procedures performed.

Table 17-1. Neurologic screening examination

- History
- General pediatric examination
  - Head shape and circumference
  - Skin lesions
- Specific neurologic observations
  - Mental state
    - Moro reflex
  - Abnormal posture
    - At rest—asymmetry
    - Position of legs (that is, frog-leg position)
    - Head retraction
    - Cortical thumb
  - Abnormal movements
    - Tremor, jitteriness
    - Lack of movement
    - Asymmetry of movement, Moro reflex
  - Power
    - Grip
    - Head lag
    - Supporting reflex
  - Tone
    - Ventral suspension
    - Upright suspension
    - Movement of individual joints
  - Cranial nerve testing

Type of test	Afferent nerves	Efferent nerves
Pupillary response	II	III
Body rotation	VIII	III, IV, VI Median longitudinal fasciculus
Facial movement (cry, eye closure)		VII
Suck	V	Motor V, VII, XII
Swallow		IX, X, XII

General pediatric examination

See also p. 95.

The general pediatric examination needs no detailing here. Of particular importance from the neurologic standpoint, however, is evidence of skin lesions, such as the hemangioma of Sturge-Weber disease, pigmented lesions of neurofibromatosis, the pale nevi of tuberous sclerosis, or the vesicles of incontinentia pigmenti (p. 582). The head shape and circumference and abnormalities of the back are of similar importance.

Specific neurologic observations

Mental state. The state of consciousness of the child should be a recorded part of

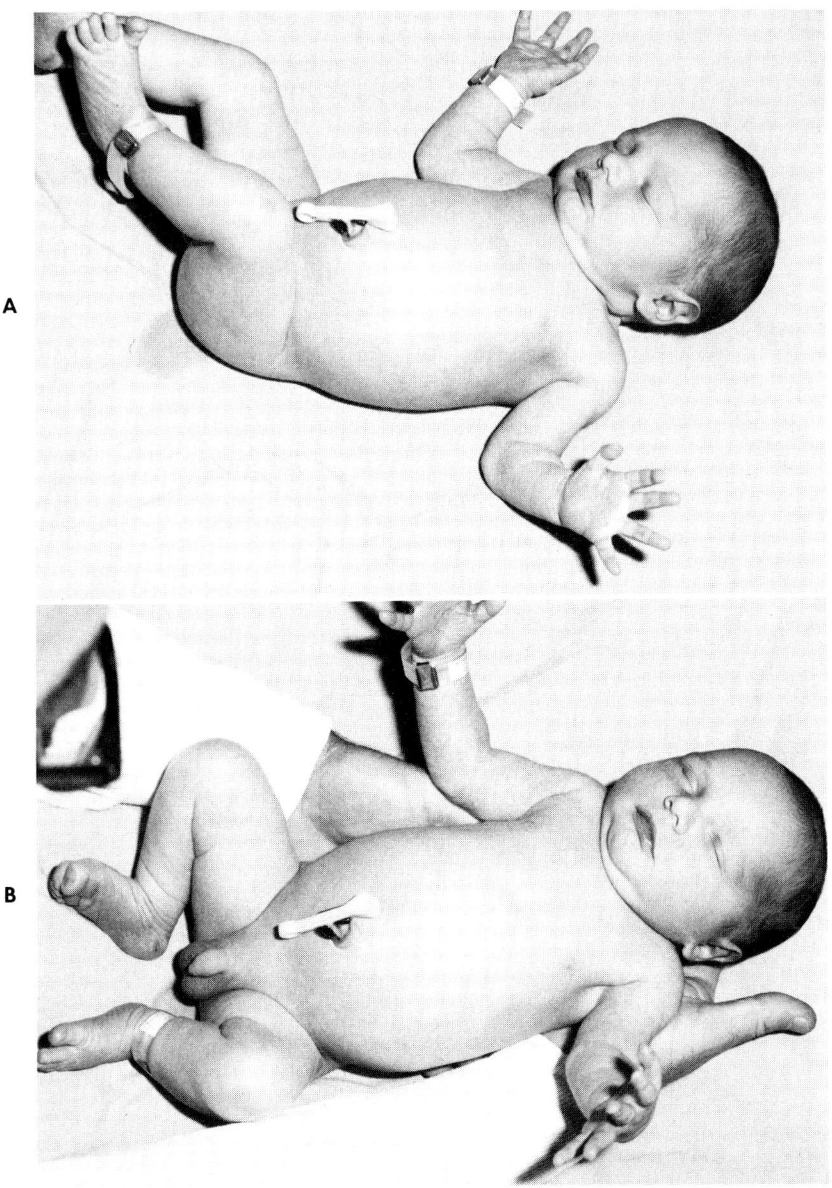

Fig. 17-1. The Moro reflex is elicited by the rapid release of the supported head. The arms abduct and fingers open as shown in **A.** In the second phase, **B,** the arms come forward in an embrace. A cry and movement of the legs accompany the reflex.

the neurologic examination. Consciousness has been divided into five stages: (1) deep sleep, eyes closed, no movements with regular respiration, (2) eyes closed with irregular respiration, no gross movements, (3) awake, eyes open and quiet, (4) eyes open or closed, gross movements, no crying, and (5) eyes open or closed, crying.

The Moro (startle) reflex affords an assessment of the state of alertness of the child (Fig. 17-1). The reflex may be depressed because of cerebral damage or drugs, or it may be depressed in the postprandial state. It may be decreased with weakness or hypotonia, and occasionally with hypertonia. The reflex may have a lower threshold with cerebral damage and hypocalcemia and in jittery babies. Performance of the Moro reflex also offers an opportunity to assess asymmetries of movement.

Abnormal posturing. The most important aspect of the neurologic examination is observation. Observation should be performed both before and after removing the infant from his crib or incubator and undressing him (Fig. 17-2). Abnormalities of posture at rest include: asymmetries from side to side, as seen in the infant with a brachial plexus lesion; asymmetries between the arms and the legs, as seen with a spinal cord lesion; the frog-leg position often seen with anterior horn cell disease, hypotonia, or paralysis; head retraction (opisthotonus) often seen with a subarachnoid hemorrhage, seizures, or metabolic disorders; and, most important of all, the cortical thumb. The cortical thumb (a closed hand with the thumb inside the fingers) is the normal position of the hand in the newborn (Fig. 17-3). However, even at this age the position is not obligatory, and the infant will periodically open the hand and extend the thumb. An obligatory cortical thumb that does not open spontaneously is the earliest sign of cortical spinal tract involvement in the infant.

Abnormal movements. Observation of the infant may reveal tremors, jitteriness, or seizures. Seizures may take varied forms (see section on seizures, p. 549), and, indeed, any sudden alteration in the state of the infant may represent a seizure. Tonic-clonic movements are relatively uncommon manifestations of seizures at this age. Tremors or jitteriness, however, are com-

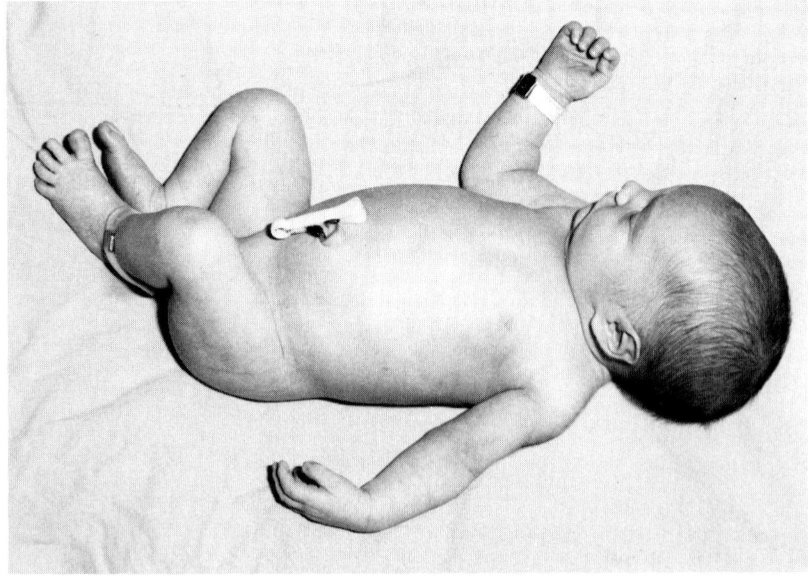

Fig. 17-2. Normal newborn at rest. Note that the posture of the arms and legs are asymmetrical. The arms are usually partially flexed; the legs are flexed at the knees and hips. Contrast this with the hypotonic infant, Fig. 17-10.

mon movements in the newborn. These movements may be provoked by exogenous stimuli, such as a startle reflex, a Moro reflex, or crying, or may be endogenous, associated with spontaneous alterations in the level of consciousness of the infant. Tremors do not occur with the infant at rest. Tremors that are high frequency, low amplitude may be seen with hypoglycemia, hypocalcemia, or may be seen in otherwise normal infants. They will usually disappear in the first days of life. Tremors of low frequency and high amplitude, however, are often associated with exaggerated reflexes and a low-threshold Moro response. There is often a correlation with the later development of choreoathetosis if the tremor persists beyond the fourth day. Characteristic coarse tremors occur as a sign of drug withdrawal in infants of addicted mothers (p. 450).

Strength. Strength and weakness are related to alertness, to physiologic maturity, and to problems in the CNS or PNS, as well as in the muscle. A detailed test of muscle strength is obviously difficult in an infant. However, an adequate screening test of strength is that of the infant's grasp. The finger inserted from the lateral aspect into the infant's palm elicits a palmar grasp. This grasp in the normal newborn should be sufficiently strong to partially support the infant's weight as he is lifted from supine to sitting position. As he pulls the infant up, the observer should feel contractions at the infant's biceps and the shoulder girdle and some contraction of the sternomastoids, so that the head does not fall completely back (Fig. 17-4). Thus, in this one maneuver, the observer can obtain a fairly good estimate of strength throughout the upper extremities and neck. Asymmetries of strength should also be noted. Strength in the lower extremities can be assessed by the supporting response, the ability of the newborn to support his weight when his feet are placed on the examining table. Stepping, placing, and the crossed

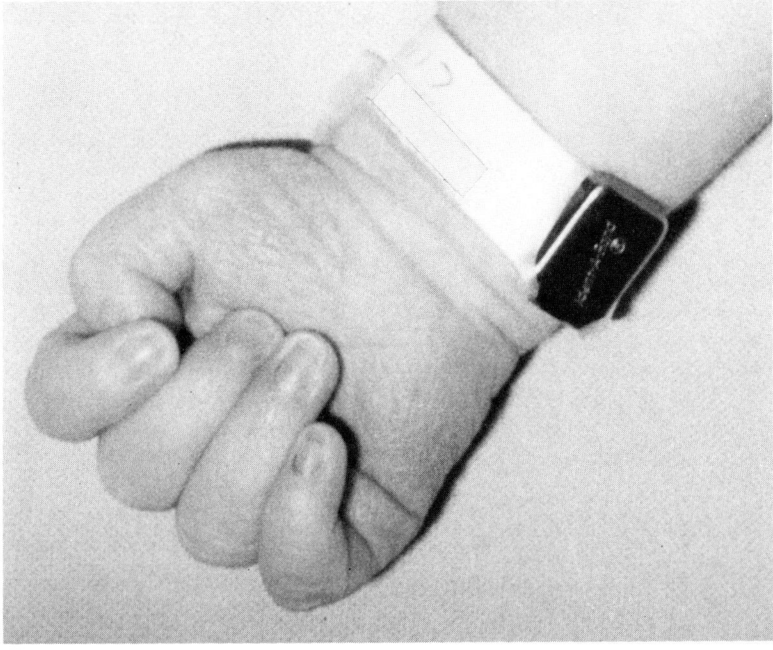

Fig. 17-3. The cortical thumb (fisting) in which the thumb is tightly enclosed within the clenched fingers. This is a common finding in the newborn, but should not be persistently present. The infant should open his hand periodically (see Figs. 17-1 and 17-2 of the same infant). *Persistent* symmetrical or asymmetrical fisting is abnormal at any age and is often the earliest sign of cortical spinal tract damage.

extensor reflexes are essential variations of similar pathways.

The spontaneous movements of the infant can give considerable information about the ability to move specific muscle groups. This information is of importance in localizing the level of a lesion of the spinal cord (see section on meningomyelocele, p. 556). Spontaneous movements can often be elicited in response to a painful stimulation with a pin.

Infants who are weak are usually hypotonic or floppy (see section on the floppy infant, p. 529).

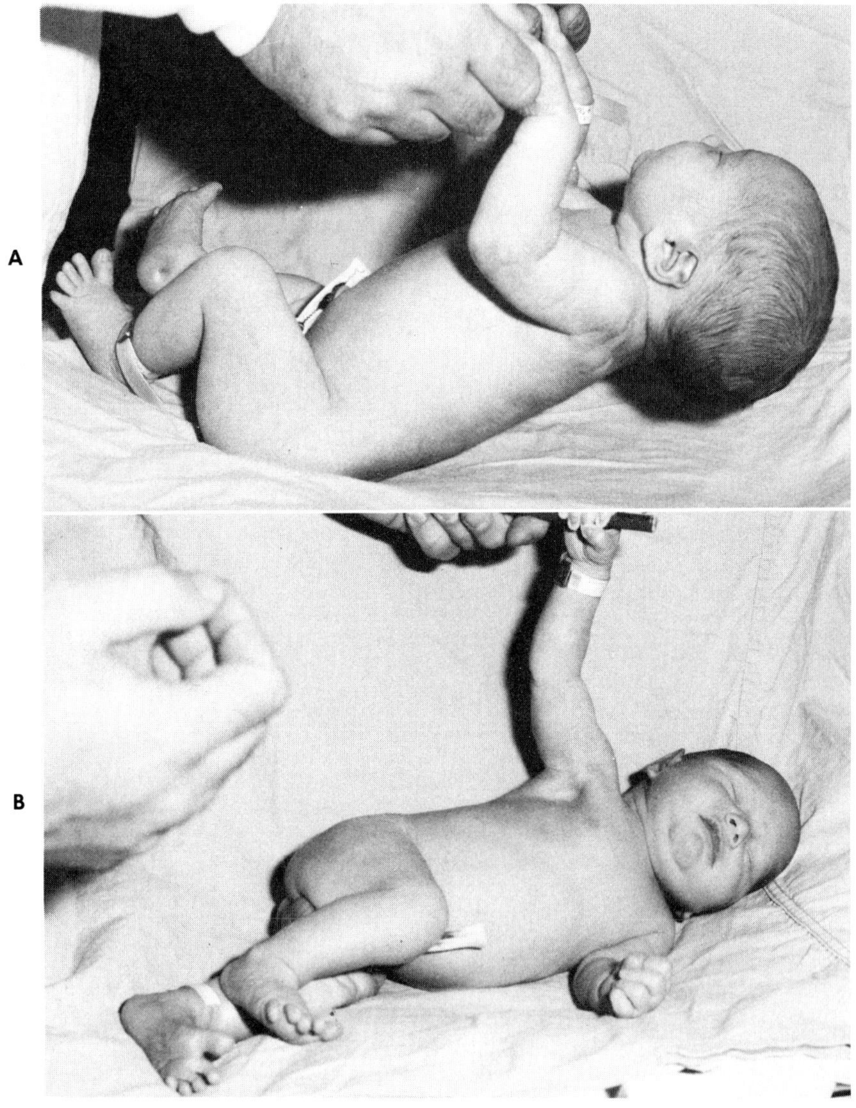

Fig. 17-4. A, Strength may be assessed by lifting the supine infant from the table. The observer's fingers are grasped by the infant; the strength of the grasp, contraction of the biceps, the shoulder girdle, and even the anterior neck muscles are seen and felt. Note this normal newborn's lack of head lag. **B,** An alternative method of testing strength in either arm is shown in this illustration. The infant is grasping a pencil. Note the tight grip and contraction of biceps as well as of the trapezius and pectorals. The infant can almost be lifted from the sheet.

Tone. The general tone of the baby can be assessed by ventral suspension (Fig. 17-5). While suspended with a hand under the abdomen, the baby should dorsiflex his back with some elevation of his head, although his feet and legs remain flexed. Hypotonia, weakness, or cerebral depression may produce a baby who looks like a limp dishrag. Upright suspension, with the baby supported by the examiner's hands under his arm (Fig. 17-6), provides good estimation of both tone and power in the shoulder girdle. An infant with decreased tone tends to slip through the examiner's hands. Tone can also be assessed by movement of individual joints (see section on hypotonia, p. 529).

Cranial nerves. Examination of the cranial nerves can be done with surprising facility, even in the newborn. Examination of vision, while not a necessary part of the screening examination, can be accomplished using opticokinetic nystagmus (p. 612). This may be performed using a large cloth tape, 6 to 8 inches across and 18 or more inches in length. On this white background are placed large, solid-colored stripes of red or black. The alternating white and colored stripes should be 2 to 3 inches in width. Movement of the tape in one direction in front of the baby's eyes should usually produce some following movement of the eyes and occasionally nystagmus back in the opposite direction. While the baby's state of alertness may cause a lack of response during a single examination, repetitive examinations should produce evidence of vision in most normal newborns. Indeed, with gradations of distance and size of stripe, visual acuity can be estimated. For screening examinations, however, the pupillary response gives evidence of intactness of the retina, optic nerve, and the third nerve.

Cranial nerves III, VI, and VIII may be assessed by holding the baby in an upright position and rotating him while he is held at arm's length. This rotation stimulates the semicircular canals, and the impulses travel through the eighth nerve up the brainstem via the medial longitudinal fasciculus and innervate the third and sixth nerve nuclei. This stimulation causes the eyes to tonically deviate in the direction of the rotation and produces nystagmus in the opposite direction when rotation is stopped. Rotation should be done in either direction.

The seventh nerve is observed through movement of the face and mouth while the infant is crying and while his eyes are

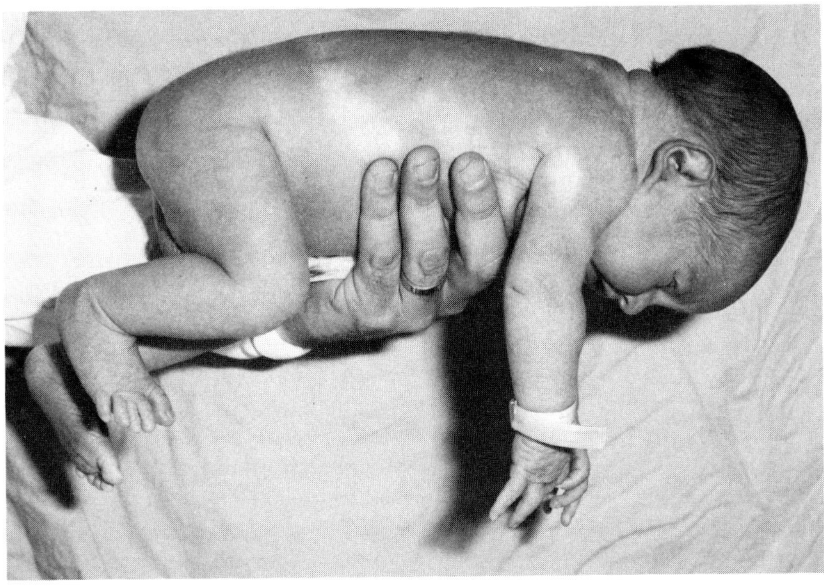

Fig. 17-5. Ventral suspension of the normal newborn infant. Note the flexion of the hip and knee, the slight dorsiflexion of the back, and the momentary ability to support the head. Contrast this with the hypotonic infant in Fig. 17-8.

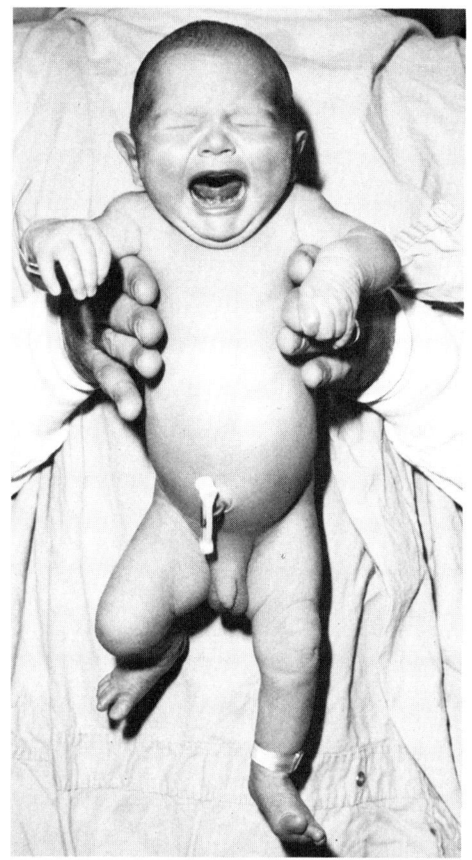

Fig. 17-6. The normal newborn infant in upright suspension. Most of the baby's weight is supported by the resistance of the infant's arms. There is no tendency to slide through the examiner's fingers. The examiner is not holding the child around the chest.

closed. The sucking response is stimulated by putting a finger in the infant's mouth; the afferent arc is the fifth nerve, and the motor efferent is motor 5, 7, and 12. Swallowing utilizes cranial nerves IX, X, and XII.

Additional aspects of the examination

In addition to these simple screening maneuvers, the neurologic examination should include: examination of the fontanelles with the infant in the upright position, for size and tenseness; examination of the cranial sutures for separation or overlap; and transillumination of the infant's head. (For the technique of transillumination, see the section on hydrocephalus, p. 539.)

Numerous reflexes have been described in the newborn. These include the tonic neck response, the magnet, Bauer, crossed extensor, placing, stepping, and many other reflexes. Most of these reflexes, while of interest, contribute little to knowledge of specific deficits within the CNS. We have, therefore, elected to omit them from routine neurologic examination.

Detailed examination. In certain situations when abnormalities are discovered during the neurologic examination, more detailed examination is necessary. Sensation should be tested accurately when one suspects a spinal cord or peripheral nerve lesion. Table 17-7 indicates the dermatomes associated with specific motor response to sensory stimuli. Fig. 17-7 shows the classic adult dermatome pattern extrapolated to infants. The examiner should be aware that nerve conduction time, both in the peripheral nerves and in the spinal cord, is greatly delayed in the newborn. When one pricks the infant with a pin, there may be a delay of as long as 2 to 3 seconds before the infant cries. The only evidence of sensation is crying or evidence on the face of awareness of the stimulus. Withdrawal of the extremity is a local reflex phenomenon and does not necessarily imply that the sensory stimulus has reached cortical awareness. The Galant (truncal incurvation) reflex is of little value as generally applied. However, truncal incurvation is segmentally innervated, and local stimulation of one area of the back may produce local trunk incurvation, indicating that that segmental arc is intact. This reflex may, therefore, be used to localize spinal cord injury.

Exogenous and endogenous factors affecting the neurologic examination. A word of caution should be given about where and when the examination is conducted. The CNS of the newborn is quite responsive to both exogenous and endogenous factors. For this reason, abnormal findings must be confirmed by repeated examinations. The timing of the examination in relationship to feeding may be of crucial importance. An infant examined in the postprandial state may be sleepy, with decreased responsiveness, and may be hypotonic as well as hyporeflexic. That same infant examined before feeding may be crying, irritable, hypertonic, and hyperreflexic,

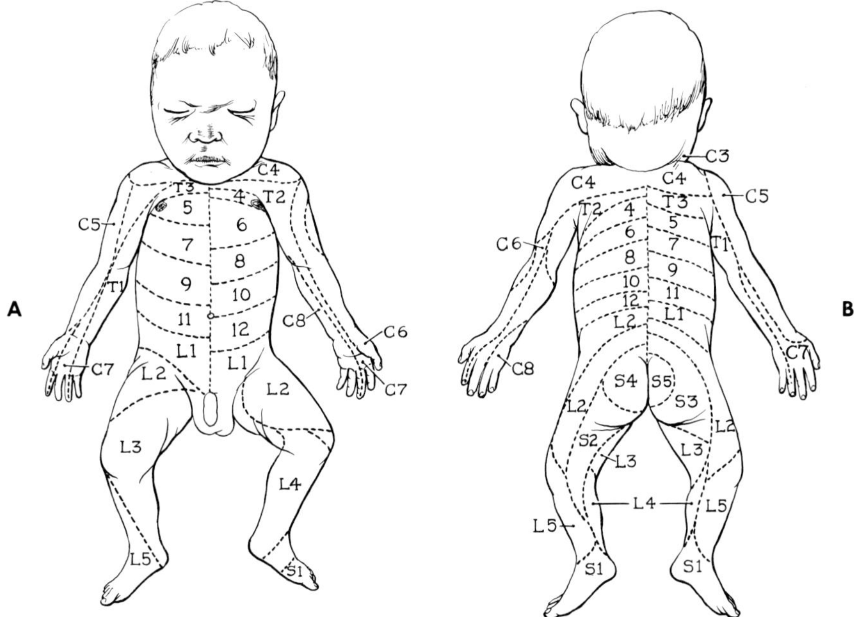

Fig. 17-7. Sensory dermatomes extrapolated from the adult to the infant. As noted on the two sides of the infant, there is considerable overlap of sensory innervation.

as well as jittery. The ambient temperature of the examining room and the temperature of the newborn may also affect the neurologic state. Hypothermia may cause depression; hyperthermia may result in irritability. The sleeping state of the infant will also alter reflexes and responsiveness. Thus one must not prognosticate on the basis of a single neurologic examination but must be willing to spend time on repeated occasions to confirm the presence of abnormalities under optimal conditions. The examiner should also be aware that the neurologic examination is age specific and may be utilized as an index of gestational age (see below). The nervous system is undergoing rapid changes in the months before and after birth, and reflexes are determined by this state of neurologic maturation.

Neurologic examination of the small infant

The neurologic status of the infant is dependent on gestational age. The difficulty of the neurologic examination is inversely related to the size of the infant. Examination of the small premature infant taxes the ingenuity of the examiner, who is forced to work within a box on a baby who may be receiving respiratory therapy and who may be wired to two or three different monitors, with several catheters in place. The examination is often, therefore, quite restricted, and an adequate opinion may not be possible. When an examination is feasible, it is important to recognize that it may be used as an estimate of gestational age. Table 17-2 gives evidence of neurologic maturation. The sick premature, like the sick full-term, may show abnormalities that are transient and of little permanent significance.

Interpretation of the neurologic examination

Definitive interpretation of the neurologic examination is fraught with hazards. Except in situations where there is definitive and unequivocal demonstrable damage, the prognosis must await confirmation over time. Hypertonicity may disappear; hypotonicity may improve. The infant with seizures may be normal during follow-up examination, and feeding problems and dysphagia may resolve.

Combinations of abnormalities, such as spasticity, hyperreflexia, and a difficult birth, are of more significance than a single

Table 17-2. Neurologic development related to gestational age

	Age in weeks 24	28	32	34	36	40
Traction	—	—	Flexion of arms		Always present	
Grasp	—	Finger grasp	Fully developed reflex	Stronger	Can be lifted off bed	
Posture	Froglike position					
	Limbs extended and rolls onto side	Limbs extended	Flexion of legs	Stronger flexion of legs	Flexion of all limbs	
Neck righting	—	—	—	Trunk follows	Rotation of head	
Tone						
Recoil	Hypotonic	Hypotonic	Slow recoil in legs	Good recoil in arms	Slow recoil in arms	Good recoil in arms
Head lag	—	Pendular head	Some attempt to flex head	Still lags, but less	Initial lag, then sudden flex	Good tone with head righting
Ventral suspension	Floppy	Floppy	Some flexion of legs	Increased flexion of legs and arms		Good flexion of legs and arms
Moro reflex	—	Complete, but easily exhausted	Complete	————→		
Pupil reaction	—	—	Present at 29 weeks	————→		
Glabella tap	—	—	Blink	————→		
Suck	Present but weak	—	Strong	Synchronized with swallowing ————→		
Head turning to light	—	—	Present			
Walking	—	Feeble	Slow on toes	Easier	Easier	Easy on heels

abnormality; but even signs seen in combination may disappear.

Asymmetries of signs are usually of more significance than symmetrical abnormalities, but even these may improve with time. Gestational age, drugs or medications, feeding, and so on may alter the neurologic state. Therefore, repeated examinations are necessary.

More detailed and sophisticated examination correlated with long-term follow-up care of infants may in the future allow better prognostication from the newborn examination than is now possible.

BIRTH TRAUMA

See also Chapter 3, p. 70.

The diagnosis of birth trauma is more often based on the condition of the child than on the demonstration of the trauma. Children who demonstrate mental or neurologic impairment without a history of neonatal trauma may, in fact, have had trauma during birth. Conversely, children who are the product of a difficult labor and delivery often show no subsequent neurologic impairment. Therefore, at the present time, we are often unable to assess the neurologic significance of trauma for the individual child and are unable to know its true incidence in the population.

Trauma to the nervous system during labor and delivery is primarily the result of compression-distortion injuries. Compression of the fetus during uterine contraction results in pressures on the fetal head of up to 200 mm Hg. Since the fetal head is compressible, this external pressure may lead to increased intracranial pressures and cerebral ischemia. Intrauterine pressure and its effects on the fetus are unfortunately still rarely monitored during labor, and therefore their role in producing cerebral damage is unknown.

Numerous factors may cause trauma to the fetal nervous system. Distortion of the fetal head during delivery (molding) is common; this distortion may cause tears of the veins bridging the dura, resulting in cortical subdural hemorrhages or in subarachnoid hemorrhage. Vertical molding may result in tears of the falx, the tentorium, or of the vein of Galen, producing posterior fossa subdural hemorrhage. Stretching of the neck with forceps or in breech deliveries may result in hemorrhage in the cervical cord or brainstem, and compression of the head may force the brain through the tentorium, leading to cerebellar lacerations. Rotation or extensions of the head and neck during delivery may lead to a laceration and spasm of the vertebral arteries, with subsequent brainstem damage. The role of these distortions and compressions on venous return, leading to anoxia, venous infarction, and hemorrhage, remains unknown.

In addition to intracranial trauma, trauma to the skull may result in fractures; trauma to the scalp may result in cephalhematomas; trauma to the spinal cord may result in paraplegia; and trauma to the brachial plexus may result in local paralysis.

Routine lumbar punctures demonstrate blood and xanthochromic fluid in 10% of normal infants, suggesting that trauma is common (Table 17-3). Indeed, it is not surprising that birth trauma occurs, but that its residua are so infrequent.

Subdural hemorrhage

Subdural hemorrhage over the cortical surface is seen more commonly in full-term infants than in prematures. It is the result of tears of the cortical bridging veins caused by molding of the skull. Premature infants have less well-developed superficial veins and are less likely to have molding; therefore, they are less likely to have subdural hemorrhages over the cortical surface.

Subdural hemorrhage over the cortical surface is occasionally found at autopsy of full-term infants. The thin clot is usually asymptomatic in the newborn and is usually spontaneously reabsorbed. Occasionally, subdural hemorrhages will form membranes and expand in size, appearing weeks or months later as cephalic enlargement, as failure to thrive, or occasionally as seizures. (The management of chronic subdural hemorrhage is discussed on p. 540.)

Subdural hemorrhage in the posterior fossa occurs in both full-term and premature infants and is usually lethal. It is secondary to marked molding with tears of the falx or tentorium.

Sublethal retrocerebellar hematomas can be suspected from changes in respiration, a high-pitched or hoarse cry, vomiting, hypotonia, and an absent Moro reflex. Rapid

Table 17-3. Spinal fluid findings in normal full-term newborns

	Day 1		Day 7	
	Range	Mean	Range	Mean
Red blood cells	0–620	23	0–48	3
Polymorphs	0–26	7	0–5	2
Lymphocytes	0–16	5	0–4	1
Protein	40–148	73	27–65	47
Sugar	38–64	48	48–62	55

From Naidoo, B. T. S.: S. Afr. Med. J. **42:** 933, 1968.

enlargement of the head occurs toward the end of the first week of life. Ventriculography demonstrates anterior and superior displacement of the fourth ventricle and a sharp cutoff of its caudal end, suggesting the diagnosis. Surgical drainage of the subdural hemorrhage may be lifesaving.

Cephalhematomas

See p. 73.

Fractures of the skull

See p. 75.

Spinal cord trauma

See also pp. 85-87.

Acute transection of the spinal cord may occur in difficult breech deliveries, with hyperflexion or extension of the body in relation to the after-coming head. Transection is most common at the C5 to C7 level. The infant appears profoundly hypotonic, with no spontaneous movements in the lower extremities. Some movement may be present in the arms and hands, depending on the exact level of the cervical cord lesion. Respirations may be abdominal, since the diaphragms are innervated from C2, C3, and C4. (See p. 86 for a discussion of the clinical manifestations.) Complete lesions above the C4 level are incompatible with life. The physician may establish a level of motor deficit by careful observations of the muscular involvement in the arms and hands. A similar sensory level may be documented by the infant's response to pain (Fig. 17-7). Spinal fluid is bloody and xanthochromic. Myelography, if performed, shows a swollen, edematous cord at the affected level. Direct observation of the cord at operation or after death reveals swelling, maceration, and hemorrhage. No therapy directed at the spinal cord is possible, but in the child who survives the neonatal period, attention must be directed toward care of the bladder and kidneys, as in children with meningomyeloceles. Physical therapy is useful in preventing contractures. Children with intact arm musculature may eventually be able to ambulate with a swing-through gait.

Complete spinal cord transection is a well-recognized entity, both clinically and pathologically, and is decreasing in frequency with improved obstetrical care. Attention is now being drawn to a less dramatic form of cervical cord and brainstem injury. This is an entity that is rarely recognized clinically.

Cervical cord and brainstem hemorrhage

Careful pathologic investigations of the brainstem and spinal cord of newborns reveal the presence of spinal injury in 10% to 33% of newborn deaths. Epidural hemorrhage is the most frequent manifestation. It is usually in the cervical area and may be seen in the premature as well as in the full-term infant. While usually not lethal of itself, the hemorrhage indicates a degree of spinal cord trauma that might result in spinal shock and impairment of respiration. Brainstem damage may result from stretch, with laceration of the cerebral peduncles, or from brainstem herniation and surface laceration of the cerebellum. There is some evidence of tears of branches of the vertebral arteries with intimal hemorrhage. These tears may result from rotations of the head and neck during delivery and lead to ischemic damage in the upper cord and brainstem. Such lesions were found in 25% of neonatal deaths. Although such lesions may be the result of traction on the body in breech deliveries or on the head in forceps deliveries, they may also be the result of fetal malposition or of compression as the infant is forced down an unrelaxed canal or against a rigid cervix.

Such cervical and brainstem lesions, if severe, may result in primary apnea or respiratory depression, with periods of apnea later complicated by the respiratory distress syndrome. Less severe involvement may result in survival with spasticity, speech defects, or strabismus. The vascular involvement may damage the cerebellum, resulting in the ataxic form of cerebral palsy. Vascular involvement of the brainstem reticular formation may later lead to the hyperactivity syndrome. Damage to the brainstem involves not only descending corticospinal tracts but also ascending tracts from the reticular activating system and thus may produce generalized cerebral depression. The floppiness seen is the sum of the depression and the corticospinal involvement. Close clinical and pathologic correlations are necessary to delineate this group of children with cervical and brainstem damage and their residual neurologic deficit.

Cerebral damage

Cerebral damage in newborns and prematures is usually attributed either to hypoxia or to hemorrhage. Recent evidence indicates that, particularly in prematures, hypoxia is usually the primary event, and the hemorrhage is secondary.

Premature infant—deep venous infarction and ventricular hemorrhage

Hypoxia may occur in utero secondary to placental dysfunction or hemorrhage or may occur during labor with placental compression or cord compression. Towbin postulates that sufficient hypoxia leads to intrauterine circulatory collapse. Venous congestion ensues, with secondary venous infarctions. Since in prematures, at 22 to 35 weeks of gestation, it is the deep veins that are most developed, the infarction involves periventricular structures. The infarction damages cerebral tissue and also vessel walls, leading to further hemorrhage. If the anoxia is minimal, it may lead to periventricular leukomalacia without hemorrhage. Sufficient hemorrhage may rupture into the ventricle, producing apnea and often leading rapidly to death. Consumption of clotting factors during the periventricular bleeding may contribute to further bleeding and to the ventricular hemorrhage. In many cases, the primary hypoxia has occurred prior to birth, and the perinatal apnea is the result rather than the cause of cerebral damage.

Events leading to periventricular and ventricular hemorrhage are less likely to occur in the full-term infant since the insult causing prematurity is rarely present, the deep venous pattern is better developed, and the periventricular germinal matrix does not require the vascular supply it did earlier in gestation.

Full-term infant—cortical venous infarction

As the infant nears term, cerebral development shifts from the deeper structures to the cortical layers. The importance of the deep veins decreases and that of the pial veins becomes more prominent. The pathogenesis of venous infarction in the full-term infant is similar to that of the premature with hypoxia, circulatory collapse, venous stasis, venous infarction, and hemorrhage, but the damage is more likely to be cortical. It is only one tenth as common as that in prematures.

Brachial plexus injuries

See p. 81.

THE FLOPPY NEONATE

The floppy newborn has often been compared to a rag doll or a limp rag (Fig. 17-8). This state is often caused by cerebral depression, hypoxia, or intracranial hemorrhage. However, there are a number of less common causes that are rarely diagnosed during the first months of life, although the condition existed since birth. If the same differential diagnosis used later in infancy were applied to the newborn, diagnosis could perhaps be made; and treatment, where indicated, could be begun.

Floppiness is caused by weakness or lack of tone and is often a combination of both. The distinction between hypotonia and weakness is important, however, because the physician's primary concern is with diseases that cause weakness. These are diseases associated with an anatomical or biochemical lesion within the motor system. They may be genetic, may require

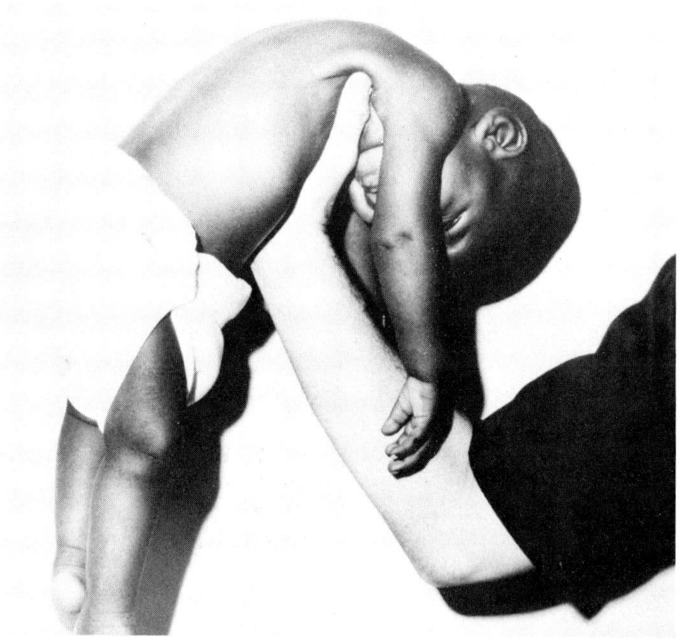

Fig. 17-8. A markedly floppy child in ventral suspension. Contrast this child with the infant shown in Fig. 17-5. This infant showed no flexion of the legs or back and no elevation of the head. The child has Werdnig-Hoffman disease.

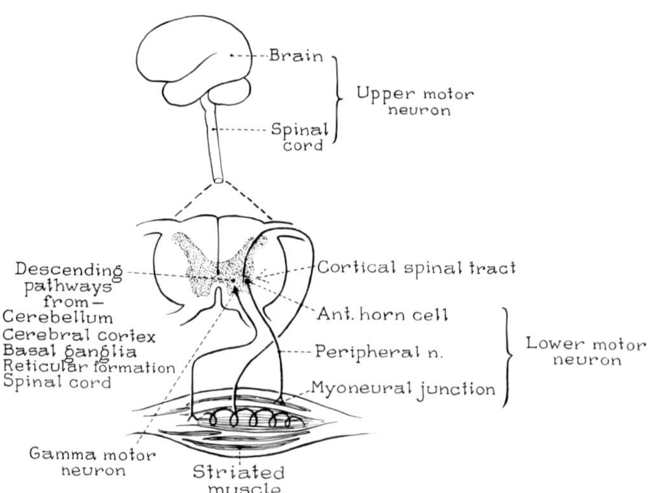

Fig. 17-9. Schematic illustration of the pathways involved in strength and in tone. The anatomical locations where strength or tone or both could be affected are shown. (See text for details.)

medical intervention, and may even be life threatening. Problems with tone alone, without weakness and without an anatomical lesion, are rarely a threat to the newborn; they often improve as the child grows older. Admittedly, even with careful examination, the distinction between weakness and hypotonia may not always be possible during the neonatal period. Fig. 17-9 illustrates the pathways involved in strength and tone and provides a framework for the classification seen in the following outlines.

CLASSIFICATION OF THE FLOPPY NEONATE WITH AN ANATOMICAL LESION

I. Weakness with depressed or absent reflexes
   A. Anterior horn cell
      1. Degeneration — Werdnig-Hoffman disease (spinal muscular atrophy)
      2. Infection
         a. Polio
         b. Coxsackievirus
   B. Peripheral nerve
      1. Peripheral neuropathies
II. Weakness with normal reflexes
   A. Neuromuscular junction
      1. Transient neonatal myasthenia gravis
      2. Congenital myasthenia gravis
   B. Muscle
      1. Myopathies—congenital
      2. Dystrophies
         a. Myotonic dystrophy
         b. Congenital myotonic dystrophy, Duchenne's disease
      3. Inflammatory—polymyositis
      4. Metabolic—glycogenosis
   C. Arthrogryposis multiplex congenita
III. Weakness with normal or exaggerated reflexes
   A. Spinal cord disease
      1. Traumatic
         a. Spinal cord laceration
         b. Epidural hemorrhage
         c. Vertical artery damage
   B. Cerebral damage
      1. Prematures—deep venous infarction
      2. Full-term infants—cortical venous infarction

CLASSIFICATION OF THE FLOPPY NEONATE WITHOUT AN ANATOMICAL LESION

I. Physiologic—prematurity
II. Generalized diseases
   A. CNS depression
      1. Sedation
      2. Acute infection
      3. Generalized illness
   B. Nutritional
      1. Rickets
      2. Scurvy
      3. Celiac disease
      4. Malnutrition
   C. Metabolic-endocrine
      1. Hypercalcemia
      2. Renal tubular acidosis
      3. Hypothyroidism
      4. Hypoadrenalism
      5. Aminoaciduria
   D. Connective tissue disease
      1. Congenital laxity of ligaments
      2. Ehlers-Danlos syndrome
      3. Osteogenesis imperfecta
      4. Marfan's syndrome
      5. Achondroplasia
      6. Mucopolysaccharidoses
III. Hypotonia with mental deficiencies
   A. Prader-Willi syndrome
   B. Down's syndrome (serotonin deficiency?)
   C. Other nonspecific mental deficiencies
IV. Benign congenital hypotonia

Clinical presentation

Weakness is defined as lack of strength or a diminution in the maximal force of muscle contraction. Strength is an active process and may be assessed by grip, by contraction of biceps and shoulder as the infant is pulled from a supine position, by the ability to support the infant under the arm, or by active withdrawal from stimuli (see section on neurologic examination, p. 517).

Weakness is the result of an anatomical or chemical defect within the motor system. The motor system is made up of four parts: the upper motoneuron (originates in neurons of the cerebral cortex and passes through the cortical spinal tracts to end on the anterior horn cell of the spinal cord) the lower motoneuron (originates in the anterior horn cell and passes through the peripheral nerve to terminate on the muscle end plate), the nerve terminal (includes muscle end plate), and the muscle (with the lower motoneuron and nerve terminal, it may be termed the motor unit). The deep tendon reflexes are helpful in locating the anatomical lesion. Lesions of the anterior horn cell or peripheral nerve usually cause hyporeflexia; infants with lesions of the neuromuscular junction or the muscle have normal or depressed reflexes; infants with lesions of the upper motoneuron have normal or increased reflexes.

Tone is the passive resistance of a muscle to stretch. It is assessed by observing the baby's resting posture, the posture of the infant when held in ventral suspension, the head lag, and the resistance of a limb to movement (see section on neurologic examination, p. 523). Tone is governed by a complex, poorly understood system. Within the muscle lie stretch receptors, the muscle spindles, which are arranged parallel to the muscle fibers. When muscle fibers are stretched, the simultaneous stretch on the muscle spindles fires receptors within the spindle. These receptors in turn cause the anterior horn cell of synergistic muscles to fire, thus contracting the stretched muscle. Contraction of the stretched muscle relaxes the spindle that is parallel to it.

The sensitivity of the muscle spindle to stretch is governed by the gamma efferent system, a separate group of neurons within the spinal cord. Descending pathways from the cortex, cerebellum, basal ganglia, and brainstem influence these neurons and thus the sensitivity of the spindle to stretch. However, since the activity of the muscle spindle on its synergistic muscle tone is affected through the anterior horn cells, peripheral nerve, and muscle in a fashion identical to strength, lesions along this pathway will produce both hypotonia and weakness.

Hypertonia is the result of lesions of the central nervous system above the level of the anterior horn cell, within the upper motoneuron. These upper motoneuron lesions will produce weakness by affecting the corticospinal tracts and will produce hypertonia by affecting the descending pathways to the gamma efferent system. Most often, infants with upper motoneuron lesions are hypotonic and gradually become hypertonic over the first 2 years of life.

Differential diagnosis of the floppy infant with weakness

The floppy, weak infant usually has an anatomical or biochemical lesion. The differential diagnosis is seen in the outline on p. 531 and is discussed below.

Weakness with depressed or absent reflexes

Anterior horn cell disease (Werdnig-Hoffman disease). Degeneration of the anterior horn cell is the most common definable cause of motor unit dysfunction. This degeneration is caused by an autosomal recessive disease termed Werdnig-Hoffman disease. The disease may begin in utero, in which case the mother notes progressive

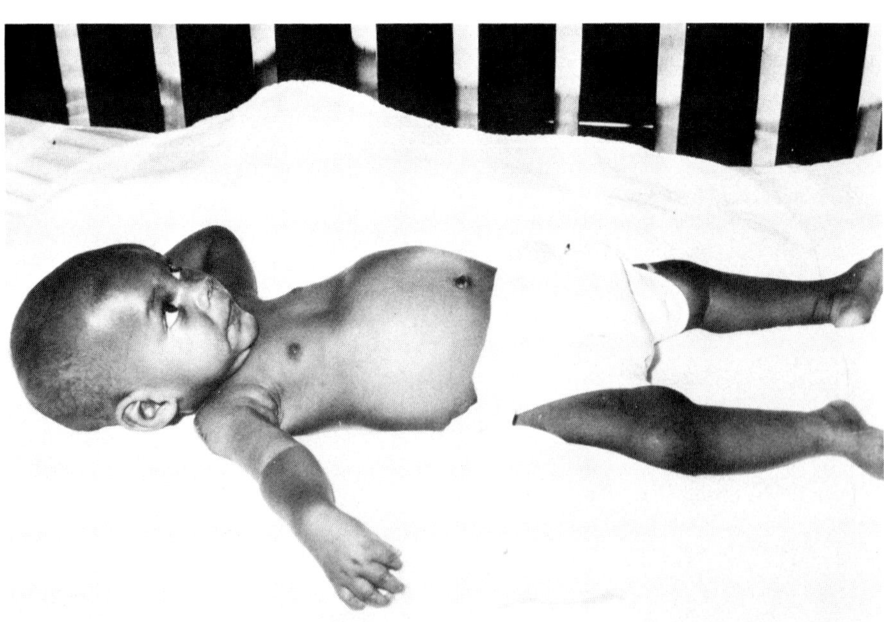

Fig. 17-10. The classic clinical picture of the infant with Werdnig-Hoffman disease, or marked hypotonia of many causes. The legs are externally rotated and slightly flexed at the knees (the frog-leg position). Note the abdominal breathing and retraction of the chest. There is minimal movement of the arms, as seen by their asymmetry. Note also the alertness of the infant.

decrease in the strength of fetal movements, or it may begin during the first year of life. The disease is usually lethal by the first year of age, but with later onset it may run a more slowly progressive course.

Clinical presentation. The classic clinical picture is that of a floppy infant who lies in a frog-leg position, with diminished spontaneous movement (Fig. 17-10). Weakness is often more proximal than distal, with relative preservation of movements in the hands and feet. Breathing is abdominal, with little or no movement of the chest. There is head lag, but facial movement is spared. Fasciculations (wormy movements) of the edges of the tongue are strongly suggestive of Werdnig-Hoffman disease. A crying infant may have movements of the tongue, but with the infant quiet, no movement of the normal tongue should be seen. Reflexes in these children are depressed or absent.

Despite their profound weakness, as these infants grow older they appear alert and interested in their environment. While motor development may be nonexistent, the observer is impressed that these children appear to have normal intelligence.

Diagnosis. The diagnosis may be suggested by the history of a similarly affected sibling, but confirmation requires evidence of denervation on electromyogram (EMG) (Table 17-4) and a muscle biopsy showing atrophy of motor units. Because of the prognostic implications for the infant and the genetic implications for the family, work-up should also document the absence of a peripheral neuropathy and the absence of a myopathy. No methods of prenatal detection are currently available.

Treatment. Therapy is supportive, with attention given to feeding techniques, to prevent aspiration and to the treatment of pneumonia, the usual cause of death. Genetic counseling of the family is important.

Other causes of anterior horn cell disease. Rare cases of intrauterine and neonatal poliomyelitis and poliolike illness have been reported. A lack of symmetry and lack of progression may serve to differentiate them from Werdnig-Hoffman disease.

Peripheral neuropathies. Peripheral neuropathies are rarely diagnosed in the neonatal period. They are important because they may be treatable and must be differentiated from anterior horn cell disease. Rare forms of congenital sensory and motor neuropathies inherited as autosomal recessive disorders have been described.

Clinical presentation. The clinical picture is similar to Werdnig-Hoffman disease, with hypotonia and weakness, decreased spontaneous movements, and areflexia. Abdominal breathing may be present. Important differential points are the absence of fasciculations in the tongue, the occurrence of facial paresis, and the relative preservation of strength in the neck

TABLE 17-4. Clinical and laboratory findings in the floppy infant

	Reflexes	EMG	Nerve conduction	Spinal fluid protein	Muscle enzyme	Muscle biopsy	Neostigmine
Anterior horn cell	Depressed	Denervation	Normal	Normal	Normal	Group atrophy	Negative
Peripheral neuropathy	Absent	Denervation	Prolonged	Increased	Normal	Group atrophy	Negative
Neuromuscular junction	Normal	Myasthenia	Normal	Normal	Normal	Normal	Positive
Muscle	Usually normal	Myopathic	Normal	Normal	Normal or increased	Specific changes	Negative
Spinal cord	Normal or increased	Normal	Normal	May be elevated	Normal	Normal	Negative
Cortex and brainstem	Normal or increased	Normal	Normal	Normal	Normal	Normal	Negative
Benign congenital hypotonic	Normal	Normal	Normal	Normal	Normal	Normal	Normal

muscles. A peripheral neuropathy involving neck musculature usually involves diaphragmatic innervation as well as intercostal innervation, and thus is lethal.

Diagnosis. The findings of elevation of spinal fluid protein, prolonged nerve conduction times, normal muscle enzymes, and *group atrophy* on muscle biopsy are the bases for the diagnosis.

Treatment. Neuropathies in infants tend to be chronic and may be nonprogressive. They may, on occasion, respond to steroid therapy.

Weakness with normal reflexes

Disease of the neuromuscular junction (myasthenia gravis). Myasthenia gravis is a disease of the neuromuscular junction. While the pathogenesis of the disease is still unknown, it appears that inadequate amounts of the neurotransmitter acetylcholine reach the muscle receptor. Therefore, with a repeated nerve stimulus (or a voluntary contraction), the muscle is inadequately stimulated, and its contractions become increasingly weak.

Two forms of myasthenia are seen in the newborn: *Transient neonatal myasthenia gravis* is seen in 12% of infants whose mothers have myasthenia gravis. However, maternal myasthenia may not be clinically evident at the time of the child's birth. This neonatal disease is presumably caused by a circulating factor transplacentally transmitted to the infant. The weakness lasts an average of 24 days (up to 47 days). After this period, the infants are healthy and without evidence of myasthenia. Subsequent infants may also be affected. *Congenital myasthenia gravis* occurs in infants of normal mothers, is rare, and is of unknown cause. The myasthenia, in these cases, is lifelong, although the severity may wax and wane.

Clinical presentation. The initial features of both forms of myasthenia are identical, but the severity of myasthenia may vary with the individual. The onset of the weakness may be delayed until the second or third day of life, and in congenital myasthenia is often not diagnosed for several months. Symptoms include a weak suck, swallowing difficulties, respiratory difficulties, hypotonia, weakness, and a feeble cry. Facial weakness, decreased blinking, ptosis, and a slack, open mouth may be seen. Abnormalities of ocular movements are uncommon.

Diagnosis. The physician must maintain a high level of suspicion since the clinical appearance of these infants is similar to that of infants with intracranial problems or myotonic dystrophy. Diagnosis may be made by the response to the intramuscular injection of neostigmine methylsulfate, 0.05 to 0.5 mg, with atropine, 0.065 mg. Within 10 minutes, a measurable increase in strength and in the ability to suck should be evident. Documentation of the infant's state before and after administration of neostigmine should be made. Edrophonium (Tensilon), 0.5 to 1 mg, may also be used, but the brevity of its action makes evaluation of the neonate difficult.

Treatment. Infants responding to intramuscularly administered neostigmine should be maintained on oral administration of neostigmine, 1 mg given 20 to 30 minutes prior to feeding. The dosage must be individually titrated. Periodic attempts to decrease the medication, with observation of its effect on function, should determine the necessary duration of therapy. Supportive methods include gavage feeding and suction. Occasionally, intubation may be necessary to preserve life.

Diseases of muscle. Myopathy is the generic term for diseases affecting the muscle. Some of the myopathies that are familial have been termed dystrophies. While inherited disorders of muscle are, by definition, present at birth, most do not become clinically significant during the neonatal period.

Congenital myopathies. In recent years new histopathologic and electron microscopic techniques have permitted the definition of a small number of congenital, inherited disorders of muscle. These disorders are known by the descriptive names of central core disease, nemaline myopathy, myotubular myopathy, and megaconial (large mitochondria revealed by electron microscopy) and pleoconial (variable-sized mitochondria) myopathy. Doubtless, others will be described.

Clinical presentation. Infants with these disorders have a variable degree of hypotonia, with minimal weakness. The weakness is nonprogressive or slowly progressive, and many of the diseases are compatible with survival into adult life with minimal disability. On rare occasions, a more severe form, lethal in infancy, has been described. Reflexes may be normal or depressed.

Diagnosis. Muscle enzymes are normal, and electrical studies of the muscle may be normal. Muscle biopsy with appropriate histochemical and electron microscopic studies is required to make the diagnosis. Biopsy is, however, rarely indicated in these infants during the neonatal period.

Dystrophies. *Myotonic dystrophy* is inherited as a dominant characteristic. It is classically seen in adolescence and adult life and is associated with mild to moderate weakness, mild mental retardation, baldness, testicular atrophy, and the slow relaxation of muscular contraction. Retrospective studies have indicated that the disease may be present in the newborn, with hypotonia and weakness, facial diplegia, and difficulties with feeding and swallowing. The manifestations may be similar to myasthenia gravis, but the infant does not respond to neostigmine. Diagnosis may be suggested by a family history of myotonic dystrophy. Percussion of the muscles, particularly the deltoid or biceps, may lead to a local contraction at the site of percussion and slow relaxation of that contraction (percussion myotonia). Electrical studies of muscle tone in the newborn may not manifest the myotonic picture seen in later life. Muscle enzymes and muscle biopsy are normal. Therapy is limited to supportive care, nasogastric feedings, and suction of secretions. Feeding difficulties appear to resolve spontaneously over the early weeks of life. Slowly progressive weakness becomes manifested during adolescence and early adult life. Mild degrees of mental retardation are also common.

Duchenne's muscular dystrophy is a sex-linked recessive disorder that does not usually become clinically evident in the first year of life. Affected siblings of patients with Duchenne's disease may have elevated muscle enzymes, particularly creatine phosphokinase (CPK). Rare forms of congenital muscular dystrophies have been reported. They may be progressive or static at the time of birth.

Inflammatory diseases of muscle. Polymyositis, or inflammatory disease of muscle tissue, is well recognized in older children and adults, although it is rarely recognized in infancy. In some adults, evidence of viral disease has been found; in children, a vasculitis is usual. The common denominator in these inflammatory conditions is weakness and an inflammatory change revealed by muscle biopsy in the absence of a family history. Similar inflammatory changes may, however, be seen in rapidly progressive dystrophies. Polymyositis in children is usually, if not always, part of a generalized vasculitis that may be revealed by muscle biopsy.

The infant with weakness and hypotonia could have an inflammatory disease of muscle. Characteristically, facial movement and respiration are not affected. The finding of elevated muscle enzymes and muscle biopsy may confirm the diagnosis and differentiate these infants from those with polyneuropathies and Werdnig-Hoffman disease. Children with polymyositis may respond dramatically to steroids.

Metabolic disease of muscle. Myopathies may be associated with metabolic or endocrine disease. Glycogen storage disease (Pompe's glycogen storage disease, type II) may be associated with glycogen deposits in the muscle and heart, profound hypotonia, and weakness (p. 425). The tongue is enlarged, but without fasciculations. The brain may also have desposits of glycogen, with resulting progressive mental retardation. Differentiation from Werdnig-Hoffman disease is made by the cardiac involvement, by the appearance of the tongue, and by muscle biopsy, with appropriate histochemical stains and biochemistry.

Myopathies may also be seen in hypothyroidism, hypoadrenalism, hyercalcemia, and renal tubular acidosis, as well as in disorders of potassium metabolism. These disorders rarely produce myopathies in the neonate, however. Enzyme studies and biopsies are usually normal, and no anatomical lesion is demonstrable.

Arthrogryposis multiplex congenita. Arthrogryposis is a condition characterized by fixed deformity of one or more joints. Club foot may thus be one of its milder manifestations. The joint fixation is secondary to lack of movement of the joint for periods of time in utero. This lack of movement may be secondary to fetal malposition or, when multiple joints are involved, secondary to intrauterine paralysis. This paralysis may be caused by anterior horn cell disease, peripheral neuropathy, or myopathies. In most cases of arthrogryposis, the underlying process has completed its course prior to birth.

Weakness with normal or increased reflexes

Upper motoneuron disease. Lesions of the corticospinal tract from the cortex to the anterior horn cell may produce a floppy infant with weakness and hypotonia. Reflexes are usually normal or increased. Over the first 2 years of life, the hypotonia gradually becomes hypertonia or athetosis.

Evaluation of the infant with weakness and hypotonia but increased reflexes should be directed toward localization of the lesion. Description of these entities is discussed in the section on trauma, pp. 85 and 528.

Spinal cord damage should produce discrete motor and sensory levels detectable on neurologic examination.

Cervical and brainstem hemorrhage and trauma may show involvement of lower cranial nerves. Localization at this level is more difficult than in the lower spinal cord because of the cerebral depression that may accompany the lesion.

Periventricular hemorrhage often appears as a depressed infant or acute collapse in the first 24 hours of life, related to intraventricular hemorrhage.

The floppy child without an anatomical lesion

Causes of pure hypotonia without weakness are shown in the outline on p. 531.

Physiologic characteristics

Tone develops with age, and premature fants are hypotonic when compared with full-term infants. Table 17-2 can be used to assess the age-specific degree of hypotonia.

Generalized diseases

Hypotonia may be seen with generalized cerebral depression from sedation given to the infant or mother. Cerebral depression may also be seen as part of acute systemic infections, unrelated to infection of the CNS, and as part of generalized illness of varied types. Therefore, no definitive statement about tone or development should be made in a sick infant with cerebral depression. The examiner must wait to confirm suspicions when the child is well.

Nutritional diseases such as rickets, scurvy, celiac disease, and malnutrition are accompanied by hypotonia. The mechanism of the hypotonia is unclear, but tone will return to normal with treatment of the underlying disease.

Metabolic and endocrine diseases may be accompanied by hypotonia and weakness, without an anatomical lesion. Hypothyroidism and hypoadrenalism, if prolonged, may produce myopathic changes on biopsy.

Connective tissue disease will alter the resistance of muscle to passive movement, thereby producing a pseudohypotonia. The most striking instance is achondroplasia, where profound hypotonia produces a pronounced pseudoretardation of motor development.

Hypotonia with mental deficiency

Hypotonia without weakness is an aspect of the Prader-Willi syndrome of obesity–hypogonadism–mental retardation as well as of Down's syndrome In Down's syndrome, the hypotonia has been ascribed to the low levels of serotonin and allegedly responds to the administration of serotonin precursors. Hypotonia may also be seen as a part of nonspecific mental deficiency; the cause is unknown but may be related to cerebral anoxia or hemorrhage.

Benign congenital hypotonia

Benign congenital hypotonia is a syndrome that is diagnosed by exclusion. Reexamination of infants carrying this diagnosis has uncovered cases of polymyositis, peripheral neuropathies, and myopathies. However, within the group of floppy infants, there are a number of children who have hypotonia and normal or depressed reflexes. Their motor development is delayed, and they eventually become functional if still somewhat hypotonic and clumsy adults. There may be a family history of double-jointedness and of delay in motor development.

Evaluation should rule out the diseases indicated in this chapter. Thus, by exclusion, the diagnosis may be strongly suspected, but improvement with time is required to confirm the diagnosis.

Summary

An orderly approach to the cause of weakness and hypotonia in infants requires consideration of anatomical lesions that could produce weakness (Table 17-4). Clinical examination supplemented by laboratory studies should permit localization of the anatomical lesion and establish the cause. Earlier consideration of the differential diagnosis may permit diagnosis in the neonatal period and therapy of entities such as myasthenia or subdural hemorrhage, which may be life threatening. Diagnosis of entities such as subarachnoid or periventricular hemorrhage may allow the development of therapeutic approaches.

THE ENLARGING HEAD

Hydrocephalus is the most common cause of a excess rate of head growth in the neonatal period, but it must be differentiated from subdural effusions and hematomas, porencephalic cysts, and megalencephaly (enlargement of the brain) and from the normal rate of growth of premature and full-term infants (C17-11). Hydrocephalus is not of itself a disease, but is the end result of a number of disease processes that produce an accumulation of cerebrospinal fluid (CSF).

Pathophysiology

CSF is produced by the choroid plexus, as well as from the brain substance, at a relatively constant rate of 0.37 ml/min (0.26 to 0.65 ml/min). CSF produced in the lateral ventricles flows through the foramen of Monro, the third ventricle, down the aqueduct to the fourth ventricle, and exits through the formina of Luschka and Magendie. The fluid then flows along the base, up the sylvian fissures, and over the surface of the hemispheres to be absorbed through valves along the sagittal sinus by bulk flow. The amount of spinal fluid made within the cerebral cortical substance and transported across the ependyma to the ventricles or absorbed by this route is still a matter of investigation. Studies using infusions of artificial CSF have indicated that there are variable pressures at which bulk absorption begins to occur. In most individuals the pressure required is around 60 mm of water; in others, the pressure may have to reach 180 mm before bulk absorption occurs. The ability of the newborn's head to expand without reaching these higher pressures may account for some forms of hydrocephalus; the arrest of hydrocephalus may occur in some infants when the sutures close firmly enough to achieve that pressure.

In addition to the increased pressures, the undamped pulsations of the choroid plexus are felt to play an important role in the dilatation of the ventricles. As the ventricles dilate, they compress the cortex, which in turn expands cranial volume. Thus the head size is only a secondary reflection of ventricular size and cortical mantle thickness. Thinning of the cortex is primarily caused by loss of white matter and lipids, with little neuronal loss until extreme thinning (less than 0.5 cm) takes place. When moderate hydrocephalus is treated, the cortex can rapidly reconstitute its normal thickness, and there may be no neurologic deficit or intellectual deficit. Only when the cortical mantle is less than 0.5 cm in thickness is it correlated with poor intellectual outcome.

Etiology

Hydrocephalus was formerly classified as obstructive or communicating. However, with the exception of hydrocephalus secondary to cortical atrophy (hydrocephalus ex vacuo) and the rare hydrocephalus secondary to overproduction of CSF by a choroid plexus papilloma, all hydrocephalus is caused by an obstruction. The obstruction may lie within the ventricular system, as in aqueductal stenosis, the Dandy-Walker syndrome, or in tumors; or it may lie outside the ventricular system, as with arachnoidal adhesions. Obstruction outside the ventricular system was formerly called communicating hydrocephalus because dye placed in the ventricle appeared in the lumbar subarachnoid space.

Overproduction—choroid plexus papillomas

Overproduction of CSF, although rare, is of major importance since it is associated with papillomas of the choroid plexus, the only curable cause of hydrocephalus. Infants with choroid plexus papillomas have a communicating hydrocephalus without focal neurologic signs. Findings of elevation of spinal fluid protein or of xanthochromia of the CSF are common and should suggest the diagnosis. Xanthochromia is caused by leakage of blood from the tumor. These tumors give an abnormal brain scan and may show a tumor stain on arteriograms. An intraventricular mass revealed by air study is pathognomonic. The tumor often produces asymmetrical enlargement of the lateral ventricles. Complete removal of the tumor will decrease the overproduction of CSF and cure the hydrocephalus.

Obstruction to CSF flow

Congenital malformations

Aqueductal stenosis. The aqueduct is a common location for obstruction producing hydrocephalus in the neonatal period. Normally, a single channel, in congenital aqueductal stenosis the aqueduct, is often found to be broken into many small channels with varying degrees of occlusion but without evidence of inflammation. Previously, aqueductal stenosis was considered a developmental abnormality, but Johnson has recently produced identical lesions in rodents by neonatal infection with mumps, influenza, and parainfluenza viruses. No pathologic evidence of the preceding infection could be demonstrated at the time the animals developed hydrocephalus. Thus "congenital" aqueductal stenosis may in some cases be caused by unrecognized viral disease.

The Dandy-Walker syndrome. The Dandy-Walker syndrome, congenital atresia of the foramina of Luschka and Magendie, produces a clinically recognizable form of hydrocephalus. The large cystic fourth ventricle produces a prominent occipital shelf, occipital transillumination, and elevation of tentorium and venous sinuses. The marked enlargement of the fourth ventricle causes either malformation or atrophy of the cerebellar vermis, leaving only residual nubbins of cerebellar hemispheres. Despite the marked atrophy of the cerebellar vermis, infants with this syndrome are not ataxic in later life.

The Arnold-Chiari malformation. The Arnold-Chiari malformation occurs in varying degrees. In its most severe and classic form, it is characterized by downward displacement of the cerebellar tonsils through the foramen magnum; downward displacement, elongation, and folding of the medulla oblongata and fourth ventricle on the cervical cord; and downward displacement of the cervical cord. It is most commonly seen in patients with spinal dysraphia, such as meningomyeloceles. Aqueductal stenosis and micropolygyria are often associated with the Arnold-Chiari malformation. While the cause of this malformation is unclear, it is not caused by traction by the fixed spinal cord, as was once proposed. The Arnold-Chiari malformation is usually asymptomatic in early life but may on occasion be related to lower cranial nerve palsies or vocal cord paralysis in the neonatal period, with ensuing respiratory tract obstruction. Symptoms may be precipitated by removal of the meningomyelocele sac, leading to impaction of the medulla and tonsils in the foramen magnum. This impaction may be prevented by ventricular drainage during and after the operation on the back of those children with meningomyeloceles.

Vein of Galen malformations. Vein of Galen malformations are another rare cause of hydrocephalus. The markedly dilated vein of Galen compresses the aqueduct, producing the picture of aqueductal stenosis. This large malformation may produce heart failure in the early days or weeks of life and produces a loud bruit that may be heard over the vertex of the skull. Arteriography delineates the malformation. Treatment usually consists of shunting rather than a direct attack on the malformation.

Inflammatory and post-inflammatory processes. Fibrosis and adhesions at the base or along the cisternal pathways will produce obstructive hydrocephalus. Adhesions may result from hemorrhage in the premature or full-term infant or may be the result of neonatal meningitis, recognized or unrecognized.

Pathology

The pathology of hydrocephalus is the progressive thinning of cortical white matter, with reduction of oligodendroglial cells and astrocytes. The neurons and axons seem quite resistant to the effects of pressure. The hydrocephalus causes greater thinning of the vertex and occipital cortex, since the basal ganglia tend to buttress the lower part of the ventricular wall. Because of the thinning at the vertex (leg area) and because fibers from the leg area undergo the greatest stretch in circumventing the dilated ventricles, patients with hydrocephalus tend to develop a paraparesis with the preservation of the arms. The compressed cerebrum shows a loss of lipids and protein from white matter, with an increase in water content. The lipid and protein loss can presumably be reconstituted with relief of the hydrocephalus. Since the neurons and axons remain intact, there may be no residual deficit.

Clinical manifestations

There are few clinical manifestations of hydrocephalus as such in the neonatal period, other than enlargement of the head. Since the head can easily enlarge, intracranial pressure is dissipated, and the signs and symptoms of increased intracranial pressure are rarely seen. Vomiting and lethargy are uncommon, and papilledema is rarely if ever seen. Neurologic disability and seizures, if present, are usually the result of the underlying disease process rather than of the hydrocephalus.

As the head enlarges, the fontanelle is tense when felt with the infant in the upright position. There is prominence of the frontal bones (in contrast to the parietal bossing classically seen in subdural hematomas), and the scalp veins become prominent. The setting sun sign, the appearance of sclera above the pupil, is a moderately late sign probably caused by pressure in the region of the superior colliculi. The posterior shelf of the Dandy-Walker malformation has been described above. The most significant clinical manifestation of hydrocephalus is enlargement of the head. Serial head measurements are the only clinical method of diagnosing progressive hydrocephalus and are far more significant than a single measurement.

Diagnosis

The most important element in the diagnosis of hydrocephalus is suspicion. Early detection can come only from serial head circumference measurements made with a metal tape. The greatest head circumference obtained should be recorded on a standard head growth chart. Measurements should be made in centimeters; although growth from 13¾ inches to 14¼ inches does not seem great, growth from 34.9 cm to 36.2 cm is more likely to alert the physician. Head circumference measurements should be a recorded part of every baby visit in the first months of life. The diagnosis of hydrocephalus is suggested when the rate of head growth is greater than the norm (that is, when the rate is crossing percentiles). The absolute head circumference is of less significance than the rate of growth. It is just as significant if the head grows from the third percentile to the fiftieth percentile as if the growth is from the seventy-fifth to greater than the ninety-fifth percentile.

A complete history and physical examination are obviously important in the initial work-up of an infant with a large head. However, unless the head circumference exceeds the ninety-seventh percentile or unless the rate of head growth is currently greater than the norm, more definitive evaluations need not be undertaken, but the infant's course should be followed.

Transillumination should also be a part of the initial outpatient evaluation of a large head. Transillumination must be done in a totally dark room, with a flashlight with a light-tight seal on the end. Sufficient time must be spent in the room to allow adequate adaptation to the dark. A rough guide to adequate adaptation is the ability to make out the baby in the dark. The whole head, including the occiput, should be transilluminated. Transillumination giving a ring greater than 1 cm around the seal (1.5 cm in the frontal area and in prematures) is considered abnormal. Abnormal transillumination is seen in chronic subdural hematomas, edema of the scalp, cortical atrophy, porencephaly, hydranencephaly, and hydrocephalus if the cortical mantle is less than 1.0 cm in thickness.

Echoencephalography offers a screening method for the evaluation of ventricular size and cortical mantle thickness. It is inexpensive and of no risk to the patient. When performed by an experienced technician, the echo can give a gross index of hydrocephalus at an early stage. Since the ventricular dilatation may be greater than suggested by the abnormalities of head circumference, echoencephalography may be an important addition to the early diagnosis of suspected hydrocephalus.

Definitive work-up includes skull films, often arteriograms, and pneumoencephalograms (PEG) or ventriculograms. Skull films may indicate the cause by calcification, elevation of the sinus, or skull shape. Arteriograms are often useful in ruling out subdural hematomas that may have been missed on subdural taps. Subdural taps should be performed in every infant with an enlarging head prior to a PEG or a ventriculogram, since the subdural hematoma, if under pressure, may cause herniation during these procedures. Air studies should be performed on every infant with hydrocephalus prior to shunting in order to find the cause of obstruction and to rule out a choroid plexus papilloma. Adequate amounts of air should be used to define the pathologic condition. We prefer to see air studies done via the lumbar route, except in patients with meningomyeloceles. Pneumoencephalography allows better definition of the posterior fossa and aqueduct and basal cisterns and may save a needle tract through the brain. Where aqueductal obstruction is demonstrated, air should be instilled into the ventricles (ventriculography) to define the problem completely.

Cisternography is a new technique for the evaluation of hydrocephalus. Radioactive material, such as technetium, is injected by a lumbar puncture, and serial brain scans follow the flow of CSF up the cord, through the basal cisterns, and over the surface of the hemispheres to its absorption at the sagittal sinus. Radioactive material enters the ventricles only if they are dilated and the aqueduct is patent. While offering a method of following the course of infants with hydrocephalus without the hazards of air studies, the usefulness of this technique in the initial work-up of hydrocephalus remains to be demonstrated.

Differential diagnosis

The differential diagnosis of the enlarging head in the neonate rests between hydrocephalus or a multitude of other less common causes (Table 17-5).

Subdural hematomas (p. 527) may be secondary to neonatal or postnatal trauma and are more common with bleeding disorders. The initial manifestations of subdural hematomas may be subtle, such as enlargement of the head with no other symptoms, or may include symptoms of increased intracranial pressure or failure to thrive. A box-like head configuration with biparietal bossing may suggest clinically that the enlargement is caused by subdural hematomas rather than hydrocephalus. Transillumination is usually abnormal in chronic subdural hematomas but may be absent during the acute phase. The diagnosis is made by subdural taps or arteriography prior to an air study for the diagnosis of hydrocephalus. The subdural space should contain less than 1 ml of clear fluid. The fluid of a subdural hematoma contains elevated protein (40 mg greater than that of the CSF), which may be xanthochromic. It

TABLE 17-5. Differential diagnosis of the enlarging head in the neonatal period

Hydrocephalus	Differentiate from
	Subdural hematomas
Overproduction	Hydranencephaly
Choroid plexus papilloma	Porencephaly
Obstruction	Megalencephaly
Aqueductal stenosis or occlusion	Familial
Congenital	Canavan's disease
Viral	Alexander's disease
Vein of Galen	Normal growth of premature and full-term infant
Familial	Growth after feeding malnourished infant
Dandy-Walker syndrome	Subgaleal hematomas
Arnold-Chiari syndrome (meningomyelocele)	Achondroplasia
Obstruction at base or absorption	Normal head in dwarf body

should be differentiated from normal subarachnoid fluid found in a porenchephalic cavity or associated with underlying cortical atrophy. The treatment of subdural hematomas is a matter of debate, but in the absence of neurologic findings or symptoms or in the absence of increasing head size there is little rationale for treatment.

Hydranencephaly is a congenital absence of the brain, but with normal coverings of dura, skull, and scalp, thus differentiating it from anencephaly. It is probably caused either by bilateral carotid occlusion in utero, with resorption of the cerebral hemispheres, or by intrauterine hydrocephalus. Hydranencephalic infants often appear normal at birth and demonstrate few neurologic abnormalities other than lack of development. A large head is a common initial manifestation. Transillumination of marked degree serves to identify these infants on initial screening, but the entity still must be differentiated from large subdural hematomas or severe hydrocephalus. Arteriograms and air studies should make the definitive diagnosis. Shunting only serves to make these infants less of a nursing problem.

Porencephaly is a cavitation of the brain that usually communicates with either the ventricle or the subarachnoid space. The cavitation is commonly the result of prenatal vascular occlusion with resorption of the dead tissue. Developmental arrests at the site of fissures (schizencephaly) produce similar clinical features. Porencephaly may be associated with hydrocephalus or with subdural fluid collections. Infants may have seizures, focal neurologic deficit, or hydrocephalus. Transillumination is often localized. Treatment of the hydrocephalus is indicated; intractable focal seizures secondary to porencephaly may respond to drainage of the cyst.

Arachnoid cysts are uncommon lesions of uncertain cause. Many of them appear to be the entrapment of CSF in the pia-arachnoid. They often mimic hydrocephalus but are usually asymmetrical. They may produce localized transillumination and local erosion of bone. When occurring in the posterior fossa, they may produce hydrocephalus by aqueductal compression. Arteriography serves to differentiate them from porencephalic cysts, but definitive diagnosis is made during surgery.

Enlargement of the head may be caused by enlargement of the brain substance, *megalencephaly*. In such cases, head growth is rarely as rapid as in hydrocephalus. Megalencephaly may be familial, with or without mental retardation, but is often associated with structural abnormalities such as overgrowth of glial cells, astrocytosis, or microgyria. Megalencephaly may be seen with storage of materials within the brain substance, as in Alexander's disease, Tay-Sachs disease in its later stages, or Canavan's disease (spongy degeneration of the white matter).

Differentiation from hydrocephalus may be suggested by the rate of head growth and may be confirmed by echoencephalography or more definitely by air studies.

Normal growth of the head of a premature from 32 to 40 weeks is almost twice as fast as that of a full-term infant, 0 to 2 months of age (Fig. 17-11). Therefore, unless the rate of head growth is plotted on an age-specific graph, the rate of head growth of small babies will appear to be excessive. This may lead to the erroneous diagnosis of hydrocephalus.

Rapid growth after feeding of malnourished child

With malnutrition, there is a relative sparing of the brain. However, small head size, small brain size, and retardation may result from severe malnutrition. The role of malnutrition in utero upon cerebral development is less well defined. With feeding of malnourished infants there may be a rapid growth in head circumference, with spreading of the sutures shown on a skull x-ray film. This is felt to be catch-up growth secondary to increase in cell size. This catch-up growth may also be seen in the head growth of babies who are SGA (Fig. 17-11, *B*).

Achondroplasia is characterized by hypotonia, developmental delay, and an enlarged head. These infants consistently have a large head, greater than the ninety-seventh percentile. However, growth usually parallels the ninety-seventh percentile, and the infants do not exhibit a tense fontanelle or dilated scalp veins characteristic of hydrocephalus. Air studies reveal

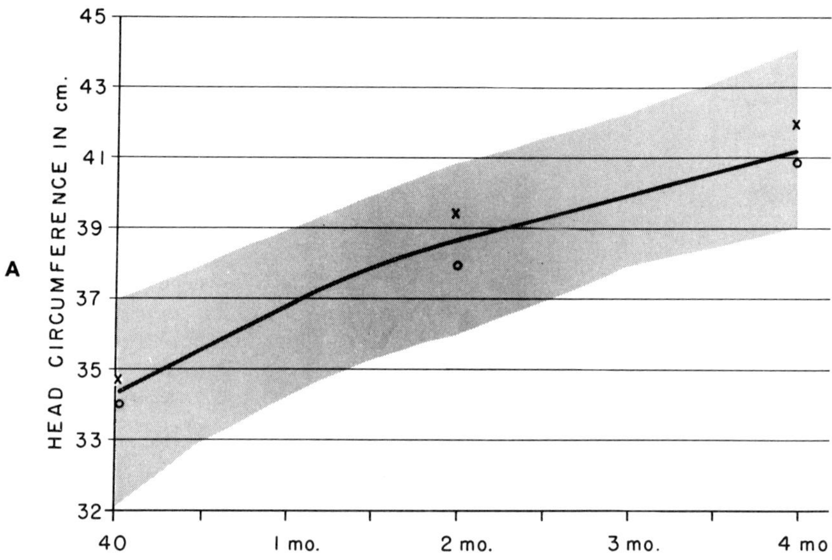

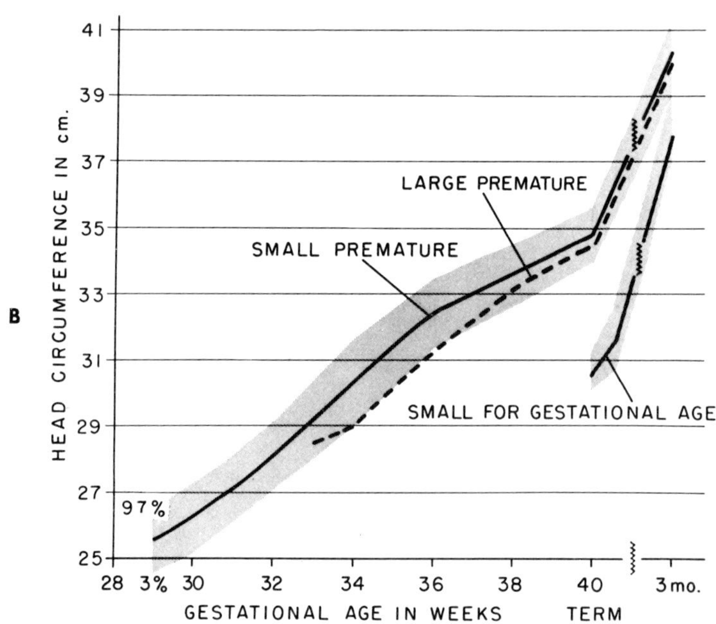

Fig. 17-11. A, Head growth of full-term infants. Birth weight greater than 2,500 gm. The solid line is a combination of males and females (redrawn from O'Neill, E. M.: Arch. Dis. Child. **36**:241, 1961). X represents males; O, females. **B,** Head growth of low birth weight infants (less than 2,500 gm): the small premature of appropriate size for gestational age (27 to 29 weeks' gestation); the large premature of appropriate size for gestational age (31 to 33 weeks' gestation); and the severely underweight or small for gestational age full-term infant (gestation greater than 38 weeks, weight less than 2.0 kg). (**A,** From Nellhaus, G.: Pediatrics **41**:106, 1968. **B,** adapted from Babson: J. Pediatr. **77**:11, 1970.)

only moderately dilated ventricles, and the infants rarely require shunting. Occasionally, the small foramen magnum does cause cervical cord compression and may interfere with CSF flow at the base. However, unless the rate of head growth continues to exceed the norm, the patient does not require evaluation or shunting. The marked hypotonia in these infants results in marked delay in the development of motor milestones. However, these infants are rarely retarded.

Dwarfs may be seen in the neonatal period with what appears to be enlarged head. This may also be seen in SGA babies where there has been relative sparing of the brain. It is important in these cases to measure head circumference in relationship to gestational age and to follow the rate of head growth rather than rely on a single measurement.

Treatment

The treatment of hydrocephalus is surgical and is less than satisfactory. It consists of shunting the fluid around the obstruction. Although shunts have been instilled from the ventricular space into virtually every orifice and space, currently most shunts are placed from the cerebral ventricles into the right atrium or into the peritoneum. Most shunts consist of varying types of tubing, with variable types of openings at either end, and with variable types of one-way valves interposed. Each of these variations carries the name of a different neurosurgeon. In most cases, the superiority of one over the other seems to be the in the eye of the inventor, and only a few are in general use.

Medical management of hydrocephalus plays only a temporizing role. Acetazolamide (Diamox), a carbonic anhydrase inhibitor, and sorbitol, a hyperosmotic agent, may be useful on occasion until a shunt is performed.

The success of shunting depends to a large extent on the experience and interest of the neurosurgeon performing the shunt. However, even in the best of hands, there are complications. The shunts may become infected at either end, and the cardiac end of the shunt may produce chronic bacteremia or septicemia. Cardiac shunts may embolize to the lungs, producing pulmonary hypertension, or may occasionally break off in the heart. All shunts may become plugged or obstructed at either end, with resultant signs of increased intracranial pressure. All shunts inserted in infancy require replacement as the infant grows, unless the hydrocephalus becomes arrested (p. 544). There are indications that shunts from the ventricle may cause aqueductal stenosis and shunt dependence.

Despite all of these complications, there is no current alternative to shunting. Shunting in infants with hydrocephalus should be performed as early as possible, once it is unequivocally determined that the head is growing at too rapid a rate. While infants with thin cortical mantles may do exceedingly well (see below), infants with thicker cortical mantles do better.

Prognosis and follow-up care

Since shunting in infants with hydrocephalus carries the risks and complications enumerated above and is obviously palliative rather than curative, one must understand the natural history of both treated and untreated hydrocephalus. Infants with uncomplicated hydrocephalus usually require shunting. In one randomized, controlled series, all but two of fifteen unoperated controls ultimately required operation. Even those two seemed to have slowly progressive hydrocephalus. Spontaneous arrest of hydrocephalus undoubtedly does occur, but the true frequency is difficult to document. Arrest of the process should be documented, not by head circumference, but by ventricular size and cortical mantle thickness. However, air studies may, of themselves, cause decompensation and should be done only when one seriously considers operation. Serial echoencephalography and perhaps periodic cisternography may offer better methods of following the course of these infants and determining when true arrest occurs.

In cases of uncomplicated hydrocephalus, the infants should be evaluated when the physician documents a progressive and definite increase in head circumference. At this time, the ventricles are usually moderately dilated, but even marked thinning of the cortical mantle should not be a deterrent to operation. It has been shown that even when the cortical mantle is less than

10 mm in thickness, the prognosis may be good (Fig. 17-12). In one series, half of the infants whose mantle was less than 10 mm in thickness at the time of operation had normal IQs.

Hydrocephalus associated with meningomyeloceles has a worse prognosis than hydrocephalus unassociated with spinal dysrhaphia. The reasons for this difference are not entirely clear. Children with hydrocephalus and meningomyeloceles, in one series, had only a 20% chance of reaching adulthood. The average IQ of the untreated survivors was less than 70. It is Lorber's recommendation that in hydrocephalus associated with meningomyelocele, if the cortical mantle is 26 to 35 mm in thickness, the patient should be watched, and only one third will require operation; whereas if the mantle thickness is less than 16 mm. operation urgently needs to be done.

Perhaps one of the differences between those in the meningomyelocele group and those in the uncomplicated hydrocephalus group is that the former are watched more closely. They are in the hospital from birth, and the physician is constantly following head size and performing definitive studies early. In this sense, perhaps we have been too vigorous and aggressive in the early diagnosis and treatment of complicated hydrocephalus. In uncomplicated hydrocephalus, patients are more likely to have large heads and definite ventricular dilation.

Arrested hydrocephalus

Arrest of the hydrocephalic process after shunting has been defined by Matson as a cessation of head growth until the head reaches approximately the ninetieth percentile. Growth after that should parallel the normal curve. The fallacy in this definition is that ventricular enlargement with mild increase in pressure may occur without abnormal enlargement of the head. The cortex, therefore, may become markedly thin, without evidence of increased intracranial pressure or increasing head size. Children with arrested hydrocephalus often show impaired intellectual performance upon reaching school age. These children may also decompensate acutely or die with infections or minor head trauma. Therefore, once the shunt has been put in, not only should head size and valve functioning be followed but also periodic echoencephalography or cisternography must also be used to be sure that the ventricles and cortical mantle remain a normal size. The physician should also be aware that following the shunting procedure, collapse of the cortex may lead to subdural hematomas, which can also produce enlargement of the head or increased pressure. In a child whose head continues to grow after shunting, subdural hematomas should be suspected.

In summary, hydrocephalus is a condition that can be diagnosed in its early

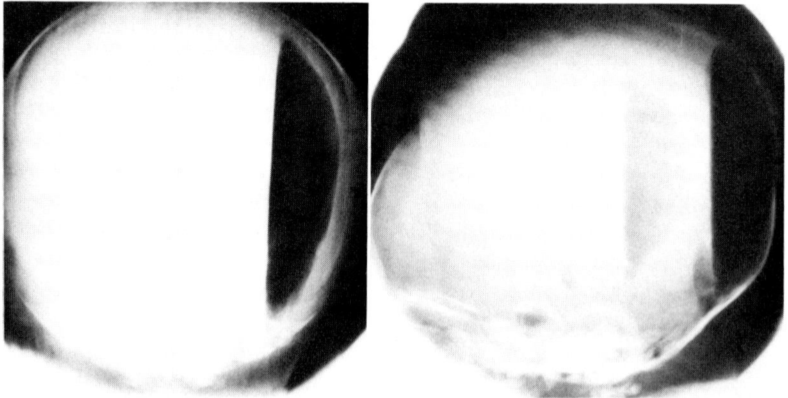

Fig. 17-12. Pneumoencephalogram of a newborn with congenital hydrocephalus. The ventricles are markedly enlarged, with virtually no cortical mantle in the left parieto-occipital area. The infant had aqueductal stenosis and a possible occlusion of the left posterior cerebral arteries. The infant was shunted at 2 days of age, and at 11 months had no demonstrable neurologic or psychologic deficit.

stages if the head circumference is measured and plotted during each of the infant's well-baby visits. While therapy is far from optimal, the prognosis for uncomplicated hydrocephalus vigorously treated is good. Hydrocephalus associated with meningomyeloceles has a less favorable prognosis, but if arrest does not occur, shunting is still indicated.

THE SMALL HEAD

Microcephaly, a small head, is always caused by microencephaly, a small brain, and the two terms have been used interchangeably. A small head circumference, *corrected for gestational age,* suggests the diagnosis. In the normally shaped head, the occipital frontal circumference is an index of cranial volume; where the head shape is abnormal, as in certain forms of craniosynostosis, the head circumference is not a valid index of cranial volume and cannot correlate with microcephaly.

Microcephaly has been defined as an occipital frontal circumference greater than 3 SD below the mean, or less than the third percentile. It has generally been equated with mental retardation. The populations used in most studies of microcephaly have had mental retardation or neurologic handicap, and a correlation between the degree of microcephaly and the degree of mental handicap has been established. However, the incidence of microcephaly in the general population and the chance of an infant with a small head having a normal I.Q. are not known. Twenty-five percent of hypopituitary dwarfs with normal IQ were microcephalic. Normal intelligence was also measured in 40% of those infants born microcephalic after exposure to the atomic bomb as fetuses. There is also variation of head circumference with race and variation of the lower limit of normal head circumference within established norms. In one series of children seen because of neurologic or cognitive handicaps, 40% were found to be microcephalic, and 14% of the microcephalic children were found to have normal intelligence. Thus, while mental retardation is often associated with a small head, a small head does not necessarily mean retardation.

Microcephaly may be either congenital or acquired. Congenital microcephaly may follow intrauterine infections with rubella or CID or congenital toxoplasmosis. These infections may be apparent from chorioretinitis or the constellation of abnormalities seen with the rubella syndrome, or they may be inapparent and suggested by IgM titers and specific antibody levels. Indeed, the high incidence of elevated CID titers among institutionalized microcephalic children who had no other evidence of CID suggests that this virus may be a relatively common cause of mental retardation in microcephalus. Congenital microcephaly is also a part of many chromosomal abnormalities and of many syndromes.

One form of microcephaly is familial and inherited as an autosomal recessive trait. The characteristic appearance of children with this form of microcephaly consists of a normal body and face, with a markedly furrowed brow. There is marked backward sloping of the forehead and a very small cranial volume. This appearance usually serves to identify the familial form and to permit genetic counseling.

Acquired microcephaly may result from perinatal infections such as herpes simplex, from anoxia and intracranial hemorrhage, and from metabolic causes, including aminoacidurias and hypothyroidism. In these patients, the head circumference is normal at birth, but the rate of brain growth is impaired, with resultant microcephaly.

Each infant with microcephaly deserves a complete evaluation. This should include serum titers for rubella, toxoplasmosis, and cytomegalovirus, IgM titers, skull x-ray films, and amino acid screening. The presence of other somatic abnormalities may lead to a chromosomal evaluation. Microcephaly must be differentiated from craniosynostosis (see below), and the cause of the microcephaly should be determined if possible. There is no treatment for microcephaly, since it is secondary to microencephaly. In some instances, however, the microencephaly can be prevented.

ABNORMALITIES OF HEAD SHAPE

Abnormalities of head shape may occur in the newborn period and may require surgical intervention. These abnormalities include the large head with frontal bossing and distended veins seen in hydrocephalus, the large head with parietal bossing seen in chronic subdural hematomas, and the small head with furrowed brow and backward sloping forehead of familial microcephaly. The broad forehead with wide bridge at the nose and hypertelorism may suggest arhinencephaly and other disorders of midline cerebral structures. One of the most common entities causing abnormalities of head shape in the neonatal period, however, is craniosynostosis.

Craniosynostosis

Craniosynostosis is the premature closure of one or more of the cranial sutures. Since the suture closure and consequent head deformity usually occurs prenatally, diagnosis often can be made within the neonatal period. The fontanelles as well as the sutures should be evaluated, since their presence or absence has great significance. The anterior fontanelle normally closes between the tenth and sixteenth month of life; the posterior fontanelle closes between the last 2 months before birth and the first 2 months following birth.

Etiology. The cause of primary (or congenital) craniosynostosis is unclear; it is thought to be a disorder of the membranous bones of the skull and not related to any local underlying growth failure of the brain. Postnatal or secondary craniosynostosis can result from rickets, hypophosphatasia, idiopathic hypercalcemia, or growth failure of the entire brain.

Pathophysiology. In the normal newborn infant the cranial bones are separate; however, during the first few hours or days of life, the cranial bones override one another. This is easily detectable by palpating ridges and feeling the mobility of the bones in relationship to one another. This mobility allows the circumference of the hard head to be molded or reduced in size as the cranial bones slide over one another during passage through the birth canal. Within several hours or days after birth, the bones are no longer overriding. Soon after birth the definite sutures are established, and the edges of the flat bones are separated by fibrous tissue. Growth in this area occurs perpendicular to the line of the suture.

The principal sutures of the infant skull are the sagittal, coronal, lamboid, and metopic. Closure of a suture inhibits growth of the skull perpendicular to the fusion. The normal increase in brain volume, however, requires expansion of the skull, which is forced to grow parallel to the fused suture. Deformity results from two factors: restriction of the growth of the vault at right angles to the involved suture and compensatory growth in the areas where the sutures are open. Closure of one of paired sutures results in inhibition of growth and flattening of the skull on that side. Closure of all sutures results in a marked distortion of skull shape as the brain expands through whatever fontanelles are opened. Closure of sutures *always* results in distortion of head shape if the underlying brain is normal. The small head with closed sutures whose shape is normal is the result of failure of the brain to grow. In these patients, closure of the sutures is secondary to failure of brain growth; failure of brain growth is *never* secondary to suture closure.

Sagittal synostosis

Sagittal synostosis is the most common form of craniosynostosis. It occurs predominantly in males and may be familial. It is seen in the neonatal period as a long, narrow head, scaphocephaly, whose circumference is often slightly greater than normal (Fig. 17-13). Sagittal synostosis is rarely associated with other somatic abnormalities and is uncommonly associated with ocular abnormalities, increased intracranial pressure, or mental retardation. Operative correction (p. 549) is purely for cosmetic purposes. The time of closure of the sutures relative to the amount of cerebral growth remaining determines the degree of cosmetic deformity. Since correction is a cosmetic procedure, it is difficult to lay down firm guidelines for operation. There is also an undocumented suspicion that many scaphocephalic heads tend to assume spontaneously a more normal shape with time.

Coronal synostosis

Unilateral and bilateral coronal synostosis are approximately equal in incidence. Coronal synostosis usually is seen as a short broad head with an increase in height. The head circumference tends to be small, although the cranial volume may be normal. The orbits may be shallow and oblique,

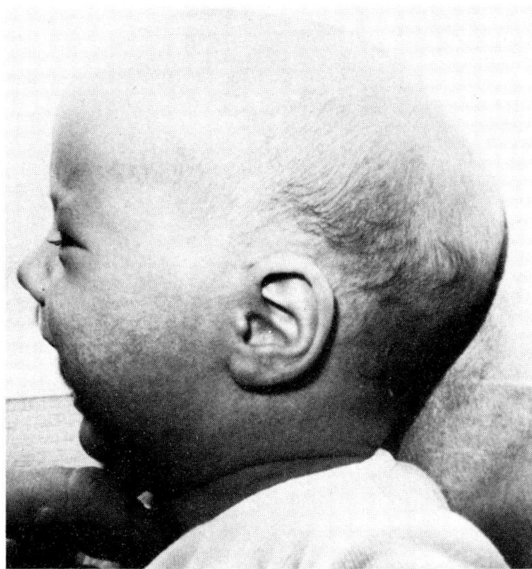

Fig. 17-13. Infant with posterior sagittal synostosis. Note the elongation of the posterior skull, which was also narrow. Ridging of the posterior sagittal suture was present.

causing proptosis. Coronal synostosis occurs predominantly in females. There is a higher incidence of developmental abnormalities and associated mental retardation with this entity than with sagittal synostosis. The stenosis is commonly associated with closure of sutures at the base, giving an appearance similar to Crouzon's disease. The short anterior fossa may lead to angulation and compression of the optic nerve, with resultant optic atrophy. The cosmetic deformity produced by coronal stenosis is more severe than that with sagittal stenosis, but the operation is still cosmetic.

Unilateral coronal synostosis produces flattening of the forehead on the affected side and accentuation of the frontal bossing on the opposite side. The orbits may be at different levels, interfering with the development of binocular vision. For this reason, operation is usually indicated. Synostosis of one coronal suture may result in severe deformity (oxycephaly) with ipsilateral involvement of the face and orbit. Other complications are exophthalmos, strabismus, nystagmus, papilledema, optic atrophy, and loss of vision. Even more serious malformation and resultant complications are present in patients with bilateral coronal synostoses or in whom multiple sutures are involved.

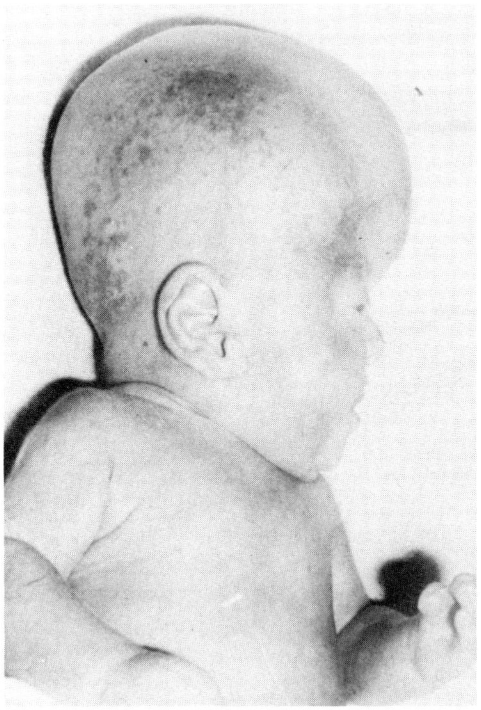

Fig. 17-14. Infant with Apert's syndrome. The shape of the head indicates closure of the lambdoid and coronal sutures. Deformities of the face are caused by closure of sutures at the base of the skull. In addition, the infant has syndactyly.

Lambdoid stenosis

Premature closure of both lambdoid sutures produces a small, flattened occiput and often broadening and increased height of the skull. Unilateral closure produces flattening on the affected side. The flattening of the occiput in a child with unilateral closure must be differentiated from positional flattening (see below). The absence of a ridge over the lambdoidal suture and skull roentgenograms (Towne's view) should adequately differentiate these entities. Operation is cosmetic.

Metopic suture

Early closure of the metopic suture during intrauterine life may produce a keel-shaped deformity of the forehead. Operation for this deformity is purely cosmetic.

Multiple sutures

Closure of multiple sutures produces varied types of severe deformity of the head (Fig. 17-14). Since there is not sufficient room for expansion of the brain, increased intracranial pressure may occur, and operations should be carried out as early as possible. While there is an increased incidence of mental retardation, many children with multiple suture closures have normal intelligence.

Diagnosis

There are several physical findings that should alert the examining physician to suspect a diagnosis of premature craniosynostosis. These findings are the presence of an irregular or asymmetric skull, detection of one area where the overriding sutures cannot be felt, the inability of the physician to move the cranial bones in relationship to one another in the early days of life, and the presence of a bony ridge along the suture line. Hypertelorism, difference in level or position of the eyes, ocular proptosis, strabismus, and optic atrophy may also be present. Signs and symptoms of increased intracranial pressure include funduscopic changes (p. 611), a cracked-pot percussion note of the skull too marked for age, bulging of any patent fontanelle, and marked irritability.

Radiographic studies are essential to determine the status of the sutures, shape of the skull, skull base, and facial structures. The affected sutures may be totally obliterated or indicated by a thin radiolucent line. Frequently there is thickening of bone along the suture, with bone bridging. It is important to recognize that the entire length of a given suture does not need to be involved. In the normal situation, the suture closes from posterior to anterior (sagittal suture) and from lateral to medial (coronal sutures). In premature synostosis the closures occur in the same directions. Consequently, prompt diagnosis may be postponed because the portion of the suture best visualized by early radiographic examination may be normal. The *devil's eye configuration,* observed on the posteroanterior radiographic projection, results from the lateral elevation of the lesser wing of the sphenoid. This finding is a clue to unilateral (if it occurs on only one side) or to bilateral coronal synostoses. Radiographic evidence of increased intracranial pressure is manifested by excessive separation of the normal sutures or a beaten silver appearance of the skull.

The question of synostosis often arises when the anterior fontanelle is thought to be too small or closed too soon. Frequently, the suspicion proves to be correct. On the other hand, the anterior fontanelle may be patent, even though the metopic, sagittal, or one or both coronal sutures are closed. Since the anterior fontanelle is open in approximately 50% of patients with each type (sagittal and unilateral or bilateral coronal) of synostosis and with multiple suture closures, it is important not to be lulled into a false sense of security simply because the anterior fontanelle remains patent.

Craniosynostosis may be an isolated defect or a component of a syndrome. When craniostenosis is suspected or proved, the pediatrician should be alerted to seek the presence of other malformations. Associated malformations include syndactyly, defects of elbow and knee joints, cardiac anomalies, and choanal atresia. Specific combinations, particularly those involving the limbs, constitute genetically distinct syndromes. The most common syndromes involving premature closure of the sutures are acrocephalosyndactyly (Apert's syndrome) and craniofacial dysostosis (Crouzon's disease). Apert's syndrome consists of acrocephaly, or pointing of the head anteriorly, irregular abnormalities of the sutures, midfacial hypoplasia, and syndactyly of the hands and, occasionally, of the feet. In this syndrome the coronal suture is primarily involved, although other sutures may be involved as well. Crouzon's disease includes shallow orbits and maxillary hypoplasia as well as premature craniosynostosis, especially of the coronal, lambdoidal, and sagittal sutures. Mental deficiency has been more frequently reported in Apert's than in Crouzon's disease.

Differential diagnosis

The differential diagnosis of the varied deformities of craniosynostosis should rarely present a problem. A small, normally shaped head with closure of the sutures always represents primary microencephaly and never requires surgery. Confusion of the distorted head shapes comes mainly from the positional flattenings. The long, narrow head of the premature is the result of the infant's lying on his side. The roentgenogram shows no ridging of the sagittal suture and no fusion of that suture. Unilateral occipital flattening may be the result of unilateral lambdoidal stenosis. More commonly, it is positional, from an infant's lying on one side of his occiput. Torticollis and bed position relative to light and activity may play a role. Often flattening is seen when there is a lack of interest in the environment, and the infant lies on the occiput with little movement. Occipital flattening should alert the physician to the possibility of developmental delay. The absence of ridging of the sutures and X-ray studies should serve to differentiate positional flattening from lambdoidal stenosis.

Treatment

The surgery of craniosynostosis is cosmetic surgery, except where multiple sutures are involved. There is little or no indication that these patients develop increased intracranial pressure; there is no evidence that the mental retardation sometimes associated with suture closure can be prevented by operation; and there is no evidence that operation prevents the optic atrophy sometimes seen with coronal stenosis. There is general agreement that the constricting effect of the total synostosis on the otherwise normal brain will cause increased intracranial pressure during the period of rapid brain growth and produce brain damage. Cosmetic indications for surgery are difficult to evaluate, particularly since the operation should ideally be done before 6 months of age, preferably between the second and third month. The operation is, thus, a prophylactic cosmetic operation, and a skilled and experienced neurosurgeon can often restore normal appearance to the infant's head.

The technique of operation is well described by Matson and involves creating new sutures parallel to the fused suture. It is important that the newly created sutures cross two suture lines (that is, in coronal stenosis the new suture must cross both the sagittal and squamosal sutures). If two sutures are not crossed, then the newly created suture will not allow sufficient expansion to correct the cosmetic deformity. The new suture line must be treated with phenol or lined wth an inert material to prevent refusion. In Matson's hands the mortality at the operation was only 0.4%; there was a 14% morbidity from wound infections, cardiac arrests, leptomeningeal cysts, and anesthetic complications. It is against this morbidity that the cosmetic indications must be weighed.

SEIZURES

Seizures in the neonate are a different entity from seizures in the older child or adult. They are different in their clinical manifestations, in their cause, in the approach to their therapy, and in their prognosis. Seizures in this period represent a medical emergency, not because they, of themselves, are life threatening, but because they are often the signal of an underlying disease process; a process that may produce irreversible cerebral damage. It is therefore, important to diagnose and treat promptly the process causing the seizure, and it is usually only of secondary importance to treat the seizure itself.

Recognition and classification

Seizures in the older child are classified by their clinical manifestations and by their site of origin, since the type of seizure may have etiologic and prognostic significance. In the newborn, most seizures are subcortical rather than cortical in origin and are classified by their cause. Major motor, tonic-clonic seizures are uncommon in this age group, and the type of seizure is rarely of importance since one cause, such as hypoglycemia, may produce varied types of seizures.

Neonatal seizures may be subtle and undoubtedly are often missed. They may be manfested by brief tonic extensions of the body, apnea, transient deviations of the eyes, clonic movements of one extremity, swallowing movements, brief losses of tone, or sucking movements. Indeed, any alteration in the state of the infant that occurs repetitively may be a seizure. Although jitteriness is often confused with seizures, the sudden symmetrical startle response followed by rapid, small-amplitude shaking is rarely a seizure but may be a signal of a similar underlying cause (see section on jitteriness, p. 551).

Pathophysiology

A seizure requires that the synchronous firing of adjacent neurons reach a critical mass in order to produce the clinical manifestations. Epileptic neurons recruit adjacent neurons to fire synchronously and thereby produce a seizure. The neonatal cortex, while having a relatively complete complement of neurons, has a paucity of dendrites, the interneuronal connections. It is therefore more difficult for the epileptic neuron of the neonate to recruit other neurons to fire synchronously. In addition, the neuronal membranes are leaky and allow sodium to enter and potassium to exit from the cell far more easily than more mature membranes. With the levels of sodium-potassium adenosine triphosphatase well below mature levels, the cell is less able to extrude sodium efficiently and become repolarized. Thus the newborn's cells remain relatively hyperpolarized, and rapid and repetitive firing of neurons does not occur at the rate seen in the more mature cortex. These reasons and perhaps others account for the paucity of cortical seizures in this age group. Subcortical structures, however, are more mature and therefore better able to sustain epileptic activity and produce a clinical seizure. This ability may explain susceptibility of the human newborn infant to such subcortical manifestations of seizures as eye movements, chewing, and respiratory arrest.

Diagnosis

Neonatal seizures are a medical emergency. Each infant must be considered to have a potentially treatable disease, regardless of his antecedent history. Each infant with seizures must be evaluated for the remediable underlying causes: hypoglycemia, hypocalcemia, hypomagnesemia, electrolyte imbalance, pyridoxine dependency, and infection. This includes an adequate history and physical examination. Blood must be drawn for glucose, calcium, phosphorus, and electrolyte determinations, as well as for culture. The physician should make use of a spinal tap to look for evidence of infection or an antecedent intracranial hemorrhage. Evaluation of the spinal fluid should include comparison of a spun-down specimen with water, to look for xanthochromia as evidence that the bloody spinal fluid is not the result of a traumatic tap. An EEG may confirm the diagnosis of seizures through the correlation of the paroxysmal electrical events with the clinical manifetsations. The EEG may also provide a means of monitoring therapy as well as prognostic information. However, therapy should not be delayed while awaiting an EEG. The major causes of seizures in the neonatal period are shown in the following outline.

CAUSES OF NEONATAL SEIZURES

A. Metabolic
    1. Hypoglycemia
        a. Transient
            (1) Diabetic mother
            (2) Low birth weight
            (3) Intracranial bleeding
            (4) Meningitis
        b. Persistent
            (1) Idiopathic
            (2) Leucine sensitive
            (3) Galactosemia
            (4) Fructosemia
            (5) Islet cell tumor
            (6) Glycogen storage disease
    2. Hypocalcemia
        a. Early
            (1) Intracranial trauma
            (2) Hypomagnesemia
            (3) Idiopathic
        b. Late
            (1) Maternal hyperparathyroidism
            (2) Neonatal hypoparathyroidism
            (3) High phosphate (cow's milk) load
    3. Hypomagnesemia
        a. With hypocalcemia
    4. Pyridoxine (B_6)
        a. Dependency
        b. Deficiency
    5. Hyponatremia and hypernatremia
        a. Inappropriate fluid therapy
        b. Inappropriate antidiuretic hormone–intracranial
        c. Salt substituted for sugar
    6. Aminoaciduria
        a. Phenylketonuria
        b. Maple syrup urine disease
        c. Hyperglycinemia
    7. Bilirubin
        a. Kernicterus
    8. Drug withdrawal
        a. Heroin
        b. Alcohol
        c. Barbiturate
    9. Hyperthermia
B. Infection
    1. Sepsis
        a. Meningitis
    2. Meningitis
        a. Bacterial
        b. Fungal
    3. Encephalitis
        a. Herpes simplex
        b. Cytomegalic inclusion disease
        c. Toxoplasmosis
        d. Coxsackie B
C. Bleeding
    1. Trauma
        a. Subarachnoid

b. Subdural
c. Thrombosis
2. Anoxia
a. Periventricular hemorrhage
b. Periventricular and intraventricular bleeding
D. Developmental anomalies
1. Cerebral dysgenesis
2. Incontinentia pigmenti

Jitteriness

Jitteriness or tremulousness in the newborn is the repetitive shaking of an extremity or extremities. The movements may be low amplitude, high frequency (fine and rapid) or may be high amplitude, low frequency (coarse and gross). These movements may be seen with crying, may occur spontaneously with changes in the sleeping state of the infant, or may be elicited with a startle or other stimulation of the infant. A mild degree of jitteriness may be normal during the first 4 days of life. The pathophysiologic mechanisms responsible for jitteriness are poorly understood. However, when the jitteriness is persistent and prolonged after an individual stimulus or when it is easily elicitable with minimal stimulus, it may be an indication of an underlying pathologic condition and may require evaluation. Jittery movements persisting after the fourth day of life, especially if they are coarse and gross, are usually abnormal.

A seizure in the newborn may be manifested by sudden spontaneous jerking of the extremity, similar to jitteriness. It may be differentiated from jitteriness by the fact that seizures cannot be elicited by stimulation, whereas in the jittery baby the responses are stimulus sensitive. Since the chemical and pathologic mechanisms underlying both seizures and jitteriness may be identical, an infant may be both jittery and have seizures.

The investigation of the infant with frequent and persistent jittery movements or in whom the jitteriness is easily elicitable is identical to that of a child having seizures, and the diagnostic evaluation should be similar (Table 17-6). In addition, drug withdrawal should be considered as the diagnosis in the infant of the mother who has been addicted to heroin, methadone, or phenobarbital. Babies who are jittery because of drug withdrawal are hypertonic and extremely irritable and tend to have a high-pitched scream. The tremors are often very coarse. Hypoglycemia and maternal thyrotoxicosis may also cause neonatal jitteriness.

The prognosis of jitteriness is dependent on the underlying cause. When chemical or metabolic abnormalities cause jitteriness, their correction should result in a normal infant. The long-term results of the jitteriness associated with drug withdrawal remain to be evalauted. When the jitteriness

Table 17-6. Neonatal seizures—work-up and therapy

Work-up
- History and physical examination
- Blood for calcium, glucose, magnesium, PO_4 and sodium determinations and for culture
- Lumbar puncture for cells, glucose and protein determinations, for culture, and for blood and xanthochromia
- EEG if possible

Specific therapy
- Glucose, 50%, 1 to 2 ml/kg, IV
- Calcium gluconate, 10%, up to 10 ml, slowly IV
- Pyridoxine, 20 to 50 mg, IV
- Magnesium sulfate, 3%, 2 to 6 ml, IV

Anticonvulsant therapy

Drug	Intravenous	Oral
Diazepam	0.2 to 2 mg	1 mg every 6 hours; increase as necessary or tolerated
Phenobarbital	10 to 20 mg/kg	Start 5 mg/kg; increase as necessary and tolerated
Diphenylhydantoin (Dilantin)	Rarely	Not more than 5 mg/kg
Paraldehyde	Up to 50 ml of 10% solution in saline	

is high amplitude and low frequency and is associated with increased tone and hyperreflexia and when it persists beyond the fourth day of life, the infant may later develop a choreoathetosis. Jitteriness and seizures are both signals of an underlying pathologic condition that must be evaluated. The results of this evaluation will indicate the prognosis of the infant.

Hypoglycemia

Hypoglycemia is the one cause of neonatal seizures likely to produce acute damage to the brain. It is therefore most important to determine if it exists. Transient hypoglycemia may occur in the infant of the diabetic or prediabetic mother; the prognosis is usually good. In contrast, symptomatic infants of nondiabetic mothers have a higher morbidity. In one series, such infants had a 40% morbidity, and only 20% of the infants were normal. Hypoglycemia may be associated with SGA babies, septicemia, meningitis, intraventricular hemorrhage, or anoxia. It may be the result, as well as the cause, of cerebral damage.

The diagnosis of hypoglycemia requires two determinations of blood glucose levels under 30 mg/100 ml (20 mg/100 ml in the premature). The use of Dextrostix may give a rapid indication of the blood glucose level. However, the inaccuracies of this method necessitate confirmation of the diagnosis by true blood glucose levels. (Further discussion of neonatal hypoglycemia is found on p. 439.)

Hypocalcemia

Serum calcium levels less than 7 to 7.5 mg/100 ml and phosphorus levels greater than 8 mg/100 ml may occur in up to 50% of newborn infants with seizures. The etiologic relationship of the hypocalcemia to the seizures is often difficult to establish. Hypocalcemia is far more common after premature or abnormal birth than after normal delivery. Since hypocalcemia may be present in asymptomatic infants, it may be difficult to be certain of its significance in the jittery baby.

In the older child, hypocalcemia may be the result of maternal hyperparathyroidism, neonatal hypoparathyroidism, or phosphate overload. Hypomagnesemia may also result in hypocalcemia, often without hyperphosphatemia. The hypocalcemia in this instance may not be correctable until magnesium is administered. (Hypocalcemia is discussed further on p. 445.) It should be emphasized that Chvostek and Trousseau signs are poorly correlated with the presence or absence of hypocalcemia. Diagnosis requires the determination of serum calcium and phosphorus levels as well as of serum protein levels. A prolonged Q-T interval on the ECG may suggest hypocalcemia.

Pyridoxine dependency and deficiency

Pyridoxine dependency is a rare cause of seizures that may occur in utero or in early neonatal life. As with other metabolic causes, the seizures are refractory to anticonvulsant medication. A history of a sibling with intractable neonatal seizures should suggest the diagnosis.

The basic defect in pyridoxine dependency may be a deficiency in the binding of the coenzyme, pyridoxal phosphate, to glutamic decarboxylase, the enzyme involved in the formation of γ-aminobutyric acid (GABA). The absence of GABA, a presumed central nervous system inhibitor, could produce convulsions. Pyridoxine deficiency is secondary to a lack of exogenous vitamin B_6. It produces seizures at several weeks of life and is associated with abnormal tryptophan metabolites in the urine. Pyridoxine dependency has no associated chemical abnormalities. A second form of transient pyridoxine dependency has been described in infants whose mothers received pyridoxine for hyperemesis gravidarum.

Diagnosis is made by the intravenous administration of 50 mg of pyridoxine, preferably while an EEG is running. Seizures will abate within several minutes. While pyridoxine dependency is a rare cause of seizures, it is treatable, and mental retardation can be prevented by early therapy. Therefore, every neonate with difficult or intractable seizures should receive a therapeutic dose of pyridoxine. Patients with dependency require continuous administration of the drug to prevent the recurrence of seizures and cerebral damage.

Hyponatremia and hypernatremia

Hyponatremia and hypernatremia are uncommon in the first days of life but may occur later in the neonatal period. An infant with hyponatremia may have symptoms of lethargy, irritability, convulsions, tremors, or other signs of seizure activity. The condition may result from water retention caused by increased excretion of antidiuretic hormone or may occur during meningitis or sepsis or after cerebral trauma. Hyponatremia may also occur from inappropriate parenteral fluid administration to the mother during labor or to the neonate. Hyponatremia secondary to diarrhea is less common than hypernatremia at this age. Sweating by the child with cystic fibrosis of the pancreas may also produce hyponatremia. Determination of the cause of the hyponatremia is important, because the hyponatremia secondary to excessive water retention should be treated with fluid restriction, whereas excess sodium loss requires sodium replacement.

Hypernatremia in the newborn infant has resulted from accidental substitution of salt for sugar in formula feeding and from the administration of high-solute formula or parenteral fluids to infants whose kidneys cannot adequately conserve water. Seizures may occur secondary to venous thrombosis or to formation of petechiae in the brain. With hypernatremia, seizures most commonly occur during rehydration, when the slow equilibration of sodium across the cell membrane leads to a marked flow of water into the brain, resulting in intracellular edema.

The seizures associated with hyponatremia respond to the administration of appropriate amounts of sodium, but like most metabolic seizures are refractory to anticonvulsant medication. Seizures occurring during rehydration of the hypernatremic child are also refractory to anticonvulsants but respond to the administration of hypertonic saline or to other hyperosmotic agents such as mannitol that serve to decrease the intracellular fluid.

Meningitis and encephalitis

See also Chapter 8, p. 141.

Seizures are rarely the initial symptom in patients with neonatal meningitis, but occur during the course of the disease in one third to one half of the patients. However, the child with neonatal seizures should have a lumbar puncture and complete examination of the CSF. Pleocytosis may follow a subarachnoid hemorrhage, but the cerebrospinal glucose concentration should remain normal. Whereas gram-negative organisms are a frequent cause of neonatal meningoencephalitis, other infectious agents such as gram-positive bacteria, cytomegalovirus, toxoplasma, herpesvirus, and other viruses should be considered.

The diagnosis of CID, toxoplasmosis, and herpesvirus may be increasingly important in the future as new forms of therapy directed toward these chronic infections become available. Recent attempts have been made to treat herpesvirus encephalitis with iododeoxyuridine and cytosine arabinoside. The effectiveness of these agents is unproved, since we do not know the natural history of herpesvirus encephalitis or systemic herpes in the newborn. Certainly, there is a high mortality and a very significant morbidity. Herpesvirus encephalitis in the newborn is usually associated with systemic herpes and is contracted during labor from a maternal genital herpes. However, herpes simplex encephalitis can occur in the absence of the systemic manifestations of herpes. The onset of seizures and progressive neurologic difficulty after the first few days of life, with or without CSF pleocytosis or elevation of protein concentration, may be compatible with herpes. A brain scan showing focal uptake is highly suggestive of herpes. Proof of herpes infection can be obtained only by brain biopsy. In general, this is a rapid infection, and prompt diagnosis and early biopsy are indicated if therapy is to be of value. Controlled studies are needed before a specific therapy can be firmly recommended.

Birth trauma and anoxia

Birth trauma and anoxia are the major causes of neonatal seizures, but the true incidence of these complications is unknown. The association of these complications with hypocalcemia and hypoglycemia has been mentioned previously. However, despite a history of traumatic birth or definite anoxia, treatable causes of seizures should be investigated before considering trauma and anoxia as the primary cause.

The interrelationship of anoxia and hemorrhage often makes a specific diagnosis difficult. Traumatic intracranial hemorrhage may result in primary apnea with secondary cerebral anoxia. Conversely, primary apnea and anoxia may produce periventricular hemorrhage, which may rupture into the ventricular system, giving subarachnoid hemorrhage. Therefore, the clinical distinction of these two entities is frequently obscure. Approximately 50% of infants who die in the neonatal period have evidence of intracranial hemorrhage and edema. The hemorrhage in the full-term infant is most commonly from traumatic tears of the tentorium or falx; in the premature infant hemorrhage is more commonly the result of intraventricular rupture of the periventricular and subependymal hemorrhages associated with anoxia. (See section on trauma, p. 527.) The occurrence of focal neurologic findings may aid in the diagnosis of these entities.

Other metabolic disorders

The child who has persistent seizures unassociated with the above causes should be screened for aminoacidurias. Ferric chloride and dinitrophenylhydrazine may give rapid indication of an aminoaciduria. Paper or column chromatography gives more definitive, although slower, results. The presence of ketonuria in the neonatal period is rare and suggests hyperglycinemia, glycogen storage disease, or maple syrup urine disease. The presence of reducing substance in the urine should be looked for with Benedict's test, which will pick up all reducing substances. If the reaction is positive, a glucose oxidase test (Dextrostix) will rule out glucosuria.

Treatment

There is little evidence that the convulsions seen in the newborn period of themselves produce damage to the brain, unless they are associated with apnea. As noted above, seizures are often the indication of underlying disease, and therapy should be directed at that underlying disease rather than at the seizures as such. The diagnostic evaluation and therapy of seizures go hand in hand (Table 17-6). Clues may be obtained from the history and physical examination. Blood should be drawn for glucose, calcium, phosphous, sodium, and magnesium determinations, as well as for culture. Looking for evidence of bleeding and of infection, the physician should perform a lumbar puncture. While the physician is awaiting the results of these tests, he should administer therapy in a diagnostic fashion. Ideally, an EEG should be obtained. The clinical correlation between the paroxysmal activity on the EEG and the clinical manifestations suggestive of seizures in the patient may aid in the diagnosis of neonatal seizures. The EEG also offers a rapid opportunity for evaluation of intravenous therapy and may also offer some aid in prognosis. However, therapy should not be delayed if an EEG is not readily available.

Since hypoglycemia is a common cause of neonatal seizures and may of itself produce cerebral damage, it should be treated first. The intravenous administration of 50% glucose, 1 to 2 ml/kg, should result in prompt cessation of seizures; if seizures persist after glucose administration, calcium gluconate in a 10% solution should be administered slowly, with monitoring of the cardiac rate. Up to 10 ml may be given. If seizures persist, 5 minutes after this therapy 25 to 50 mg of pyridoxine should be administered. If pyridoxine dependency is the cause of the seizures, they should stop within several minutes.

It should be noted that calcium is a cerebral depressant; therefore, the fact that seizures stop after calcium administration does not necessarily mean that hypocalcemia was the cause of the seizures. The diagnosis of hypocalcemia can be made only by the chemical determination of calcium and phosphorus, as indicated above, and by evidence of prolongation of the Q-T interval on the ECG. Continued seizures should be treated with magnesium sulfate, 2 to 6 ml of a 2% to 3% solution administered intravenously or 1 ml of a 50% solution adminstered intramuscularly.

Anticonvulsants

Anticonvulsants should be used only in the child who has not responded to the above-mentioned specific therapy. In general, convulsions in the neonatal period are *overtreated* with anticonvulsants. If seizures are persistent, interfering with respiration or with the feeding and care of the child, they should be treated with anticonvulsant medications. Severe and persistent seizures should be treated intravenously. Less severe seizures or infrequent seizures may be treated intramuscularly or orally.

The dosage and therapy of anticonvulsants in the neonatal period are shown in Table 17-6. Diazepam (Valium) is an effective agent for the treatment of status epilepticus in the adult. Little is known about the metabolism of this drug in the neonatal period, and less is known about the appropriate dosage. Dosages that have been effective in the newborn range from 0.08 to 2.7 mg/kg administered intravenously over several minutes. Respiratory arrest has been seen when this drug was administered to infants who had previously received barbiturates. Phenobarbital may be used in the treatment of status epilepticus at a dosage of 15 mg/kg intravenously given over several minutes. Respiratory depression may also occasionally complicate this form of therapy. Infrequent or less severe seizures may be treated with intramuscular administration of phenobarbital, 5 to 7 mg/kg. For severe or persistent seizures that have not responded to the above medications, paraldehyde given intravenously is often a safe and effective form of therapy. Paraldehyde is excreted primarily by the lungs, and while not producing respiratory depression, may on occasion produce a pneumonitis. It should not be used in infants with respiratory disease. Paraldehyde may be diluted as a 3% to 10% solution in 0.25 N saline and injected slowly at a rate sufficient to control the seizures. Higher concentrations of paraldehyde may be given but should not be used in plastic apparatus. A total dosage of 1.0 to 5 ml of undiluted paraldehyde may be safely used.

Once the seizures of an infant in status epilepticus are stopped with the above medications, intramuscular administration of anticonvulsants should be started immediately to prevent recurrence of seizures. All infants with seizures not caused by one of the metabolic causes listed above or by infection should receive prolonged anticonvulsant medication for 1 to 2 years or until their EEG has been normal for a period of time. Diphenylhydantoin (Dilantin) should be used with caution in the neonatal period, since clinical manifestations of intoxication cannot be seen in the young infant and since the drug may produce irreversible cerebellar damage if given in too high doses for prolonged periods. Therefore, unless the blood level is monitored, diphenylhydantoin should be used with extreme caution and in low dosage.

Prognosis

There is a high mortality, up to 40%, among infants having seizures in the neonatal period. However, two thirds to three fourths of the survivors of the neonatal period are normal at follow-up. Cerebral trauma and anoxia account for two thirds of neonatal deaths from seizures. Developmental anomalies are relatively uncommon as the cause of seizures in this age group. Seizures starting in the first 24 hours of life are most often related to anoxia or trauma and have a high mortality and morbidity. Seizures starting on the second to seventh day of life and lasting 24 hours to 7 days still had a good outlook, and three fourths of the survivors were normal. It should be emphasized that most of the series reported in the literature place little emphasis on the metabolic causes of seizures; therefore, it is possible that the morbidity may be further improved.

Summary

Seizures in the neonatal period are a medical emergency, not because of the seizures as such, but because they may indicate an underlying treatable cause of neurologic impairment. Evaluation and therapy should be initially directed to the infectious (p. 141) and metabolic causes, including hypoglycemia, hypocalcemia, pyridoxine dependency, and hypomagnesemia. In the neonate with persistent seizures, anticonvulsants may be used. While neonatal seizures have a high mortality, there is a significant chance that the survivors will be normal.

DEVELOPMENTAL ABNORMALITIES

Defects in closure of the neuraxis

Defects in closure of the cranium present a clinical spectrum from anencephaly and complete craniorachischisis to dermal sinuses of the head. Defects of the spinal column run from complete spinal rachischisis to spina bifida occulta and also include such entities as diastematomyelia, spinal lipomas, and pilonidal sinuses. Defects in closure of the neuraxis are the most common of the major structural abnormalities of the newborn nervous system.

Classification of abnormalities of closure of the spinal cord—spina bifidas

Defects in closure of the spinal canal, termed spina bifidas, may be associated with abnormalities of the cord and meninges of varying severity. They are classified below.

Meningocele. Meningocele is a cystic dilatation of the meninges associated with spina bifida and a defect of the overlying skin. The spinal cord and nerve roots are normal. There is no neurologic deficit.

Meningomyelocele. Meningomyelocele is a lesion identical to the meningocele, but with associated abnormalities of the spinal cord and nerve roots. There is neurologic deficit below the level of the lesion. The extent of the deficit depends on the location of the lesion (see below).

Myeloschisis (spina bifida aperta). Myeloschisis is a spina bifida with exposure of the spinal cord and roots and with no cystic covering of meninges. This defect may be small or may extend the whole length of the spinal axis. The clinical significance is identical to that of meningomyelocele.

Spina bifida occulta. Spina bifida occulta is nonfusion of one or more posterior arches of the spine, usually lumbosacral. A common abnormality found at L5 in 30% of adults, it is of consequence only when associated with underlying abnormalities or when found at other levels. Significant associated abnormalities are usually signaled by either a hemangioma, a patch of abnormal hair, a dimple or a lipoma in the lumbosacral area (Fig. 17-15). The underlying abnormalities include diastematomyelia, spinal lipomas or dermoids, and dermal sinuses (p. 558).

Embryology

Several theories of the embryology of the spina bifidas have been proposed. One of the more recent theories suggests that damage to ectoderm produces a bleb of fluid from the neural cleft, which results in embryonic scarring. The degree of damage

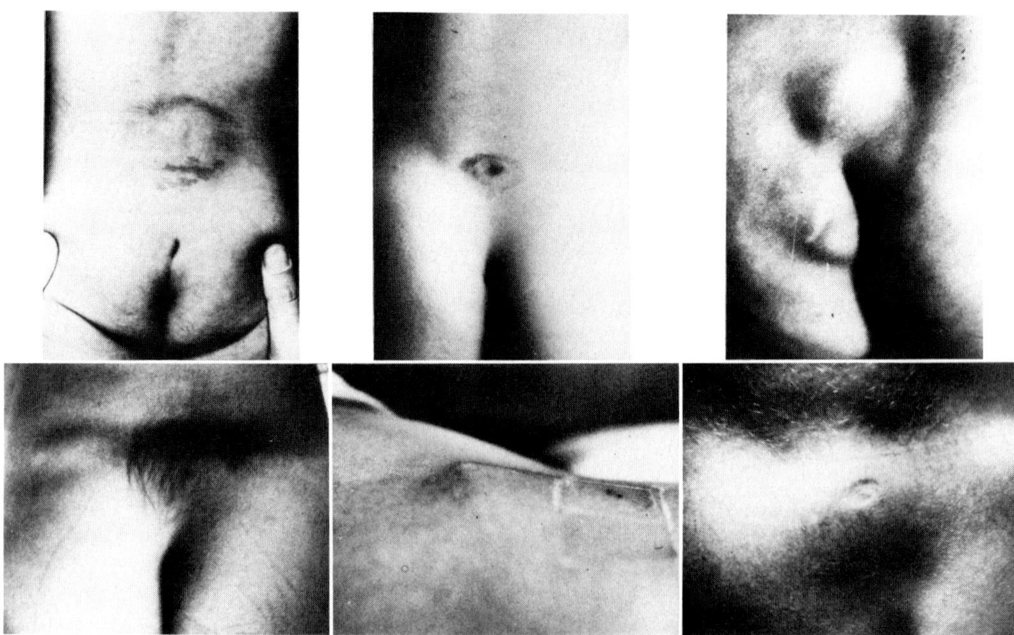

Fig. 17-15. Lesions of the back associated with spina bifida occulta and spinal cord problems. *Top: Left,* lipoma with hairy patch above hemangioma; *center,* hemangioma; *right,* lipoma. All had tethered cords and intradural lipomas. *Bottom: Left,* patch of fine hair; *center,* bony spur; *right,* midline scar. Bottom left and center were associated with diastematomyelia.

to ectodermal and mesodermal tissue and the success of the healing and scarring process determine the resultant defect.

Myelomeningoceles and myeloschisis

Clinical manifestations. The degree of neurologic deficit associated with these defects is determined by the level of the lesion. Accurate diagnosis and prognosis for ambulation can be determined to a large degree at birth by careful sensory and motor testing of the infant. The sensory level, in general, gives an approximation of the motor level in these children (Table 17-7) but may be several segments lower. The prognosis and plans for therapy can be predicted with a high degree of certainty at birth (Table 17-8).

Treatment. A newborn infant with a meningomyelocele presents the pediatrician with difficult decisions of what to tell parents and whether or not to recommend surgical closure of the defect on the back. Closure of the back, while usually not technically difficult, carries significant implications. It greatly increases the chances of the infant's survival but in doing so obligates the profession to total care of the child and places a considerable emotional and financial burden on the family for the numerous operations and the rehabilitation that will be required. It also involves appreciable suffering of the infant. Furthermore, the decision to operate must be made promptly, for there is reasonable evidence to suggest that the operation ideally should take place within the first 24 hours to prevent further deterioration of the spinal cord and roots.

Numerous factors may influence the decision. These should include the size of the lesion and the technical feasibility of closure, the location of the lesion and the prognosis for ambulation of the child, the presence or absence of associated abnormalities (such as hydrocephalus, kyphosis, or other major structural abnormalities),

TABLE 17-7. Motor examination of lower extremities in children with meningomyeloceles

Movement	Spinal segment: Lumbar	Spinal segment: Sacral	Muscle
Hip			
Flexion	1, 2, 3, 4		Iliopsoas Rectus femoris
Adduction	2, 3, 4		Adductors
Adduction	4, 5,	1	Gluteus medius
Extension	4, 5,	1, 2	Gluteus maximus Obturator
Knee			
Extension	2, 3, 4		Quadriceps
Flexion	5	1, 2	Hamstrings
Foot			
Dorsiflexion	4, 5	1	Tibialis anterior
Plantar flexion	5	1,2	Soleus, gastrocnemius

TABLE 17-8. Deficit and prognosis of meningomyeloceles as related to site of lesion

Motor/sensory level	Maximum motor deficit	Prognosis for ambulation	Risk of hydrocephalus
L5–S1	Dorsiflexion and plantar flexion of feet, weakness of glutei	Will ambulate with or without short leg braces; outlook good	60%
L3–L4	Involvement of quadriceps and hamstrings, plus above	May be able to ambulate with long leg braces and crutches; paralytic hip dislocation	86%
L1 and L2 or above	Complete paraplegia	No functional ambulation	96%

the presence of personnel and facilities to provide adequate care for the infant, and the infant's family structure and the attitudes of the family toward the defect and its consequences. Keeping these factors in mind, the physician must weigh the consequences of the three possible courses of action.

1. *Immediate closure of the defect.* If the defect is closed immediately, the infant will have approximately a 90% chance of survival. The chance of developing hydrocephalus requiring repetitive shunt procedures will depend on the site of the lesion (Table 17-8). Urologic complications requiring an ileal loop will occur in about 90%. Fecal soiling can be controlled with rigorous management. Orthopedic care involving braces and transplants of muscles, tendons, and cortex will depend on the site of the lesion, as will the prognosis for ambulation. Psychologic help and social-work assistance will be required for these children. Closure of the defect obligates the physician and society to provide optimal care in each of these areas for the survivors. Despite this care, the function of the child with spinal cord involvement will only approximate normal. The degree of that approximation is predictable at birth.

2. *Passive euthanasia.* Many physicians faced with an infant with a meningomyelocele wish that the problem would go away. However, it has been said that the problem does not go away; only the physician goes away. Even if these infants receive no treatment, a number of them will survive. Feeding, antibiotics, and care of the sac will each increase the quantity of survivors without affecting their quality. Figures on the natural history of untreated meningomyeloceles are difficult to find. One series suggests that 40% are stillborn or die within the first week of life. Forty percent of the survivors die by 2 months of age, another 30% die by 2 years of age, and 30% survive. Causes of death are not listed, but many of the late deaths are related to mental deterioration secondary to hydrocephalus and to renal deterioration secondary to the neurogenic bladder. Thus, lack of therapy results in fewer infants surviving, while still allowing the survival of a number of infants who are less functionally able to compete than if they had received therapy. Death may occur soon after birth, but for many death occurs weeks, months, or years later.

3. *Active euthanasia.* This solution to the problem has many moral objections and is presently illegal.

The quality of survival is of paramount importance and the preservation of existing function in the lower extremities requires early operation to close the spinal defect. Where a high lesion has produced complete paraplegia, early operation does little to improve the quality of survival, although treatment of hydrocephalus and the neurogenic bladder will require treatment at the appropriate time. While closure of the spinal defect takes precedence, evaluation of the hydrocephalus and of the renal and bladder status, and orthopedic consultation should all take place in the early weeks of life.

An infant born with a meningomyelocele should be transferred immediately to the care of a physician experienced in dealing with the problem. The decision on whether or not to operate on these infants requires the experience of someone who has worked with and followed the course of such infants. The techniques of closure and exploration of the sac may require both neurosurgeons and plastic surgeons, and an orthopedic surgeon may be needed at the initial operation to deal with spinal anomalies. Both survival itself and the quality of that survival may be determined during this neonatal period. After closure of the sac, the infant's course must be closely followed for the development of hydrocephalus. Hydrocephalus may cause bulging of the wound and its breakdown, as well as thinning of the cortex. Evaluation and shunting for hydrocephalus are discussed in the section on the enlarging head (p. 543). An intravenous pyelogram and voiding cystourethrogram should also be performed as soon as feasible in the neonatal period. Hydronephrosis may be present at birth, and urinary infection may be a continuing problem. It should be emphasized that the neonatal care of these infants is only the first step in the continuous, interdisciplinary, lifelong care that will be required.

Diastematomyelia

Diastematomyelia is a division of the spinal cord or roots by a bony spicule or fibrous or cartilaginous band that pierces the cord in an anteroposterior diameter. This lesion is often associated with a spina bifida occulta at one or more levels, and is usually accompanied by a cutaneous lesion such as a hemangioma, a patch of long, fine hair, a lipoma, or a dimple (Fig. 17-15).

At birth, there is no neurologic deficit associated with the diastematomyelia; but as the infant grows, the spinal cord is not able to ascend because of the bone. Traction on the spinal cord produces neurologic deficit. The deficit may range from persistent enuresis to a neurogenic bladder with hydronephrosis. Pain in the legs, weakness, or growth failure of a foot or leg may all be later manifestations. The cutaneous manifestations should suggest the diagnosis. Spine films show a spina bifida and usually show widening of the canal. A midline bony defect confirms the diagnosis. (Fig. 17-16). Infants with cutaneous lesions should be followed every 2 to 3 months, and a myelogram should be done if any neurologic deficit appears. Treatment consists of removal of the bony spicule and release of any tethering of the spinal cord. Operation is prophylactic rather than curative; an established neurologic deficit may be permanent.

Dermal sinuses and dermoids

Dermal sinuses may occur anywhere along the midline of the back or head but are most common in the occipital area of the skull and in the lumbar region. The sinus is 1 to 2 mm in diameter and may be accompanied by hemangioma or a tuft of hair. These sinuses are to be differentiated from the common superficial dimples seen at the upper end of the gluteal crease. The dermal sinus may extend variable depths into the skin and may continue into the intraspinal space. The sinus often passes unnoticed until it shows redness and swelling associated with infection or is carefully looked for in the patient with meningitis. Roentgenograms of the spine may show a spina bifida, and there may be widening of the spinal canal if an associated dermoid or lipoma is present. If a sinus is associated with meningitis or with superficial infection or if there is neurologic deficit, the sinus should be removed. Excision should follow the sinus tract to its end and should include laminectomy if there is intraspinal extension.

Lipomas

Lipomeningoceles are large, amorphous accumulations of fatty tissue beneath the

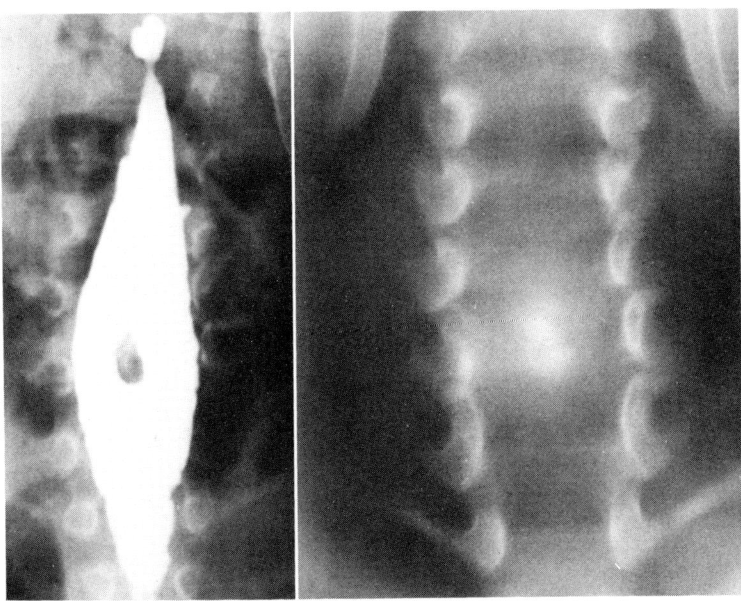

Fig. 17-16. Tomogram of the spine of an infant with diastematomyelia. The bony spur protruding through the spinal canal and widening of the canal at that area is shown. Myelogram of the same patient. The spinal cord split around the spur and re-fused. Same patient as in Fig. 17-15, bottom center. The patient was asymptomatic.

skin that may be associated with meningeal defects and may resemble meningomyeloceles. Smaller subcutaneous lipomas may be associated with spina bifida occulta. They may occur at any level of the subcutaneous tissue and may involve the cord itself. It is the intraspinal extensions of these lipomas that become neurologically significant. Widening of the spinal canal shown on a roentgenogram or the development of a neurologic defect suggests the intraspinal process. Operation is prophylactic, and, as in diastematomyelia, neurologic deficit may not be reversible. Therefore, these infants must be followed frequently and surgery performed at the earliest sign of neurologic involvement.

Encephaloceles

Encephalocele is the name given to cranial anomalies that are similar to the spina bifidas. The term includes craniomeningoceles, encephalomeningoceles, and cranium bifida. These lesions may occur anywhere along the midline of the head, including the nose, the nasopharynx, and the orbit, but are most common in the occipital area. It is usually not possible to determine the extent of brain involvement prior to surgery. The size of the lesion should not be a deterrant to surgery, since large lesions may be meningoceles, or small lesions may contain cerebral tissue. Roentgenograms of the defect and ventriculograms or pneumoencephalograms are indicated prior to surgery. Surgery should be undertaken as soon as feasible in the neonatal period to prevent infection and to facilitate care and feeding of the child. Operation is similar to that undertaken for the closure of the back in meningomyeloceles. These children should be evaluated for other structural anomalies of the cervical spine or back and should be followed closely in the postoperative period for the development of hydrocephalus.

ACUTE METABOLIC DISEASE

See also Chapter 14.

Acute metabolic disease in the neonatal period is uncommon, but its prompt recognition may determine the mental outcome of the infant or may even be lifesaving. The hallmark is the abrupt onset of lethargy, vomiting, and coma in a previously well infant. These findings are often accompanied by seizures. Onset may be in the first hours or days of life. This constellation of symptoms also suggests the diagnosis of sepsis, meningitis, or intracranial hemorrhage. Immediate evaluation of such an infant should include blood cultures and lumbar puncture. Urinalysis for acetonuria will often lead to the diagnosis of ketoacidosis found in many of the metabolic diseases. Ketoacidosis is uncommon in the first month of life, even with starvation, vomiting, or diarrhea. Its presence should, therefore, suggest the possibility of a metabolic disorder. Specific diagnosis requires the prompt performance of metabolic screening procedures and chromatography of serum and urinary amino acids. For some diseases, such as hyperammonemia, chromatography will be normal, and diagnosis requires specific testing. Acute therapy in most of these diseases consists of removal of protein from the diet and the administration of glucose and intravenous fluids while awaiting the diagnosis. Exchange transfusions may occasionally be lifesaving. A family history of siblings or relatives with acute neonatal disease should increase suspicion of a metabolic disorder. Detailed discussion of each of the metabolic disorders that may include seizures and other neurologic manifestations is found in Chapters 14, p. 408, and 15, p. 439.

PROGNOSIS OF NEUROLOGIC ABNORMALITIES IN THE NEWBORN

The neurologic examination of the newborn, if carefully done, is sensitive enough to detect minor abnormalities as well as gross disturbances in function. However, our current state of knowledge permits prognosis only where major CNS dysfunction is demonstrated. The long-term significance of most neurologic abnormalities in the newborn is unclear. This problem is shown in two studies. Parmalee found that three fourths of the premature babies who were considered to have abnormal neurologic examinations in the newborn period had either doubtful or normal examinations at 2 to 4 years of age. Prechtl found that three fourths of children with abnormal neurologic signs in the newborn period continued to have abnormal signs between 2 and 4 years of age. The discrepancy lies in the selection of patients and in the classification of what is abnormal, both in the newborn and at a later stage. In attempting to make a prognosis, one must distinguish between the SGA infant and the true premature. The SGA infant appears to have a considerably higher incidence of neurologic deficit than the true premature. Most of the previous studies of prognosis are of doubtful value, since no such distinction was made. Drillin now divides low birth weight infants into three groups: low birth weight caused by factors early in pregnancy, such as rubella or other infections; low birth weight caused by factors late in pregnancy, including infection, hemorrhage, and hypertension; and low birth weight without definable cause (true prematures). The types of abnormalities found in each group and the subsequent prognosis are considerably different. For example, the children with rubella early in pregnancy have a high incidence of multiple abnormalities, microcephaly, and retardation. Rubella occurring in the second trimester may produce no congenital abnormalities but may result in hearing loss or minimal cerebral dysfunction. Fetal malnutrition in the SGA babies may result in varying degrees of abnormalities of CNS development. The occurrence of insults at critical periods of CNS development may alter both the quality and quantity of CNS function. Schulte has demonstrated that infants born of toxemic mothers may have abnormalities in cortical-evoked responses and may show abnormalities of tone and strength. The significance of these abnormalities is unknown. Prechtl has shown that the hyperexcitable syndrome, which consists of tremulousness of the limbs, hyperkinesis, hypertonia, and hyperreflexia persisting beyond the fourth day of life, is often associated with the development of choreoathetosis. Apathetic babies with poor tone and reflexes and CNS depression also have a high incidence of future neurologic abnormalities. Asymmetrical abnormalities of reflexes, tone, and strength may be associated with hemiparesis; but often the hemiparesis will disappear with time, and subsequent learning disorders or retardation may become evident. The EEG has been used to indicate the prognosis of infants with seizures. However, except in the hands of sophisticated electroencephalographers, this tool is of doubtful value. Even more sophisticated testing with evoked responses may give clearer evidence of CNS function and prognosis. At the present time, one should be exceedingly careful about making prognostic statements on the basis of a single neurologic examination. Careful follow-up with repeated developmental and neurologic examinations is the only method of providing an accurate prognosis.

JOHN M. FREEMAN
EDWIN C. MYER

BIBLIOGRAPHY

Barwick, D. D., and Walton, J. N.: Polymyositis, Am. J. Med. **35**:646, 1963.

Bazelon, M., Paine, R. S., Cowie, V. A., and others: Reversal of hypotonia in infants with Down's syndrome by administration of 5-hydroxytryptophane, Lancet **1**:1130, 1967.

Bejsovec, M., Kulenoa, Z., and Ponca, E.: Familial intrauterine convulsions in pyridoxine dependency, Arch. Dis. Child. **42**:201, 1967.

Blattner, R. J.: Arthrogryposis multiplex congenita, J. Pediatr. **71**:367, 1967.

Cutler, R. W. P., and others: Formation and absorption of cerebrospinal fluid in man, Brain **91**:707, 1968.

DeLevie, M., and Nogrady, M. B.: Rapid brain growth upon restoration of adequate nutrition causing false radiologic evidence of increased intracranial pressure, J. Pediatr. **76**:523, 1970.

Dobbing, J.: Undernutrition and the developing brain, Am. J. Dis. Child. **20**:411, 1970.

Dodge, P. R., Gamstorp, I., Byers, R. K., and Russell, P.: Myotonic dystrophy in infancy and childhood, Pediatrics **35**:3, 1965.

Dodge, P. R., and Porter, P.: Demonstration of intracranial pathology by transillumination, Arch. Neurol. **5**:594, 1961.

Drillien, C. M.: Etiology and prognosis of small for date babies, Pediatr. Clin. North Am. **17**:9, 1970.

Dubowitz, L. M. S., Dubowitz, V., and Goldberg, C.: Clinical assessment of gestational age in the newborn, J. Pediatr. **77**:1, 1970.

Dubowitz, V.: The floppy infant, Clinics in Developmental Medicine, No. 31, London, 1969, William Heinemann, Ltd.

Dubowitz, V.: Infantile muscular atrophy, Brain **87**:707, 1964.

Freeman, J. M.: Neonatal seizures; diagnosis and management, J. Pediatr. **77**:701, 1970.

Freeman, J. M., editor: A practical approach to the problems of meningomyeloceles, Baltimore, 1972, University Park Press.

Freeman, J. M., and Borkowf, S.: Craniostenosis, Pediatr. **30**:57, 1962.

Gilles, F. H., and Shillito, J.: Infantile hydrocephalus; retrocerebellar subdural hemotoma, J. Pediatr. **76**:529, 1970.

Gold, A. P., Ransohoff, J., and Carter, S.: Vein of

Galen malformation, Acta Neurol. Scand. **40** (Suppl. 11):1, 1964.

Harcke, H. T., Jr., and others: Perinatal cerebral intraventricular hemorrhage, J. Pediatr. **80**:37, 1972.

Haworth, J. C., and Zachary, R. B.: Congenital dermal sinuses in children; their relationship to Pilonidal sinus, Lancet **2**:10, 1955.

Illingworths, R. S.: The development of the infant and young child; normal and abnormal, ed. 4, Baltimore, 1970, The Williams & Wilkins Co., p. 117.

James, A. E., and others: CSF imaging (cisternography) in pediatric patients, Ann. Radiol. (Paris) **14**:591, 1971.

Johnson, R. T., and Johnson, K. P.: Hydrocephalus as a sequela of experimental mixoviruses, Exp. Mol. Pathol. **10**:68, 1969.

Knobloch, H., and others: Prognostic and etiologic factors in hypoglycemia, J. Pediatr. **70**:876, 1967.

Landau, W. M.: Spasticity and rigidity, Recent Adv. in Neurol. **6**:1, 1969.

Laurence, K. M.: The survival of untreated spina bifida cystica, Dev. Med. Child Neurol. Suppl. **2**:10, 1966.

Laurence, K. M., and Coates, S.: The natural history of hydrocephalus, Arch. Dis. Child. **37**:345, 1962.

Lorber, J.: Medical and surgical aspects in the treatment of congenital hydrocephalus, Neuropaediatric **2**:239, 1971.

Lorber, J.: The prognosis of encephalocele, Dev. Med. Child Neurol. **13**(Suppl.):75, 1967.

Lorber, J.: Results of treatment of myelomeningocele, Dev. Med. Child Neurol. **13**:279, 1971.

Lorber, J., and Zachary, R. B.: Primary congenital hydrocephalus, Arch. Dis. Child. **43**:516, 1968.

Martin, H. P.: Microcephaly and mental retardation, Am. J. Dis. Child. **119**:128, 1970.

Millichap, J. G., and Dodge, P. R.: Myasthenia gravis, Neurology (Minneap.) **10**:1007, 1960.

Morris-Jones, P. H., Houston, I. B., and Evans, R. C.: Prognosis of the neurologic complication of acute hypernatremia, Lancet **2**:1385, 1967.

Padget, D. H.: Spina bifida and embryonic neuroschisis; a causal relationship, Johns Hopkins Med. J. **123**:233, 1968.

Paine, R. S.: The future of the "floppy infant"; a follow-up study of 133 patients, Dev. Med. Child Neurol. **5**:115, 1963.

Parmalee, A. H., and others: Neurological evaluation of the premature infant, Biol. Neonat. **15**: 65, 1970.

Paunier, L., and others: Primary hypomagnesemia with secondary hypocalcemia in an infant, Pediatrics **41**:385, 1968.

Prechtl, H.: Prognostic values of neurological signs, Proc. R. Soc. Med. **58**:3, 1965.

Prechtl, H., and Beintema, D.: The neurological examination of the full term newborn infants, Clinics in Developmental Medicine, No. 12, London, 1964, National Spastics Society.

Prichard, J. S.: The character and significance of epileptic seizures in infancy. In Kellaway, P., and Petersen, I., editors: Neurologic and encephalographic correlative studies in infancy, New York, 1964, Grune & Stratton, Inc., p. 273.

Rabe, E. F.: The hypotonic infant, J. Pediatr. **64**: 422, 1964.

Rabe, E. F.: Subdural effusion in infants, Pediatr. Clin. North Am. **14**:831, 1967.

Rose, A. L., and Lombroso, C. T.: Neonatal seizure states, Pediatrics **45**:404, 1970.

Scarf, J. E.: Treatment of hydrocephalus; an historical and critical review of methods and results, J. Neurol. Neurosurg. Psychiatry **26**:1, 1963.

Schick, R. W., and Matson, D. D.: What is arrested hydrocephalus, J. Pediatr. **58**:791, 1961.

Schulte, F., and others: Maternal toxemia, fetal malnutrition and motor behavior in newborn, Pediatrics **48**:871, 1971.

Schulte, F. J., and Schwenzel, W.: Motor control and muscle tone in the newborn period; electromyographic studies, Biol. Neonat. **8**:198, 1965.

Shillito, J., and Matson, D. D.: Craniosynostosis, Pediatrics **41**:829, 1968.

Shulman, S. T., and others: Transection of the spinal cord, Arch. Dis. Child. **46**:291, 1971.

Sieben, R. L., Hamida, M. B., and Shulman, K.: Multiple cranial nerve deficits associated with the Arnold-Chiari malformations, Neurology (Minneap.) **21**:673, 1971.

Smith, B. T., and Masotti, R. E.: Intravenous diazepam in the treatment of prolonged seizure activity in neonates and infants, Dev. Med. Child Neurol. **13**:630, 1971.

Taksuji, N., Brown, B., and Brob, D.: Neonatal myasthenia gravis, Pediatrics **45**:488, 1970.

Tasker, W., and Chutorian, A. M.: Chronic polyneuritis of childhood, J. Pediatr. **74**:699, 1969.

Thomas, A., and Dargassies, S. A.: The neurologic examination of the infant, Little Club Clinics in Developmental Medicine, No. 1, London, 1960, National Spastics Society.

Towbin, A.: The central nervous system damage in human fetus and newborn infant, Am J. Dis. Child. **119**:529, 1970.

Towbin, A.: Central nervous system damage in the premature related to the occurrence of mental retardation in physical trauma as an etiological agent. In Angle, C. R., and Bering, E. A., editors: Mental retardation, Washington, D. C., 1970, U. S. Government Printing Office, p. 213.

Towbin, A.: Cerebral intraventricular hemorrhage and subependymal matrix infarction in the fetus and premature newborn, Am. J. Pathol. **52**:121, 1968.

Zellweger, H., and others: Severe congenital muscular dystrophy, Am. J. Dis. Child. **114**:591. 1967.

18 Special management of craniofacial problems*

Craniofacial malformations constitute a special category of birth defects. The malformation may be life threatening if it affects respiration or deglutition. The condition may prevent normal growth and, if untreated, can produce secondary defects, as in premature cranial synostoses. If the organs of speech and hearing are malformed, the patient's most human ability, to communicate by speech, is jeopardized. A defect of the face is not only a somatic problem but soon becomes a social problem because of the premium placed on facial appearance. All of these factors make the infant significantly different to his parents from the normal child almost at birth.

In the first hours after the birth of an infant with a craniofacial defect, the attending physician who is himself usually disturbed by the malformation finds that he must quickly attend to the immediate needs of the infant and to the needs of the anxious and profoundly upset parents. The physician who ordinarily may see few, if any, similar cases in his practice is faced with the concurrent problems of identification of the malformation and clinical management of respiratory and feeding problems. The physician must also assume a continuing role, with an obligation to become sufficiently informed and skilled, as an ombundsman for the infant with a birth defect and his family from the first hours of life through the ultimate course of habilitation that may involve several disciplines. What is done for the infant in the perinatal period and the counsel that is given to his parents may have long-term consequences for the future of the patient.

*This work was supported in part by a grant from the National Institutes of Health (DE-2872) and Maternal and Child Health Services, Department of Health, Education, and Welfare.

OVERVIEW OF BIRTH DEFECTS

Incidence of malformations

The accuracy of reports on the frequency of malformations as a percentage of total birth figures is dependent on a definition of what constitutes a malformation, the experience of the examiner, and other factors. In a follow-up study Babbott and Ingalls reported that only about 60% of malformed live babies had a malformation noted on their birth certificates. Underreporting of malformations can be ascribed to inexperienced examiners, the conditions under which examinations of the newborn are performed, or the physician's desire to spare the infant and the family any stigma.

Deficiencies in reporting on birth certificates are both quantitative and qualitative. Meskin and Pruzansky found that only 70.6% of the three major facial cleft types were reported at birth. Cleft lip in combination with cleft palate was reported most frequently (86%), whereas isolated cleft palate, a less striking defect, was reported least often (52%). In the latter category, the subtype of incomplete cleft of the soft palate was reported on the birth certificate in only 14% of the cases that were referred to a cleft palate clinic in subsequent years.

Figures derived from birth and death certificates are not uniform, since the frequency of malformations vary depending on the populations studied. Based on evaluation in the newborn period by teams of pediatricians, roentgenologists, and pathologists, McIntosh and associates estimated a malformation incidence of 3.2%. Nishimura and associates studied embryos aborted for social reasons and found that certain malformations were 10 times more frequent among them than in newborn infants. Stevenson reported that more than half of aborted fetuses are grossly abnormal. The frequency of chromosomal abnormalities in tissues of spontaneous abortions was 22%, an incidence 50 times that in live-born infants. The incidence of malformations in stillborns has been estimated as 17% to 20%. Malformation rates among infants dying in the perinatal period are much higher than among survivors. Among children dying unexpectedly in early life, approximately 18% die of congenital malformations. The incidence of anomalies in multiple births is 3 times that in the general population.

Oral-facial clefts rank among the more common congenital malformations. Cleft lip with or without cleft palate occurs in about 1 (range, 0.6 to 1.3) per 1,000 Caucasian births. The incidence is higher in Orientals and lower among black persons. Genetically and in other respects, isolated cleft palate seems to be a separate entity from cleft lip with or without cleft palate. The incidence of isolated cleft palate among Caucasians and black persons is between 1 per 2,000 and 1 per 2,500. Cleft uvula, an incomplete form of cleft palate, has an incidence of 1 per 80 Caucasians, with a higher frequency in American Indians and Orientals (1 in 10) but a lower frequency in black persons (1 in 300). Similar statistics are not available for the other malformations considered in this chapter.

Etiology

Among the first questions asked by the parents of an infant with congenital malformation are: "Why did this happen?" and "will it happen again?" To help the physician cope with this complex problem some general, though brief, comments on etiology are in order. Based on the present state of knowledge, it is now recognized that development involves a continuous interaction between genes and environmental factors. In the case of a single mutant gene, the major cause of malformations is genetic; for example, the dominantly inherited trait brachydactyly. Conversely, an extrinsic factor such as a teratogenic drug, thalidomide, can also be a primary cause. Yet in both cases it is recognized that mutant genes can be modified by environmental factors, and genetic factors can alter the response to extrinsic insults.

Table 18-1 is a list of some of the drugs implicated as teratogens. This list emphasizes the importance of the antenatal history as a guide to neonatal complications. Women in the first trimester of pregnancy should take no drugs unless clearly needed for the health of the mother or the future child or both. Factors other than drugs are also known to be harmful to the fetus. Maternal infections such as rubella, toxoplasmosis, and cytomegalic inclusion disease often go unrecognized in the mother but can cause extensive damage to the fetus. Radiation is capable of arresting development and producing malformations. The risks probably rise sharply with the dose. Rugh advocates termination of pregnancy if 25 rads or more have been received by the conceptus between the third and eighth postconception weeks. Single radiographic exposures of a fetus from 3 months onward are associated with an increase in the frequency of childhood leukemia and probably with other neoplasms.

The status of knowledge regarding the etiology and the basis for genetic counseling concerning the special clinical entities included in this chapter are discussed separately.

Significance of associated malformations

The presence of one developmental abnormality should alert the pediatrician to search for associated malformations. Certain clusters of malformations within a region of the body are recognized. Microtia, for example, may be associated with malformations of the temporal bone, facial bones, facial nerve, and oropharyngeal structures. Identification of such constellations is important in the organization of the sequence of care and treatment for the malformation.

The findings of low-set, rotated, or malformed ears, excess posterior skin, abnormal dermatoglyphics, or involvement of numerous systems suggest chromosomal aberration. The statistically higher frequency

TABLE 18-1. Recognized fetal and neonatal effects of maternal medication

Maternal medication	Fetal or neonatal effect
Quinine	Thrombocytopenia
Bishydroxycoumarin (Dicumarol)	Fetal bleeding and death
Antithyroid drugs	Neonatal goiter
Vitamin K analogues	Jaundice and kernicterus
Sulfonamides	Kernicterus
Novobiocin	Hyperbilirubinemia
Narcotics	Neonatal convulsions and tremors, death
Reserpine	Nasal congestion, drowsiness, death
Hexamethonium bromide	Neonatal ileus
Thiazides	Thrombocytopenia with or without agranulocytosis
Anticonvulsants	? Cleft palate
Lysergic acid diethylamide (LSD)	? Abnormal development of extremities, chromosomal breaks
Thalidomide	Extremities, eye, ear, cerebrovascular, gastrointestinal, and genitourinary abnormalities
6MP Bulsulfon Busulfan (Myleran) Chlorambucil	Suppression of cellular metabolism and proliferation Multiple anomalies and abortions
Testosterone Progesterone Diethylstilbestrol	Musculinization Adenocarcinoma of the vagina of offspring
Cortisone Hydrocortisone Adrenocorticotropic hormone (ACTH)	Cleft palate
Phenmetrazine hydrochloride (Preludin)	? Diaphragmatic hernia
Tetracycline	Deposition in bone Inhibition of bone growth in premature infants Discoloration of teeth
Chloramphenicol	Death (gray matter syndrome)
Streptomycin	? Eighth nerve deafness
Chloroquine	Retinal damage
Vitamin D	? Idiopathic hypercalcemia

of cardiac malformations and facial clefts suggests the need for careful patient evaluation.

Single minor malformations

It has been estimated that 14% of newborn babies have a single minor malformation detectable by surface examination. These minor external malformations are most common in areas of complex and variable features such as the face, auricles, hands, and feet. These minor variants are also frequently associated with specific syndromes so that when observed, they may lead to erroneous diagnosis and consequent family anxiety. *Inner epicanthic folds* of varying degree are found in 30% of Caucasian babies during the first 3 years of life. Some families show this trait as a single entity in more than one generation.

Brushfield's spots are found in about 20% of normal newborn babies, compared with 80% of babies with Down's syndrome. *Slanted and low-set ears* with underdeveloped helices are not unusual in the premature infant. Darwinian tubercles are a very frequent finding. *A unilateral single upper palmar simian crease* is found in about 4% of normal Caucasians, and it is present on both palms in less than 1% of normal individuals. *A single crease on a short incurved fifth digit* is of little significance if present alone. Other examples are saddle nose with an upturned tip (retroussé nose), mild to moderate inbowing of the lower limbs with tibial torsion, mild syndactyly of the second and third toes, toenail hypoplasia, and hydrocele of the testicles. These findings are all common in the newborn. When a single minor abnormality is found during examination of a newborn, it is of prime importance to look at the other members of the family before ascribing any serious significance to it. The recurrence of a minor defect in that family and its presence in numerous members of the family may diminish its importance and significance.

Types of malformations and rationale for care

Craniofacial malformation can be a threat to survival in the neonatal period or may seriously impede normal growth and development in subsequent years. Certain craniofacial malformations such as micrognathia (Pierre Robin syndrome) and choanal atresia affect the vital functions of respiration and feeding and are life-threatening in the immediate newborn period. Other malformations, such as craniostenosis, are also life threatening, but in the later stages of development.

In planning treatment and in counseling the family, one should know something about the natural history of the clinical entity. Some conditions improve in time, some grow worse, and some will not be changed. In the Pierre Robin syndrome, if the infant can survive the immediate postnatal threat of respiratory and feeding difficulties, the prognosis for continued growth of the jaws and for resolution of the symptoms and facial deformity is excellent. In view of this favorable outlook, plastic surgery to correct the micrognathia in childhood is unwarranted. In contrast, certain types of craniostenosis if untreated will grow worse in time, resulting in increased intracranial pressure, mental retardation, and blindness. Early recognition and surgical intervention are, therefore, crucial. A third pattern in which no substantial change occurs with time is demonstrated in mandibulofacial dysostosis. In such instances, elective surgical reconstruction may be undertaken during the earlier school years to facilitate the child's acceptance and improve his self-image.

Family's reaction

The birth of an infant with a malformation precipitates an immediate and continuing stress for the family. The long-term effect of this experience on the psychodynamics of the family is coming under increasing scrutiny by behavioral scientists. Part of the immediate problem may stem from the failure of professional personnel to recognize the unspoken fears and nebulous anxieties experienced by the family. In part this results from the transfer of care from obstetrician to pediatrician or family physician and then to the specialist, such as the plastic surgeon. The obstetrician may be the first to inform the parents about the malformation. He may minimize the deformity or leave the fuller explanation to the pediatrician, since the obstetrician will not be the infant's primary physician and often does not have complete medical information about the infant's present and future condition. The pediatrician, on the other hand, may never bring up the subject of the parents' initial reaction on the assumption that the problem has already been discussed with the obstetrician. Although there may not be a time lapse between the transfer from obstetrical to pediatric care, there may be a large void centering around the psychologic impact of this birth, which is not filled by either physician.

When the baby is finally turned over to him, the pediatrician may feel that he should not take responsibility for the discussion of the parents' emotional response, but that the responsibility should be relegated rightfully to the psychiatrically oriented specialists, who have had a wide exposure to this particular patient population. There is a valid argument against this reasoning. The emotional reaction of the parents is a critical one in the future family structure, but in no sense an abnormal one. The parents' reaction is a natural, human reaction to tragedy, no different from that in response to profound illness or death, with which the physician knows he must rightfully deal. If their emotional reaction is discussed openly and faced promptly, a rational basis for continued and reinforced counseling may be established that may preclude the development of more complex problems. In addition, although the infant's physician may turn to specialists in a center for the treatment of craniofacial malformations for advice and consultation, he should remain the advocate for the infant in the continuing relationship with the clinic's diagnostic and therapeutic procedures. In this relationship, he maintains responsibility for both routine and acute medical matters. He will observe the growth and development of the child in the environment of his home, school, and community.

If the pediatrician is the first to talk with the parents, he must consider how and when to tell the father and when to show the infant to him, how to plan with the father about when and how to tell the mother, and when to show the infant to the mother. The pediatrician should hold the infant, showing acceptance and concern. If the pediatrician and the mother look at the baby together, he can often get clues about what is most disturbing to the mother about the malformation. At some time after the immediate newborn period, but before much time has passed, the pediatrician should explain the meaning of facial disfigurement to the family and should encourage the parents, particularly the mother, to grieve and mourn the loss of the image of the anticipated perfect child. These observations and those throughout the early days of the infant's life may indicate to the physician the factors that shape the family's trauma or that lead to the family's adaptive responses. At this time, a detailed examination of the infant to rule out the presence of other malformation helps to define the extent of the infant's defect to the parents.

MEDICAL MANAGEMENT OF CRANIOFACIAL ANOMALIES

Only a few of many craniofacial malformations are discussed in detail in this section. The principles of management, however, can be applied to all malformations of the oral-facial-pharyngeal area. The treatment, and occasionally even the diagnosis, of a visible malformation requires attention over years. This chapter deals with problems occurring only in the neonatal period. The following conditions are discussed in detail: choanal atresia, the Pierre Robin syndrome (micrognathia), cleft lip and palate, malformations of the tongue (aglossia, microglossia, macroglossia, and ankyloglossia), and neonatal teeth.

Choanal atresia

See also p. 373.

The most common congenital abnormality of the nasal passages is choanal atresia, which may be complete or incomplete, and unilateral or bilateral. The incidence of choanal atresia is not known, since unilateral involvement is not life threatening and is not detected. Although the majority of the cases are sporadic, a few familial cases have been reported. The findings of two cases of concordant twins and of one family with unilateral choanal atresia in three consecutive generations suggest a genetic component.

Pathology. The obstructing membrane is a vestigial structure that usually begins to disappear at the end of the fifth week of intrauterine life. If the atresia is anterior to the choana, it is usually bony, the remnants of the vestigial structure or the bucconasal membrane. If the atresia is posterior, at the choanal orifice, it is usually membranous, derived from the buccopharyngeal membrane.

Clinical presentation. When only one side is affected, the infant usually does not have severe symptoms at birth. If both sides are blocked by a membrane or bony septum, the infant may suffer from severe asphyxia immediately after birth and may succumb from suffocation (p. 65). The same condition does not produce the same symptoms in all infants, since most, but not all, normal newborn infants are obligatory nose-breathers. The infants with bilateral choanal atresia who are unable to mouth-breathe will make vigorous attempts to inspire with a sucking action of the lips and will become cyanotic very soon after birth. As a routine matter, the examination of every newborn infant should demonstrate the patency of the choanae by insertion of a catheter with ease for a distance of 3 to 4 cm, first into one nostril and then into the other ventromedially along the floor of the nose to the nasopharynx. The instillation via catheter of a radiopaque material into each nostril while the infant is in the supine position may occasionally be necessary to outline the nasal cavity and position of the block radiographically.

The infant with bilateral choanal atresia who is able to mouth-breathe at once will experience difficulty only when sucking and swallowing and, therefore, will become cyanotic when he attempts to nurse. Additional clues in the newborn infant that aid in detection of bilateral choanal atresia are persistent breathing through the mouth, cyanosis when the mouth is closed, and return to normal color when the infant cries. Unilateral atresia will usually be asymptomatic in the newborn unless an upper respiratory tract infection occurs, with profuse unilateral nasal discharge.

Treatment. If bilateral choanal atresia is present, an airway must be promptly provided. In an emergency situation in the delivery room or in the newborn nursery, the pediatrician should either prop the jaws open with a suitable device or introduce an airway device into the nasopharynx. Once the airway through the mouth is established, the infant can be fed by gavage until he learns to breathe, as well as eat, without the assisted airway. This adaptation usually requires 2 or 3 weeks (normal babies are obligatory nose-breathers for 2 to 3 months). With this regimen, operation can be delayed for weeks, months, or even years. Immediate surgical intervention for bilateral choanal atresia has been advocated by others.

Pierre Robin syndrome

The infant with the Pierre Robin syndrome presents both an immediate and a relatively prolonged management problem for the physician and nursing staff during the neonatal period. Low birth weight is common, and mortality is high.

Most cases of the Pierre Robin syndrome are sporadic, but more than one familial case has been reported. An isolated sign, such as micrognathia or cleft palate, has been reported in parents. It has been suggested that the distribution of cases in families is compatible with dominant inheritance showing variable expressivity and reduced penetrance. However, suggestions such as irregularly dominant, polygenic, multifactorial, or even autosomal recessive inheritance have not been ruled out.

Pathology. The pathophysiology of the syndrome can be related to the small mandible, which in turn produces a glossoptosis with resultant obstruction or constriction of the airway, cyanosis, and feeding difficulty. The intrusion of the tongue into the nasal cavity, as well as its displacement posteriorly into the pharyngeal airway, can obstruct the nasal and pharyngeal passage. Although cleft palate is not included as a characteristic in some series of patients reported in the literature, the abnormal distal and superior displacement of the tongue (Fig. 18-1), characteristic of this syndrome, is usually dependent on the presence of a cleft palate.

It is significant that other forms of micrognathia, such as that observed in mandibulofacial dysostosis and hemifacial microsomia, do not as a rule present similar obstructive problems. The possibility of feeding and respiratory difficulties in such cases, however, should not be discounted, and alertness for these problems should be maintained during the perinatal period.

Etiology. Early mandibular hypoplasia, before 9 weeks' gestation, may be the primary defect in this syndrome. Since the buccal cavity is small because of the small mandible, the tongue must rest posteriorly in the mouth and thereby impair the closure of the posterior palatal shelves that ordinarily grow over the tongue mass to meet in the midline.

Clinical presentation. The appearance of the infant with the Pierre Robin syndrome is striking (Fig. 18-2). The infant is often small and cyanotic and makes marked respiratory efforts. The face appears bird-like. The signs and symptoms of children with the Pierre Robin syndrome may range from clinically normal to mild to severe respiratory or feeding difficulties or both. The frequency of respiratory difficulty and feeding problems with consequent failure to thrive is not known, since the patients with milder symptoms escape undetected.

Associated defects encountered in the

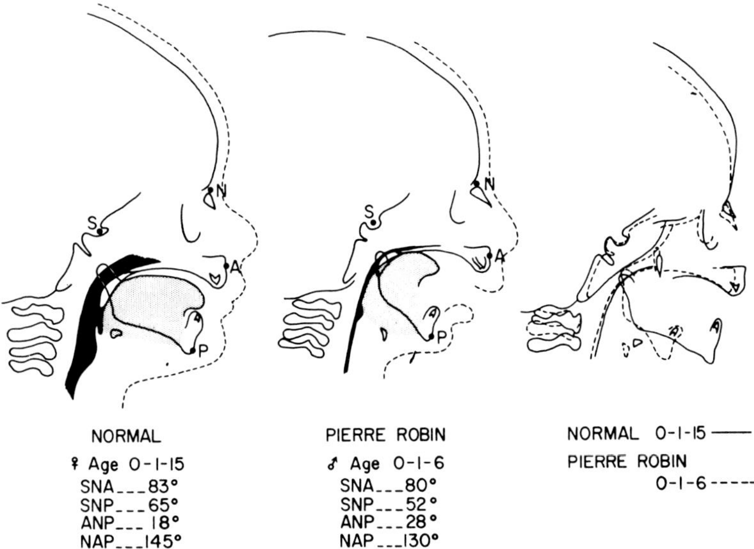

Fig. 18-1. Tracings of lateral cephalometric radiographs demonstrating a normal infant (age 1 month and 15 days), an infant with the Pierre Robin syndrome (age 1 month and 6 days), and the tracings of the two superimposed on the cranial base. Note the difference in the size of the airway shown in black. In the Pierre Robin syndrome, the airway is reduced by the glossoptosis in which the tongue is retruded backward and upward, obstructing the nasopharyngeal space. The superimposed tracings demonstrate that the primary skeletal difference resides in the reduced size of the mandible in the Pierre Robin syndrome. Anthropometric measures of the facial skeletal profile are appended.

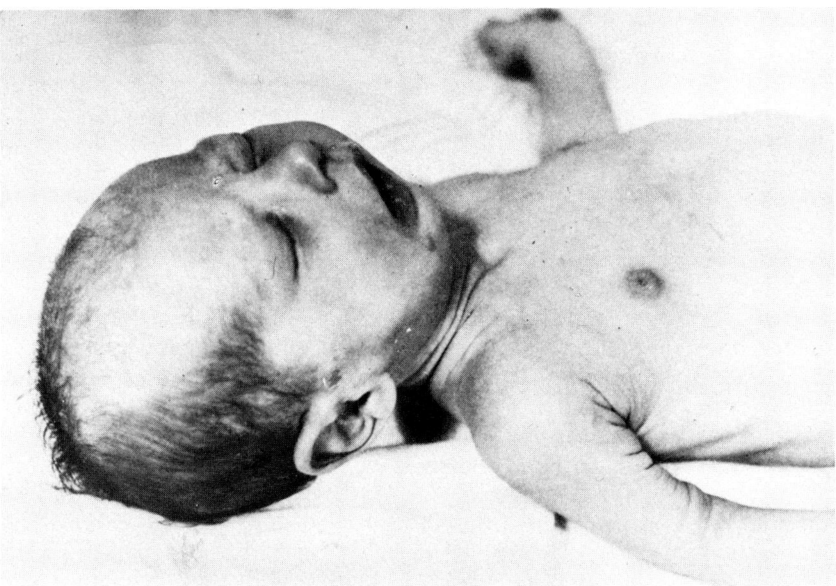

Fig. 18-2. Three-month-old infant with Pierre Robin syndrome. The bird-like appearance with micrognathia is evident. The infant is emaciated. There is suprasternal and intercostal retraction.

Pierre Robin syndrome involve the cardiovascular system, the central nervous system, the ears, the eyes, and the extremities. As is true when any single malformation is discovered, the child with the Pierre Robin syndrome merits a meticulous examination for associated malformations.

Management problems. The main problem, usually noted at birth, is the *obstruction of the pharyngeal airway* by the glossoptotic tongue, causing episodes of cyanosis, with difficulty breathing and swallowing. The airway obstruction, more marked during inspiration, usually requires treatment in order to avoid suffocation or central nervous system damage caused by hypoxic episodes. *Feeding* is difficult because of the posterior position of the balled tongue in the throat. The introduction of milk further obstructs the airway, making it even more difficult for the baby to breathe, which adds to the danger of aspiration. For reasons not clearly understood, some of these infants vomit excessively. Because of poor oral intake, frequent emesis, and chronic exhaustion from respiratory effort, these infants, who generally start life below average in weight, do not grow or gain steadily in the first months of life. *Cor pulmonale* resulting from hypoventilation caused by upper airway obstruction, as observed in children with hypertrophied tonsils and adenoids, has been reported in the Pierre Robin syndrome. Signs of cor pulmonale may include: (1) noisy, stertorous respiration and stridor when the infant is in the supine position, (2) intermittent somnolence, (3) pulmonary hypertension, (4) right heart failure, (5) ECG changes of right atrial and right ventricular hypertrophy and strain, (6) arterial hypoxia and hypercapnia, and (7) radiographic findings of cardiomegaly, dilatation of the pulmonary artery, and often pulmonary edema.

There is a wide spectrum of variation within the syndrome. Some patients have severe respiratory obstruction; in others, the severity is complicated by associated malformations; in many the course is relatively moderate to mild, with only occasional respiratory embarrassment. The severity of the respiratory and feeding problem can be roughly related to the degree of mandibular hypoplasia, tongue size, and airway obstruction as visualized on the lateral radiographic projection.

Treatment. The infant with the Pierre Robin syndrome should be placed in a special care nursery unit as soon as possible. The interval between birth and intensive monitoring of the infant may be critical in avoiding brain damage or death. The major and continuing problems of *respiratory complications* and *feeding difficulties* require the coordinated collaboration of the pediatrician with the nursing staff, as well as with various specialists.

As soon as *respiratory distress* is recognized, the infant should be placed in the prone (or partially prone) position so that his tongue falls forward and obstruction of the airway is relieved. He should always be kept in the prone position and suctioned frequently, if necessary. His respirations should be monitored closely, with an apnea monitor if available. If the baby's distress is not relieved sufficiently by these simple measures, other steps should be taken to ensure an adequate airway. Occasionally, the insertion of a Berman airway will keep the tongue from falling backward. Additional treatment may be necessary, such as suturing the ventral surface of the tongue to the lower lip temporarily (Beverly Douglas procedure, which pulls the tongue forward). Descriptions of numerous splints and traction devices have appeared in the literature; none, however, has been widely accepted or very useful.

The infant in moderate to severe respiratory distress should be monitored by frequent blood gas studies of the Po_2 and Pco_2. Hypercapnea, indicated by elevated Pco_2, is an early indication of respiratory obstruction. Arterial pH above 7.3, Po_2 in the range of 50 to 80 mm Hg, and Pco_2 in the range of 30 to 40 mm Hg usually indicate adequate ventilation. For emergency use an infant laryngoscope and endotracheal tube, a tongue suture kit, and tracheostomy set should be at the infant's bedside at all times. All of the infants with the Pierre Robin syndrome, whether in mild or severe respiratory distress, should have radiographs of the nasal and cervical airway for a proper evaluation. The physician dealing with the newborn should acquaint himself with the appearance of the size of the mouth, nose, pharynx, and larynx of an infant.

If at all possible, *tracheostomy* should be avoided, since clinical observation of infants who have undergone this procedure suggests that they may do very poorly on a long-range basis. There are situations, however, in which a tracheostomy is necessary to save the infant's life. Two clear indications are unrelieved upper airway obstruction and inability to control secretions. Severe respiratory tract infection may cause these complications. Other indications are unsuccessful trial of less traumatic procedures; the presence of an additional medical problem, such as severe cardiac or central nervous system disease caused by an associated malformation; the progressive development of significant hypoxia or hypercapnia; and severe feeding difficulties with repeated episodes of aspiration. Delay in performing a tracheostomy, when there are clear indications for the procedure, results in causing the infant increased debilitation, leading to further airway obstruction, and more hypoxic episodes, which may lead to central nervous system damage and possibly to death. The tracheostomy should be performed in the operating room with the airway previously established either by an endotracheal tube or a bronchoscope. It is imperative that the infant remain in the intensive care unit after the procedure. After the tracheostomy is performed, the infant must have constant, attentive nursing care, continual tracheal toilet, and close observation of vital signs. A roentgenogram of the neck and chest should be obtained immediately after the procedure to determine the exact location of the tube and to detect the presence of mediastinal emphysema or pneumothorax.

If a child with micrognathia, either isolated or as part of any syndrome, requires a surgical procedure for some other associated condition, special attention to anesthesia and airway management is mandatory, since such patients are difficult to intubate.

Feeding problems and consequent failure to thrive are the other major sources of difficulty in the first days of life in the infant with the Pierre Robin syndrome. Feeding of infants with mandibular hypoplasia requires great patience and much time. Usually, the infant can be fed in the prone position or supported in an upright position and fed with a lamb's nipple, a winged nipple, or "premie" nipple (Fig. 18-3). The Takagi feeding method, using a curved bottle with a lamb's nipple is designed especially for the prone position (Fig. 18-4). According to proponents, once feeding in the prone position is accomplished, the infants show rapid and progressive improvement in oral and pharyngeal function and develop compensatory posture of tongue and related structures so as to maintain an adequate pharyngeal airway in the variety of head and neck postures. The necessary period of maintaining the prone feeding procedure is, consequently, relatively short.

When the infant is fed in the upright position, the airway can be improved and

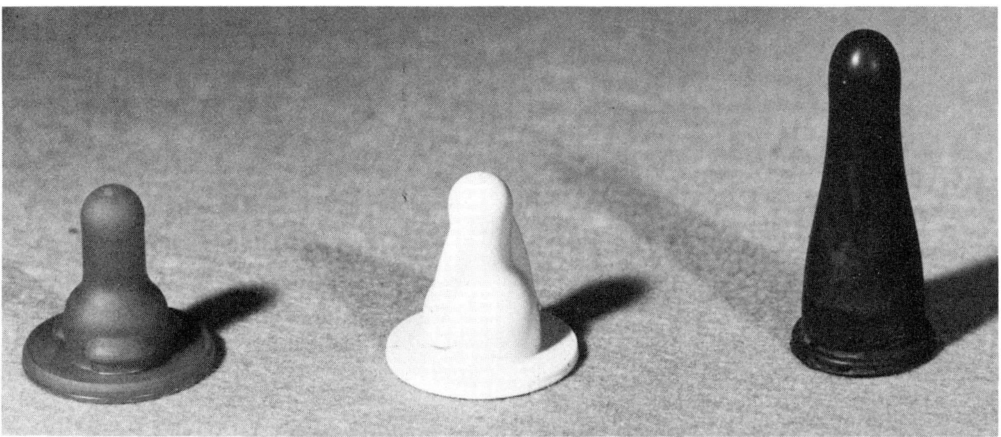

Fig. 18-3. Types of nipples used for feeding the infant with the Pierre Robin syndrome. The nipple on the left is a "premie" nipple. A winged nipple is in the middle. On the right is a lamb's nipple.

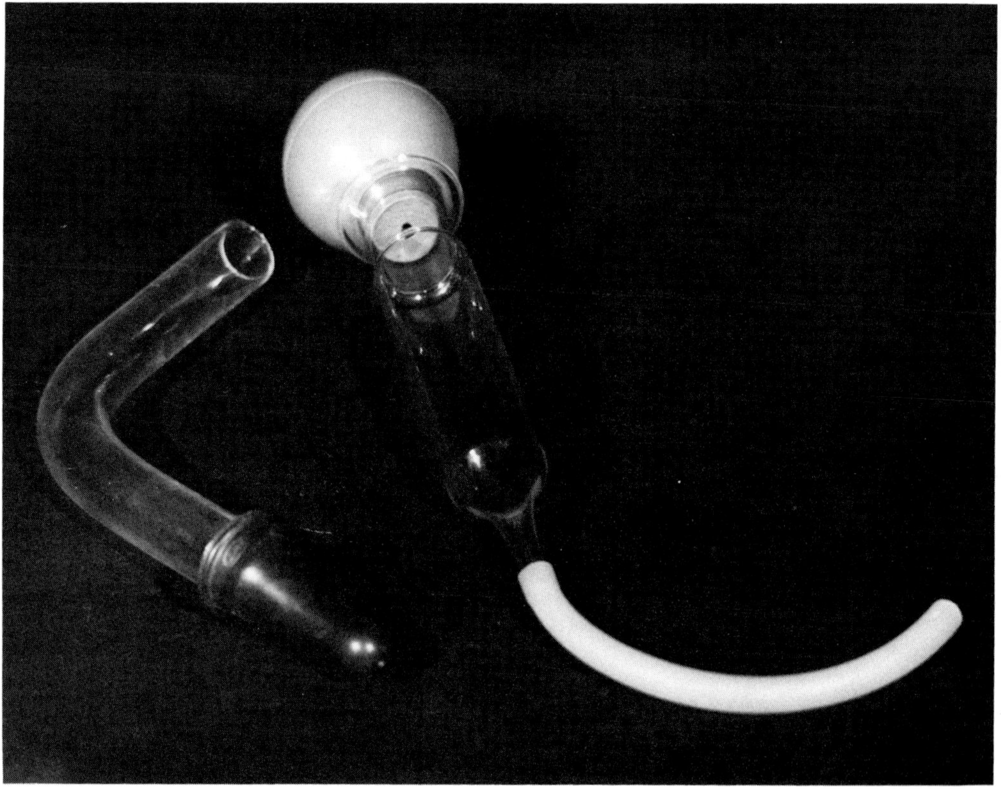

Fig. 18-4. Feeding devices employed for infants with Pierre Robin syndrome. Left, the Takagi curved bottle with a lamb's nipple. Right, a syringe with curved rubber tubing.

feeding made easier if the mandible is pushed forward by the thumb and index finger on both angles. If these feeding measures are unsuccessful, the nursing and medical staff may have to resort to feeding by gavage or even by gastrostomy tube. Formulas of increased caloric value can be used for these infants who have so much difficulty taking even small amounts.

A third, but much less frequent, complication is *cor pulmonale.* This cause of heart failure in children can be permanently cured by removal of the airway obstruction as discussed above.

Prognosis. If the infants can be assisted to breathe and feed in the early days and months of life, growth of the mandible will progress so that the tongue can rest in the usual position by 3 or 4 months of age. An essentially normal profile is achieved by 4 to 6 years of age, although the mandible has distinctive characteristics that are present on x-ray examination even in adulthood.

Cleft lip and palate

Cleft palate is a complex anomaly that may affect oral functions such as feeding, deglutition, and respiration. Since the function of speech, one of the most human functions, is an acquired skill overlaid on basic oral-pharyngeal acts, its development may be impaired or delayed by a malformation affecting labial-oral structures and velopharyngeal valving. Infants with cleft palate are also more susceptible to middle ear dysfunction and to associated malformations of craniofacial and other organ and tissue systems.

Etiology. Fogh-Andersen was the first to suggest that cleft lip with or without cleft palate was a genetically different malformation from isolated cleft palate. Children with isolated cleft palate weigh less at birth and have a higher frequency of associated malformations than do children with cleft lip and palate. The sex distribution also varies in that males predominate in the cleft lip and palate group while the frequency of

TABLE 18-2. Approximate risk of recurrence of cleft lip and cleft palate

		Risk for next child (average, in percent)	
Parents	Siblings	Cleft lip with or without cleft palate	Cleft palate
Not affected	One affected	4	2
Not affected	Two affected	10	2
One affected	Not affected	4	6
One affected	One affected	15	15

Adapted from Curtis, E., Fraser, F. C., and Waarburton, D.: Am. J. Dis. Child. **102**:853, 1961; and Fraser, F. C.: Pediatr. Clin. North Am. **5**:475, 1958.

isolated cleft palate is greater in females.

The mixture of entities that constitute oral-facial clefts can be regarded as products of disturbed intrauterine development generally occurring during the latter part of the first trimester of pregnancy. Experimental and clinical evidence implicates a variety of mechanisms. Etiologic factors may be rare mutant genes with relatively simple mendelian inheritance, as in clefts and lip pits. Chromosomal-determined aberrations, as in the trisomy D, and specific environmental teratogens including drugs, such as the anticonvulsants, have been implicated in a small proportion of cases. The great majority of cases are probably caused by the interaction of many genetic and environmental differences, each with a relatively small effect; they constitute the multifactorial group.

Genetic counseling. Recognition of patients with specific syndromes is important for counseling with respect to recurrence risks. For example, the syndrome of cleft lip–cleft palate and congenital lip fistulas is transmitted as an autosomal dominant trait, with 80% penetrance of any component of the syndrome. An affected individual has a 22% to 39% chance of having an affected child with a cleft lip with or without lip pits. On the other hand, the risk rate for recurrence of trisomy D is minimal if the parents are not carriers of the translocation. After elimination of mutant genes, chromosomal aberrations, or environmental agents, the risk rates shown in Table 18-2 based on empirical data may be applied to the greater number of cases within the multifactorial group.

Feeding the infant. Since clefts of the soft palate may not be ascertained during the initial examination, regurgitation of fluids through the nose while the infant is feeding should alert the physician to repeat his examination of the palate, including the palpation for a submucous cleft of the hard palate, which can contribute to incompetence of the velopharyngeal valve. Absence of the normal separation between the oral and nasal cavities requires modification in feeding techniques. Breast feeding should not be attempted. In the initial feedings after birth or following lip surgery, an Asepto syringe with rubber tubing may be used in feeding (Fig. 18-4). Gavage feedings are seldom necessary. Placing the infant in a sitting position and using a soft nipple with a slightly larger opening are generally effective. The impaired sucking function is compensated for by the effectiveness of the tongue stroking the nipple. Care should be taken not to force excessive quantities of milk or to use too large an opening in the nipple. Air swallowing may be a significant complication requiring more frequent burping.

Infants with bilateral clefts of the lip and palate or with wide clefts require the use of a lamb's nipple to provide a broader surface for compression. With minor modifications and patience, it is usually possible to avoid using palatal obturators or special cleft palate feeding devices. For the parents' sake, it is desirable not to emphasize further their baby's difference by resorting to unusual devices if possible. Persistent feeding difficulties may be caused by improper technique or the presence of other congenital anomalies, particularly disorders of the central nervous system.

Otitis media. Serous otitis media is common in infants with clefts. On the basis of available evidence, myringotomy with indwelling plastic catheters cannot be recommended as a routine preventive measure at this time. It may be indicated under special circumstances.

Lip repair. Lip repair may be carried out during early infancy, but palatal procedures should be deferred to a later date. Repair of the lip should be regarded as an elective procedure, with the timing dependent on the health of the infant, the severity of the defect, and the special qualifications of the surgeon. Generally, 10-lb weight and 10-gm hemoglobin level are minimal requirements. General anesthesia is indicated for careful reconstruction of the lip and nose. Some surgeons elect to operate early with the infant under local anesthesia and are satisfied with limited repair of the lip as a basis for further reconstruction at a later date.

Prognosis. The prognosis for satisfactory cosmetic and functional habilitation through surgery and dental care is quite good. Vigilance in monitoring otologic disease and upper respiratory tract infections is essential. Where possible, the adenoid should be preserved, since it facilitates velopharyngeal valving. With gradual involution of the adenoid, the infant is able to develop compensatory muscular activity. This compensation may not be possible if the adenoid is abruptly removed.

The physician's contribution during this neonatal period as a counselor to the parents and in the care of the infant is critical in dealing with subsequent emotional considerations of the child and the parents and in preparing the child for habilitation through surgery.

Craniosynostosis

See p. 546.

Malformations of the tongue

Aglossia and microglossia

Malformations of the tongue range from complete absence of the tongue to macroglossia. They occur less frequently than malformations of other oral structures. In aglossia congenita the tongue may be completely absent, but usually is present as a small nubbin located posteriorly in the mouth. The anterior part (two thirds) of the tongue is absent, and the posterior part is represented by a mobile rudiment. The epiglottis may be absent.

Associated malformations are common. The appearance of children with aglossia has been described as birdlike. The face is usually sharp and narrow, with a receding chin, caused by hypoplasia of the mandible and a narrow mandibular arch. Involvement of the extremities varies from bilateral peromelia to agenesis of a single digit, syndactyly, and absence of fingernails.

Tongue anomalies usually do not cause breathing problems in the newborn period, but these infants may have difficulty in feeding. In the baby with aglossia, milk must enter the mouth under the influence of gravity through a large hole in a feeding nipple. The infant assists the force of gravity by suction and compression of the nipple, which he accomplishes by raising and lowering the floor of the mouth. Compression cannot be very effective, since there is no closure of the nipple and the floor of the mouth cannot push against the hard palate. Once the food leaves the mouth, the bolus is swallowed normally. These infants show no nasal regurgitation, choking or coughing.

The parents should be informed that children with aglossia are usually slow in learning to talk. With speech therapy, these children have demonstrated a capacity to develop reasonably intelligible speech. However, there will be some sounds that cannot be properly formed without the tongue.

Macroglossia

The presence of an enlarged tongue is usually caused by lymphangioma or hemangiolymphoangioma. More rarely, the enlargement is caused by a true muscular hypertrophy or by congenital hemifacial hypertrophy. A symptom complex, the *macroglossia-omphalocele (Beckwith) syndrome,* includes high birth weight, accelerated postnatal growth, facial nevus flammeus, abnormal pinnae, a diaphragmatic anomaly, and possibly neonatal hypoglycemia. Some conditions exist in which the tongue seems large either because the surrounding structures are small, as in the Pierre Robin syndrome, or because the tongue simply protrudes from the mouth, as in Down's syndrome, cretinism, and Hurler's syndrome. In the normal healthy newborn, there is a relative macroglossia, with the tongue protruding between the alveolar processes.

Macroglossia, except when it is caused by a tumor, usually causes no breathing or feeding problem unless enlargement is so great that the tongue cannot be contained in the mouth. In such instances, the problem may be exacerbated by an upper respiratory tract infection that impedes nasal breathing. Treatment of a tumor is surgical extirpation. In cases not caused by tumor some relative adjustment does occur as the child grows older and other oral structures catch up and confine the tongue so that its relative size is decreased. The tongue in normal infants is proportionately larger than other oral structures because it grows at a relatively faster rate and because, in the newborn infant, it is not confined by teeth.

Ankyloglossia

Ankyloglossia (tongue-tie) results when the lingual frenulum extends to near the tip of the tongue and interferes with its free protrusion. If the attachment reaches the anterior border, a notch may be visible in the tongue tip. Ankyloglossia only very rarely interferes with function and never necessitates immediate treatment. It is no longer customary to clip the frenulum at birth, since the incision may serve as a source of infection and since the frenulum usually stretches with time. The decision for frenulectomy should be deferred until the child is able to speak and a more complete assessment of tongue-tip place is possible.

Neonatal and natal teeth

Approximately 1 in 2,000 normal newborns has teeth erupted at birth or shortly thereafter, usually two in the position of the mandibular central incisors. Fully erupted teeth at the time of birth are frequently seen in infants with Hallermann-Streiff syndrome. Teeth may cause complications in the neonatal period, including difficulty in nursing. The tongue, which is relatively large in the newborn period, lies between the alveolar processes at this time and as a result may become lacerated, or the tip of the tongue may be amputated. If the teeth are loose, there is a serious danger of exfoliation and aspiration. Since almost 90% of the natal or neonatal teeth are part of the normal deciduous set, which have erupted prematurely, a radiograph should be taken before a decision is made for extraction.

CONSTANCE U. BATTLE
HERMINE PASHAYAN
SAMUEL PRUZANSKY

BIBLOGRAPHY

Ardran, G. M., and Kemp, F. H.: The nasal and cervical airway in sleep in the neonatal period, Am. J. of Roentgenol. Radium Ther. Nucl. Med. **108**:537, 1970.

Babbott, J. G., and Ingalls, T. H.: Field studies of selected congenital malformations occurring in Pennsylvania, Am. J. Public Health **52**:2009, 1962.

Bluestone, C. D.: Eustachian tube obstruction in the infant with cleft palate, Ann. Otol. Rhinol. Laryngol. **80** (Suppl. 2):1, 1971.

Bronstein, I. P., Abelson, S. M., Jaffe, R. H., and von Bonin, G.: Macroglossia in children, Am. J. Dis. Child. **54**:1328, 1937.

Carroll, D. B., Peterson, R. A., Worton, E. W., and Birnbaum, L. M.: Hereditary factors in the Pierre Robin syndrome, Brit. J. Plast. Surg. **24**: 43, 1971.

Crow, M. L., Holder, T. M., McCoy, F. J., and Chandler, R. A.: The use of temporary gastrostomy to prevent aspiration in Pierre Robin syndrome, Plast. Reconstr. Surg. **35**:494, 1965.

Curtis, E., Fraser, F. C., and Waarburton, D.: Congenital cleft lip and palate; risk figures for counseling, Am. J. Dis. Child. **102**:853, 1961.

Dennison, W. M.: The Pierre Robin syndrome, Pediatrics **36**:336, 1965.

Fogh-Anderson, P.: Inheritance of harelip and cleft palate, Copenhagen, 1942, Arnold Busck.

Fraser, F. C.: Genetic counselling in some common pediatric diseases, Pediatr. Clin. North Amer. **5**:475. 1958.

Fraser, F. C.: The genetics of cleft lip and cleft palate, Am. J. Hum. Genet. **22**:336, 1970.

Fulford, G. E., Ardran, G M., and Kemp, F. H: Aglossia congenita and cineradiographic findings, Arch. Dis. Child. **31**:400, 1956.

Gorlin, R. J., Cervenka, J., and Pruzansky, S.: Facial clefting and its syndromes, Birth Defects: Orig. Art. Series **7**:3, 1971.

Grahne, B., and Kaltiokallio, K.: Congenital choanal atresia and its heredity, Acta Otolaryngol. (Stockh.) **62**:193, 1966.

Gunter, G. S., and Wakefield, A. R.: Early management of the Pierre Robin syndrome, Cleft Palate J. **7**:495, 1970.

Gurney, W.: Congenital amputee. In Greene, M., and Haggerty, R. J., editors: Ambulatory pediatrics, Philadelphia, 1968, W. B. Saunders Co.

Herbst, A. L., Ulfelder, H., and Poskanzer, D. C.: Adenocarcinoma of the vagina; association of material stilbestrol therapy with tumor appearance in young women, N. Engl. J. Med. **284**: 878, 1971.

Hooley, J. R.: The infant's mouth, J. Am. Dent. Assoc. **75**:95, 1967.

Jeresaty, R. M., Huszar, R J., and Basu, S.: Pierre Robin syndrome; cause of respiratory obstruction, cor pulmonale, and pulmonary edema, Am. J. Dent. Assoc. **117**:710, 1969.

Kelln, E. E., Bennett, C. G., and Klingberg, W. G.: Aglossia-adactylia syndrome, Am. J. Dent. Assoc. **116**:549, 1968.

Kennell, J. H., and Rolnick, A. R.: Discussing problems in newborn babies with their parents, Pediatrics **26**:832, 1960.

Lis, E. F.: Management of children with cleft lip and cleft palate. In Green, M., and Haggerty, R. J., editors: Ambulatory pediatrics, Philadelphia, 1968, W. B. Saunders Co.

McIntosh, R., Merritt, K. K., Richards, M. R., Samuels, M H., and Bellows, M. T.: The incidence of congenital malformations; a study of 5,964 pregnancies, Pediatrics **14**:505, 1954.

Meskin, L. H., and Pruzansky, S.: Validity of the birth certificate in the epidemiologic assessment of facial clefts, J. Dent. Res. **46**:1456, 1967.

Moyson, F.: A plea against tracheostomy in the Pierre Robin syndrome, Brit. J. Plast. Surg. **14**: 187, 1961.

Nishimura, H., Takano, K., Tanimura, T., Yasuda, M., and Uchida, T.: High incidence of several malformations in the early human embryos as compared with infants, Biol. Neonate **10**:93, 1966.

Paradise, J. L., Bluestone, C. D., and Felder, H.: The universality of otitis media in fifty infants with cleft palate, Pediatrics **44**:35, 1969.

Proctor, B., and Proctor, C.: Congenital lesions of the head and neck, Otolaryngol. Clin. North Am. **3**:221, 1970.

Pruzansky, S.: Not all dwarfed mandibles are alike, Birth Defects: Orig. Art. Series **5**(2): 120, 1969.

Rugh, R.: Radiation teratology in mice and a review of what is known in man, Brit. J. Radiol. **41**:717, 1968.

Smith, D. W.: Recognizable patterns of human malformation. In Major problems in clinical pediatrics, vol. 7, Philadelphia, 1970, W. B. Saunders Co.

Smith, J. L., and Stowe, F. R.: The Pierre Robin syndrome (glossoptosis, micrognathia, cleft palate); a review of 39 cases with emphasis on associated ocular lesions, Pediatrics **27**:128, 1961.

Solnit, A. J., and Stark, M. H.: Mourning and the birth of a defective child, Psychoanalytic Study Child **16**:523, 1961.

Stevenson, A. C.: Frequency of congenital and hereditary disease; with special reference to mutation, Brit. Med. Bull. **17**:254, 1961.

Takagi, Y., McCalla, J. L., and Bosma, J. F.: Prone feeding of infants with the Pierre Robin syndrome, Cleft Palate J. **3**:232, 1966.

Weinberg, B., Christensen, R., Logan, W., Bosma, J., and Wornall, A.: Severe hypoplasia of the tongue, J. Speech Hear. Disord. **34**:157, 1969.

19 Special orthopedic problems

CONGENITAL HIP DISLOCATION

The history of congenital hip dislocation dates back to Hippocrates' initial description and classification. Congenital hip dislocation is one of the most challenging and important congenital abnormalities of the musculoskeletal system. It is almost as common as club foot, and yet not as obvious at birth. Congenital hip dislocation demands a specific method of examination for its detection; unless treated early and definitively, it will lead to a painful and crippling deformity in adult life.

A brief description of terms is a prerequisite for discussion of this defect. Dislocation (luxation) refers to the femoral head being completely outside the socket, or acetabulum, but still within the stretched and elongated capsule. Subluxation of the femoral head refers to the head riding on the edge of the acetabulum. Such a defect is easily reduced and is stable when the hip is flexed and abducted, but is subluxated when the hip is extended and adducted. When the infant's hip is either dislocated or subluxated, the bony development of the acetabulum becomes progressively abnormal, leading to acetabular dysplasia. Our discussion focuses only on the more common variety of congenital hip dislocation—that is, the dislocation characterized by its postnatal appearance—and does not focus on the less common teratologic hip dislocation arising as part of a generalized congenital abnormality such as arthrogryposis multiplex (p. 535) and spina bifida (p. 556).

Incidence and etiology. There is considerable variation in the incidence of congenital hip dislocation in different parts of the world. In England and Sweden the frequency has been estimated at approximately 1 case per 1,000 live births. The incidence in northern Italy, southern France, and Japan may be three times as high. The highest incidence has been reported in the Lapps and certain American Indians and may be related to swadling with hips extended and adducted in the first few months of life.

Both environmental and genetic factors play a role in the causation of congenital hip dislocation. The sex ratio is approximately one male to seven females and may be related to estrogenic hormone metabolism. Another genetic factor that may predispose children to congenital hip dislocation is primary acetabular dysplasia with poor covering of the femoral head. Such dysplasia may be seen on the unaffected side in some 30% of unilateral cases of hip dislocation and is probably present but poorly recognized in many bilateral cases. Acetabular dysplasia may be found in one or both parents of affected children, and its genetic determination is probably multifactorial. Generalized joint laxity with capsular relaxation has been demonstrated in families of some affected children, and the causal relationship between this laxity and hip instability has been postulated.

The most important environmental factor determining the incidence of congenital hip dislocation is prenatal and relates to the intrauterine breech posture with hips flexed and knees partially extended. There is a significantly higher incidence of congenital hip dislocation in breech presentations. No adequate explanation has been postulated that fully explains the involvement of the left hip three times more frequently than the right hip and why this condition is bilateral in only one out of every four children. Likewise, the rarity of this disease in the black population remains an enigma.

Pathology. The significant pathologic findings are time dependent and initially consist only of abnormal laxity of the capsule, with elongation of the ligamentum teres and a femoral head, which may be small but is of normal configuration. Without therapeutic intervention, growth and weight bearing stimulate further pathologic changes in the infant's hip. The femoral head becomes further displaced upward and backward to lie on the ilium. The capsule elongates, extending across the acetabulum, and eventually adheres to the floor of the fossa, while the hip adductor muscles become progressively shortened. The acetabulum becomes shallower and more oblique; and with persistent dislocation, a secondary or false acetabulum may develop on the ilium posterior to the original fossa. The femoral head also becomes small with persistent dislocation, and its shape changes. All of these changes constitute increasing obstacles to subsequent reduction of the congenitally dislocated hip.

Diagnosis. Early diagnosis and appropriate therapeutic intervention is essential to avoid crippling deformity. Caffey and Coleman have emphasized that apart from demonstrating definite dislocation or malformation or both, roentgenographic studies have little to offer diagnostically during the neonatal period. Diagnosis depends on clinical evaluation; such evaluation will identify more than 95% of infants with congenital hip dislocation. This evaluation, now called the Ortolani maneuver, is performed by placing the infant on his back with his knees bent and hips flexed to 90° and fully abducted. When the hip is reduced by abduction, one can appreciate a click as the femoral head slides across the posterior of the aectabulum and enters the socket. With adduction of the hip, the femoral head redislocates out of the acetabulum with a palpable click, which can be best appreciated with the thumb on the lesser trochanter and the index finger on the greater trochanter. During this examination the infant should be relaxed and the hip adductors not tight. Furthermore, entry and exit clicks must be differentiated from the clicks associated with a tight ileotibial band or a gluteal tendon sliding over the greater trochanter and the knee click of a subluxating patella or a discoid meniscus. While the Ortolani test is considered diagnostic for congenital hip dislocation, it has several shortcomings that limit its use during the immediate neonatal period: (1) as the hips are abducted and dislocated, the femoral head may slide so smoothly over the low rim of the acetabulum that a click is not appreciated; (2) a truly dislocated hip may not reduce and cannot, therefore, provide the characteristic exit and entrance clicks; and (3) infants with congenitally unstable hips (that is, subluxated or subluxatable), may escape detection only to dislocate in the future. Barlow's test, a modification of the Ortolani maneuver, should therefore be carried out on all newborn infants and will, when combined with the latter maneuver, detect almost all congenitally abnormal hips. To perform this test the infant is placed on his back with hips flexed to 90° and the knees fully flexed. The index finger of each hand is applied over the greater trochanter and the thumbs opposite the lesser trochanter in the femoral triangle. The hips are brought into midabduction and thumb pressure applied posteriorly over the lesser trochanter; an unstable hip will dislocate across the posterior lip of the acetabulum. With release of thumb pressure, the femoral head will be reduced back into the hip socket. With the passage of time other physical findings appear. These findings include asymmetry of the skin folds of the thigh, shortening of the involved extremity, limitation of passive abduction of the hip in the 90° flexed position, apparent shortening of the femur as shown by differences in the knee levels with the hips flexed at right angles and the infant in the supine position (Galeazzi's sign), and piston mobility of the telescoping sign. Other physical findings associated with posture and gait are not applicable to the neonate.

Treatment. The orthopedic treatment of congenital dislocation and subluxation of the hip varies with the age of the affected individual, and we will consider only therapy that is applicable to the neonate. Initially, all unstable hips, either subluxated or dislocated, should be gently reduced, which is usually not difficult at this age, and maintained in a stable position of flexion and abduction by some device such as the Frejka pillow, orthopedic splints, or multiple diapers. The treatment of the subluxable (dislocatable) hip is more controversial, since 75% of these hips will revert to normality during the first few weeks of life without therapeutic intervention. However, these hips should likewise be maintained in a stable position of flexion and abduction. Occasionally, a dislocated hip is too unstable to be kept reduced by any simple device, and in such infants a plaster hip spica cast is indicated. A period of 3 to 4 months is usually required before the capsule becomes tighter and the femoral head stimulates development of the acetabulum. The hips should be periodically assessed both clinically and radiographically. The crippling sequelea of congenital dislocation and subluxation of the hip can be virtually eliminated by alert and adequate diagnosis and treatment in the neonatal period.

CONGENITAL KNEE DISLOCATION

Congenital knee dislocation is a comparatively rare disorder that most often is a manifestation of arthrogryposis (p. 535) and consists of anterior dislocation of the knee. More commonly, congenital hyperextension of the knee (genurecurvatum) occurs without dislocation and is seen in normal infants. Both conditions are more common in the female and following breech presentation, suggesting an etiologic relationship with congenital dislocation. The completely dislocated knee usually requires surgical correction, while genurecurvatum almost always spontaneously improves. Some orthopedic surgeons have advocated plaster casting for this latter abnormality.

CONGENITAL PATELLA DISLOCATION

Patella dislocation rarely occurs. The patella is usually displaced laterally, and this can occur either with or without congenital dislocation of the knee. This abnormality may be bilateral. An attempt should be made to replace the patella and to apply a dressing to maintain it in the correct position. However, early reconstructive surgery is frequently indicated.

CONGENITAL SHOULDER DISLOCATION

Congenital shoulder dislocation is extremely rare. The head of the humerus may lie beneath the spine of scapula, with the arm in a position of abduction and internal rotation. This condition is frequently associated with other congenital malformations. It is often difficult to differentiate between congenital dislocation, dislocation caused by birth trauma, and subluxation secondary to obstetrical paralysis. Orthopedic surgical intervention is necessary.

CONGENITAL DISLOCATION OF THE RADIUS

Congenital dislocation of the radius, a rare abnormality, is usually not detected early, because there is relatively little deformity and frequently no disability. The radial head dislocates laterally and as a result of overgrowth increases in length. Reconstructive surgery has little to offer since it seldom improves function.

PSEUDARTHROSIS

Pseudarthrosis is a rare but serious abnormality that most frequently involves the tibia. The tibia, which has failed to grow normally in width, becomes angulated in its lower third, resulting in an anterior bowing of the leg before birth. It is frequently seen in children with neurofibromatosis, but the exact etiologic relationship is unknown. The thin sclerotic bone at the site of the angulation is unstable, and a pathologic fracture occurs at birth or shortly thereafter. Since the abnormal bone is avascular at this site, the fracture fails to unite and a pseudarthrosis develops, with a resultant increase in the angular deformity. Congenital pseudarthrosis may affect the clavicle but is often asymptomatic. Extensive orthopedic surgical manipulation is necessary for correction of this musculoskeletal abnormality.

INTRAUTERINE AMPUTATION AND CONGENITAL RING CONSTRICTIONS

Absence of the distal part of a limb at birth is called a congenital amputation. The defect may be minimal as in the absence of a single digit, or it may involve a complete extremity. These amputations may be associated with annular constricting bands. Shallow constricting bands may be seen without any abnormalities or may have associated distal malformations, such as clubbing of feet, lymphedema, and syndactyly. A great deal of controversy surrounds the origin of both congenital amputations and annular constricting bands. Hippocrates was the first to suggest that such deformities were caused by mechanical factors acting in utero. However, Streeter's observations in the 1930s cast doubt on the earlier speculations and suggested that such abnormalities were the result of defective germ plasm. While Streeter's hypothesis is still accepted by many, more recent studies by Torpin and by Baker and Rudolph have established the importance of intrauterine mechanical factors. These investigators demonstrated that early rupture of the amnion without damage to the chorionic sac does occur and that the outer surface of the amnion produced mesodermal fibrinous strings (amniotic bands) that provide an opportunity for entanglement of fetal parts, often with disastrous results.

Diagnosis. The clinical recognition of congenital amputation secondary to amniotic bands becomes extremely important when one faces distraught parents seeking genetic counseling or reassurance or both. Not all congenital malformations involving the extremities are secondary to amniotic bands, and a clinical classification of such abnormalities is useful. These malformations may be either endogenous (defective germ plasm) or exogenous (external factors acting on normal germ plasm). The endogenous defects may be either genetic or teratologic. The genetic abnormalities are easily recognized and include such malformations as arrested development of an extremity, polydactylism, claw hand, and so on. In addition to the musculoskeletal malformations, these genetic abnormalities usually have associated specific organ system malformations. The teratologic malformations are secondary to noxious agents such as irradiation, chemicals, drugs, infective agents, and so on; careful clinical and epidemiologic investigations facilitate their recognition. The exogenous malformations (that is, those caused by amniotic bands) have certain characteristics that facilitate their recognition: (1) the absent limbs or digits are usually multiple and unilateral; (2) the abnormal limbs and digits are frequently associated with proximal constricting bands, which usually have the associated distal abnormalities of clubbing of the feet, lymphedema, and syndactyly; and (3) the most common sites of involvement are fingers, toes, the ankle, legs, forearm, and arm, in that order.

Treatment. Therapy of infants with congenital amputation involving an extremity consists of providing the infant with an artificial limb fitted at a young age. Most constricting bands do not require treatment; however, the deeper bands may be surgically divided and excised through a Z-plasty incision in an attempt to minimize future circulatory embarrassment.

SUPERNUMERARY DIGITS

Supernumerary digits involving the hands and feet are more common in black infants and may be developed to varying degrees of completeness. The most common and least serious supernumerary digit is the small incomplete digit united to one side of the hand or foot by a tiny soft tissue pedicle. This may be removed by simple ligation in the early neonatal period. Rarely, the duplication may involve one or more phalanges and may even include an extra metacarpal. The decision as to which digit or portion of a digit should be removed must be made on the basis of function as well as appearance and frequently is best deferred until the child is old enough to demonstrate such function adequately.

CLUBFOOT

Clubfoot may be congenital or acquired. Talipes (derived from the Latin *talus* ankle bone, and *pes,* foot) is the generic name used to designate these foot and ankle deformities, which are conventionally described according to the position of the foot: (1) varus, or inversion, (2) valgus, or eversion, (3) equinus, or plantar flexion, and (4) calcaneus, or dorsiflexion.

Equinovarus deformities are the most common and represent more than 95% of all congenital clubfeet. This abnormality occurs with a frequency of 1 case per 1,000 live births; the condition is more common in males (2:1) and is bilateral in 50% of infants. All degrees of the equinovarus deformity exist, and the condition is often present in the fetus when the foot begins to form. Pathologically, the muscles on the posterior and medial aspect of the leg are shortened, and the distal portions of the tibia and fibula usually show slight inward rotation (tibial torsion). In most instances the individual bones of the feet are normal at birth, and only their relationship to each other is affected. Talipes calcaneovalgus deformities are the second most common variety of clubfoot. This is generally a mild and transient deformity involving a pathologically normal foot and is probably secondary to intrauterine malposition rather than a true developmental abnormality. The other varieties of club feet are extremely rare.

The therapeutic approach to children with clubfeet is similar regardless of the type. It consists of determining if the abnormality in the foot can be passively brought to the opposite position. If this maneuver proves successful, simple exercises started early will correct the deformity. If the foot abnormality is fixed and cannot be passively overcome, orthopedic treatment consisting of plaster cast or splinting or both is required. Forceful manipulation and surgery are rarely required.

Talipes varus (metatarsus primus varus)

Talipes varus involves a varus, or adduction, deformity of the first metatarsal in relation to the other four metatarsals. The medial border of the forefoot is curved inward, and there is a wide space between the first and second toe. If treated early by the application of a series of corrective plaster casts, the deformity is rapidly overcome.

Metatarsus varus (metatarsus adductus)

In metatarsus varus the forefoot, involving all five metatarsals, is adducted and inverted at the tarsometatarsal joint. The normal position of the heel and ankle readily distinguishes this condition from congenital clubfoot. Metatarsus varus is usually associated with internal tibial torsion. This deformity is quite common (2:1,000 live births) and is generally bilateral. In most cases, the forefoot deformity is mild and flexible, and the prognosis is good with simple stretching and the avoidance of sleeping in the face-down position with the feet curved in. If the deformity is marked and fixed, treatment involves the application of a series of plaster casts molding the foot into adduction and pronation.

WILLIAM T. SPECK

BIBLIOGRAPHY

Baker, C. J., and Rudolph, A. J.: Congenital ring constrictions and intrauterine amputations, Am. J. Dis. Child. **121**:393, 1971.

Carter, C. O., and Wilkinson, J. A.: Genetic and environmental factors in the etiology of congenital dislocation of the hip, Clin. Orthop. **33**:119, 1964.

Palmen, K.: Preluxation of the hip joint, Acta Pediatr. Scand. **50**:129, 1961.

Torpin, R.: Amniochorionic mesoblastic fibrous strings and amnionic bands, Am. J. Obstet. Gynecol. **91**:65, 1965.

von Rosen, S.: Diagnosis and treatment of congenital dislocation of the hip joint in the newborn, J. Bone Joint Surg. (Brit.) **44B**:284, 1962.

20 Diseases of the skin*

The skin of the newborn infant may present a variety of lesions: some innocent, temporary, and the result of a physiologic reaction; others the result of episodic disease; and still others indicative of a serious, potentially fatal underlying disorder. The definitive diagnosis of specific skin lesions requires an understanding of the physiologic characteristics and peculiarities of neonatal skin, a recognition of primary skin lesions, and knowledge of their significance.

BIOLOGY OF FETAL AND NEONATAL SKIN

Structure of the epidermis

Human skin has two distinct interdependent components, the epidermis and the dermis, which together provide a regenerating protective coat. The epidermis has marked regional variations in thickness, color, permeability, and surface chemical components. It consists of a highly structured compact layering of keratinocytes and melanocytes. Recently there has been recognition of a third distinct cell type, the Langerhans cell, the function of which is unknown.

The young keratinocytes are columnar basal cells that produce and contain a filamentous protein, keratin. They lie adjacent to the dermis, separated from it by a narrow basement membrane. The basal keratinocytes divide and migrate toward the surface. Their cellular structure is replaced by keratin, and the cells become dehydrated and flattened, forming a tough, resilient, anuclear, relatively impermeable membrane. In infants these cells of the stratum corneum are more uniform in size than those in children or adults.

Another important component of the epidermis is the melanocyte, a cell of neural crest origin capable of producing melanin. The melanocytes in the basal layer contain melanin at about the fourth month of fetal age. Melanin protects against ultraviolet radiation damage to vital nuclear elements. Melanin granules (melanosomes) are formed in the melanocytic cytoplasm and move via the dendritic processes toward the basal cell. As the basal keratinocyte matures, its melanin is dispersed as a fine intracellular granular dust that may be visualized in the horny layer.

The epidermal attachment to the dermis is less adherent in the early weeks of life, resulting in a greater propensity to blister formation in the newborn infant. In addition, melanin production is low; the newborn infant is not as pigmented as the older child and is more sensitive to sunlight. The stratum corneum is also more permeable to chemical agents during this period of life. Nachman and Esterly assessed permeability by comparing the skin blanching response in infants of varying gestational ages to the topical application of a 10% phenylephrine (Neo-Synephrine) solution. The skin of the youngest infants (28 to 34 weeks) had the most rapid and prolonged response, whereas the skin of full-term infants in most instances failed to blanch even on the first day of life.

*This study was supported in part by a grant from the National Institutes of Health (DE 2872), U. S. Public Health Service, Department of Health, Education and Welfare.

The appendages

The appendages derive from invaginations of epidermal germinative buds into the dermis. They include hair, sebaceous glands, apocrine glands, eccrine glands, and nails. The arrector pili muscle is attached to the hair follicle.

Lanugo (fine, soft, immature hair) frequently covers the scalp and brow in the premature infant; the scalp line may be poorly demarcated. Lanugo may also cover the face; scalp hair is usually somewhat coarser and more mature earlier in dark-haired infants. The growth phases of the hair follicle are usually synchronous at birth; 80% of the follicles are in the resting state. During the first few months of life the synchrony between hair loss and regrowth is disturbed, and hair may become coarse and thick, acquiring an adult distribution, or there may be a temporary alopecia. There are also sex differences in hair growth; boys' hair grows faster than girls' hair. In both sexes, scalp hair growth is slower at the crown. The outline below shows disorders associated with abnormal amounts and morphologic characteristics of hair.

- I. Disorders with hypertrichosis
  - A. Generalized
    1. Congenital lipodystrophy
    2. Cornelia de Lange syndrome
    3. Craniofacial dysostosis with dental, eye, and cardiac anomalies
    4. Hypertrichosis lanuginosa universalis
    5. Hypertrichosis with gingival fibromatosis
    6. Leprechaunism
    7. Mucopolysaccharidoses
  - B. Localized
    1. Congenital hemihypertrophy with hypertrichosis
    2. Hairy ears
    3. Hairy elbows syndrome
    4. Hairy nevi
    5. Ring chromosome E (low hairline)
    6. Trisomy 18 (back and forehead)
    7. Turner's syndrome (low occipital hairline)
- II. Disorders with hypotrichosis
  - A. Anhidrotic (hypohidrotic) ectodermal dysplasia
  - B. Atrichia with papular lesions
  - C. Combined immunodeficiency syndrome with short-limbed dwarfism
  - D. Congenital alopecia
  - E. EEC syndrome (ectrodactyly, ectodermal dysplasia, cleft lip-palate)
  - F. Goltz's syndrome
  - G. Hallerman-Streiff syndrome (oculomandibulodyscephaly)
  - H. Hidrotic ectodermal dysplasia
  - I. Hypotrichosis, syndactyly, and retinitis pigmentosa
  - J. Incontinentia pigmenti
  - K. Keratosis follicular spinulosa decalvans
  - L. Ocular-dental-digital dysplasia
  - M. Oral-facial-digital syndrome
  - N. Progeria
  - O. Rothmund-Thomson syndrome
  - P. Seckel's syndrome
  - Q. Trisomy A
- III. Disorders with hair of abnormal morphology
  - A. Structural defects
    1. Arginosuccinicaciduria—monilotheix, trichorrhexis nodosa
    2. Hereditary trichodysplasia (Marie Unna hypotrichosis)—twisted hair
    3. Menkes syndrome
    4. Monilotheix
    5. Netherton's syndrome—multiple defects
    6. Pili annulati
    7. Pili torti
    8. Pili torti and nerve deafness
    9. Trichorrhexis nodosa
  - B. Abnormal color, caliber, and fragility
    1. Cartilage-hair hypoplasia—small caliber
    2. Citrullinemia—fragile, atrophic bulbs
    3. Congenital trichomegaly with dwarfism, mental retardation, and retinal pigmentation—long brows and lashes
    4. Dyskeratosis congenita—sparse and fine
    5. Hartnup disease—fine, fragile hair
    6. Hereditary enamel hypoplasia and kinky hair—abnormal curliness
    7. Homocystinuria—fine, fragile hair
    8. Marinesco—Sjögren syndrome—fragile, brittle, rough hair
    9. Phenylketonuria—fine, light-colored hair
    10. Pierre Robin syndrome—fine, light-colored hair
    11. Trichorinophalangeal syndrome—thin hair
    12. Trisomy 21—fine, light-colored, atrophic bulbs
    13. Tyrosinemia—fine, light-colored hair
    14. Woolly hair—abnormal curliness

Nails are fully formed at birth. Syndromes associated with nail defects are presented in the outline below.

SYNDROMES ASSOCIATED WITH NAIL DEFECTS*

- I. Total or partial absence of nails; nail hypoplasia or dysplasia
  - A. Acrodermatitis enteropathica

*Data from Smith, 1970; Pardo-Costello, 1960; Zaias, 1971; Samman, 1968; Gorlin, 1964.

B. Anhidrotic (hypohidrotic) ectodermal dysplasia
C. Anonychia and ectrodactyly
D. Apert's syndrome (acrocephalosyndactyly)
E. Cartilage-hair hypoplasia
F. Deafness and nail dystrophy (Feinmesser; Robinson)
G. Dyskeratosis congenita
H. Ellis-van Creveld syndrome
I. Enamel hypoplasia and curly hair
J. Epidermolysis bullosa
K. Focal dermal hypoplasia (Goltz's syndrome)
L. Glossopalatine ankylosis, microglossia, hypodontia, and anomalies of the extremities (Gorlin-Pindborg)
M. Incontinetia pigmenti
N. Larsen's syndrome
O. Long-arm 21 deletion syndrome
P. Nail-patella syndrome
R. Popliteal web syndrome
S. Progeria
T. Pyknodysostosis (Maroteaux-Lamy)
U. Rothmund-Thomson syndrome
V. Skin hypoplasia—nail dystrophy (Basan)
W. Trisomy 13
X. Trisonmy 18
Y. Turner's syndrome

II. Hypertrophic or abnormally large nails
A. Congential hemihypertrophy
B. Familial hyperpigmentation with dystrophy of the nails (Touraine and Soulignac)
C. Pachyonychia congenita
D. Rubinstein-Taybi syndrome
Q. Otopalatodigital syndrome

The eccrine sweat glands are distributed over all the skin. They arise from an epidermal downgrowth at about the sixth week of embryogenesis and are innervated by a sympathetic cholinergic mechanism. During the first 24 hours of life, full-term infants usually do not sweat; at about the third day sweating begins on the face. Palmar sweating begins later. Sweating varies markedly with ambient and body temperature, crying, eating, and fever.

The sebaceous glands differentiate primarily from the epithelial portion of the hair follicle at about 13 to 15 weeks of life and almost immediately produce sebum in all hairy areas. The gland develops as a solid outpouching from the upper third of the hair follicle. These solid buds become filled with liquid centrally where the cells disintegrate; acini and ducts develop, opening most frequently into the canal between the hair follicle wall and hair shaft. The rapid growth and activity of sebaceous glands up to and immediately after birth is governed, in part, by maternal androgens and, possibly, also by endogenous steroid production by the fetus. Androgens are the only hormones that unequivocally have a stimulating effect on the sebaceous glands; estrogens depress their growth. In normal infants maternal androgens are responsible for what Beare and Rook call the miniature puberty of the newborn, with its attendant infantile acne and transient development of secondary sexual characteristics. Shortly after birth the sebaceous glands of the normal infant begin a period of quiescence that lasts until puberty. Ectopic glands occur occasionally on the lips, buccal mucosa, esophagus, and vagina.

The apocrine glands are relatively large organs that originate from and empty into the hair follicle. Embryologically, they develop somewhat later than the eccrine glands. Apocrine development is advanced by 7 or 8 fetal months, when the glands begin to produce a milky white fluid containing water, lipids, protein, reducing sugars, ferric iron, and ammonia; in the newborn infant the acini are well formed. The biologic function of the gland is unknown.

Structure of the dermis

The dermis has a symbiotic relation to and may exert a controlling influence on the epidermis. It is a metabolically active tissue that contains fibrous elements, amorphous ground substance, free cells, nerves, blood vessels, and lymphatic vessels. The fibrinous elements are collagen and elastic tissue. Collagen makes up more than 90% of the connective tissue of the dermis. As age increases, collagen becomes progressively less soluble. The morphologic characteristics and chemical and physical properties of cutaneous elastic fibers are different from collagen, but there is little quantitative knowledge about the elastic content of newborn skin. Clinical changes in cutaneous elasticity may be related to the spatial arrangement of elastic tissue or collagen fibers in the skin and to a qualitative change in the elastic fiber rather than to the quantity of elastin present in the dermis. The fibroblasts are the most numerous cells of the dermis. They produce collagen and the mucopolysaccharides of the ground substance. Mast cells (which produce heparin and histamine), histiocytes, macrophages, lymphocytes, neutrophils, and an occasional plasma cell and eosinophil are also present in the dermis. The major mucopolysaccharides in the ground substance of skin are hyaluronic acid and dermatan sulfate (chondroitin sulphate B).

The blood and lymphatic vessels

The development of the vascular supply of the skin is closely related to its size. The physiologic requirements of skin vary considerably; skin blood flows range from 0.1 to 150 ml/100 ml of tissue per minute. The vascular network supplying the skin develops in early embryonic life from the mesoderm. The dermis and epidermis are served by networks of anastomosing arteries at three levels: a subepidermal (or papillary) plexus, a dermal (or subpapillary) plexus, and a third plexus at the junction of the dermis and subcutaneous panniculus (fascial network). The subpapillary network is disorderly at birth and gradually develops its adult structure during the first 17 weeks of postnatal life. The veins form five plexuses. Direct arteriovenous anastomoses are present in abundance, with glomerular organs probably responsible for thermoregulatory shunting. The appendages also have special vascular networks.

Vasomotor tone is controlled by a delicate and complex series of nervous and pharmacologic mechanisms that involve the sympathetic nervous system, norepinephrine, acetylcholine, and histamine and may also involve serotonin, vasoactive polypeptides, corticosteroids, and prostaglandins. The nervous control of thermoregulation also involves the hypothalamus, higher centers, sympathetic and sensory nerves, and the axon reflex. The venous circulation is similarly controlled.

Cutaneous innervation

The nerve networks in the dermis develop at a very early embryologic age and appear to be distributed in random fashion. The most superficial nerves have the smallest diameter and are the least myelinated. At the papillary level, sensory nerves cannot be distinguished from autonomic nerve fibers with the light or electron microscope. In addition to the dermal nerve network, which may show considerable regional variation, nerve fibers may serve particular regions or structures such as hair follicles, eccrine glands, arrector pili muscles, and the subepidermal zone. The sebaceous glands are not innervated.

Cutaneous nerves serve overlapping cutaneous areas; one nerve impulse does not necessarily stimulate one spot on the cerebral cortex. Sensation is probably the product of several factors, including spatial and temporal patterns of nerve stimulation in skin and spinal cord, local chemical factors in the skin, previous experience, the state of cortical arousal, and genetic factors relating to nerve stimulation threshold. Special neurologic structures include a dense perifollicular nerve network with exquisite tactile sensory properties and mucocutaneous end-organs highly concentrated in erogenous zones. Meissner's tactile organs are found in newborn skin as undeveloped structures that mature after birth. The Merkel-Ranvier corpuscles are important for two-point tactile discrimination on palms and fingertips; they are disc-shaped terminals that are seen during the twenty-eighth week of fetal life. After birth these receptors undergo little alteration. Vater-Pacini bodies are found around the digits, palms, and genitals; they are fully formed and numerous at birth.

The arrector pili muscle and arterioles are innervated by sympathetic nerves, and norepinephrine acts as the neurotransmitter. The eccrine glands are innervated by sympathetic fibers, but acetylcholine acts as the neurotransmitter. Parasympathetic fibers may accompany the sensory nerves in the vessel walls and cause vasodilation. The axon reflex is poorly developed in the newborn infant; in the neonate of low birth weight, axon reflex sweating may be difficult to elicit.

NORMAL SKIN IN THE NEWBORN INFANT

The gross appearance of the skin at birth is related, in part, to the maturity of the infant. In the normal full-term infant, the skin is soft, wrinkled, velvety, and covered with a greasy yellow-white material, the vernix caseosa, a mixture of desquamating cells and sebum with a pH of 7.4. Removal of the vernix is followed by desquamation of the epidermis in the majority of infants. The fetal epidermis is rich in glycogen. Glycogen, present in the basal layer at the sixth fetal month, diminishes as normal keratogenesis progresses, but may reaccumulate at the site of an injury. The pH of the newborn skin surface is 5.7 on the dorsa of the arms and 6.4 in areas where the vernix accumulates, such as the groin, scalp, and forehead. Skin surface lipids in the first 2 weeks of life are low in cholesterol and high in wax esters (compared with childhood values). Free fatty acids and triglycerides slowly decrease during postnatal and childhood development.

Within a few hours of birth, the skin develops an intense red color, which may remain for a period of several hours. With fading of this erythema, bluish mottling (livedo reticularis) becomes evident, particularly when the infant is exposed to a cool environment. Localized mild edema may also be present over the pubis and the dorsa of the hands and feet, possibly an additional manifestation of an unstable peripheral circulation.

Although the body surface tends to be less pigmented during the neonatal period than later in life, certain areas such as the linea alba, the areolas, and the scrotum are often deeply pigmented as a result of high circulating levels of maternal and placental hormones. Palpable nodules of breast tissue, active secretion by mammary glands, and a hyperplastic vaginal epithelium are additional normal end-organ responses to these hormones.

The premature infant's skin may be readily distinguished from the full-term infant's skin. At birth the skin is more transparent and gelatinous and tends to be free of wrinkles. The premature infant may be covered with a fine lanugo, which in the full-term infant has been lost or in some areas replaced by vellus hair. Sexual hormonal effects are less conspicuous in the premature infant; the scrotum is less rugose and pigmented, the labia majora are less prominent, nipples and areolas are less pigmented, and breast tissue is less palpable.

EPHEMERAL CUTANEOUS LESIONS

A number of benign and ephemeral lesions are commonly observed in a normal nursery population.

Milia

About 40% of infants have multiple yellow-white 1-mm cysts (milia) scattered over the cheeks, forehead, nose, and nasolabial folds. These may be few or numerous, but they are frequently distributed in clusters. Histologically, milia are keratogenous cysts similar to Epstein's pearls in the oral cavity. All of these lesions usually disappear spontaneously within the first few weeks of life.

Pigmentary lesions

The most frequently encountered pigmented lesion is the mongolian spot, which occurs in over 50% of black, Oriental, and American Indian infants and in 1% to 5% of Caucasian infants. Although the majority of these lesions are found in the lumbosacral area, occurrence at other sites is not uncommon. The pigmentation is macular and gray-blue, may cover an area 10 cm or larger in diameter, and results from an infiltrate of melanocytes deep in the dermis. These lesions gradually disappear during the first few years of life. With the exception of the bathing trunk nevus (a developmental defect resulting in a massive nevus of the trunk), other melanocytic nevi usually develop in the older infant or child. Lentigines (freckles) and cafe au lait spots also have their onset in later infancy or early childhood, although occasionally the latter may be present at birth. Abnormal hyperpigmentation of the areolas and genitals may be evidence for the existence of an in utero glucocorticoid insufficiency associated with defects in the biosynthesis of hydrocortisone.

Macular hemangiomas (salmon patches)

Macular hemangiomas are present in 30% to 50% of normal newborn infants. They are usually found on the nape, the eyelids, and the glabella. In a prospective study of affected infants most of the facial lesions were not present at 1 year of age, but those on the neck were more persistent. Surveys of adult populations confirm the persistence of the nuchal lesions in about one fourth of the population.

Harlequin color change

Harlequin color change is a phenomenon observed in the immediate neonatal period and is more common in the low birth weight infant. When the infant is placed on his side, a sharp midline demarcation bisects the body into a pale upper half and an intensely red, dependent half. The peak frequency of attacks in one series occurred on the second, third, and fourth days, but episodes were observed during the first 3 weeks of life. These episodes are of no pathologic significance. They have been attributed to a temporary imbalance in the autonomic regulatory mechanism of the cutaneous vessels; there are no accompanying changes in respiratory rate, muscle tone, or response to external stimuli.

Erythema toxicum

This benign and self-limited eruption usually occurs within the first 2 days of life, but lesions may appear until the fourteenth day. The incidence of affected full-term newborn infants in a normal nursery population varies from 30% to 70%. The disorder is less common with decreasing birth weight and gestational age. These lesions may vary considerably in character and number; they may be firm, shotty, 1 to 3 mm in diameter, pale yellow to white papules or pustules on an erythematous base, erythematous macules (up to 3 cm), or a splotchy erythema. There are no related systemic symptoms, and their cause is unknown. A microscopic examination of a Wright- or Giemsa-stained smear of these lesions demonstrates numerous eosinophils; Gram stains are negative for bacteria, and cultures are sterile. No treatment is necessary.

Miliaria

Miliaria is related to an eccrine gland disturbance. The lesions are of two types: superficial, thin-walled vesicles without inflammation (miliaria crystallina) and small, erythematous, grouped papules (miliaria rubra). Lesions occur in the intertriginous areas and over the face and scalp. During the first week of life, these lesions may be exacerbated by a warm and humid environment. Miliaria is often confused with erythema toxicum; rapid resolution of the lesions differentiates them from pyoderma. No treatment is indicated.

Acne neonatorum

Acne neonatorum is an uncommon but distressing facial eruption (most often of male infants) that may occur during the first week of life. The condition resembles acne in the adolescent patient; comedones, papules, pustules, and rarely, nodules may be present. The duration of acne neonatorum may vary, but usually it clears spontaneously during the first year of life. Elevation of urinary 17-ketosteroid levels in the infant has been reported but has not been a consistent finding. Conservative treatment with mild topical preparations to produce drying and peeling should suffice. Occasionally, the infant may be left with pitted scarring.

THE SCALY BABY

There are three causes for excessive scaliness in the newborn infant. Two of these, physiologic epidermal desquamation of the normal newborn infant and the desquamation seen in dysmature infants, are probably not of particular significance. However, ichthyosis, the third cause, is a chronic and heritable disease.

Physiologic desquamation and dysmaturity

The normal infant with accentuated physiologic desquamation usually has a gestational age of between 40 and 42 weeks; peak shedding occurs on approximately the eighth day of life. These infants are otherwise normal in physical appearance and behavior. In contrast, the dysmature infant has several distinctive characteristics. His weight will be low for his length. The body is lean with thin extremities and little subcutaneous fat. The skin is parchmentlike, scaly and stained with meconium, as are the nails and umbilical cord; the hair is abundant, and the nails are abnormally long. There may be an elevation of the serum nonprotein nitrogen, bilirubin, and hemoglobin levels, as well as albuminuria and glycosuria. In both of these groups of neonates, the normal infant with accentuated physiologic scaling and the dysmature infant, desquamation is a transient phenomenon, and the integument continues to serve its intended protective function. However, the infant with ichthyosis may have serious difficulty early in life because of impaired epicutaneous barrier function and the subsequent risks of secondary infection.

Ichthyosis

Of the four major types of ichthyosis, three may be symptomatic during the first month of life: X-linked ichthyosis, nonbullous congenital ichthyosiform erythroderma (lamellar ichthyosis), and bullous congenital ichthyosiform erythroderma (epidermolytic hyperkeratosis). The diagnosis depends on an analysis of the morphologic features, the histologic pattern, and pedigree information. The fourth type of ichthyosis, ichthyosis vulgaris, is the most common and benign form and rarely has its onset before the third month of life. In addition to the terms used above, two descriptive terms are applied to severely scaling newborn infants: the halequin fetus and the collodion baby.

Harlequin fetus

The harlequin fetus is the most severe form of ichthyosis. Several reports of affected siblings suggest that it is the result of an autosomal recessive type of inheritance; it may be an extreme form of nonbullous congenital ichthyosiform erythroderma. Virtually all of the affected infants die within the first hours or days of life despite treatment. The skin is hard, thick, and gray or yellow, with deep crevices running both transversely and vertically. The fissures are most prominent over areas of movement. Rigidity of the skin about the eyes results in marked ectropion, although the globe is usually normal. The ears and nose are undeveloped, flattened, and distorted, and the lips are everted and gaping, thus producing a "fish mouth" deformity. The nails and hair may be hypoplastic or absent. Extreme inelasticity of the skin is associated with flexion deformity of all of the joints. The hands and feet are ischemic, hard, and waxy in appearance, with poorly developed distal digits. These infants do not survive after the first week or two of life.

Collodion baby

The collodion baby (lamellar exfoliation of the newborn) is less severe and more common than the harlequin fetus and probably represents a phenotypic expression of several genotypes. This disorder usually evolves into a nonbullous congenital ichthyosiform erythroderma (recessive type), but collodion type of skin has also been observed in patients with X-linked ichthyosis. Rarely, shedding of the collodion-like membrane may reveal a normal underlying integument. A significant number of these babies are premature. The infant is covered with a cellophane-like membrane, which may by its tautness distort the facial features and the distal extremities. Less commonly, only a part of the integument is involved. The membrane is shiny and brownish yellow, resembling an envelope of collodion or oiled parchment, which may be perforated by hair. Fissuring and peeling begin shortly after birth, and large sheets may desquamate, revealing erythema of variable intensity. Once the membrane has fissured, no respiratory difficulties are encountered. Complete shedding of the collodion membrane may take several months. Pedigree information and histopathologic examination of skin sections are additional aids in the delineation of the specific type of ichthyosis.

X-linked ichthyosis

The patient with X-linked ichthyosis, if affected at birth, may have collodion membranes or only hyperkeratosis. In several studies 17% to 36% of the subjects had manifestations of the disease at birth, and 84% to 94% were affected by 3 months of age. The scales are characteristically large, thick, and ochre and are prominent over the neck, anterior trunk, and anterior extremities. Sparing of palms and soles and partial sparing of the flexures are helpful diagnostic features. Usually the axillas or the antecubital fossae or both are involved early in life. Systemic manifestations are generally absent, and complications are rare. Skin biopsy is helpful (although the histologic pattern resembles that of nonbullous congenital ichthyosiform erythroderma), showing hyperkeratosis, a well-developed granular layer, hypertrophic epidermis, and a perivascular lymphocytic infiltrate. This form of ichthyosis is present only in males and not in heterozygous females. Recently, deep corneal opacities have been described as a consistent finding. Since the female carriers also have these lesions, corneal opacities may eventually prove to be a reliable genetic marker.

Nonbullous congenital ichthyosiform erythroderma (CIE)

A brilliant and generalized erythema characterizes the scaly infant with nonbullous CIE. Affected babies are commonly of low birth weight. Hyperkeratosis is universal, involving the flexural areas as well as other body surfaces, but scaling in the neonatal period is less prominent than later in childhood. The palms and soles may show only increased skin markings or may be considerably thickened. Ectropion, often severe later in life, is not a problem during the neonatal period. Maceration of the skin in intertriginous areas may serve as an entry point for bacterial organisms. CIE has a recessive mode of inheritance. Since nonbullous CIE can occur as the cutaneous feature of several rare syndromes, affected infants must be thoroughly evaluated, particularly for central nervous system abnormalities. The epidermis in CIE has a decreased turnover time.

Bullous congenital ichthyosiform erythroderma

The infant with bullous CIE has recurrent bullous lesions, as well as erythema, dryness, and peeling. During the neonatal period, bullae may occur over widespread areas, resulting in extensive denudation with secondary infection, sepsis, and death. These skin lesions may be confused with those of Ritter's disease or epidermolysis bullosa. The histopathologic picture in bullous CIE is diagnostic; it shows vacuolization of the epidermis, abnormally large, clumped keratin granules, hyperkeratosis, and an increased granular layer. The judicious use of steroids administered systemically in conjunction with antibiotics may be lifesaving during the first months of life. As the infant grows older, the bullous lesions become less prominent.

VESICOBULLOUS ERUPTIONS

Blistering eruptions in the neonatal period may be caused by infections, congenital diseases, or infiltrative processes, or they may be of unknown origin. The proper management of such infants depends on knowledge of the cause of the disease or, when this is not known, on an understanding of the pathogenesis of the type of blister encountered. The latter is often dependent on determining at what level within the skin the blister has occurred.

Blister sites may be either epidermal or subepidermal. In the epidermis the blister can be very high (subcorneal), midepidermal, or basal. The midepidermal blister may be formed by primary separation of intercellular contacts (acantholysis), by secondary edematous disruption of intercellular contacts (spongiosis), or by intracellular injury as seen in viral infections. The diagnosis of a blistering disease usually requires a family history, an immediate past history of the infant and mother, laboratory studies relative to finding an infectious agent, evaluation of the infant's general state of health, consideration of the morphologic characteristics of the eruption, and a biopsy of the involved skin. The biopsy should be obtained from a fresh, typical, small lesion and preferably should include some normal surrounding skin.

Treatment of erosive lesions with steroids and antibiotics should be tempered by two considerations: awareness that knowledge of the metabolism and toxicity of these substances in the neonatal infant is incomplete and that increased permeability of the skin may result in excessive absorption.

BACTERIAL AND YEAST INFECTIONS

The colonization of the newborn infant's skin begins at birth, and the organisms acquired at birth are similar to those found on adult skin. *Staphylococcus epidermidis* (coagulase negative) predominates, but diphtheroids, streptococci, and coliform bacteria are also found. The newborn skin affords an excellent culture medium for *Staphylococcus aureus;* the groin and other skin sites may become colonized before the umbilicus. *Candida albicans* is not usually found on normal skin but may be present in the oral mucosa or in the diaper area as a result of fecal contamination.

Bullous impetigo of the newborn

The lesions of impetigo usually appear after the first few days of life. This is in contrast to the congenital blistering diseases that may be present at birth. The blisters vary in size and may appear on any body surface. They soon rupture, leaving a red, moist, denuded area. When the epidermis sheds in large sheets, Ritter's disease should be suspected. The organism most frequently involved is S. *aureus*. Certain phage types (for example, type 71) are frequently associated with these lesions. The diagnosis is made by Gram stain and culture of the blister fluid. In atypical cases, skin biopsy may be helpful by showing the characteristic intraepidermal (subcorneal or midepidermal) bulla filled with polymorphonuclear leukocytes. Blood cultures should be obtained from affected infants. Contacts and nursery personnel should be investigated for a source of the infecting organism. The infant should be placed in isolation and observed carefully for early signs of sepsis. A high index of suspicion during examination of other infants in the nursery is the most effective means of preventing epidemic spread of this infection (see also Chapter 8, p. 134).

Topical therapy consists of compresses of sterile water or physiologic saline. Local antibiotics may also be indicated. Systemic antibiotics are indicated to cover the principal etiologic possibilities until the results of culture are available. Fluid and electrolyte replacement therapy may be required if the disease is extensive. Recovery is usually complete in a few weeks, and there is little residual scarring.

Ritter's disease

Ritter's disease (also known as toxic epidermal necrolysis, Lyell's disease, and the scalded skin syndrome) is an extremely severe bullous eruption that has been reported at all ages. The eponym Ritter's disease has been used for infants up to a few weeks of age; the term Lyell's disease, or toxic epidermal necrolysis, is used for older children and adults.

The eruption is heralded by a bright erythema that gives the appearance of scalded skin. Large flaccid bullae follow and become confluent, and the skin sheds in sheets. Frequently, the entire epidermis is shed from a limb like a glove. Conjunctivitis and ulcerations of the oral mucosa may also occur. The infant may appear toxic and sustain severe fluid losses.

The infecting organism in Ritter's disease is most often S. *aureus,* phage type 71 or 55/71. The scalded skin syndrome has been reproduced in newborn mice by strains of S. *aureus* isolated from affected patients. A delta toxin, common to isolates from affected patients, has recently been shown to cause this dermonecrosis. Drugs may serve as the etiologic agent in the older child and adult. Histologic examination of the skin demonstrates a midepidermal blister characterized by cellular death and acantholysis; there is a striking absence of inflammatory infiltrate. Subepidermal bullae may also be seen. Treatment includes prompt systemic administration of antibiotics and fluid and electrolyte replacement.

Viral lesions

The vesicles of variola, vaccinia, vericella, herpes zoster, and herpes simplex have similar histologic patterns (Chapter 8). The causative virus may be found in early lesions; aspirated fluid may be a source of virus when it is cultured on the appropriate medium. The vesicle occurs in the midepidermis. There is acantholysis and marked destruction of individual cells. This results in the ballooning type of degeneration characteristic of viral vesicles. Eosinophilic mononuclear and multinucleated balloon cells may be seen on a smear carefully prepared by scraping the base of a fresh vesicle and staining with Giemsa stain (the Tzanck test). These balloon cells are most frequently seen in the herpes group (varicella-zoster and simplex) and are uncommon in the pox group (variola and vaccinia). A young viral blister may also be identified according to the type of viral inclusion body found in the degenerated cells.

HEREDITARY BLISTERING DISEASES

Epidermolysis bullosa

Epidermolysis bullosa refers to a group of hereditary defects that are characterized by intraepidermal or subepidermal blisters produced by minor degrees of trauma. Epidermolysis bullosa may be grouped into two major types: those lesions that result in complete healing without scarring and those that inevitably produce scars. Nonscarring epidermolysis bullosa has two modes of transmission: autosomal recessive (epidermolysis bullosa letalis) and autosomal dominant (epidermolysis bullosa simplex). The term nonscarring refers to the manner in which an uncomplicated blister may heal. Unfortunately, in the recessive form few blisters heal without complications, and scarring may result as a secondary phenomenon.

Epidermolysis bullosa letalis is usually present at birth. Sheets of epidermis loosen after minimal trauma, leaving moist erosions anywhere on the body. The nails are frequently lost. Anal and esophageal lesions also occur. Many lesions heal spontaneously, but large lesions may become infected and ulcerate. Septicemia and refractory anemia complicate the clinical course. The life span of the majority of patient is short. The blisters form between the basement membrane of the epidermis and the plasma membrane of the basal cells, lying therefore at the junction between dermis and epidermis. The cause of separation is unknown. Treatment is usually protective and palliative. Systemic administration of corticosteroids may prolong life in selected critical cases.

The autosomal dominant form of nonscarring epidermolysis bullosa may be present at birth or may appear shortly thereafter in areas of trauma related to delivery. The legs, feet, and scalp show erosions that heal slowly. The bullae may contain blood. Secondary infection is common. Nails are usually not involved. In contrast to the recessive form, the infants are usually in good general health. In all forms of epidermolysis bullosa, blisters may be readily elicited by gentle rubbing. Mild trauma will result in a blister within a few hours, and the resulting fresh lesions may be used for histopathologic examination. The diagnostic blister of the dominant form results from acute distintegration of basal cells. Cytolysis starts in the perinuclear region and spreads centrifugally to involve the entire basal cell. The cause is unknown. Treatment is aimed at protecting the skin from trauma, keeping lesions clean, and eradicating secondary infection. Systemic administration of steroids is rarely needed, and the prognosis is good.

Scarring epidermolysis bullosa (dystrophic epidermolysis bullosa) has both a recessive and a dominant form. Recessive scarring epidermolysis bullosa may occur in consanguineous families. Hemorrhagic erosions and blisters may be present at birth, especially about the feet. In contrast to the nonscarring group, milia may mark the site of healed blisters. Usually trauma precedes blister formation. The toe and finger lesions heal with fusion of digits and loss of nails, which results in a characteristic mittenlike envelope of the hands. As the fingers fuse (this usually takes several years), the hands and arms become fixed in a flexed position, and contractures develop. Repeated episodes of blistering, infection and scar formation lead to severe deformities, loss of hair, buccal mucosal scarring, dysphagia, and retarded physical and sexual development. Visceral amyloidosis, hyperglobulinemic purpura, and clotting abnormalities are associated with this severe, life-limiting disease. The electron microscopic changes in all of the scarring forms are identical and diagnostic. There is a sharp separation just beneath the basement membrane (subepidermal bulla), and the normal basal layer anchoring fibers are absent. The defect probably involves the connective tissue of the dermis immediately adjacent to the basement membrane of the epidermis. Recent studies have demonstrated elevated levels of collagenase in this area.

Treatment for scarring epidermolysis bullosa is essentially the same as that for the nonscarring forms. Systemic administration of corticosteroids may be helpful, and in selected patients, surgery may be indicated for correction of flexion deformities of fused digits. Iron therapy is necessary to treat the anemia. Topical administration of steroids has been useful in some cases.

The dominant form of scarring epidermolysis bullosa is less severe than the recessive type. Lesions may be present at birth, but often they appear later and are usually limited to hands, feet, and sacrum. Nails may be lost, but deforming scars and contractures are not frequent. Red plaques rather than blisters may result from injury. The lesions heal with soft wrinkled scars; keloids may occur in predisposed individuals. Hypopigmentation and hyperpigmentation and milia are often found at old blister sites. The general health is usually unimpaired.

Incontinentia pigmenti

Incontinentia pigmenti is a hereditary disorder that affects the skin, skeletal system, heart, eye, and central nervous system. Its mode of inheritance is probably as an X-linked dominant trait. Almost all of the patients are female, but a few documented affected males have been reported. The cutaneous lesions are usually present at birth and have three morphologic stages. Initially, there are inflammatory bullae, which are arranged linearly and appear in crops. These are replaced by pigmented, warty excrescences, which gradually resolve to form flat pigmented patterns of whorls and lines. These bizarre pigmented lesions represent the third and end stage, although pigmentation may occasionally accompany some of the early lesions. The blistering lesions occur on the trunk or limbs or both and vary in density from few to many. Nails and hair may also be affected. There is often a transient peripheral eosinophilia during the bullous phase of the disease. The diagnosis should be considered when inflammatory bullae arranged in lines are seen in a newborn female infant; ocular and skeletal abnormalities also may be present at this time. Faulty dentition, microcephaly, and abnormalities of the central nervous system can occur but are not apparent during the neonatal period. Biopsy of a small blister demonstrates a subcorneal vesicle filled with numerous eosinophils suggestive of an inflammatory dermatitis. The differential diagnosis includes erythema toxicum neonatorum and other bullous diseases. The clinical evolution of the cutaneous process and the presence of pigment-laden macrophages in the upper dermis of end-stage lesions establishes the diagnosis. No specific therapy is required for the skin lesions; if inflammation becomes excessive during the bullous phase, treatment with compresses and topical steroids may be helpful.

OTHER BULLOUS DISEASES

Acrodermatitis enteropathica

Acrodermatitis enteropathica is a rare disorder, probably inherited as an autosomal recessive trait. It is characterized by an acute vesicobullous eruption occurring around the mouth, genitals, and on the peripheral extremities. Secondary infection with *Candida* is a common complication. The onset may be as early as the third week of life, but more frequently it occurs later in infancy. Failure to thrive, hair loss, marked irritability, and paronychial lesions are additional features of the disease. Chronic severe diarrhea is the most serious manifiestation and may be life threatening. The disease may be the result of a defect in the metabolism of tryptophan or the synthesis of essential fatty acids or both. The pathogenesis has not been established. Diiodohydroxyquinoline (Diodoquin) is effective in controlling the disease but is required for protracted periods of time.

Dermatitis herpetiformis

Dermatitis herpetiformis is rarely found in the first month of life. The clear, tense blisters appear in crops in an otherwise healthy infant (boys more than girls), usually on the genitals, buttocks, and face. The lesions are highly pruritic and resemble impetigo. In contrast to impetigo, the lesions are usually sterile, and the blisters are located below the epidermis. The disease generally recurs periodically until spontaneous resolution occurs within several years. During the acute phases, sulfapyridine or dapsone administered in high doses may prevent blister formation.

Candidiasis

See also p. 157.

Cutaneous candidiasis in infancy may be a mild episodic disease or a chronic disorder, or it may result in disseminated infection and death. The latter two forms are often associated with multiple endocrinopathies or a defect in the immune response or both. Candidiasis in the first 4 weeks of life is usually benign and is most often localized to the oral cavity (thrush) or the diaper area. If maternal vaginal organisms are acquired during the birth process, the infant may manifest symptomatic mouth lesions or become an intestinal carrier. Fecal contamination is the usual source of the organism in candidal diaper dermatitis. Paronychial lesions may also occur, particularly in thumb-sucking infants. Rarely, cutaneous or systemic candidiasis may be present at birth as a result of transplacental or ascending infection.

The early cutaneous lesions are vesicular, with an areola of erythema; these rapidly become pustular and confluent, forming a moist erosion surrounded by satellite pustules. In the chronic mucocutaneous or granulomatous forms (rare in the neonatal period), the scalp, lips, hands, and nails may be sites of chronically scaling, heaped-up lesions. The diagnosis is aided by identification of budding yeast spores on Gram stain or of spores and pseudohyphae on a potassium hydroxide preparation. Growth of the organism is rapid on Sabouraud's or Mycosel agar.

Treatment depends on the extent of involvement. Specific candidicidal agents include nystatin and amphotericin B. The latter may be administered topically. Systemic administration of amphotericin B or 5 fluorocytosine should be reserved for those patients with evidence of severe disseminated disease involving more than the gastrointestinal tract and skin.

PIGMENTARY ABNORMALITIES

The melanocyte system of the newborn skin is not usually at maximal functional maturity. As a result, all babies, even black, Indian, or Chinese, may look pink or tan at birth. Within the first few weeks, racial color becomes more evident because melanin production has been stimulated by exposure to light. For purposes of classification, it is useful to think of pigmentary changes as diffuse or localized.

Diffuse hyperpigmentation

The intensity of pigmentation must be considered in the light of the infant's genetic and racial background. What may be hyperpigmentation in one infant obviously may be normal for another. Diffuse hyperpigmentation in the newborn is a very unusual occurrence. It may be caused by a gene whose main effect is on the melanocyte, by a hereditary disease that has secondary pigmentary consequences, by an endocrinopathy, or by a nutritional disorder or hepatic disease. Although in such cases, hyperpigmentation may be described as diffuse, it may in fact be accentuated in certain areas such as the face, over the bony prominences, or in the flexural creases.

Localized hyperpigmentation

Flat lesions

Cafe au lait patches. Cafe au lait patches may occasionally be seen in the newborn period. The lesion is flat, light brown in Caucasians to dark brown in blacks. Single lesions are found in 19% of normal children. They have no special significance. Lesions that are 4 to 6 cm in length and greater than 6 in number and that are frequently accompanied by axillary freckling are found in neurofibromatosis. The cafe au lait lesion is often the first to appear in neurofibromatosis, but the pigmented lesions may increase slowly in number so that auxilliary genetic and histologic information is required to establish a diagnosis. Twenty-six percent of patients with tuberous sclerosis also show cafe au lait spots. These are identical in appearance to those seen in neurofibromatosis but are very frequently accompanied by white macules (see below).

Albright's syndrome. In Albright's syndrome, the pigmented lesion is usually unilateral, elongated, and large (more than 10 cm), with a ragged, irregular ("coast of Maine") border. When the epidermis of a melanotic plaque is incubated with DOPA, an increased number of melanocytes and giant pigment granules are seen in melanocytes and keratinocytes of the affected areas in neurofibromatosis but not in the cafe au lait spot in normal individuals or those of Albright's syndrome.

Flat melanocytic nevi. Flat melanocytic nevi (junction nevi) are found in about 3% of newborn white infants and about 16% of black infants. Usually they are very few in number and are brown or black; in general they are smaller than 1 cm, but they may be larger. Occasionally, they may involve a nail bed, resulting in a pigmented nail. Junction nevi increase with age. In certain syndromes, such as neurofibromatosis, tuberous sclerosis, lentiginosis, xeroderma pigmentosum, and bathing trunk nevi, there are increased numbers of flat melanocytic nevi present at birth. Histologic examination of the lesion is usually diagnostic. It is not necessary to remove these lesions routinely. A large speckled or very black lesion can be removed surgically and the defect grafted.

Peutz-Jeghers syndrome. The cutaneous features of the Peutz-Jeghers syndrome may be present at birth or develop soon thereafter. These consist of pigmented macules, somewhat darker than freckles, around the nose and mouth. The lips and oral mucosa are often involved, as are the hands, fingertips, and nails. Macular hyperpigmentation is the only visible sign of this autosomal dominant disorder until adolescence, when the patient begins to suffer from attacks of intussusception, evidence of coexisting small bowel polyposis.

Xeroderma pigmentosum. Xeroderma pigmentosum is transmitted by an autosomal recessive gene and results in marked hypersensitivity to ultraviolet light. Soon after birth and depending on the rapidity and intensity of light exposure, the infant develops erythema, speckled hyperpigmentation, atrophy, actinic keratoses, and all known types of cutaneous malignancy. The outcome is usually fatal by the second decade of life, as a result of metastatic disease. Cleaver has recently shown that the underlying abnormality is probably caused by a deficiency in an endonuclease that is responsible for the repair of DNA damaged by ultraviolet light.

Postinflammatory hyperpigmentation. Hyperpigmentation may secondarily result from any banal inflammatory process in the skin and thus may have a multitude of causes, including primary irritant dermatitis, infectious processes, panniculitis, and hereditary diseases such as epidermolysis bullosa. The hyperpigmentation may result from an increase in melanosome production, increased melanin deposits in basal cells, increased number of keratinocytes, increase in the thickness of the stratum corneum, or deposits of melanin in dermal melanophages.

Raised lesions

The most important of the congenital melanocytic nevi is the *giant hairy (bathing trunk) nevus.* About 10% of these patients develop malignant melanoma in the lesion. They are present at birth, are probably not hereditary, and may occupy 15% to 35% of the body surface, most often involving the trunk. The pigmentation is light brown to deep black. The affected skin may be leathery in consistency. Almost invariably, numerous junction nevi, other dermal nevi, and cafe au lait spots coexist elsewhere on the body. Leptomeningeal melanocytosis has been documented in many of these patients, and this latter finding may be manifested as seizures.

The melanocytic invasion may involve subcutaneous tissue, fascia, or even underlying muscle. Because of the significant incidence of malignant degeneration in these nevi and of the hideous deformity and the intense pruritic element that may accompany them, it is desirable to remove these lesions surgically as soon as possible. The infant should be old enough to withstand major surgery. *Intradermal* or *compound* (involving both epidermal junction and dermis) *nevi,* circumscribed, hairy, and pigmented, may be present at birth. They occur everywhere but on the palms and soles and are usually raised, warty, and dome shaped. Histologically, the melanocytic nevus cells are found localized to the upper dermis and around the appendages and contain variable amounts of pigment. Usually, the diagnosis presents no problem, nor does their surgical removal for cosmetic purposes.

Occasionally, one may see a *blue nevus* (so called because of its Prussian-blue color) at birth. Lund and Kraus have called these lesions dermal melanocytomas. They are usually 1 to 3 cm in diameter, oval, dome-shaped tumors found on the upper half of the body. They grow very slowly and have little or no known tendency to become malignant but may be difficult to differentiate clinically from vascular tumors. Excisional biopsy is at once diagnostic and curative of the condition.

Incontinentia pigmenti and urticaria pigmentosa (mastocytosis)

Both of these conditions, which start as blistering diseases, may result in hyperpigmentation as a terminal feature of the process. They have been discussed elsewhere.

Hypopigmentation

Diffuse or localized loss of cutaneous pigment in the neonatal infant may be caused by heredity or by developmental disorder or may be acquired as a result of a nutritional disorder or postinflammatory changes. Decrease in cutaneous melanin may be caused by an absence or destruction of melanocytes or by a defect in one of four biologic processes: formation of melanosomes, formation of melanin, transfer of melanosomes into keratinocytes, and transport of melanosomes by keratinocytes.

Albinism (complete albinism, oculocutaneous albinism)

Albinism, which occurs in all races, has an incidence of between 1:5,000 to 1:25,000; the phenotypic picture is caused by an autosomal recessive gene. The affected infant usually has markedly reduced skin pigment, yellow or white hair, pink pupils, gray irides, photophobia, and cutaneous photosensitivity. Melanocytic nevi can develop in albinism, and these may or may not be pigmented. In blacks, the skin may be tan; freckles can appear on exposure to light. The usual eye findings are nystagmus and a central scotoma with reduced visual acuity. Other associated abnormalities reported in albinism are small stature, mental retardation, and coagulation disorders.

The biochemical defect responsible for this disease is caused by a deficiency of tyrosinase, the enzyme responsible for converting tyrosine to DOPA, an early step in the formation of melanin (p. 582). As a result of this biochemical deficiency, the melanosomes do not pigment and therefore never become melanin granules. Structurally, the melanosomes appear to be normal. Treatment is aimed at protection from ultraviolet light, since early actinic keratoses and squamous cell carcinoma are common occurrences in these patients.

Piebaldness (partial albinism)

Piebaldism is an inherited disease caused by an autosomal dominant gene. It is present at birth but may not be evident in fair-skinned infants because of a lack of contrast in skin color. The differential diagnosis may include vitiligo, achromic nevus, nevus anemicus, and the amelanotic macules of tuberous sclerosis and Addison's disease. In piebaldism, the hair and skin are affected. The amelanotic areas usually involve the widow's peak and anterior scalp, forehead to the base of the nose, the chin, thorax, trunk, back, midarm, and midleg. There are normal islands of pigment within the hypomelanotic areas, and the distribution pattern is fairly constant. Examination of an amelanotic area by electron microscopy shows an absence of melanocytes or shows melanocytes with markedly deformed melanosomes. Repigmentation does not take place.

Phenylketonuria

A hereditary lack of phenylalanine hydroxylase is transmitted by an autosomal recessive gene. This biochemical defect results in a variety of neurologic and cutaneous abnormalities, which include mental retardation, seizures, diffuse hypopigmentation, eczema, and photosensitivity (Chapter 14, p. 408).

Chédiak-Higashi syndrome

The Chédiak-Higashi syndrome is a rare disorder transmitted by an autosomal recessive gene. Its clinical features include a diffuse to moderate reduction in cutaneous and ocular pigment, photophobia, hepatosplenomegally, and recalcitrant, recurrent infections. The leukocytes and other cells contain large granules, and this finding has its parallel in the melanocyte, which produces giant melanosomes. It is not known why there is a clinical pigmentary deficiency, but it appears to have little to do with true albinism. Windhorst and others have speculated that the basic defect is a structural defect in the lipoprotein matrix that gives rise to the melanosome (and granulocytic lysosomes). Thus the melanin granule is either too easily destroyed or cannot be transferred to the keratinocyte (melanocytic impaction). The diagnosis may be made by the characteristic family history, physical findings, laboratory demonstration of abnormal leukocytes and melanonsomes, and the usual course, which leads to death in childhood. Death results from a lymphomalike process or infection. Hodgkin's disease has recently been reported as the fatal outcome in one case.

Klein-Waardenburg's syndrome

Klein-Waardenburg's syndrome is inherited as an autosomal dominant condition; the most constant features are lateral displacement of the inner canthi of the eyes, a prominently broad nasal root, confluent eyebrows, loss of pigment in the iris (heterochromia iridis) and fundus, congenital deafness, a white forelock, and cutaneous hypochromia. The clinical picture is quite striking, and the diagnosis is usually not difficult. Although it is usually limited to small areas, the hypopigmentation may be severe and extensive enough to resemble that of partial albinism.

Nevus anemicus

Nevus anemicus is a pale, mottled, hand-sized area appearing on the trunk, frequently in patients with neurofibromatosis. The lesions contain normal amounts of pigment but appear pale. There is no decrease in the number of vessels in the affected area, but the vascular tone is increased because of an excess local accumulation of catecholamines. There is no effective treatment.

Nevus achromicus

Present at birth, nevus achromicus is a unilateral (usually), somewhat hypopigmented, irregular-shaped, bizarre, streaky lesion. The hypopigmented area is quite uniform in color, and, in contrast to nevus anemicus, the vessels within it react normally to rubbing. The melanocytes in the affected epidermis seem to have nonfunctioning or partially functioning melanocytes.

White spots in tuberous sclerosis

Ninety percent of infants with tuberous sclerosis have white macules that become apparent at birth or soon after. They are about the size and shape of a European mountain ash leaflet. In fair-skinned infants the vitiliginous areas may be easily demonstrated by examining the skin with a Wood's lamp. They are variable in number and tend to affect the trunk and buttocks. The white macule of tuberous sclerosis has melanocytes with poorly pigmented melanosomes.

ANGIOMAS

Cutaneous hemangiomas are exceedingly common developmental nevoid lesions involving the dermal and subcutaneous vasculature. They are either superficial (approximately 68%), subcutaneous (15%), or mixed (20%). The terms capillary and cavernous refer to the histopathologic pattern apparent on biopsy. Capillary hemangiomas show only dilated vessels, with or without endothelial proliferation, and cavernous hemangiomas have large, dilated, blood-filled cavities with a compressed endothelial lining.

Port-wine stain or nevus flammeus

Nevus flammeus is present at birth and should be considered a relatively permanent developmental defect. These lesions may be only a few millimeters in diameter or may cover extensive areas, occasionally involving up to one half of the body surface. They do not proliferate after birth; the apparent increase in size is caused by growth of the child. A nevus flammeus may be localized to any body surface, but facial lesions are probably the most common. Port-wine nevi are usually sharply demarcated and flat, but they may have a pebbly or slightly thickened surface. Variation in color ranges from pale pink to purple. The most successful modality of treatment is the use of a cosmetic opaque cream (such as Covermark) that blends with the surrounding skin.

Most port-wine nevi occur as isolated defects and do not indicate involvement of other organs; however, occasionally the nevus flammeus may be a clue to the presence of certain vascular syndromes. The *Sturge-Weber syndrome* (encephalofacial angiomatosis) consists of a facial port-wine nevus in the cutaneous distribution of the trigeminal nerve, convulsions, hemiparesis contralateral to the facial lesion, and ipsilateral intracranial calcification. Ocular manifestations are frequent and include buphthalmos, glaucoma, angioma of the choroid, hemianoptic defects, and optic atrophy (Chapter 21). In a few cases the vascular defect may affect other organs. Roentgenograms of the skull of the older child show pathognomonic "tramline," double-contoured calcification in the cerebral cortex on the same side as the nevus flammeus. Electroencephalography shows unilateral depression of cortical activity, with or without spike discharges.

The prognosis depends on the extent of cerebral involvement, rapidity of progression, and response to treatment. Anticonvulsant therapy and neurosurgical procedures have been of value in some patients.

Klippel-Trenaunay-Weber syndrome

Klippel-Trenaunay-Weber syndrome is characterized by a cutaneous vascular nevus, venous varicosities, and overgrowth of the bony structures and soft tissues of a limb. The vascular lesions are usually apparent at birth, and boys are more frequently affected than girls. The hemangioma may be of the capillary or cavernous type and is often associated with arteriovenous shunts and lymphoangiomatous anomalies. Polydactyly, syndactyly, and oligodactyly have been associated findings. Complications include severe edema, phlebitis, thrombosis, ulceration, and hyperhidrosis of the affected area. The prognosis depends on the extent of involvement, which should be carefully assessed by complete peripheral vascular studies. A surgical approach may be effective in preventing severe limb hypertrophy in occasional patients.

Macular capillary hemangiomas also occur with moderate frequency in trisomy 13, Rubenstein-Taybi syndrome (broad thumbs and toes, slanted palpebral fissures, and hypoplastic maxilla) and in the Wiedemann-Beckwith syndrome (macroglossia, omphalocele, macrostomia, and cytomegaly of the fetal adrenal gland).

Strawberry (nevus) hemangioma

The strawberry hemangioma is a raised, circumscribed, soft, bright red tumor that is lobulated and compressible. When a subcutaneous component is present, it consists of a bluish red mass with less well-defined borders. If the entire nevus is deeply situated, the overlying skin may appear normal or show only a blue discoloration. The histologic pattern will depend on whether the angioma is purely capillary, cavernous, or mixed in type.

Approximately 20% to 30% of raised angiomatous nevi are present at birth, and roughly 90% are evident by the second month of age. The remainder have their onset between the second and ninth month of life. Girls are affected more often than boys. The most common site is the face, and the majority of infants have a single lesion. Virtually all of these lesions show some increase in size during the first 6 months of life, often with an initial rapid growth spurt. The phase of active expansion, particularly in larger nevi, may result in ulceration, which is usually of no consequence unless complicated by secondary infection or hemorrhage.

If left untreated, most of the hemangiomas in this group will involute spontaneously. Knowledge of the course of these lesions has led most physicians to follow an expectant rather than aggressive approach to therapy. Regression may be anticipated when pale gray areas appear on the previously bright red surface of the lesion. Approximately 50% of hemangiomas disappear by 5 years of age and 70% by 7 years of age. Rapidity and completeness of resolution seems unrelated to the size of the lesion or age of appearance. In some patients there are no residual skin changes; others show variable degrees of atrophy and telangiectasis. Lesions that ulcerate tend to scar and may, therefore, eventuate in a poorer cosmetic result. Profuse hemorrhage is rare unless there is an accompanying thrombocytopenia or coagulation defect. Minor degrees of hemorrhage can usually be managed by compression bandages.

The vast majority of patients with strawberry hemangiomas require no treatment other than careful follow-up to detect possible complications and to provide much needed reassurance to parents. However, under certain circumstances intervention may be indicated. Such situations include rapid growth of a lesion that compromises a vital structure or marked tissue destruction and associated symptomatic thrombocytopenia. Surgical excision is often the best means of approach, but an acceptable cosmetic result is not always achieved. A short intensive course of orally administered corticosteroids may be effective in young infants if severity of involvement warrants radical therapy.

Kasabach-Merritt syndrome

The association of thrombocytopenia with hemangiomas is known as the *Kasabach-Merritt syndrome.* This phenomenon is most frequently seen in early infancy, and in one author's series of 72 cases from the literature and two of his own, the median age of hospital admission for this problem was 5 weeks. Most, but not all, of the hemangiomas associated with thrombocytopenia are very large. Multiple coagulation defects in addition to thrombocytopenia have also been reported in association with hemangiomas. These defects include deficiency of factors II, V, and VII and hypofibrinogenenia.

In contrast to the infant with a hemangioma and normal hematologic findings, the infant with a Kasabach-Merritt syndrome should be hospitalized and treated promptly. The emergence of petechiae or ecchymoses in the adjacent skin or overt bleeding is an indication for fresh blood or platelet-rich transfusions. Surgical extirpation of the lesion or a course of irradiation to the hemangioma usually results in alleviation of the thrombocytopenia. Splenectomy is not indicated. Corticosteroid therapy has occasionally been successful. A few of these infants have recovered without treatment, following spontaneous involution of the hemangioma.

Miliary hemangiomatosis (diffuse neonatal hemangiomatosis)

A number of infants have been reported with multiple hemangiomas in several visceral organs. Some have had a myriad of small cutaneous lesions, most commonly in association with lesions of the gastrointestinal tract, liver, central nervous system, and lungs. Despite supportive therapy, affected infants often die early in life from intractable high output failure (p. 322), gastrointestinal hemorrhage, respiratory tract obstruction, or severe neurologic deficiency caused by extensive compression of neural lesions.

Blue rubber bleb nevus syndrome

The blue rubber bleb nevus syndrome is a rare disorder consisting of multiple cavernous hemangiomas of the skin and bowel. Cutaneous lesions are sometimes present at birth, and their appearance is characteristic, as the descriptive name of this syndrome suggests. The lesions are blue to purple, rubbery, compressible protuberances, which vary in size from a few millimeters to 3 to 4 cm in diameter. They are diffusely distributed over the body surface and may be sparse or number in the hundreds. Gastrointestinal lesions are common in the small bowel but may also involve the colon. Occasionally, lesions in the liver, spleen, and central nervous system have also been noted. Severe anemia may result from recurrent episodes of gastrointestinal bleeding. Neither the skin nor the bowel lesions regress spontaneously. Surgery is sometimes palliative, but it is frequently impossible to resect all of the affected bowel.

Cavernous hemangiomas have also been reported as a congenital feature of Riley-Smith syndrome and Leroy's syndrome (I-cell disease). *Maffucci's syndrome* (cavernous hemangiomas and dyschondroplasia) and *Gorham's disease* (cavernous hemangiomas and disappearing bones) are not usually apparent in the neonatal period.

Lymphangiomas are hamartomatous malformations composed of dilated lymph channels that are lined by normal lymphatic endothelium. They may be superficial or cavernous and are often associated with anomalies of the regional lymphatic vessels.

Lymphangioma circumscriptum

Lymphangioma circumscriptum is probably the commonest type of lymphangioma and may be present at birth or appear in early childhood. Areas of predilection are the oral mucosa, the proximal limbs, and the axillary folds. The tumor consists of clustered, small, thick-walled vesicles resembling frog spawn and is often skin colored but is in some instances of a blue cast because of a hemangiomatous component. Treatment is by excision; however, larger lesions may require full-thickness skin grafting. Recurrence has been noted even in full-thickness grafts.

Simple lymphangioma

Simple lymphangioma appears in infancy as a solitary, skin-colored, dermal or subcutaneous nodule. Following trauma it may exude serous fluid. Occasionally, it has been associated with more extensive lymphatic involvement. Uncomplicated lesions may be removed by simple excision.

Cavernous lymphangioma

Cavernous lymphangioma is a diffuse, soft-tissue mass consisting of large, cystic dilatations of lymphatics in the dermis, subcutaneous tissue, and in the intermuscular septa. Surgery is impractical in most cases.

Cystic hygroma

Cystic hygroma is a benign, multilocular tumor usually found in the neck region. The tumors tend to increase in size and should be treated by surgical excision (p. 567).

VERRUCOUS NEVI

Verrucous nevi are a group of lesions that may occur in the neonatal period. Most of them consist of an overgrowth of keratinocytes, while some may have an identifiable differentiation to one of the appendages normally found in skin. They vary considerably in their size, clinical appearance, histologic characteristics, and evolution, and have a low potential toward malignant degeneration.

Clinically, epidermal nevi may take the following forms.

1. A string of pigmented papillomas, a few centimeters in length, found anywhere on the body.
2. Long unilateral streaks involving a limb or up to half the body (nevus unius lateralis). The nails may be deformed by the process.
3. Large, cerebriform, linear, ochre-orange lesions involving the scalp and associated with black verrucous linear lesions elsewhere (including the mucous membranes). Pigmentary disorders and vascular nevi are often found in these patients.
4. A diffuse scaly eruption with a feathered or whorled, marbled appearance (ichthyosis hystrix).
5. Velvety hyperkeratotic areas over the extensor surfaces of hands and feet as well as in the skin folds and associated with profound mental retardation (benign congenital acanthosis nigricans).
6. A small papillomatous yellow or pink growth on the scalp, forehead, or face (simple sebaceous nevus and papilliferous syringocystadenoma). Since a significant incidence of basal cell epitheliomas develop in these lesions, they should be studied histologically. Once the diagnosis has been established, they should be removed surgically.

The treatment of large verrucous epidermal nevi is generally unsatisfactory. The only effective treatment requires removal of the lesion, together with its underlying dermis. In localized lesions this may be accomplished by electrodesiccation and plastic repair; but this treatment is not recommended in the neonatal period, since lesions may develop over a period of years. The scars that result from surgery may be as cosmetically unsatisfactory as the original lesions, and an extension of the nevus may appear beyond the repaired area. In the older child salicylic acid (3% in cold cream) may keep the lesion soft, and water-dispersible bath oils provide some palliative relief. When the nails are involved, no treatment is effective, and aside from filing or avulsion of the affected nails, none is suggested.

The epidermal nevus syndrome

Solomon, Fretzin, and DeWald reviewed the associated findings in 23 patients with epidermal nevi, including all of the types described above. In more than two thirds of these patients they found associated skeletal defects, vascular anomalies, and serious central nervous system disease. (A greater likelihood of associated anomalies existed if the lesions were large.) The anomalies found included kyphoscoliosis, vertebral defects, short limbs, osseous hypertrophy, angiomas of skin and central nervous system, mental retardation, and convulsive disorders. On discovering the existence of an epidermal nevus, the physician must take a careful family history (the genetic background to this syndrome is not clear) and perform a thorough physical examination. Particular emphasis should be placed on the musculoskeletal and nervous system, as well as on the skin. If indicated, periodic ECGs, psychologic testing, and radiographic examination of the long bones, pelvis, and vertebral column is desirable.

ECZEMA

The term eczema is a source of confusion. For the purposes of this discussion it is useful to think of eczema as a genus of skin disorder of which there are several species (for example, eczematous contact dermatitis). There are four phases of eczema, any one of which may persist as the dominant feature, dependig on the age of the patient, the local physiologic characteristics of the skin involved, and the persistence of the underlying cause. The initial stage is *erythema*, which proceeds to microvesicle formation, *weeping*, or oozing. The epidermal response to the injurious process then causes a burst of rapid epidermal mitotic activity that leads to *scaling*. Finally, *lichenification* (thickening of the skin) and *pigmentary disturbances* supervene. In the young infant, the first three stages predominate; lichenification is not seen.

Although the eczematous eruption itself is not difficult to recognize, it may be quite difficult to distinguish one type of eczema from another, particularly because the histologic features in most of them are identical. The most common causes of eczema in the adult are least common in the newborn. Indeed, eczema is a much less common disorder in the neonatal period than in the infant older than 2 months.

During the neonatal period eczema may be considered under two broad categories: exogenous and endogenous. The exogenous causes include primary irritant contact dermatitis and infection. The endogenous group may be divided into those causes in which the skin's role is predominant and others in which the eruption reflects a serious systemic disease.

Primary irritancy (as opposed to allergy) is probably the most common exogenous cause of eczema in the newborn. The distribution of the eruption varies somewhat, depending on the precipitating agent. Saliva may be irritating to the face and fecal excretions irritating to the buttocks. Detergent bubble bath, antiseptic proprietary agents, and harsh soaps containing mercury, phenol, tars, salicylic acid, or sulphur may cause an acute eczematous diaper dermatitis, which may become generalized. Precise information about what has been applied to the skin is imperative in making an accurate diagnosis.

When exogenous agents have been ruled out as a cause of the eruption and the infant is otherwise quite well, several diagnoses may be entertained. One of these is *seborrheic eczema (seborrheic dermatitis)*. This refers to a condition characterized by greasy scaling associated with patchy redness, fissuring, and occasional weeping, usually involving the scalp, ears, and perineal folds. There is controversy as to whether seborrheic eczema is a distinct entity or whether it presages the advent of atopic dermatitis. Since many cases of seborrheic eczema evolve into typical atopic dermatitis, perhaps it would be more accurate to consider the greasy scaliness as one of the morphologic components of the eczematous process, such as redness and weeping. Some infants never progress beyond the seborrheic phase of the dermatitis or develop the other features of atopic dermatitis, which in its classical form is rarely seen in the first month. *Cradle cap* is probably a minor variant of seborrheic eczema. The usual course of seborrheic eczema is one of rapid regression after 1 or 2 weeks of therapy. Occasionally, the process becomes more widespread to involve the entire body, resulting in a full-blown exfoliative dermatitis lasting 3 or 4 months. This has been called *Leiner's disease*. Scaling may also result from Ritter's disease or congenital ichthyosiform erythroderma (p. 590).

From the preceding discussion, it should be clear that the term diaper dermatitis may have a variety of causes. The proper management of a diaper dermatitis should include culture of the exudate for bacteria and yeast, the discontinuance of all ointments containing irritants, and conservative treatment (see below) for 1 or 2 weeks. If no improvement follows, a biopsy may be indicated.

Eczema may also be caused by a number of systemic conditions (discussed elsewhere), including histiocytosis X, Wiskott-Aldrich syndrome, ataxia-telangiectasia, sex-linked agammaglobulinemia, phenylketonuria, gluten-sensitive enteropathy, and long arm 18 deletion syndrome. It is especially noteworthy that practically all patients with anhidrotic ectodermal dysplasia have an eczematous eruption identical to atopic dermatitis.

Topical treatment of eczema

When bacterial or fungal infection exists, appropriate antibacterial or antifungal therapy is indicated, based on the results of culture and sensitivity studies. Weeping lesions should be treated by compressing or bathing in tepid water; protective ointments (such as simple zinc oxide paste) and nonmedicated powders (such as talc) should be applied after each diaper change; soiled ointments and pastes should be removed with mineral oil. A more extensive eruption may be treated for short periods with 1% hydrocortisone cream. A scaly eruption in the scalp may be treated by frequent shampooing with a sulfur- or salicylic acid–containing shampoo. Bathing should be done in tepid water containing a water-dispersible oil. It must be stressed that infants with diffuse dermatitis lose heat readily and are intolerant of even mild changes in environmental temperature or humidity. For these reasons humidification of the bedroom in winter and air conditioning in summer are desirable.

SUBCUTANEOUS AND INFILTRATIVE DERMATOSES

Juvenile xanthogranuloma

One fifth of infants with juvenile xanthogranuloma are affected at birth, and two thirds have onset of lesions before 6 months of age. There is no predilection for race or sex; no familial predisposition has been noted for this self-limiting disorder, which usually remains confined to the skin. The skin lesions are often restricted to the head, neck, and upper trunk and typically are reddish yellow, small papules, which may enlarge to become nodules. Involution may leave a flat atrophic pigmented scar. Serum lipids are normal, but histologically the lesions result from an infiltrate of fat-laden histiocytes, giant cells, and mixed inflammatory cells. Ocular lesions represent the most frequent complication (although, rarely, involvement of other organs may occur) and may result in ocular tumors, unilateral glaucoma, hyphema, uveitis, heterochromia iridis, and proptosis. Ophthalmologic consultation is required for management of the ocular lesions, but the best treatment for the skin lesons is expectant observation.

Mastocytosis

Mast cell disease may be present at birth and result in a solitary mast cell tumor, a disseminated maculopapular or nodular eruption, a bullous eruption, or a diffuse infiltration in the skin. The disseminated form may be complicated by mast cell infiltrates in internal organs. The most common form is the firm, soltary mast cell tumor. These are generally ovoid, pink or tan hue, and rarely exceed 6 cm in diameter. The lesions are conspicuous by their tendency to form wheals when rubbed and, in the newborn, to develop overlying blisters. Solitary lesions involute spontaneously within months to years. The maculopapular or nodular forms often become manifest in later infancy. Systemic manifestations of histamine release and residual cutaneous brown patches may be present. Treatment of disseminated forms should aim at control of the manifestations of excess histamine release, avoidance of drugs known to cause histamine release (for example, codeine, morphine and its derivatives, and polymyxin B), and frequent monitoring for spread of the disease. Infrequently occurring coagulopathies may need correction. Some of the distressing cutaneous symptoms, such as dermographism and pruritis, may be palliated with cyproheptadine. Hot water bathing and vigorous toweling must be avoided. The prognosis for most cases of mastocytosis, even in its disseminated cutaneous form, is good. The genetics of this condition is not clear. A few pedigrees have been reported with more than one affected family member.

Subcutaneous fat necrosis and sclerema neonatorum

Both subcutaneous fat necrosis and sclerema neonatorum occur within the first 3 months of life. Recently it has been suggested that they may be variants of the same basic disorder of fat metabolism. Sclerema neonatorum usually affects the preterm or debilitated newborn. It is manifested by diffuse hardening of the subcutaneous tissue, resulting in a tight, smooth skin that feels bound to the underlying structures. The skin is cold and stony hard. The joints become immobile and the face masklike. The affected infant may also have multiple congenital anomalies or develop sepsis, pneumonia, or severe gastroenteritis. Central nervous system abnormalities, autonomic dysfunction, and respiratory distress frequently complicate the course of the disease. The mortality is high, but the cutaneous changes rarely last longer than 2 weeks if the infant survives. Systemic administration of steroids has been used in severely ill infants, but they have not been demonstrated to be effective.

The lesions of subcutaneous fat necrosis are localized and sharply circumscribed. They may appear as small nodules or large plaques and are found on the cheeks, buttocks, back, arms, and thighs. The affected tissue is hard, may appear reddish or violaceous, and occasionally has the texture of orange peel. Histologically, there is a granulomatous reaction in the fat, with foreign body giant cells, fibroblasts, lymphocytes, and histiocytes. Resolution of the lesion results in fibrosis. Several studies have led to the suggestion that the ratio of saturated to unsaturated fatty acids in the affected area is altered in the direction of an increase in palmitin and stearin. Precipitating causes of fat necrosis include cold exposure, trauma, asphyxia, and peripheral circulatory collapse. Usually the lesions resolve in several weeks or months without symptoms. Complications include calcium deposits in the lesion, leading to ulceration and drainage. Accompanying systemic findings may include refusal to feed, irritability, fever, and failure to thrive. Systemic administration of steroids is not indicated. Local drainage of calcified areas may lessen subsequent scarring.

Cold panniculitis

Cold-induced fat necrosis of the cheeks may occur in the small infant. Warm, red, indurated plaques appear a few hours to a few days following the episode of cold exposure. The lesions resolve in 2 to 3 weeks. An ice cube applied to normal skin of these patients for 2 minutes will result in formation of a nodule at the site of application. The induced nodule appears in 3 to 72 hours and parallels the course of the spontaneous lesion. The histologic picture is one of perivascular inflammation and aggregation of lipids from rupture of fat cells. Postinflammatory hyperpigmentation may mark the site of a healed nodule.

MISCELLANEOUS CONGENITAL DISEASES AFFECTING THE SKIN

A multitude of hereditary diseases affect the skin. Some of these have been discussed earlier in this chapter, and some are discussed elsewhere in this text. The limitations of space do not permit extensive discussion of others, but it is appropriate to review some congenital diseases that have particular outstanding cutaneous findings.

Focal dermal hypoplasia (Goltz's syndrome)

Focal dermal hypoplasia is a profound mesodermal and ectodermal deficiency syndrome that appears to be inherited as a sex-linked or simple dominant, mutant gene. It is not clear whether the gene is on the X chromosome or one of the autosomes. The cutaneous features of the process are linear streaks of atrophy, yellow-brown or red excrescences—some papillomatous and others looking like partially deflated balloons, perioral and perianal papillomas, pigmentary variability, telangiectasia, sweating deficits as well as excesses, hyperkeratosis, abnormalities in the quality and density of hair, and vascular instability. Histologically, there is almost complete absence of the dermis and its appendages; herniations of fat that lie just beneath the epidermis result in the characteristic yellowish, sacklike nodules and papules. Associated with the cutaneous features are a host of other abnormalities, including skeletal defects (spinal anomalies, microcrania, asymmetry of facial bones, absence of digits, syndactyly, phocomelia, and rib, scapular, clavicular, and pelvic anomalies), ocular anomalies (ranging from enophthalmia to minor pigmentary defects of the iris), dental anomalies, renal defects, central nervous system defects (mental retardation, seizures), and a variety of other soft tissue abnormalities affecting heart, stomach, rectum and muscle.

Cutis laxa (generalized elastolysis)

Congenital cutis laxa (there is also an adult form) is a rare disorder that is probably inherited as an autosomal recessive trait. Infants with cutis laxa have diminished resilience of the skin, which hangs in folds and results in a bloodhound appearance, at once pathetic and aged. The joints do not show hypermobility, and there is no tendency to increased brusing. Elastic tissue may be greatly diminished in the dermis and is of poor quality. The collagen has normal tensile properties. Elastic fibers elsewhere in the body also seem to be affected, resulting in inguinal, diaphragmatic, and ventral hernias, pulmonary emphysema, and aortic aneurysm.

Cutis hyperelastica (Ehlers-Danlos syndrome)

Cutis hyperelastica is inherited as an autosomal dominant trait. It is frequently confused with cutis laxa, but there are many differences between the two disorders. The skin of patients with Ehlers-Danlos skin is hyperextensible when stretched but snaps back with normal resiliency. In contrast to cutis laxa, the skin does not hang in redundant folds; the joints are hyperextensible; there is a tendency to easy bruising; and the elastic tissue defect (if any exists) is poorly defined. Characteristic lesions in the older child are flabby atrophic scars about the knees and elbows. Associated findings have included hypertelorism, frontal bossing, and myopia. Involvement of gastrointestinal tract may lead to episodes of acute blood loss; aortic aneurysms may also develop.

THE ECTODERMAL DYSPLASIAS

Anhidrotic (hypohidrotic) ectodermal dysplasia

Absence of sweating, hypotrichosis, and defective dentition are the most striking features of this disorder, which is usually inherited in an X-linked dominant fashion. The existence of females with the full syndrome suggests that an autosomal recessive gene may cause the same phenotype. The facies is distinctive because of frontal bossing and depression of the bridge of the nose. Eyebrows and lashes are absent or sparse. The skin around the eyes is wrinkled and frequently hyperpigmented. The skin elsewhere is thin, dry, and hypopigmented, and the cutaneous vasculature is prominent. The scalp and body hair is sparse, the ears and chin prominent. The lips are thick and everted and may show pseudorhagades. Dental anomalies range from total anodontia to hypodontia with defective teeth.

The most striking physiologic abnormality is the absence of sweating, which can be demonstrated by application to the palm of 1 drop of 5% O-phthalaldehyde in xylene and confirmed by skin biopsy. Other glandular structures may also be absent or hypoplastic. Less constant ancillary findings include conductive hearing loss, gonadal abnormalities, stenotic lacrimal puncta, corneal dysplasia, and cataracts. Mental development is usually normal, but some degree of retardation has been seen in selected patients.

The most serious constitutional effect of anhidrotic ectodermal dysplasia is the marked heat intolerance caused by an inability to adequately regulate the body temperature by sweating. Undiagnosed infants often undergo extensive investigation for unexplained bouts of fever. Prudent observation of such infants, however, will rapidly disclose correlation of fever with fluctuations in environmental temperature. Every effort should be made to moderate extreme environmental temperatures by air conditioning. Deficient lacrimation can be palliated by the regular use of artificial tears. The nasal mucosa must also be protected by intermittent saline irrigations and application of petrolatum. It is imperative that these children have a thorough dental evaluation during the first years of life, and prostheses should be provided even for toddlers so that adequate nutrition is maintained. Reconstructive procedures can be performed later in life to improve the facial configuration. A wig may be required for patients with extremely scant scalp hair.

The incidence of atopic diseases—asthma, allergic rhinitis, and atopic dermatitis—is increased significantly in anhidrotic ectodermal dysplasia. Atopic manifestations should be managed as they would be in otherwise normal infants and children.

Other causes of ectodermal dysplasia include hidrotic ectodermal dysplasia, the EEC syndrome (ectrodactyly, ectodermal dysplasia, and cleft palate), Ellis van Creveld syndrome, and congenital ectodermal dysplasia of the face. Isolated lack of sweat glands occurs in familial and congenital familial anhidrosis.

PRINCIPLES OF THERAPY

Punch biopsy technique

Punch biopsy may provide valuable information and is a frequently used diagnostic procedure. It is advisable to have someone hold the infant while a second person performs the procedure. Biopsy should be avoided around the eyelids and their margins, the tip and bridge of the nose, the cupid's bow of the lips, the columella of the upper lip, and the nipples. Hairy areas should be shaved. The site should be washed with soap and water. Seventy percent alcohol is acceptable but should not be used around the eyes or genitalia.

The area is infiltrated with 0.5 to 1 cc of 1% lidocaine hydrochloride without epinephrine. A sharp 3 mm punch is firmly pressed against the lesion and gently rotated until a slight give is felt. The punch is then removed. Very little effort is required to penetrate newborn skin. Considerable gentleness is required so that the epidermis is not torn away from the dermis in performing the biopsy, particularly in the blistering diseases. It is desirable to obtain some subcutaneous fat with each biopsy. Newborn fat will generally separate quite readily. One may cut the plug away from the underlying tissue with a sharp scissors. The tissue should not be squeezed. Usually no sutures are necessary, and a simple dressing will suffice for the healing period.

The specimen should be placed in a bottle containing 10% aqueous buffered formaldehyde solution (Formalin), the cap closed, and the bottle agitated to ensure that the skin plug is immersed in the formaldehyde solution. The bottle should then be labeled as to name, date, and site of biopsy. Clinical information should be included with the specimen sent to the pathologist. It is often desirable in a general pathology laboratory to inform the pathologist that a skin biopsy from an infant is being forwarded so that special care may be taken in the processing. Tiny specimens are easily lost during the gross examination or in the automated tissue-processing devices.

General principles

Treatment of the skin of the newborn infant requires adjustment from the adult dosage of topical medicaments. The following guidelines are useful.

1. Minor fleeting erythematous macular or papular eruptions occur at the end of the first month. Their cause is unknown, and the best treatment is undiluted patience.
2. The more severe a dermatitis, the more vulnerable is the skin and therefore the more conservative should be the topical therapy.
3. In order to treat with confidence, one should know the natural course of a skin disease and so advise the parents.
4. Systemic complications of diffuse cutaneous eruptions occur more readily in infants; they should be anticipated and treated early.
5. If lesions are in different stages, treat only the most acute.
6. It is best to know and use a few topical remedies. Plain tap water is one of the safest and most helpful treatments for any acute dermatitis.
7. Pruritus is often more trying for parents than the infant. Environmental control of temperature and humidity and mild sedation is quite helpful for uncomplicated pruritus.
8. The passage of time is the most effective treatment of small, uncomplicated cavernous hemangiomas.
9. Hexachlorophene should not be used on damaged skin, if at all.
10. Normal skin does not need extensive lubrication. If lubrication is desirable, it is better to use a cream than an oil (for example, hydrophilic ointment).
11. Removal of a protective paste from the perineal area should be done gently with mineral oil, not by scrubbing with soap and water.
12. Lotions, pastes, talc, and ointments should not be used on weeping lesions.
13. Occlusive dressings (such as polyethylene film, Saran Wrap) should not be used in this age group.
14. Daily shampoos are not harmful if used to treat seborrheic dermatitis.
15. Exposure to sunlight should be very gradual, especially in fair-skinned infants.
16. Topical anesthetics, proteolytic enzymes, and tar ointments are rarely indicated in this age group.

NANCY B. ESTERLY
LAWRENCE M. SOLOMON

BIBLIOGRAPHY

Barman, J. M., Pecoraro, V., Astore, I., and Ferrer, J.: The first stage in the natural history of the human scalp hair cycle, J. Invest. Dermatol. **48**:138, 1967.

Carr, A., Hodgman, J. E., Freedman, R. J., and Levan, W. E.: Relationship between erythema toxicum and maturity, Am. J. Dis. Child. **112**: 129, 1966.

Cash, R., and Berger, C. W.: Acrodermatitis enteropathica; defective metabolism of unsutured fatty acids, J. Pediatr. **74**:717, 1969.

Champion, R. H.: Disorders of sweat glands. In Rook, A., Wilkinson, D. S., and Ebling, F. J. G., editors: Textbook of dermatology, Philadelphia, 1968, F. A. Davis Co., p. 1317.

Cleaver, J. E.: DNA damage and repair in light-sensitive human skin diseases, J. Invest. Dermatol. **54**:181, 1970.

Esterly, N. B.: The ichthyosiform dermatoses, Pediatrics **42**:990, 1968.

Fost, N. C., and Esterly, N. B.: Successful treatment of juvenile hemangiomas with prednisone, J. Pediatr. **72**:351, 1968.

Gordon, J.: Miliary sebaceous cysts and blisters in the healthy newborn, Arch. Dis. Child. **24**:286, 1949.

Green, M., and Behrendt, H.: Sweating capacity of neonates, Am. J. Dis. Child. **118**:725, 1969.

Griffiths, A. D.: Skin desquamation in the newborn, Biol. Neonate **10**:127, 1966.

Harris, J. R., and Schick, B.: Erythema neonatorum, Am. J. Dis. Child. **92**:27, 1956.

Holden, K. R., and Alexander, F.: Diffuse neonatal hemangiomatosis, Pediatrics **46**:411, 1970.

Horsefield, G. J., and Yardley, H. J.: Sclerema neonatorum, J. Invest. Dermatol. **44**:326, 1965.

Levin, S. E., Bakst, C. M., and Isserow, L.: Sclerema neonatorum treated with corticosteroids, Br. Med. J. **2**:1533, 1961.

Lund, H. A., and Kraus, J. M.: Melanotic tumors of the skin; fascile 3, atlas of tumor pathology, Washington, D. C., 1962, Armed Forces Institute of Pathology.

Maxwell and Esterly, N. B.: Cutis laxa, Am. J. Dis. Child. **117**:479, 1969.

Melish, M. E., and Glascow, L.: The staphylococcal scalded-skin syndrome; experimental model, N. Engl. J. Med. **282**:1114, 1970.

Mortensen, O., and Strougard-Andresen, P.: Harlequin color change in the newborn, Acta Obstet. Gynecol. Scand. **38**:352, 1959.

Nachman, R. L., and Esterly, N. B.: Increased skin permeability in preterm infants, J. Pediatr. **79**: 623, 1971.

Perera, P., Kurban, A. K., and Ryan, T. J.: The development of the cutaneous microvascular system in the newborn, Br. J. Dermatol **82**:86m 1970.

Pratt, A. G.: Birthmarks in infants, Arch. Dermatol. **67**:302, 1953.

Reed, W. B., Becker, S. W., Sr., Becker, S. W., Jr., and Nickel, W. R.: Giant pigmented nevi, melanoma and leptomeningeal melanocytosis, Arch. Dermatol. **91**:100, 1965.

Reed, W. B., Lopez, D. A., and Landing, B.: Clinical spectrum of anhidrotic ectodermal dysplasia, Arch. Dermatol. **102**:134, 1970.

Rostenburg, A., Jr., and Solomon, L. M.: Atopic dermatitis and infantile eczema. In Samter, M., editor: Immunologic diseases, ed. 2, Boston, 1971, Little, Brown and Co., p. 920.

Simpson, J. R.: Natural history of cavernous haemangiomata, Lancet **2**:1057, 1959.

Smeenk, G.: Two families with collodion babies, Br. J. Dermatol. **78**:81, 1966.

Solomon, L. M.: Epidermal nevi. In Madden, S., and Brown, T. H., editors: Current dermatology management, St. Louis, 1970, The C. V. Mosby Co.

Solomon, L. M., and Beerman, H.: Cold panniculitis, Arch. Dermatol. **88**:897, 1963.

Solomon, L. M., Fretzin, D. F., and DeWald, R. L.: The epidermal nevus syndrome, Arch. Dermatol. **97**:273, 1968.

Somerville, D. A.: The effect of age on the normal bacterial flora of the skin, Br. J. Dermatol. **81**: 14, 1969.

Tromovitch, T. A., Abrams, A. A., and Jacobs, P. H.: Acne in infancy, Am. J. Dis. Child. **106**: 230, 1963.

Varadi, D. P., and Hall, D. A.: Cutaneous elastin in Ehlers-Danlos syndrome, Nature **208**:1224, 1965.

Weary, P. E., Graham, G. F. and Selder, R. F., Jr.: Subcutaneous fat necrosis of the newborn, South. Med. J. **59**:960, 1966.

Wessells, N. K.: Differentiation of epidermis and epidermal derivatives, N. Engl. J. Med. **277**:21, 1967.

Whitehouse, D.: Diagnostic value of the cafe-au-lait spot in children, Arch. Dis. Child. **41**:316, 1966.

Wilkes, T., Freedman, R. I., Hodgman, J., and Levan, N. E.: The sensitivity of the axon reflex in term and premature infants, J. Invest. Dermatol. **47**:491, 1966.

Windhorst, D. B., Zelickson, A. S., and Good, R. A.: A human pigmentary dilution based on a heritable subcellular structural defect—the Chediak-Higashi syndrome, J. Invest. Dermatol. **50**:9, 1968.

Winkelmann, R. K.: The cutaneous innervation of the human newborn prepuce, J. Invest. Dermatol. **26**:53, 1956.

21 Ophthalmology

This chapter is designed to aid the pediatrician or general practitioner in diagnosing the most important eye diseases of the newborn infant. Developing the ability to recognize diseases early in their course is stressed. Blinding diseases such as congenital glaucoma, ophthalmia neonatorum, exposure of the cornea, or ocular infections will rapidly destroy useful vision unless diagnosed and treated. Malignant orbital tumors and retinoblastoma can threaten the life of the neonate. Ocular findings may lead to a diagnosis of a general pathologic condition, such as galactosemia and rubella. The infant usually has contact with only one physician during his neonatal period. It is important, therefore, for the pediatrician or general practitioner to recognize the subtle eye findings that may help save the eye or the life of his patient.

The importance of this ability is emphasized when one realizes that distinct ocular complaints are usually taken directly to the ophthalmologist, whereas subtle changes usually go unrecognized unless they are found by the primary physician. A detailed examination is described for detection of an occult ocular pathologic condition. The minimum ocular examination suggested for all neonates is outlined below.

No attempt is made to make the examiner an ocular specialist, since ophthalmic consultation is frequently available following the discovery of important ocular diseases. Therefore, we do not cover the entire field of pediatric ophthalmology. Certain detailed aspects of examination and treatment are included, however, for use in localities where ophthalmic consultation may not be readily available.

The eyes at birth are not completely developed either physiologically or anatomically. They will constantly change during the neonatal period. Thus a particular expected ocular reflex or response at an early period may be distinctly abnormal at a later, more mature phase. It is important, then, that the physician recognize the normal findings during different phases of the infant's growth in order to understand what is abnormal. A section on normal ocular findings is included and is given considerable stress for this purpose.

EXAMINATION OF THE EYE AND ORBITS

The complete ophthalmologic examination that follows occupies a period of 30 to 45 minutes. This may be a period of time that is difficult to fit into the examiner's busy day for every neonate; it can be shortened for the routine examination of all neonates (see outline below). A detailed examination is described for each part of the eye so that a maximum amount of information may be obtained for those patients where a subtle pathologic condition necessitates a thorough examination or where history indicates the potential for a pathologic condition in one specific segment of the eye.

MINIMAL OCULAR EXAMINATION SEQUENCE

A. History (including family history), length and possible abnormality of pregnancy, labor, and delivery
B. External examination
    1. Proportional relationships of globes and orbits to surrounding facial structures
    2. Equality of orbits, globes, and corneas to fellow eye
    3. Symmetry and normal contour of lids
    4. Ptosis

5. Ocular motility (including fixation and following response)
6. Pupil size, regularity and response to light
7. Palpation of the orbital rim and eyelids
8. Palpation of the lacrimal sac
9. Inspection of the lid margins and lashes
10. Inspection of the conjunctival sac (note conjunctival and scleral color)
11. Cornea, size and clarity to the limbus

C. Internal examination
1. Inspection of anterior chamber depth
2. Iris, color and clarity of trabeculation
3. Dilatation of the pupils with 1% cyclopentolate (Cyclogyl) hydrochloride and 10% phenylephrine (Neo-Synephrine) hydrochloride
4. Normal black pupil with direct illumination and clear red reflex through the ophthalmoscope
5. Vitreous clarity
6. Disc size, contour and sharpness of detail
7. Vessels, normal distribution and ratio
8. Macular area pigmentation
9. Peripheral retina

An adequate ocular examination should begin with a careful history. A family history of ocular diseases is of considerable importance. For example, a family history of retinoblastoma necessitates a thorough, frequent search of the fundus for the onset of this dominantly inherited malignant disease. Important additional information includes maternal diseases such as rubella, injuries, or unusual medication during the prenatal period. It is important to note the length and possible abnormalities of pregnancy, labor, and delivery; and specific attention should be directed to those areas that are suggested by the pertinent history. For example, prematurity suggests the possibility of retrolental fibroplasia, and difficult delivery with obstetrical forceps suggests the possibility of direct ocular trauma.

The examination will be easier and more complete if it is done under comfortable circumstances. The best examining surface is waist high in a room where the light is bright but can be easily darkened for the intraocular examinations. A blanket should be available to swaddle the infant, and a nurse or assistant should be available to hold the infant's head or expose the eye. Irritating and forceful studies should be deferred until all general observations have been made. A great deal can be learned if the examiner takes a few moments to observe the infant while he is undisturbed and comfortable. Observations of spontaneous general and ocular activity are considerably more reliable while the infant is being held or is nursing and are totally unreliable when he is screaming and crying (Fig. 21-1).

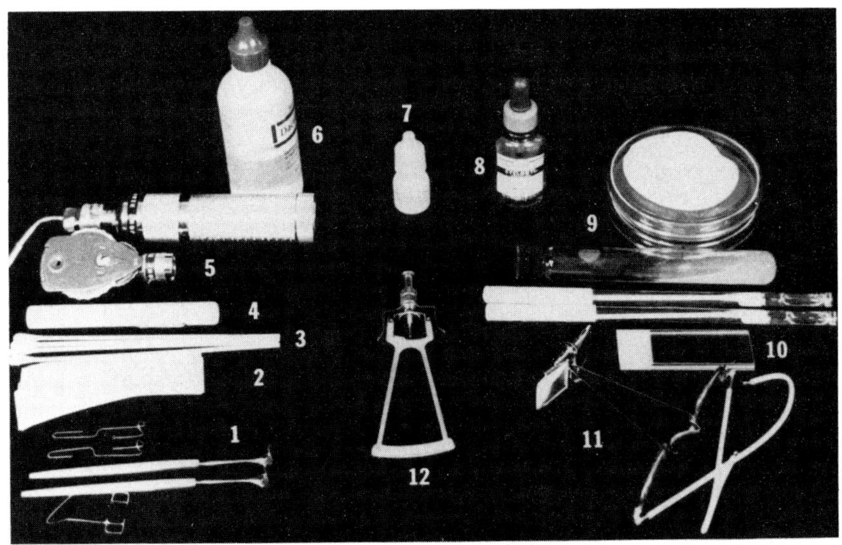

Fig. 21-1. Equipment for ocular examination: *1,* Eye speculum, paper clip retractors or Desmarre retractors; *2,* fluorescein strips; *3,* sterile cotton tipped applicator; *4,* penlight or otoscope; *5,* ophthalmoscope; *6,* saline or 5% dextrose irrigation; *7,* 10% phenylephrine, ophthalmic; *8,* 1% cyclopentolate, ophthalmic; *9,* culture tubes and plates, sterile swabs; *10,* glass microscope slides; *11,* loupe; and *12,* Schiøtz tonometer.

A useful pattern for the ophthalmic examination is as follows. The general facial configuration and the external configuration of the orbit are inspected first. The orbital contents should be proportional and symmetrical when compared with the overall craniofacial configuration. The lids are examined grossly and are appraised for symmetry and for both horizontal and vertical position. The spontaneous opening and closing of the eyes is assessed. If a ptosis is present, particular attention should be paid to the size of the pupils. Miosis (a small pupil) on the side of the ptosis is suggestive of Horner's syndrome. A rapid up and down movement of the lid during nursing indicates a Marcus Gunn (jaw-winking) syndrome.

The eyes should be examined for spontaneous range of motion and for conjugate movement. This is best done while the infant is undisturbed and nursing. Fixation and following of a brightly colored object, the nursing bottle, or a bright light in a dimly lit room should be noted for each eye separately and both eyes together.

A gross estimate of vision can be obtained at this time. The pupils should first be inspected to see if they are normally round and equal in diameter. A penlight or ophthalmoscope with transilluminating head is used to shine direct light at the pupil, first in one eye and then in the other. Normally, each pupil will constrict to both direct and contralateral stimulation. First, the reaction of the illuminated pupil is observed. It should constrict briskly (the response in the neonate may not be as rapid as that in an older child) and should remain constricted as long as the illumination is maintained. If it does not constrict, the contralateral pupil's reaction to the direct illumination of the first eye should be studied. If the contralateral pupil constricts, the directly illuminated eye must have intact photoreceptors and optic nerve pathways. Failure of constriction in the directly illuminated eye may be the result of the absence of useful vision or inflammation of the iris, which prevents pupillary movement. If neither the illuminated pupil nor the contralateral pupil constricts (and the contralateral pupil constricts on subsequent direct illumination), the first eye is deficient in vision and may be blind. Each eye should be tested similarly for both direct and consensual reaction.

Direct light stimulation to one eye should normally produce direct and consensual pupillary constriction. If the light is rapidly shifted to the opposite eye after pupillary constriction, both pupils should remain constricted for as long as the stimulation continues. If, however, the shift of light should be followed by dilatation of the newly directly stimulated eye, the phenomenon of pupillary escape (the Marcus Gunn pupil) has occurred. This indicates decreased vision in the eye whose pupil dilates.

Rarely, the pupillary reflexes will be completely normal but the child still will not see, because of intracranial abnormalities, particularly in the occipital cortex. This phenomenon is called cortical blindness.

The normal neonate frequently has small, 2-mm pupils that may show some tendency to change size symmetrically and rhythmically (hippus). The phenomenon of hippus rarely has clinical significance.

The pupillary space should be uniformly black. A white reflection of any amount is abnormal and indicates an opacity within the lens, vitreous, or retina (p. 634).

Examinations that may be annoying to the infant may now be carried out. The lid margins should be inspected for regularity of contour and for the presence of the lacrimal puncta. The lacrimal puncta are seen as two minute holes in the lid margins posterior and medial to the lashes and a short distance laterally from the inner corner of the eye. The puncta should lie next to the globe but should not be turned either in or out.

Palpation of the orbit should include examination of the orbital margin, the contents of the upper and lower lids, and the round contour of the globes. The orbital rims should be sharp in outline. In the newborn, they are initially round and increase more in vertical diameter with the normal growth pattern. The area of the lacrimal sac is palpated for abnormal masses or increase in size and should be pressed against the bones of the nose and medial orbital wall. Expression of mucopurulent or purulent material from the lacrimal puncta should be noted.

To see the lash structures the examiner

should view them with magnification, such as an ocular loupe (which gives 2× to 3× magnification), or through the ophthalmoscope with the +10 diopter lens in place. Normally, the lashes are directed outward in an orderly row. Abnormalities are distichiasis, or an additional row of lashes posterior to the gray line; entropion, an inward turning of the lid; and trichiasis, an inward turning of the lashes. Lashes that contact the cornea are dangerous. Continued irritation will eventually predispose the eye to infections of the cornea.

The lids should be separated and the conjunctival sac inspected. Lid separation may be accomplished by the use of a pediatric ocular speculum, lid retracters, or the fingers (Fig. 21-2). A useful lid retractor may be fashioned from a paper clip. The paper clip is straightened out, leaving the two bent ends. One of the ends is bent back upon itself approximately ¼ inch from the tip, making a small, hook-shaped process with a rounded tip. All instruments that are introduced into the eye should, of course, be sterilized. The bulbar and palpebral conjunctiva should then be examined for the normal, moist, pinkish appearance. Redness or exudate is abnormal and often indicates infection, which can be confirmed by smear and culture. The conjunctiva of the lids overlying the tarsal plates should be examined by eversion of the lids. Eversion usually occurs quite readily when the lids are separated with fingers, particularly if the infant is attempting to squeeze his lids shut. If eversion of the lids does not occur readily, further attempts should probably not be pursued if the examiner is not an ophthalmologist, since stretching or tearing of the delicate lid structures may occur.

The normal white sclera is inspected for changes of color. Normally, a bluish discoloration is present in prematures and other small babies, because of their very thin sclera. The cornea is inspected with a penlight. Magnification with a loupe or with an ophthalmoscope's +10 diopter lens in place is again employed. In prematures and in full-term infants during the first few days of life, the cornea may be somewhat less than transparent, with a slight hazy appearance. This is thought to be the result

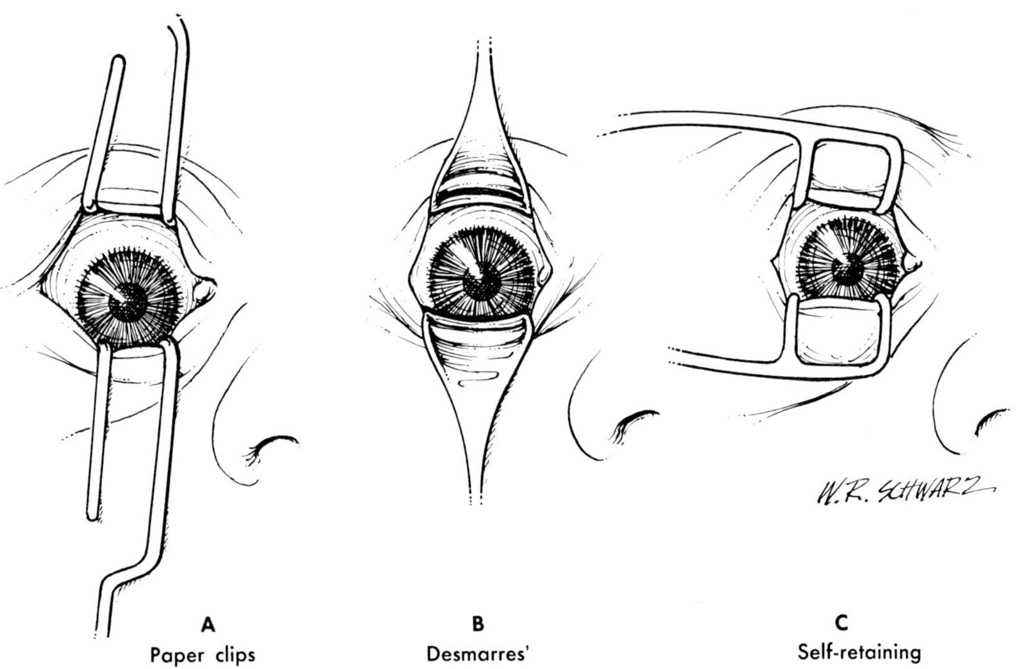

Fig. 21-2. Ophthalmic lid retractors available for eye examinations. Illustrations show the proper application and retraction. *A*, Made from ordinary paper clips; **B**, manual Desmarres' retractor; **C**, self-retaining lid retractor.

of corneal edema, and it eventually disappears. The surface of the cornea should have good luster, and the whole cornea should be absolutely transparent. A change in luster usually indicates a break or an unevenness in the anterior surface of the cornea, such as an abrasion of the cornea or corneal edema. Transparency should be complete to the extreme periphery of the cornea. Any opacity or translucency is abnormal after the first few days of life. Changes in transparency or opacification of the periphery of the cornea is associated with a local mesodermal abnormality, which may be complicated by congenital glaucoma. The horizontal diameter of the cornea should be approximately 10 mm. However, we have measured a number of apparently normal corneas that are between 9 and 10 mm in full-term infants. The average adult cornea measures 12 mm in the horizontal diameter, and this dimension is achieved during the first year of life. The corneas should be equal in size. An accurate measurement of the cornea is unnecessary at this time. If congenital glaucoma is suspected, however, because of corneal haze or enlargement or because of photophobia or tearing, an accurate measurement of corneal diameter and intraocular pressure with the infant under general anesthesia is required.

Next, the anterior chamber should be inspected. This is the aqueous-filled area between the cornea and the iris. It should be clear. The depth of the anterior chamber is the distance between the posterior surface of the cornea and the anterior surface of the iris. The simplest method of estimating the depth of the anterior chamber involves illuminating the iris at a right angle to the observer's line of sight; that is, the light source is directed from the temporal side in the plane of the iris (Fig. 21-3). Normally, the neonate has a moderately shallow chamber. As a result of flattening of the lens and the increase in corneal diameter during growth, the anterior chamber increases in depth and the iris flattens during the first year of life.

Normal irises are equal in color. Iris pigmentation is normally incomplete for the first 6 months of life; both irises develop pigmentation at the same time. The normal Caucasian iris lacking pigment is blue or blue-gray for the first few weeks or months of life, whereas the darkly pigmented Caucasians and darker races may show pigmentation at birth or within the first week. Heterochromia, or dissimilarity in pigmentation between the two eyes, may indicate a normal hereditary pattern, congenital Horner's syndrome, or several syndromes, which are discussed later in this chapter. These may not develop until the end of the neonatal period or even later in life when full pigmentation of the normal iris occurs.

The normal lens should be clear and appear black in direct light. The red reflex through the ophthalmoscope should show no dullness or irregularities.

The fundus examination should be conducted in a dimly lit room with the infant's pupils dilated. The pupils may be safely dilated in a newborn infant as well as in prematures by the use of one drop of 1% cyclopentolate (Cyclogyl) and one drop of 10% phenylephrine (Neo-Synephrine). Dark irises take somewhat longer than an average of 20 minutes to dilate fully. Drops may be

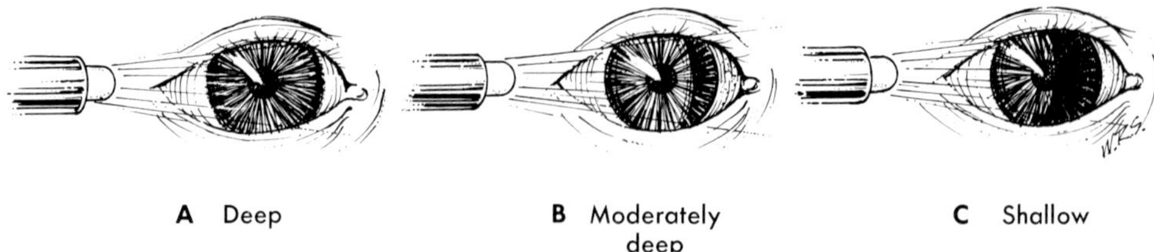

A Deep **B** Moderately deep **C** Shallow

Fig. 21-3. Method of estimating the depth of the anterior chamber with a handlight. *A*, Deep anterior chamber—the iris is flat and completely illuminated by a light at right angles at the lateral canthus. *B*, If the anterior chamber is moderately shallow (less distance from the cornea to the iris), the domed shape of the iris casts a crescentlike shadow nasally; the shallower the depth, the more shadow. *C*, With an extremely shallow anterior chamber the entire nasal iris is in shadow.

repeated once or twice if the pupils do not dilate well. Infants with cardiac irregularities, those with extremely flattened anterior chambers, and those with changing neurologic signs should not have their pupils dilated. In actual practice, the vast majority of neonates, especially prematures, can and should have their pupils dilated. Visualizing the fundus of the newborn eye is difficult under any circumstances and is nearly impossible with undilated pupils. The examination with the ophthalmoscope requires the use of an assistant and a small lid speculum to overcome the squeezing of the lids, the inevitable result of shining a strong light in the infant's eye.

Each eye should first be studied with the ophthalmoscope with a +10 diopter lens in place, beginning approximately 5 inches in front of the eye. Because of the sharp plane of focus of a +10 diopter lens, only one plane of depth may be studied with the ophthalmoscope at a given distance from the eye. Thus the ophthalmoscope may be used in a tomographic fashion, first to study the cornea, then the anterior chamber and iris, then the pupil and lens, and finally the anterior vitreous. Each are focused individually as one moves closer to the patient.

With the lenses in the ophthalmoscope changed, the posterior vitreous and the fundus are then seen and studied in detail. In eyes of near-adult antero-posterior length, the fundus will be focused with a zero of low-power lens. Most newborn eyes, especially those of prematures, have short anteroposterior lengths, and their fundi are seen clearly with plus diopter lenses (black numbers on the ophthalmoscope).

The optic nerve is the largest and most readily recognized structure in the posterior pole. Its diameter with the usual ophthalmoscope should be approximately one half to three fourths the diameter of the total area illuminated at one time. The optic disc is usually round and sharp in outline. It may normally be somewhat oval in its vertical diameter. Excessive elongation, especially inferiorly, may indicate a defect or coloboma of the disc. The disc appears to be larger in size in the myopic infant and smaller in the hyperopic infant. The optic nerve head or disc has been described as being somewhat more pale in the neonate than in the adult; however, this may be artifact, caused by external pressure placed on the globe by the examiner or his assistant, which transmits pressure to the small vessels of the disc, which collapse, producing an apparent pallor. The retinal vessels should exit from the disc in the superior and inferior quadrants and should be smooth in outline as they curve diagonally and branch dichotomously to cover the full extent of the retina. Branches usually leave the main vessel at an angle of less than 90°. The arterioles and venules of the retinal circulation should be examined for size, regularity, color, and the presence or absence of pulsation. These should be followed from the disc to the periphery as far as possible in each meridian of the clock. The macular area of the retina, which subserves precise vision and color vision, is located approximately 1½ disc diameters temporal to the disc and is identified normally by a slightly reddish brown color and by the pattern of surrounding blood vessels, which appear to radiate toward it. In prematures, the normal macular coloration may be absent, and in all neonates the foveal reflex is absent until approximately 4 months of age. The normal reddish brown pigment of the macula should be approximately ½ disc diameter in size and should show uniform regularity. Pigment mottling or stippling in the macula or elsewhere is abnormal. The examination of the retina should be continued from the macula as far toward the periphery as possible, examining the regularity of the normal pink-orange color. The far periphery of the retina, especially in the premature infant, appears pale gray and is hazy in appearance. This appearance often falsely suggests a retinal detachment. Premature and newborn infants have completely developed pigment epithelium but incompletely developed uveal pigment in the choroid. This gives a pale appearance to the fundus and offers a better view of the choroidal blood vessels, which appear as distinct, closely packed, red, linear structures. They are broader and shorter than retinal vessels.

Abnormalities of the fundus are located by anatomical location from the disc, and size is related to fractions or multiples of the disc diameter. Areas of the fundus that appear to be out of focus in comparison to the rest of the surrounding fundus may indicate an elevation or tumor of the retina or underlying tumors of the choroid. Small rapid motions of the fundus while the examination is in progress may indicate the presence of nystagmus, which was not obvious during external inspection.

NORMAL OCULAR FINDINGS

The eye of the newborn infant differs from the adult eye primarily in function, although structural differences are also present. The growth of the eye parallels that of the brain. Thus growth continues at a rapid rate for the first 3 years of life, especially during the first year. The anteroposterior dimension of the eye at birth is about 16.5 mm and grows to a maximum of about 24 mm in adulthood. Seventy percent of the adult eye volume is obtained by the age of 4 years. Normal values in the neonate fall within a very wide range, and possibilities of abnormality in size may frequently be substantiated only by comparison in proportion to nearby structures or by relationship to measured values in the fellow eye.

The full-term infant's lid apertures are usually quite narrow, often being widely separated by prominent epicanthal folds. The term telecanthus indicates a disproportionate broadening of the medial canthal angles, a frequent finding in most neonates. Hypertelorism indicates a broadening of the distance between the two pupils. The latter is infrequent and abnormal. Measurements between the two medial canthi may vary from 18 to 22 mm. Horizontal measurement of the lid apertures varies considerably from 17 to 27 mm. These measurements should be nearly identical in the two eyes of any patient (Table 21-1).

Reflex tearing to irritants should be present shortly after birth. However, emotional tearing does not usually begin until about 3 weeks of age and is universally complete at 2 to 3 months. The latter tearing usually appears concomitantly with the onset of activity of the sebaceous glands of the skin. The newborn infant possesses a strong blink reflex to light and to stimulation of the lids, lashes, or cornea. The reflex response to a threatening gesture does not appear until 7 or 8 weeks of age.

The eyes should, for the most part, appear straight from birth. Changes in ocular position should be conjugate during the first few weeks of life. Conjugate gaze is determined by observing the light reflex from a hand light, held in front of the examiner's face, to be in an equal position on the patient's pupils. Erratic, purposeless, and independent movements of the two eyes are, however, normally observed during this period. These movements are comparable to the peripheral muscle activity seen in the extremities at the same time.

Since the macula of the newborn infant is structurally immature at birth, the capacity for central acute vision is lacking. The newborn infant, therefore, possesses only peripheral vision.

Retinal function is present at birth or shortly thereafter; whether it is perceived or cortically integrated as vision is yet unknown. Electroretinograms in newborns have shown an initial absence of electrical activity of the retina, followed by positive electrical activity, especially to strong stimuli, several hours after birth. We know by the pupillary response to light and by optokinetic responses that impulses travel the visual pathways at birth and participate in visual motor function.

Optokinetics describes the reflex ocular response to a moving target. A pursuit motion occurs as the target moves across the visual field and is followed by a rapid return motion in the opposite direction in order to regain fixation. This is similar to

TABLE 21-1. Ocular measurements

Measurement	Full-term newborn	Premature newborn (1,000-1,300 gm)
Intermedial canthal distance	18-22 mm	12-16 mm
Medial canthus to lateral canthus	17-27 mm	12-16 mm
Anteroposterior diameter of eye at birth	16 mm	16 mm
Horizontal diameter of cornea	10 mm (average) 9.0 mm (lower limits)	7½-8 mm (lower limits)

what occurs while watching telephone poles or fence posts while one is traveling in a fast-moving automobile. By the use of the optokinetic reflex, it has been determined that the infant is able to receive visual stimuli as early as 1½ hours after birth, and it has been estimated that the visual acuity of the newborn is approximately 20/700.

From birth and thereafter, a rapid turning of the head on the shoulders produces an opposite movement of the eyes—a doll's eye sign. The stimulation of tonic neck muscle reflexes makes the eyes move so that it appears that the eyes remain approximately in place as the head turns. The doll's eye movement occurs in blind as well as in normal eyes. At 2 weeks of age, the vestibuloocular reflex is superimposed. This is elicited by holding the infant vertically and rotating his body. A turning motion to the right produces a simultaneous movement of the eyes in the opposite direction. This is followed by a quick return movement of the eyes just as the rotation stops. This is a vestibular type of nystagmus. The absence of rotational nystagmus is an early indicator of gross neurologic abnormality.

The macula provides central precise vision. The center of the macula is termed the fovea; movement of the eyes in order to project the object of regard onto the fovea is called fixation. The ability to maintain a somewhat unsteady gaze occurs shortly after birth, particularly if a strong light stimulus is used. However, the ability to maintain steady gaze or fixation by following an object and its movement is achieved only weakly at 5 to 6 weeks of age. At first the "following" reflex, in which the eyes pursue a moving visual stimulus, is extremely weak and occurs for only a few degrees of eye movement without any further attempt on the infant's part to locate or direct his eyes toward the target. By 3 months of age the following reflex is fully active. At this time the infant maintains fixation and pursuit movements instantaneously in both vertical and horizontal directions. At approximately 4 months, central fixation is associated with the motor activity of grasping. Fusion of the two eyes with convergence ability is present at 6 months of age. The latter functions require visual acuity of approximately 20/40 to 20/60. Visual acuity cannot be measured in the neonatal period.

Prematurity

Prematurity imposes a number of anatomical and functional handicaps in the newborn infant, not the least of which involve the ocular structures. At 28 weeks' gestation, the normal developmental pupillary membrane is still present and is just beginning to atrophy. The lacrimal canaliculi are growing within the lids but are not yet open. The globe is only 10 to 14 mm in diameter. At the disc, Bergmeister's papilla and the hyaloid artery are beginning to atrophy. The anterior and posterior hyaloid systems surrounding the lens frequently are still present at this age. These structures begin to atrophy at the 28-week stage and continue their disappearance during the eighth month of gestation or during the premature's early extrauterine existence.

The lens has been noted to have a transient period of cataractous changes in a significant number of premature infants. These have been observed during the second week after birth and persist for approx-

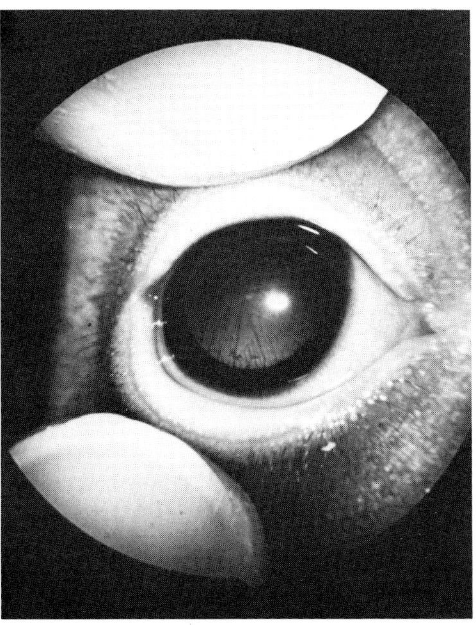

Fig. 21-4. Persistent pupillary membrane in a premature infant. Note the remnants of vascular loops of the anterior hyaloid system anterior to the lens. This will continue to atrophy during the first months of extrauterine life.

imately 2 weeks. These transient opacities of the lens are thought to be the result of a transient metabolic deficiency, possibly similar to that occurring in galactosemia. At 32 weeks' gestation the fetal nucleus of the lens is complete, but the lens may be hazy or translucent for some weeks. All of the retinal layers are developed, but they are thick and gray from the equator to the periphery.

The eyelids are usually separated by this period, but the last stages of separation may still be in progress. The horizontal corneal diameter may be 7½ to 8 mm, and the distance separating the two canthi may be 14 to 16 mm, with the horizontal lid measurement being approximately 12 to 14 mm.

THE BLIND INFANT

The pediatrician or general practitioner is usually called upon as the first examiner of a blind infant. This may be an infant whose eyes appeared normal during external inspection. A normal ocular examination does not rule out the possibility of blindness resulting from abnormalities lying within the remaining visual pathways between the eye and the occipital cortex. Tests of use in indicating the presence or absence of normal neural pathways include pupillary responses and doll's eye or rotational nystagmus or both, which are normal responses indicating intact subcortical reflexes. The presence of optokinetic nystagmus implies at least one intact visual cortex. Fixation, following, and eye-hand coordination indicate bilaterally intact visual cortical pathways. Electroretinography and oculoencephalography (the visually evoked response) may be the only means of detecting an intact retinal function and receipt of stimulation from the retina at the cortex, respectively (see outline below).

EXAMINATION OF THE BLIND INFANT

A. Subcortical reflexes
   1. Pupillary response
   2. Doll's eye movement
   3. Rotational or vestibular nystagmus
B. Visual cortical pathways
   1. Optokinetic nystagmus
   2. Fixation
   3. Following eye movements
   4. Eye-hand coordination
C. Electrical responses
   1. Electroretinography
   2. Visually evoked responses (oculoencephalography)
   3. Electrooculography

BIRTH TRAUMA

See also pp. 77-79.

Eye injuries may be associated with labor and delivery and are found in increasing amounts proportional to the length of labor and difficulty of delivery. Lid petechiae and hemorrhages are frequently found in face presentations and less frequently in vertex presentations (p. 77). These usually clear quite rapidly without treatment. Subconjunctival hemorrhages are also frequently seen and require no treatment (p. 78). These findings should, however, increase the suspicions of associated intraocular injuries. Forceps deliveries, particularly when associated with improper application, may produce lacerations of the lid or the globe (p. 78). The presence of a forceps mark or lid laceration requires a careful complete examination of the orbit for associated injuries. Forceps application may also produce ruptures in Descemet's membrane of the cornea (p. 79). These ruptures are seen only with magnification and appear as diagonal lines in the posterior cornea. They are rapidly followed by excess hydration of the cornea, with a subsequent cloudy appearance that must be differentiated from congenital glaucoma, infections of the cornea, or diseases associated with cloudy cornea, such as the mucopolysaccharidoses. Prolonged labor or forceful delivery with forceps may also produce bleeding into the anterior chamber. Retinal hemorrhages are frequently seen following delivery (p. 79). These are usually small and multiple and are scattered throughout the retina as small red dots. Notation should be made of any hemorrhage near or in the macular area, since it may possibly be related to subnormal visual acuity and strabismus at a later date. Retrobulbar hemorrhage may produce protrusion or proptosis of the globe and must be differentiated from a retrobulbar tumor. Rarely, the eye may be completely prolapsed, especially when the orbit is shallow; this constitutes an emergency because of exposure of the cornea and stress on the optic nerve and blood supply.

OCULAR INJURIES

Of prime importance in the treatment of ocular injuries is a full and careful evaluation of the extent of damage, with special reference to the globe itself. Ocular injuries caused by trauma in the neonatal period must be treated with the same meticulous care that is required in the adult. Because of the diminutive size of the neonate's eye, treatment usually requires microscopic evaluation and repair with the infant under general anesthesia. Lid lacerations should be given precise primary repair in order to minimize permanent deformity. Involvement of the lacrimal canaliculi, the lid margin, and the lacrimal gland requires special attention. Avulsion for tissue loss of the lids constitutes an urgent requirement for repair to prevent exposure injuries of the cornea.

Blunt injury in the neonate may produce blood in the anterior chamber (hyphema), rupture of the globe, dislocation of the lens vitreous hemorrhage, contusion cataract, scleral rupture, traumatic retinal detachment, retinal hemorrhages or edema, rupture of the choroid, and arterial or venous occlusion in the retina. Thermal and chemical burns may occur about the eyes and must be treated with the same care as in the adult. Treatment of these injuries is best handled by the ophthalmologist after the usual first-aid measures of cooling and protective covering. Of immediate and highest priority in the first-aid management of the chemical burn of the eye is copious irrigation with any available noninjurious fluid, such as tap water, milk, or normal saline solution.

Corneal abrasions are probably more frequent than is realized in the infant and are suggested by a symptom of tearing in one eye. The use of eye bandages during phototherapy has increased the incidence of this complication. Diagnosis is made by staining the cornea with a fluorescein-impregnated paper strip. This is done by moistening a sterile fluorescein strip with a drop of sterile saline solution and touching its tip to the lower conjunctival fornix. The area of corneal abrasion turns light green in ordinary illumination but is best seen in a light with a cobalt blue filter. A corneal abrasion is also suggested when a small shadow cast by the irregular epithelium is seen on the iris surface. The shadow moves with movement of the examining light. Treatment required for healing in most cases is the simple instillation of antibiotic drops for a few days.

Lacerations may involve the conjunctiva, the cornea, or the sclera. All conjunctival lacerations should be presumed to be associated with a laceration of the globe until proved otherwise. Lacerations of the cornea or sclera require immediate evaluation and surgical repair, even when they are tiny, as in the case of a perforation from a diaper pin.

Orbital or ocular foreign bodies require specialized precise localization in order to determine the proper therapeutic approach. Fortunately, they are rare in the neonate.

ABNORMAL FACIES

See also Chapter 18.

Eye abnormalities associated with congenital abnormalities of the face, skull, or head as a whole are briefly reviewed in this section. Many abnormalities are sufficiently extensive that it is impossible to correct them totally. Treatment is therefore limited to those areas that are presently amenable to surgical correction, such as the plastic repair of eyelids, nasal and aural deficiencies, and strabismus surgery.

Apert's syndrome

Acrocephalosyndactyly is a systemic deformity probably caused by a general mesodermal disturbance occurring about the seventh or eighth week of embryonic life. Oxycephaly affecting primarily the anterior portion of the skull creates high frontal bones, hypertelorism, and shallow orbits. The condition is sometimes associated with proptosis sufficient to produce corneal exposure and ulceration, exotropia, and ophthalmoplegia. The remainder of the syndrome shows syndactyly in varying degrees (from partial webbing to complete fusion of the fingers and toes), skeletal deformities of the limbs, and varying degrees of mental deficiency (p. 547).

Cornelia de Lange syndrome

The typical facial appearance in infants with the Cornelia de Lange syndrome is composed of a low hairline, eyebrows that are joined in the middle (synophrys), long eyelashes, and a small upturned nose. Skeletal deformities may be present, ranging from syndactyly to phocomelia. Eye disorders less frequently include hypertelorism and antimongoloid slant, strabismus, nystagmus, ptosis, high myopia, and pupillary abnormalities.

Cretinism (congenital hypothyroidism)

Swollen eyelids, hypertelorism, and an enlarged tongue constitute an early suggestive triad (p. 459).

Crouzon's disease

Craniofacial dysostosis is a hereditary abnormality formed, in part, by premature union of the coronary and lambdoidal sutures, combined with hypoplasia of the maxillary area of the face. This is manifest by prominence at the superior portion of the frontal bone, hypoplasia of the superior maxilla, and shortened orbital cavities, with a prognathic jaw. Ocular defects consists of exophthalmos, exotropia, and progressive optic atrophy.

Facial clefts

Typical facial clefts are caused by a failure of fusion between the maxillary and lateral nasal processes during fetal development. This creates a line of cleavage between the medial end of the lower lid and the upper lid. Such colobomas may vary in extent from a very small notch to almost total absence of the entire lower lid. Atypical clefts, presumably caused by pressure of amniotic bands, may occur in any direction on the face and may produce a great variety of anomalies. All facial clefts involving colobomas of the lids that prevent lid closure, and therefore cause corneal exposure, require immediate measures to prevent damage to the exposed cornea.

Goldenhar's syndrome

Goldenhar's syndrome is a rare syndrome of oculoauricular dysplasia, characterized by epibulbar dermoid cysts, accessory auricular appendages, and aural fistulas. The characteristic unilateral triad may also be associated with micrognathia, macrostomia, and multiple vertebral anomalies. Other ocular abnormalities less frequently seen include microphthalmia, microcornea, and coloboma of the upper lid. A genetic cause is uncertain.

Greig's hypertelorism

Greig's syndrome is a congenital dysostosis, which is the result of an anomaly in the development of the cranial bones. There is a gross broadening and depression of the nasal bridge, with a prominent forehead. The orbits are widely displaced and are accompanied frequently by external strabismus. Optic atrophy may occur. Proptosis is rare. The mentality is usually normal. There is maxlllary hypoplasia.

Hallerman-Streiff syndrome

Mandibulooculofacial dyscephaly is marked by hypoplasia of the mandibles, a thin, prominent nose, described as a parrot beak, and bilateral microphthalmia often associated with cataracts or microcornea or both. Glaucoma may complicate the eye findings at a later period. This syndrome may be confined to the above findings or may be more severe and associated with more generalized anomalies, including atrophy of the facial skin, hypotrichosis, and marked dwafism with dental and nasal abnormalities, which together give the infant an aged, wrinkled appearance. All cases have been sporadic in their appearance. The causative factors are unknown.

Hemifacial atrophy of Romberg

This unilateral deformity is characterized by hypoplasia of the external ear, occasional extra appendages, and an atrophic middle ear. The maxillary, malar, and palatine bones are most often smaller and flatter with hemiatrophy of the mandible and absence of the zygomatic arch. The soft tissues of the face are hypoplastic and flat, and the fifth and seventh cranial nerves may be paretic. Ocular complications commonly include Horner's syndrome and an antimongoloid slant to the outer canthus. Other associated abnormalities that have been reported are anophthalmia, heterochromia iridis, ptosis, oculomotor palsies, and nystagmus. The cause of this condition is unknown.

Mandibulofacial dysostosis

Also known as Treacher Collins' or Franceschetti's syndrome, this anomaly is a result of inadequate differentiation of the maxillary mesoderm derived from the first branchial arch and is inherited as an irregular autosomal dominant trait. The amount of expression of this abnormality is variable. It is characterized by an antimongoloid obliquity of the fissures, with atypical colobomas of the outer portion of the lower lids. Extraocular abnormalities are hypoplasia of the malar bone and mandible, malformations of the external ears and occasionally of the middle ear, macrostomia with a high palate and dental abnormalities, blind fistulas between the angle of the mouth and the ear, and tongue-shaped projections of the hairline onto the cheek. Treacher Collins' syndrome is differentiated from Goldenhar's syndrome by presence in the former of lateral lower lid colobomas, while ocular dermoid cysts and upper lid colobomas occur in the latter.

Nuclear aplasia

Facial diplegia, or Möbius syndrome, is characterized by a combination of bilateral central paresis of the sixth and seventh cranial nerves. This paresis creates a failure of lateral movements of both eyes, producing esotropia and associated bilateral facial paresis. The syndrome is inherited as an autosomal dominant trait.

Pierre Robin syndrome

The Pierre Robin syndrome is characterized by micrognathia, glossoptosis, and cleft palate. The ocular abnormalities include retinal detachment, microphthalmia, congenital glaucoma, cataracts, and high myopia. (See also p. 568.)

Sturge-Weber syndrome

The association of capillary angiomas of the upper part of the face, the eye, and the leptomeninges forms a triad of signs also called the encephalooculofacial angiomatosis. The capillary angioma or port-wine stain of the face (nevus flammeus) is typically unilateral and may or may not be confined to the distribution of the first or second division of the trigeminal nerve. Only those angiomas that include the forehead and the upper lid have been implicated in patients with ocular disease. The associated choroidal angioma is frequently located near the disc. The choroidal angioma is usually rather indistinct and difficult to visualize without indirect ophthalmoscopy and fluorescein angiography of the fundus. If present, it may lead to macular edema and decreased visual acuity. There is no apparent hereditary pattern. Congenital glaucoma frequently occurs and, if unrecognized, can lead to irreversible blindness.

Waardenburg syndrome

The Waardenburg syndrome is transmitted as an autosomal dominant trait and is associated with lateral displacement of the medial canthi, hyperplasia of the medial part of the eyebrows frequently coalescing in the midline, white forelock, heterochromia iridis, and nerve deafness. The fundus may also participate in the heterochromia.

Chromosomal aberrations and deletions

The trisomies

Syndromes associated with trisomy of the smaller chromosomes present multiple anomalies that include both facial and ocular findings.

Trisomy 13. Trisomy D, or Patau's syndrome, is manifested by cleft palate, hairlip, polydactyly, umbilical hernia, and malformations of the heart and of the central nervous system. Ocular findings are microphthalmia, colobomas of the iris or choroid, and the occasional presence of intraocular cartilage.

Trisomy 18. Trisomy E is characterized by micrognathia, flexed fingers with the index finger overlapping the third finger, generalized hypertonicity of skeletal muscles, mental retardation, ventricular septal defect, umbilical hernia, rocker-bottom feet, and malrotation of the gut. Ocular abnormalities include corneal opacities, ptosis, strabismus, inner epicanthal folds, and abnormal orbital ridges. Congenital optic atrophy has also been reported.

Trisomy 21. Down's syndrome, or mongolism, is a well-recognized entity consisting of mongoloid facies, mental retardation, small obese habitus, and large tongue. The ocular abnormalities associated with this entity are epicanthus, hypertelorism, mongoloid slant of the palpebral fissures, and congenital cataracts. Brushfield's spots are found, frequently at birth, on the unusually thin, lightly colored irides of 85% of mongoloid patients. The monogoloid iris, as well as the infant as a whole, is unusually, and sometimes dangerously, susceptible to the action of atropine.

MONGOLOID SLANT

Down's syndrome
Penta-X syndrome
Laurence-Moon-Biedl syndrome
Chromosome 18p− syndrome
Chromosome 18q− syndrome

ANTIMONGOLOID SLANT

Cerebral gigantism
Cornelia de Lange syndrome
Rubinstein-Taybi syndrome
Treacher Collins' syndrome
Chromosome 4p− syndrome
Chromosome 5p− syndrome (cri du chat)
Chromosome 13q− syndrome

Chromosomal deletions

The loss of deoxyribonucleic acid from within a chromosome leads to a variety of syndromes, each more or less characteristic of the specific chromosome involved.

Partial deletion of the short arm of chromosomes 4 (4p−) and 5 (5p−). Infants with chromosome 4p− syndrome have low birth weights, are retarded, and may have spastic diplegia or quadriplegia. They resemble those with the syndrome of partial deletion of the short arm of chromosome 5 (5p−) because of the additional presence of microcephaly, abnormal ears, micrognathia, inguinal hernia, simian crease, and low dermal ridge count. In addition, chromosomes 4p− and 5p− syndromes are characterized by antimongoloid palpebral apertures, hypertelorism, ptosis, strabismus, epicanthus, and broad nasal roots. Other features of chromosome 4p− syndrome absent in chromosome 5p− syndrome include midline scalp defect, ocular colobomas, beak-shaped nose, carplike mouth, cleft palate, preauricular or presacral dimple or sinus, hypospadias, and cryptorchidism. Chromosome 5p− syndrome is characterized by a catlike cry (cri du chat). In addition to the above-mentioned features, this syndrome is also characterized by decreased tear secretion, refractive errors, tortuous retinal arterioles and venules, optic atrophy, and pupillary supersensitivity to methacholine.

Partial deletion of the long arm of chromosome 13 (13q−). Patients with this syndrome have a unique facial configuration with microcephaly, trigonocephaly, micrognathia, large, malformed ears, a wide nasal bridge with hypertelorism, and protruding upper incisors. Ocular abnormalities, which may be profound, include epicanthus, microphthalmia, iris coloboma, ptosis, cataract, antimongoloid palpebral apertures, and most significant, retinoblastoma. Although this malignant neoplasm of the retina is inherited characteristically as an autosomal dominant trait, it has been reported in 6 of 11 patients with chromosome 13q− syndrome. Other findings include urogenital, thumb, and congenital cardiac defects.

Partial deletion of the short arm (18p−) and of the long arm (18q−) of chromosome 18. Chromosome 18p− and 18q− syndromes are characterized by mental retardation, short stature, hypertelorism, epicanthal folds, and strabismus. Patients with chromosome 18p− syndrome also have micrognathia, dental caries, moon facies, webbed neck, ptosis, flat bridge of the nose, eccentric pupils, cataract, corneal opacities, and monogloid or antimongoloid palpebral apertures. In two cases cyclopia has occurred. Patients with chromosome 18q− syndrome also have microcephaly, midface retraction, urogenital and cardiac anomalies, optic atrophy, nystagmus, narrow palpebral apertures, myopic astigmatism, ophthalmoscopic abnormalities, oval pupils, glaucoma, microcornea, and mongoloid or antimongoloid palpebral apertures.

ABNORMAL EYELIDS

Colobomas

Colobomas of the lids are defects that may vary from being only a small notch of the lid borders to involving the entire length of the lid, either in partial or complete thickness (Fig. 21-5). Most lid colobomas are found in the medial aspect of the upper lid. When the lower lid is involved, the defect is more often in its lateral aspect. The cause of lid colobomas is unknown; they are thought, however, to be either the localized failure of adhesion of the lid folds, resulting in a lag of growth, or caused by the mechanical effects of am-

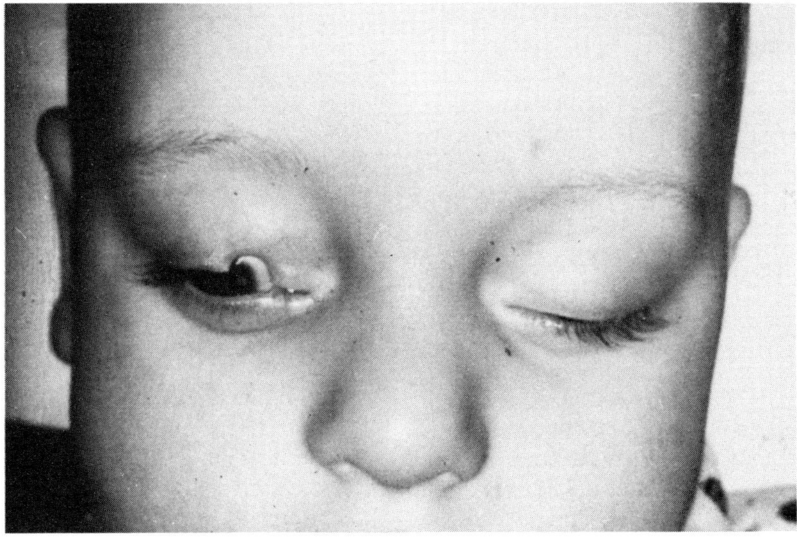

Fig. 21-5. Atypical coloboma of right upper lid.

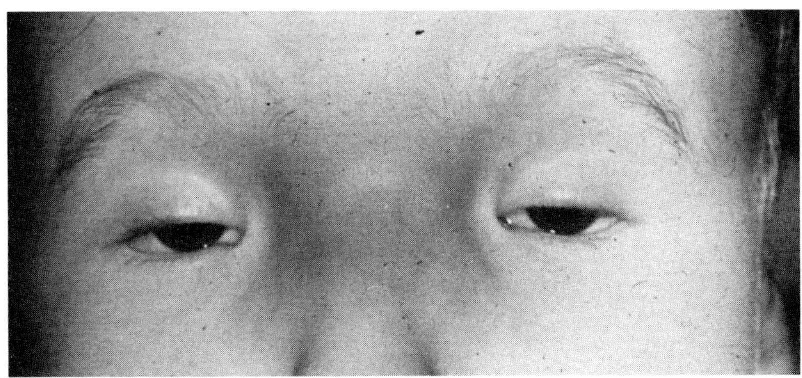

Fig. 21-6. Congenital blepharophimosis, ptosis, and epicanthus inversus (bilateral).

niotic bands. Lid colobomas are of extreme importance when they prevent adequate lid closure, thus exposing the cornea. Subsequent thickening, opacification, infection, ulceration, or perforation of the cornea may occur. Surgical correction of small colobomas is accomplished by removing a V-shaped wedge that includes the coloboma, with subsequent primary closure of the full-thickness defect. Larger colobomatous defects require more extensive plastic repair in which the lid is mobilized at the lateral canthus and the lateral lid is swung medially to meet the inner margin of the defect. Occasionally, large defects may be repaired by transfer of a segment of the lower lid to bridge the defect in the upper lid, and vice versa.

LID COLOBOMAS

Isolated colobomas
Treacher Collins' syndrome (lower lid)
Goldenhar's syndrome (upper lid)
Turner's syndrome (rare)

Syndromes with colobomas of the lids are Treacher Collins' syndrome, Goldenhar's syndrome, and Turner's syndrome.

Congenital blepharophimosis

Blepharophimosis indicates eyelids that are too narrow horizontally as well as vertically (Fig. 21-6). There is usually an associated ptosis and wide epicanthus. Blepharophimosis is also associated occasionally with microphthalmia. Lid fissure measurements are usually reduced to approximately two-thirds their normal values, while the space between the medial canthi is considerably widened. This condition is relatively rare, and the cause is usually unknown. Autosomal dominant transmission has occurred. Treatment is usually required in the form of surgical repair; the medial and lateral canthal angles are widened where possible. Ptosis surgery is used, where indicated, to strengthen the weakened upper lid levators.

Epicanthus

Epicanthus is the most commonly encountered lid abnormality. A skin fold originating in the upper lid extends over the medial end of the upper lid, the medial canthus, and the caruncle and ends in the skin of the lower lid. This appears to be an autosomal dominant characteristic and is normally found in mongolians. It is a frequent occurrence in the neonatal period of persons of other races and gradually disappears as the growth of the bridge of the nose obliterates the excess skin in this area. Epicanthus inversus is similar, except that the predominance of the skin fold arises in the lower lid and runs diagonally upward toward the root of the nose to overlie the medial canthus. A plastic surgical technique may be employed later in life to obliterate this extra skin fold, especially if the fold is sufficiently prominent to simulate the appearance of esotropia. This pseudoesotropia is commonly encountered during the first year of life.

LID TUMORS

Hemangiomas

Hemangiomas of the lid are a relatively frequent occurrence in infancy, with an incidence of approximately 1% in full-term newborns. Approximately 20% of hemangiomas are noted at the time of birth, the remainder becoming apparent usually after the first several weeks or not arising until as late as the second decade of life. The incidence is greater (5%) in premature infants. In the era prior to the judicious use of oxygen therapy for prematurity, the incidence was considerably higher, suggesting a common cause with that of retrolental fibroplasia.

Capillary hemangiomas, the most frequently encountered of the vascular tumors, may progress at a rapid rate during the first 5 to 6 months of life, producing a considerable enlargement and reddish blue discoloration of the upper or lower lid. Such tumors gradually reduce in size and may completely disappear by the second year. Treatment should be confined to expectant observations, since resolution is usually the rule. However, the alarming rate of growth that may occasionally occur in these tumors may force the institution of therapy, especially when the lesion produces gross cosmetic defects or interference with vision. Chronic obstruction of the pupillary axis will produce amblyopia.

Therapy usually produces imperfect results. Surgical removal is difficult and often incomplete. X-rays produce radiation effects to the growth centers of the surrounding bone and possible damage to the eye. Sclerosing solutions risk damage to the periocular tissues. Carbon dioxide snow or other freezing techniques may produce cutaneous scarring. Where disproportionate growth of the hemangioma occurs, the use of systemic corticosteroid therapy has shown good (although often transient) results in arresting the progression or in producing some resolution.

Lymphangiomas

Lymphangiomas are slowly progressive, diffuse, soft tumors of the lids that may be present at birth or that may gradually become apparent during the first several years of life. They tend to grow slowly, with cessation of growth in early adulthood. Approximately 25% of all lymphangiomas occur in the orbital or periorbital region. Of these, 80% are found in the lids. There may be sufficient vascularization to make differentiation from hemangiomas difficult except by histologic study. Because of edema and hemorrhage, these tumors tend to increase in size more dramatically than do hemangiomas. Surgical removal and repair is done when the tumor is cosmetically unacceptable. Recurrence is frequent.

Dermoid cysts

Dermoid cysts are of congenital ectodermal origin and develop in the brow, the lid, or the orbit at the closure site of an embryonic cleft. They usually occur in the lateral third of the brow or upper lid. They are soft, and the overlying skin is freely moveable, while the cyst remains attached to the periosteum at the site of the embryonic cleft. Roentgenograms of the area are important, since these cysts frequently have connections with the cranial cavity, paranasal sinuses, or the orbit. The treatment is surgical removal.

Neurofibromatosis

Neurofibromatosis (von Recklinghausen's disease) is a congenital, autosomal dominant disease that produces tumors of proliferating Schwann cells. The presence of cafe au lait spots in the patient or parents should alert the examiner to the possibility of this disease. Lid involvement may rarely occur in the neonatal period. This produces a tumor, initially small and gradually enlarging, composed of wormlike tissue of the lids with overlying elephantiasis of the skin. Massive deformity of the periorbital tissue can occur. Radical excision, done for cosmetic purposes, is usually incomplete and at times is accompanied by a recurrence that is larger than the original lesion. This tumor is considered further in the section on orbital tumors.

SPARSE EYEBROWS AND EYELASHES

The amount of upper facial hair, including the eyebrows and eyelashes, shows considerable variation in the neonate, conforming either to familial or to racial characteristics. In Eskimos and Mongols the eyebrows and eyelashes are normally less dense than in other races. Abnormally, the absence of eyebrows or eyelashes may occur as a congenial anomaly, usually as a part of a general alopecia. The absence of eyebrows occurs concomitantly with cryptophthalmos, where the skin is continuous over the orbits and there are no eyelids. Generalized facial hypotrichosis occurs in ectodermal dysplasia, in the Hallerman-Streiff syndrome, and may occur unilaterally in congenital facial hemiatrophy of Romberg. Cartilage-hair hypoplasia, an autosomal recessive type of short-limb dwarfism, is also characterized by sparse, thin, and lightly pigmented hair and lashes.

HYPERTRICHOSIS

Excessive hair on the lids and forehead occurs not infrequently as a dominant characteristic in males and may, on occasion, be quite extreme. Abnormalities in hair distribution may point to specific diagnoses. Simple synophrys is present in the Waardenburg syndrome as an autosomal dominant characteristic. Distichiasis is the presence of an additional row of lashes posterior to the gray line (the tarsal edge or center of the lid margin). Districhiasis may refer to the presence of two lashes growing from the same follicle. Tristichiasis is the presence of a third row of eyelashes, one or two of which are posterior to the center of the lid margin. These two conditions usually are associated with contact of the lashes with the cornea, producing corneal irritation and abrasions. Hypertrichosis involving the brows, forehead, and upper lid are seen in the Cornelia de Lange syndrome, a pathologic dwarfism associated with multiple congenital anomalies, also described as typus degenerativus amstelodamensis. Hypertrichosis lanuginosa is a condition in which the fetal lanugo persists into adult life, creating an abundant covering of hair of the eyebrows, forehead, and eyelids as well as of the remainder of the body. This anomaly also occurs as an autosomal dominant hereditary characteristic. A rare condition has been reported in which there is reduplication of the eyebrows bilaterally, the second pair occurring a short distance above the normally placed brows, with no apparent connection. The latter anomaly has been called duplicitas supercilia.

PTOSIS

Ptosis (sleepy eye) is defined as an upper lid that cannot or does not rise to a normal level (see list below). Lid position can be evaluated only in the undisturbed neonate. The examiner can usually induce momentary ocular fixation by using a hand light in a moderately darkened room. The lids should normally be elevated to a point midway between the pupil and the upper margin of the cornea in the position of primary gaze. Ptosis is the result of dysfunction of the levator palpebrae, which can be either partial or complete. Complete dysfunction is present when no elevation of the lid occurs on upper gaze. Ptosis may be present either unilaterally or bilaterally, with any gradation of function in either situation. If one is sufficiently patient, exact measurements may be taken by measuring a distance between the light reflex on the cornea and the margin of the upper lid.

Ptosis that is the result of absence of normal levator function will have additional signs; for example, the normal upper lid fold may be absent, and the upper lid lashes will tend to point in a more downward position.

PTOSIS

Congenital ptosis
Congenital myasthenia gravis
Congenital Horner's syndrome
Möbius syndrome
Smith-Lemli-Opitz syndrome
Turner's syndrome (rare)
DeToni-Franconi syndrome (infrequent)
Chromosome 4p− syndrome
Chromosome 5p− syndrome (cri du chat)
Chromosome 13q− syndrome
Trisomy 18
Transient neonatal myasthenia gravis

In the presence of a unilateral ptosis (Fig. 21-7), comparison of pupillary size with that of the opposite eye is an important factor in diagnosing Horner's syndrome. Congenital Horner's syndrome occurs as a result of birth trauma (p. 78). Diagnosis is confirmed when one drop of 10% phenylephrine instilled into the conjunctiva produces marked elevation of an affected lid in approximately 15 to 20 minutes. Heterochromia becames apparent only during the process of pigmentation of the irises.

Ptosis may also be the result of a Marcus Gunn syndrome. The patient with this condition shows a marked movement of the affected upper lid during nursing activity. The jaw-winking portion of the syndrome is thought to decrease or disappear in early adulthood. However, the ptosis remains. Surgical correction of the Marcus Gunn ptosis is frequently unsatisfactory because of the continued presence of the jaw-winking phenomenon, even though the ptosis may be improved by shortening of the levator palpebrae muscle. The syndrome is caused by anomalous innervation of the levator palpebrae muscle (abnormal connections of the motor fibers of the pterygoid, lingual, and levator palpebrae muscles). There is a relatively toneless levator palpebrae muscle unless the jaw or tongue are additionally activated.

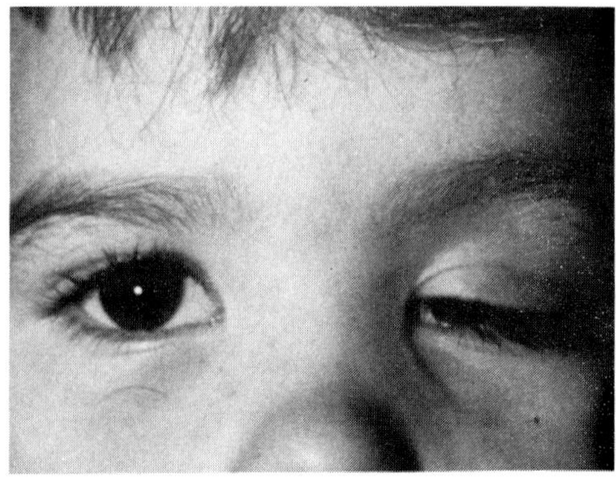

Fig. 21-7. Congenital ptosis of left upper lid.

A temporary apparent ptosis (so-called protective ptosis) may be seen as the result of corneal or conjunctival irritation or infection and in conditions, such as congenital glaucoma, causing photophobia. These conditions should always be considered and ruled out before diagnosing other forms of ptosis, since they are the more important, and often correctable, ocular diseases.

CLOSED EYES

Eyes that have spontaneously opened at birth but then subsequently close may do so because of infection or irritation. Lid anomalies producing a failure of spontaneous lid opening present from birth are anophthalmia and cryptophthalmos. Anophthalmia, in which there is total absence or a minute rudiment of the globe, occurs rarely. This may occur as a failure of development of the optic vesicle and is usually bilateral. Marked microphthalmia may simulate true anophthalmia, in which case colobomatous signs of incomplete embryonic fissure closure may be seen in either eye. The contralateral eye in this situation may be normal in size; for example, showing only a fundus or iris coloboma inferiorly. In most cases, anophthalmia is accompanied by other congenital anomalies, such as central nervous system defects and retardation. Since lid formation is not dependent on ocular formation, the lids are present with lashes and lacrimal puncta. However, the lids remain closed and sunken without the support of the eye. The lacrimal gland is present and is capable of producing tears. Occurrence in most cases is sporadic in nature. However, there have been some cases of familial incidence with varied types of mendelian inheritance. Treatment is only cosmetic and is usually accomplished by the use of gradually enlarging plastic molds of the conjunctival sac in order to stretch the lids and sac sufficiently to hold a cosmetic prosthetic shell.

In cryptophthalmos, the eyelids fail to form their normal cleavage. Uninterrupted skin runs from the forehead to the malar area. The eyelids and eyelashes are usually absent. However, the eye can be palpated beneath the skin of the lids and may even be seen to move with the stimulation of a strong light. The anterior segment of the eye is invariably disorganized into fibrovascular tissue adherent to the subcuticular tissue of the lids. The conjunctival sac is absent. Therefore, attempts to separate the lids from the ocular structures usually results in incision of the ocular tissues concomitant with the incision of the eyelids. Surgical correction is therefore not advisable in most circumstances.

THE PURULENT EYE

An eye infection is one of the most serious problems encountered in the newborn. This problem usually occurs during a period when the pediatrician or general practitioner has the prime responsibility for the patients' care and, if undiagnosed and untreated, may rapidly proceed to loss of one or both eyes. Thus the recognition and differentiation of ophthalmia neonatorum requires vigilance and early treatment or consultation. Acute purulent conjunctivitis is a chemical or bacterial inflammation of the conjunctiva characterized by cellular infiltration and exudation.

Chemical conjunctivitis

Today the most common cause of ophthalmia neonatorum, referred to in some areas as the "sticky eye," is the result of instillation of 1% silver nitrate into the eye at birth. In spite of its disadvantages and occasional irritation, the Credé prophylaxis is statistically the most effective, least troublesome method of prevention of gonococcal conjunctivitis. The rate of occurrence of this chemical conjunctivitis is estimated at approximately 10% of all newborns and probably is enhanced by the prolonged contact of the silver nitrate with the conjunctival sac or by excessive concentration of the silver nitrate. This is the only conjunctivitis generally present from the first day and is usually unilateral in occurrence. The lids are slightly swollen, the conjunctiva is congested and chemotic (edematous), and purulence is not observed. This condition clears spontaneously in 3 to 4 days if no secondary bacterial infection occurs. A sulfonamide such as 10% sodium sulfacetamide drops 4 times a day may be used locally to prevent secondary infection. Secondary bacterial infection is suggested if the disease persists beyond this time or increases in severity. Cultures with sensitivity tests identify the organism and appropriate treatment.

Gonorrheal conjunctivitis

See also p. 130.

Conjunctivitis caused by *Neisseria gonorrhoeae* is an acute, severe, purulent conjunctivitis with an incubation period of 2 to 5 days. The rate of occurrence in the United States today is less than 0.03% as the result of the legal requirement of silver nitrate or penicillin instillation at birth. There have been reports of resistance to the Credé prophylaxis. (See Chapter 8, pp. 135-136 for detailed discussion.)

Inclusion blennorrhea

Inclusion conjunctivitis (p. 135) is another form of ophthalmia neonatorum. Differentiation from gonococcal conjunctivitis is aided by the longer incubation period, by the primary involvement of the inferior conjunctival fornix, and by the smear. In gonococcal conjunctivitis, there is involvement of both the superior and inferior fornices. The usual cultures and Gram stain are unproductive in inclusion blennorrhea. Demonstration of the typical basophilic inclusion bodies in the epithelial cells is made with Giemsa-stained smears of the conjunctival scraping of the lower lid.

Nongonococcal bacterial conjunctivitis

Ophthalmia neonatorum may also occur as the result of any of a number of common pathogens, among which are pathogenic staphylococci, pneumococci, streptococci, coliform bacteria, and influenzal bacteria (p. 135).

THE WATERY EYE

Epiphora (excess tearing) is usually not present until after the first 3 weeks of life, since the major portion of the lacrimal gland is not functional until that time. With the onset of emotional tearing at 3 to 4 weeks, epiphora is a frequent symptom. Although the most usual causes of epiphora are blockage of the lacrimal ducts, the possibility of congenital glaucoma is the most important disease to be considered in the differential diagnosis of this symptom. Congenital absence of the entire lacrimal drainage apparatus occurs as an extremely rare phenomenon. More frequent obstructions of the lacrimal drainage systems are, in the order of their occurrence: obstruction of the nasolacrimal duct, obstruction at the common canaliculus, and congenital absence of the lid puncta. Stenosis of the nasolacrimal duct, which becomes more obstructed by a recurrent mild inflammation, produces excess tearing for several weeks, followed by apparent improvement, only, in all likelihood, to recur at a later date.

Constant epiphora is present with total obstruction of the lacrimal drainage apparatus and usually is the result of a persistent membrane at the lower end of the nasolacrimal duct. This condition creates a stagnant pooling of tears in the lacrimal sac, which contributes to chronic or recurrent dacryocystitis. This is heralded by a purulent exudate in the medial canthal area of the conjunctiva. If severe, dacryocystitis will produce a swelling and induration of the lacrimal sac, medial and inferior to the medial canthus. Treatment of the nasolacrimal infection is usually accomplished with the local instillation of antibiotic drops or ointment. If especially severe, systemic administration of medication may be required. Repeated massage of the nasolacrimal sac at the root of the nose by the mother at home may serve to encourage the opening of the nasolacrimal duct. If the epiphora continues beyond the age of 3 to 6 months, the passage of a lacrimal probe through the nasolacrimal duct to the nose may suffice to produce an adequate opening. Recurrent probings are often necessary. With obstruction of the puncta, the common canaliculus, or major obstructions in the lacrimal sac, probing is insufficient. A surgical procedure, usually accomplished later in life, is needed to bypass the tears from the conjunctival sac to the nose. Occasionally, minor surgical unroofing of a congenitally closed punctum will be sufficient.

Trigeminal irritation

Reflex stimulation of tearing may be produced by any stimulation of the fifth cranial nerve. Therefore, epiphora may occur as the result of corneal abrasion, corneal foreign body, or irritation by nasal and facial lesions that irritate the fifth cranial nerve. Chronic nasal congestion may also produce epiphora as the result of mechanical blockage of the nasolacrimal duct.

Congenital glaucoma

The presence of epiphora in the neonate should always suggest the possibility of congenital glaucoma, especially when epiphora is combined with photophobia. Congenital glaucoma is, fortunately, not very common. However, the devastating effects of the uncontrolled pressure that occurs without adequate surgical treatment are of sufficient important to keep this disease uppermost in the mind of the examining physician. The obvious signs of enlarged corneal diameters and a cloudy cornea occurring at birth are not likely to be missed by the examiner if these signs are present at birth. However, the onset of the glaucoma may be sufficiently delayed so that the eyes may remain normal for the first weeks or months of life. The usual initial symptoms prior to corneal changes include epiphora, photophobia, and blepharospasm. Persistent symptoms of this nature, which are not the result of corneal abrasion or foreign body, require specific evaluation for increased intraocular pressure. Early diagnosis must be made by examination, with the infant *under general anesthesia,* for precise measurement of corneal diameters and of intraocular pressures by ocular tonometry. Congenital glaucoma is discussed in more detail in the section on the the large eye (p. 629).

THE DRY EYE

Recognition of alacrima in the infant is important in the prevention of corneal abrasions, infections, and perforations, which are the inevitable end results of the dry eye. During the first month, the infant with alacrima of any cause may not appear to be different from the normal infant, since tear production is normally minimal at this period. The usual time of discovery is at 6 months of age or later, after the lack of tears has produced changes such as scarring or ulceration in the corneal epithelium. The tear film, with alacrima, is minimal but present. At 1 to 2 months of age early symptoms that are suggestive of a dry eye are conjunctival hyperemia and photophobia. Instead of the ample tears expected with conjunctival irritation, there is usually a sticky mucoid secretion, and the cornea shows a punctate staining with fluorescein. Treatment includes the frequent use of artificial tears such as 1% methylcellulose (as often as every 15 to 30 minutes), punctum occlusion, or tarsorrhaphy.

Congenital absence of the lacrimal secretion

Isolated congenital lack of tears, usually bilateral, is a rare anomaly. The cause is unknown but has been suggested to be either the result of hypoplasia of the lacrimal gland or the absence of innervation of the lacrimal gland structures. Treatment includes the frequent use of artificial tears and prevention of secondary infection.

Familial dysautonomia

The ocular findings in the Riley-Day syndrome are characteristic of this disease and may produce the initial criteria for diagnosis. There is a lack of lacrimation, corneal hypesthesia, and exodeviation (divergence of the eyes). These ocular changes, plus constriction of the pupil by instillation of 2.5% solution of methacholine (Mecholyl), comprise the diagnostic criteria. Major systemic symptoms usually have their onset at approximately age 2. The multiplicity of congental systemic alterations (abnormal swallowing mechanism, inappropriate blood pressure and respiratory control) and the ocular findings in this syndrome are probably the result of sympathetic and parasympathetic imbalance of an undefined type.

Additional ocular findings are myopia, anisometropia (different refractive error in the two eyes), and occasionally ptosis. Tortuosity of the retinal vessels has also been noted in a majority of the patients examined for this finding, but its pathogenesis is unknown. The concomitant occurrence of alacrima and corneal hypesthesia make the cornea particulraly susceptible to corneal abrasion, infection, and ulceration. Thus corneal scarring is a frequent secondary finding in familial dysautonomia.

THE RED EYE

Conjunctival and corneal irritation from any source produces hyperemia of the conjunctiva. Probably the most frequent source of conjunctival irritation in the newborn is corneal abrasion produced by fingernails or clothing. These are of small importance and usually require little in the way of therapy, except an antibiotic eyedrop and sometimes a firm patch for 1 to 2 days. However, conjunctival hyperemia may also be the initial symptom of ocular infection or congenital glaucoma, and these may be devastating to the eye if left undiagnosed.

Blood in the anterior chamber of the eye, called a hyphema, requires ophthalmologic consultation. A hyphema occurring shortly after birth may be the result of excessive birth trauma, vascular anomalies of the iris, or the presence of blood dyscrasias. The appearance of the eye with hyphema varies with the amount of blood present in the anterior chamber. The eye may grossly show a level of red blood cells behind the cornea; there may be a diffuse, hazy red appearance; or the area of the anterior chamber may be quite black and opaque. Other diseases that are associated with anterior chamber hyphema are retinoblastoma, juvenile xanthogranuloma, and rarely retrolental fibroplasia and persistent hyperplastic primary vitreous (PHPV).

Bleeding abnormalities should also be considered and evaluated by appropriate laboratory evaluation.

ABNORMAL ORBITS

Abnormal spatial relationships between the two orbits, creating excessively wide or excessively narrow intraorbital distances, are frequent. The cause of these abnormalities is not homogenous but constitutes a wide variety of related cranial abnormalities. The probable cause is the disproportionate growth or lack of development of the body and lesser wing of the sphenoid, the ethmoid sinuses, and the maxillary processes.

Hypotelorism (a narrowing of the intraorbital distance) is usually a secondary phenomenon associated with scaphocephaly (a boat-shaped cranium caused by premature closure of the sagittal suture). Hypertelorism (a widening of the intraorbital distance) is normal in the early fetus and may persist as a genetic trait. Hypertelorism may occur as an associated finding in other diseases. (See lists below.)

HYPOTELORISM

Cebocephaly
Ocular-dental-digital dysplasia
Trisomy 13
Scaphocephaly

HYPERTELORISM

Apert's syndrome
Cerebral gigantism
Cerebrohepatorenal syndrome
Chromosome 18p− and 18q− syndromes
Crouzon's disease
Infantile hypercalcemia
Greig's hypertelorism
Median cleft face syndrome
Male Turner's syndrome
Smith-Lemli-Opitz syndrome
Chromosome 4p− syndrome
Chromosome 5p− syndrome (cri du chat)
Chromosome 13q− syndrome
Chromosome 21q− syndrome

ORBITAL TUMORS

The contents of the orbit are confined to a conical shape by its bony walls. The apex of the orbit faces posteriorly where the extraocular muscles originate and where the vascular and nerve structures enter the orbit. Superiorly, a thin bony wall separates the orbit from the frontal lobe and the frontal sinus. The medial wall is formed by the ethmoid sinuses and the nasal cavity. The inferior wall is formed by the thin bony wall separating the maxillary sinus and forming the inferior orbital fissure. The lateral wall is formed by heavier bony structures composed of the zygoma, the greater wing of the sphenoid, and the lateral extension of the frontal bone. The bony structures of the lateral wall do not cover the orbital contents as far anteriorly as the remaining sides of the orbit, leaving the eye exposed to trauma more on its lateral side. At the apex of the orbit is the junction of the anterior and middle cranial fossae. At the base of the cone, anteriorly, the orbital rims form a sharp circular outline in the neonate.

Tumors within the orbital cavity can most easily expand anteriorly, producing proptosis or exophthalmos. Tumors located within the cone of extraocular muscles produce a symmetrical anterior displacement, whereas tumors located outside the cone of extraocular muscles displace the eye out and away from the area of origin of the tumor. Thus a tumor in the inferior portion of the orbit will displace the eye up and forward, whereas a tumor located medially will displace the eye laterally and forward. Proptosis may also occur from venous engorgement of the orbital cavity, such as that produced by a carotid-cavernous fistula. Unfortunately, the presence of a cephalic bruit is often heard in an infant and is not pathognomonic of carotid-cavernous sinus fistulas. The diagnosis of proptosis may be additionally confirmed by sighting the eyes and lids from above, over the prominence of the eyebrows. Here one sees a more anterior protrusion of the orbital contents when compared with the contents of the opposite side. The proptosed eye frequently has a widened palpebral fissure.

A false diagnosis of proptosis may occur with a slight ptosis of one eye, giving the opposite eye an appearance of a wider palpebral fissure in the normal eye. Marked enlargement of the eye, as occurs in congenital glaucoma, makes the eye appear proptotic because of the increased size of the globe. Facial abnormalities with shallow orbits, as in Crouzon's disease, simulate exophthalmos because of the normal amount of orbital structures in an abnormally shallow orbit. Since the extraocular muscles are retractors of the globe, a paralysis of all the extraocular muscles may produce a proptosis of as much as 2 mm without increase in orbital contents by a tumor. If the tumor is located anterior to the equator of the globe, the tumor can extend anteriorly into the lids without producing proptosis. A diffuse extensive tumor can produce sufficient general changes so that the eye will become fixed, whereas a localized tumor produces proptosis usually without interfering with rotation of the eye.

Orbital tumors may be primary from

both ectodermal and mesodermal tissues or may arise by metastasis from distant body tissues. They may also arise from the intracranial cavity or paranasal sinuses and enter the orbit by growing through bony defects in the orbital wall.

Roentgenograms are valuable in the diagnosis of orbital disease. Posteroanterior, lateral, Waters', and Caldwell projections are required for estimating the orbital depth and the integrity of the bony walls.

Orbital hematoma

Bleeding into the orbital contents may occur as the result of birth trauma. This bleeding produces a unilateral proptosis that tends to increase gradually in size during the first 3 or 4 hours after birth. Ecchymoses of the lids may be associated findings at birth or may occur 1 to 2 days later. Differential diagnosis includes dermoid cysts, teratoma, and other congenital tumors of the orbit. Treatment is usually not required, since absorption of the hematoma usually takes place over a 1- to 2-week period. It is important during this period to ensure that the cornea is not abraded and that the retinal circulation is not compromised. If examination with the direct ophthalmoscope shows compression of the arterial or venous supply at the disc, a surgical decompression of the orbit is required.

Hemangioma

Cavernous hemangioma is the most common primary orbital tumor producing exophthalmos. In infants the hemangioma is usually not well encapsulated and frequently involves the lower lid as well as the orbit. Although observation of lid involvement assists in making the diagnosis, a biopsy is frequently required to rule out other orbital tumors. Treatment is usually deferred until after the age of 2 years, at which time spontaneous regression often occurs (as described in the section on hemangiomas of the lids). The use of systemic corticosteroid therapy has been advocated when excessive growth has produced dangerous compression of the orbital structures.

Dermoid cysts

Dermoid cysts are thought to arise from a congenital nest of primitive ectoderm at the site of closure of a fetal cleft. They usually contain connective tissue, sebaceous glands, hair follicles, and smooth muscle. They are often located near the orbital rim, where they are attached to bone at suture sites. Because of their location, a proptosis, combined with vertical or horizontal displacement and irregular lid swelling, is produced. Roentgenographic examination may provide evidence of teeth or show dehiscences in the bony wall where the cyst is attached. Treatment is surgical excision, which may prove difficult because of extension of the demoid cyst through the bony suture into surrounding structures. Trauma, such as that occurring at birth, may produce a hemorrhage into the dermoid cyst. This occurs rarely, but under such circumstances differentiation from a primary hematoma of the orbit is difficult.

Teratoma

Teratoma is a primary orbital tumor composed of mesodermal and ectodermal elements. It may differentiate into a variety of tissues containing cartilage, connective tissue, skin, hair, and sebaceous glands, or even endodermal epithelium. Bone is a frequent component and may be identified by orbital roentgenograms. Orbital teratomas that are present at birth produce a striking picture of massive proptosis. Treatment is early excision of the orbital contents (exenteration) both for cosmetic value and for the possible carcinomatous and sarcomatous changes that may occur within the tumor.

Rhabdomyosarcoma

Rhabdomyosarcoma is the most common malignant tumor of the orbit in children (Fig. 21-8). Although it may be found in the neonatal period, the average of occurrence is 6 to 10 years. Rhabdomyosarcoma occurs in the orbit more frequently than elsewhere in the body. It produces an exophthalmos with vertical or horizontal displacement, frequently with a palpable mass in the lid or the brow and with progressive protrusion of the eye. Diagnosis is usually made by biopsy. Accepted treatment has included surgical exenteration of the orbit, followed by irradiation. Recent evidence suggests that irradiation alone may be curative.

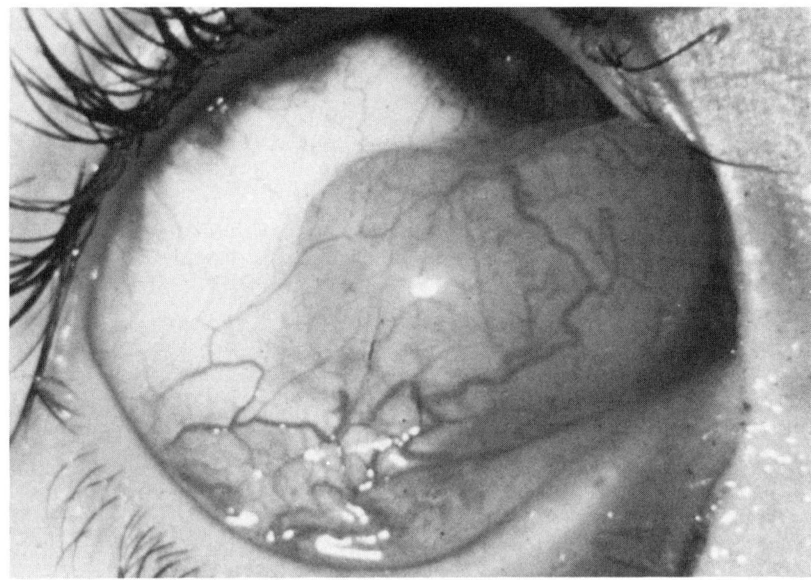

Fig. 21-8. Rhabdomyosarcoma of right orbit.

Neuroblastoma (sympathicoblastoma)

This very malignant tumor frequently originates in the adrenal gland. It may first be noticed as a unilateral or bilateral proptosis caused by metastasis to the orbit. Exophthalmos is progressive, and associated hemorrhage into the neoplastic tissue produces characteristic ecchymoses of the lid, which may assist in diagnosis. The orbital metastasis is often the initial sign of the disease before the primary tumor is discovered. Curative treatment is not available. Exenteration of the orbit has been done in some instances in order to palliate the extensive exophthalmos.

Hyperthyroid exophthalmos

This rare neonatal sequela of hyperthyroidism has been found in the newborn infant as the result of maternal Graves' disease during the last trimester of pregnancy (p. 466). Under these circumstances, the infant is born with classical hyperthyroidism, including exophathlmos, upper lid retraction, and extraocular muscle involvement. Symptoms usually subside during the first 2 months of life.

Lymphoma

Proptosis caused by lymphomatous lesions of the orbit is rare in the neonatal period. Diagnosis is made by biopsy, and the prognosis with radiation treatment is usually rather good.

Orbital cellulitis

Cellulitis of the orbital tissues is rare in the neonate but is a common cause of proptosis in older children and in adults. This infection is often located originally in the paranasal sinuses and produces massive swelling of the orbital contents. The possibility of its occurrence is enhanced by a highly virulent upper respiratory tract, sinus infection, or a puncture wound of the orbit. The disease is characterized by rapid onset of progressive proptosis, often with redness of the lids and chemosis of the conjunctiva, and systemic signs of toxicity and hyperpyrexia. Rapid loss of vision, caused by compression of the orbital structures, can occur. Treatment includes surgical drainage of the purulent infection and systemic administration of antibiotics.

Neurofibromatosis

Neurofibromatosis (von Recklinghausen's disease) is also rarely seen during the neonatal period. However, plexiform neuromas of the lids and orbit have been reported in the first 3 months of life. The typical "bag of worms" tissue may produce proptosis and irregular enlargement of one or both lids. The overlying tissue becomes hypertrophic and resembles elephantiasis of the skin. Surgical treatment of the plexiform neuroma is frequently attempted for cosmetic benefits. The extension of the tumor is usually diffuse, and complete removal is difficult, if not impossible. Recurrence is frequently seen. Neurofibromatosis disease has also been associated with glioma of the optic nerve, a slowly growing tumor producing its appearance during the first 10 years of life. Invasion of the optic nerve by the glioma results in visual loss.

Letterer-Siwe disease

Letterer-Siwe disease, sometimes referred to as aleukemic reticulosis or histiocytosis, is the most severe form of lymphogranuloma. The condition usually affects children under 2 years of age and nearly always has a fatal outcome. Reticuloendothelial cells are seen to proliferate in the skin, lymph nodes, and spleen, as well as in the tissue of the orbit, producing proptosis. Hepatosplenomegaly and generalized lymphadenopathy with bone lesions and anemia are typical findings. Diagnosis is made from biopsy of skin lesions or of lymph nodes. There is no current effective therapy for this disease.

Congenital deformities producing proptosis

An orbital encephalocele or meningocele producing proptosis or orbital cyst formation may be evident at birth or may be delayed until later years. This results from a defect in the wall between the cranial cavity and the orbit and is usually located at the suture lines. Pressure within the cranium causes herniation of brain tissue or of meninges or of both into the orbit, most often at the inner angle of the orbit at the root of the nose. Diagnosis is made by identifying the bony defect in association with the area of the orbital cyst. Clinically, an encephalocele is suggested by the presence of a pulsating, fluctuant cyst that can be somewhat reduced with digital pressure or that increases with coughing or crying. Excessive manipulation of the encephalocele may produce slowing of the pulse or respiration and convulsions. The sign of slowly progressive proptosis, with pulsation synchronous with the vascular pulse or accentuated with coughing, is diagnostic. Neurosurgical correction is difficult and has a high morbidity and mortality.

THE SMALL EYE

Microphthalmia indicates a variety of conditions in which the diameter of the neonatal eye is less than two thirds of the normal 16 mm. Pure congenital microphthalmia is a relatively rare condition with the abnormally small eye as the only clinical finding. It is associated with three features of significance: a high degree of hypermetropia, hypoplasia of the macula, and the late occurrence of glaucoma. It has been reported in both recessive and dominant transmissions. Colobomatous microphthalmia occurs when the embryonic cleft of the optic vesicle fails to close and is typically associated with other ocular anomalies such as colobomas of the iris, the ciliary body, the choroid, or the optic nerve. These may be transmitted as autosomal dominant or X-linked traits. D group deletions or trisomy also produces these abnormalities. A third group of anomalies, termed complicated microphthalmia, is the result of associated genetic malformations inherited as autosomal dominant, autosomal recessive, or X-linked recessive traits. It may also occur secondary to prenatal infections, such as rubella or toxoplasmosis. Microphthalmia and congenital cataract are the two most frequent clinical ocular findings in rubella infection of the embryo. Complicated micropthalmia is also associated with other ocular abnormalities such as Norrie's disease. (See list below.)

MICROPHTHALMIA

Microphthalmia with cataract
Microphthalmia with coloboma
Hallerman-Streiff syndrome
Rubella syndrome
Trisomy 13
Ocular-dental-digital dysplasia
Trisomy 18 (infrequent)
De Toni-Fanconi syndrome (infrequent)
Congenital toxoplasmosis (infrequent)
Pierre Robin syndrome (rare)
Treacher Collins' syndrome (rare)
Chromosome 13q− syndrome
Goldenhar's syndrome

THE LARGE EYE

The presence of an abnormally enlarged eye present in the neonatal period is a rel-

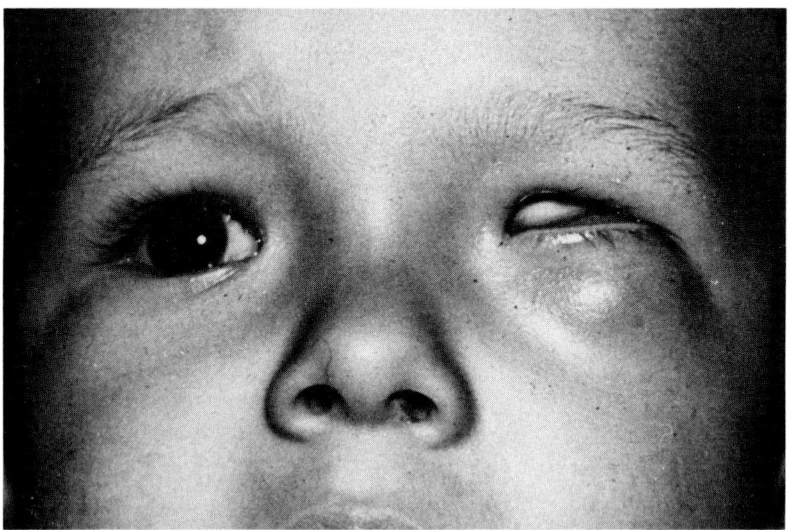

Fig. 21-9. Congenital microphthalmia with large cyst of left eye.

atively rare occurrence but is extremely important to recognize. Only two entities can cause this abnormality: colobomatous microphthalmia with an associated large cyst (Fig. 21-9) and congenital glaucoma. Colobomatous microphthalmia with cyst results from a failure of closure of the embryonic optic vesicle. Tissue that was originally destined to become intraocular in nature is thus located outside the eye in the orbit in a cystic structure. This may become sufficiently large that proptosis occurs, and the microphthalmic eye simulates an enlarged eye.

Congenital glaucoma, often transmitted as a recessive trait when it is the only abnormality, most commonly produces abnormal signs during the first year of life. Early recognition is most important in order to prevent progressive damage to the eye from the increased intraocular pressure (Fig. 21-10). The most frequent symptoms of congenital glaucoma are tearing, photophobia, and blepharospasm. In the neonatal period, tearing may be absent from the triad of symptoms. These symptoms should always suggest the possibility of congenital glaucoma, even though more common problems, such as corneal abrasion, foreign body, or ocular infection, could be present.

Clouding or haziness of the cornea occurs with further advancement of the disease. This results from stretching and overhydration of the cornea. The normal clouding of the cornea, which may be present in the newborn for the first several days of life, should be carefully observed for complete resolution. As the disease progresses, the increased tension produces further stretching of the eye, creating increased corneal and ocular diameters. A corneal diameter of more than 12 mm should suggest glaucoma. (The normal corneal diameter is 10 to 11 mm, increasing to about 11.5 or 12 mm at 1 year of age.)

Once the suspicion of glaucoma has arisen at any age, the infant should be examined under general anesthesia by an ophthalmologist. Preanesthetic medication should consist only of atropine given systemically. The anesthetic agent of choice is diethyl ether. If the diagnosis is confirmed, a surgical procedure should be performed on the anterior chamber angle (goniotomy) while the infant is still under anesthesia, since medical therapy is ineffective.

If the diagnosis of congenital glaucoma has been made early in its course, the percentage of successful recoveries is high; however, if there is considerable enlargement of the eye, the possibility of reducing intraocular pressure and achieving useful vision is greatly decreased.

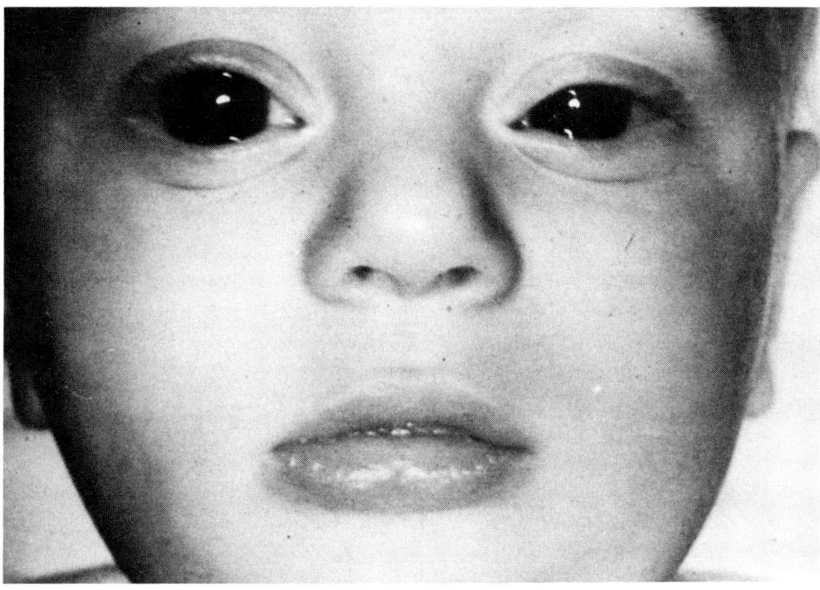

Fig. 21-10. Bilateral congenital glaucoma (buphthalmos), right eye greater than left.

Buphthalmos (an enlarged eye caused by glaucoma) may also be secondary to a variety of diseases having obstruction of the aqueous drainage mechanism in the anterior chamber angle. The list below gives diseases associated with glaucoma.

GLAUCOMA

Isolated (congenital)
Rubella syndrome
Hallerman-Streiff syndrome
Rieger's anomaly
Lowe's syndrome
Persistent hyperplastic primary vitreous (rare)
Aniridia
Sturge-Weber syndrome
Homocystinuria (infrequent)
Marfan's syndrome (infrequent)
Weill-Marchesani syndrome (infrequent)
Neurofibromatosis (infrequent)
Ocular-dental-digital syndrome (infrequent)

STRABISMUS

Clinically significant strabismus is encountered less frequently in the neonatal period than in the remainder of the first decade of life. Its recognition is important, however, since therapy, when indicated, must begin early. Few, if any, patients with congenitally crossed eyes, for example, will spontaneously "grow out" of this problem with the passage of time. Crossed eyes (esotropia) may occur as the result of dominant inheritance (congenital), of paralysis of the lateral rectus muscles, or of refractive errors (usually hyperopia) or may be secondary to any type of disease that reduces visual acuity in one eye. Exotropia (wall eyes) is seen rarely in the neonate (in congenital anomalies such as Greig's hypertelorism). The usual forms of exotropia do not appear until 1 to 2 years of age or later.

The diagnosis of strabismus can be made by the Hirschberg test, an evaluation of the pupillary light reflex on both corneas while the patient fixes binocularly on a small light source held before his face and directed toward his pupils. The pupillary light reflex, if the patient is properly fixing with both eyes on the light source, should be positioned in the same part of the pupillary space of each eye. If the light reflex is centered in one eye and deviated to the lateral side of the pupil or cornea of the fellow eye, esotropia is present. A rough estimation of the visual acuity can be made by determining the fixation pattern of each eye while the infant's eyes fix on a light. If one eye fixes on the light centrally and steadily at all times and the other does not, the latter is certain to have poor acuity.

When strabismus is present, a careful ocular examination is required to rule out the possibility that an intraocular pathologic condition has caused the strabismus. Pathologic conditions that may create esotropia are corneal opacities, cataracts, and diseases of the fundus that have reduced or destroyed macular vision, such as infections (for example, toxoplasmosis) or tumors (for example, retinoblastoma). *Fundus examination with the patient's pupils dilated is mandatory.*

Congenital esotropia may be present while the neonate is still in the nursery or may become evident during the first few weeks of life. In this condition, results of the ocular examination are otherwise normal, and visual acuity is usually equal in the two eyes. Amblyopia may develop from congenital esotropia, although it does so less frequently than in the accommodative type, which appears at a later date in childhood.

Esotropia caused by the paralysis of the lateral rectus muscles may occur as the result of birth trauma and is diagnosed by failure of an eye to deviate laterally beyond the midline. The examination of lateral rotation is best accomplished by occlusion of one eye and observation of the opposite eye. Congenital esotropia also shows weakness of lateral gaze when both eyes are tested simultaneously but shows normal lateral rotations with one eye occluded.

Pseudostrabismus is the term given to infants who appear cross eyed because the bridge of the nose is wide and the epicanthal folds on either side cover most of the sclera on the medial side of the cornea. True stabismus is ruled out by observation of the corneal light reflex, which is found to be symmetrically placed in both pupils.

The treatment of strabismus begins with an adequate ocular examination and a careful cycloplegic refraction. Aims in the treatment of strabismus include the prevention of strabismic amblyopia, the improvement or correction of the cosmetic appearance, and if possible the creation of binocular vision. It is important to remember that the chances of improving amblyopia and strabismus are better the earlier therapy is begun. Treatment, which includes a variety of procedures (drops, patching, glasses, surgery, and so on) should be completed before the child is of school age so that the child is not handicapped by a visual or cosmetic defect.

THE CLOUDY CORNEA

The normal premature infant may have a slightly hazy cornea for the first 7 days of life, and the normal full-term infant occasionally has a similar appearance for the first 48 hours after delivery. This is thought to be caused by a temporary excess hydration of the cornea.

The presence of a persistently hazy or cloudy cornea should immediately suggest congenital glaucoma, as discussed in the previous section. Once this has been ruled out, the following diseases are suggested.

The mucopolysaccharidoses

In the mucopolysaccharidoses, various combinations of acid mucopolysaccharides are excessively deposited in the body tissues (see Chapter 14, p. 433). They are accumulated, as well, in the stroma of the cornea in types I (Hurler's syndrome), IV (Morquio's syndrome), V (Scheie's syndrome), and VI (Maroteaux-Lamy's syndrome). Because of progressive accumulation, corneal clouding is often minimal or invisible in the early periods of life, but it increases with age. Exact pathogenesis of this corneal clouding is not as yet known. Electron microscopic studies have recently shown that the stromal fibroblasts are considerably enlarged because of the presence of inclusion material in their cytoplasm. These cells may produce sufficient anatomical disturbance in the stroma to produce changes in the refractive index with scattering of light. The appearance in the neonatal period includes fine gray punctate opacities in the peripheral stroma, which may cause a faint and diffuse opalescence. Other ocular lesions that are associated with mucopolysaccharidoses can cause an irreversible loss of vision; for example, pigmentary degeneration of the retina and optic atrophy. Therefore, the fundus should be examined through a dilated pupil in all such cases. Corneal transplantation as a method of improving visual acuity is recommended only if abnormal mental, retinal, and optic nerve functions are not associated findings. Differential diagnosis of ground-glass corneal opacification includes congenital glaucoma, rubella keratopathy, severe birth trauma to the cornea, and congenital hereditary corneal dystrophy. Diagnosis is made by identification of the abnormal mucopolysaccharides in the urine. Intraocular pressure determinations with the infant under general anesthesia are needed to rule out congenital glaucoma. Serologic tests rule out rubella, and slit-lamp determination of stromal thickness rules out congenital hereditary corneal dystrophy.

Rubella keratopathy

Rubella embryopathy may appear at birth with a cloudy or opaque cornea that is small or of normal size without an increase in intraocular pressure (p. 154). This has often been confused with the congenital glaucoma of rubella; however, the disturbance appears to be a local corneal defect that exhibits no progressive increase in corneal size. The opacities may vary from mild to severe and may be transient or permanent.

Congenital glaucoma may be differentiated from this condition by the associated increase in intraocular pressure and by the increase in corneal diameter. True congenital glaucoma, of course, may also be one of the manifestations of rubella embryopathy.

Congenital hereditary stationary dystrophy

Congential hereditary stationary dystrophy is a rare corneal dystrophy that appears at birth as a ground-glass appearance of the cornea. The corneal thickness is frequently three to four times normal and is virtually diagnostic of this disease. Intraocular pressure is occasionally mildly elevated in this syndrome, making the differentiation from congenital glaucoma difficult. In congenital hereditary stationary dystrophy, however, progressive corneal enlargement does not occur, and the photophobia and lacrimation of isolated congenital glaucoma are not present.

THE ABNORMALLY COLORED SCLERA

The sclera of the full-term neonate is normally glistening white, as it is in the adult. The overlying conjunctiva and conjunctival vessels produce a superimposed filmy and vascular pattern. A generalized bluish discoloration of the underdeveloped sclera is normally present in early prematures. Rarely, a congenital, idiopathic weakness in a small area of the sclera will produce a bulging called a staphyloma. The light blue color is caused by thinness of the sclera, which transmits the color of the underlying uveal tissue. Osteogenesis imperfecta may be associated with a similar bluish discoloration of the sclera in the full-term neonate, because of inadequately developed scleral collagen.

DISEASES OF THE INTERNAL EYE

Aniridia, iris colobomas, and persistent pupillary membranes

Aniridia, or absence of the iris, is a rare congenital anomaly, usually bilateral, which is almost invariably associated with poor vision. Aniridia is an inaccurate term, since a small rudimentary cuff of peripheral iris is always present grossly or microscopically. Associated findings with aniridia include: severe congenital glaucoma in greater than 50% of cases, a corneal pannus, cataract, and dislocation of the lens. Aplasia of the macula is also frequently found with aniridia and causes the nystagmus and poor visual acuity. Aniridia may result from an autosomal dominant genetic transmission or may be sporadic. The sporadic variety of aniridia is associated with Wilms' tumor in approximately 10% of cases.

Simple iris coloboma is one of the most common congenital abnormalities seen in the eye. Typical colobomas occur in the inferior nasal quadrant, the area of closure of the embryonic cleft (Fig. 21-11). Atypical colobomas may occur in any quadrant and may rarely be multiple. A coloboma may vary in amount from a small notch in the pupil to the absence of an entire segment of the iris. It is usually not associated with visual difficulties. Since iris colobomas are associated with an abnormal closure of the embryonic cleft, however, they may also be associated with a coloboma of the ciliary body, choroid, retina, or optic nerve. When the optic nerve or macula is involved in the coloboma, visual difficulty occurs. Thus it is always wise to look for a pathologic condition of the fundus when an iris coloboma is detected.

Although iris coloboma usually appears as a single ocular finding and although it has previously been listed as a single dominant transmission, it may represent a mild or variable expression of colobomatous mi-

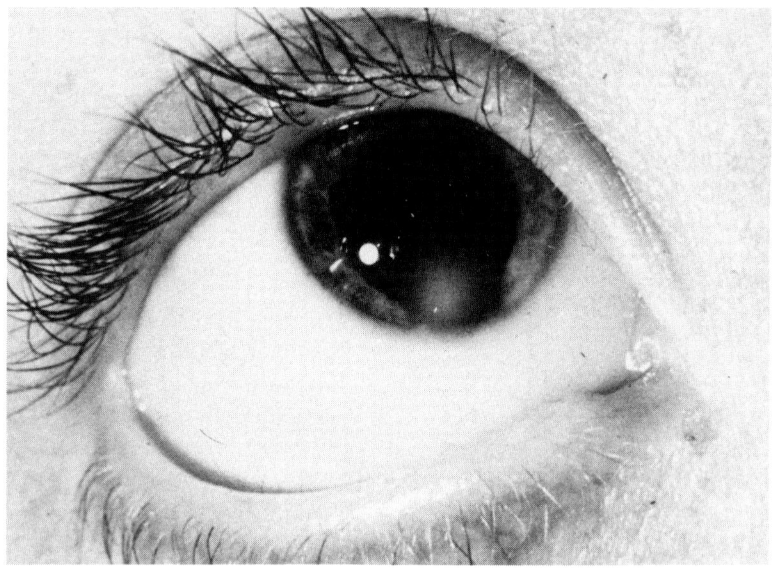

FIG. 21-11. Typical iris coloboma with inferonasal iris defect.

crophthalmia with its several modes of inheritance.

IRIS COLOBOMAS

Isolated congenital colobomas
Congenital colobomatous microphthalmia
Trisomy 13
Trisomy 18
Rieger's syndrome
Iris coloboma and anal atresia syndrome
Lowe's syndrome (infrequent)
Goldenhar's syndrome (infrequent)
Rubinstein-Taybi syndrome (infrequent)
Chromosome 13q− syndrome

Although not associated with aniridia or colobomas, persistent pupillary membranes may be seen in the neonate, particularly in the premature. These are remnants of the anterior fetal vascular coat of the lens that have failed to undergo atrophy in the seventh month of gestation. A filmy lacework of fibers radiates from the pupillary rim over the center of the lens and may persist into adulthood or, more frequently, continue to atrophy. Disappearance during the first few months of existence is the rule.

The unusually colored iris

Heterochromia indicates a difference in pigmentation between the two irises. Since many infants do not develop iris pigmentation until after the neonatal period, this is infrequently seen and is of little diagnostic value in this group. However, in Caucasians with darkly colored irises and in the darkly pigmented races, some iris pigmentation is established at birth or shortly thereafter, and these neonates occasionally show abnormalities in pigmentation. Heterochromia may occur as an isolated autosomal dominant trait. Heterochromia is also associated with several syndromes; and, if they are present, they may be helpful in establishing the diagnosis. The hemifacial atrophy of Romberg is occasionally associated with lack of pigmentation on the side of the face that is atrophic; the Waardenburg syndrome is typically associated with heterochromia; and congenital Horner's syndrome produces heterochromia, usually after the neonatal period, as the result of failure of development of normal pigmentation in the iris on the sympathetically denervated side.

The white pupil

A white pupil (also called a cat's eye reflex) denotes an ocular abnormality of the lens, the vitreous, or the fundus. An understanding of the etiology of diseases associated with a white pupil is helpful in searching for genetic factors and in requesting pertinent laboratory data that may be diagnostic, as in galactosemia. Knowledge of available treatment encourages early correction before permanent visual loss occurs

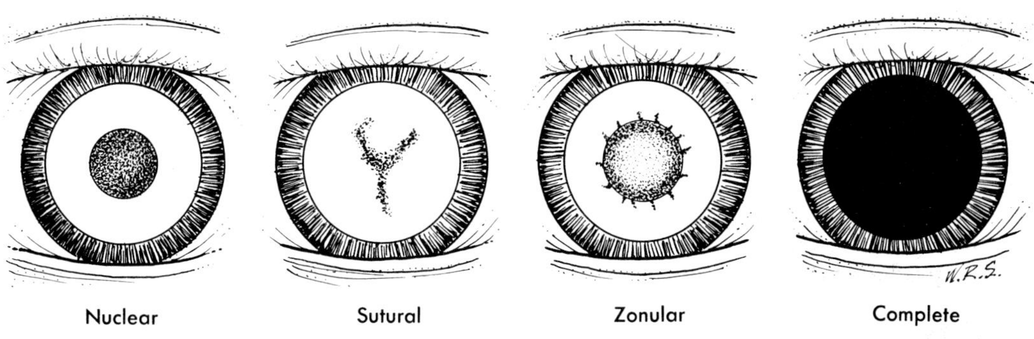

FIG. 21-12. The appearance of the red reflex with various cataracts. With the ophthalmoscope set at 0, the pupil is observed with the examiner standing approximately 1 foot from the infant. The normal eye is seen to have a clear round red reflex. Lens opacities (cataracts) interrupt the red reflex, producing black opacities as shown.

or before secondary complications produce irreversible ocular damage.

Examination of the white pupil

Since the infant sleeps much of the time and since the pupils are small, the casual observation of the white pupil is often delayed in discovery until the infant becomes more alert and active. Including the observation of a red fundus as a part of the normal neonatal examination of the pupil provides an early clue that an abnormality exists. However, nothing takes the place of ophthalmoscopy through dilated pupils.

The initial examination may be made using a handlight, the light of the otoscope, or an ophthalmoscope. This is done with a maximally dilated pupil. With the light source held close to the eye, the pupillary reflex is evaluated for whitish discoloration; and if a discoloration is present, the percentage of involvement of the pupillary area is estimated. With a +1 or +2 lens in the ophthalmoscope, a red reflex is obtained by observing the pupillary area from a position that is approximately a foot away from the eye. When an extensive pathologic condition of the cornea, lens, or vitreous totally obstructs the reflection of light from the red fundus, the fundus reflex in the pupil is black. With lesser degrees of opacification or lesser amounts of diseased tissue, the reflex is dull red. Irregular densities, such as those occurring in an incomplete cataract, produce a correspondingly irregular reflex (Fig. 21-12). White lesions in the fundus itself (retina and choroid) provide a white reflex, rather than a black or red one. The site of the abnormality may often be localized initially by focusing through the pupil with the ophthalmoscope and the +10 diopter lens in place. Abnormalities of the lens are seen to focus immediately adjacent to the plane of the pupil, whereas abnormalities of the vitreous come into focus more deeply behind the pupil. In moving slightly to the side while viewing the opacity, the examiner can see that the more deeply it is placed behind the pupil, the greater the apparent relative movement of the opacity in relationship to the pupil. Accurate examination of this area can be accomplished only by ophthalmic slit-lamp examination with the infant under adequate sedation or general anesthesia. The importance of this examination and its aid to diagnosis and treatment far outweigh the risks of sedation or general anesthesia.

The lens (cataracts)

A large number of morphologic types of cataracts are known, but only a brief description may be presented here. The size and shape of the cataract (lens opacification) depends on the area of the lens that is being formed at the time the damage or developmental effects are occurring. The lens grows continually during life, laying down new lens fibers on its external surface, much like an onion. Damage that occurs in the early fetal period produces opacifications in the very center of the lens. Such nuclear cataracts have clear layers in the periphery of the lens. Later periods of damage produce ringlike opacifications surrounded by central and peripheral clear areas (zonular cataracts). Recent damage produces peripheral opacifications near the surface of the lens (cortical cataracts). Very dense opacities cause greater visual disturbance, especially if they are located in the central anterior-to-posterior axis, whereas peripheral opacities near the equator or the lateral periphery of the lens produce little or no visual disturbance.

Etiology. Causes of cataracts may be grouped somewhat arbitrarily under the following headings: genetic, viral, inborn errors of metabolism, trauma, associated with other eye malformations, and generalized syndromes. The following discussion begins with the most frequently encountered cataracts. The remaining causative factors are shown in Table 21-2, with evaluation as to frequency of occurrence.

Congenital cataracts of genetic origin. Genetically determined cataracts often occur as isolated abnormalities. They are frequently present at birth but occasionally originate during childhood. The primary mode of transmission is autosomal dominant. Recessive and X-linked transmission has infrequently been recorded. Examination of the pedigree frequently reveals the genetic cause; however, the specific pathogenesis of genetic cataracts is not known.

Rubella. The rubella embryopathy syndrome is composed of multiple congenital anomalies that result from maternal viremia during the first trimester of pregnancy. Cataracts are present in approxi-

TABLE 21-2. Neonatal cataracts

Type	Incidence of occurrence in the syndrome
Genetic	
Dominant	
Recessive	
X-linked recessive	
Viral	
Rubella	50% incidence
Cytomegalic inclusion disease	Infrequent
Inborn errors of metabolism	
Galactosemia	50% incidence
Galactokinase deficiency	Frequent
Lowe's syndrome	Frequent
Trauma	
Birth trauma	Infrequent
Blunt trauma	Frequent
Perforating injuries	Frequent
Battered child syndrome	Infrequent
Endocrine	
Congenital hypoparathyroidism	Frequent
Albright's hereditary osteodystrophy	Infrequent
Neurologic	
Marinesco-Sjögren syndrome	Infrequent
Smith-Lemli-Opitz syndrome	Rare
Miscellaneous	
Aniridia (sporadic or associated with Wilm's tumor)	Infrequent
Treacher Collins' syndrome	Infrequent
Pierre Robin syndrome	Infrequent
Rubinstein-Taybi syndrome	Infrequent
Hallerman-Streiff syndrome	Frequent
Chromosomal anomalies	
Trisomy 13	Infrequent
Trisomy 18	Infrequent
Turner's syndrome	Infrequent
Associated with other eye malformations	
Microphthalmia	Frequent
Rieger's anomaly	Infrequent

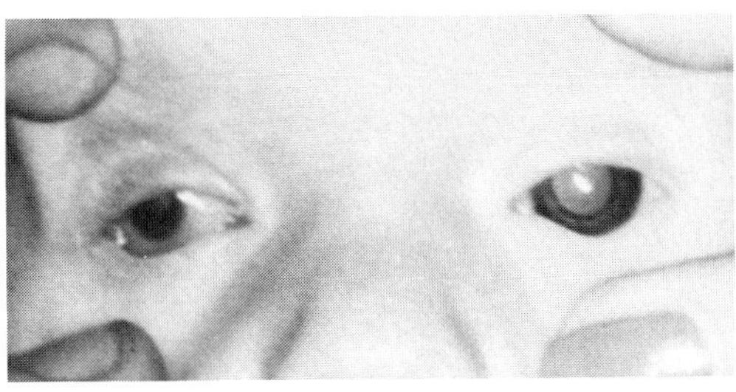

Fig. 21-13. Rubella syndrome with cataract of the left eye and microphthalmia of the right eye.

mately 50% of these patients (Fig. 21-13). They may be nuclear (confined to the center of the lens) or complete (involving all layers of the lens). The rubella virus is known to remain dormant in lens material in the offspring, in some instances for several months to several years of life. Microphthalmia and anterior uveitis may also be present in the same eye. The pupil is usually small and sometimes difficult to dilate because of atrophy of the iris structures. The iris, therefore, transilluminates abnormally. Congenital glaucoma also occurs in 10% to 25% of patients with congenital rubella; and if it is present at birth, it causes an enlarged, hazy cornea. A cloudy, edematous, or white cornea, however, may also be found with normal intraocular pressure as part of the rubella embryopathy. Rubella retinopathy may be found later in life. It is a pigmentary degeneration of the retina without demonstrable effect on visual function.

Galactosemia. Galactosemia is a hereditary inborn error of metabolism with deficiency of the enzyme galactose-1-phosphate uridyl-transferase and accumulation of galactose-1-phosphate, galactose and galactitol (p. 423). The affected neonate may be normal at birth. Subsequently, cataracts may appear during the first 2 months of life. The cataracts may be zonular or may appear as the classically described drop of oil (vacuoles) in the center of the lens. The latter description results from the imbibition of water that occurs in association with accumulation of galactose and galactitol in the lens.

Diagnosis is made by the finding of galactosuria or the absence of galactose-1-phosphate uridyl-transferase in red blood cells. Early diagnosis and a regimen of a galactose-free diet will prevent the development or further progression of cataracts. Occasional resolution of the lens opacity may also occur if the infant receives the appropriate diet.

Treatment. All congenital cataracts require early evaluation by an ophthalmologist. Most dense cataracts need surgical treatment for prevention of amblyopia or strabismus. Small central cataracts may be effectively treated by long-term dilatation of the pupil to expose the optically clear periphery of the lens. If dilatation is inadequate, a removal of a portion of the iris (optic iridectomy) for the same purpose may be performed surgically. It should be remembered also that the visual effects of lens extraction without a corrective lens will be no better than leaving the cataract in its original state. Newer concepts of congenital cataract surgery suggest that early removal of the lens (within the first few months of life if the cataract is complete), followed by contact lens application, provides the best hope of preventing amblyopia.

Pendular nystagmus may be present in association with bilateral cataracts and may continue after surgery. This type of nystagmus is a broad to-and-fro excursion of the eyes that is approximately equal in both directions. It is usually the result, not the cause, of poor visual acuity. Treatment of bilateral dense congenital cataracts by surgical removal and subsequent correction with contact lenses may prevent the development of or may reverse pendular nystagmus.

Diseases of the vitreous and retina producing a white pupil

Diseases of the posterior portion of the eye, which may be sufficiently severe in their involvement of the vitreous or retina to produce a white reflex in the pupil, are: retinoblastoma, retrolental fibroplasia, PHPV, Norrie's disease, incontinentia pigmenti, and retinal dysplasia. In addition, any lesion creating a white area in the fundus, such as a coloboma or medullated nerve fibers, may create a white pupillary reflex.

Retinoblastoma. Retinoblastoma is the most frequent malignant tumor affecting the neonatal eye. This malignancy usually produces a white pupil only when it is of sufficient size to involve a large area of the posterior segment of the eye.

Retinoblastoma occurs in approximately 1 out of every 25,000 to 30,000 births, with no predilection for race or sex. The tumor usually arises sporadically or is inherited through an autosomal dominant mutation that exhibits approximately 80% penetrance. The inherited variety may be gradually increasing in frequency because of a greater survival rate of patients whose retinoblastoma has been treated. Unilateral tumors are usually sporadic and may represent a somatic mutation. Bilateral retinoblastomas are customarily inheritable. An affected individual who has survived the hereditary form of retinoblastoma will have about a 40% risk that each of his offspring will be similarly affected. An individual surviving a sporadic unilateral variety of tumor will have about a 10% chance or less that each offspring will be affected. Those surviving sporadic bilateral involvement appear to have a 40% chance that each offspring will be affected. Empirical risk figures suggest that normal parents having one affected child will have about a 6% chance that any subsequent child will be affected. However, if they have two affected children, the risk increases to 40% for each additional child, since the hereditary nature of the tumor has been established by the presence of a second affected offspring.

Clinical presentation. The tumor originates in the retina and grows anteriorly into the vitreous by direct extension or by seeding and may also grow posteriorly into the choroid. Early in its course it produces decreased vision and strabismus, and with further growth subsequently produces a white pupil (Fig. 21-14), which is frequently detected by the parents. Any cross-eyed infant requires a fundus examination, with the pupils dilated, to rule out retinoblastoma. With further enlargement, the tumor produces secondary glaucoma, which may be associated with pain and photophobia or symptoms identical to congenital glaucoma. With extension into the anterior chamber, an opaque layer of white cells (hypopyon) or spontaneous bleeding (hyphema) may occur.

Diagnosis. The diagnosis of retinoblastoma is supported by finding one or more solid white masses in the fundus of the eye. Multiple tumors are present in a high percentage of cases. Small whitish opacities in the vitreous, representing an anterior seeding of the tumor, may be present. Additional confirmatory findings are the presence of calcification in the intraocular area, as shown radiologically (found in

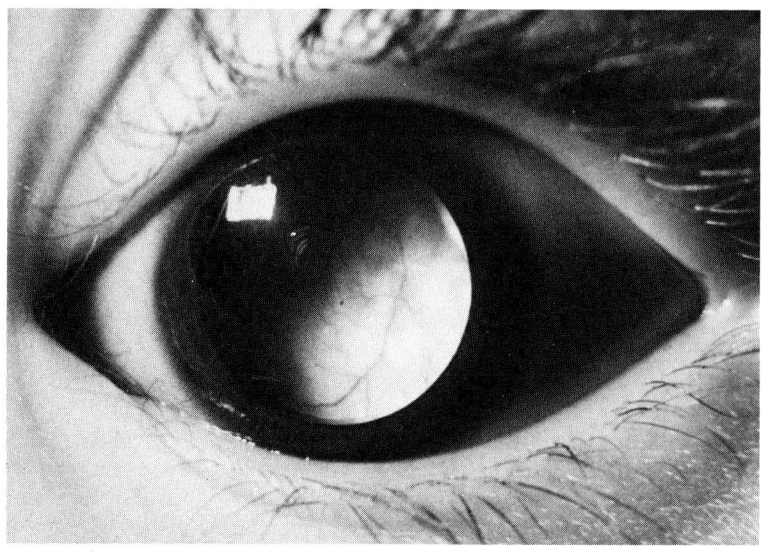

Fig. 21-14. Leukokoria, advanced retinoblastoma.

75% of cases), and the clinical impression that the intraocular mass is solid, as shown by transillumination of the globe or by ultrasonography. Differential diagnosis may be exceedingly difficult if the tumor is advanced or atypical and may require enucleation for histologic study and positive identification. PHPV may be confused with retinoblastoma (p. 641).

Treatment. The management of retinoblastoma is determined by its size and location. Examination should be performed with the infant under anesthesia, and accurate relationships of all lesions should be plotted on retinal drawings. Reese's classification is used for grading the severity and prognosis of the disease. This classification has five groupings. The most favorable, group I, includes small, single or multiple tumors in the posterior half of the fundus. The most unfavorable, group V, includes tumors involving over half of the retina or seeding of the tumor into the vitreous. Intermediate groups are graded upward in severity according to increasing size and more anterior location of the tumor.

The standard treatment of retinoblastoma has been enucleation when the tumor is unilateral. Since one mode of spread of the disease is by way of direct extension along the optic nerve, the removal of as much optic nerve as possible in the process of enucleation is important. Recently, however, unilateral (and bilateral) tumors in groups I, II, and III have been treated by therapeutic x-irradiation. With advanced bilateral disease, the more involved eye is enucleated for histologic identification, and the remaining eye is treated with radiation plus such chemotherapeutic agents as triethylene melamine. Treatment modalities also include radioactive applicators for small isolated recurrent tumors in accessible locations. Light coagulation, cryotherapy, and diathermy have also been used successfully for control of localized recurrences. Chemotherapeutic agents, such as triethylene melamine, have been used in a palliative way, in combination with irradiation for orbital spread or distant metastases. Treatment can produce regression of the tumor, in some cases to total disappearance. In larger tumors, a reduction in size occurs. Color of the tumor changes from pinkish white to grayish or glistening white. Often, a regressed tumor has the appearance of cottage cheese.

Prognosis. With prompt, adequate treatment, group I patients have approximately a 95% chance for 5-year survival. With advanced disease or evidence of extension beyond the globe, the cure rate is markedly reduced (below 30% 5-year survival).

Retrolental fibroplasia. Retrolental fibroplasia occurs in premature infants treated with oxygen above ambient levels (Chapter 5, p. 107). From 1940 to 1950 the use of high oxygen concentrations in incubators was common for most premature infants. During this period of time, the incidence of retrolental fibroplasia was markedly increased. Subsequent to this time, oxygen concentrations were used more judiciously, and the rate of occurrence decreased. However, the recent advent of treating the respiratory distress syndrome with high oxygen concentrations, in an effort to increase the survival rate of premature infants, has again increased the occurrence rate of retrolental fibroplasia.

Pathogenesis. The pathogenesis of this disease is incompletely known, but increased arterial oxygen tensions are known to produce severe vascular constriction in the immature retina. When an infant is returned to normal levels of oxygen, those retinal areas that would have been supplied by the constricted vessels become hypoxic. Apparently, this stimulates vascular proliferation into the hypoxic area in an attempt to increase oxygenation. The new vascular tissue results in leakage, hemorrhage, and fibrous proliferation.

Prematurity is the most nearly constant feature of this disease. The smaller the infant, the greater is the chance for the disease to be produced. The normal retina develops relatively late in fetal development. At 3½ months' gestation, only the posterior half of the retina is well differentiated. At 4 months' gestation, the central retinal vessels appear at the disc and begin to vascularize the retina. By the seventh month, the peripheral retina is still relatively immature, and the retinal vessels have reached only the equator of the globe. By the eighth month, vascularization is complete except for the temporal periphery of the retina. Differentiation of the retina, as well as the completion of the vascular supply, lags behind in the temporal retina as compared with the remainder of the eye; thus the temporal retina becomes more vulnerable to the effects of high arterial oxygen concentration and is the area most likely to show the effects of retrolental fibroplasia.

Pathology. The active stage of the disease usually begins during the first month after birth. Following the acute period of vasoconstriction, which occurs during oxygen administration, retinal vessels become dilated and tortuous. After removal of the infant from oxygen therapy, the areas of incompletely formed retina develop neovascularization with tufts or arcades of newly formed, thin-walled anastomosing vessels. Small retinal hemorrhages develop from the neovascular sites and subsequently become fibrotic. Massive vitreous hemorrhage may also occur from the areas of neovascularization. The diseased, contracted vitreous produces traction and areas of retinal detachment. Further tearing of neovascular tissue occurs, with production of additional retinal and vitreous hemorrhages. With marked advancement of the disease, the entire retina and its newly formed fibroblastic and neovascular tissue become detached and are pulled forward to lie just posterior to the lens, hence the name of the disease. Spontaneous regression may occur at any point during this process up to the point of fibrosis and extensive vitreous traction. There is, as yet, no way to predict accurately how often and to what extent regression will occur. In approximately 25% of patients, retrolental fibroplasia progresses to the severe stage, with production of a retrolental mass of fibroblastic tissue.

With cessation of the active process, the eye is left with a cicatricial aftermath, which may be mild to severe, depending on the extent of the active process. Minor changes include tortuosity of the vessels and a slightly pale fundus with occasional irregular pigmentation. Myopia is common. A more advanced form shows retinal vessels that are distorted or pulled to the temporal side of the retina (Fig. 21-15). A still more advanced form shows a peripheral opaque mass in the temporal periphery, with a fold of retinal tissue extending from the optic disc to the peripheral mass. In this fold of tissue, most of the major retinal blood vessels are incorporated. Where proliferation has been more marked, the retina becomes detached, and portions or all of the retina are pulled anteriorly. The most severe form is manifested by microphthalmia, a dense retrolental mass, and cataractous changes in the lens. The anterior chamber is frequently shallow, and the cornea may be cloudy as the result of secondary glaucoma. Vision is severely reduced. This latter, major form of involvement usually takes 4 to 5 months to evolve.

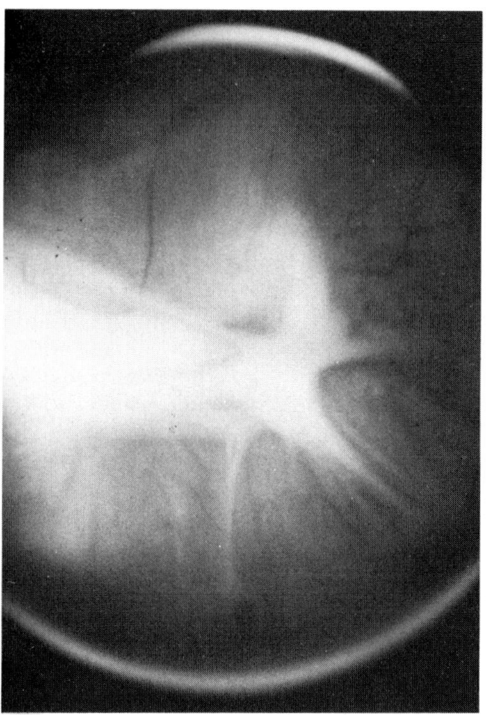

Fig. 21-15. Retrolental fibroplasia, moderately advanced, with gliotic retina drawn into upper temporal fold.

Clinical presentation. Unfortunately, there is no method of determining which infant may or may not develop retrolental fibroplasia when exposed to increased ambient oxygen concentrations. Vascular constriction or tortuosity or both were thought to be of some prognostic value; however, recent evidence suggests that these signs are of little help in regulating oxygen concentration. Arterial oxygen tension must be monitored when oxygen is administered during the neonatal period. In infants with respiratory distress syndrome, arterial oxygen concentrations may not be elevated in spite of high incubator concentrations during the major period of pulmonary involvement. However, with beginning recovery, arterial oxygen tensions may rapidly rise, with subsequent increased risk of toxicity to the retina.

Prevention. Prevention is based on avoiding the toxic arterial oxygen concentrations. Unfortunately, the exact level or duration of elevated arterial Po_2 that is toxic to the retina is not yet known, but the arterial oxygen tensions should usually be kept below 80 mm Hg.

Persistent hyperplastic primary vitreous. PHPV is a congenital anomaly that produces a white pupil at birth or shortly thereafter. This disease results from the failure of reabsorption of the embryonic hyaloid system (the primary vitreous). This embryonic system develops as a complex network of vessels growing anteriorly from the disc to surround the developing lens (the tunica vasculosa lentis). This vascular scaffolding supplies the posterior eye and lens during its early formation and is replaced by the clear secondary vitreous when the eye further matures. During the fifth to eighth months of gestation, the hyaloid vascular system atrophies almost completely, leaving a small, nearly transparent canal running from the disc to the posterior surface of the lens (Cloquet's canal). Failure of complete atrophy of this vascular system may leave a number of possible remnants that may be seen at birth. At the disc, a small protrusion of mesodermal tissue, which extends a short distance into the vitreous, is called Bergmeister's papilla. Remnants of the hyaloid artery may be seen extending from the disc to the posterior central area of the lens. A small remnant of the tunica vasculosa lentis on the posterior central area of the lens is called a Mittendorf dot. A persistence and hyperplasia of the entire system is called PHPV.

Clinical presentation. PHPV may appear at birth as a sheet of white tissue immediately behind the lens. It is usually most dense at the center of the lens and thins out toward the periphery. As a result of this vascular origin, vessels frequently are seen to radiate from its center. The retrolental mass, therefore, may be pinkish white. When the pupil is dilated, the ciliary processes may be seen being drawn centrally along the posterior surface of the lens toward the central mass.

PHPV is nearly always unilateral and occurs in full-term infants without history of oxygen therapy. The involved eye is usually microphthalmic. The anterior chamber is frequently shallow because fibrous contraction of the primary vitreous pulls the ciliary body centrally. In turn, the lens is forced forward. With continued organization and contraction of the primary vitreous, the lens capsule may be involved, and cataract formation may occur. At this stage in development of the disease, glaucoma may occur, as well as posterior chamber hemorrhages and hemorrhages into the lens. Retinal detachment occurs in the final stages, with continued vitreous traction.

Diagnosis. Differentiation of PHPV from retrolental fibroplasia is usually possible because of the unilateral involvement and occurrence of PHPV in a full-term infant. Retrolental fibroplasia is present bilaterally in a premature infant who has had oxygen therapy. Differentiation from retinoblastoma may be somewhat difficult but is aided by the presence of visible ciliary processes in the periphery of the dilated pupil and the presence of vascular elements in the central portion of the retrolental mass. Also, retinoblastomas do not occur in microphthalmic eyes. The absence of radiologic evidence of calcification within the eye may be of additional value. However, because of the progressive and changing nature of PHPV, it may closely simulate retinoblastoma and may require enucleation for differentiation.

Treatment. Therapy of PHPV is ineffective in most circumstances, but experimental attempts at surgery have recently been made.

Prognosis. Since the macula is poorly developed in microphthalmic eyes, even anatomically successful surgery for PHPV may not result in useful vision.

Retinal dysplasia. Retinal dysplasia is a congenital anomaly of full-term infants, is usually bilateral, and is associated with microphthalmic eyes. Retinal dysplasia may occur as part of a group of congenital anomalies, including defects of the central nervous system, cardiovascular system, and skeletal system of sufficient degree to produce early death of the infant. Such a syndrome should always suggest the possibility of trisomy 13. When the dysplasia is advanced, a white retrolental mass may be produced. Milder forms of dysplasia occur as developmental abnormalities but are often detected only by histologic techniques. In such cases, results of chromosome analysis are usually normal.

Norrie's disease. Norrie's disease is a rare genetic disorder that is transmitted as an X-linked recessive trait. It is characterized by the presence of bilateral massive retinal detachments, resulting in a white pupil, often, but not always, combined with deafness and mental retardation. Organization of the retinal detachment may disrupt the lens, producing cataract, or may affect the anterior chamber angle, producing congenital glaucoma. The usual result is atrophy of the globe (phthisis bulbi).

The dislocated lens

The discovery of a dislocated lens (ectopia lentis) in the neonatal period is helpful in the identification of systemic disease processes that are associated with this abnormality. Lens dislocation may be present in the following diseases during the neonatal period, or it may not assume its dislocated position until the first or second decade of life: homocystinuria, sulfite oxidase deficiency, hyperlysinemia, Marfan's syndrome, and Weill-Marchesani syndrome. It occurs as the result of a laxity, absence, or defect of the zonular attachments that suspend the lens from the ciliary body.

Ectopia lentis may be suggested by iridodonesis, or tremulousness of the iris, which results from the lack of normal support the lens gives to the posterior surface of the iris. Identification of an eccentric location of the lens is made by wide dilatation of the pupil and visualization of a portion of the equator of the lens in the pupillary space (Fig. 21-16). Treatment of the dislocated lens is usually not necessary during the neonatal period, unless it is complicated by cataract formation or glaucoma. The glaucoma may be caused either by complications of the cataract formation or by blockage of aqueous flow through the pupil.

The abnormal fundus

Observing the neonatal eye *through a dilated pupil* should be a routine part of the examination in every infant. When one views the fundus with the direct ophthalmoscope, the appearance of a flat, two-dimensional surface is obtained. However, this represents a three-dimensional organization of tissue where several successive layers are viewed simultaneously as the result of their transparency. The retinal ves-

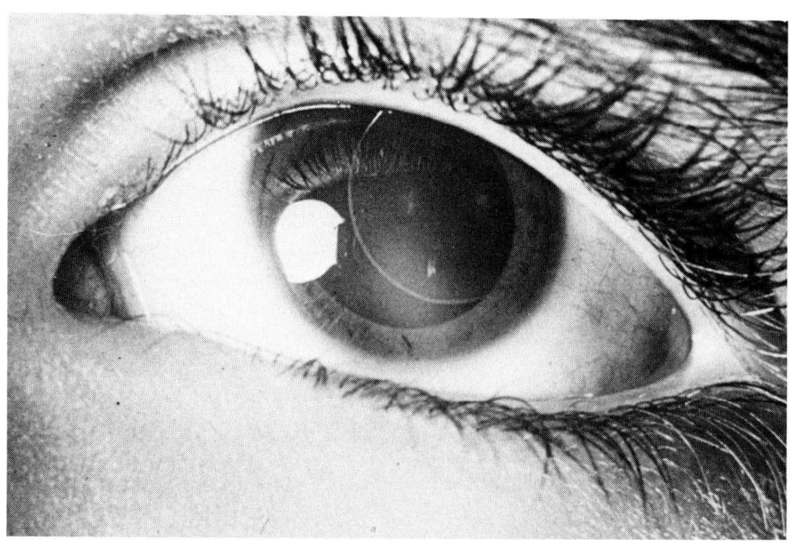

Fig. 21-16. Ectopia lentis (dislocated lens) of left eye.

sels lie near the surface of the retina. Deep to the vessels the retina is a nearly transparent layer of tissue with a sheen to its inner surface. The retina becomes visible only when abnormalities are present. It resembles a pale ghostlike sheet when it is detached. Retinal edema gives a slightly raised opalescent appearance. Infection obscures the underlying structures by a fuzzy-white thickening of the retinal tissue itself.

During the neonatal period, the fundus is nearly transparent because of the lack of uveal pigmentation. It is well to remember, therefore, that in all pathologic processes characterized by either a lack or an excess of pigment, these defects may be only minimally suggested and may become progressively more evident as the normal uveal pigmentation becomes complete after the first 6 months of life. The choroid is the deepest layer normally visible by the ophthalmoscope. Pathologic processes that prevent its development or that destroy areas of choroid will, therefore, expose areas of bare sclera that will appear glistening white with the ophthalmoscope.

Pathologic conditions of the retina are discussed as follows: hereditary abnormalities, congenital disorders, infectious diseases, and finally, acquired pathologic conditions.

Hereditary abnormalities

Retinoschisis is a hereditary abnormality in which the superficial layers of the retina are split from the deeper layers and are elevated into the vitreous. This splitting creates a veillike appearance in front of the retina. Visual function is absent in the affected tissue. Retinoschisis is a progressive, degenerative disorder, which has an X-linked recessive transmission. Macular changes and vitreous hemorrhages can occur as associated findings. Both lead to loss of vision.

Fundus albipunctatus is characterized by gray or white mottling of the fundus. This is a stationary form of retinal degeneration, transmitted as an autosomal recessive trait. Visual acuity, color vision, and visual fields are normal in patients with this disorder.

Retinitis pigmentosa is a pigmentary degeneration of the retina, which typically makes its appearance in the early teens or even later. In severe form it may rarely appear in the neonatal period. The ophthalmoscopic findings are the result of retinal pigment epithelial degeneration, with migration of the pigment to form irregular black deposits resembling bony spicules.

Leber's congenital amaurosis occasionally produces symptoms of blindness shortly after birth but usually occurs later in childhood. Typical findings are a salt-and-pepper appearance of the fundus, with a grayish cast to the retina. Electroretinography reveals severely deficient retinal function. Although autosomal recessive transmission is most common, autosomal dominance characterizes some forms of congenital amaurosis.

The diagnosis of *albinism* in the neonatal period is extremely difficult to substantiate as the result of the normal paucity of the uveal pigment during this period. The diagnosis may be suggested when pigmentation of the skin, hair, and irises fails to progress during the first several months in comparison with parents and siblings. Lack of pigmentation is more apparent in darker races. The fundus remains quite pale and shows a prominent appearance of its choroidal vessels. Photophobia, pendular nystagmus, and abnormal transillumination of the irises are characteristic of albinism. Severely reduced vision is the result of macular dysfunction.

Congenital disorders

Retinal folds presumably occur as the result of overgrowth of retinal tissue in comparison with ocular size, thereby preventing total attachment of all retinal tissue to the underlying pigment epithelium and choroid. A white fold or ridge of retinal tissue may be seen running from the disc, typically inferotemporally, to the periphery. Occasionally, the macular area may be involved.

Congenital grouped pigmentation is a rare finding of unknown cause in which small areas of the retina, one disc diameter or less in size, show hyperpigmentation. These areas are typically paired or grouped and are usually kidney shaped. They have no clinical significance but should not be confused with old inflammatory scars.

Infectious diseases

Intrauterine ocular infections occur as the result of maternal infections that cross the placental barrier (see Chapter 8). Chorioretinitis occurs in patients with rubella and occasionally in patients with influenza and congenital syphilis. An irregularity of the retinal pigment develops, with what appears to be a salt-and-pepper type of distribution. Congenital cytomegalic inclusion disease may include chorioretinal lesions in any form, from large, whitish, necrotic lesions in the posterior pole to the more typical multiple, small, peripheral white areas that tend to enlarge or coalesce as the disease progresses. Congenital toxoplasmosis, in its severe form, may lead to large chorioretinal scars in the macular area. The chorioretinal scars appear as large white areas of exposed sclera, with prominent, darkly pigmented borders. The treatment of the eye manifestations of congenital toxoplasmosis is not established. Large doses of systemically administered steroids are advocated for evidence of progressive extension of the retinal infection. Pyrimethamine (Daraprim), sulfadiazine, and folinic acid, previously thought to be effective in combination, are still recommended by some.

Acquired fundus pathologic conditions

The retina of the premature infant is incompletely formed at birth and continues its development during the first few months of neonatal life. The periphery of the fundus from the equator to the ora serrata (the junction of the retina and the ciliary body) appears pale or grayish white, and the overlying vitreous may be somewhat hazy in appearance. These are normal findings, which gradually give way to the normal reddish pink color of the fundus as the retina progressively differentiates.

Birth trauma may produce a pathologic condition of the retina (p. 79). A *battered infant* may have scattered retinal hemorrhages, vitreous hemorrhage, or areas of retinal edema. *Retrolental fibroplasia* has been discussed in the previous section dealing with the white pupil. A fold of retina extending from the disc to the temporal periphery, indicating marked involvement, is sometimes difficult to differentiate morphologically from a congenital retinal fold.

The abnormal macula

Abnormal appearance of the macula may occur in Best's vitelline degeneration of the macula. This is an autosomal dominant disorder that rarely occurs in the neonatal period as cystlike changes in the macular retina, which rapidly coalesce and become yellowish. Its appearance has been likened to an egg yolk. This macular degeneration, curiously, produces little initial reduction in visual acuity. It gradually undergoes further atrophic degeneration, with decrease in visual acuity at a much later period.

Several of the storage diseases produce an abnormal appearance of the macula, and abnormalities in the macula may be useful in detecting these disorders (see Chapter 14). The abnormal appearance of the macula is produced by accumulation of the stored material in the ganglion cells of the retina. This produces a decrease in transparency of the retina except at the very center of the macula, where no ganglion cells exist. Therefore, the center of the macula retains its normal cherry red appearance in sharp contrast to the surrounding grayish retina. Sphingolipidoses that may produce a cherry red spot are Tay-Sachs disease, in which a cherry red spot may be present shortly after birth or may develop during the first year, and Niemann-Pick disease (infantile), in which approximately 50% of patients develop a cherry red spot in the macula during the neonatal period. Of the so-called mucolipidoses, Farber's disease has been noted to show a grayish discoloration of the macula at 6 to 8 weeks of age and G_{M1} generalized gangliosidosis has been found to demonstrate a cherry red spot in the macula in approximately 30% of patients prior to 2 months of age. The mucopolysaccharidoses are characterized by abnormal deposition of mucopolysaccharides in the cornea, but the macula is normal.

TABLE 21-3. Neonatal macular changes

Condition	Defect
Tay-Sachs disease	Cherry red spot
Niemann-Pick disease	Cherry red spot
G_{M1} generalized gangliosidosis	Cherry red spot
Farber's disease	Gray macula
Best's vitelline degeneration	Cystic macula (rare)
Toxoplasmosis	Chorioretinal scar
Coloboma	Absence of retina and choroid

Optic disc abnormalities

All transmissions of the visual pathways must exit the eye through the optic disc. Estimations of pallor or optic atrophy can be relied on only if careful attention is paid to preventing pressure on the orbital structures from being transmitted to the eye itself during examination of the disc. Disc margins in the neonate should be as clear and distinct as they are in the adult.

Persistence of hyaloid artery

Persistence of the central hyaloid artery is a common developmental abnormality. Its persistence in the premature infant is sufficiently frequent to be considered normal. It occurs in some 3% of full-term infants. Most frequently, it is a fine thread of nearly transparent tissue or, rarely, it may be patent and contain blood. It usually continues to undergo atrophic degeneration during the neonatal period and early life, with rare persistence into adulthood.

Bergmeister's papilla

The persistence of the mesodermal supporting elements of the hyaloid vascular system at the disc may leave a small protuberance of gray-white tissue extending from the disc forward into the vitreous. A small knuckle of a retinal vessel may course into this area and return to the disc before supplying the normal retina, or the papilla may be associated with one or several small, round pearly gray cysts of remaining glial tissue. Vision is usually unimpaired.

Medullated nerve fibers

Normal myelination of the optic nerve fibers occurs in fetal development in reverse direction to the growth of the axons themselves. Development of medullated sheaths, therefore, progresses from the geniculate bodies through the optic tracts, optic chiasm, and optic nerves to end normally just posterior to the optic disc. This process is usually complete at birth or within the first month of extrauterine life. Occasionally, medullation of the nerve fibers proceeds through the disc and onto the retinal surface. This appears as a glistening, white, opaque area, involving the peripheral portion of the disc and extending into segments of the nearby retina. Sometimes there is no continuity between the disc and the medullated nerve fibers of the retina. The edges of the medullated areas are feathered, and the involved areas are sometimes arcuate. This process is stable after the first several months of life, and visual acuity is not often impaired, except for an enlarged area of the blind spot when measured in adults.

Conus or congenital crescent

The sharp margins of the optic disc are created by the abrupt ending of the choroid and pigment epithelium at the disc borders. On occasion, one quadrant of the disc fails to have these structures extend to the immediate edge of the disc; instead, they stop short in a sloping margin, which is crescent shaped. This allows the underlying sclera to be visible as a whitish crescent adjacent to the disc. This crescent is sometimes bordered by a darkly pigmented line. Two thirds of congenital crescents occur below the disc. Most eyes with congenital crescents are associated with defective vision in the form of hypermetropic astigmatism. A congenital conus should be differentiated from a myopic conus, or crescent, in that the former is present at birth and is stationary throughout life, whereas the latter develops as the eye becomes excessively myopic and is usually temporal.

Coloboma of the disc

Coloboma of the disc is formed by a failure of adequate closure of the embryonic optic vesicle. A coloboma of the iris or choroid has a similar pathogenesis. In this condition the disc may appear enlarged and elongated, usually inferiorly or temporally. The coloboma may include the macular area. The blood vessels may be distributed normally or may be displaced to the periphery of the disc and appear to be somewhat disorganized in their initial direction from the disc. Colobomas of the disc are usually associated with defective vision.

Optic pit

Occasionally, the surface of the optic disc shows a hole or pit. This pit is usually situated near the lower temporal quadrant of the disc at its border and may vary in size, shape, and depth. It is thought to be a minimal coloboma of the disc. Frequently, visual defects are present with this finding. Later in life, they are manifested as enlargement of the blind spot, sector field defects, or involvement of the papillomacular bundle, with production of a partial paracentral or central scotoma. In association with a pit of the optic disc, serous fluid may elevate the macula and cause reduction in visual acuity later in life.

Oblique discs

The optic nerve usually enters the posterior aspect of the eye from a slightly nasal angle. If this angle is accentuated, the nerve head or disc may be tilted obliquely, with its temporal margin considerably more posteriorly located than its nasal margin. This gives the disc an ovoid appearance, with its longest diameter in the vertical meridian. This abnormality is also frequently associated with poor visual acuity.

Hypoplasia of the optic nerve

Hypoplasia of the optic disc is a rare anomaly in which part of all of the optic nerve fibers fail to develop and reach the disc. In this condition the optic disc is smaller than normal (the normal disc is approximately one half to three fourths of the diameter of the area of fundus viewed with the direct ophthalmoscope). The disc is pale, and the retinal vessels are usually attenuated. This may occur unilaterally or bilaterally. If the condition is bilateral, the child is usually blind, or nearly so.

Congenital optic atrophy

Congenital optic atrophy is a condition of unknown cause in which the nerve fibers have been formed and have subsequently atrophied. The disc is pale and has a normal size and configuration. The child is usually blind, or vision is exceedingly poor and associated with nystagmus. The condition remains static and is not usually associated with other central nervous system disturbances.

JOHN E. READ
MORTON F. GOLDBERG

BIBLIOGRAPHY

Abbassi, V., Lowe, C. U., and Calcagno, P. L.: Oculo-cerebro-renal syndrome; a review, Am. J. Dis. Child. **115**:145, February, 1968.

Baum, J. D., and Bulpitt, C. J.: Retinal and conjunctival haemorrhage in the newborn, Arch. Dis. Child. **45**:344, 1970.

Cogan, D. G., and Kuwabara, T.: The sphingolipidoses and the eye, Arch. Ophthalmol. **79**: 437, April, 1968.

de Venecia, G., and Lobeck, C. C.: Successful treatment of eyelid hemangioma with prednisone, Arch. Ophthalmol. **84**:98, July 1970.

Duke-Elder, S.: System of ophthalmology. Vol. 3, Normal and abnormal development. Part 2, Congenital Deformities. St. Louis, 1963, The C. V. Mosby Co.

Ellsworth, R. M.: The practical management of retinoblastoma, Trans. Am. Ophthalmol. Soc. **67**:462, 1969.

Emery, J. M., Green, W. R., Wyllie, R. G., and Howell, R. R.: G_{M1}-gangliosidosis; ocular and pathological manifestations, Arch. Ophthalmol. **85**:177, February 1971.

Fontaine, M.: Manifestations oculaires de la prématurité. Arch. Ophthalmol. (Paris) **31**:383, April 1971.

Forbes, G. B., and Forbes, G. M.: Silver nitrate and the eyes of the newborn; Credé's contribution to preventive medicine, Am. J. Dis. Child. **121**:1, January 1971.

Francois, J.: General anomalies and diseases associated with congenital cataracts. In Congenital cataracts, Springfield, Ill., 1963, Charles C Thomas, Publisher, Chapter 12.

Fraumeni, J. F., Jr., and Glass, A. G.: Wilms tumor and congenital aniridia, J.A.M.A. **206**: 825, October 21, 1968.

Friendly, D. S.: Ocular manifestations of physical child abuse, Trans. Am. Acad. Ophthalmol. Otolaryngol. **75**:381, March-April 1971.

Gitzelmann, R.: Hereditary galactokinase deficiency; a newly recognized cause of juvenile cataracts, Pediatr. Res. **1**:14, January 1967.

Goldberg, M. F.: Waardenburg's syndrome with fundus and other anomalies, Arch. Ophthalmol. **76**:797, December 1966.

Goldberg, M. F., Cotlier, E., Fichenscher, L. G., Kenyon, K., Enat, R., and Borowsky, S. A.: Macular cherry-red spot, corneal clouding and β-galactose deficiency; clinical, biochemical and electron microscopic study of a new autosomal recessive storage disease, Arch. Int. Med. **128**: 387, September 1971.

Goldberg, M. F., Maumenee, A. E., and McKusick, V. A.: Corneal dystrophies associated with abnormalities of mucopolysaccharide metabolism, Arch. Ophthalmol. **74**:516, October 1965.

Goldberg, M. F., Payne, J. W., and Brunt, P. W.: Ophthalmologic studies of familial dysautonomia; the Riley-Day syndrome, Arch. Ophthalmol. **80**:732, December 1968.

Khodadoust, A. A., Mohsen, Z., and Biggs, S. L.: Optic disc in normal newborns, Amer. J. Ophthalmol. **66**:502, September 1968.

Knox, D. L.: Examination of the cortically blind infant, Am. J. Ophthalmol. **58**:617, October 1964.

Liebman, S. D., and Gellis, S. S.: The pediatrician's ophthalmology, St. Louis, 1966, The C. V. Mosby Co.

McCormick, A. Q.: Transient cataracts in premature infants; a new clinical entity, Can. J. Ophthalmol. 3:202, 1968.

Newell, F. W.: Opthalmology; principles and concepts, ed. 2, St. Louis, 1969, The C. V. Mosby Co.

Parks, M. M.: Growth of the eye and development of vision. In Liebman, S. D., and Gellis, S. S., editors: The pediatrician's ophthalmology, St. Louis, 1966, The C. V. Mosby Co., Chapter 2.

Reese, A. B.: Tumors of the eye, ed. 2, New York, 1963, Harper & Row, Publishers, p. 403.

Sagerman, R. H., Cassady, R. J., and Tretter, P.: Radiation therapy for rhabdomyosarcoma of the orbit, Trans. Am. Acad. Ophthalmol. Otolaryngol. 72:849, September-October 1968.

Scheie, H. G., and Albert, D. M.: Adler's textbook of ophthalmology, Philadelphia, 1969, W. B. Saunders Co., p. 106.

Smith, D. W.: Recognizable patterns of human malformations; genetic, embryologic and clinical aspects; major problems in clinical pediatrics, vol. 3, Philadelphia, 1970, W. B. Saunders Co.

Smith, G. F., Berg, J. M., and McCreary, B. D.: de Lange syndrome. In The First Conference on the Clinical Delineation of Birth Defects. Part II. National Foundation, March of Dimes Birth Defects: Original Article Series 5(2):18, February 1969.

Spranger, J. W., and Wiedemann, H. R.: The genetic mucolopidoses; diagnosis and differential diagnosis, Humangenetik 9:113, 1970.

Summitt, R. L.: Familial Goldenhar syndrome. In The First Conference on the Clinical Delineation of Birth Defects. Part II. National Foundation, March of Dimes Birth Defects: Original Article Series 5(2):106, February 1969.

Symposium on Surgical and Medical Management of Congenital Anomalies of the Eye, Transactions of the New Orleans Academy of Ophthalmology, St. Louis, 1968, The C. V. Mosby Co.

Vogel, F.: Genetic prognosis in retinoblastoma. In Sorsby, A., editor: Modern trends in ophthalmology, London, 1967, Butterworth & Co. (Publishers) Ltd., Chapter 3.

Walsh, T. J., Smith, J. L., and Shipley, T.: Neurologic blindness in infancy. In Smith, J. L., editor: Neuro-ophthalmology Symposium of the University of Miami and Bascom Palmer Eye Institute, vol. 3, St. Louis, 1967, The C. V. Mosby Co., Chapter 9.

Wilson, W. A., and Donnell, G. N.: Cataracts in galactosemia, Arch. Ophthalmol. 60:215, August 1958.

Appendix of normal tables

BLOOD PRESSURE

Table 1. Average systolic, diastolic, and mean blood pressures during the first twelve hours of life in normal newborn infants grouped according to birth weight

Birth weight		Hour 1	2	3	4	5	6	7	8	9	10	11	12
1,001 to 2,000 gm	Systolic	49	49	51	52	53	52	52	52	51	51	49	50
	Diastolic	26	27	28	29	31	31	31	31	31	30	29	30
	Mean	35	36	37	39	40	40	39	39	38	37	37	38
2,001 to 3,000 gm	Systolic	59	57	60	60	61	58	64	60	63	61	60	59
	Diastolic	32	32	32	32	33	34	37	34	38	35	35	35
	Mean	43	41	43	43	44	43	45	43	44	44	43	42
Over 3,000 gm	Systolic	70	67	65	65	66	66	67	67	68	70	66	66
	Diastolic	44	41	39	41	40	41	41	41	44	43	41	41
	Mean	53	51	50	50	51	50	50	51	53	54	51	50

Kitterman, J. A., Phibbs, R. H., and Tooley, W. H.: Pediatrics **44**:959, 1969.

URINE AND STOOL

Table 2. Time of first voiding by 500 full-term infants

	Number	Percent	Cumulative percent
Delivery room	85	17.0	17.0
Hours			
12	253	50.6	67.6
12–24	124	24.8	92.4
24–48	35	7.0	99.4
Over 48	3*	0.6	100.0
Total	500	100.0	

Sherry, S. N., and Kramer, I.: J. Pediatr. **46**:189, 1955.
*These patients voided at 50, 50, and 51 hours.

Table 3. Time of passage of first urine in 200 premature infants

Time	Number	Percent
Delivery room	45	21.5
Hours		
0–12	86	43.0
12–24	52	26.0
24–48	17	9.5
Over 48 hours		

Kramer, I., and Sherry, S. N.: J. Pediatr. **51**:374, 1957.

Table 4. Time of passage of first stool by 500 full-term infants

	Number	Percent	Cumulative percent
Delivery room	136	27.2	27.2
Hours			
12	209	41.8	69.0
12–24	125	25.0	94.0
24–48	29	5.8	99.8
Over 48	1*	0.2	100.0
Total	500	100.0	

Sherry, S. N., and Kramer, I.: J. Pediatr. **46**:158, 1955.
*Sixty-two hours.

Table 5. Time of passage of first stool in 200 premature infants

Time	Number	Percent
Delivery room	26	13.0
Hours		
0–12	63	31.5
12–24	71	35.5
24–48	28	14.0
Over 48 hours	12	6.0

Kramer, I., and Sherry, S. N.: J. Pediatr. **51**:373, 1957. From the Department of Pediatrics, Sinai Hospital of Baltimore, Incorporated.

BLOOD GASES AND ACID BASE

Table 6. Acid base status

Determination	Vigorous term infants, vaginal delivery	Birth	1st hr	3rd hr	24 hr	2 days	3 days
pH	Umbilical artery	7.26					
	Umbilical vein	7.29					
pCO_2 mm Hg	Arterial	54.5	38.8	38.3	33.6	34	35
	Venous	42.8					
O_2 sat	Arterial	19.8	93.8	94.7	93.2		
	Venous	47.6					
pH	Left atrial		7.30	7.34	7.41	7.39 (temporal artery)	7.38 (temporal artery)
CO_2 content, mEq/L			20.6	21.9	21.4		
	Premratures						
	Capillary						
pH	<1250 gm				7.36	7.35	7.35
pCO_2 mm Hg					38	44	37
pH	>1250				7.39	7.39	7.38
pCO_2 mm Hg					38	39	38

Schaffer, A. J.: Diseases of the newborn, ed. 3, Philadelphia, 1971, W. B. Saunders Co. Data of Weisbort, and others: J. Pediatr. **52**:395, 1958; and Bucci, and others: Biol. Neonate **8**:81, 1965.

CHEMISTRY

Table 7. Normal blood chemistry values, term infants

Determination	Sample source	Cord	1-12 hr	12-24 hr	24-48 hr	48-72 hr
Sodium, mEq/L*	Capillary	147 (126–166)	143 (124–156)	145 (132–159)	148 (134–160)	149 (139–162)
Potassium, mEq/L		7.8 (5.6–12)	6.4 (5.3–7.3)	6.3 (5.3–8.9)	6.0 (5.2–7.3)	5.9 (5.0–7.7)
Chloride, mEq/L		103 (98–110)	100.7 (90–111)	103 (87–114)	102 (92–114)	103 (93–112)
Calcium, mg/100 ml		9.3 (8.2–11.1)	8.4 (7.3–9.2)	7.8 (6.9–9.4)	8.0 (6.1–9.9)	7.9 (5.9–9.7)
Phosphorus, mg/100 ml		5.6 (3.7–8.1)	6.1 (3.5–8.6)	5.7 (2.9–8.1)	5.9 (3.0–8.7)	5.8 (2.8–7.6)
Blood urea, mg/100 ml		29 (21–40)	27 (8–34)	33 (9–63)	32 (13–77)	31 (13–68)
Total protein, gm/100 ml		6.1 (4.8–7.3)	6.6 (5.6–8.5)	6.6 (5.8–8.2)	6.9 (5.9–8.2)	7.2 (6.0–8.5)
Blood sugar, mg/100 ml		73 (45–96)	63 (40–97)	63 (42–104)	56 (30–91)	59 (40–90)
Lactic acid, mg/100 ml		19.5 (11–30)	14.6 (11–24)	14.0 (10–23)	14.3 (9–22)	13.5 (7–21)
Lactate, mm/L†		2.0–3.0	2.0			

Schaffer, A. J.: Diseases of the newborn, ed. 3, Philadelphia, 1971, W. B. Saunders Co.
*Acharya and Payne: Arch. Dis. Child. **40**:430, 1965.
†Daniel, Adamsons, and James: Pediatrics **37**:942, 1966.

Table 8. Normal blood chemistry values (average), low birth weight infants, capillary blood, first day

Determination	<1,000	1,001-1,500	1,501-2,000	2,001-2,500
Sodium, mEq/L	138	133	135	134
Potassium, mEq/L	6.4	6.0	5.4	5.6
Chloride, mEq/L	100	101	105	104
Total CO_2, mEq/L	19	20	20	20
Urea, mg/100 ml	22	21	16	16
TSP, gm/100 ml	4.8	4.8	5.2	5.3

Schaffer, A. J.: Diseases of the newborn, ed. 3, Philadelphia, 1971, W. B. Saunders Co.
Data from Pincus, and others: Pediatrics **18**:939, 1956.

Table 9. Levels of sugar in whole blood in normal full-term infants

Group		No.	Mat.	At delivery: Umbilical: Vein	Artery	Prior to milk feedings: Age (hours): ½	1	1½	2	2½	3	4	6	9	12	24	References
I		46															
Blood sugar	Mean		108	80	68	60	51	50	52	56	56		56	52	52		Creery and Parkinson, 1953
mg/100 ml	SE		4.2	2.6	4.3	2.5	2.4	2.0	1.8	1.8	2.0		1.6	1.4	1.8		
	Range		68	49	40	27	21	19	30	34	30		32-82	30-73	10-75		
			154	126	118	110	87	79	77	90	90			Normal	vaginal		
II		32	Birth														
Blood sugar	Mean			76 (vein and artery)		77	71		64			63	63	Normal			Farquhar, 1954
mg/100 ml	SE			2.6		3.5	3.7		2.4			2.0	2.0	vaginal			
	Range			43-105		44-128	39-121		39-102			31-87	38-90				
IIIa		13	Vaginal, no fluid to mother														
True blood sugar	Mean		85	66		55	55		48			55	47	Normal			Cornblath and others, 1961
mg/100 ml	SE		4.6	3.5		5.8	5.2		3.5			3.5	3.9				
	Range		63-121	44-84		34-90	35-89		22-73			30-71	27-28				
IVb		7	Cesarean section, saline IV to mother														
	Mean		85	64		75	76		70			60	57			54	
	SE		11.2	6.0		6.6	11.8		8.5			9.7	5.3			5.0	
	Range		46-131	38-90		58-107	34-136		45-108			47-101	35-76			43-76	
Vc		23	Cesarean section, glucose IV to mother														
	Mean		149	107		72	67		57			60	53			67	
	SE		17.3	12.6		8.0	8.5		6.1			4.3	3.7			5.7	
	Range		77-354	61-204		31-125	28-117		35-115			27-90	32-77			35-109	
IIId		8	Vaginal, glucose IV to mother														
	Mean		127	89		54	47		41			50	51				
	SE		20.1	12.9		8.4	8.3		5.8			4.8	7.0				
	Range		80-250	54-163		27-98	16-82		19-71			34-80	29-81				

Cornblath, M., and Schwartz, R.: Diseases of carbohydrate metabolism, Philadelphia, 1966, W. B. Saunders Co.

Table 10. Levels of sugar in whole blood in low birth weight infants

Group		At birth Cord	Age (hours) 0-3	4-6	12	18	24	30	36	42	48	References
I												
True blood sugar	Mean	71	47		45	43	43	44	41	46	50	Ward, 1953
mg/100 ml	SE	6.0										
	Range	24-140	26-72		18-107	15-62	16-60	18-90	25-60	18-78	19-80	
No. determinations		21	20		23	23	14	15	10	14	14	Somogyi
IIa												
Blood glucose	Mean		41	47	48	45		44				Baens and others, 1963
mg/100 ml	SE		2.6	2.5	3.1	2.5		1.7				
	Range		24-72	21-70	25-89	23-84		18-73				
No. determinations			20	26	22	37		49				Glucose oxidase

Group		Age (days) 0	1	2	3	4	5	6	7	8	9	10	11	12	13	References
III																
True blood sugar	Mean	45	53	55	60	60	58	63	63	66	65	71	65	63	64	Fast: 2-3 hr
mg/100 ml	SE	1.8	1.6	2.0	1.9	2.0	1.4	1.7	1.9	2.1	2.1	2.9	1.7	2.3	2.0	Norval, 1950
	Range	←						15 to 115 mg/100 ml							→	
No. determinations		33 →							28	25	24	23	23	23	22	Somogyi
IIb									**7-13 days**		**14-20**	**21-27**	**28-55**			
Blood glucose	Mean		44	39	40	42	43	43	45		56	52	48			Fast 3½-4 hr
mg/100 ml	SE		1.7	1.9	1.9	2.1	2.1	2.2	1.6		2.8	2.9	2.5			Baens and others, 1963
	Range		18-73	15-73	20-64	21-79	18-78	22-83	28-61		23-98	18-77	22-83			
No. determinations			49	45	43	32	33	33	40		33	26	43			Glucose oxidase

Cornblath, M., and Schwartz, R.: Disorders of carbohydrate metabolism, Philadelphia, 1966, W. B. Saunders Co.

HEMATOLOGY

Table 11. Mean red cell values during gestation

Age (in weeks)	Hb (gm/ 100 ml)	Hemato-crit (%)	RBC (10^6/ mm^3)	Mean corpuscle vol (μ^3)	Mean corpuscle Hb ($\gamma\gamma$)	Mean corpuscle Hb conc (%)	Nuc RBC (% of RBCs)	Retic (%)	Diam (μ)
12	8.0–10.0	33	1.5	180	60	34	5.0–8.0	40	10.5
16	10.0	35	2.0	140	45	33	2.0–4.0	10–25	9.5
20	11.0	37	2.5	135	44	33	1.0	10–20	9.0
24	14.0	40	3.5	123	38	31	1.0	5–10	8.8
28	14.5	45	4.0	120	40	31	0.5	5–10	8.7
34	15.0	47	4.4	118	38	32	0.2	3–10	8.5

Oski, F. A., and Naiman, J. L.: Hematologic problems in the newborn, ed. 2, Philadelphia, 1972, W. B. Saunders Co.

Table 12. Normal hematology of the full-term newborn infant (venous blood)

	Cord blood	Day 1	Day 2	Day 7	Day 20	Day 45	Day 75
Hemoglobin (gm/100 ml)	16.8	18.4	17.8	17.0	15.9	12.7	11.4
Range	13.7–20.1				11.3–20.5	9.5–15.9	9.6–13.2
	(14.0)*	(14.5)	(14.0)	(14.0)		(10.0)	(10.0)
Hematocrit (%)	53	58	55	54			
	(44)	(48)	(45)	(45)			
Reticulocyte count (%)	3–7	3–7	1–3	0–1	0–1	0–1	0–1
Nucleated RBC/mm^3	500	200	0–5	0	0	0	0
(% per 100 WBC)	(10%)	(7%)					
Per 100 RBC	.1	.05	0	0			
RBC morphology		Macrocytes					

*Values given in the parentheses indicate anemia.

TABLE 13. Postnatal hematologic values*

		1-3 days	4-7 days	2 weeks	4 weeks	6 weeks	8 weeks
<1,200 gm birth weight	Hgb	15.6	16.4	15.5	11.3	8.5	7.8
	Retic	8.4	3.9	1.9	4.1	5.4	6.1
	Plat	148,000 ±61,000	163,000 ±69,000	162,000	158,000	210,000	212,000
	Leuk	14,800 ±10,200	12,200 ±7,000	15,800	13,200	10,800	9,900
	Seg	46	32	41	28	23	23
	Band	10.7	9.7	8.0	5.9	5.8	4.4
	Juv	2.0	3.9	5.3	3.6	2.6	2.0
	Lymph	32	43	39	55	61	65
	Monos	5	7	5	4	6	3
	Eos	0.4	6.2	1.0	3.7	2.0	3.8
	Nuc/RBC	16.7	1.1	0.1	1.0	2.7	2.0
>1,200–<1,500 gm birth weight	Hgb	20.2	18.0	17.1	12.0	9.1	8.3
	Retic	2.7	1.2	0.9	1.0	2.2	2.7
	Plat	151,000 ±35,000	134,000 ±49,000	153,000	189,000	212,000	244,000
	Leuk	10,800 ±4,000	8,900 ±2,900	14,300	11,000	10,500	9,100
	Seg	47	31	33	26	20	25
	Band	11.9	10.5	5.9	3.0	1.4	2.1
	Juv	5.1	2.4	2.7	1.8	1.7	1.6
	Lymph	34	48	52	59	69	64
	Monos	3	6	3	4	5	5
	Eos	1.3	2.2	2.5	5.1	2.6	2.3
	Nuc/RBC	19.8	0.8	0	0.4	1.4	1.0

*Wolff and Goodfellow: Pediatrics **16**:753, 1955.

TABLE 14. The white blood cell count and the differential count during the first two weeks of life

Age	Leukocytes	Neutrophils Total	Neutrophils Seg	Neutrophils Band	Eosinophils	Basophils	Lymphocytes	Monocytes
Birth								
Mean	18,100	11,000	9,400	1,600	400	100	5,500	1,050
Range	9.0–30.0	6.0–26			20–850	0–640	2.0–11.0	0.4–3.1
Mean %	—	61	52	9	2.2	0.6	31	5.8
7 days								
Mean	12,200	5,500	4,700	830	500	50	5,000	1,100
Range	5.0–21.0	1.5–10.0			70–1,100	0–250	2.0–17.0	0.3–2.7
Mean %	—	45	39	6	4.1	0.4	41	9.1
14 days								
Mean	11,400	4,500	3,900	630	350	50	5,500	1,000
Range	5.0–20.0	1.0–9.5			70–1,000	0–230	2.0–17.0	0.2–2.4
Mean %	—	40	34	5.5	3.1	0.4	48	8.8

Altman, P. L., and Dittmer, D. S.: Blood and other body fluids, Washington, D. C., 1961, Federation of American Societies for Experimental Biology.

TABLE 15. Venous platelet counts in normal low birth weight infants

Day	No. of infants	Mean mm³	Range 1,000's
0	60	203,000	80–356
3	47	207,000	61–335
5	14	233,000	100–502
7	52	319,000	124–678
10	40	399,000	172–680
14	50	386,000	147–670
21	47	388,000	201–720
28	40	384,000	212–625

Appleyard, W. J., and Bunton, W. A.: Biol. Neonate **17**:30, 1971.

TABLE 16. Platelet counts in full-term infants

Day	Mean	Range
Cord	200,000	100,000–280,000
1	192,000	100,000–260,000
3	213,000	80,000–320,000
7	248,000	100,000–300,000
14	252,000	

TABLE 17. Normal percentile values for micro-ESR in 100 low birth weight infants 3 days of age or less

	ESR (mm per 1 hr)	
Percentile	Male*	Female†
10	1.0	1.0
25	1.8	1.8
50	2.5	3.0
75	3.3	4.0
90	4.0	6.0
95	6.0	6.0
99	8.8	8.3

Evans, H., and others: J. Pediatr. **76**:448, 1970.
*Hematocrit: median 57%, range 43% to 78%.
†Hematocrit: median 54%, range 41% to 77%.

TABLE 18. Normal percentile values for micro-ESR in 30 low birth weight infants, median age 28 days, range 9 to 56 days

Percentile	ESR (mm per 1 hr)
10	3.0
25	3.8
50	5.5
90	9.5
95	11.0

Evans, H., and others: J. Pediatr. **76**:450, 1970.
Hematocrit: median 35%, range 25% to 58%.

Table 19. The bone marrow differential during the first week of life

	0-24 hours (%)	7 days (%)	Adult (%)
Myeloblasts	0–2	0–3	0.3–50
Promyelocytes	0.5–6.0	0.5–7.0	1.0–8.0
Myelocytes	1.0–9.0	1.0–11.0	5.5–22.5
Metamyelocytes	4.5–25.0	7.0–35.0	13.0–32.0
Band forms	10.0–40.0	11.0–45.0	—
Erythroblasts	0–1.0	0–0.5	1.0–8.0
Proerythroblasts	0.5–9.0	0–0.5	2.0–10.0
Normoblasts	18.0–41.0	0–15.0	7.0–32.0
Myeloid: erythroid ratio	1.5:1.0	6.5:1.0	3.5:1.0

Oski, F. A., and Naiman, J. L.: Hematologic problems in the newborn, ed. 2, Philadelphia, 1972, W. B. Saunders Co. Adapted from Shapiro and Bassen (1941) and Gairdner and others (1952).

Table 20. Serum iron and iron-binding capacity in the newborn and mother

Serum iron (µg/100 ml)		Total iron-binding capacity (µg/100 ml)		
Infant	Mother	Infant	Mother	Author
173	98	259	470	Hagberg (1953)
147	80	226	446	Laurell (1947)
193 (145–240)	—	240 (147–468)	—	Sturgeon (1954)
159 (106–227)	—	—	—	Vahlquist and others (1941)

Oski, F. A., and Naiman, J. L.: Hematologic problems in the newborn, ed. 2, Philadelphia, 1972, W. B. Saunders Co.

TABLE 21. Coagulation factor and test values in normal pregnant women and newborn infants

Category	Fibrinogen (mg/100 ml)	Factors									Euglobulin lysis time (min)	Partial thrombo-plastin time* (sec)	Prothrombin time (sec)	Thrombin time (sec)
		II (%)	V (%)	VII (%)	VIII (%)	IX (%)	X (%)	XI (%)	XII (%)	XIII (titer)				
Normal adult or child	190–420	100	100	100	100	100	100	100	100	1/16	90–300	37–50	12–14	8–10
Term pregnancy	483	92	108	170	196	130	130	69	—	1/16	278	44	13	8.0
Premature (1,500-2,500 gm) cord blood	233	25	67	37	80	Dec†	29	—	—	1/8	214	90	17(12–21)	14(11–17)
Term infant cord blood	216	41	92	56	100	27	55	36	—	1/8	84	71	16(13–20)	12(10–16)
Term infant, 48 hours	210	46	105	20	100	Dec	45	39	25	—	105	65	17.5(12–21)	13(10–16)

Adapted from Hathaway, W. E.: Pediatr. Clin. North Am. **17**:929, 1970.
Note: All levels expressed as means or ranges; if no reference is noted, the value is derived from unpublished data from the author's laboratory.
*Kaolin PTT.
†Dec = decreased.

Table 22. Haptoglobin levels in low birth weight infants

Gestation, weeks	Days after birth					
	0	5	10	15	21	28
<32	10 (3)	—	—	—	—	—
32–34	—	18.5 (2)	51.6 (3)	42.6 (3)	12 (1)	12 (1)
34–36	9.8 (9)	14.9 (11)	11.4 (10)	11.6 (9)	7.1 (7)	16.5 (4)
36–38	13.0 (7)	18.3 (3)	16.6 (5)	16.3 (2)	11 (1)	7.5 (1)
38+	9.3 (8)	28.3 (6)	20.9 (4)	10.1 (5)	9.2 (3)	7.0 (1)
Total	10.5 (27)	19.6 (22)	19.5 (22)	16.1 (19)	8.3 (12)	13.2 (7)

Philip, A. G. S.: Biol. Neonate **19**:322, 1971.
Haptoglobin levels are measured as mg% MetHb binding capacity. Numbers in parenthesis indicate number of samples from which mean values were derived.

Table 23. Haptoglobin levels in full-term infants

	Birth	Fifth day
Haptoglobin (mg/100 ml Hgb binding capacity)	23.9 (10.6–50.0)	52.3 (14.8–100.0)

Table 24. Mean complement levels of sera of newborn infants of different birth weights and the maternal sera, compared with a normal adult standard serum

Group	Complement component levels (mean ± 1 standard error of mean)								
	Ratio to standard serum[3]						mg/100 ml[4]		
	CH_{50}[1]	C1q	C2	C3(B_{1C})	C4	C4(B_{1E})	C1q	B_{1C}	B_{1E}
1. <1,000 g	0.6±0.1 (7)[2]	0.5±0.1 (7)	1.2±0.1 (2)	0.6±0.1 (7)	0.5±0.1 (7)	0.6±0.2 (7)	1.1±0.2	89±16	9±3
2. 1,000-1,500 g	0.7±0.1 (7)	0.4±0.02 (9)	0.4±0.2 (3)	0.7±0.1 (9)	1.4±0.3 (7)	0.8±0.1 (9)	1.1±0.1	94±10	12±2
3. 1,500-2,000 g	0.7±0.3 (5)	0.7±0.1 (8)	1.2±0.5 (4)	0.9±0.2 (7)	1.0±0.6 (4)	1.0±0.3 (8)	1.6±0.3	141±24	15±4
4. 2,000-2,500 g	0.9±0.2 (5)	0.8±0.1 (5)	1.0±0.2 (5)	1.0±0.2 (5)	1.2±0.4 (5)	1.4±0.3 (5)	1.9±0.3	151±33	21±5
5. >2,500 g	0.9±0.1 (8)	0.9±0.5 (11)	1.0±0.2 (6)	1.0±0.1 (11)	1.4±0.2 (7)	1.0±0.1 (11)	2.2±0.1	160±13	16±2
6. Mother	1.5±0.1 (24)	0.9±0.04 (25)	1.2±0.2 (18)	1.8±0.1 (27)	1.9±0.2 (23)	2.3±0.1 (26)	2.3±0.1	254±12	35±2
7. Normal standard	1.0	1.0	1.0	1.0	1.0	1.0	2.5	145.2	15.2

Sawyer, M. K., and others: Biol. Neonate **19**:148, 1971.
[1]Total hemolytic complement expressed in 50% hemolytic units.
[2]Number in parenthesis refers to number in group.
[3]Determined by titration assay.
[4]Determined bv radial immunodiffusion assay.

TABLE 25. Thyroid function

	Birth	24 hr	48 hr	1 wk	2 wk	4 wk
PBI (μg/100 ml)	4.3–9.5	7.3–12.9	9.6–16.8	7.3–14.5	4.0–11.0	4.0–11.0
BEI (μg/100 ml)	5.5 (4.5–6.5)	—	—	9.8 (7.8–12.0)	7.8 (7.0–8.2)	4.8 (4.0–5.5)
T_3 uptake (%)	3.0 (22–32)	—	—	38 (30–45)	38 (28–48)	25 (18–32)
TSH 24 hr uptake (%) μV/ml	—	46–96	24–96	5–47	—	13–30
Free T_4	2.4–8.4	—	—	4.0–13.2	—	—

DRUGS

TABLE 26. Drugs

Drug	Dosage	Comments
Adrenergics		
Epinephrine	1:1,000 aqueous solution SC 0.01 ml/kg/dose	Repeat every 2-4 hr as needed
Isoproterenol (Isuprel)	1 mg in 100-500 ml of D5W	Slow infusion of 0.1-0.4 mg/kg/min
Antibiotics		
Ampicillin	IM, IV 100-200 mg/kg/day every 12 hr for first 3 days of life; every 6-8 hr after 3 days	(See Table 8-2, p. 133)
Bacitracin	IM or IV 500 units/kg/day; 4 doses per day; ointment (500 units/gm) 3-4 times per day	
Carbenicillin	IV 100-200 mg/kg/day; divided 4 doses	
Chloramphenicol (Chloromycetin)	Premature: 10-25 mg/kg/day; 3-4 doses Full-term: 50/mg/kg/day; 3-4 doses	
Clindamycin	PO 8-20 mg/kg/day; 4 doses; parenteral dose after 1 mo of age is 10-15 mg/kg/day, 3-4 divided doses	
Colistimethate	Premature: IM 5 mg/kg/day; 2 doses Full-term: IM 8 mg/kg/day; 3 doses	
Colistin sulfate	Premature and full-term: PO 8 mg/kg/day; 4 doses	
Erythromycin	IM or IV 30-50 mg/kg/day; 4 doses PO 50 mg/kg/day	
Gentamicin	Premature: IM 5 mg/kg/day; 2 doses Full-term: 5 mg/kg/day; 3 doses Intrathecal 0.5-1.0 mg in 1 ml saline daily for 3-5 days	
Kanamycin	IM 15 mg/kg/day; 2 doses	
Methicillin (Staphcillin)	Premature: IM 100 mg/kg/day; 2 doses Full-term: IV 200 mg/kg/day; 2 doses	
Nafcillin	Same as methicillin	
Neomycin	PO 100 mg/kg/day; 4 doses; topical ointment; 4 times a day	
Oxacillin	Same as methicillin	
Penicillin	IM or IV aqueous 100,000 μ/kg/day; 2-4 doses	
Benzathine penicillin G	IM 50,000 μ/kg congenital syphilis	
Polymyxin	IM or IV 3-4 mg/kg/day Intrathecal 1-2 mg/day for 3-5 days	
Streptomycin	IM 20-40 mg/kg/day; 2-4 doses	
Antifungal		
Amphotericin B	IV 0.25-1.0 mg/kg/day; dilute to 1.0 mg/10 ml, infuse slowly	
Nystatin (Mycostatin)	PO 100,000-200,000 μ daily Ointment: 3 doses for 7-10 days	

Continued.

Table 26. Drugs—cont'd

Drug	Dosage	Comments
5-Fluorocytosine	IV 1,500-4,500 mg/m²/day; 2 doses	
Antituberculous		
Isoniazid	PO Prophylaxis: 10 mg/kg/day Therapeutic: 15-20 mg/kg/day	
Streptomycin	See antibiotics	
Rifampin	PO 10-20 mg/kg/day	
Chemotherapeutics		
Sulfisoxazole (Gantrisin)	PO 100-150 mg/kg/day; 4 doses	
Anticoagulants		
Heparin	IV Initial: 50 units/kg Maintenance: 50-100 units/kg every 4 hr; titrate to maintain clotting times at 20-30 minutes	
Anticonvulsants		
Phenobarbital	PO, IM, IV 5-10 mg/kg/day; 4-6 doses acutely; 2 doses, prophylaxis for seizures	
Diphenylhydantoin sodium (Dilantin)	PO, IM, IV 3-5 mg/kg/day; 3 doses	
Paraldehyde	PO, IM, 0.15 ml/kg every 4-6 hr as necessary; IV, titrate a drip dose of a 4% solution	
Diazepam (Valium)	PO, IM, IV 0.1-0.8 mg/kg/day	
Antidotes		
Atropine	SC 0.01 mg/kg; may repeat every 2 hr	
Methylene blue	IV 1% solution 0.1-0.2 ml/kg	Slow infusion
Nalorphine hydrochloride	IM, IV 0.1-0.2 mg/kg/dose	
Naloxone hydrochloride	IV, IM, SC .005 mg/kg/dose	
Protamine	IV 1.0 mg for every 10 mg heparin	
Blood derivative		
Albumin	IV 1.0 gm/kg/day	
Blood		
Packed RBC	IV 5-10 ml/kg	
Whole blood	IV 10-20 ml/kg	
Fibrinogen	IV 50 mg/kg; repeat as needed	
Gammaglobulin	IM Prophylaxis: 0.22 ml/kg Attenuate: 0.05 ml/kg Agammaglobulinemia: 1 ml/kg every 2-4 weeks	
Plasma	IV 20 ml/kg; as necessary	
Calcium salts		
Calcium chloride (27%)	PO 1-2 gm/day; 250 mg/kg/day	
Calcium gluconate (9%)	IV 0.5-1.0 gm/kg/day in 2-3 doses; dilute to 10% solution PO 0.5-1.0 gm/dose; 2-4 times daily	
Calcium lactate (13%)	PO 0.5 gm/kg/day in 4 doses	
Cardiovascular drugs		
Antiarrhythmics		
Lidocaine	IV 1-2 mg/kg/dose; single dose over 5 minutes	(See p. 281 for recurrences)
Propranolol	.05-.15 mg/kg	½ dose IV; not to exceed 1 mg/min (p. 280)
Antihypertensives		
Hydralazine hydrochloride (Apresoline)	PO 0.75 mg/kg/day; 4 doses IV or IM 0.20 mg/kg every 12-24 hr when used with reserpine IV or IM 1.7-3.5 mg/kg in 4 divided doses when used alone	
Magnesium sulfate	IM 0.2 ml/kg/dose, 50% solution every 4-6 hr	(See p. 336)
Reserpine	IM 0.07 mg/kg—hypertension	
Diazoxide	IV 5 mg/kg; single dose for fulminant hypertension	
Cardiotonics		
Digoxin	Premature: PO 0.03-.04 mg/kg Full-term: PO 0.05-.07 mg/kg	Divided in 3 doses (every 6-12 hr)

TABLE 26. Drugs—cont'd

Drug	Dosage	Comments
	IM or IV 2/3 of oral dose	More rapidly in emergencies
Cholinergic blocking agents		
Atropine	See antedotes	
Belladonna tincture	PO 0.1 ml (0.03 mg atropine) every 4 hr	
Cholinesterase inhibitors		
Neostigmine	PO 6-8 mg/day; 4-8 doses	
Pyridostigmine (Mestinon)	PO 1.0-2.0 mg, every 4-12 hr IM 0.1-0.4 mg, every 4-8 hr	
Edrophonium chloride (Tensilon)	IM, SC: test dose 0.1 ml	
Diuretics		
Acetazolamide (Diamox)	PO, IV 5 mg/kg/day; 3 doses	
Meralluride (Mercuhydrin)	IM 0.1 ml/5 kg	May be repeated daily for 1-2 wk
Chlorothiazide (Diuril)	PO 20 mg/kg/day	Divided in 2 doses
Ethacrynic acid (Edecrin)	IV, PO 1 mg/kg/dose, over 5-10 min	
Furosemide	IV, IM 1-3 mg/kg/dose, over 2 min	
Spironalactone (Aldactone)	PO 1.5-3.0 mg/kg/day	Divided in 3 doses
Endocrine		
Adrenal		
ACTH	IM 3-5 units/kg/day; 4 doses	
Cortisone	PO 0.5-2 mg/kg/day; 4 doses	
Desoxycorticosterone (DOCA)	IM 1-5 mg/day	
Dexamethasone (Decadron)	IM, IV 0.5-1.0 mg; 3-4 doses	
Hydrocortisone	PO 3-10 mg/kg/day; 4 doses IM, IV 25-50 mg, every 6 hr as needed	
Prednisone	PO 1-3 mg/kg/day	
Pancreas		
Glucagon	IM, IV 30-100 μg/kg; repeat every 6-12 hr	
Pituitary		
Vasopressin (Pitressin)	SC 1-3 ml/day; 3 doses	
Thyroid		
Desiccated thyroid	PO Initial dose: 8 mg/day	(See p. 465 for increments)
Triiodothyronine (T_3)	PO 5 μg/day	(See p. 465 for increments)
Methimazole	PO 0.4 mg/kg/day	3 doses
Propylthiouracil	PO 10 mg/kg/day	3 doses
Lugol's solution	PO one drop 3 times a day	
Enzymes		
Pancreatin	PO 0.3-0.5 gm with feedings	
Iron		
Ferrous sulfate	Premature: prophylaxis 2 mg/kg/day PO treatment: 6 mg/kg/day	
Narcotics		
Meperidine (Demerol)	IV, IM 0.5-1 mg/kg/dose	May repeat after 1 hr
Morphine	SC 0.05-0.1 mg/kg/dose	May repeat after 1 hr
Sedatives		
Barbiturate	See Anticonvulsants, phenobarbital	
Chloral hydrate	PO 25-50 mg/kg/day	
Paraldehyde	See Anticonvulsants, paraldehyde	
Benadryl	PO 5 mg/kg/day; 4-6 doses	
Tranquilizers		
Chlorpromazine (Thorazine)	PO, IM, IV 2.0-2.5 mg/kg/day	
Diazepam (Valium)	PO, IM, IV 0.1-0.8 mg/kg/24 hr	(See p. 452 for addicted infants)
Promethazine (Phenergan)	PO, IM 0.5 mg/kg/dose	Repeat every 4-6 hr
Vitamins		
A	PO 600-1,000 IU	
B_1 (thiamine)	PO 0.5-1.0 mg daily	

Continued.

Table 26. Drugs—cont'd

Drug	Dosage	Comments
	Treatment: 10 mg every 6-8 hr	
B_2 (riboflavin)	PO 0.5 mg daily	
B_6 (pyridoxine)	PO 1-2 mg daily	
B_{12} (cyanocobalamin)	PO 1-2 μg daily	
C (ascorbic acid)	PO 25-50 mg/day	
	Treatment: PO or IM 100 mg every 4 hr	
D	PO 400 IU/day	
E	PO 9 mg/day	
K	IM 1.0 mg; single dose	
	Treatment: 2.5-5.0 mg every 6-12 hr	
Miscellaneous		
Actinomycin D	IV 75 mg/kg, divided into 5 daily doses	
Atabrine	PO 5 mg/kg; 2 doses	
Pyrimethamine (Daraprim)	IV 0.05-1.0 mg/kg/day	
Silver nitrate	Ophthalmic, 1 drop 2% solution each eye	
Mannitol	IV 200-400 mg/kg/dose	Infuse over 1 hr
Curare	IV 0.15-0.3 mg/kg/dose	Repeat as needed
Paregoric	PO 3-6 drops every 3-4 hr	
Methadone	PO 0.3 to 0.4 mg/kg/day	
Pentamidine	IM 4 mg/kg/day for 10-14 days	
Chloroquine	PO 10 mg/kg/day	
	IV 5 mg/kg/day	
Quinine	PO 20-30 mg/kg/day; 3 doses for 7-10 days	

Index

C

E

P

R

W

X

Y

Z